Computed Tomography
of the
Head, Neck, and Spine

Computed Tomography
of the
Head, Neck, and Spine

Edited by

Richard E. Latchaw, M.D.

Professor of Radiology and Neurological Surgery
University of Pittsburgh
Chief, Division of Neuroradiology
Department of Radiology
University Health Center of Pittsburgh

YEAR BOOK MEDICAL PUBLISHERS
CHICAGO

0 9 8 7 6 5 4 3 2

Library of Congress Cataloging in Publication Data
Main entry under title:

Computed tomography of the head, neck, and spine.

   Includes bibliographical references and index.
   1. Central nervous system—Diseases—Diagnosis.
2. Tomography.   3. Head—Radiography.   4. Neck—
Radiography.   5. Spine—Radiography.   I. Latchaw,
Richard E.   [DNLM: 1. Tomography, X-ray computed.
2. Head—Radiography.   3. Neck—Radiography.   4. Spine—
Radiography.   WE 141 C738]
RC386.6.T64C65   1984   616.8′047572   84-3715
ISBN 0-8151-5329-5

Sponsoring editors: Daniel J. Doody, James D. Ryan
Editing supervisor: Frances M. Perveiler
Copyeditor: Kareen Snider
Production project manager: Sharon W. Pepping
Proofroom supervisor: Shirley E. Taylor

Contributors

MICHAEL BRANT-ZAWADZKI, M.D.
Associate Professor of Radiology
University of California at San Francisco
San Francisco, California

R. NICK BRYAN, M.D., PH.D.
Professor of Radiology
Baylor College of Medicine
Director of Neuroradiology
The Methodist Hospital
Houston, Texas

HUGH D. CURTIN, M.D.
Associate Professor of Radiology
University of Pittsburgh
Chief of Radiology
Eye and Ear Hospital
Pittsburgh, Pennsylvania

MONY J. DE LEON ED.D.
Research Assistant Professor
Department of Psychiatry
New York University Medical School
New York, New York

CHARLES R. FITZ, M.D.
Associate Professor of Radiology
University of Toronto
Chief, Division of Special Procedures
Department of Radiology
Hospital for Sick Children
Toronto, Ontario, Canada

AJAX E. GEORGE, M.D.
Professor of Radiology (Neuroradiology)
New York University Medical School
New York, New York

ROBERT I. GROSSMAN, M.D.
Associate Professor of Radiology and Neurological Surgery
Hospital of the University of Pennsylvania
Philadelphia, Pennsylvania

DAVID GUR, SC.D.
Professor of Radiation Health and Radiology
University of Pittsburgh
Pittsburgh, Pennsylvania

L. ANNE HAYMAN, M.D.
Associate Professor of Radiology
Harvard University
Boston, Massachusetts

VINCENT C. HINCK, M.D.
Professor of Radiology
Baylor College of Medicine
Houston, Texas

BARRY L. HOROWITZ, M.D.
Clinical Assistant Professor of Radiology
Baylor College of Medicine
Houston, Texas

JOSEPH A. HORTON, M.D.
Associate Professor of Radiology
University of Pittsburgh
Pittsburgh, Pennsylvania

CHARLES K. KEYSER, M.D.
Fellow in Radiology
The Cleveland Clinic Foundation
Cleveland, Ohio

RICHARD E. LATCHAW, M.D.
Professor of Radiology and Neurological Surgery
University of Pittsburgh
Chief, Division of Neuroradiology
Department of Radiology
University Health Center of Pittsburgh
Pittsburgh, Pennsylvania

L. DADE LUNSFORD, M.D.
Assistant Professor of Radiology and Neurological Surgery
University of Pittsburgh
Pittsburgh, Pennsylvania

CHARLES W. McCLUGGAGE, M.D.
Assistant Professor of Radiology
Baylor College of Medicine
Houston, Texas

JOHN D. MEYER, M.D.
Department of Radiology
Northside Hospital
Atlanta, Georgia
Formerly Assistant Chief of the
    Division of Neuroradiology
Department of Radiology
University Health Center of Pittsburgh
Pittsburgh, Pennsylvania

MICHAEL T. MODIC, M.D.
Head, Section of Nuclear Magnetic Resonance
The Cleveland Clinic Foundation
Cleveland, Ohio

ROBERT M. QUENCER, M.D.
Professor of Radiology and Neurosurgery
University of Miami School of Medicine
Chief, Section of Neuroradiology
Jackson Memorial Medical Center
Miami, Florida

HELEN M. N. ROPPOLO, M.D.
Clinical Associate Professor of Radiology
University of Pittsburgh
Pittsburgh, Pennsylvania

WILLIAM E. ROTHFUS, M.D.
Assistant Professor of Radiology
University of Pittsburgh
Pittsburgh, Pennsylvania

KATHERINE A. SHAFFER, M.D.
Associate Professor of Radiology
Medical College of Wisconsin
Milwaukee, Wisconsin

SAUL TAYLOR, M.D.
Assistant Professor of Radiology
University of Minnesota
Minneapolis, Minnesota
Staff Radiologist
St. Paul-Ramsey Medical Center
St. Paul, Minnesota

MEREDITH A. WEINSTEIN, M.D.
Head, Section of Neuroradiological Imaging
The Cleveland Clinic Foundation
Cleveland, Ohio

SIDNEY K. WOLFSON, JR., M.D.
Professor of Neurological Surgery
University of Pittsburgh
Director of Peripheral Vascular Diagnostic Laboratory
Director of Surgical Research
Montefiore Hospital
Pittsburgh, Pennsylvania

HOWARD YONAS, M.D.
Associate Professor of Neurological Surgery
University of Pittsburgh
Pittsburgh, Pennsylvania

ROBERT A. ZIMMERMAN, M.D.
Professor of Radiology
Hospital of the University of Pennsylvania
Pittsburgh, Pennsylvania

Preface

COMPUTED TOMOGRAPHY has become an increasingly important and efficacious diagnostic modality over the last decade. Major technological advances that have propelled CT scanning into the forefront of the diagnostic armamentarium include increased spatial and contrast resolution, computer programs for rapid-sequence dynamic scanning, and software for high quality reformatted images in multiple projections. New techniques for diagnosis using the CT scanner are now possible, such as the determination of cerebral blood flow to small areas of cerebral tissue using inhaled stable xenon as a contrast agent. The CT scanner has also provided major advances in therapy, such as the accurate localization of intracranial targets for stereotactic neurosurgery. Such new advances in both hardware and software have made the CT scanner the most important radiologic invention since the discovery of the x-ray tube. This is a very exciting time for the diagnostician, because the anatomical accuracy and histologic specificity of diagnosis are far better than they have ever been in the history of x-ray procedures. Likewise, it is the perfect time to bring forth a book dedicated to both a description of diseases of the head, neck, and spine and an exposition of the diversity of functions of the CT scanner.

While an attempt has been made to discuss most of the disease states of the head, neck, and spine that are applicable to CT scanning, there has been no attempt to be rigorous in describing all pathologic entities. Other volumes, either longer or dedicated to specific regions of the body or pathologic categories, might be far more specific about the CT scan findings of certain diseases. Rather, we have had a number of goals and objectives that do not necessarily correlate with length or specificity of description.

First, there has been an attempt to describe logical approaches to the diagnosis of lesions of the head, neck, and spine by CT scanning. The particular approach that is used when confronting an unknown lesion seen on a CT scan, including an evaluation of the density characteristics of the lesion, the pattern of enhancement with contrast material, and the location and spread of the disease process, is paramount in arriving at either a specific diagnosis or the determination of a particular pathologic category of disease. A volume that only listed the CT scan characteristics of a series of lesions would not adequately fulfill its function as an instrument to teach appropriate CT scan analysis.

Second, a major goal has been the correlation of anatomy, pathology, physiology, and therapy. Not only is the CT scanner an instrument for the exquisite demonstration of anatomy and pathology, but it is also the source of much physiologic information derived from patterns of contrast enhancement, appearance and progression of edema, and determination of blood flow and tissue perfusion. Not only may therapeutic procedures actually be performed on the CT scanner, but multiple projections of pathologic lesions will directly influence the surgeon or radiation therapist in his attempt to obliterate the lesion.

Third, an attempt has been made to ask the questions "how" and "why" lesions are seen as they are on the CT scan. Rather than only listing specific CT scan findings, there has been a concerted effort to explain why those appearances occur.

vii

Such a discussion is vital in understanding the differential diagnosis of a given lesion and the reasons for a specific diagnosis.

Fourth, attempts have been made to grapple with controversial aspects of CT scan diagnosis in the head, neck, and spine. For example, there is controversy regarding the most efficacious but least morbid way of examining the spine in a patient suffering from herniated disc, spondylosis, or spinal stenosis. Some authorities advocate the use of the plain scan, while others suggest scanning after myelography. Because there is no absolute position in this controversial area, both approaches are discussed.

Lastly, future trends and new techniques using the CT scanner are discussed. New computer programs allow for reformatted images in oblique projections, which add greatly to the therapy of a lesion. Software manipulations such as three-dimensional imaging or the determination of the effective atomic number of a lesion may contribute substantially to both diagnosis and therapy. Cerebral blood flow determination using the CT scanner during stable xenon inhalation, a technique just being developed, will allow determination of tissue perfusion in volumes of the brain measuring 3 mm or less. Such future trends will greatly advance the diagnostic and therapeutic efficacy of the CT scanner.

The organization of this book reflects the correlation with and emphasis on physiology and therapy, in addition to the more typical anatomical and pathologic descriptions. Section I is devoted to physiology and is divided into two chapters. The first discusses the evaluation of the blood-brain barrier using a group of contrast agents. The second is devoted to the determination of cerebral blood flow and in particular the developing technique of cerebral blood flow determination using the CT scanner during xenon inhalation. Section XI is dedicated to direct therapy utilizing the CT scanner. The most dramatic therapeutic use of the CT scanner is its role in stereotactic neurosurgery, giving exquisitely fine anatomical localization of intracranial targets. Sections II through X are devoted to clinical problems and specific disease states, but again emphasizing correlation of physiology and therapeutic implications with anatomical and pathologic considerations.

Specific sections reflect the overall philosophy of this volume. There is little in the chapter on dementia regarding the obvious anatomical changes of cerebral atrophy, including increased ventricular and sulcal size. Rather, there is an in-depth discussion of new techniques for correlating cognitive change with morphological data. The four chapters in Section IX, CT in Otolaryngology, are not meant to be all-inclusive of diseases of the ear, nose, and throat. Of greater importance is the emphasis on the use of multiple CT projections, the understanding of fine anatomical detail in these complex regions, and correlation of pathology with CT-derived anatomical data. Because a specific diagnosis frequently rests on histologic examination of a lesion in these areas, emphases are placed on both an appropriate radiographic approach and anatomical-pathologic correlation.

In summary, this book is devoted to the teaching of useful approaches to the diagnosis of disease states of the head, neck, and spine. These approaches will not only aid in questions of differential diagnosis, but in the planning of appropriate therapy. This book is also devoted to demonstrating the diversity of the CT scanner, which is not only a major technology for demonstrating morphological detail, but is moving towards new horizons in physiology and therapy.

RICHARD E. LATCHAW, M.D.

Acknowledgments

IT IS ALWAYS DIFFICULT to give a series of acknowledgments at the beginning of a book, because invariably someone who has added greatly to the success of a project will be overlooked. Many individuals at the University Health Center of Pittsburgh have been instrumental in the production of this volume, including CT scan technologists and coordinators, film librarians, and members of the secretarial staff. Many such individuals contributed greatly to the production of high quality scans and their assembly into a meaningful product. All of my coauthors at universities outside of UHCP will likewise have many debts of gratitude to unsung individuals who have made their chapters possible. Rather than attempting to name all the individuals who have influenced the production of this volume, I would simply like to acknowledge a few people without whose help the writing of this book would have been impossible.

First and foremost is my secretary, Ms. Joan Roberge. For 3 years, Joan has helped shoulder the responsibility of organizing this volume, editing manuscripts, typing and retyping multiple chapters, and helping in the organization of the 1,500 photographs in this book—a truly remarkable job and my heartfelt thanks! Praise must also go to Ms. Margaret Havran and Ms. Deborah Clark, who as secretaries in the Neuroradiology Division have likewise been responsible for the production of many of the chapters appearing in this volume.

The success of a radiology book of this type is highly dependent upon the quality of the photography and artistic work that illuminate the written concepts. Mr. Robert Coulter has been tireless in the production of the overwhelming majority of images appearing in chapters by my colleagues at this Health Center. The production of photographs of CT scans is a difficult process, far more difficult than the production of photographic material derived from routine x-rays because of the large number of gray scales that must be captured to reflect all of the information contained in a high quality CT scan. One of our important goals has been to display as much visual information as possible in the conversion of a high quality CT image to a picture on a printed page. Bob has responded to this challenge in a way that has insured the highest quality CT images possible. My thanks to him for his perseverance and devotion to quality. Jon Coulter is responsible for the gorgeous drawings appearing in many of the chapters from UHCP. Such artistry greatly aids in the appreciation of complex anatomy. We have been fortunate to have an artist of Jon's calibre to help us on this project.

A final word of thanks must go to my wife, Joan, and my two boys, Andy and Greg. Too often we forget the role of family members, who bear the brunt of the sacrifice of vacations and family activities while the professional insists on working on "the book." I owe a great deal to these three people who have been so supportive during this project.

RICHARD E. LATCHAW, M.D.

Contents

Physiology

1

Water-Soluble Iodinated Contrast Media

L. Anne Hayman, M.D.
Vincent C. Hinck, M.D.

TYPES OF WATER-SOLUBLE CONTRAST MEDIA

Water-soluble iodinated contrast medium was first used in humans in 1927 by Egas Moniz. In his initial experiments, he percutaneously injected a 70% solution of strontium bromide into the carotid arteries of six patients, but obtained no suitable radiographs. However, the second patient in the series experienced severe pain during the injection; the fourth patient suffered a severe reaction and fever; and the sixth patient died 8 hours after the injection from a cerebral thrombosis.

Given these results, if Moniz were a modern-day radiologist, it is highly unlikely that he would have been permitted to continue his research and ultimately test the 25% solution of sodium iodide that enabled demonstration of the internal carotid artery and its branches. Because sodium iodide caused pain on injection, a colloidal preparation of thorium dioxide was introduced for carotid angiography. This radioactive agent, retained by the liver and at sites of extravasation that occurred during injection, induced fibrosis and neoplasia over time and was abandoned.[1]

Ionic monomers.—Thorium dioxide was supplanted by iodinated water-soluble compounds, which were originally introduced in 1928 for *intravenous* administration to visualize the urinary collecting system. None of these compounds (iodopyracet, sodium methiodal, and sodium iodomethamate) are in use today because of their toxic side effects. They were replaced in the early 1950s by ionic triiodo compounds, which are better tolerated and are commonly used today. Figure 1–1 shows the four variations of the triiodo structure of these ionic monomeric contrast agents. All of these agents are sodium or meglumine salts of a substituted monomeric triiodobenzoic acid and completely dissociate into ions in solution. There is evidence to suggest that varying the side chains that are attached to each

molecule may significantly affect the behavior of these compounds in the clinical setting.[1] The compounds added to stabilize the solution also influence the reactions that will be manifested in clinical use. These media are referred to as *ionic* contrast media. They have a relatively high osmolarity, because each molecule of the salt has one cation (sodium or meglumine) and one anion (the iodinated benzoate radical) in solution. Only the anion has clinical relevance. The osmotic effect of the cation is undesirable.[2]

Nonionic monomers.—In 1969, Almen[3] proposed several chemical formulations that would produce fewer or no ions when in solution. Some of these compounds form the group of *nonionic* water-soluble contrast media. Note that the iodinated benzoic acid seen in Figure 1–2 has been converted into a molecule that will not dissociate in solution. The first of these agents, metrizamide, was introduced into the United States in 1978. It will soon be removed from the U.S. market when many of the agents listed in Figure 1–2 become available for myelography and angiography.

Ionic dimers.—Another way in which the osmolality of the contrast agent has been reduced is by connecting the two triiodobenzoic acid molecules (Fig 1–3). The meglumine salt of iothalamic acid (Dimeray) was introduced for use in myelography before metrizamide became available. It was withdrawn from the market after a short time, because a number of serious neurotoxic reactions occurred. Dimeray was the first *ionic dimer* used in the United States. It had a lower osmolarity than conventional ionic agents, because it dissociated into three particles (one large iodinated dimeric anion and two cations) rather than the four particles (two anions and two cations), which would have resulted if a solution containing six iodine atoms were prepared using the ionic formula demonstrated in Figure 1–1.

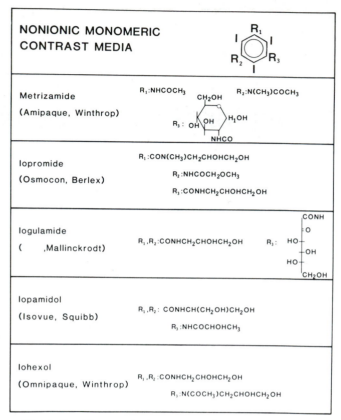

IONIC MONOMERIC CONTRAST MEDIA	
Diatrizoate (Hypaque, Winthrop Renografin, Squibb)	$R:NHCOCH_3$
Iothalamate (Conray, Mallinckrodt)	$R:CONHCH_3$
Ioglicate (Rayvist, Berlex)	$R:CONHCH_2CONHCH_3$
Metrizoate (Isopaque, Winthrop)	$R:N(CH_3)COCH_3$

Fig 1–1.—Four ionic monomeric contrast media. All share the structure pictured in the category heading. They differ in the composition of the R chain that is pictured with each contrast medium. Diatrizoate, iothalamate, and metrizoate are available on the U.S. market. Ioglicate is about to be introduced.

Another contrast medium that is an ionic dimer is Ioxaglate. It will be introduced to the U.S. market by Mallinckrodt for use as an angiographic agent. The reduced osmolality of this medium appears to moderate the burning sensation that accompanies intracarotid injection of ionic contrast media. It does not reduce the retinal irritation produced by contrast injection.[4]

NONIONIC DIMERS.—Two of these agents (Fig 1–4) that are currently being developed are Iotasul for lymphangiography and Iotrol for myelography. These agents have the basic structure of ionic dimers, but they eliminate the cations by substituting two radicals.

All of these new dimers and the nonionic agents have succeeded in reducing the number of particles in solution from that originally encountered in solutions of the traditional monoacid ionic agents (see Fig 1–1) that contain the same amount of iodine. In reality, some of the new agents have an osmolality that is reduced to one third of that found in the ionic agents, although theoretically their structure should have reduced the osmolality less dramatically (Fig 1–5). This "exaggerated" effect can be ascribed to the fact that these molecules not only have fewer particles in solution, but also aggregate in solution, thereby further diminishing the particle count and further reducing osmolality.[2]

With the development of these new compounds, the radiologist will be confronted with the need to select the safest and least costly contrast medium for a given procedure, to evaluate image quality with each agent,

NONIONIC MONOMERIC CONTRAST MEDIA	
Metrizamide (Amipaque, Winthrop)	$R_1:NHCOCH_3$ $R_2:N(CH_3)COCH_3$ R_3: (sugar ring)
Iopromide (Osmocon, Berlex)	$R_1:CON(CH_3)CH_2CHOHCH_2OH$ $R_2:NHCOCH_2OCH_3$ $R_3:CONHCH_2CHOHCH_2OH$
Iogulamide (, Mallinckrodt)	$R_1,R_2:CONHCH_2CHOHCH_2OH$ $R_3:$ (chain)
Iopamidol (Isovue, Squibb)	$R_1,R_2: CONHCH(CH_2OH)CH_2OH$ $R_3:NHCOCHOHCH_3$
Iohexol (Omnipaque, Winthrop)	$R_1,R_2:CONHCH_2CHOHCH_2OH$ $R_3:N(COCH_3)CH_2CHOHCH_2OH$

Fig 1–2.—Five nonionic monomeric contrast media. All share the structure pictured in the category heading. They differ in composition of the three R chains that are pictured with each of the contrast media. Metrizamide is the only agent currently available on the U.S. market. It will soon be supplanted by the other agents listed.

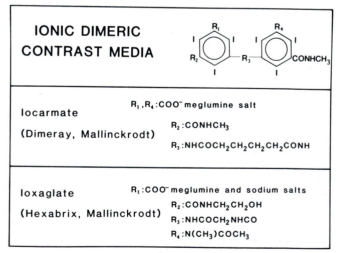

IONIC DIMERIC CONTRAST MEDIA	
Iocarmate (Dimeray, Mallinckrodt)	$R_1,R_4:COO^-$ meglumine salt $R_2:CONHCH_3$ $R_3:NHCOCH_2CH_2CH_2CH_2CONH$
Ioxaglate (Hexabrix, Mallinckrodt)	$R_1:COO^-$ meglumine and sodium salts $R_2:CONHCH_2CH_2OH$ $R_3:NHCOCH_2NHCO$ $R_4:N(CH_3)COCH_3$

Fig 1–3.—Two ionic dimeric contrast media. Both share the structure pictured in the category heading. They differ in composition of the three R chains that are pictured with each of them. Iocarmate was removed from the U.S. market, and ioxaglate is about to be introduced to the U.S. market.

NONIONIC DIMERIC CONTRAST MEDIA

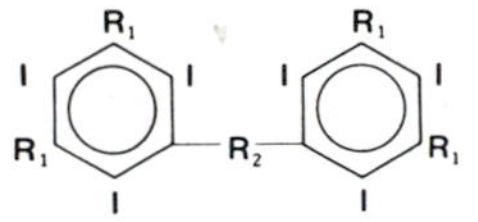

Iotrol
(Isocon, Berlex)

R₁:CONHCH(CH₂OH)CHOHCH₂OH

R₂:N(CH₃)COCH₂CON(CH₃)

Iotasul
(Lymphocon,Berlex)

R₁:CON(CH₃)CH₂CHOHCH₂OH

R₂:NHCOCH₂CH₂SCH₂CH₂CONH

Fig 1–4.—Two nonionic dimeric contrast media. Both share the structure pictured in the category heading. They differ in composition of the two R chains that are pictured with each of them. Both of these agents are about to be introduced to the U.S. market. Iotrol is under development as a myelographic contrast medium, whereas iotasul may be suitable for lymphography.

	Myelography	Angiography	Intravenous	Lymphography
Metrizamide (Amipaque)	*			
Iopromide (Osmocon)		√	√	
Iogulamide	√			
Iopamidol (Isovue)	√	√		
Iohexol (Omnipaque)	√	√		
Diatrizoate (Hypaque)		√	√	
Iothalamate (Conray)		√	√	
Ioglicate (Rayvist)		√	√	
Metrizoate (Isopaque)			√	
Iotrol (Isocon)	√			
Iotasul (Lymphocon)				√
Iocarmate (Dimeray)	**			
Ioxaglate (Hexabrix)		√		

Fig 1–6.—Neuroradiologic uses for water-soluble iodinated contrast media (* indicates the agent will be removed from the U.S. market; ** indicates the agent has been removed from the U.S. market).

phatic, or intravascular) and, of course, that the information gleaned from each approach is quite different from that developed by the others. Accordingly, discussion of the physiology and the practical clinical implications of the contrast agents will be divided into three sections discussing the available media for intrathecal, intravascular, and intralymphatic applications, respectively.

PHYSIOLOGY OF WATER-SOLUBLE CONTRAST MEDIA INTRODUCED TO THE SUBARACHNOID SPACE

Normal Nervous System

Water-soluble contrast media are now introduced routinely into the subarachnoid space to define contours of the spinal cord, nerve root sheaths, and/or the cisterns surrounding the brain. Ionic contrast media were the first water-soluble agents to be used clinically for this purpose. They were introduced by the Europeans, but were limited to studies of the lumbar canal, because above this level they caused many side effects.[18] For this reason, they were never used in the United States. The incidence of side effects was reduced with the introduction of an ionic dimer (Dimeray), which, though it contained the same amount of iodine, had a lower osmolality than the ionic media (see Fig 1–5). As we have already noted, Dimeray was withdrawn from the U.S. market and metrizamide, a nonionic monomer, became the water-soluble agent of choice for examination of the subarachnoid space and the cerebral intraventricular compartments. Metrizamide produces neurotoxic side effects (seizures, changes in mood or perception, nausea, and vomiting) that are dose related[19] and that occur 4 to 10 hours after injection into the lumbar subarachnoid space. They ap-

and possibly to encounter a new spectrum of complications. Preliminary uses for the new contrast media discussed can be found in Figure 1–6.

Experience teaches that the side effects caused by a given water-soluble contrast agent will vary according to route of administration (i.e., intrathecal, intralym-

Generic Name	Trade Name	Mol. Wt.	mgI/ml	mOsmol/kg	Refs.
Metrizamide	Amipaque	789	170	300	6,13,14
Iopromide	Osmocon	791	300	600	*
Iogulamide		881	250	817	*
			300	1085	
Iopamidol	Isovue	777	200	413	7,15
			280	570	
Iohexol	Omnipaque	821	300	700	12
Diatrizoate	Hypaque	614	292	1520	11,13
	Renografin		400	1909	
Iothalamate	Conray	614	280	1500	5,13
Ioglicate	Rayvist	671	300	1790	*
Metrizoate	Isopaque	628	280	1460	13
Iotrol	Isocon	1626	300	300	17
Iotasul	Lymphocon	1608	300		16
Iocarmate	Dimeray	1254	280	1040	5
Ioxaglate	Hexabrix	1269	280	490	8,9,10
			320	600	

* Information obtained from confidential company sources

Fig 1–5.—The physical characteristics of water-soluble iodinated contrast media. References 5 through 17, as indicated in this figure, are found at the end of the chapter. Each reference pertains to the specific contrast medium for which it is listed.

pear to be related to entry of contrast agent into the brain substance (documented as computed tomographic [CT] contrast enhancement of the cortical surfaces after intrathecal administration). However, because patients who are clinically asymptomatic after intrathecal contrast injection have been noted on CT to display brain and spinal cord "blush" (i.e., CNS contrast entry), other factors than just tissue penetrance must be involved in the production of these toxic side effects, which appear to be more frequent in elderly patients and rarely occur in children.[20,21] Caille and coworkers[22] have suggested that the amount of medium in the cisterns and thus available to diffuse into the tissue is an important factor influencing toxicity seen after intrathecal injection.

Canine experiments have shown that the concentration of radiolabeled metrizamide in the brain correlates with the neurotoxic symptoms that can be observed clinically. Research has shown that puppies receiving the same dose of metrizamide as adult dogs will have a brain metrizamide concentration that is 2,500 times lower than the adult. This may explain why fewer neurotoxic side effects from metrizamide are noted in infants and children when compared with those in adult patients.[23] This reduced brain concentration of metrizamide appears to be due to two factors. First, the current clinical guideline for the maximum dose in infants and children is approximately twice that of the adult dose on a per-kg body weight basis. However, this increase does not fully correct for the greatly increased proportion of body weight contributed by the brain in children. When the recommended maximum dosages are recorrected on a *brain* weight basis, the maximum clinical dose recommended for children is less than 50% of the maximum adult dose. This failure to correct for brain weight differences is partially responsible for the reduced brain concentrations, but it does not fully account for the 2,500-fold decrease in brain metrizamide concentration. Physiologic differences are undoubtedly at work.

It is possible that there is an increased cerebrospinal fluid (CSF) clearance of metrizamide in the puppy compared with the adult dog. This would prevent prolonged contact of the metrizamide with the puppy brain. Another explanation would be to postulate differences in the brain itself that enable increase of metrizamide penetration in the adult dog. Further studies will be needed to determine precisely why these age-related differences occur.

While metrizamide penetration of the brain is well documented, the precise tissue compartment in which it is located is unknown. In rabbits, intraventricular perfusion studies using ^{125}I-labeled metrizamide were undertaken to determine its distribution, but it was not

possible to distinguish between interstitial and intracellular components.[24] The presence of metrizamide in the extracellular fluid is *assumed,* because other compounds of similar molecular weight and size have been shown to enter the brain from the CSF by diffusing from the region of high CSF concentration at the brain surface to the lower concentration in the interstitial spaces. That the diffusion of metrizamide from the cisterns into the brain is altered by the composition of the brain surface has been demonstrated by CT scans. In surface areas composed of white matter (i.e., spinal cord, brain stem, corpus callosum, and nerve roots), the penetration of the medium is diffuse. These areas never achieve the high concentrations found in gray matter zones that are in direct contact with the CSF (i.e., cerebellar cortex, cerebral cortex, the putamen of the thalamus, the hypothalamus, and inferior surfaces of the basal ganglia). These latter regions equilibrate with the cisternal metrizamide so readily that the brain CSF boundaries are obliterated at CT (Fig 1–7).[25]

The theory that metrizamide freely diffuses into brain extracellular space has been proposed by Winkler and Sackett[26] on the basis of experiments performed with other labeled tracers. The problem of where the metrizamide is located is complicated by the fact that there may be *two* extracellular compartments within the brain. Levin and associates[27] observed that tracers in the CSF equilibrated in an extracellular space that contains 14% to 14.7% of brain fluid. The same tracer given by the venous route equilibrated in a smaller, presumably perivascular space, which contained 1.9% to 5% of the brain fluid. There were no demonstrable connections between these extracellular compartments.

There is indirect evidence that extracellular compartments of the brain may communicate when the animal is dehydrated. In this situation, extracellular fluid is drawn into the cerebral vessels to counteract the increased blood osmolarity produced by the dehydration.[28] If the CSF contains metrizamide, the augmented brain penetration caused by this "bulk flow" may increase the brain concentration of the media and hence the incidence of toxic symptoms. This mechanism has been verified by a prospective study in which metrizamide myelogram patients who were hydrated had fewer side effects than those who fasted overnight.[29]

We do not know how injected metrizamide is cleared from the CSF in normal subjects. There are three theories:

1. The first postulates that the rate of metrizamide clearance from the CSF is closely related to the rate of CSF absorption by the arachnoid granulations.[30] Hence, changes in degree of hydration or level of CSF

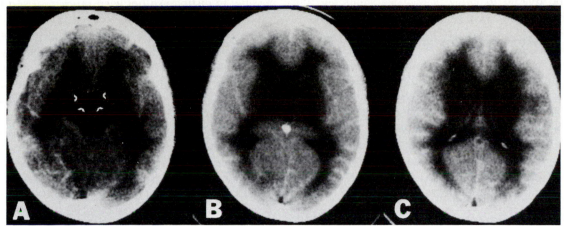

Fig 1–7.—CT scans of a 59-year-old woman 6 hours after metrizamide (290 mgI/ml, 11 ml) administered by lumbar puncture for a cervical myelogram inadvertently entered the cranial cisterns. Within 8 hours, the patient was mute and semicomatose. Her condition returned to normal over 48 hours. Premedication with diphenylhydantoin (Dilantin) presumably averted overt seizure activity. **A,** note the general shape of suprasellar cistern still preserved *(arrows)* as contrast agent penetrates basal (surface) aspect of basal ganglia, hypothalamic area, and the adjacent frontal and temporal cortex surrounding third ventricle. Note cerebral peduncles are surrounded by contrast medium, yet their Hounsfield measurements are 10 to 30 units below those of the enhanced cortex. **B, C,** note the gyral type of pattern at leading edge of the diffusion margin has almost disappeared.

pressure (which would affect CSF absorption) would alter metrizamide clearance.

2. The second theory proposes reabsorption by cerebral vessels as another important factor in removal of the metrizamide. Autoradiographic findings (after giving huge doses of marker) indicate that clearance is different in gray and white matter. This may be due to the difference in density of vessels in the two tissues (Fig 1–8). There were marked age-related differences in the distribution of labeled metrizamide when adult and 6-day-old dogs were compared.[31]

3. The third theory postulates that the bulk flow of fluid *from* the center of the brain *to* its surface prevents contraflow penetration of the contrast medium into the brain's depths and "washes it out" of the gray matter. This "flow" is postulated to be decreased in older subjects, thus perhaps accounting for the increased incidence of symptoms they experience after intrathecal metrizamide administration.

The following evidence, however, suggests that there is *no* bulk flow of CSF in *normal* brain: (1) Hydrostatic pressure in the perineuronal fluid space is lower than systemic blood pressure and spinal CSF pressure; (2) the entry of tracers from CSF into brain is not affected by changes in CSF pressure.[32, 33] Under *normal* conditions, brain entry of most CSF tracers appears to occur by diffusion (sink action) at a rate determined by the tracer's diffusion constant. If, however, the tracer is injected through a cannula *into* the brain, it is transported away from the injection site by bulk flow, probably along perivascular channels. *Bulk flow* can-

not, however, be demonstrated if the tracer is injected after the edema caused by cannula insertion has resolved.[34]

Indeed, the bulk flow theory may explain why the brain blush has not been observed in patients and ani-

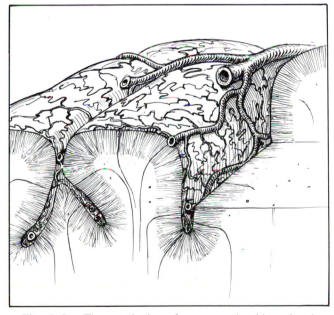

Fig 1–8.—The cortical surface vessels. Line drawing shows the angiographically invisible small arterial branches that form the pial vascular network. From the network, innumerable small vessels arise and penetrate the cortical gray matter. Each of them is surrounded by the CSF-filled perivascular space of Virchow-Robin. Note that only an occasional penetrating vessel continues into the white matter.

mals with acutely damaged brain. Evidence for bulk flow in the normal brain is at present controversial.

Abnormal Nervous System

INFARCTION.—There is little experimental or clinical information available concerning the penetration of intrathecally administered contrast medium into the abnormal CNS. Drayer has shown that metrizamide will not enter an area of acutely devitalized dog brain.[35] Perhaps (1) cytotoxic edema reduces the volume of extracellular space into which the contrast agent can diffuse, or (2) the vasogenic edema that follows infarction creates a "bulk flow" away from the lesion.[26]

HYDROMYELIA/SYRINGOMYELIA.—Cavitation of the spinal cord, including hydromyelia and syringomyelia, has been studied using metrizamide CT. Observations of the lesion immediately after instillation of the contrast medium and again 6 to 11 hours later showed delayed enhancement of the cavity. This supports the theory that the fluid in some syrinx cavities arises in the subarachnoid space and passes through the spinal cord into the cavity.[36] Slow filling of the cyst through a very small central canal is a less likely explanation when one considers that metrizamide penetrates normal spinal cord tissue (Fig 1–9).[37]

HYDROCEPHALUS.—The CT findings of communicating hydrocephalus have been studied on delayed scans after ventricular injection of metrizamide. Opacification of low attenuation areas adjacent to the dilated ventricles documents pathologic entry of the agent through the abnormally fenestrated ependymal lining of the ventricle. From here it passes into the enlarged periventricular extracellular spaces of the brain.[38] Following ventricular instillation of metrizamide in 17 children with known or suspected obstructive hydrocephalus, CT showed transependymal diffusion equally throughout the white and gray matter. This persisted for up to 6 days after instillation in cases in which adequate shunting was not performed (Fig 1–10).[39] The uniform distribution of the metrizamide seems to indicate that absorption by the numerous vessels of the gray matter did not occur in these children.

Delayed scans after instillation of intrathecal metrizamide in elderly patients with a triad of acute-onset dementia, broad-based gait, and incontinence (i.e., normal pressure hydrocephalus or NPH) showed patterns of media transit identical to those reported in radionuclide cisternography.[40] Because the latter test does not reliably predict which patients will show clinical improvement following a shunt procedure,[41] water-soluble contrast media are rarely used to investigate NPH.

MISCELLANEOUS.—The authors discovered no information in the literature concerning the CT enhancement patterns found after injection of metrizamide into the CSF of patients or animals with brain or spinal tumors. The dearth of such clinical reports is surprising, because spinal punctures are frequently performed on patients whose small intracerebral tumors have been defined by CT prior to tap. Theoretically, the zones of vasogenic edema surrounding the tumor would prevent contrast medium from entering the edematous region.

There is virtually no information in the literature concerning the interactions of metrizamide with other types of brain abnormality. This is particularly surprising in regard to pseudotumor cerebri, because spinal tap is part of the treatment, and the brain in this disease has an unusual form of edema that may be primarily cytotoxic. The degree of metrizamide brain penetration in these patients could be measured by CT scans. This information might reveal how the reduction in extracellular space affected the CT brain blush (i.e., the brain penetration of the contrast medium).

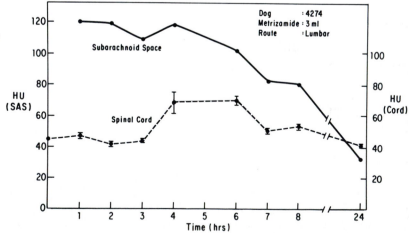

Fig 1–9.—Graph of CT units in the subarachnoid space (SAS) and spinal cord after injection of intrathecal metrizamide. Note the rise in hounsfield units (HU) within the spinal cord. (Courtesy of Philip Dubois, M.D., Duke University.)

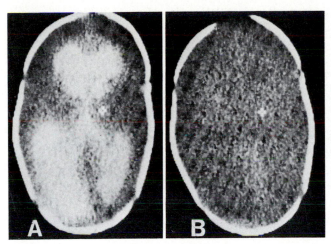

Fig 1–10.—CT scans in a 1-month-old child with aqueductal stenosis. **A,** scan shows transependymal absorption of the contrast medium into the periventricular white matter. (The brain density was 8 HU greater than on the precontrast scan.) **B,** repeat CT scan 48 hours later shows metrizamide throughout the brain with slightly less in the ventricles and the cortical rims. (The brain density was 11 HU greater than the precontrast scan.) The brain and ventricles showed no residual metrizamide 7 days after injection. It is worthwhile noting that this pattern may not be representative of the adult brain, which is composed of myelinated central white matter and has a lower water content than does that of a 1-month-old infant. (From Fitz C.R., Harwood-Nash D.C., Chuang S., et al.: Metrizamide ventriculography and computed tomography in infants and children. *Neuroradiology* 16:6–9, 1978. Used by permission.)

PHYSIOLOGY OF WATER-SOLUBLE CONTRAST MEDIA INTRODUCED TO THE VASCULAR SYSTEM

Normal Nervous System

In the United States at the present time, only ionic contrast media are approved for intravascular use in angiography, CT, and digital angiography. The high cost of the nonionic agents (which is mainly due to expensive but necessary purification procedures)[42] has limited their use as intravascular contrast agents even though the nonionic agents are better tolerated by experimental animals (Fig 1–11).

INTRAARTERIAL ROUTE.—Contrast media are currently ranked as to toxicity according to the amount of blood brain barrier (BBB) damage induced in normal brain tissue by very prolonged or repeated intracarotid injections. This is at best an arbitrary test, because none of the ionic media in Figure 1–1 cause BBB damage in the normal brain at the formulations, injection rates, and doses used clinically. A nonionic agent, iopamidol, with the same iodine content as an ionic agent, iothalamate, can be given as a prolonged (1.5 ml/second for *30 seconds*) intracarotid injection in dogs without inducing the BBB disruption that would be seen if iothalamate were used.[43] This presumably can be ascribed to the marked difference in the osmolalities of these agents (see Fig 1–5).[44] Whether or not this reduction in osmolality is of sufficient clinical advantage remains to be seen. The high cost of nonionic agents and the fact that they are clearly superior to ionic media only when given as 30-second carotid injections may limit the application of nonionic media in carotid angiography.

Rarely, a situation arises in which an ionic contrast agent with an extremely high osmolality is unintentionally injected at cerebral arteriography. The highly concentrated contrast medium induces changes on CT that are primarily the result of osmotic insult to the BBB. Sage and coworkers[45] reported a case in which 10 ml of Renografin 76 (osmolality of 1,940 milliosmols (mOsm)/kg H_2O) was inadvertently used for a selective right carotid injection. Figure 1–12 shows the contrast enhancement and edema on a 45- to 60-minute delayed scan. The patient experienced a focal left body seizure that subsided without treatment, but the EEG was abnormal 2 hours later. The mild left central facial weakness, initially noted 15 minutes after the seizure, re-

Contrast Agent	LD$_{50}$(g of Iodine/kg body weight)
Sodium meglumine ioglicate	8.72 (8.04–9.27)
Sodium meglumine ioxaglate	8.41 (7.70–9.13)
Metrizamide	12.97 (11.99–14.03)
Iohexol	~13
Iopromide	12.92 (11.70–14.22)
Nonionic dimer	16.05 (14.24–18.37)

Fig 1–11.—The lethal dose (LD$_{50}$: that dose producing death in 50% of test rats) for various intravenous water-soluble contrast agents. The 95% confidence limits are given in parentheses. (From Mutzel W.: Properties of conventional contrast media, in *Contrast Media Computed Tomography.* Amsterdam, Excerpta Medica, 1981, pp. 19–30. Used by permission.)

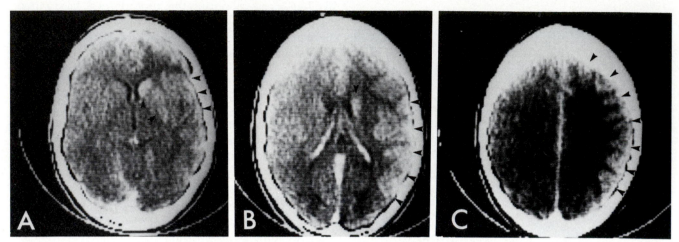

Fig 1–12.—Blood-brain barrier disruption of the right hemisphere of an adult after inadvertent intracarotid injection of Renografin 76 is seen on 45- to 60-minute delayed CT scans at three different levels (**A, B, C**). Note enhancement of the cortex (**A, B, C,** *lateral arrowheads*) and basal ganglia (**A, B,** *medial arrowheads*) and edema of the white matter. Transient seizures and neurologic deficits were noted. (From Sage M.R., Drayer B.P., Dubois P.J., et al.: Increased permeability of the blood-brain barrier after carotid renografin-76. *A.J.N.R.* 2:272–274, 1981. Used by permission.

solved 3 hours later.[45] There were no permanent neurologic deficits.

Permanent damage can, however, be induced by intraarterial injection of concentrated ionic media. A very high dose of Renografin 76 given to a neurologically normal 20-month-old child during cardiac angiography preceded the onset of seizure, coma, and death. The CT scans at 1, 3, and 7 days after angiography showed persistent enhancement of both gray and white matter (Fig 1–13). The anuria that developed caused extremely high blood iodine levels for a prolonged period. Dialysis reduced the blood levels, but the abnormal brain enhancement could still be seen on CT 7 days later. The microscopic location of the contrast medium within the brain could not be determined. However, its persistence 7 days after the arteriography seems to indicate that "binding" of unknown nature and significance had occurred.

Use of the newer nonionic water-soluble agents instead of the standard ionic agents (e.g., Renografin 76) for cardiac and arch angiography would eliminate the possibility that extremely hyperosmolar contrast media might inadvertently reach the brain and harm the patient. It is possible that the nonionic agents may be intrinsically less harmful than the ionic media for reasons other than the reduction in osmolality. Hydrophilic agents have been shown to be better tolerated in vivo than lipophilic agents. This generalization can only be made about compounds with a similar structure. Therefore, the evaluation of structurally dissimilar contrast media by their butanol coefficients (Fig 1–14) may not be predictive of toxicity.[44] (The butanol coefficient may be defined as a property of the contrast medium that measures the degree to which it is soluble in lipid and water at a given pH.)

INTRAVENOUS ROUTE.—The rate of entry and distribution of contrast medium in normal brain after maintaining a constant, prolonged (4-hour) contrast blood level by intravenous infusion has been calculated in the rabbit using labeled diatrizoate (an ionic contrast medium) and labeled metrizamide (a nonionic contrast medium). Regardless of the blood levels, there was no difference between these two agents as to *distribution* in normal brain tissue, both being generally more concentrated in gray than in white matter. Also, there was no difference in the slow rate and limited extent of entry of the contrast media. Both agents entered the brain and appeared to move through the gray matter by diffusion. They occupied a volume equal to 0.5% to 2.0% of the brain water.[24] This is the same size as the compartment that equilibrates with intravenously administered radioactive sodium, iodide, mannitol, chromium ethylenediamine tetraacetic acid (EDTA), or sucrose. While the ultrastructural site of this space is unknown, the Virchow-Robin space (that region around intracerebral vessels and inside the glial sheaths) has been proposed (Fig 1–15).[46]

If this site is correct, the contrast medium appears to have crossed normal, tight endothelial junctions that are the primary barrier against large particles (i.e., those with a diameter larger than 1.5 ng). Horseradish peroxidase with a molecular weight of 44,000 and albumin-bound Evans blue with a molecular weight of 69,000 are examples of commonly employed large molecules that are excluded from the perivascular space.

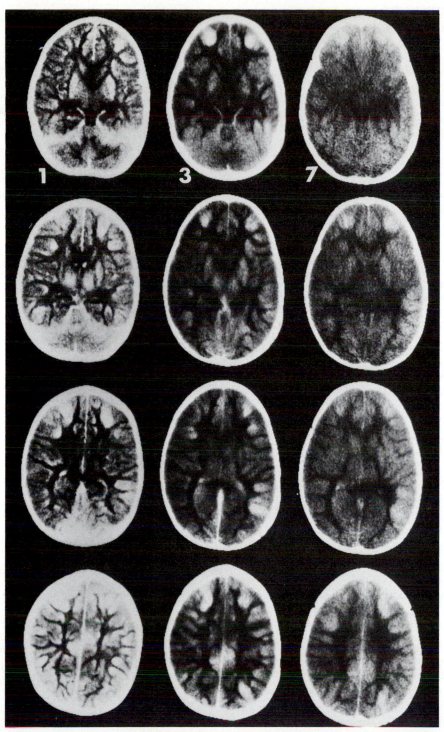

Fig 1–13.—Serial CT scans of a 20-month-old child after receiving an extremely high dose of Renografin 76 during cardiac angiography, which induced generalized BBB disruption, seizure, coma, renal failure, and death. The *left column* of scans, 1 day after angiography, shows intense enhancement of all gray matter structures. Some focal areas of particularly striking enhancement may have been caused by the additional BBB damage resulting from the seizures. The *center column* of CT scans, 3 days after angiography, continues to show enhancement of the brain in spite of dialysis to reduce the blood iodine level. The *right column* of scans, 7 days after angiography, shows persistent diffuse enhancement from contrast medium extravasation. No hemorrhage was present in the enhanced areas at autopsy. (Courtesy of Robert Peister, M.D., Philadelphia.)

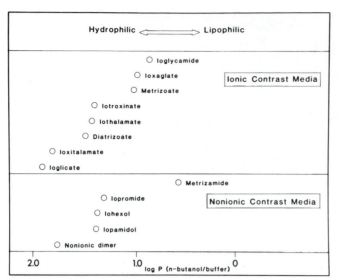

Fig 1–14.—Butanol/buffer partition coefficients of water-soluble ionic and nonionic contrast media (n − butanol buffer, pH 7.6). Among *similar* compounds, those that are lipophilic produce more neurotoxic symptoms. The comparison of dissimilar contrast media on the basis of this measurement appears unproductive. (From Mutzel W.: Properties of conventional contrast media, in *Contrast Media Computed Tomography.* Amsterdam, Excerpta Medica, 1981, pp. 19–30. Used by permission.)

Thus, it is possible that the smaller molecules of the contrast agents enter the perivascular space from the vessels (see Fig 1–15). If one assumes that there is only one extracellular compartment, the intravenous medium diffuses into the same space in the brain as the intrathecally administered agents. *If* this is true, we are left to wonder why one does not routinely encounter observable neurotoxic side effects in patients given intravenous ionic contrast media, because ionic agents have devastating effects when they enter the brain (even in very low concentration) after intrathecal injection. Remember that it took only small amounts of an ionic contrast medium used in the lumbar subarachnoid region to induce such severe side effects that it was banned as a myelographic agent in the United States.

The extravasation of intravenously administered ionic contrast material documented in the previously cited animal study has been shown by CT to occur in normal human brain. The enhancement observed of brain after intravenous contrast cannot be explained by the volume of the vascular bed.[47] It appears to represent contrast medium that has escaped from the normal cerebral circulation.*

---

*This precludes the use of iodinated contrast agents for measuring cerebral blood flow, because the enhancement on CT represents not only the intravascular pool, but also an unknown amount of extravascular medium. This is a particularly significant problem in evaluating areas of abnormal brain (which are, after all, the regions of clinical interest).

There is no rational way to rate the neurotoxicity of intravenously administered contrast media, because minimal amounts of both nonionic and ionic agents enter the normal brain. Even in very high doses (1.1 gm iodine/kg body weight), the contrast agent rapidly equilibrates with the plasma osmolality of approximately 280 to 300 mOsm/kg H_2O.[48] Hence, the neurologic symptoms seen in normal animals after prolonged or repeated intracarotid injections of contrast media are not seen after intravenous contrast. A previous report in dogs, which claimed to show generalized and focal BBB damage caused by high doses of intravenous contrast media,[49] could not be substantiated when it was repeated in dogs who were not under general anesthesia.[50]

Another (as yet untried) more precise way to rank vascular contrast media would be to measure the *rate constant* of brain entry for each agent and calculate the *Km*, which is a working measurement of each agent's BBB permeability.[46] Furthermore, the site at which the agents equilibrate could be determined by careful film and microscopic autoradiography using tritium-labeled contrast media.

All of the parameters listed could then be remeasured in normal brain of various ages and in abnormal brain to determine how the changes of extracellular fluid composition and alterations in glia and neurons caused by pathology contribute to the overall toxicity of each contrast agent. Until standardized techniques are developed and applied to various contrast media, our

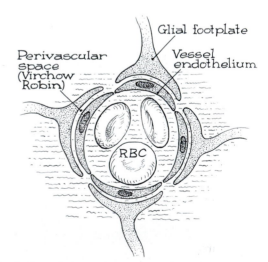

Fig 1–15.—Schematic cross section of a penetrating cerebral vessel such as seen in Figure 1–7. The endothelial cells are connected at "tight junction points," which prevent the entry of large molecules into the *perivascular* space. Because contrast media are relatively small molecules that equilibrate with a small percentage of the brain water after intravenous infusion, it has been postulated that they may be free to enter the *Virchow-Robin* spaces. (*RBC* = red blood cell.)

understanding of these compounds will remain, as presently, severely circumscribed.

Before moving on to discuss lesions that can be detected on CT scan through enhancement, it should be noted that the BBB is easily penetrated by contrast media in the region of the pineal gland, the posterior half of the pituitary gland, the choroid of the eye, the choroid plexus of the ventricles, and the dura.[43] Therefore, these areas normally display intense contrast enhancement on CT.

Abnormal Nervous System

There is a profusion of experimental and clinical data in the literature concerning alteration of the BBB in the abnormal brain.[51] Detection of this alteration by intravenous infusion of water-soluble contrast media before CT scanning has provided the basis for many publications over the past 6 or 7 years. The enormous interest evident in this area can be ascribed to the fact that most neurologic disorders are associated with an increased permeability of CNS vessels, which is important to the pathophysiology, diagnosis, treatment, and perhaps even to the etiology of the disorders discussed. The advances made in the last several years will be discussed by category.

Infarction

Many clinical and experimental CT studies have examined the behavior of ionic vascular contrast media given after cerebral infarction. There are three contrast CT patterns that can be seen alone or in combination after an infarction. Each of these will be discussed separately. The *first* is absence of normal gray matter enhancement, which can be seen throughout the evolution of the infarction. In the early stages, it indicates that the iodine transporting cerebral circulation does not adequately perfuse that portion of the brain. Later, it indicates a cystic or gliotic area traversed by capillaries that have developed a mature BBB. Absence of normal gray matter enhancement is a reliable sign of permanent cerebral destruction.[52]

The *second* pattern is only seen on scans done within 24 hours after onset of or sudden worsening of ischemic symptoms. The immediate contrast scan shows a variety of patterns that are not predictive of the ultimate viability of the tissue. The 3-hour delayed contrast CT scan has a characteristic pattern of slowly increasing, diffuse, heterogeneous enhancement that involves both white and gray matter without regard for differences in their vascular anatomy. In one study, three of the seven patients reported with this CT pattern were on heparin therapy or had a clotting disorder. These three and one other in the series subsequently developed massive confluent hemorrhagic infarction in areas that showed delayed CT enhancement. This pattern of enhancement

may predict which patients run the risk of developing hemorrhagic infarctions. The contrast extravasation may represent accumulation in the zones of vasogenic edema that precede the hemorrhage (Fig 1–16).[53]

The *third* pattern is characterized by *immediate* contrast enhancement, which persists or intensifies on delayed CT scans. When this pattern is seen *4 or more days after the onset* of cerebral ischemia, most of it can be attributed to extravasation of contrast medium into damaged areas containing proliferating immature capillaries.[52, 54] It resolves when the new capillaries are surrounded by glial foot processes and develop an effective BBB.[55] Capillary maturation throughout the lesion can be a lengthy process, particularly in larger infarcts. Hence, enhancement may be seen as late as 150 days following cerebral infarction. Enhancement caused by this mechanism is not necessarily related to vasogenic edema, because it can be observed long after the mass effect caused by edema has resolved.

While capillary proliferation adequately explains CT enhancement seen 4 or more days after infarction, it does not explain the persistent enhancement that has been reported by one study in patients after a very recent transient ischemic attack.*[56] Animal studies indicate that enhancement in such cases may be due to extravasation of the contrast medium into compromised but viable brain substance that is found *adjacent* to zones of cerebral infarction. Cats with acute middle cerebral artery infarction that were given intravenous ^{125}I-labeled Conray, technetium pertechnetate, or chlormerodrin Hg 203 showed tracer was surrounding *or possibly within* viable neurons at the periphery of the infarct 2 hours after the infusion.[57, 58] The Conray and technetium studies were not supplemented by autoradiography. However, these tracers accumulated in areas of brain adjacent to the infarct at a time when dysautoregulation (which theoretically might increase tissue radioactivity by increasing the relative volume of tracer-containing blood) had subsided.[59] Therefore, evaluation of infarct size by measuring volume of enhancing tissue is unreliable, because enhancement may indicate areas of transiently compromised viable brain.

In view of the above animal evidence of contrast extravasation into viable brain that surrounds infarcted brain, one would expect neurotoxic side effects from the contrast media to occur. Multiple studies have been done to detect contrast medium-induced side effects. Clinical observations indicate that patients with persistent gray matter enhancement on contrast CT after what appear to be transient ischemic attacks experience

---

*It is difficult to determine if areas of brain that were functionally silent or possessed abilities that are difficult to quantitate clinically may have been infarcted, thus producing the enhancement seen in the "transient ischemia" patients reported in this study.

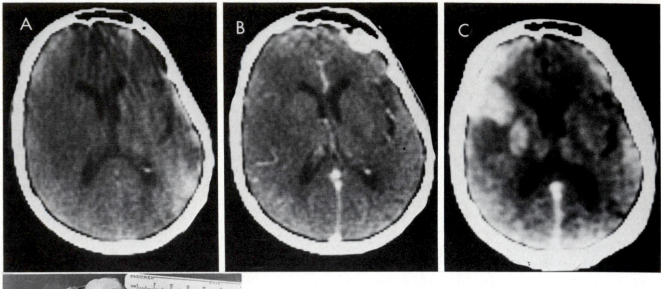

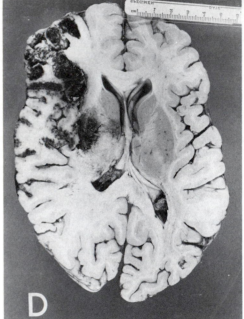

Fig 1–16.—Series of CT scans done 20 hours after cerebral embolization during a bout of atrial fibrillation: **A,** precontrast CT: obliteration of right Sylvian fissure; compression of right lateral ventricle. **B,** immediate high-dose contrast CT: absence of gray matter enhancement in right operculum and posterior lateral right thalamus. **C,** filtered delayed high-dose contrast scan 3 hours later showing wedge *enhancement* that includes lentiform area and adjacent cortex. In addition, an adjacent zone of cortical nonenhancement is seen. The mass effect did not increase as enhancement developed. **D,** autopsy specimen obtained 8 days later. Hemorrhagic infarction is seen in the area of delayed enhancement, and anemic infarction (with a very small punctate zone of hemorrhage) in areas showing no gray matter enhancement. (From Hayman L.A., Evans R.A., Bastion F.O., et al.: Delayed high dose contrast CT: Identifying patients at risk of massive hemorrhagic infarction. *A.J.N.R.* 2:139–147, 1981. Used by permission.)

no clinically apparent reaction after a 42-gm iodine infusion.[60] The authors have prospectively observed a series of 40 consecutive patients with cerebral infarction who received a high dose of contrast containing 80 gm of iodine without experiencing any detectable clinical deterioration. This is particularly interesting, because the number of infarctions in a given series that enhance can be increased by using higher doses of iodine.[61]

A large retrospective study has been done to examine the effect of contrast administration upon recovery from cerebral infarction. It suffered from the usual severe methodological handicaps of a retrospective study. Nevertheless, *it failed to demonstrate any statistically significant deleterious effect from the contrast agent.* The lack of correlation was surprising, because, according to the protocol, contrast medium (sodium iothalamate) was administered to patients with large infarctions and considerable mass effect (i.e., those with a poor prognosis) and withheld from those with normal preinfusion scans (i.e., those with an excellent prognosis).[62, 63] The authors of that study concluded that, although statistical proof was lacking, the *possibility* that contrast material *may* adversely affect potentially viable neuronal tissue should be kept in mind. The absence of documented contrast-induced side effects in these patients should cause us to consider a theory that relates the toxicity of *vascular* contrast media to factors other than accumulation in the brain.

In summary, when the third pattern is found 0 to 4 days after infarction, it can be explained by extravasation of contrast medium from compromised vessels into areas that may not become necrotic. This occurs principally in gray matter, because, as we have already noted, the majority of cerebral vessels are in gray matter. Gradually, *no sooner than 4 days* after ischemia, the third pattern of contrast CT enhancement can be ascribed to extravasation of contrast media from immature capillaries. In the early stages, it also tends to predominate in gray matter, because reanastomosis of iodine containing circulation with the developing immature capillaries occurs more readily in the gray matter than in the sparsely vascularized white matter.

In theory, a *fourth* pattern of CT enhancement may occur. A very large increase in the blood volume caused by vasodilation in areas adjacent to an acute infarct might produce enhancement on the immediate contrast scan that would diminish or disappear on the delayed scan (as the blood iodine concentration diminished).[52] This pattern has not been reported in clinical material, perhaps because it is obscured by simultaneous extravasation, which creates the third pattern of CT enhancement.

The administration of contrast material to patients with cerebral infarction has advanced our understanding of the events that occur in human infarction, but it appears to have no value in the therapeutic context, because enhancement does not appear to correlate with prognosis. To determine whether such a correlation exists would require a large series of patients in which all important parameters (i.e., age, sex, etiology, location and extent of infarction, presence or absence of collaterals, and a standardized mode of therapy) were precisely controlled.

Neoplasm

One of the most important uses for intravenous ionic contrast media in neuroradiology has been to enhance the CT visibility of CNS neoplasms. In 1975, Gado and associates[64] demonstrated that CT enhancement in two patients with intracranial neoplasms could not be explained by increased blood volume in the lesion. He did this by measuring the tissue-blood enhancement ratio and surmised that extravasation of contrast agent into the tumor was the cause of the tumor enhancement recorded by CT. Impairment of the BBB (which normally prevents the escape of all but a very small proportion of the intravascular contrast medium) is a well known feature of neoplastic vessels. With the exception of low-grade gliomas, necrotic neoplasms, and patients on corticosteroid therapy,[65] contrast administration commonly causes enhancement of neoplasms on CT. However, those neoplasms that have minimal BBB deficiency require higher doses of contrast agent to produce prolonged high blood-iodine levels before they

become visible (i.e., on *delayed* CT scans) (Fig 1–17).[66-69]

Multiple clinical papers have shown that traditional doses of intravenous contrast medium given immediately before CT sometimes fail to demonstrate BBB leakage (i.e., contrast enhancement).[66-69] One study of patients being followed by contrast CT after chemotherapy and radiotherapy for cranial tumors found that BBB damage was not detected in 11.5% of *treated* cases unless a 90-minute delayed scan was done.[67] Takeda and coworkers[70] have analyzed the dynamics of CT enhancement of 31 neoplasms by performing immediate CT scans followed by scans 1 and 2 hours after intravenous administration of contrast medium. They calculated tissue-blood contrast ratio and noted differences between meningiomas, pituitary adenomas, and neurinomas. They postulated that the mechanism of BBB disruption (i.e., increased pinocytosis or vascular endothelial fenestration) was different in each type of tumor. This resulted in different tissue-blood contrast ratios.

The precise location of the contrast medium that extravasates from the tumor vessels is not known. An autoradiographic study using intravenous tritium-labeled methotrexate (a chemotherapeutic agent) in mice with intracerebral implants of ependymoblastoma has shown vascular and interstitial tracer within the neoplasm 2 and 10 minutes after injection. Sixty minutes after injection, however, intracellular methotrexate was identified in the center of the neoplasm. Peripheral and infiltrating neoplastic cells showed comparatively little intracellular methotrexate. Uptake was higher in the edematous brain surrounding the neoplasm than in normal brain, but not as high as that found in the neoplasm per se.[71] These results are intriguing, because the molecular weight of the methotrexate is similar to that of the currently used ionic contrast agents. In fact, Neuwelt and coworkers[72] have shown that the concentrations of methotrexate and ionic contrast media can be correlated in brain after osmotic BBB disruption.[72] If the autoradiography of methotrexate were comparable to that of contrast media, the initial CT enhancement of neoplasms might be explained by the vascular and interstitial component alluded to above, and the findings on delayed CT scan might be related to the intracellular entry of the contrast agent. Until contrast medium extravasation in neoplasms is autoradiographed, these issues will remain the subject of speculation.

The incidence of intravenous contrast medium-induced seizures is increased by six to 19 *hundred*fold in patients with brain metastases compared with (presumably neurologically normal) patients receiving intravenous contrast infusion for pyelograms.[73-76] The risk of seizures after contrast administration in the neoplasia group is increased thirty *hundred*fold over the standard

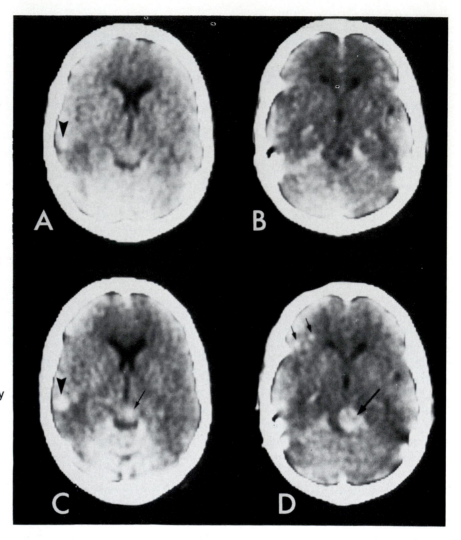

Fig 1–17.—A, B, immediate conventional dose postinfusion scans showing a subtle left temporal metastasis *(arrowhead)* from adenocarcinoma of the lung and surrounding focal cerebral edema. A scan 1 hour later failed to show the lesion. **C, D,** one-hour delay high-contrast dose (80 gml) scan of the same patient 1 day later showing additional lesions in brain stem and left frontal lobe *(arrows)*. Visualization of the left temporal lesion *(arrowhead)* is improved considerably. The large brain stem lesion was not visible on the immediate high-dose scan done that same day. (From Hayman L.A., Evans R.A., Hinck V.C., et al.: Delayed high iodine dose contrast computed tomography: Cranial neoplasms. *Radiology* 136:677–684, 1980. Used by permission.)

pyelogram group if the patient with a brain tumor also has a neoplasia-related seizure history and/or is undergoing (or has undergone) CNS antineoplastic therapy. Clearly, these patients have a seizure focus that predates contrast administration, and the administration of contrast medium triggers a seizure. Unlike the seizures induced in patients receiving intrathecal contrast material, the entry of the agent into the brain after the intravenous infusion does not appear to be the precipitating factor. Witness the fact that in Scott's series,[75] three of the seven patients with contrast-induced seizures had no detectable enhancement on CT. Conversely, there was no correlation between seizure induction and the presence of massive CT enhancement of metastases in Pagani and coworkers' series[73] of 188 cases.

Fischer[77] has postulated that the vasogenic edema associated with brain neoplasms produces local slowing of the circulation around these lesions, and this phenomenon has been well documented on contrast CT scans.[78]

Fischer believes that the prolonged exposure of the vascular endothelium to contrast medium gives the chemical an opportunity to exert a *direct* "permeability changing effect," thus causing seizures in patients with metastatic disease. The pattern was indeed detected by Pagani and associates[73] in several patients (Fig 1–18), but they did not suffer seizures. It would appear, therefore, that extravasation of contrast medium, manifested as cortical enhancement, was not the cause of contrast-induced seizures in this group.[73]

The intra-arterial injection of contrast material in patients with brain neoplasm is primarily directed at defining the vascularity of the lesion and its immediately surrounding area in order to gauge the location and extent of tumor and to thereby assist in planning the neurosurgical approach. In recent studies, patients with intracerebral neoplasms have been given an intracarotid infusion of 25% mannitol (to disrupt the BBB) and then an infusion of chemotherapeutic agent. Interposed 2 minutes after the infusion of mannitol, a high dose of

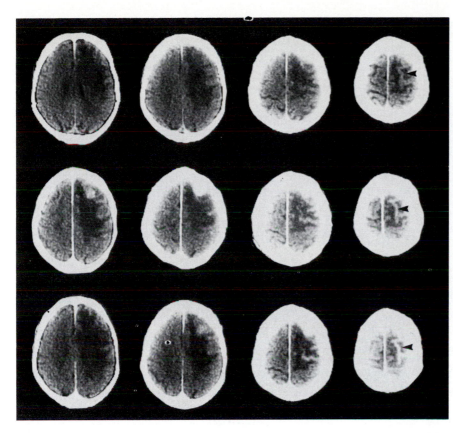

Fig 1–18.—Noncontrast CT scans of an 83-year-old man with edema secondary to a metastasis in the left cerebral hemisphere *(top row).* A high-dose contrast CT scan done 1 hour after infusion reveals the metastatic focus. An *arrow* indicates enhancement of the motor cortex *(center row),* which intensified on the 2-hour delayed scans *(bottom row).* Despite the persistent accumulation of contrast medium in the motor cortex, the patient did not seize. (Window settings are adjusted to maximize enhancement. The intensity of the contrast enhancement should be compared with the normal cortex of the right hemisphere.) (From Pagani J.J., Hayman L.A., Bigelow R.H., et al.: Diazepam prophylaxis of contrast media-induced seizures during computed tomography of patients with brain metastases. *A.J.N.R.* 4:67–72, 1983. Used by permission.)

ionic contrast medium (containing approximately 80 gm of iodine) has been given intravenously. Amazingly intense enhancement has been seen in both normal brain and neoplasm in areas perfused by the carotid that received the mannitol injection. Enhancement with CT after osmotic insult to the BBB persisted longer than that seen using the same dose of contrast agent in absence of the osmotic insult (Fig 1–19).[79] Despite the exceptionally high, prolonged levels of intracerebral contrast agent to which the normal brain tissue was subjected, the incidence of seizure induction in the high-risk patients reported by Neuwelt[72] does not appear to have been greater than that reported by others who have examined similar high-risk subjects.[73]

As we have seen, the intra-arterial injection of contrast media with an osmolality similar to 25% mannitol (e.g., Renografin 76) induces seizures (see Fig 1–12) and death if given in sufficiently large doses (see Fig 1–13). It is surprising that osmotic disruption of the cerebral BBB with the intracarotid injection of mannitol induced no EEG changes or visible seizures.[72] This must mean that the osmotic disruption caused by the contrast medium is insufficient alone to cause the toxic manifestations noted.

It is equally interesting that the intravenous infusion of a high dose of ionic contrast agent (containing approximately 80 gm of iodine) 2 minutes after intracarot-

id mannitol did not produce a higher incidence of neurotoxic side effects, because it did produce amazingly high contrast levels in the brain. These observations support Pagani's suggestion that the amount of extravasation of intravascular media per se is not the key to neurotoxicity as it appears to be with intrathecally administered contrast media.

One theory to explain the data would be to suggest that damaging the BBB sets in motion a chain of events that alters the extracellular fluid, glia, and neurons and that these changes in turn protect the brain from the effects of the contrast medium. The changes must, of course, occur (or be substantially underway) within 2 minutes after disruption of the BBB, because, as indicated above, massive CT contrast enhancement has been recorded when the intravenous contrast infusion was started 2 minutes after BBB disruption.

These changes would not have had time to develop if it was the contrast agent per se that disrupted the BBB, because intracarotid injections of hyperosmolar contrast media *simultaneously* produce BBB disruption and contrast extravasation. Protective mechanisms would not, in such circumstances, have had a chance to become activated. This theory (of protective changes rapidly induced by BBB disruption prior to contrast extravasation) could also explain why intrathecally administered contrast material that enters the brain at much lower

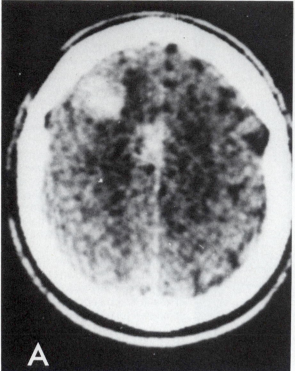

Fig 1–19.—A, thirty-minute delayed contrast scan showing extravasation of contrast medium into two areas of a malignant neoplasm in the right hemisphere. **B,** repeat 30-minute delayed contrast scan several days later. Scan was obtained after intracarotid mannitol was infused to disrupt the BBB. The contrast medium was given 2 minutes after the mannitol infusion. Note the extensive extravasation of contrast medium in tumor and adjacent motor cortex. The patient did not seize. (From Neuwelt E.A., Diehl J.T., Vu L.H., et al.: Monitoring of methotrexate delivery in patients with malignant brain tumors after osmotic blood-brain barrier disruption. *Ann. Intern. Med.* 94:449–453, 1981.)

concentrations (as documented on CT) causes seizures. In the case of intrathecal administration, the protective BBB mechanisms are not invoked before the contrast agent contacts the normal brain tissue.

Another, but less likely, possibility is that contrast medium that enters the brain from the vascular system enters a space different from the one occupied by contrast medium that enters from the subarachnoid space.[27]

While it is not clear how contrast agents trigger seizures, it has been shown that giving adequate levels of diphenylhydantoin does not prevent seizures induced by intravenously administered contrast media in high-risk tumor patients. However, it does appear to protect "normal" brain patients who receive subarachnoid nonionic contrast for myelographic studies. Prophylactic doses of diazapam, on the other hand, have been found to significantly reduce the incidence of seizures caused by intravenous contrast administration.[73] Considerable work has yet to be done to determine precisely how toxic side effects are induced by different agents given by the intravascular and intrathecal routes.

Infection

The pattern of CT enhancement following intravenous infusion of ionic contrast agents in subjects with *bacterial* cerebritis and abscess has been studied in both patients and laboratory animals. The early detection of these lesions has enabled timely therapy, thereby reducing the mortality rate in this condition.[80] Enzmann and coworkers[81] studied the CT contrast patterns in dogs after injection of α-streptococcus into the brain (traumatic abscess formation). He identified four stages of CT enhancement: (1) *Early cerebritis* appeared as an ill-defined area of enhancement (contrast extravasation), which intensified and enlarged on delayed CT scans 1 hour after bolus infusion of contrast agent. (2) *Late cerebritis* appeared as an area of ring enhancement that filled in centrally on delayed CT scans. The enhancement achieved greatest intensity 10 to 20 minutes after the contrast infusion and plateaued during the remainder of the 60-minute scan session. (3) *Early capsule formation* appeared as a smaller width of ring enhancement than that described above. The intensity of enhancement peaked 5 to 10 minutes after infusion and began to fade after 30 minutes. (4) *Late capsule formation* appeared as a still smaller ring or nodule, which no longer filled centrally on delayed scans. The enhancement intensity was greatest early and faded rapidly. The fact that the pattern of CT enhancement changes over time (i.e., amount and timing of entry and resorption of contrast agent) indicates an orderly progression of pathophysiologic processes that could be mapped. This is important, because patients with cerebritis may respond well to medical management with antibiotics and corticosteroids and not require surgical intervention. Britt and colleagues[82] suggest that these patients can be recognized as having a ring-shaped enhancing pattern that fills in on 30-minute postcontrast scans. Conversely, the patients with abscesses requiring surgical therapy will have enhancing rings that do not fill in on delayed contrast CT scans.

The CT pattern in immunosuppressed patients with brain abscesses is atypical. The ring enhancement is absent, presumably because of an alteration in host response to infection. It is a poor prognostic sign.[83] Immunologically compromised patients may also be infected with papovavirus, which is thought to produce progressive multifocal leukoencephalopathy. Enhancement with CT has been reported in some of these patients.[84]

It has been noted that medical therapy with corticosteroids reduces lesion enhancement on CT and that lesion enhancement will intensify after corticosteroids are withdrawn. These findings have no apparent clinical significance. In fact, lesion enhancement appears to persist after antibiotic therapy has obliterated a focus of infection.[80]

The CT enhancement seen after cerebral infection is caused by contrast extravasation from the new vessels found at the boundary zone surrounding cerebritis and abscess. These vessels develop more slowly if an experimental lesion is induced with septic emboli (i.e., the usual route of nontraumatic clinical infections) rather than by direct traumatic injection, because the embolic lesions are associated with infarction.[82]

Pathologic correlation of other types of brain infection with contrast CT patterns has not yet been reported in laboratory animals. Tuberculous, cysticercotic, and fungal lesions seen on CT scans of patients resemble pyogenic abscess, presumably because they also induce neovascularity with a deficient BBB.[85]

An unusual contrast CT scan appearance in a case of herpes simplex viral encephalitis has been reported in an infant. It was associated with persistent, apparently irreversible contrast enhancement (i.e., extravasation) in the gray matter of the brain. The infant's poor con-

dition precluded determining if this contrast retention ("binding") contributed to clinical deterioration.[86]

Congenital

Angiography and CT with and without contrast infusion are the primary diagnostic methods of evaluating patients for congenital vascular malformation and aneurysm. Noncontrast CT is superior to angiography in detecting small hemorrhages, small areas of adjacent infarction, subarachnoid blood, and calcification. Contrast CT can provide information not revealed by the arteriogram concerning thrombosed or partially thrombosed lesions. Thrombosed areas can be visible on contrast CT for three reasons: (1) The scanner is sensitive to smaller amounts of contrast entering the lesion than are detectable at angiography. (2) Small vessels in the walls of giant aneurysms have a defective BBB, which allows contrast extravasation.[87] (3) Areas of resolving hemorrhage have new vessels with an immature BBB, which allow contrast extravasation. Contrast CT scan can also detect zones of ischemic infarction in uninvolved adjacent brain that can appear "normal" on the noncontrast scan.[88]

Trauma

In general, contrast CT and arteriography are not necessary in the evaluation of patients examined after acute trauma unless an underlying brain disorder is suspected clinically. The noncontrast scan adequately detects cerebral contusions as well as intra- and extracerebral blood. The authors have noted one case in which a high dose of contrast material was given to a patient within 48 hours after acute head trauma, and extremely intense gray matter enhancement was seen on immediate scan (Fig 1–20). A scan 3 hours later demonstrated contrast extravasation within a zone of edema. This was not associated with alteration of clinical status of the patient, who was alert and oriented throughout. Intraventricular pressure, which was recorded throughout the period, was not altered. This case suggests that preexistence of a BBB defect created by acute brain concussion may protect the patient from the effects of massive contrast extravasation. (See Neoplasm in this section for a discussion of this theory.)

Contrast administration is necessary for the occasional patient in whom the unenhanced scan shows an isodense mass that could represent resolving subacute subdural hematoma. This situation is encountered less frequently with newer generation scanners. When it does occur, bolus infusion of contrast medium can be used to enhance the brain surfaces and thereby differentiate subdural collection from brain swelling.[89]

Amendola and Ostrum[90] reported that some subdural

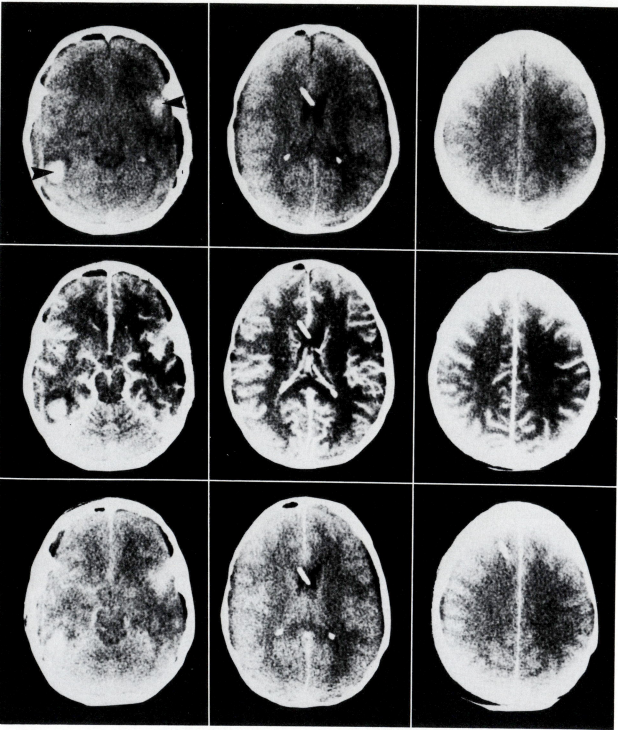

Fig 1–20.—*Top row,* CT scan 48 hours after head trauma showing two intracerebral hematomas *(arrowheads)* and an intraventricular pressure cannula. *Center row,* CT scans immediately after intravenous ionic contrast medium (diatrizoate) infusion show *extremely* intense enhancement of gray matter structures presumably caused by the cerebral concussion. *(Bottom row),* CT scan 3 hours later shows residual enhancement of a broad area surrounding the gray matter and enhancement of the crescent of edema formerly seen anterior to the right temporal hematoma. No neurologic sequelae or change in intracranial pressure were noted during or 24 hours after these scans.

collections enhance on delayed contrast CT (Fig 1–21). The etiology of delayed subdural enhancement is unknown. It may indicate that a membrane has formed, and the subdural collection must be removed surgically. However, electron microscopy of the inner surface of the normal dura has revealed that it has no tight junctions[91] to prevent contrast medium from entering the CSF or, theoretically, the subdural collection. Surgical pathologic correlation would be necessary to resolve the mechanism by which delayed subdural enhancement occurs.

Miscellaneous

OSMOTIC BRAIN INJURY.—The degree of osmotically induced BBB disruption can be quantitated by serially measuring intensity of enhancement on serial CT scans after intravenous infusion of Renografin 60.[92] Animal experiments have been done that suggest nonionic agents such as metrizamide may not be as effective as the traditional high-osmolality ionic agents in producing contrast enhancement on CT. Neuwelt and associates[93] examined phenobarbitol-sedated dogs after 25% mannitol was injected into the carotid artery to disrupt the BBB. He showed that the CT enhancement produced by meglumine iothalamate (Conray 60) was greater and persisted longer after intravascular administration than the enhancement caused by metrizamide. Similar studies comparing CT enhancement after intravascular administration of ionic and nonionic media must be done in patients with commonly encountered clinical types of brain lesions before one can conclude that the nonionic agents (e.g., metrizamide) do not produce equivalent CT brain enhancement.

RADIATION AND DRUG-INDUCED BRAIN INJURY.— Normal brain exposed to prophylactic intrathecal methotrexate and/or radiotherapy can develop necrosis of deep hemispheric white matter that may be fatal. These areas can be detected on contrast CT scans as enhancing foci.[94] These areas may be mistaken as neoplastic foci and biopsied. The CT appearance in the early stages of this condition is poorly documented.

Marked CT contrast enhancement of the spinal cord and roots have been reported in children who received 1,200 to 2,400 rad to the spine 1 month to 4½ years

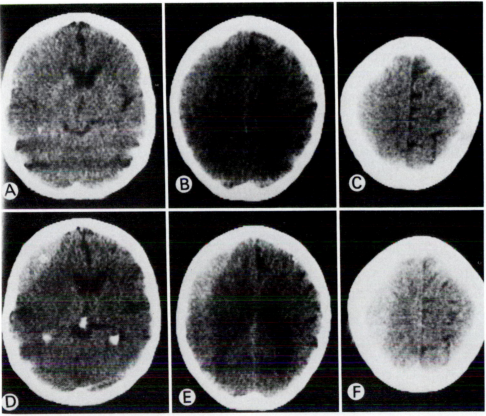

Fig 1–21—A, B, C, CT scans 5 minutes after administration of contrast media in a 65-year-old man. Effacement of sulci in the right hemisphere is evident. **D, E, F,** delayed scans 6 hours later showing contrast extravasation into the right frontal subdural hematoma. (From Amendola M.A., Ostrum B.J.: Diagnosis of isodense subdural hematomas by computed tomography. *A.J.R.* 129:693–697, 1977. Used by permission.)

prior to the scan. Subclinical damage to the BBB has been postulated as the cause of this phenomenon.[95]

MULTIPLE SCLEROSIS.—Disruption of the BBB occurs in vessels of the white matter and, less commonly, in the cortical and subcortical regions of the brain in patients with acute and relapsing multiple sclerosis. The number of lesions detected by CT can be dramatically increased if high intravenous doses of contrast medium are used and the scan is delayed for 1 hour. This allows time for the maximum amount of ionic contrast medium to accumulate in lesions having minimal BBB damage.[96, 97] Chronic multiple sclerosis lesions can usually be identified as nonenhancing low-density zones in the white matter. Occasionally, a chronic lesion will be isodense on noncontrast scans, but identified as a zone of nonenhancement surrounded by normal diffuse white matter enhancement in delayed contrast scans (Fig 1–22).[96]

PHYSIOLOGY OF WATER-SOLUBLE CONTRAST MEDIA INTRODUCED TO THE LYMPHATIC SYSTEM

A new water-soluble contrast agent, Iotasul (see Fig 1–4), has been tested in dogs. Injection of this agent into the tissues of the neck resulted in opacification of the regional lymphatic system.[16] This agent, used with CT, could have a substantial impact on the staging of tumor spread. The difficulty in producing the substance lies mainly in purifying the product. Once this problem has been solved, this agent will be subjected to clinical tests in humans.

SUMMARY

The authors have tried to recapitulate the development of water-soluble contrast agents, review present knowledge concerning the physiology of existing contrast media, and define four important areas that merit further investigation. In summary, these are to (1) define the BBB for contrast media directly instead of relying on extrapolated data obtained by using markers of different molecular size and characteristics, (2) determine why intrathecal administration is more toxic than intravascular administration, (3) isolate those factors, other than osmolarity, that cause the neurotoxic side effects of contrast media, and (4) determine the macro- and microscopic location of those contrast molecules that enter both normal brain (at all ages) and abnormal brain.

REFERENCES

1. Fischer H.W.: Contrast media, in Newton T.H., Potts D.G. (eds.): *Radiology of the Skull and Brain: Angiography.* St. Louis, C.V. Mosby Co., 1974, vol. 2, book 1, pp. 893–894.
2. Grainger R.G.: Osmolality of intravascular radiological contrast media. *Br. J. Radiol.* 53:739–746, 1980.
3. Almen T.: Contrast agent design: Some aspects on the synthesis of water soluble contrast agents of low osmolality. *J. Theor. Biol.* 24:216–226, 1969.
4. Hayman L.A., Tang R., Pagani J.J., et al.: A comparison of visual phenomena and pain following carotid injection of Conray and Hexabrix, in preparation.
5. Amundsen P., Miller R.E., Skucas J. (eds.): Water solu-

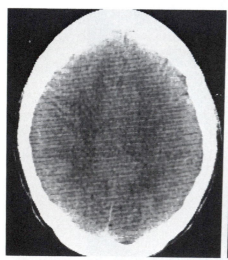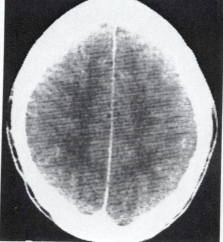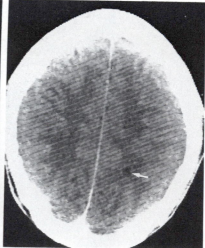

Fig 1–22.—Low-density multiple sclerosis plaque seen only on high-dose delayed scan. **A,** unenhanced scan appears normal. **B,** immediate standard contrast CT scan appears normal. **C,** one-hour delayed scan after a high dose of contrast medium in the patient shows small low-density plaque in the left centrum semiovale *(arrow).* (From Vineula F.V., Fox A.J., Debrun G.M., et al.: New perspectives in computed tomography of multiple sclerosis. *A.J.R.* 139: 123–127, 1982. Used by permission.)

ble myelographic agents, in Miller R. (ed.): *Radiographic Contrast Agents*. Baltimore, University Park Press, 1977, pp. 437–445.

6. Bertoni J.M., Schwartzman R.J., vanHorn G., et al.: Asterixis and encephalopath following metrizamide myelography: Investigations into possible mechanisms and review of the literature. *Ann. Neurol.* 9:366–370, 1981.

7. Bonati F., Felder E.E., Tirone P.: Iopamidol: New preclinical and clinical data. *Invest. Radiol.* 15:s310–s316, 1980.

8. Grainger R.G.: Intravascular contrast media: The past, the present, and the future. *Br. J. Radiol.* 55:1–18, 1982.

9. Gonsette R.E.: Animal experiments and clinical experiences in cerebral angiography with a new contrast agent (ioxaglic acid) with a low hyperosmolality. *Ann. Radiol.* 21:271–273, 1978.

10. Gonsette R.E., Liesenborgh L.: New contrast media in cerebral angiography: Animal experiments and preliminary clinical studies. *Invest. Radiol.* 15(suppl. 6):270–274, 1980.

11. Hoppe J.O., Archer S.: X-ray contrast media for cardiovascular angiography. *Angiology* 11:244–254, 1960.

12. Lindgren E.: Iohexol. *Acta Radiol. Suppl.* 362:9–11, 1980.

13. Olin T.B., Redman H.C.: Experimental evaluation of contrast media in the vertebral circulation. *Acta Radiol. Suppl.* 270:216–227, 1967.

14. *Physician's Desk Reference*, ed. 34. Oradell, N.J. Medical Economics Company, 1980, pp. 2039–2041.

15. Pitre D., Felder E.: Development, chemistry and physical properties of Iopamidol and its analogues. *Invest. Radiol.* 15:s301–s309, 1980.

16. Siefert H.M., Mutzel W., Schobel C., et al.: Iotosul: A water-soluble contrast agent for direct and indirect lymphography. *Lymphology* 13:150–157, 1980.

17. Sovak M., Ranganathan R., Speck U.: Nonionic dimer: Development and initial testing of an intrathecal contrast agent. *Radiology* 142:115–118, 1982.

18. Skalpe I.O.: Adverse effects of water-soluble contrast media in myelography, cisternography, and ventriculography. *Acta Radiol. Suppl.* 355:359–370, 1977.

19. Peeters F.L.: Myelography with metrizamide. *Radiol. Clin.* 46:203–213, 1977.

20. Drayer B.P., Rosenbaum A.E., Reigel D.B., et al.: Metrizamide computed tomography cisternography: Pediatric applications. *Radiology* 124:349–357, 1977.

21. Sleven D.: Winthrop Laboratories regarding FDA approval for intrathecal metrizamide use in children (personal communication).

22. Caille J.M., Guibert-Tranier F., Howa J.M., et al.: Cerebral penetration following metrizamide myelography. *J. Neuroradiol.* 7:3–12, 1980.

23. Hayman L.A., Pagani J.J., Anderson G.M., et al.: Intrathecal ^{3}H labelled metrizamide in normal dog brain: I. Age related brain concentration. *A.J.N.R.* 4:1091–1096, 1983.

24. Fenstermacher J.D., Bradbury M.W., duBoulay G., et al.: The distribution of ^{125}I-metrizamide and ^{125}I-diatri-

zoate between blood, brain and cerebrospinal fluid in the rabbit. *Neuroradiology* 19:171–180, 1980.

25. Hayman L.A., Hinck V.C., Pagani J.J., et al.: Regional differences in permeability of the cisternal spaces of the normal brain (in preparation).

26. Winkler S.S., Sackett J.F.: Explanation of metrizamide brain penetration: A review. *J. Comput. Assist. Tomogr.* 4:191–193, 1980.

27. Levin E., Arieff A., Kleeman C.R.: Evidence of different compartments in the brain for extracellular markers. *Am. J. Physiol.* 21:1319–1325, 1971.

28. Weed L.H., McKibben S.: Pressure changes in the cerebrospinal fluid following intravenous injection of solutions of various concentrations. *Am. J. Physiol.* 48:512–530, 1919.

29. Eldevick O.P., Nakken K.O., Haughton V.M.: The effect of dehydration on the side effects of metrizamide myelography. *Radiology* 129:715–716, 1978.

30. Potts D.G., Gomez D.G., Abbott G.F.: Possible causes of complications of myelography with water-soluble contrast medium. *Acta Radiol. Suppl.* 355:390–402, 1977.

31. Hayman L.A., Anderson G.M., Betoni J.M., et al.: Intrathecal ^{3}H labelled metrizamide in normal dog brain: II. Autoradiography (in preparation).

32. Cuypers J., Matakas F., Potolicchio S.J. Jr.: Effect of central venous pressure on brain tissue pressure and brain volume. *J. Neurosurg.* 45:89–94, 1976.

33. Matakas F., Stechele S., Keller F.: Microcalcifications in the cerebral extracellular space, in Cervol-Navarro J. (ed.): *Advances in Neurology*. New York, Raven Press, 1978, pp. 125–131.

34. Cserr H.F., Ostrach L.H.: Bulk flow of interstitial fluid after intracranial injection of blue dextran 2000. *Exp. Neurol.* 45:50–60, 1974.

35. Drayer B.D., Dujovny M., Boehnkem W., et al.: The capacity for computed tomography diagnosis of cerebral infarction. *Radiology* 125:393–402, 1977.

36. Barnett H.J.M., Fox A., Vinuela F., et al.: Delayed metrizamide CT observations in syringomyelia, abstracted. *Ann. Neurol.* 8:116, 1980.

37. Dubois P.J., Drayer B.P., Sage M., et al.: Intramedullary penetrance of metrizamide in the dog spinal cord. *A.J.N.R.* 2:313–317, 1981.

38. Hiratsuka H., Fujiwara K., Okada K., et al.: Modification of periventricular hypodensity in hydrocephalus with ventricular reflux in metrizamide CT cisternography. *J. Comput. Assist. Tomogr.* 3:204–208, 1979.

39. Fitz C.R., Harwood-Nash D.C., Chuang S., et al.: Metrizamide ventriculography and computed tomography in infants and children. *Neuroradiology* 16:6–9, 1978.

40. Hindmarsh T.: Computed cisternography for evaluation of CSF flow dynamics. *Acta Radiol. Suppl.* 355:269–279, 1977.

41. Symonn L., Hinzpeter T.: The enigma of normal pressure hydrocephalus: Tests to select patients for surgery and predict shunt function. *Clin. Neurosurg.* 24:285–315, 1976.

42. Bettmann M.A.: Angiographic contrast agents: Conven-

tional and new media compared. *A.J.R.* 139:787–794, 1982.

43. Sage M.R.: Comparison of blood brain barrier disruption following intra-carotid iopamidol and methylglucamine iothalamate. *A.J.N.R.*, to be published.

44. Mutzel W.: Properties of conventional contrast media, in Felix R., Kazner E., Wegener O.H. (eds.): *Contrast Media in Computed Tomography.* Amsterdam, Excerpta Medica, 1981, pp. 19–30.

45. Sage M.R., Drayer B.P., Dubois P.J., et al.: Increased permeability of the blood-brain barrier after carotid Renografin-76. *A.J.N.R.* 2:272–274, 1981.

46. Bradbury M.: *The Concept of a Blood-Brain Barrier.* New York, John Wiley & Sons, 1979, pp. 38–58.

47. Caille J.M., Billerey J., Renou A.M., et al.: Cerebral blood volume and water extraction from cerebral parenchyma by hyperosmolar contrast media. *Neuroradiology* 16:579–582, 1978.

48. Feldman S., Hayman L.A., Hulse M.: Pharmacokinetics of low and high dose intravenous diatrizoate contrast media. *Invest. Radiol.* 19:54–57, 1984.

49. Zamani A., Kido D., Morris J., et al.: Permeability of the blood brain barrier to different doses of diatrizoate megulamine-60. *A.J.N.R.* 3:631–634, 1982.

50. Hayman L.A., Pagani J.J., Serur J., et al.: Relative impermeability of the blood barrier to intravenous high iodine dose meglumine diatrizoate in the normal dog (submitted to *A.J.N.R.*).

51. Sage M.R.: Blood-brain barrier: Phenomenon of increasing importance to the imaging clinician. *A.J.N.R.* 3:127–138, 1982.

52. Hayman L.A., Sakai F., Meyer J.S., et al.: Iodine enhanced CT patterns after cerebral arterial embolization in baboons. *A.J.N.R.* 1:233–238, 1980.

53. Hayman L.A., Evans R.A., Bastion F.O., et al.: Delayed high dose contrast CT: Identifying patients at risk of massive hemorrhagic infarction. *A.J.N.R.* 2:139–147, 1981.

54. DiChiro G., Timins E.L., Jones A.E., et al.: Radionuclide scanning and microangiography of evolving and completed brain infarction: A correlative study in monkeys. *Neurology* 24:418–423, 1974.

55. Cancilla P.A., Frommes S.P., Kahn L.E., et al.: Regeneration of cerebral microvessels: A morphologic and histochemical study after local freeze-injury. *Lab. Invest.* 40:74–82, 1979.

56. Kinkel W.R., Jacobs L., Kinkel P.R.: Grey matter enhancement: A computerized tomographic sign of cerebral hypoxia. *Neurology* 30:810–819, 1980.

57. Dudley A.W., Lunzer S., Heyman A.: Localization of radioisotope (Chloromerodrin Hg-203) in experimental cerebral infarction. *Stroke* 1:143–148, 1970.

58. Anderson D.C., Coss D.T., Jacobson R.L., et al.: Tissue pertechnetate and iodinated contrast material in ischemic stroke. *Stroke* 11:617–622, 1980.

59. O'Brien M.D., Jordan M.M., Waltz A.G.: Ischemic cerebral edema and the blood brain barrier. *Arch. Neurol.* 30:461–465, 1974.

60. Kinkel W.: Personal communication, 1980. (Harry M. Dent Neurologic Institute, Millard Fillmore Hospital, 3 Gates Circle, Buffalo, NY 14209.)

61. Valk J.: High dose contrast injections and cerebral infarctions, in *Computed Tomography and Cerebral Infarctions With an Introduction to Practice and Principles of CT Scan Reading.* New York, Raven Press, 1980, pp. 45–46.

62. Kendall B.E., Pullicino P.: Intravascular contrast injection in ischemic lesions: II. Effect on prognosis. *Neuroradiology* 19:241–243, 1980.

63. Pullicino P., Kendall B.E.: Contrast enhancement in ischemic lesions: I. Relationship to prognosis. *Neuroradiology* 19:235–239, 1980.

64. Gado M.H., Phelps M.E., Coleman R.E.: An extravascular component of contrast enhancement in cranial computed tomography: II. Contrast enhancement and the blood-tissue barrier. *Radiology* 117:595–597, 1975.

65. Crocker E.F., Zimmerman R.A., Phelps M.E., et al.: The effect of steroids on the extravascular distribution of radiographic contrast material and technetium pertechnetate in brain tumors as determined by computed tomography. *Radiology* 119:471–474, 1976.

66. Davis J.M., Davis K.R., Newhouse J., et al.: Expanded high iodine dose in computed cranial tomography: A preliminary report. *Radiology* 131:373–380, 1979.

67. Shalen P.R., Hayman L.A., Wallace S., et al.: Protocol for delayed contrast enhancement in computed tomography for cerebral neoplasia. *Radiology* 139:397–402, 1981.

68. Hayman L.A., Evans R.A., Hinck V.C.: Delayed high iodine dose contrast computed tomography: Cranial neoplasms. *Radiology* 136:677–684, 1980.

69. Raininko R., Majurin M.L., Virtama P., et al.: Value of high contrast medium dose in brain CT. *J. Comput. Assist. Tomogr.* 6:54–57, 1982.

70. Takeda N., Tanaka R., Nakai O., et al.: Dynamics of contrast enhancement in delayed computed tomography of brain tumors: Tissue-blood ratio and differential diagnosis. *Radiology* 142:663–668, 1982.

71. Tator C.H.: Chemotherapy of brain tumors: Uptake of tritiated methotrexate by a transplantable intracerebral ependymoblastoma in mice. *J. Neurosurg.* 37:1–8, 1972.

72. Neuwelt E.A., Maravilla K.R., Frenkel E.P., et al.: Osmotic blood-brain barrier disruption: Computerized tomographic monitoring of chemotherapeutic agent delivery. *J. Clin. Invest.* 64:684–688, 1979.

73. Pagani J.J., Hayman L.A., Bigelow R.H., et al.: Diazepam prophylaxis of contrast media-induced seizures during computed tomography of patients with brain metastases. *A.J.N.R.* 4:67–72, 1983.

74. LoZito J.C.: Convulsions: A complication of contrast enhancement in computerized tomography. *Arch. Neurol.* 34:649–650, 1977.

75. Scott W.R.: Seizures: A reaction to contrast media for computed tomography of the brain. *Radiology* 137:359–361, 1980.

76. Pagani J.J., Hayman L.A., Bigelow R.H., et al.: Prophylactic diazepam in prevention of contrast media associated seizures in glioma patients undergoing cerebral computed tomography. *A.J.N.R.* 4:67–72, 1983.

77. Fischer H.W.: Occurrence of seizure during cranial computed tomography, opinion. *Radiology* 137:563–564, 1980.

78. Penn R.D., Walser R., Kurtz D., et al.: Tumor volume, luxury perfusion, and regional blood volume changes in man visualized by subtraction computerized tomography. *J. Neurosurg.* 44:449–457, 1976.

79. Neuwelt E.A., Diehl J.T., Vu L.H., et al.: Monitoring of methotrexate delivery in patients with malignant brain tumors after osmotic blood-brain barrier disruption. *Ann. Intern. Med.* 94:449–453, 1981.

80. Whelan M.A., Hilal S.K.: Computed tomography as a guide in the diagnosis and followup of brain abscesses. *Radiology* 135:663–671, 1980.

81. Enzmann D.R., Britt R.H., Yeager A.S.: Experimental brain abscess evolution: Computed tomographic and neuropathologic correlation. *Radiology* 133:113–122, 1979.

82. Britt R.H., Enzmann D.R., Yeager A.S.: Neuropathological and computerized tomographic findings in experimental brain abscess. *J. Neurosurg.* 55:590–603, 1981.

83. Enzmann D.R., Brant-Zawadzki M., Britt R.H.: CT of central nervous system infections in immunocompromised patients. *A.J.R.* 135:263–267, 1980.

84. Heinz E.R., Drayer B.P., Haenggeli C.A., et al.: Computed tomography in white matter disease. *Radiology* 130:371–378, 1979.

85. Whelan M.A., Stern J.: Intracranial tuberculoma. *Radiology* 138:75–81, 1981.

86. Junck L., Enzmann D.R., DeArmond S.J., et al.: Prolonged brain retention of contrast agent in neonatal herpes simplex encephalitis. *Radiology* 140:123–126, 1981.

87. Pinto R.S. Kricheff I.I., Butler A.R., et al.: Correlation of computed tomographic, angiographic and neuropathological changes in giant cerebral aneurysms. *Radiology* 132:85–92, 1979.

88. Hayman L.A., Fox A.J., Evans R.A.: Effectiveness of contrast regimens in CT detection of vascular malformations of the brain. *A.J.N.R.* 2:421–425, 1981.

89. Hayman L.A., Evans R.A., Hinck V.C.: Rapid high-dose contrast computed tomography of isodense subdural hematoma and cerebral swelling. *Radiology* 131:381–383, 1979.

90. Amendola M.A., Ostrum B.J.: Diagnosis of isodense subdural hematomas by computed tomography. *A.J.R.* 129:693–697, 1977.

91. Nabeshima S., Reese T.S., Landis D.M., et al.: Junctions in the meninges and marginal glia. *J. Comp. Neurol.* 164:127–169, 1975.

92. Drayer B.P., Schmeckel D.E., Hedlund L.W., et al.: Radiographic quantitation of reversible blood-brain barrier disruption in vivo. *Radiology* 143:85–89, 1982.

93. Neuwelt E.A., Maravilla K.R., Frenkel E.P., et al.: Use of enhanced computerized tomography to evaluate osmotic blood-brain barrier disruption. *Neurosurgery* 6:49–56, 1980.

94. Shalen P.R., Ostrow P.T., Glass P.J.: Enhancement of the white matter following prophylactic therapy of the central nervous system for leukemia: Radiation effects and methotrexate leukoencephalopathy. *Radiology* 140:409–412, 1981.

95. Pettersson H., Harwood-Nash D.C.F., Fitz C.R., et al.: Contrast enhancement of the irradiated spinal cord in children. *A.J.N.R.* 2:581–584, 1981.

96. Vinuela F.V., Fox A.J., Debrun G.M., et al.: New perspectives in computed tomography of multiple sclerosis. *A.J.R.* 139:123–127, 1982.

97. Sears E.S., McCammon A., Bigelow R., et al.: Maximizing the harvest of contrast enhancing lesions in multiple sclerosis. *Neurology* 32:815–820, 1982.

2

Cerebral Blood Flow Determination

Sidney K. Wolfson, Jr., M.D.
David Gur, Sc. D.
Howard Yonas, M.D.

IN THE FOREGOING chapter, we learned about the characteristics of the cerebral vasculature with respect to the transfer of materials between the intravascular compartment and brain tissue. Most importantly, we have seen that there is a special selectivity possessed by cerebral capillaries, which restricts the passage of many materials that diffuse easily in other body tissues. The subject of this chapter depends upon the fact that many substances do cross the "blood-brain barrier" (BBB) freely, including some that are radiodense. While lack of ability to leave the vascular bed renders a radiodense or radiopaque medium capable of clearly outlining the limits of the vascular space and of estimating transit time of blood across a given vascular bed, the presence of the ability to cross the BBB renders it useful in estimating the volume flow rate of the blood perfusing and nourishing the tissue itself. One such freely diffusible, radiodense substance is stable xenon gas, a natural constituent of the atmosphere. We shall see that using it in conjunction with CT gives xenon unique qualities with respect to highly detailed cerebral blood flow measurements. In fact, it may be possible to provide anatomical maps in both two and three dimensions with precision and resolution approaching that of CT itself. These developments are exceedingly important, because it is becoming more and more clear that an understanding of the physiologic changes accompanying or preceding morphological changes is necessary for the correct interpretation of the morphological changes themselves. Obviously, such knowledge could provide a basis for treatment. As anatomical resolution improves, this is becoming even more significant, because we can now begin to see elemental functional units and need to have an appreciation of their workings beyond a mere knowledge of presence and size. Hence, the existing interest in cerebral blood flow (CBF) measurement has been supplemented by efforts to identify met-abolic events and relate them to specific anatomical elements. Both blood flow and metabolism have been studied by a variety of newer methods that involve tomographic measurements.

Although great effort has already been expended in the development of methodology for CBF measurement, uncertainties remain regarding both physiologic variations and the altered patterns of disease. This is especially true for local cerebral blood flow (LCBF) as it relates to neuroanatomical structures: gray/white matter, nuclei, ganglia, tracts, etc. Information is needed about flow in specific functional centers in relation to metabolism, nerve transmission, information and motor integration, and projected excitatory and inhibitory influences.

While global and hemispheric measurements[1] and cortical studies[2-4] have been made in man, detailed mapping of brain blood flow has been restricted to invasive or acute experiments in animals. The most detailed measurements have utilized radionuclide-labeled microemboli (e.g., microspheres[5, 6]) or chemical substances that are diffusible and thus equilibrate in tissue (e.g., iodoantipyrine[7-9]). Both require the immediate death of the subject after a very limited number of measurements. Because of these limitations, such work has usually been carried out with small, common animals, mainly rodents, although some reports have involved larger animals.[7, 10] These methods do have the advantage of higher resolution, especially true for the autoradiographic techniques, but, of course, suffer the serious disadvantage of the limited number of measurements (often only one) before the need to kill the subject and perform rapid, crucial manipulation of the brain tissue. A widely used method is H_2 clearance.[11, 12] This requires the penetration of the region of interest (ROI) by a needle electrode, which, no matter how delicate, of necessity alters local microscopic anatomy and function and also limits the number of simultaneous discrete regions of interest (ROIs) in the study.

In spite of these problems, much valuable information has been obtained about normal CBF, effects of physiologic stimuli upon its regulation, and the changes brought about by conditions such as ischemia (focal or hemispheric), edema, altered blood circulation (e.g., hemorrhage), tumors and degenerative disease, and specific neurologic insults. Thus, we have learned about the autoregulation of CBF, the response to pharmacologic and physiologic stimuli (e.g., P_{O_2}, P_{CO_2}) and to neurophysiologic work. We also have been able to appreciate the responses to ischemia of collateral circulation and the pattern of damage or infarction to be expected after a specific vascular accident. In fact, LCBF is not constant in any region of the brain and varies appropriately as the metabolism and function of a region alters. Motor activation of a hand is seen to immediately increase flow within the appropriate region of the motor strip on the opposite side, as does visual stimulation activate the occipital region.[13, 14] Deprivation of a specific sensory input has also been coupled with a significant reduction of flow from baseline values in the appropriate regions that subserved that sensory function. In diseased states such as Huntington's chorea, when neuronal activity may be focally reduced in the caudate nucleus, local flow reductions have been defined even in the preclinical situation with positron emission tomography (see below) before atrophy is apparent on the CT scan. This ability to interpret the nature of local metabolism through local flow data is valid in normal or chronic-diseased states where flow information is "coupled" to metabolism. The ability to study normal and diseased brain function through a noninvasive and widely available local flow methodology would appear to have broad application for the study of brain function in both normal and diseased states.

One of the major clinical and investigative areas where LCBF information is expected to be of great importance is obviously that of cerebral ischemia involving occlusive vascular disease, where the major problem is a reduction of cerebral blood flow below metabolic needs. Laboratory studies have defined a wide range of flow values that are consistent with normal neuronal function. A value of 55 ml/100 gm/minute is a normal average regional flow value.[1, 15] With higher resolution studies, gray matter and white matter are shown to receive 80 ml/100 gm/minute and 20 ml/100 gm/minute respectively.[16, 17] Stimulation and deprivation studies have been shown to cause a local variation of 20% to 30% of flow above and below these baseline values.[13, 18] The threshold for normal neuronal function appears to be about 18 ml/100 gm/minute for a region of mixed

gray and white matter. While reversibility of a functional loss is seen to occur after hours at values in the high teens, lower flow values, especially less than 8 to 10 ml/100 gm/minute are consistent with only a brief period of reversibility before infarction will inevitably occur.[19, 20]

Sophisticated experiments and clinical need alike demand that repeated precise measurements of blood flow be possible; that these measurements include deeply seated structures with equal facility to superficial; that they have anatomical resolution on a par with the functional elements of interest (e.g., tracts and nuclei); and finally, that they be noninvasive so as not to disturb the organism under study and not impose significant risk or discomfort in the case of human subjects.

The methods referred to thus far do not satisfy the immediately preceding criteria. In this chapter, we shall describe several more recently developed techniques that do meet the criteria (more or less). For completeness, we will also briefly discuss the older methods that have contributed so much to present knowledge. Most of the emphasis will be upon an LCBF technique developed in our laboratories that we believe fully meets the above criteria and that makes use of CT technology, thus imposing minimal additional elevation of both cost and technical requirements, but taking a quantum step toward improving anatomical resolution and ease of performance. The recent developments include emission tomography of both single photon[21–23] and positron[24, 25] varieties, and the stable Xe/CT LCBF method as developed in our laboratory and applied by ourselves[26–30] and others.[31–35] The older methods are H_2 clearance and ^{14}C iodoantipyrene autoradiography (which are not clinically applicable) and ^{133}Xe regional cerebral blood flow, which has been extensively applied to clinical problems. Nuclear magnetic resonance will not be discussed in relation to blood flow, because its current capabilities are very limited at the level of tissue perfusion.[36]

CBF METHODS

While this book is intended to provide the reader with a discriminating overview of the important roles of CT in clinical medicine, a reasonably complete treatment of each covered subject is required so as to provide the reader with a reasonable basis for consideration and understanding of the material at hand. Thus, we have undertaken a brief, but broad in scope, review of relevant subject matter that extends to the nonclinical methods included in the ensuing section. All of the flow methods to be described depend upon application of the Fick principle, which, simply stated, defines the change in amount of an indicator in tissue as the difference between its rate of absorption and its rate of dissipation.

H₂ Clearance

This is an invasive laboratory method for monitoring CBF that has had a limited clinical (intraoperative) use. The method is simple and inexpensive, requires easily obtainable equipment, and provides for multiple in vivo determinations of blood flow from any tissue into which small electrodes can be implanted. Much basic physiologic research has been carried out using H₂ clearance. Kety[37] indicated that H₂ is an inert gas, not present in the body normally, and that it would thus be suitable for a blood flow tracer. When Mishray and Clark[38] recorded H₂ oxidation potentials from platinum (Pt) electrodes implanted in cerebral tissue, they provided the means for implementing such a method. By recording current generated at the platinum electrode by H₂ oxidation, Hyman[39] was able to correlate electrical phenomena with H₂ concentration. Aukland and associates[40, 41] really described the first use of H₂ polarography in measurement of CBF. The use of the technique rapidly took hold, and other authors applied it in the ensuing years.[42–44] The H₂ clearance technique has been applied to man as an adjunct to surgical procedures, but mainly has been a laboratory method used for a wide range of blood flow phenomena including middle cerebral arterial occlusion,[45] autoregulation and spinal cord trauma,[46] and brain ischemia,[47] among others. While it was originally believed that the volume of tissue represented by the method is as small as 1 cu mm (depending on electrode size), some evidence exists that H₂ generated as far as 2 to 5 mm from the electrode might contribute to the measured current.[48, 49] Disadvantages or restriction of its use include the fact that implantation of electrodes may cause local injury and, thus, alteration of blood flow;[50] the correct mathematical treatment of the result is not clear, because the clearance curves are often polyexponential, raising questions as to whether a single exponential clearance rate is valid;[49] arterial concentration may not fall rapidly to zero as assumed; and Pt electrodes are sensitive to O₂ concentration, which could cause errors, especially in the case of severely ischemic tissue.[48]

Autoradiography and Labeled Microspheres

Both of these methods depend upon the deposition of a radioactive label in tissue during the early moments after injection into the bloodstream. In the case of microspheres, the tracer forms emboli in a small but evenly distributed sample of tissue. These emboli remain in place until the subject is sacrificed at the end of the study.[5, 6] At this point, the tissue is cut into volumes of about 1 cu cm for deep well counting.

The most widely used autoradiographic method utilizes ^{14}C iodoantipyrine, which diffuses into tissue and then remains fixed, because blood perfusion is ended by acute decapitation.[7, 10] High-resolution autoradiographs are produced by thin sectioning of brain and contact exposure of x-ray film over a period of time. These methods obviously have no clinical or human investigative application and, although of importance physiologically, will not be described further.

Regional Cerebral Blood Flow (rCBF) with Diffusible Radioemitters

There is a whole family of methods involving radiolabeled, inert diffusible gases that have been studied by other investigators.[2–4, 51, 52] These include ^{85}Kr and ^{133}Xe and depend, again, upon the relationship between blood flow and the rate of gas diffusion into or out of tissue. The gas may be administered by intracarotid injection or by inhalation and is monitored by external collimated scintillation counters. These methods usually extract blood flow information from tissue clearance or washout curves after cessation of indicator administration, although they can also use data acquired during absorption or washin. Because of the size of the counters, such curves from brain contain at least two components having widely different blood flow rates and different solubilities for the indicator. These components represent gray and white matter. In order for the method to be noninvasive, the indicator must be administered by inhalation, and the monitoring must be external to the skin. These methodological limitations result in restriction upon the type of computation and upon the precision and resolution of the results. The interaction of the physics of ^{133}Xe photon emission and of the need to detect external to the skin has several undesired effects. Because of self-absorption, the detected signal is limited to relatively superficial levels, and because skin, muscle, and bone are interposed between the detector and tissue of interest, at least one additional flow compartment must be considered when analyzing the measured clearance curves. A serious limitation of this method is the need to define the relative solubility of the indicator (e.g., ^{133}Xe) in blood and in tissue. The parameter generally used, λ or blood/brain partition coefficient, must be available from some prior study, because it cannot be estimated by the external scintillation counting method. Usually, normative values, either published or determined for gray and white matter in separate cadaver or animal tissue experiments, are applied to the measured tissue and blood clearance data. This is a disadvantage, because λ has been found to vary in disease[53] and even may vary from one normal to the next. Certainly, tumor tissue Xe solubility will not be characteristic of either gray or white matter, so flow estimates for tumor would be subject to serious errors.

A three-compartment model has been proposed,[54] but this requires prolonged periods of recording clearance of indicators (40 minutes). It has been possible to separate the fast components or gray matter flow from the slower components (white matter, bone, muscle, and skin) after only 10 minutes of recording. The fast component then is the only accurate output. Because the tissue of greatest interest with respect to blood flow and metabolism is gray matter, which encompasses nuclei and ganglia as well as cerebral cortex, this approach has considerable merit.

In an effort to obtain more detailed information, as many as 100 or more collimated detectors have been fitted to helmets so as to record multiple data simultaneously during a single washout curve.[4] These and other studies (see Fig 2–6) have demonstrated changes in carotid blood flow correlated with function such as muscular and mental activity in normal individuals and changes with disease and with aging. There is a general decrease in flow with age, and selected regional reductions are seen with dementias and with localized ischemic disease.

Emission Tomography

Single Photon Emission Computed Tomography (SPECT)

The ^{133}Xe tomography technique was described by Lassen and associates[21, 22] and by other investigators using the same or other radionuclides such as ^{81}Kr.[23] This method, generally called SPECT, overcomes two of the major limitations of traditional two-dimensional rCBF methods: that of being restricted to the superficial layer of the tissue under study and that of the occurrence of the error mentioned above caused by counts originating in overlying skin, muscle, and bone. Thus, while previous information was available only from cerebral cortex (and only that portion of cortex exposed on the brain convexity to the exclusion of that present in fissures and sulci), it is now possible to apply tomographic techniques and provide information from deeper structures. This is accomplished by choosing appropriate radionuclides and increasing detector sensitivity so as to detect photons reaching the surface from all depths. Because the path direction of the photon is known by virtue of the collimated detector, and its likelihood of exiting the head depends upon its energy and the medium through which it courses, the source of the signal can be established by analyzing many crossing paths similar to the approach used in CT. A large number of collimated detectors are placed concentrically about the skull, or a smaller array is rotated and computerized methods are employed in calculating values at depth. This technique

permits use of more traditional radionuclides of longer half-lives without the need to manufacture them on the spot as with positron emission tomography (see below). More recently, simplified equipment (rotating gamma camera) has been employed, which promises to make this method more widely available. This technique has limitations in resolution, but does have the important advantage of use for both blood flow and metabolism. However, techniques for measuring positron-emitting radionuclides, also useful for metabolic studies, are more numerous (see below). The SPECT method has been used to study CBF in patients with cerebrovascular disease and tumors.[55] In these and in normal subjects, there has been good agreement with two-dimensional rCBF studies.

Positron Emission Tomography (PET)

This method has received wide interest in recent years, because it potentially provides a means of displaying information, obtained noninvasively, about blood flow and metabolism simultaneously and at varying tissue levels. The method utilizes, as chemical markers, certain radionuclides (e.g., $^{15}O_2$, $^{13}N_2$, ^{11}C, ^{18}F, and ^{77}Kr) that spontaneously disintegrate with the emission of positively charged particles (positron). Positrons travel only very short distances in tissue before losing enough kinetic energy to encounter electrons with which they collide, resulting in the phenomenon of mutual annihilation where the masses of the positron and electron are converted to energy. The result is two photons, each having energy of 0.511×10^6 electron volts (0.511 meV) and traveling in very nearly opposite directions (180°). A ring of detectors records this event and, because of known path and travel times, can associate the disintegration of the biochemical label with a precise anatomical site within the tomogram or "slice" under study. The number of such events over time at a given locus reveals the concentration of the specific radionuclide and its chemical substance at that locus. This becomes a very useful tool, because it allows the investigator to measure uptake of important metabolites (glucose, O_2, etc.) as well as local blood volume and flow—the information being presented as a functional image of a brain or other tissue slice.

There are considerations that limit the usefulness of even this exciting development. Because of the range of movement of the original positron before annihilation and the fact that the photons are not emitted at exactly 180° angles, the spacial resolution is only about 1 cm (full width, half maximum), and significant improvement in resolution is constrained by theoretical limits inherent in the method. Thus, events localized to smaller functional units (nuclei and tracts) cannot be resolved. The radionuclides exhibiting *positron emission* are all evanescent, typically having half-lives of 2 to 20 minutes, necessitating their manufacture or generation in very close proximity to the point of use. Because this usually requires a cyclotron or similar device, it often poses serious logistic as well as financial problems. Both the tomograph and cyclotron are very expensive. Even though the agents have very short lives, they do persist in tissue long enough to prevent immediate or rapid serial remeasurement, and very fast events cannot be followed. In spite of these limitations, a significant number of units have been installed, and an impressive number of very exciting studies are underway. However, PET does not hold promise for the routine management of clinical problems, except at a very limited number of sites.

Stable Xenon/CT (LCBF)

The suggestion that xenon gas might be useful as a radio-enhancing agent[56] led to the realization that it could also be used for measurement of CBF if the x-ray device, in this case CT scanner, were employed as a densitometer during a dynamic Xe inhalation sequence. Xenon, with an atomic number of 54, has radiodensity characteristics similar to those of iodine (atomic number 53). Unlike iodine, it is diffusible throughout the body tissues, including brain, readily crossing the BBB. This is an obvious fact, given the wide use of ^{133}Xe as a radionuclide tracer in both two- and three-dimensional emission CBF studies (above). Kelcz and coworkers[57] defined the CT enhancement characteristics of stable Xe while, at approximately the same time, Drayer and associates[26] of this laboratory reported early experiments with actual blood flow measurements. Subsequently, we have continued work to bring this method to an advanced and clinically useful technique for measuring LCBF both in tomographic "slices" and in three-dimensional solid constructions for a series of such slices.[27-30] To avoid confusion, we hasten to point out that this solid or three-dimensional flow image is not the "three-dimensional" image as referred to in connection with SPECT or PET, where a slice (with thickness) that penetrates completely through the brain is considered three-dimensional. We are referring to the multi-level "slicing" technique, where a solid, of equal (cubic) or near equal (rectangular) dimension is created from a series of four or more adjacent slices (see following: Three-Dimensional Flow Mapping). During the development period of about 4 years, a significant number of other investigators have worked in parallel ways and made substantial contributions to the technique,[31-35] so that we now believe it to be unquestionably important both for investigation (clinical and animal) and for routine management of patients with ischemic or other intracranial disease. We shall briefly describe the method and its principles and provide several illustrations of its use.

DESCRIPTION OF STABLE Xe/CT METHOD

In common with other methods, the stable Xe/CT LCBF technique makes use of the Fick principle, which states simply that the quantity of a diffusible indicator present in a tissue at the end of a time period is the difference between the quantity absorbed by the tissue and the quantity removed or washed out of the tissue during that period. From this, it follows that the concentration of indicator is a function of its quantity and of the volume of tissue or, at steady state, is the difference between the rate of delivery and the rate of removal. In the case of a highly diffusible indicator (such as Xe gas) that is transported via the bloodstream, knowledge of the time-dependent changes in blood and tissue concentration and the relative solubility of the indicator in blood and tissue (blood/brain partition coefficient; λ) permits the calculation of the blood flow rate to the tissue under scrutiny. This could be a whole or hemibrain or, as we shall see, it could be as little as one CT unit (voxel). The time-tested equation of Kety and Schmidt[1] as shown below is used to define the relationship.

$$C(t) = \sum_i w_i \lambda_i k_i \int_o^t C_a(u)e^{-k_i(t-u)}\,du \qquad (1)$$

$$F = \lambda k \qquad (2)$$

$$F = \frac{\lambda k}{m} \qquad (3)$$

where:

$C(t)$	=	indicator concentration in tissue (brain)
w_i	=	weight factor
λ_i	=	blood brain partition coefficient
k_i	=	flow rate constant
$C_a(u)$	=	indicator concentration in arterial blood
F	=	blood flow
m	=	equilibration factor (a value of 1 implies instantaneous equilibration between blood and tissue)

Because present CT technology permits us to obtain rapid scans of brain (or other tissue) sections that are 5 mm thick, require only 4 to 6 seconds per scan, and can be repeated immediately with table incrementation, it is possible to scan three to six levels of brain and repeat at intervals of 1 to 3 minutes. If this is done while the subject breathes a suitable Xe/air or Xe/O$_2$ gas mixture or after cessation of Xe breathing, then the buildup or washout of Xe can be appreciated as a function of the measured enhancement of the CT image. Conveniently, CT now resolves soft-tissue volumes as small as 0.5×1.5 mm (voxels), which are presented as an average density on a two-dimensional image (pixels), one such image representing each slice taken. Thus, the Xe/CT method is not troubled by interference from overlying skin, muscle, or bone, and the anatomical source of each enhancement value is identified by the locus of the voxel.

Figure 2–1 illustrates the changes in CT enhancement at three locations (ROIs) of a baboon brain while the animal breathes a 61% Xe/O_2 mixture. The cursors were placed so as to sample gray matter (fast-flow region), white matter (slow-flow region), and the center of an experimentally induced cerebral infarction (zero-flow region). One readily sees that the fast-flow ROI equilibrated with blood Xe level within 2 minutes, while the slow-flow or white matter ROI had not yet equilibrated after 6 minutes. Actually, complete equilibration requires about 25 to 30 minutes as illustrated in Figure 2–2.

In practice, the study is carried out as follows: The awake patient is placed on the CT table with the head

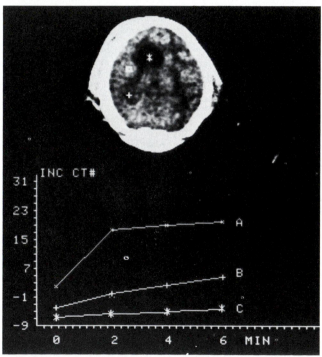

Fig 2–1.—Time-dependent changes in tissue enhancement of the baboon brain during 61% Xe inhalation. *Curve A* is a plot of the degree of enhancement (Hounsfield units) from an ROI located in a fast-flow or gray matter region. *Curve B* is an ROI selected from slow-flow or white matter, while *curve C* is located within an infarct caused by lateral lenticulostriate artery occlusion. While there is an obvious absence of enhancement in the infarct, the most important point is that the equilibration of Xe with tissue is virtually complete in 2 minutes in fast-flow regions, while it is only partially so after 6 minutes in slow-flow regions. (From Gur D., Yonas H., Wolfson S.K. Jr., et al.: Xenon and iodine enhanced cerebral CT: A closer look. *Stroke* 12:573–576, 1981. Used by permission.)

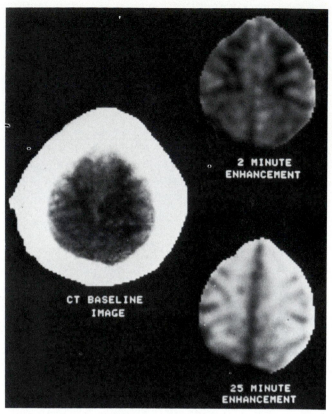

Fig 2–2.—Brain enhancement over time in the baboon. Note the reversal of more dense regions brought out by *25 minutes* equilibration when compared to 2 minutes inhalation of 60% Xe. The white matter regions, having a greater solubility for Xe, but requiring longer to equilibrate, ultimately become more radiodense than the more rapidly equilibrating but lower solubility gray matter regions. (From Gur D., Wolfson S.K. Jr., Yonas H., et al.: Progress in cerebrovascular disease: Local cerebral blood flow in xenon enhanced CT. *Stroke* 13:750–758, 1982. Used by permission.)

partially encircled by an evacuable "bean bag" (Vac-Pac, Olympic Medical Supply Co., Seattle) placed within the plastic head holder. After explaining the procedure and establishing a comfortable position, the subject is asked to keep the head perfectly still for about 10 minutes (4 to 6 minutes is essential). One or two baseline sequences of scans are taken in planes parallel to the orbitomeatal line (similar to the usual CT technique). The patient breathes air or O_2 via a special face mask or a mouthpiece with nose clip. The mask or breathing tube is arranged for to and fro airway ventilation as illustrated in Figure 2–3. If an endotrachial tube is in place, it is simply connected instead of the mask. There are three non-rebreathing (check) valves, two of which are just downstream of the "T." A small volume of the last expired air is thus trapped in the space between valves. This air remains in place

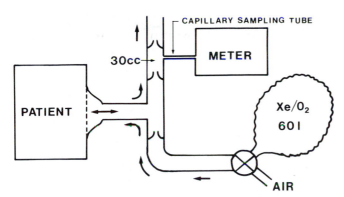

Fig 2–3.—Xe breathing circuit. The 60-L bag may contain either Xe/O₂ or Xe air in concentrations between 30% and 60% Xe. The present clinical protocol calls for 30% to 35% Xe. Expired gas is aspirated at high velocity via the capillary and permits the thermal conductivity meter to generate expired gas Xe concentration curves. End-tidal Xe levels are easily identified and used for the blood flow computations.

throughout inspiration and is sampled by a capillary suction tube and drawn through a thermal conductivity meter calibrated for Xe/O₂ or Xe/air mixtures. A newer method, under study, involves intermittent sampling in phase with the ventilatory cycle. This eliminates one of the expiratory check valves, reducing airway resistance. When it is established that the baseline scans are good (radiologic technique, slice orientation, etc.), the breathing gas is switched to the predetermined Xe/O₂ or air mixture (usually 30% to 35% Xe). A preprogramed scanning sequence is invoked so as to provide scanning series at the desired levels, repeated at approximately 1.3, 2, 3, and 5 minutes after the initiation of Xe breathing. At the end of scanning, the breathing mixture is switched back to O₂ or air. The entire procedure requires 30 minutes. The actual measurements are made in about 15 minutes, with 5 to 6 minutes of Xe breathing.

At the end of the session, the computer will construct images of the CT slices before and at four times during Xe inhalation. There is time-dependent Xe enhancement data for each volume unit (voxel or on the x-ray film, pixel). Difference between the baseline and Xe-enhanced scans is proportional to the tissue Xe concentration. The output of the airway Xe meter is a function of the end-tidal (arterial) Xe concentration. These data may be solved for both λ and for k as defined in equation (1) using multivariable analysis techniques. Blood flow in ml/minute/unit volume of tissue is calculated from equation (2). When instantaneous diffusion equilibration cannot be assumed, equation (3) is used. The factor m increases to a maximum value of 1 as the equilibration state is approached. When the method is applied to animal studies, including a new cerebral infarct

model in the baboon,[58] the technique is as above with certain departures required by the inability to obtain voluntary cooperation, especially with respect to motion. For example, baboons are anesthetized, intubated, and paralyzed.

Xe/CT BLOOD FLOW IMAGING

Two-Dimensional Flow Mapping

We have been able to produce blood flow maps with good anatomical correlation between blood flow images and CT anatomy. Goodness-of-fit studies, comparison of normals with gross anatomical slices, and, in the infarct model, the relationship of blood flow values to the pathologically identified infarct boundaries have all contributed to our impression of the method's validity. Figure 2–4 illustrates how flow may be represented on a gray (or color) scale with values computed for each pixel-sized unit (0.8 × 0.8 mm). When compared to the actual gross pathologic slice, the interdigitation of high- and low-flow regions of the map closely follows the distribution of gray and white matter throughout the gyri and central regions of cerebrum and brain stem.

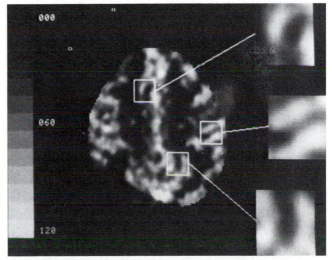

Fig 2–4.—Map of normal blood flow in the baboon. Blood flow values are obtained by using multivariable analysis techniques to solve for λ and k in equation (1), which are then applied to equation (2) or (3). Input data such as that illustrated in Figure 2–1 are combined with end-tidal Xe levels as monitored by a thermal conductivity meter. The result is a flow value for each pixel of the original scan. After application of smoothing techniques, the image is constructed by reference to a gray scale such as that at the left of the illustration. Levels of flow are represented by 256 shades: 0 = black, maximum flow = white. We have been able to produce anatomically well-correlated images with a resolution of 4- to 5-mm full width, half maximum. The data can as easily be displayed on a color scale with a total of 4,096 different hues and shades. In practice, 64 flow levels have been discriminated.

Sensitivity to Physiologic Change

The responsiveness of the method to physiologic flow variations was assessed in a baboon experiment by increasing the inspired (P_I) CO_2 or causing hypoventilation of the anesthetized animal so as to raise the Pa_{CO_2} and by causing hyperventilation to lower the Pa_{CO_2}. The computed blood flow values revealed the wide swings in tissue perfusion to be expected when going from a Pa_{CO_2} of 30 torr to 60 torr. A typical response is illustrated in Figure 2–5, where marked changes are seen in the difference between the upper and lower flow maps corresponding to Pa_{CO_2} of 38 torr and 58 torr. Increases in blood flow with increased Pa_{CO_2} are readily appreciated, especially in gray matter regions.

The first human illustrations (Fig 2–6) are of a normal subject both at rest and while performing a motor task. Of note in the resting flow map is the even distribution

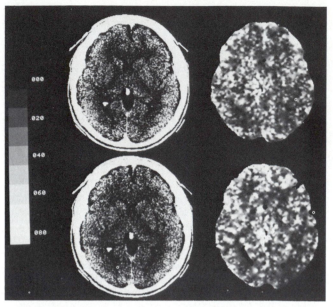

Fig 2–6.—Xe/CT LCBF study of normal subject at rest and during left hand movement. The *upper images* are of CT scan *(left)* and LCBF map *(right)* at rest. In the *lower images,* the subject is actively opening and clenching his left fist. A definite increase in local blood flow is seen in the area of right motor cortex of the lower flow map.

of flow patterns throughout the hemispheres and the fact that the high- and low-flow regions generally follow the gray and white matter distribution of normal anatomy. Zero flow is seen in ventricles, cysterns, sulci, etc. Tables 2–1 and 2–2 show the actual pixel flow values through the ROI of the motor area on Figure 2–6. The mean flows for this entire region (8.8 × 8.8 × 5 mm) dramatically illustrate the sensitivity of the method. At rest, flow was 30.0 ± 8.5 ml/100 gm/min-

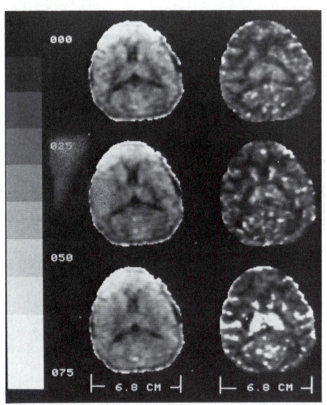

Fig 2–5.—Sensitivity to varying physiologic parameters. The three *leftmost images* are Xe-enhanced CT scans of the same level of a baboon brain. The animal was hyper-hypoventilated to produce Pa_{CO_2} of 38, 44, and 55 torr *(top to bottom).* The corresponding LCBF map is displayed just to the right of each CT scan. Readily apparent is the change in flow values of various structures, especially in gray matter caused by varying Pa_{CO_2}. The gray scale units are ml/100 gm/minute. (From Gur D., Good W.F., Wolfson S.K. Jr., et al.: In vivo mapping of local cerebral blood flow by xenon enhanced CT. *Science* 215:1267–1268, 1982. Used by permission.)

TABLE 2–1.—PRINTOUT OF ACTUAL FLOW VALUES* FOR AN 8.8 × 8.8 × 5-MM ROI OF THE RIGHT ANTERIOR CENTRAL GYRUS VICINITY IN A RESTING HEALTHY VOLUNTEER SUBJECT†‡

	HOR COL										
ROW	68	69	70	71	72	73	74	75	76	77	78
94	23	22	22	24	25	23	22	22	22	21	19
95	27	26	25	26	26	24	24	25	26	26	25
96	32	30	30	29	27	26	26	27	28	29	31
97	39	35	33	32	29	27	27	28	29	31	34
98	45	40	37	34	31	29	28	28	30	32	32
99	48	43	39	36	32	30	28	27	28	29	28
100	45	41	40	37	34	31	28	25	24	24	24
101	40	38	39	38	36	33	28	24	21	19	19
102	39	37	38	40	39	35	28	21	18	16	15
103	34	35	40	45	45	41	31	20	16	15	13
104	30	34	44	51	53	49	36	22	14	13	11

*Ml/100 gm/minutes, pixel by pixel.
†File = IMG1:8307532.BF; block = 4.
‡N = 121; x̄ = 30.0 ± 8.5; high value = 53; low value = 11.

TABLE 2–2.—PRINTOUT OF THE SAME ROI AS IN TABLE 2–1 WHILE THE SUBJECT REPETITIVELY OPENS AND CLOSES HIS LEFT FIST*†‡

	HOR COL										
ROW	68	69	70	71	72	73	74	75	76	77	78
94	30	41	52	64	79	81	74	80	83	73	84
95	28	38	49	62	76	74	59	68	84	77	62
96	28	32	46	60	70	64	53	62	81	80	55
97	29	29	46	65	72	69	65	70	82	80	55
98	37	41	61	77	78	75	74	77	84	80	57
99	46	58	80	88	80	73	73	79	84	79	62
100	62	88	103	95	80	68	69	76	80	74	60
101	81	101	99	89	75	63	62	68	77	75	62
102	69	75	74	70	61	52	49	57	75	80	70
103	40	44	49	51	47	40	37	46	62	70	69
104	24	25	31	37	38	37	38	42	48	56	66

*Examination of individual values and mean values clearly reveals pronounced increase in blood flow.
†File = IMGl:8307536.BF; block = 4.
‡N = 121; $\bar{x}$ = 63.4 ± 17.9; high value = 103; low value = 24.

ute with a range of 53 to 11. During hand activity, the values increased to 63.4 ± 17.9 ml/100 gm/minute, range: 24 to 103. This kind of change has been reported by others[4] using rCBF and PET techniques, but Xe/CT LCBF opens a new dimension in resolution and depth of measurements.

Mapping over Time

If good registration (anatomical coincidence of successive studies) is maintained, a program can be invoked that will seek and plot mean blood flow values for ROIs selected from any flow map entered into the data. Values are plotted for all ROIs selected and for each study done (each time). Thus, graphs over time are automatically produced once ROIs are designated. This technique is illustrated in Figure 2–7. This kind of display and analysis is of great value in the study of flow changes surrounding (both anatomically and temporally) an event such as vessel occlusion.

Three-Dimensional Flow Mapping

As described above, a typical Xe study involves repeated rapid scanning of one to six slices with automatic table incrementation. For three-dimensional work, five or six 5-mm slices are taken, but the table increment is only 2 or 3 mm, providing considerable overlap. Flow is computed for all slices as usual. By using a cursor, the observer may select an ROI on one slice that will be projected through all. As illustrated in Figure 2–8, A, flow values for pixel-size units of planes through the z axis are calculated using a simple linear interpolation algorithm. Intervening pixels are weighted in favor of the nearest actual slice, and all flow values are stored in a three-dimensional array from which the solid image is constructed. The result is seen in Figure 2–8, B. This

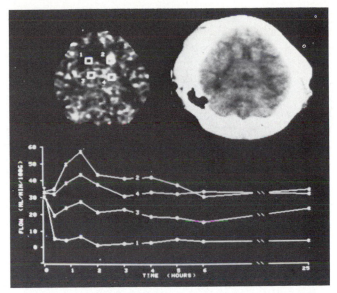

Fig 2–7.—Graphic display of simultaneous blood flow changes (LCBF). The baboon had right lateral lenticulostriate occlusion (method of Yonas[58]) immediately after the initial LCBF study. The *upper left image* is the flow map from the 25-minute postocclusion study, and the corresponding baseline CT is shown at *right*. The four ROIs were chosen so that each pair had approximately the same flow before occlusion, but represented (on the right) regions within and on the edge of the ischemic zone.

solid may be "cut," under computer control, to reveal flow maps for interior structures and in planes not parallel to the original scans (e.g., coronal, sagittal, or any angle).

LCBF as a Laboratory Tool

There is a broad application for Xe/CT blood flow studies in the laboratory. High Xe concentration and radiation exposure are possible in animals with small heads (e.g., baboon). This provides an ideal situation for LCBF determination. The ability to paralyze the subject with the resulting lack of movement adds significantly to the degree of resolution that such studies can provide. Flow studies in nonhuman primates, with 40% to 50% Xe/O_2 mixtures have defined exquisite anatomical detail of the normal variation of gray and white matter where cortical ribbon normally measures only 2 mm across.[29, 59] Disturbances of flow with experimental stroke caused by embolic or direct vessel occlusive procedures are readily defined, as are variations of flow as CO_2 is varied.[59] We believe that the application of LCBF by Xe/CT should have a broad and exciting application to experimental work that involves any disturbance of flow. In our hands, excellent results have been obtained in study of experimental cerebral infarction provided by lateral lenticulostriate (LLS) occlusion in the baboon.[58] Because of the good control of all exper-

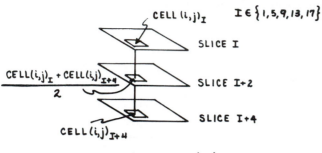

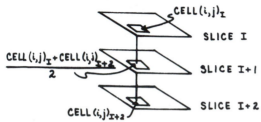

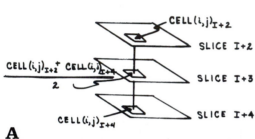

A

Fig 2–8.—Three-dimensional blood flow images. **A,** the method of weighted linear interpolation used to obtain the solid-flow image of a baboon brain as constructed in **B.** Four to six *(five in this case)* adjacent and overlapping CT slices are acquired during Xe inhalation using the dynamic scanning feature of the CT unit. The cerebral infarction caused by lateral lenticulostriate occlusion in this baboon is readily seen as a zero- to very low-flow region involving basal ganglia and internal capsule.

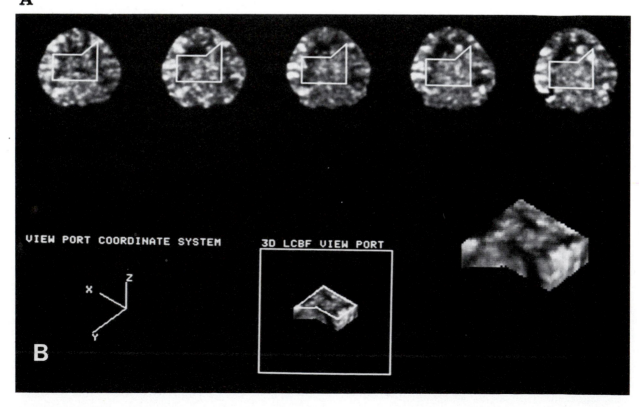

B

imental parameters, we were able to get near perfect registration of the successive images over a 25-hour period after acute LLS artery occlusion. The computer could then plot curves of blood flow for multiple ROIs over this period (see Fig 2–7). The figure speaks for itself and opens the door to many investigations.

Effects of Xe Inhalation

Anesthetic Properties

Xenon is an inert atmospheric constituent that has definite anesthetic properties.[60–62] Anesthesia is usually manifest only in concentrations higher than 50% P_IXe. In one study carried out in our laboratory on healthy volunteers (Table 2–3), Xe/O_2 mixtures (28% to 47% Xe) were administered for 3 to 6 minutes via a face mask.[63] In general, the gas was reasonably well tolerated. The most common symptoms were lightheadedness, euphoria, heavy feeling, and tingling of extremities. One subject of that study and one other at a later time did have more severe symptoms, including brief loss of consciousness (40% Xe) and headache. It is interesting that both of these individuals were senior investigators in the Xe blood flow project. Other investigators have reported greater tolerance at concentrations up to 70% to 80%[64–67] in studies on patients as opposed to normal volunteers. In fact, one investigator has reported *no* adverse side effects to 65% Xe breathing in a very carefully monitored study.[67] Our subsequent experience with patients[68–70] tends to confirm a very low incidence of significant neurologic side effects.

Effect upon Blood Flow

Prolonged Xe breathing will cause reduction of blood flow of 10% to 20% from baseline levels.[29] The degree

to which this occurs is largely dependent upon dose and duration of Xe breathing. We have found that 8 to 10 minutes of 35% Xe may reduce blood flow by 15% to 25%, but no appreciable effect is noticed in the first few minutes. Results of microsphere studies suggest a small increase (5% to 10%) in the first few minutes.

Motion of Subject

This has the potential to be a most serious problem. When one includes (as need be) the baseline studies, the subject's head must remain perfectly still for a minimum of about 10 minutes. Misregistration can occur with an accumulated movement of only 1 to 2 mm. Obtunded and unconscious patients are usually no problem. Similarly, alert and cooperative patients can be easily studied. We have used an evacuable "bean bag" (Vac-Pac, Olympic Medical Supply Co., Seattle) to aid the cooperative patient in his effort to remain still and to brace against involuntary movement in some potentially uncooperative patients such as those with advanced Alzheimer's disease (AD). The plastic filler material is radiolucent in the scanner. A different approach to this problem is to increase slice thickness to 1 cm. This would, of course, reduce anatomical resolution and decrease the method's applicability to smaller structures. Finally, it is possible to make computational correction for rotational misregistration, but this approach is not applicable to axial linear motion (craniad or caudad).

Radiation Dose

The familiar trade-off between signal-to-noise ratio and radiation level is certainly not absent in work with stable Xe enhancement. The limitation of study to specific slices limits exposure of adjacent structures, because the CT beam is well collimated. Yet, repeated scans of the slices under study do result in significant dose to those tissues. While in vivo autoradiographic technique keeps radiation dose to a minimum, the computational method causes the accuracy of the resulting flow estimate to hang on single datum for tissue enhancement. The usual multilevel study requires a minimum of one baseline and two enhanced scans. We prefer to average two baseline scans and to record at least 3 to 4 enhanced scans during Xe inhalation. This results in at least 15 to 20 rad to the slice itself, but much lower levels are absorbed by organs outside the scan field. The whole body dose is thus more comparable to that received when a radionuclide study (e.g., ^{133}Xe) is carried out.

CLINICAL EXPERIENCE

The stable Xe/CT technique has been applied clinically at a number of institutions for study and diagnosis

TABLE 2–3.—Xe ADMINISTRATION IN HEALTHY VOLUNTEERS

SUBJECT	FIXe (%)/TIME*	SYMPTOMS† DURING Xe BREATHING	AFTER Xe BREATHING
1	30/4	4,5,6	11
2	32/4	4,5,6	11
3	35/6	2,4,5,6,8	11
4	35/4	3,4,5,7	11
5	40/3	2,3,5,6,7	11
6	35/4	2,3,4,5	12
7	28/5	3	11
8	28/4	3	11
9	34/5	4,6	11
10	47/3	4,6	11
11	27/6	3,6	11
12	39/4	3,5,6,9,10	11

*Duration of inhalation of the indicated mixture.
†1, None; 2, anxiety during buildup; 3, euphoria; 4, heavy feeling; 5, tingling extremities; 6, lightheadedness; 7, profuse perspiration; 8, headache; 9, unpleasant dysesthesias; 10, loss of consciousness; 11, lightheaded less than 2 hr; and 12, lightheaded more than 2 hr.

of many conditions.[31-34, 53, 67-72] The results are varied and depend somewhat upon the group and the methodology employed. Although beginning research in this area in 1977 at the University of Pittsburgh, we found that development and refinement were effectively carried out in animals (nonhuman primates). This conservative approach did not provide for human study until we satisfied the ideal clinical method criteria listed in the introduction. We believe that in exchange for the effort on the part of patient and investigator, and in view of the radiation exposure, data should be superior to that otherwise obtainable. The method has now been used to study a variety of clinical problems. In our hands, these have been mostly of an ischemic nature, thus far in about 50 patients. Some examples of other conditions will also be illustrated, however. Recently, we have used General Electric scanners of both CT/T 8800 and 9800 series; American Science and Engineering and EMI scanners were employed in earlier work.

Ischemic Syndromes

Primary Ischemic Problems: Flow Augmentation

Implicit in ischemia is abnormal blood flow and reduced tissue perfusion. The LCBF method, therefore, can be expected to find one of its greatest applications in this area. This has indeed been the case, as attested by the numerous reports cited in the previous section. Because Xe/CT LCBF is a noninvasive functional or physiologic test, it can be expected to provide information that is not available from strictly anatomical studies such as angiography. Such factors as the recanalization of previously occluded vessels, the participation of microvascular collateralization, and the persistence of an ischemic zone late in the course of major vessel occlusion should be amenable to study by Xe/CT LCBF. Moreover, the functional aspect of Xe/CT LCBF should be helpful in deciding whether blood flow augmentation procedures are indicated. In the ensuing pages, illustrated case reports will serve both to exhibit the results of the LCBF technique and to show how it can be applied.

BILATERAL CAROTID OCCLUSION WITH LOW FLOW.— A 72-year-old right-handed woman had a number of increasingly frequent episodes of vertigo and dysarthria over a 2-month period. One year previously, she was found to have asymptomatic bilateral carotid bruits with bilateral carotid stenosis and had been treated by left and right carotid endarterectomy. This patient had bilateral infarction in both hemispheres subsequent to the procedure and was left with a spastic left hemiparesis and expressive aphasia. A digital subtraction angiogram was performed because of the recent onset of vertebrobasilar symptoms (Fig 2–9,A). It demonstrated bilateral carotid occlusion and filling of both anterior circulatory distributions via the vertebrobasilar system. The dominant left vertebral artery was also compromised by a stenosis at the origin. An Xe/CT LCBF study (see Fig 2–9,B) demonstrated progressively reducing blood flow from the occipital lobes forward, most profound in the left frontal lobe. Left superficial temporal to middle cerebral artery bypass was performed. The postoperative LCBF study (see Fig 2–9,C) demonstrated significant improvement in the regions that were previously most ischemic. Six weeks postoperatively, the patient had had no further vertebrobasilar or mental symptoms.

UNILATERAL CAROTID OCCLUSION WITH ADEQUATE FLOW.—Four months prior to admission, a 46-year-old, right-handed man awoke with numbness of the left hand, which he said resolved over the next few days. He denied weakness at any time, but did notice clumsiness of his left hand since the episode. His physical examination and past medical history were not remarkable except for a slight left pronator drift with accentuated deep tendon reflexes on the left. The initial CT scan (Fig 2–10) demonstrated an area of infarction within the anterior distribution of the middle cerebral artery without basal ganglia involvement. Angiography disclosed an occlusion of the right internal carotid artery with rapid filling of the right middle cerebral artery via the anterior communicating artery complex. The Xe/CT LCBF study showed symmetrically high flow in both the proximal (caudate nucleus and putamen) and in the distal middle cerebral artery distribution. Because the LCBF study did not demonstrate a persistent compromise of flow to the right hemisphere, surgical intervention was not necessary.

OLD CEREBRAL INFARCT WITH ADEQUATE LCBF.—A 50-year-old white man developed a left-sided weakness and numbness 1 year before admission. Over a period of 1 month, he had recovered all but fine dexterity of the left hand. Angiography had demonstrated a high-grade right middle cerebral artery narrowing suggestive of a dissecting aneurysm. The patient was symptom-free for 9 months under aspirin and dipyridamole (Persantine) treatment. He then awoke with left-sided focal seizure activity. There was no new focal neurologic deficit following this episode, but angiography once again demonstrated proximal middle cerebral artery stenosis with delayed filling of the distal middle cerebral artery distribution.

Diphenylhydantoin therapy was initiated, and the patient remained stable for 3 months, at which point he was referred with a question of need for flow augmentation. Physical abnormalities at the time of referral were clumsiness of fine finger movements on the left

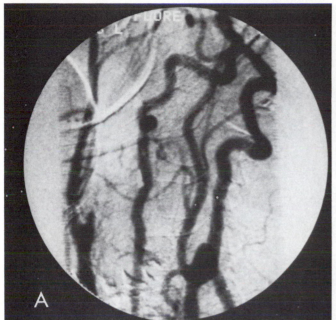

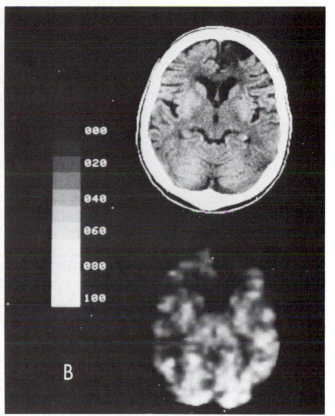

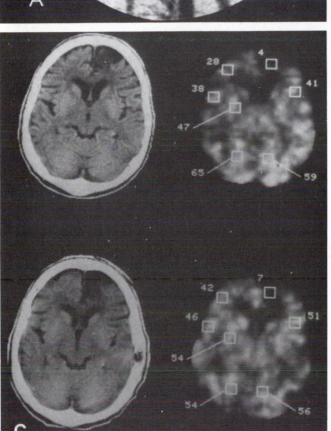

Fig 2–9.—Bilateral carotid occlusion. **A,** digital subtraction angiogram that clearly indicates bilateral internal carotid artery occlusion. It also shows a very prominent, patent left vertebral artery. **B,** the old left frontal infarction in both CT scan *(upper)* and LCBF *(lower)*. Of more importance is the gradual reduction of local flow worsening from occipital to frontal regions where CT anatomy is retained. **C,** improvement in LCBF noted after the flow augmentation procedure *(lower* scan and LCBF) compared with preoperative studies *(upper* scan and LCBF). (From Yonas H., Good W.F., Gur D., et al.: Mapping cerebral blood flow by xenon-enhanced computerized tomography. *Radiology,* to be published. Used by permission.)

side and pronation of the left hand. Deep tendon reflexes were also increased on the left. A CT scan demonstrated moderate, diffuse atrophy within the distal right middle cerebral artery distribution (Fig 2–11). The Xe/CT blood flow map (34% Xe) showed flow val-

ues within the normal range in the lentiform and thalamic nuclei bilaterally. Atrophic regions within the insular cortex had appropriate low-flow values, while a central island of retained, normal-appearing gray matter was shown to have normal flow values compared with

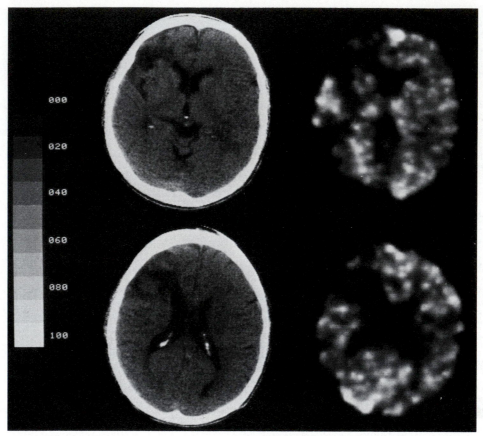

Fig 2–10.—Unilateral carotid occlusion with adequate flow in surviving tissue. This 46-year-old patient had angiographically demonstrated old left internal carotid artery occlusion. The CT scan shows infarction in the region of the anterior distribution of the middle cerebral artery, but sparing basal ganglia. The LCBF maps confirm the infarction, but demonstrate good flow in the remainder of the middle cerebral artery territory. (Patient's left is on reader's left.)

the left hemisphere. Consistent flow values were demonstrated in the two brain levels studied. A repeat angiogram the following day demonstrated a recanalization of the right middle cerebral artery and rapid filling of the distal middle cerebral artery vessels. Following these studies, the patient has remained asymptomatic for 12 months without surgical intervention.

OLD CEREBRAL INFARCT WITH TRANSIENT ISCHEMIC ATTACKS (TIA).—A 38-year-old woman had a 6-year history of recurrent ischemic attacks within the left middle cerebral artery distribution. Angiography 4 and 6 years previously had demonstrated proximal anterior and middle cerebral artery stenosis and delayed filling of the middle cerebral artery distribution. Until 1 month prior to admission, this woman had been relatively asymptomatic on anticoagulation therapy with warfarin sodium (Coumadin). Despite adequate anticoagulant level, the ischemic attacks had then recurred, and the woman was referred for an extracranial/intracranial bypass procedure to augment flow in the left middle cerebral artery distribution.

An angiogram with carotid and vertebral injections of contrast media demonstrated slow filling of the middle cerebral artery region on the left side. Filling was delayed and via leptomeningeal and medullary collaterals in a "moyamoya" pattern (Fig 2–12,A). The preoperative CT scan (see Fig 2–12,B) showed an old and relatively small infarction within the left anterior cerebral artery distribution, with a normal-appearing tissue volume and architecture in the remainder of the hemisphere. Despite the normal anatomical appearance by CT of tissues within the middle cerebral artery distribution and appropriate gray and white matter enhancement patterns, the Xe/CT blood flow study (33% Xe) showed that flow values were reduced within the entire left middle cerebral artery distribution (see Fig 2–12). The patient subsequently underwent an extracranial/intracranial bypass procedure and has remained asymptomatic for 6 months on antiplatelet therapy.

OLD CEREBRAL INFARCTION COMPLICATED BY RECENT MASSIVE INFARCT.—A 60-year-old white woman who had undergone a massive middle cerebral artery

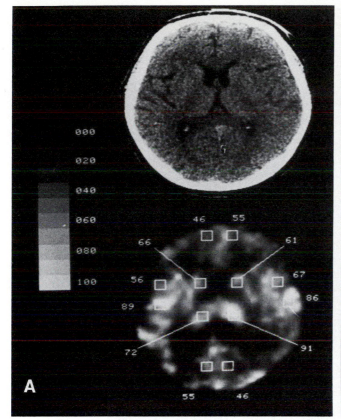
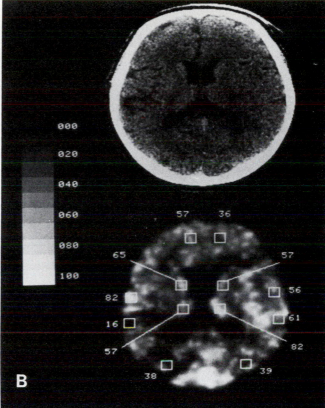
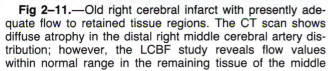

Fig 2–11.—Old right cerebral infarct with presently adequate flow to retained tissue regions. The CT scan shows diffuse atrophy in the distal right middle cerebral artery distribution; however, the LCBF study reveals flow values within normal range in the remaining tissue of the middle cerebral artery watershed. These were consistent at the two levels studied (**A** and **B**). (From Yonas H., Wolfson S.K. Jr., Gur D., et al.: Clinical experience with the use of xenon-enhanced CT blood flow mapping in cerebral vascular disease. *Stroke* 15:(in press), 1984. Used by permission.)

territory infarction 1 year earlier was referred for evaluation. Noninvasive studies had suggested that the left middle cerebral artery might still be patent, although severely compromised. Because this woman had gained a significant degree of independent function, an angiogram was performed, which showed that the left internal carotid artery was, in fact, occluded. One hour later, the patient had a grand mal seizure. Although seizure activity subsided, the patient did not awaken, and a CT scan obtained 6 hours after the event did not reveal a new abnormality. Because the patient remained unresponsive but without seizures for the next 48 hours, a Xe/CT blood flow study was performed. The baseline CT scan now demonstrated a new region of low density within the right lentiform nuclei, in addition to the known left middle cerebral artery infarction (Fig 2–13). The Xe/CT blood flow study (35% Xe) verified the absence of flow within this area as well as in the region of the old infarction. There was profound reduction of cerebral blood flow within the frontal lobes, although they appeared anatomically intact on the baseline CT scan. Flow values were also markedly reduced within the region immediately behind the area of the old left-side infarction. It is interesting to speculate whether these reductions of flow in (CT) normal-appearing structures are due to further compromise of perfusion or to a functional reduction of metabolism because of loss of neurologic substrata. It is likely that a LCBF study, had it been performed at the time of the 6-hour postictal CT, would have provided a clearer picture even earlier.

From the foregoing illustrations, it becomes clear that somewhat similar histories can lead to quite different indications for treatment, depending upon what the functional circulatory status is at the time of examination. In the first four cases, we saw an assortment of severe ischemic disease ranging from the total occlusion of both internal carotid arteries to the presence of middle cerebral artery stenosis and delayed filling. In each case, the LCBF study gave current functional information that defined both the degree of reduced perfusion or its absence and pinpointed the problem to various anatomical regions. The study added support to the de-

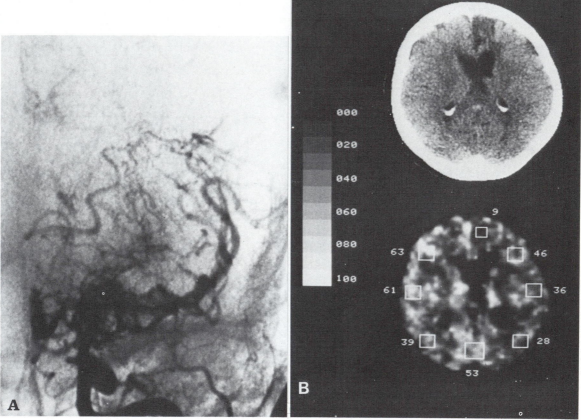

Fig 2–12.—Old cerebral infarct with recent episodes of TIA. **A,** occlusion of anterior cerebral artery and delayed filling of middle cerebral artery on the left side resembling a "moyamoya" pattern. **B,** the LCBF study showing reduced flow in the entire left middle cerebral artery distribution. Note that the flow values, ml/100 gm/minute, printed next to the corresponding ROIs are markedly reduced on the left as compared with right. (Patient's left is on the reader's right.) (From Yonas H., Wolfson S.K. Jr., Gur D., et al.: Clinical experience with the use of xenon-enhanced CT blood flow mapping in cerebral vascular disease. *Stroke* 15:(in press), 1984. Used by permission.)

cision to augment or not to augment blood flow surgically, and holds promise to give us a noninvasive test that ultimately may provide all the needed information for these decisions. The fifth case is somewhat different in that a catastrophic event occurred acutely, and the LCBF was able to give us precise information about the profound reduction in blood flow to large critical regions long before changes in CT could be expected. In the next several cases, we shall see that LCBF can also aid in understanding secondary ischemic processes.

Secondary Ischemic Problems

LATE VASOSPASM SECONDARY TO HEMORRHAGE FROM ANEURYSM.—A 37-year-old white man presented with the sudden onset of a severe headache associated with moderate numbness and weakness of his left arm. A CT scan showed retained blood within the deep insular region on the right side, and angiography verified the presence of a right middle cerebral artery aneurysm.

There was only moderate narrowing of the vessels. Three days later, the patient was referred for possible surgical treatment when it was apparent that the weakness in his left side was becoming more profound. A CT scan demonstrated only a small area of low density within the distal right middle cerebral artery distribution. The patient was treated with aggressive blood volume expansion, and his blood pressure was maintained within a normal range over the following 3 days; this resulted in stabilization and some improvement of the left-sided hemiparesis. However, repeat angiography demonstrated severe vasospasm of the internal carotid artery on the right side, with delayed filling of the distal branches of the middle cerebral artery (Fig 2–14,A). An Xe/CT blood flow study (31% Xe) obtained the following morning showed reduced flow throughout the entire right hemisphere and supported the angiographic diagnosis of severe vascular compromise (see Fig 2–14,B). Flow values were also reduced within the right

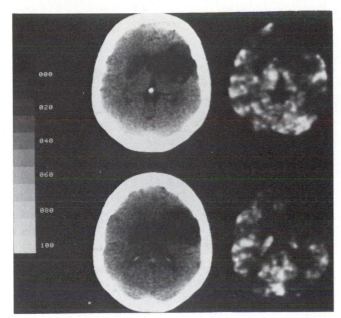

Fig 2–13.—Recent massive infarct following angiography in a patient with large old infarcts. This patient was in poor neurologic status that was not predicted by the CT scan; the scan was actually too recent after the event to be expected to reveal recent tissue death. The LCBF study shows large areas of reduced flow where there is apparent tissue retention on CT. These changes, while not fully explained, did agree with the poor physical condition of this patient. (From Yonas H., Wolfson S.K. Jr., Gur D., et al.: Clinical experience with the use of xenon-enhanced CT blood flow mapping in cerebral vascular disease. *Stroke* 15:(in press), 1984. Used by permission.)

thalamus and occipital lobe. Surgery was performed 5 days later, by which time the patient's clinical condition had improved markedly. The aneurysm was clipped in an uneventful fashion, and there was no increase in neurologic deficit postoperatively.

VEGETATIVE STATE: COMA VIGIL.—An 18-year-old white man had undergone a successful renal transplantation 18 months previously. He was readmitted to the hospital 2 months prior to this blood flow study because of the rapid onset of shortness of breath and fever. A massive pulmonary infection of an undefined etiology had developed, which resulted in rapid deterioration and finally cardiac arrest. A prolonged resuscitative effort did restart cardiac function, but the patient remained in a vegetative state with no evidence of normal cortical electrical activity on EEG or somatosensory evoked potential testing. The brain stem evoked potentials were normal and correlated with the clinical findings of intact brain stem reflexes, including spontaneous eye movements and repetitive yawning and chewing. The enhanced CT scan after 90 seconds of Xe inhalation demonstrated only a thin cortical gray matter ribbon consistent with the expected pathologic picture of postischemic pseudolaminar necrosis (Fig 2–15,B).

The cerebral blood flow study derived from the above and subsequent enhanced CT images disclosed relatively normal CBF values within the brain stem, but with only scattered patches of moderate blood flow through the hemispheres (see Fig 2–15,C).

BRAIN DEATH.—A 53-year-old white woman was found unconscious just prior to admission, following a

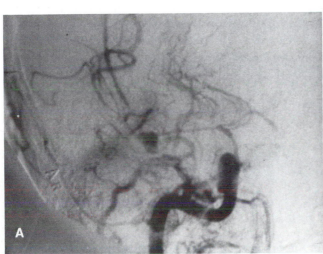

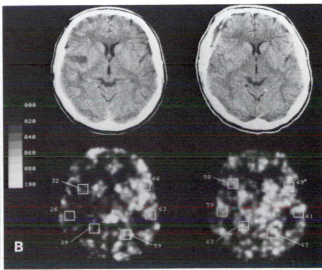

Fig 2–14.—Vasospasm (late) secondary to leaking middle cerebral artery aneurysm. **A,** spasm of right internal carotid and middle cerebral arteries with delayed filling of the distal branches of middle cerebral artery. **B,** on *left,* LCBF study confirming the pronounced reduction of flow throughout the right hemisphere including the right thalamus and occipital lobe; on *right,* postoperative LCBF study showing restoration of normal blood flow.

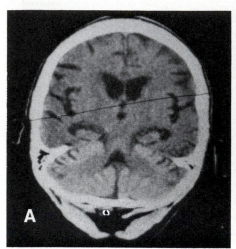 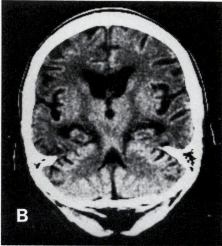 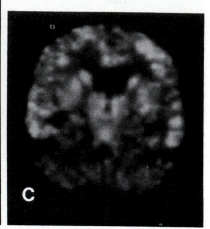

Fig 2–15.—Vegetative state. This 18-year-old patient had cardiac arrest and was resuscitated, but remained comatose with intact brain stem reflexes: "coma-vigil." **A,** baseline CT scan. **B,** enhanced CT scan taken from the flow study. **B** reveals Xe uptake only by a thin cortical ribbon and brain stem as expected in postischemic laminar necrosis. **C,** LCBF showing normal brain stem flow, but many patchy areas of "normal" flow amid a generally depressed hemispheric flow.

1-week history of left-sided retro-orbital eye pain and double vision. Upon arrival, she was comatose, and CT demonstrated acute hydrocephalus with blood throughout the ventricular system and encasing the entire brain. A dramatic clinical improvement followed the placement of bilateral external ventriculostomies. The next morning, she had no focal deficit and a normal sensorium. Angiography demonstrated a left-sided internal carotid/posterior communicating artery aneurysm. The aneurysm was operated upon, and the patient remained stable without focal deficit for 2 days. On the fifth postbleed day, she became lethargic. A CT scan revealed diffuse brain swelling, and angiography demonstrated diffuse and severe vasospasm. The patient was aggressively treated for vasospasm, but she became progressively less responsive. Finally on the seventh postbleed day, she was once again comatose with a loss of cortical and brain stem responses. The LCBF study did not show significant hemispheric, brain stem, or cerebellar blood flow (Fig 2–16). Later that evening, the patient fulfilled all clinical criteria for brain death.

Discussion of LCBF in Ischemia

Cerebral occlusive disease, in which the reduction of flow is the major pathologic mechanism, may be seen to have three broad subdivisions: (1) a relatively reversible reduction of flow, (2) the acute infarction process, and (3) a chronic postinfarction situation in which there may or may not be a persistence of reduced flow to remaining viable tissue. Patients in the first group may have TIA and present a question of whether the epi-

sodic disturbances (TIA) are due to embolic or hemodynamic causes. Regional flow studies in a group of patients with TIA have been shown to be helpful in defining a group of patients who do have a localized reduction of flow and for whom extracranial-to-intracranial (EC/IC) bypass procedures have appeared to have been of assistance.[73] Recent work with PET[74] has also defined the existence of a reduced-flow region in which metabolism is slightly reduced and in which improved metabolism and flow have been noted after EC/IC bypass. Baron termed this situation "misery perfusion." The ability to localize relative flow reduction in a region of retained tissue integrity is an example of how the Xe-enhanced CT studies should serve as a useful clinical guide to the indication for the augmentation of CBF. The second and fourth cases described under Primary Ischemic Problems above are examples of this, while the first and third cases show how Xe/CT LCBF revealed that the ischemic event was not followed by reduced flow in viable tissue. The LCBF studies aided in this differentiation.

Acute ischemia presents a complex problem in which CBF studies alone appear to provide only limited guidance. Combined blood flow and metabolism studies using PET have shown that flow and metabolism are severely reduced following a major vessel occlusion such as commonly occurs with an embolus to the middle cerebral artery. This is the situation in over half the individuals studied within hours of a cerebral vascular occlusive accident. A significant number, however, rapidly go on to a phase of hyperemia while metabolism remains impaired. This has been attributed to fragmen-

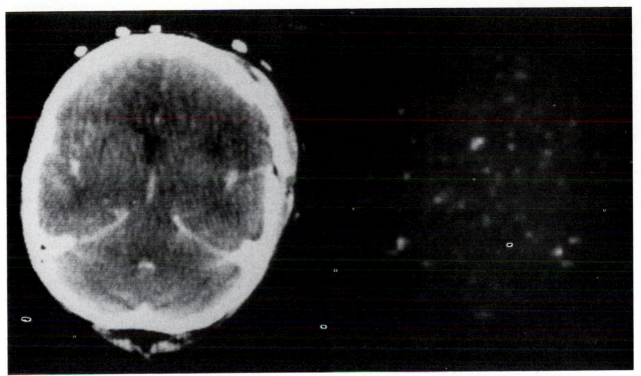

Fig 2–16.—Brain death. The baseline CT scan is on the *left*. There is virtually no flow in any portion of the LCBF map *(right)*. The LCBF map of this illustration was deliberately overexposed so as to be easily viewed. The actual flow is thus considerably less than it appears. The original image is almost invisible. This patient fulfilled all criteria for brain death shortly after this study was done.

tation of the embolus after the infarction is produced, resulting in reperfusion of the injured region. Seven to 10 days later, a second phase of hyperemia appears about the infarction. This hyperemic rim, presumably due to neovascularization, presents a major difficulty to regional flow studies such as ^{133}Xe rCBF, which "see" the rim and are unable to define the area of reduced or absent flow just below it. Tomographic flow studies including Xe/CT do allow better definition in this situation and improved understanding of the nature of the ischemic insult. Yet, in the face of "uncoupling" of flow and metabolism, the interpretation of flow data alone needs to be made very cautiously. Effective therapies designed to improve CBF and reduce intracranial pressure can be followed and guided with an available tomographic means of local CBF determination.

The individual who has suffered a stroke from a proximal occlusive disease may be a candidate for CBF augmentation. An EC/IC bypass may enable viable tissue with an insufficient blood flow to return to function. This region of ischemic "penumbra," in which presumably "idling" neurons are said to exist, has been the subject of a great deal of experimental and clinical effort. While studies with PET have helped define such regions of "misery perfusion," CT enhanced-Xe LCBF studies with their higher degree of spatial resolution may be better suited for this purpose and will certainly be more readily available than PET. The retention of tissue integrity seen on the baseline CT scan associated with reduced LCBF is a useful guide for clinicians trying to decide if flow augmentation might be of benefit.

Head Trauma

Another area in which flow measurements should prove to be of value is in the study and management of patients with closed-head injury. Presently the evaluation of such patients initially does involve obtaining a CT scan to define a degree of anatomical distortion. In children, the ability to couple this study with flow should prove to be particularly useful. This is of relevance to this age group because these injuries are associated with a tendency to lose vasoregulation, so that the resulting problem of increased intracranial pressure is often caused by elevated blood volume and reduced CBF. Therapies in children that are currently directed toward the management of this phenomena should benefit from the study of blood volume transit provided by iodine bolus CT studies and CBF provided by Xe-enhanced CT studies.

Seizure Disorders

Patients with seizure disorders, especially if bilateral, may benefit from the careful appraisal of local CBF. The ability to do multiple-level flow studies with three-dimensional reconstruction through both temporal lobe regions may offer a new approach for the diagnosis and localization of a seizure focus. This is especially true for patients who are nonresponsive to medication and where localization is needed if the surgeon is to be ideally guided to the source of the disorder. This is an area for extensive clinical investigation.

Degenerative and Other Syndromes

Nervous activity depends upon specific metabolic processes for both impulse transmission and for synthesis of chemical substances such as neurotransmitters. These are energy-consuming processes that create the need for generous supplies of oxygen and metabolites and hence of arterial blood. From this follows the concept of blood flow coupled to metabolic rate that was mentioned above. When there is a primary failure of blood supply, from whatever cause, metabolism and the functions that depend upon it suffer. Examples of this are the subject of the foregoing section. Is the converse true? It is certainly reasonable to suppose that as the metabolic activity diminishes as a result of some disruptive condition, the blood flowing through the affected tissue might diminish correspondingly. Indeed, there are examples of this occurring. The elegant system of autoregulation and chemical regulation of normal brain tissue really demonstrates how the cerebral circulation is organized so that, ordinarily, blood flow responds to events within tissue rather than the converse. If there is a change in the central circulation (e.g., fall or rise in blood pressure), but no change in the brain requirement for nourishment, the autoregulation supervenes to maintain a constant flow (and source of nourishment). On the other hand, if increased activity demands increased blood flow, this will occur, being mediated by the increase in Pa_{CO_2} produced as a result of the increased level of activity. Figure 2–6 is an illustration of how this can be perceived by Xe/CT LCBF. The upper images are the Xe-enhanced CT scans and flow maps of a healthy volunteer at rest. In the lower images, the subject is actively opening and closing his left fist with a corresponding increase in blood flow of the right parietal (motor) region (refer to preceeding section on Sensitivity to Physiologic Change for more complete description).

In conditions that are primarily of a functional or even of a degenerative nature, one might then expect to see appropriate changes in LCBF that either precede, coincide with, or result from the disease process. These flow changes, if present, would aid both in diag-

nosis and in understanding the pathogenesis of the condition. Included in this group would be dementia, both senile and nonsenile, depression, demyelinating diseases, and metabolically linked problems such as Pick's disease. Using existing techniques such as ^{133}Xe rCBF and PET, investigators have observed blood flow in some of these conditions. A few examples include the effort by Freyhan and associates[75] to look at global and hemispheric flow (N_2O method) in "psychoses and senility." Studies have reported CBF lowered in various dementias including AD,[71, 76–78] and a recent report from this institution using the Xe/CT LCBF method describes changes in multiple sclerosis.[72] The remaining cases to be illustrated come from this group. We and others have had limited experience in studying these patients using Xe/CT, but it is certainly a most stimulating area.

Acute Progressive Dementia

A 38-year-old engineer had a 6-week history of rapidly progressing dementia. At the time of admission, he was in a stuporous state. A cortical biopsy was performed, and the tissue (frontal lobe near coronal suture) appeared histologically normal. An LCBF study done at that time (Fig 2–17) revealed extremely low thalamic flow. A gray-scale map of blood/brain partition coefficient (λ) was also imaged and shows that the thalamic tissue has assumed the Xe solubility qualities of white matter. The interesting question arises as to whether the nuclear component of the thalamus has been severely damaged, leaving only the white matter substratum, or has the flow diminished consequent to withdrawal of activating input? The cause of either is unknown and will have to await histologic verification if the opportunity arises in this case.

Alzheimer's Disease

The first patient is illustrated in Figure 2–18. He was a 64-year-old white man with a known 12-year history of AD with a progressive decline of mental function. He was hospitalized for the last several years of his illness. At the time he had the LCBF study done, the patient was totally unable to communicate. An autopsy was performed, which confirmed the diagnosis. Examination of the scans and flow maps reveals marked atrophy evidenced both by massive ventricular enlargement and by widening of fissures and sulci. The reader's attention should be drawn to the fact that while the greatest flow reductions are in region where atrophy is greatest, there are significant, even profound reductions of CBF where there is retained and sometimes hyperdense CT anatomy.

The second patient is a 59-year-old right-handed man who formerly operated a printing business. His family started noticing a disorder of mentation. He was admit-

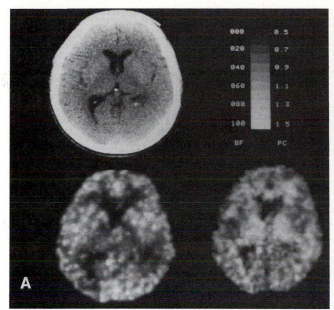 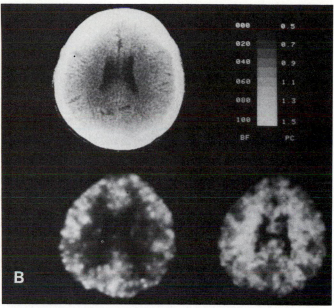

Fig 2–17.—Acute progressive dementia. Shown are two levels (slices) **(A** and **B)** in a patient with rapidly progressive dementia. In each case, *top left* is CT scan, *bottom left* is LCBF, and *bottom right* is blood/brain partition coefficient (λ) image. Flow map *(BF)* and λ map *(PC)* refer to the gray scale shown. Notable are the very low thalamic flow and the λ map showing thalamic tissue solubility very similar to white matter (elevated partition coefficient).

ted for treatment of mental depression, and diagnosis of AD was made. He had been hospitalized for the past 4 years, during which there was a progressive decline in his mentation. At the time of LCBF study, he was mute and had to be fed by nasogastric tube. Figure 2–19 again illustrates the profound atrophy, but also the significant reduction in flow in the left frontoparietal region where there is retained CT anatomy.

We have embarked upon a detailed longitudinal study of AD in relation to other senile-type dementias and normal aging. The method of LCBF is only a part of this study, but we think that its role in this group of diseases will be multiple. In diagnosis, it should aid in differentiating between AD and multiinfarct dementia, where flow deficits will follow vascular anatomy. The pattern of flow changes may also have a characteristic that can become a diagnostic aid. Finally, the temporal and spacial relationship to neurologic deficits may play a role in the study of pathogenesis.

Multiple Sclerosis (MS)

This condition is representative of a number of selective degenerative (in this case demyelinating) diseases that could have associated blood flow aberrations although they have not been described as prominent features of the pathologic picture. Especially important would be the finding that changes in tissue perfusion occur early or even precede the neurologic changes. Eidelman and associates[72] have undertaken a study of Xe/CT LCBF in patients with this condition. While this study is exceedingly preliminary, we are fortunate in having several cases to review. In Figure 2–20, we see the baseline scan and LCBF flow map of a woman in the early years of her fourth decade who has an immunologically confirmed diagnosis of about 5 years' duration. She has minimal neurologic findings, restricted

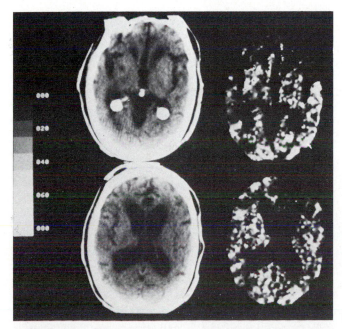

Fig 2–18.—CT scans and gray scale blood flow maps in a patient with advanced AD. Note that regions of reduced flow do not always correspond to regions of atrophy or of tissue dropout. Xe was administered at 35% for 6 minutes.

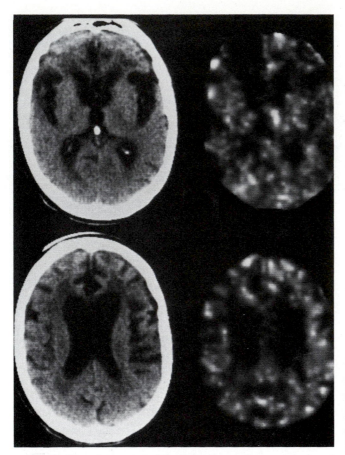

Fig 2–19.—Advanced AD. This is another example of this condition that again illustrates profound atrophy, but reduced flow in areas of retained CT anatomy. The most prominent reductions of flow are present in the left frontal and temporal regions. Comparison of this figure with Figure 2–17 also reveals differences in techniques of flow display. This image is smoother and provides a more natural appearance, reflecting improvements in the LCBF methodology.

mainly to changes of affect. The CT scan is normal, but the LCBF map shows reduction in flow of the right caudate nucleus, although flow in other areas appears normal. Similar and even more profound dissociations between CT anatomy and LCBF have been found in several other patients. Another case is a 40-year-old woman with advanced, long-standing MS. Severe affective deficiencies were present as well as a left spastic hemiparesis. Markedly reduced flow was seen in the right parieto-occipital region as well as subnormal values in the basal ganglia. These areas all were seen to have reasonably normal CT anatomy. While the LCBF changes were easily detected, the flow maps themselves did not reproduce well enough for publication. If these findings are consistent in future work, it may open a new mode of study and new possibilities for pathogenesis in this and related conditions.

GENERAL DISCUSSION

Each of the tomographic blood flow methods described above have obvious advantages and sometimes more obscure disadvantages. Both pros and cons of emission tomography were discussed above and also extensively in the literature cited. The Xe/CT LCBF method is, in common with the others, completely noninvasive. It cannot be used for rapidly repetitious determinations, because it requires a period of gaseous indicator inhalation (washin) and exhalation (washout). Fast phenomena cannot be studied directly. On the other hand, unlike both PET and SPECT, flow changes of small structures can be appreciated (4 to 5 mm full width, half maximum, flow values calculated on a *pixel* by *pixel* basis).

The value of m (see preceding, Description of Stable Xe/CT Method) for different tissues and techniques, the effect of improving signal-to-noise ratio, and the interrelationships of the amount of enhancement, Xe con-

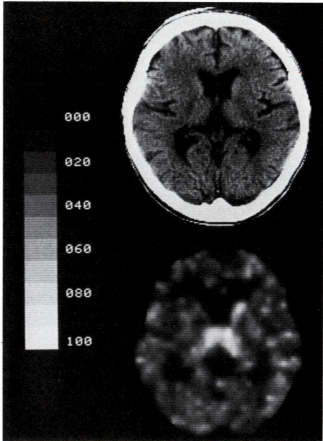

Fig 2–20.—Multiple sclerosis of 5 years in a young person. Although diagnosis is immunologically confirmed, this patient's symptoms are minimal. The CT scan is normal, but the LCBF map shows reduced flow in the right caudate nucleus.

centration, scan sequence and number of scans, the merits of single vs. multicompartmental analysis, among other considerations, are of great importance in understanding the significance and anatomical resolving power of the technique. These considerations have been described and analyzed elsewhere by ourselves and others[30, 35] and cannot be adequately addressed here. The Xe/CT flow method provides the ability to measure and to image blood/brain partition coefficient (λ) as well as blood flow. Besides containing information about the type of tissue, λ also may provide clues about the metabolic state and about changes in tissue composition as a result of disease (see Fig 2–17). While normal metabolism has been inferred from normal CT anatomy, the degree of functional disturbance required to alter radiodensity is unknown. As we have seen previously, reduced flow can exist in tissue with a normal CT appearance. These speculations are interesting, but remain to be studied. The ability to estimate λ directly from the CBF study has other important advantages. It frees the computation from dependence upon "normative" values measured at another time in a different specimen. The use of "normative" values is an obvious disadvantage when abnormal tissue or foreign tissue such as tumor is involved. For a specific tumor, λ is never available, so tumor blood flow estimates using normal gray, white, or average values is almost always in error. While the positron-emitting radionuclides of PET can be used as metabolic markers or tracers and can be measured at the same time as blood flow, the literature reveals that flow and metabolism are seldom measured simultaneously in practice. This is apparently due to the technical difficulties encountered when this is attempted.

Although free of the need to take precautions with respect to gaseous radionuclides as with most SPECT, the method does expose the subject to ionizing radiation. The dose for thyroid gland, for example, is higher than that absorbed by other blood flow techniques (e.g., ^{133}Xe), but the dose to other critical organs (e.g., gonads) is comparable or lower (see preceding, Radiation Dose). The brain is relatively radioinsensitive, and the more sensitive eyes (cornea and lens) are usually left out of the scan field. Based both upon the anesthesia literature of the 1950s and upon our experience and that of others, it appears that the concentration of Xe required for satisfactory blood flow studies (30% to 35%) does not cause significant side effects for most subjects (see preceding, Anesthetic Properties).

The cost of sophisticated CT scanners is comparable to costs involved in PET and greater than those generally encountered with SPECT. Yet, only a small portion of these costs need accrue to the LCBF studies, because the extensive equipment is already available in a well equipped medical center. Equipment that must be dedicated to the CBF application (breathing apparatus, recorder, Xe meter, etc.) is much less expensive and readily obtained. A prominent manufacturer of CT equipment (General Electric) is, at this writing, developing a software package with an associated hardware unit (principally a breathing apparatus with Xe monitor) that will be available for their 9800 series scanners and that will nearly fully automate the LCBF measurement, producing flow maps 10 to 20 minutes after a dynamic CT examination is completed. This will make the method available to a very large number of clinical centers at minimal cost and should be in use by the time this book is published.

In theory, the CT slices could be made in any plane. Practical considerations render it difficult to cut scan slices very far from the horizontal, because positioning and holding the patient for this is not easily achieved. The three-dimensional capability is therefore useful for studying structures whose long axis is in a plane different from the CT slices taken or when blood flow maps are to be compared with pathologic slices made in other planes such as coronal or sagittal. Thus, in our blood flow study of senile dementia, we are using data obtained in conventional transaxial planes to construct maps in coronal planes so as to correspond with those to be ultimately studied by the neuropathologist and neurochemist.

In summary, a method of imaging blood flow to the brain has been described. This method, Xe/CT LCBF, has been discussed in relation to other tomographic blood flow methods, and its use is illustrated. We are of the opinion that Xe/CT has been shown to be an effective blood flow method of high utility, and one that has promise of widespread application because of its relatively high anatomical resolution, low cost, and ease of procedure.

ACKNOWLEDGMENT

The Xe/CT LCBF work has been supported, in part, by grants from the American Heart Association, Western Pennsylvania Affiliate, and the U.S. Public Health Service (HL 27208); by an American Heart Association established investigatorship (D. Gur); and by institutional funds of Childrens Hospital of Pittsburgh, Montefiore Hospital Association of Western Pennsylvania, and Presbyterian-University Hospital of Pittsburgh.

The authors are indebted to a host of individuals for collaboration, technical assistance, and contribution of patient material. These include but are not limited to F. Boller, E.E. Cook, B. Drayer, M. Dujovny, B.H. Eidelman, D.L. Jackson, P.J. Jannetta, R.E. Latchaw, J. Moossy, G. Rao, O.M. Reinmuth, R. Sclabassi, J.

Vries, and J. Willy. A special thank you to Darlene Woomer for typing and correcting the manuscript.

REFERENCES

1. Kety S.S., Schmidt C.F.: The nitrous oxide method for the quantitative determination of cerebral blood flow in man: Theory, procedure, and normal values. *J. Clin. Invest.* 27:476–483, 1948.
2. Mallett B.L., Veall N.: The measurement of regional cerebral clearance rates in man using xenon-133 inhalation and extracranial recording. *Clin. Sci.* 29:179–191, 1965.
3. Obrist W.D., Thompson H.K., Wang H.S., et al.: Regional cerebral blood flow estimated by ^{133}xenon inhalation. *Stroke* 6:245–256, 1975.
4. Lassen N., Ingvar D.H., Skinhoj E.: Brain function and blood flow. Changes in the amount of blood flowing in areas of the human cerebral cortex, reflecting changes in the activity of those areas, are graphically revealed with the aid of radioactive isotopes. *Scientific American* 239:62–71, 1978.
5. Wagner H.N., Rhodes B.A., Sasaki Y., et al.: Studies of the circulation with radioactive microspheres. *Invest. Radiol.* 4:374–386, 1969.
6. Dull W.P., Jackson D.L., Rosenblat T.I., et al.: Relative error and variability in blood flow measurements with radiolabeled microspheres. *Am. J. Physiol.* 243:H371–H378, 1982.
7. Reivich M., Jehle J., Sokoloff L., et al.: Measurement of regional cerebral blood flow with antipyrine-^{14}C in awake cats. *J. Appl. Physiol.* 27:296–300, 1969.
8. Eklof B., Lassen N.A., Nilsson L.: Regional cerebral blood flow in the rat measured by the tissue sampling technique: A critical evaluation using four indicators C^{14}-antipyrine, C^{14}-ethanol, H^{3}-water and xenon^{133}. *Acta Physiol. Scand.* 91:1–10, 1974.
9. Kennedy C., Des Rosiers M.H., Sakurada O., et al.: Metabolic mapping of the primary visual system of the monkey by means of the autoradiographic [^{14}C] deoxyglucose technique. *Proc. Natl. Acad. Sci. U.S.A.* 73:4230, 1976.
10. Sakurada O., Kennedy C., Jehle J., et al.: Measurement of local cerebral blood flow with iodo[^{14}C]antipyrine. *Am. J. Physiol.* 234:H59–H66, 1978.
11. Symon L., Pasztor E., Branston N.M.: The distribution and density of reduced cerebral blood flow following acute middle cerebral artery occlusion: An experimental study by the technique of hydrogen clearance in baboons. *Stroke* 5:335–364, 1974.
12. Young W.: H$_2$ clearance measurement of blood flow: A review of technique and polarographic principles. *Stroke* 11:552–564, 1980.
13. Ingvar D.H.: Brain activation patterns revealed by measurements of regional cerebral blood flow, in Desmedt J.E. (ed.): *Cognitive Components in Cerebral Event-Related Potentials and Selective Attention Progress in Clinical Neurology.* Basel, Switzerland, Karger, 1979, vol. 6, pp. 200–215.
14. Ingvar D.H., Philipson L.: Distribution of cerebral blood flow in the dominant hemisphere during motor ideation and motor performance. *Ann. Neurol.* 2:230–237, 1977.
15. Kety S.S., Schmidt C.F.: The determination of cerebral blood flow in man by the use of nitrous oxide in low concentrations. *Am. J. Physiol.* 143:53–65, 1945.
16. Gelmers H.J.: *Regional Cerebral Blood Flow: Regulation, Measurement and Changes in Diseases.* Assen, The Netherlands, Van Grocum, 1978.
17. Hoedt-Rasmussen K.: Regional cerebral blood flow: The intra-arterial injection method. *Acta Neurol. Scand.* 43(suppl. 27):17–79, 1967.
18. Larsen B., Orgogozo J.M., Rougier A., et al.: Value of intracranial regional cerebral blood flow study (rCBF) to the selection for neurosurgical intervention of focal epilepsy. *Acta Neurol. Scand.* 60(suppl. 72):554–555, 1979.
19. Sundt T.M., Sharbrough F.W., Anderson R.E., et al.: Cerebral blood flow measurements and electroencephalogram during carotid endartectomy. *J. Neurosurg.* 41:310–320, 1974.
20. Morawetz R.B., DeGirolami U., Ojemann R.G., et al.: Cerebral blood flow determined by hydrogen clearance during middle cerebral artery occlusion in unanesthetized monkeys. *Stroke* 9:143–149, 1978.
21. Stokely E.M., Sveinsdottir E., Lassen N.A., et al.: A single photon dynamic computer assisted tomograph (DCAT) for imaging brain function in multiple cross sections. *J. Comput. Assist. Tomogr.* 4:230–240, 1980.
22. Lassen N.A., Henriksen L., Paulson O.: Regional cerebral blood flow in stroke by ^{133}xenon inhalation and emission tomography. *Stroke* 12:284–288, 1981.
23. Fukuyama H., Akiguchi I., Kameyama M., et al.: A krypton-81m single photon emission tomography on the collateral circulation in carotid occlusion: The role of the circle of Willis and leptomeningeal anastomoses. *J. Cereb. Blood Flow Metab.* 3:S143–S144, 1983.
24. Phelps M.E.: Positron computed tomography studies of cerebral glucose metabolism in man: Theory and application in nuclear medicine. *Semin. Nucl. Med.* 11:32–49, 1981.
25. Alavi A., Reivich M., Greenberg J., et al.: Mapping of functional activity in the brain with ^{18}F-fluorodeoxyglucose. *Semin. Nucl. Med.* 11:24–31, 1981.
26. Drayer B.P., Wolfson S.K. Jr., Reinmuth O.M., et al.: Xenon enhanced computed tomography for the analysis of cerebral integrity, perfusion, and blood flow. *Stroke* 9:123–130, 1978.
27. Wolfson S.K. Jr., Drayer B.P., Boehnke M., et al.: Regional cerebral blood flow by xenon enhanced computed tomography. *Proc. Annu. Meet. Am. Assoc. Neurol. Surgeons* (New Orleans). 1978, pp. 1–3.
28. Gur D., Yonas H., Herbert D., et al.: Xenon enhanced dynamic computed tomography: Multilevel cerebral blood flow studies. *J. Comput. Assist. Tomogr.* 5:334–340, 1981.
29. Gur D., Wolfson S.K. Jr., Yonas H., et al.: Progress in cerebrovascular disease: Local cerebral blood flow by xenon enhanced CT. *Stroke* 13:750–758, 1982.
30. Good W., Gur D., Shabason L., et al.: Errors associated with single-scan determinations of regional cerebral blood

flow by xenon enhanced CT. *Phys. Med. Biol.* 27:531–537, 1982.

31. Meyer J.S., Hayman L.A., Sakai F., et al.: High resolution three dimensional measurement of localized cerebral blood flow by CT scanning and stable xenon clearance: Effect of cerebral infarction and ischemia. *Trans. Am. Neurol. Assoc.* 104:85–89, 1979.

32. Ono H., Ono K., Mori K.: Mapping of CBF distribution by dynamic Xe-enhanced CT scan method. *J. Cereb. Blood Flow Metab.* 1:50–51, 1981.

33. Sakai F., Gotoh F., Ebihara S., et al.: Xenon enhanced CT method for the measurement of local cerebral blood flow in man. *J. Cereb. Blood Flow Metab.* 1:29–30, 1981.

34. Segawa H., Wakai S., Tamura A., et al.: CBF study by CT with Xe enhancement: Experience in 30 cases. *J. Cereb. Blood Flow Metab.* 1:52–53, 1981.

35. Rottenberg D.A., Lu H.C., Kearfott K.J.: The in vivo autoradiographic measurement of regional cerebral blood flow using stable xenon and computerized tomography: The effect of tissue heterogeneity and computerized tomography noise. *J. Cereb. Blood Flow Metab.* 2:173–178, 1982.

36. Nunnally R.L., Peshock R.M., Rehr R.B.: Fluorine-19 [^{19}F] NMR in vivo: Potential for flow and perfusion measurements. *Proc. Ann. Meet. Society of Nuclear Magnetic Resonance in Medicine* (San Francisco). August 1983, p. 266.

37. Kety S.S.: The theory and applications of the exchange of inert gas at the lungs and tissues. *Pharmacol. Rev.* 3:1–41, 1951.

38. Mishray G.A., Clark L.C.: Use of the platinum black cathode for local blood flow measurements in vivo. *Proc. Intl. Cong. Physiol.* (Brussels). 20:650, 1956.

39. Hyman E.S.: Linear system for quantitating hydrogen at a platinum electrode. *Circ. Res.* 9:1093–1097, 1961.

40. Aukland K.: Hydrogen polarography in measurement of local blood flow: Theoretical and empirical basis. *Acta Neurol. Scand.* 41(suppl. 14):42–44, 1965.

41. Aukland, K., Bower B.F., Berliner R.W.: Measurement of local blood flow with hydrogen gas. *Circ. Res.* 14:164–187, 1964.

42. Fieschi C., Bozzao L., Agnoli A.: Regional clearance of hydrogen as a measure of blood flow. *Acta Neurol. Scand.* 41(suppl. 14):46–52, 1965.

43. Gotoh F., Meyer J.S., Tomita M.: Hydrogen method for determining cerebral blood flow in man. *Arch. Neurol.* 15:549–559, 1966.

44. Neely W.A., Turner M.D., Hardy J.D., et al.: Use of the hydrogen electrode to measure tissue blood flow. *J. Surg. Res.* 5:363–369, 1965.

45. Symon L.: Regional vascular reactivity in the middle cerebral arterial distribution: An experimental study in baboons. *J. Neurosurg.* 33:532–541, 1970.

46. Senter H.J., Venes J.L.: Altered blood flow and secondary injury in experimental spinal cord trauma. *J. Neurosurg.* 49:569–578, 1978.

47. Lubbers D.W., Leniger-Follert E.: Capillary flow in the brain cortex during changes in oxygen supply and state of activation, in *Cerebral Vascular Smooth Muscle and Its Control* (CIBA Foundation Symposium 56). Amsterdam-New York, Elsevier, Excerpta Medica, 1978, pp. 22–47.

48. Stosseck K., Lubbers D.W., Cottin N.: Determination of local blood flow (microflow) by electrochemically generated hydrogen: Construction and application of the measuring probe. *Pflugers. Arch. Eur. J. Physiol.* 348:225–238, 1974.

49. Halsey J.H., Capra N.F., McFarland R.S.: Use of hydrogen for measurement of regional cerebral blood flow: Problem of intercompartmental diffusion. *Stroke* 8:351–357, 1977.

50. Brock M., Ingvar D.H., Sem Jacobsen C.W.: Regional blood flow in deep structures of the brain measured in acute cat experiments by means of a new beta-sensitive semiconductor needle detector. *Exp. Brain Res.* 4:126–137, 1967.

51. Ingvar D.H., Cronqvist S., Ekberg R., et al.: Normal values of regional cerebral blood flow in man, including flow and weight estimates of gray and white matter. *Acta Neurol. Scand.* 41(suppl. 14):72–78, 1965.

52. Ueda H., Hatano S., Koide T., et al.: External measurement of regional cerebral blood flow in man by common carotid arterial injection of radioactive krypton-85 saline solution. *Jpn. Heart J.* 9:349–358, 1968.

53. Segawa H., Susumu W., Tamura A., et al.: Computed tomographic measurement of local cerebral blood flow by xenon enhancement. *Stroke* 14:356–362, 1983.

54. Obrist W.D., Thompson H.K. Jr., King C.H., et al.: Determination of regional cerebral blood flow by inhalation of 133-xenon. *Circ. Res.* 20:124–135, 1967.

55. Paulson O.B., Lassen N.A., Henriksen L., et al.: Regional cerebral blood flow distribution evaluated by emission computer tomography with ^{133}xenon and ^{123}I-isopropyl-amphetamine. *J. Cereb. Blood Flow Metab.* 3:S162–S163, 1983.

56. Winkler S.S., Sacket J.F., Holden J.E., et al.: Xenon inhalation as an adjunct to computerized tomography of the brain: Preliminary study. *Radiology* 12:15–18, 1977.

57. Kelcz F., Hilal S.K., Hartwell P., et al.: Computed tomographic measurement of xenon brain-blood partition coefficient and implication for regional cerebral blood flow: A preliminary report. *Radiology* 127:385–392, 1978.

58. Yonas H., Wolfson S.K. Jr., Dujovny M., et al.: Selective lenticulostriate occlusion in the primate: A highly focal cerebral ischemia model. *Stroke* 12:567–572, 1981.

59. Gur D., Good W.F., Wolfson S.K. Jr., et al.: In vivo mapping of local cerebral blood flow by xenon enhanced CT. *Science* 215:1267–1268, 1982.

60. Morris L.E., Knott J.R., Pittinger C.B.: Electroencephalographic and blood gas observations in human surgical patients during xenon anesthesia. *Anesthesiology* 16:312–319, 1955.

61. Cullen S.C., Gross E.G.: The anesthetic properties of xenon in animals and human beings with additional observations on krypton. *Science* 113:580–582, 1951.

62. Lawrence J.H., Loomis W.F., Tobias C.A., et al.: Preliminary observations on the narcotic effect of xenon with a review of values for solubilities of gases in water and oils. *J. Physiol.* 105:197–204, 1946.

63. Yonas H., Grundy B., Gur D., et al.: Side effects of xenon inhalation. *J. Comput. Assist. Tomogr.* 5:591–2, 1981.

64. Meyer J.S., Hayman L.A., Yamamoto M., et al.: Local cerebral blood flow measured by CT after stable xenon inhalation. *Am. J. Roentgenol.* 135:239–251, 1980.

65. Coin C.G., Coin J.T.: Contrast enhancement by xenon gas in computed tomography of the spinal cord and brain: Preliminary observations. *J. Comput. Assist. Tomogr.* 4:217–221, 1980.

66. Haughton V.M., Donegan J.H., Walsh P.R., et al.: A clinical evaluation of xenon enhancement for computed tomography. *Invest. Radiol.* 15:160–163, 1980.

67. Dhawan V., Goldiner P., Ray C. Jr., et al.: Mass spectrometric measurement of end-tidal xenon concentration for clinical stable xenon/computerized tomography cerebral blood flow studies. *Biomed. Mass. Spectrom.* 9:241–245, 1982.

68. Yonas H., Wolfson S.K. Jr., Gur D., et al.: Clinical experience with the use of xenon-enhanced CT blood flow mapping in cerebral vascular disease. *Stroke* 15:(in press), 1984.

69. Yonas H., Good W.F., Gur D., et al.: Mapping cerebral blood flow by xenon-enhanced computerized tomography. *Radiology,* to be published.

70. Wolfson S.K. Jr., Gur D., Yonas H., et al.: Two- and three-dimensional imaging of local cerebral blood flow by xenon CT. *Ann. Biomed. Eng.,* to be published.

71. Meyer J.S., Shaw T., Okayasu H., et al.: Multi-infarct and Alzheimer dementias differentiated from normal aging by xenon contrast CT CBF measurements. *J. Cereb. Blood Flow Metab.* 3:S506–S507, 1983.

72. Eidelman B.H., Yonas H., Latchaw R.E., et al.: Cerebral blood flow in multiple sclerosis (in preparation).

73. Schmiedek P., Gratzl O., Spetzler R., et al.: Selection of patients for extra-intracranial arterial bypass surgery based on rCBF measurements. *J. Neurosurg.* 44:303–312, 1976.

74. Baron J.C., Bousser M.G., Rey A., et al.: Reversal of focal "misery perfusion syndrome" by extra-intracranial arterial bypass in hemodynamic cerebral ischemia. *Stroke* 12:454–459, 1981.

75. Freyhan F.A., Woodford R.B., Kety S.S.: Cerebral blood flow and metabolism in psychoses of senility. *J. Nerv. Ment. Dis.* 113:449–456, 1951.

76. Ingvar D.H., Brun A., Hagberg B., et al.: Regional cerebral blood flow in the dominant hemisphere in confirmed cases of Alzheimer's disease, Pick's disease, and multi-infarct dementia: Relationship to clinical symptomatology and neuropathological findings, in Katzman R., Terry R.D., Bick K.L. (eds.): *Alzheimer's Disease: Senile Dementia and Related Disorders (Aging, Vol. 7).* New York, Raven Press, 1978, pp. 203–211.

77. Phelps M.E., Mazziotta J.C., Huang S.: Study of cerebral function with positron computed tomography. *J. Cereb. Blood Flow Metab.* 2:113–162, 1982.

78. Obrist W.D., Chivian E., Cronqvist S., et al.: Regional cerebral blood flow in senile and presenile dementia. *Neurology* 20:315–322, 1970.

Trauma and Vascular Abnormalities

3

Cranial Trauma

JOSEPH A. HORTON, M.D.

TO UNDERSTAND the CT of trauma and its sequelae, it is necessary first to examine the CT appearance of blood, both acutely and over time. Initially, extravasated blood falls into the density range of 50 to 60 Hounsfield units (HU),[1, 2] while normal brain occupies the range of 18 to 30 HU. For this reason, acute hematomas are usually easy to identify (Figs 3–1 and 3–2). It was initially thought that the iron in hemoglobin and/or the calcium in serum were responsible for the increased density, but measurements of the attenuation values of solutions of iron and calcium in high physiologic concentrations failed to confirm this. What made this failure all the more puzzling was the fact that some subdural collections even showed a hematocrit,[3] suggesting that erythrocytes were somehow responsible.

Resolution of the problem hinged upon scanning solutions of globin and of albumin. New and Aronow[4] showed that physiologic concentrations of hemoglobin were in the appropriate density range, but because iron does not significantly increase the density in these concentrations, the protein or protein-heme combination is responsible. Subacutely, the clot may contract, further increasing its density, but this effect is short-lived. Soon proteolysis begins, and hematoma protein is degraded and absorbed.[5] After passing through the state of isodensity (same density as that of adjacent brain), the hematoma's attenuation ultimately falls to near that of cerebrospinal fluid (CSF).

As one would predict from the above discussion, anemic patients may present diagnostic dilemmas: their acute hematomas may lack enough globin to be denser than brain.[6] This group may present with iso- or even hypodense acute hematomas.

SUBDURAL HEMATOMA

Acute subdural hematoma (SDH) (Figs 3–1 and 3–3) generally results from traumatic tearing of the veins bridging the space between the dura and the brain surface.[7, 8] Fractures may or may not be present.* On occasion, SDH may have a nontraumatic etiology, such as the too-rapid decompression of obstructive hydrocephalus (Fig 3–4). In this, the brain surface recedes from the dura faster than the parenchyma can reexpand after having been compressed by distended ventricles. The resulting traction on bridging veins can tear them and result in an SDH.

An SDH assumes a crescentic shape,[14] because it occupies the crescent-shaped potential space between the brain surface and the dura (Fig 3–5). Although at a single level the actual thickness of the hematoma may seem small, there is no mechanical barrier to its spread, and it can cover most or all of the hemisphere. The total hematoma volume can therefore become quite large without seeming to be so on individual sections.

The degree of shift reflects the magnitude of mass effect. In addition to the extracerebral collection, trauma to underlying brain can produce parenchymal swelling in at least two ways.[15] Edema can result from direct trauma, producing diffuse swelling. But more ominous is a loss of autoregulation of blood flow. This can, in turn, increase the cerebral blood volume, itself giving rise to a swollen cerebral hemisphere that is *not lucent*. Patients with this syndrome characteristically do very poorly. Determination of cerebral blood flow (see Chapter 2) may help in the identification and therapy of this group of patients.

Over time, several changes characterize the conservatively managed SDH[14] that is not spontaneously reabsorbed. The acutely crescentic shape evolves through a straight-edged collection to a biconvex one. This results from formation of a subdural membrane around the clot. The hematoma's density, that of blood

---

*Fractures and shifted calcified pineal glands are the only useful plain film radiographic changes in the trauma patient. Correlation between the presence or absence of a fracture and the existence and severity of underlying pathology in the form of hematomas, contusion, and/or cerebral edema is very questionable.[9–13]

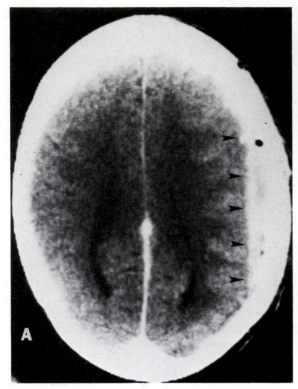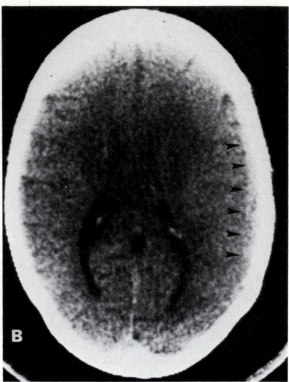

Fig 3–1.—Hematoma: time course. Acute **(A)** and 2-week **(B)** scans show a decrease in the size and density of the subdural hematoma *(arrowheads).* Acutely, the slight mass effect is reflected by effacement of the ipsilateral ven-

tricle. The effacement could easily be within normal limits of ventricular asymmetry; the later scan shows the ventricle's true size.

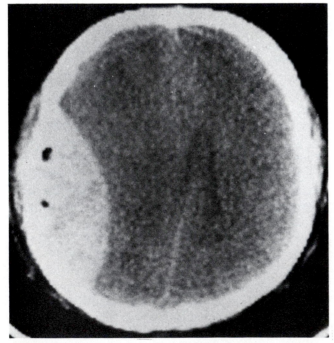

Fig 3–2.—Acute epidural hematoma. The biconvex shape and high density is characteristic of an epidural hematoma. Diffuse but marked midline shift is of a magnitude about equal to the size of the hematoma.

acutely, gradually lessens to hypodensity (less dense than brain) as a result of protein absorption. The membrane is porous and allows seepage of protein as well as its absorption. Particulate material (cells) are removed, but the dynamics of fluid accumulation and persistence may allow an extracerebral collection to persist indefinitely. Occasionally, a resolving SDH that has been decreasing in density will suddenly increase in density with or without a hematocrit-like level. Such a change represents rebleeding,[3, 5] the dense lower level containing erythrocytes.

As the SDH matures from hyperdensity to hypodensity, it logically must pass through a stage during which it is isodense. The same situation can be seen occasionally in patients who are severely anemic: an acute SDH in an anemic patient may have a density less than or equal to that of normal brain (Fig 3–6). It might also be invisible unless a contrast-enhanced scan is performed.

Whatever the cause of the isodense extracerebral collection (IECC), its diagnosis is not simple, because the classic clue, a dense crescent adjacent to cortex, is absent. Matters are made even more difficult by two other factors. First, chronic SDHs may accumulate slowly under low pressure, but present as an apo-

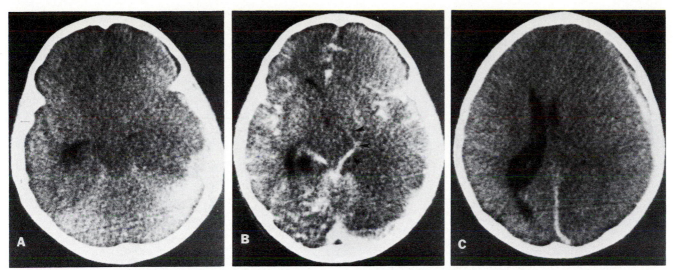

Fig 3–3.—SDH, severe brain edema, brain death. Three successive cuts from inferior to superior **(A, B, C)** demonstrate that the subarachnoid space is totally effaced from a combination of SDH and brain swelling. Note, however, that the brain density is essentially normal, indicating cerebral hyperperfusion secondary to loss of autoregulation, an ominous finding. *Arrowheads* **(B)** point to the severely deviated midbrain, indicating herniation of the left uncus and hippocampus.

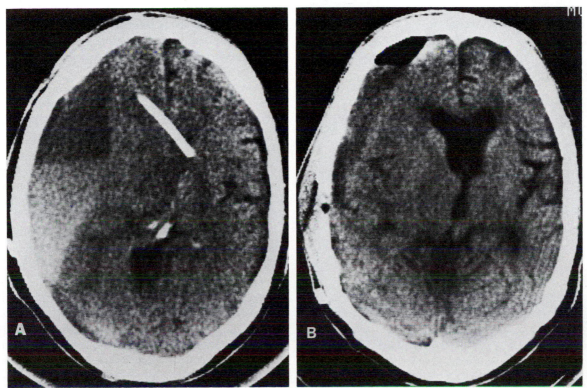

Fig 3–4.—SDH following decompressive shunting. **A,** the elderly patient has undergone rapid decompressive shunting for obstructive hydrocephalus, resulting in the formation of a large right SDH. Note the hematocrit level in the massive extracerebral collection, indicating acute bleeding; red blood cells are hemolyzed early. **B,** nine days later, after surgical removal of more than half of the collection, the lateral and third ventricles have begun to return to their full dilated proportion. Now the extracerebral collection is both smaller and less dense; no hematocrit is present.

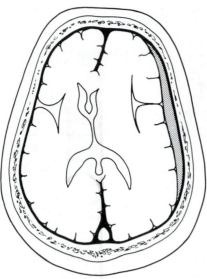 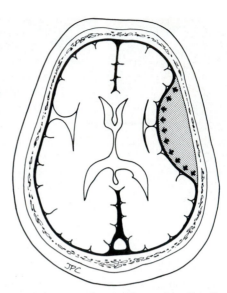

Fig 3–5.—Subdural and epidural hematomas. In the *left* illustration, a subdural collection *(shaded)*, finding no natural boundaries to prevent its spread, interposes itself widely between the brain and dura. Although it appears smaller than the epidural collection (*right* figure, *shaded* part), it would be present on many more sections and therefore oc-cupy a larger volume. The epidural collection, on the other hand, is formed by stripping dura from the skull. *Arrows* show the direction of the force exerted on the dura by the expanding hematoma. It therefore is much more confined than is a subdural collection.

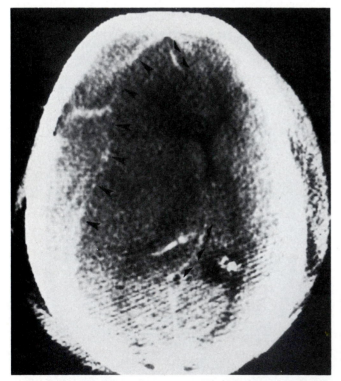

Fig 3–6.—Virtually isodense acute SDH. This patient's hematocrit was 19 as a result of her extensive liver disease. While awaiting a liver transplant, she fell, striking her head. This premortem CT scan shows a huge, mostly isodense SDH *(large arrowheads)*. It is certain that this was an acute event, because a scan done 2 days earlier as a baseline study was normal. *Small arrowheads* point to the deviated falx both anteriorly and posteriorly.

plectic event at a time distant from the insult. Thus, the history may be misleading. A unilateral IECC may present purely as a hemispheric mass effect on the unenhanced scan. Contrast enhancement fails to opacify an intracerebral mass, but it identifies the subdural membrane.

Second, chronic SDHs frequently are bilateral, so a midline shift can be absent in the face of large, approximately equal collections. Some clues *do* help to make the diagnosis of bilateral IECC. First, a brain that looks "too good" for patient's age or social history, e.g., alcoholics, should cause suspicion of an IECC (Fig 3–7). One should be very wary of a CT scan on, for example, a 70-year-old patient whose ventricles and sulci look like those of a healthy 20-year-old. Secondly, the liberal use of contrast material will often be definitive. It may demonstrate the subdural "membranes" separating the IECC from the brain. The membrane is not always present, but when it is, visualization can be diagnostic. What is considered to be the so-called subdural membrane can actually be cortical veins (Figs 3–8, 3–9, and 3–10).* In addition, normal gray matter enhances immediately (within one circulation time), while an IECC has no immediate change in density at all. Thus, the separation of enhanced cerebral cortex from the inner table of the skull can be demonstrated. Finally, a delayed enhanced scan may show a slow increase in den-

---

*We consider this to be exactly analogous to a recently reported sign of left lower lobe atelectasis by Lacombe P. and associates.[16]

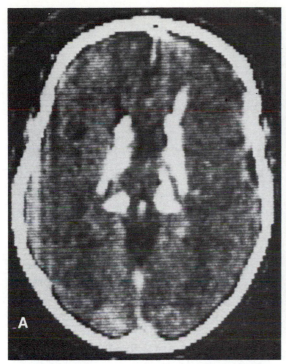
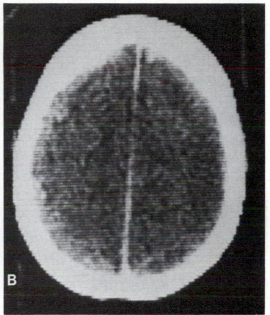

Fig 3–7.—Large bilateral isodense SDH. The ventricular system **(A)** and cortical sulci **(B)** look much too small for this 72-year-old alcoholic man. Idiopathic calcification of basal ganglia is present. At angiography, bilateral 4- to 5-cm thick lentiform extracerebral collections were present (not shown). After evacuation, ventricles and subarachnoid space resumed their anticipated generous size.

sity of the IECC.[17] Exactly analogous to visualization of SDHs by radionuclide scanning, there is leakage of contrast material into the collection from vessels lacking the equivalent of a normal blood-brain barrier. In fact, at 6 hours the SDH: blood iodine ratio is 20:1. For this reason, scanning at 4 to 6 hours after contrast injection may show an extracerebral collection that was isodense initially but became dense after time.

Statistical analyses have shown that the numerical properties of an IECC are different from those of normal brain.[18–20] Using a ranking technique, it has been possible to identify otherwise invisible occurrences of IECC. While a detailed discussion of the ranking algorithm is not possible in this work, its implementation is, in principle, not difficult, nor would one expect the calculations to be particularly time consuming.

Subdural "hygroma" is a very flexibly used term, perhaps only applied correctly to a subdural CSF collection resulting from an arachnoid tear.[21] It can produce the same diffuse mass effect as an SDH, but is lucent acutely, while a classic acute SDH is dense. Confusion arises when attempting to differentiate an old, lucent SDH from a hygroma. While the SDH is still more proteinaceous than CSF, it may appear to be as lucent, and differentiation may not be possible (see Fig 3–8).

EPIDURAL HEMATOMA

Epidural hematoma (EH) is an extracerebral blood collection that usually results from traumatic disruption of a meningeal artery with bleeding between the dura and the skull.[22] Classically, an EH is seen in patients whose trauma has resulted in a fracture, usually crossing the groove for the middle meningeal artery. Because the dura is firmly adherent to the inner table, the epidural space is not a potential space in the same sense as is the subdural space. Forming an SDH only requires a source of blood under minimal pressure. On the other hand, to form an EH, the dura must be stripped from the inner table, usually at increased pressure. This requires some time to accumulate, resulting in a latent period that precedes the decline in neurologic status.

A second proposed mechanism holds that the traumatic event flexes the skull and thus strips dural attachments, instantaneously providing a potential space.[23, 24] We believe this to be unlikely, because depressed skull fractures—the injuries with maximum flexion of the skull—rarely are associated with EH.

The shape of an EH reflects the stripping mechanism. As shown in Figures 3–2 and 3–5, forces directed medially against the dura cause the medial border of

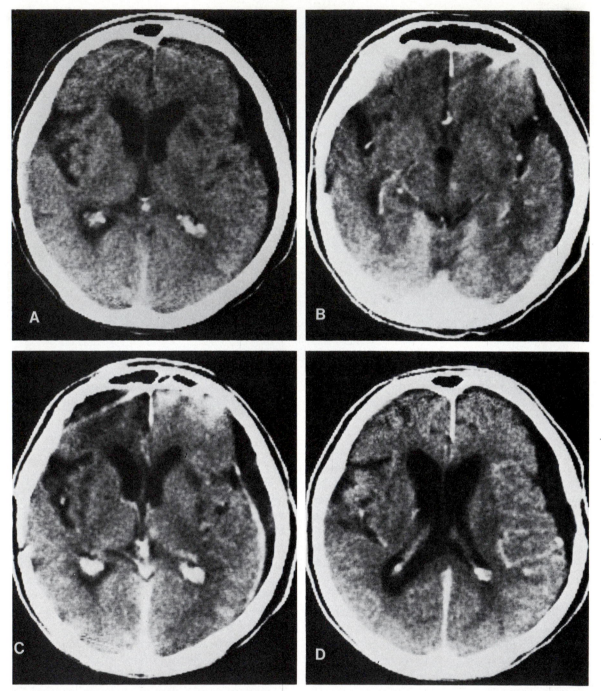

Fig 3–8.—Chronic SDH vs. hygroma: plain **(A)** and contrast enhanced **(B–D)** CT images. A lucent crescentic collection overlies the left hemisphere **(A).** While the enhanced CT image corresponding to the unenhanced one suggests a "membrane" **(C),** the sections immediately above **(D)** and below **(B)** that level fail to show it. The "membrane" is a vein, probably that of Labbé.

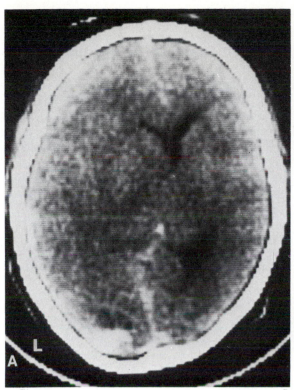
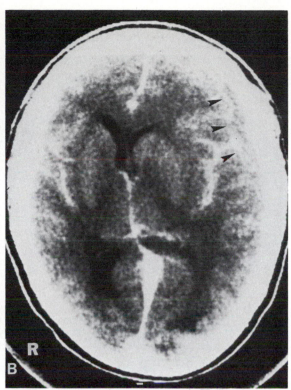

Fig 3–9.—Rare acute isodense SDH. Unenhanced and enhanced images from different scanners on the same day. Image **A** (patient's left *(L)* is on reader's left) shows left-sided mass effect with midline shift to right. Enhanced image **B** (patient's left is on reader's right; patient's right = *R*) shows separation of brain surface as located by cortical veins *(arrowheads)* from inner table. Patient had a hematocrit of 22%.

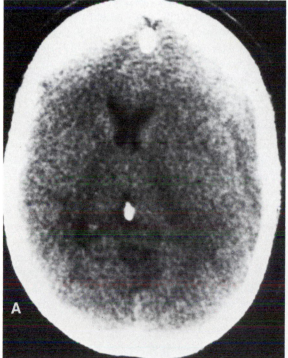
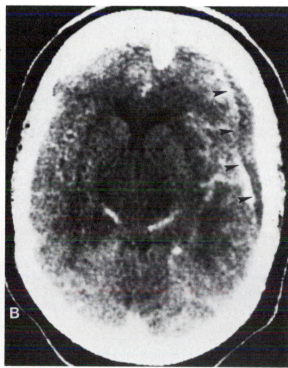

Fig 3–10.—Isodense SDH. A subtle mass effect shifts the frontal horns to the left and compresses the left trigone **(A)**. Contrast administration **(B)** opacifies vessels on the surface of the brain *(arrowheads)*, which is separated from the inner table by the isodense SDH. This has previously been considered to represent a subdural "membrane," but this is not always so.

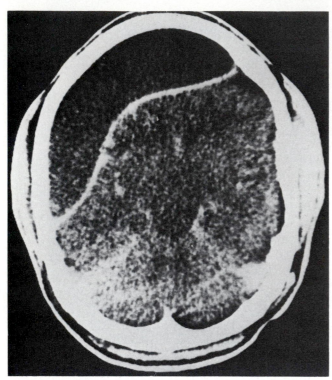

Fig 3–11.—Very old EH. The patient was examined for other reasons (headaches). A head injury in the distant past was noted. CT examination reveals a large lucent extracerebral collection that *crosses the midline* anteriorly. An epidural collection may cross the midline, while a subdural mass is stopped by the falx.

the hematoma to be convex to the brain. Forces directed at the edge of the collection increase its size by stripping more dura.

Unlike SDH, which spreads quickly through the unrestrained potential subdural space, EH tends to remain localized. It usually *appears* to be larger than an SDH, but in most cases is probably just the opposite.

Rarely, a venous EH can result from a tear of the venous sinus adjacent to the inner table of the skull. These take longer (days) to collect.[25] Delayed arterial EH has also been reported.[26]

The CT appearance of EH is predictable. The collections have a biconvex appearance and are acutely dense unless the patient is severely anemic. Because they are *epi*dural, they can cross the points of attachment of the falx and tentorium (Fig 3–11). Most are formed from trauma to the middle meningeal artery and are therefore over the temporal and posterior frontal lobes.

Rarely, an EH or even SDH may arise along an orbital roof or other horizontal structure. When this occurs, axial sections may convey the appearance of an irregularly mottled brain with contusional hemorrhage. Coronal or sagittal images will resolve the issue.[27]

If an EH is not enlarging, is not life-threatening, and is not producing neurologic deficit, it might be treated conservatively. Our unpublished experience with these cases shows that in some cases absorption can occur over time, but not until after the epidural collection has become isodense with the brain. Because the collection does become more lucent, contrast enhanced scans are necessary for follow-up. The shape of a conservatively managed EH gradually changes from biconvex to crescentic prior to complete absorption, secondary to reexpansion of the underlying brain.

INTRAPARENCHYMAL HEMORRHAGE

Several distinct mechanisms can be responsible for traumatic hemorrhage into the brain. The best known mechanism is the coup-contrecoup injury (Fig 3–12), in which the moving skull comes to an abrupt stop, but the enclosed brain continues to move for another moment. The brain then comes to an equally abrupt stop against the inner table. That part of the brain located 180° away from the impact site is cavitated from being pulled suddenly from its dura, but on recoil is caused to strike it with great force. Injury to the brain at the primary impact site is referred to as the coup injury, that on the opposite side as the contrecoup. Both can result in hemorrhage, but contrecoup is more frequent (Figs 3–13, 3–14, and 3–15).

Shearing forces, which result from asymmetric pressure to the brain, are exerted on the white matter and deep gray matter.[28] Such shearing injuries result in local hemorrhage in both white and deep gray matter, most commonly at the subcortical gray-white interface (Fig 3–16) and in the corpus callosum.

Again, CT appearances can be explained logically from the causal mechanisms. If a local skull fracture is present, it is reasonable to assume an underlying coup injury, hemorrhagic or not. Remembering that contrecoup hematoma is a likelihood, the side opposite to the coup may show one or more hematomas. Acutely, these parenchymal hemorrhages tend to be round, discrete, well-marginated areas of increased density (see Fig 3–16). Local mass effect is usually present from the hemorrhage itself as well as accompanying edema. As in SDH, changes in cerebral blood flow may play a role in swelling.

Birth offers still another mechanism of injury. Perinatal cerebellar hematomas are not uncommon (see Fig 3–16).[29, 30] Their formation has been attributed to extreme flexion of the occipital bone about its midline suture—the "occipital hinge." Forceps are not required to produce them, but they are more common in assisted deliveries. One could argue that because forceps would be used only to facilitate an other-

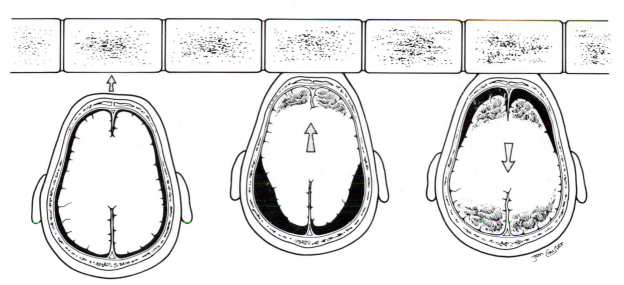

Fig 3–12.—Coup-contrecoup injury mechanism. The figure on the *left* represents the normal brain before the head strikes a solid object. The figure in the *middle* demonstrates the primary or coup injury, that on the *right* the secondary or contrecoup. See text for explanation.

wise difficult delivery, the hematomas might have occurred in any case from the skull traversing a small birth canal.

In a contused (bruised) brain, hemorrhage is a result of the coup-contrecoup forces previously described. Rather than a focal hemorrhage, however, there is a mixture of petechial hemorrhage and swelling, resulting in an isodense-to-hyperdense appearance. Contrast enhancement may be dramatic (Fig 3–17). If present, it may conform to gyri if the injury is not massive, but may be more extensive or deeper if the injury is not focal, secondary to diffuse shearing forces. Enhance-

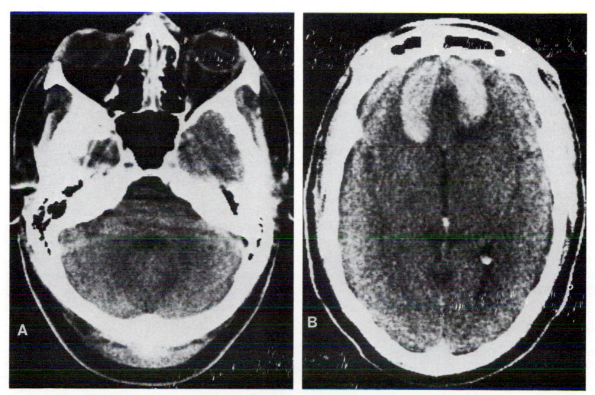

Fig 3–13.—Coup-contrecoup. Occipital scalp swelling **(A)** results from the coup injury, bifrontal polar hematomas from the contrecoup **(B).**

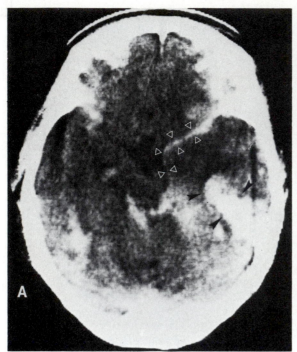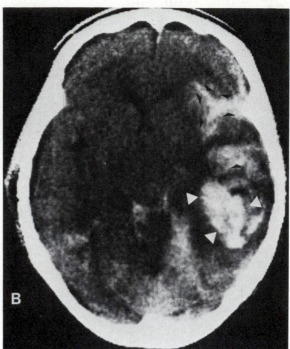

Fig 3–14.—The coup-contrecoup; scans at the levels of the suprasellar cisterns **(A)** and frontal horns **(B)**. The right scalp hematoma reflects the coup injury. Contralateral intracerebral **(A,** *black arrowheads;* **B,** *large white arrowheads*) and subarachnoid **(B,** *small black arrowheads*) hemorrhage results from the contrecoup. Blood in the subarachnoid space outlines the herniated medial temporal lobe surface **(A,** *open arrowheads*), indicating downward transtentorial herniation of the temporal lobe uncus.

ment results from a local loss of autoregulation of brain vasculature as well as incompetence of the blood-brain barrier.

Intracerebral hematomas need not be acute;[31–35] multiple petechial hemorrhages may coalesce to form a rapidly enlarging ecchymosis. This may be associated with an acute or subacute deterioration in the patient's status. Follow-up scanning is indispensable. Over time, intraparenchymal hemorrhage undergoes liquefaction, as does SDH. Pathologically, the loculated hematoma is dark in color, resembling crankcase oil; ultimately, encephalomalacia results.

Whatever the cause—extracerebral hematoma, intraparenchymal hemorrhage, edema, primary brain swelling from increase in blood volume, or a combination of these—displaced brain can cause herniation[36, 37] and secondary vessel compromise. This in turn can lead ultimately to infarction.

INTRAVENTRICULAR HEMORRHAGE

Traumatic intraventricular hemorrhage can arise from one of two mechanisms. The most common is extension of traumatic intraparenchymal hemorrhage.[38] The ependymal surface does not offer a significant barrier to extension of bleeding. The second mechanism is shear-ing of subependymal veins.[28] This can occur in the same way that shearing injuries of white and deep gray matter result.

The CT appearance is straightforward. Dense blood is seen in one or more ventricles and usually conforms to the ventricles' shapes. If blood has entered the aqueduct of Sylvius, an obstructive hydrocephalus almost always follows. Finally, a fluid level is seen if the blood remains liquefied in the face of dilution by CSF.

Intraventricular hemorrhage, from whatever cause, usually produces a local obstructive hydrocephalus. If only lateral ventricular hemorrhage is present, a local lateral ventricular dilatation may occur, but this is rare. More common is blood in the third ventricle obstructing the aqueduct of Sylvius and causing dilatation of both lateral ventricles and the third ventricle. If not relieved, this can result in a rapid increase in intracranial pressure and ultimately in brain death. Acute ventricular lavage and decompressive shunting may produce dramatic improvement.

SKULL FRACTURE

Identifying skull fractures with routine radiography is made difficult by the fact that the skull is roughly spherical. Depressed fractures can be seen directly on

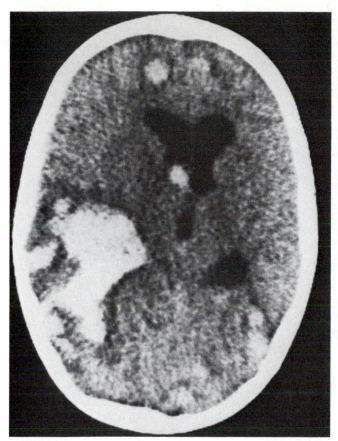

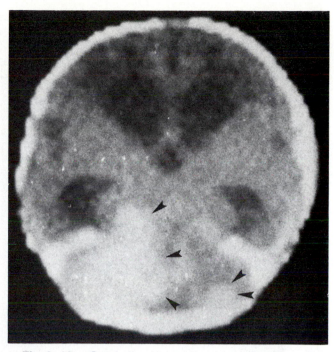

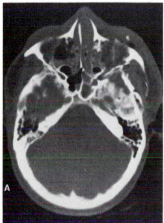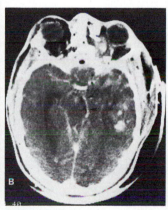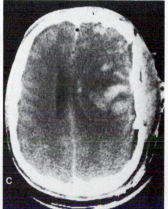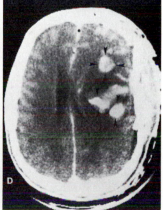

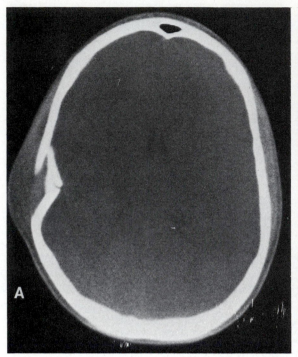

Fig 3–18.—Depressed skull fracture. At least two fragments are tented inward and are surrounded by a large scalp hematoma (**A,** bone window). Note the conspicuous *absence* of an SDH or EH (**B,** brain window). For reasons that are not yet entirely clear, depressed fractures are only rarely associated with hematomas.

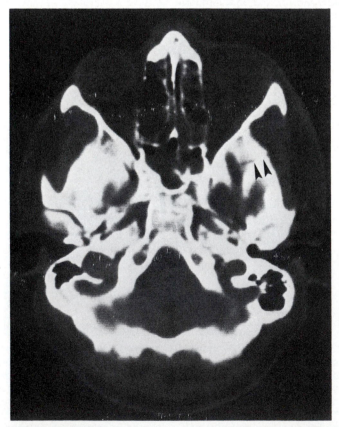

Fig 3–19.—Skull base fracture at floor of middle fossa. Basal fractures *(arrowheads)* are exceedingly difficult to show on routine skull films. Axial CT makes the task simple.

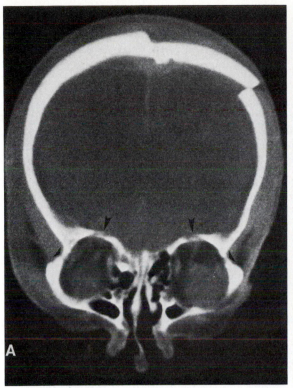
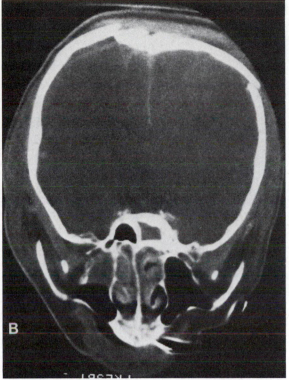

Fig 3–20.—Complex biparietal fracture; supine coronal views, top-bottom reversal. Fragments override and the vertex edges are depressed. This raised the question of patency of the superior sagittal sinus. Carotid angiography (not shown) demonstrated it to be patent. Also note bloody opaci-fication of the left sphenoid sinus and an air-blood level in the right maxillary antrum **(B)**. There are fractures of the orbital roofs (**A,** *large arrowheads*) and lateral orbital walls (**A,** *small arrowheads*).

plain films only if they are severe; slightly depressed fractures can be seen only by indirect signs. Immediate identification of fractures, sutural diastases, and depressed fragments are permitted by CT (Figs 3–18 to 3–20).[15, 35, 39] Visualization requires the use of a "bone window," namely a large window width (1,000 to 4,000) and high window levels (800 to 2,000).

Fractures can have long-term sequelae. Leaks of CSF through the ear (CSF otorrhea) and nose (CSF rhinorrhea) result from the combination of arachnoid tears and bony nonunions. Basilar-petrous skull fractures lead to CSF otorrhea, while fractures through the paranasal sinuses and/or cribriform plate are associated with rhinorrhea.

The CSF leak itself is unpleasant, but a more serious complication, meningitis, can occur if the rent does not spontaneously close or is not repaired. Identification of the leaking site hinges upon metrizamide cisternography. Multiple positions may be required to demonstrate leakage of the contrast through the fracture site into a paranasal sinus (Fig 3–21).

If a fracture crosses or overlies a dural sinus, then hemorrhage from a torn sinus (epidural or subdural) or thrombosis of that sinus must be considered a possibil-

ity. Angiography is then required to confirm or exclude sinus patency (see Fig 3–20).

Penetrating injuries of the calvaria usually result from projectiles, but occasionally from sharp objects, e.g., knives. Immediate damage is done by the projectile itself, including bony fractures and laceration of brain, sometimes with hematoma formation. The offending agent is frequently lead and therefore exceedingly radiopaque (Fig 3–22). Unfortunately, "spray" artifact may completely obscure brain detail in the area.

Delayed sequelae consist of encephalomalacia and infection in and near the projectile's trajectory. Encephalomalacia results from failure of healing and repair of the injured brain. When the projectile enters the head, it carried with it pieces of skin, sebaceous material, and hair. These, not the bullet itself, are responsible for infection (Fig 3–23). Slower-moving penetrating objects like knives may contribute primarily to the infection.

Sometimes a fracture and associated dural tear fail to heal, but the underlying arachnoid tissue either remains intact or heals normally. Subject to constant repetitive CSF pulsations, the arachnoid pouch extends through the dural rent. This leptomeningeal cyst erodes the margins of the skull to produce a gaping calvarial

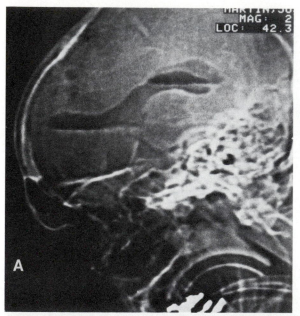

Fig 3–21.—Complex injury with extensive pneumocephalus. Pneumocephalus usually results from fracture through a sinus. Both lateral ventricles contain air, but one air-fluid level is fortuitously in line with an extracerebral gas collection (CT scoutview, **A**). Axial sections **(B, C)** show massive gas collections in the head, both within ventricles and subarachnoid spaces. At a later time, following placement of intrathecal metrizamide, there is immediate and extraordinarily *dense* opacification of the sphenoid sinus (**D**, *arrowheads*), the site of air entry.

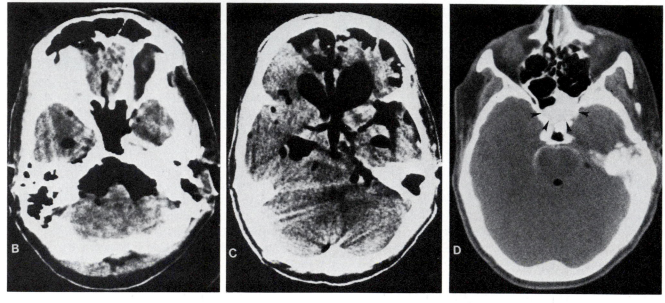

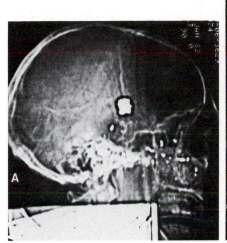

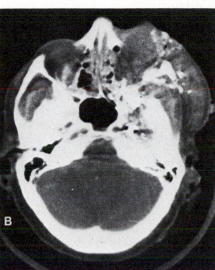

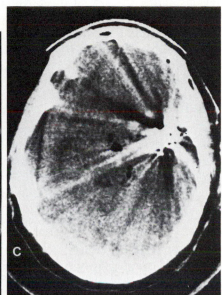

Fig 3–22.—Gunshot wound of head and face. The scout-view **(A)** demonstrates the main bullet fragment as well as numerous smaller ones in the head and face. Axial section through the lower orbits **(B)** shows disruption of the left bony orbit and globe with bullet fragments in the middle fossa. Ethmoidal hematoma results from fracture of the lamina papyracea. Photograph **C** shows the effect of the excessively radiodense bullet on the CT image. So much distortion and "spray" artifact is present that the image is severely degraded.

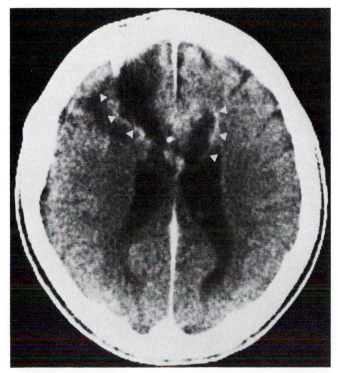

Fig 3–23.—Gunshot wound with ependymitis. Not the bullet, but the scalp, hair, and sebaceous debris carried into the head by the projectile causes infection. The injury was self-inflicted, fired into the front of the head. A week later, fever and an increased white blood cell count suggested infection. Contrast CT showed enhancement of the bullet track and anterior ependyma *(arrowheads.* CSF pleocytosis with positive culture confirmed infection.

defect and associated soft-tissue mass that communicates with the subarachnoid space.

END RESULTS

If trauma to the brain has been focal, localized encephalomalacia may result. This appears as a nonenhancing lucent area of brain, often accompanied by dilatation of sulci in the vicinity of the abnormality. Often there will be local dilatation of the ventricle nearest to the traumatic lesion. This can, in fact, be so pronounced as to result in a porencephalic extension of the ventricle. More diffuse trauma can result in generalized atrophy of one or both hemispheres, with enlargement of sulci and ventricles.

An extracerebral collection may result in chronic "hematoma fluid" (see Fig 3–11). Except for knowing the time course, distinguishing such a collection from a subdural hygroma by CT scans alone is impossible.

PEDIATRICS

Children are certainly no less prone to accidents than are adults. In fact, accidents are the main cause of death in children through 15 years of age.[40] The radiologic manifestation of injury to the skull and brain are the same as they are for adults. Children differ, however, in their vulnerability to serious sequelae from unusual and unexpected trauma. In this category are birth injuries[30] and the parent-infant trauma syndrome (PITS).[41–44]

Considering the size of the birth canal and the tension it exerts on the rather flexible head of the infant, it is remarkable that we see so few instances of birth trauma to the CNS. Nevertheless, the head is occasionally injured. Subdural, epidural, and intraparenchymal hematomas have been shown to occur and are more common in the posterior fossa.[45, 46] It has been suggested that this is related to a folding motion of the posterior synchondrosis at delivery. Most reported cases are *not* related to the use of obstetric forceps. Clinical manifestations include jaundice and signs of hypovolemia and intracranial mass. The CT findings are typical of those of hemorrhage in any age group.

REFERENCES

1. Bergstrom M., Ericson K., Levander B., et al.: Variation with time of the attenuation values of intracranial hematomas. *J. Comput. Assist. Tomogr.* 1:57–63, 1977.
2. Scotti G., Terbrugge K., Melancon D., et al.: Evaluation of the age of subdural hematomas by computerized tomography. *J. Neurosurg.* 47:311–315, 1977.
3. Kao M.-C.: Sedimentation level in chronic subdural hematoma visible on computerized tomography. *J. Neurosurg.* 58:246–251, 1983.
4. New P.J.F., Aronow S.: Attenuation measurements of whole blood and blood fractions in computed tomography. *Radiology* 121:635–640, 1976.
5. Bergstrom M., Ericson K., Levander B., et al.: Computed tomography of cranial subdural and epidural hematomas: Variation of attenuation related to time and clinical events such as rebleeding. *J. Comput. Assist. Tomogr.* 1:449–455, 1977.
6. Rieth K.G., Schwartz F.T., Davis D.O.: Acute isodense epidural hematoma on computed tomography. *J. Comput. Assist. Tomogr.* 3:691–693, 1979.
7. Slager U.T.: Mechanical trauma and the effects of space occupying lesions, in *Basic Neuropathology.* Baltimore, Williams & Wilkins Co., 1970, pp. 67–68.
8. Ingvar S., Ask-Upmark E.: Contribution to the knowledge of subdural hematomas. *Acta Med. Scand.* 94(fasc. I-II):225–240, 1938.
9. Masters F.J.: Evaluation of head trauma: Efficacy of skull films. *A.J.R.* 135:539–547, 1980.
10. Bell R.F., Loop J.W.: The utility and futility of radiographic skull examinations for trauma. *N. Engl. J. Med.* 284:236–239, 1974.
11. Cromwell L.D., Mack L.A., Loop J.W.: CT scoutview for skull fracture: Substitute for skull films? *A.J.N.R.* 3:421–423, 1982.
12. Cummins R.O.: Clinicians' reasons for overuse of skull radiographs. *A.J.R.* 135:549–552, 1980.
13. de Campo J., Petty P.G.: How useful is the skull x-ray examination in trauma? *Med. J. Aust.* 2:553–555, 1980.
14. Norman O.: Angiographic differentiation between acute and chronic subdural and extradural haematomas. *Acta Radiol.* 46:371–378, 1956.
15. French B.N., Dublin A.B.: The value of computerized tomography in the management of 1000 consecutive head injuries. *Surg. Neurol.* 7:171–183, 1977.
16. Lacombe P., Lallemand D., Garel L., et al.: Pulmonary vascular nodules: New sign of left lower lobe collapse in children. *A.J.R.* 139:873–878, 1982.
17. Messina A.V.: Computed tomography: Contrast media within subdural hematomas: A preliminary report. *Radiology* 119:725–726, 1976.
18. Reid M.H., Dublin A.B.: Statistical detection of nonvisible isodense subdural fluid collections. *J. Comput. Assist. Tomogr.* 3:491–496, 1979.
19. Snedecor G.W., Cochran W.G.: *Statistical Methods,* ed. 6. Ames, Iowa, Iowa State University Press, 1967, pp. 128–130.
20. Wilcoxon F.: Individual comparisons by ranking methods. *Biometrics Bulletin* 1:80–83, 1945.
21. Jaeckle K.A., Allen J.H.: Subdural hygroma: Diagnosis with computed tomography. *Comput. Tomogr.* 3:201–206, 1979.
22. Ford L.E., McLaurin R.L.: Mechanisms of extradural hematomas. *J. Neurosurg.* 20:760–769, 1963.
23. Jacobson W.H.A.: On middle meningeal haemorrhage. *Guy's Hosp. Rep.* 43:147–308, 1886.
24. Frank E., Berger T.S., Tew J.M.: Bilateral epidural hematomas. *Surg. Neurol.* 17:218–222, 1982.
25. Bullock R., Van Dellen J.R.: Chronic extradural hematoma. *Surg. Neurol.* 18:300–302, 1982.
26. Rappaport Z.H., Shaked I., Tadmor R.: Delayed epidural hematoma demonstrated by computed tomography: Case report. *Neurosurgery* 10:487–489, 1982.
27. Rieth K.G., Davis D.O.: Subdural hematomas: An unusual appearance on computed tomography. *J. Comput. Assist. Tomogr.* 3:331–334, 1979.
28. Zimmerman R.A., Bilaniuk L.T., Genneralli T.: Computed tomography of the cerebral white matter. *Radiology* 127:393–396, 1978.
29. Martin R., Roessmann U., Fanaroff A.: Massive intracerebellar hemorrhage in low-birth-weight infants. *J. Pediatr.* 89:290–293, 1976.
30. Takagi T., Fukuoka H., Wakabayashi S., et al.: Posterior fossa subdural hemorrhage in the newborn as a result of birth trauma. *Childs Brain* 9:102–113, 1982.
31. Diaz F.G., Yock D.H., Larson D., et al.: Early diagnosis of delayed posttraumatic intracerebral hematomas. *J. Neurosurg.* 50:217–223, 1979.
32. Kishore P.R.S., Lipper, M.H., Domingues da Silva, A.A., et al.: Delayed sequelae of head injury. *Comput. Tomogr.* 4:287–295, 1980.
33. Roberson F.C., Kishore P.R.S., Miller J.D., et al.: The value of serial computerized tomography in the management of severe head injury. *Surg. Neurol.* 12:161–167, 1979.
34. Koo A.H., LaRoque R.L.: Evaluation of head trauma by computed tomography. *Radiology* 123:345–350, 1977.
35. Dublin A.B., French B.N., Rennick J.M.: Computed tomography in head trauma. *Radiology* 122:365–369, 1977.
36. Osborn A.G.: Diagnosis of descending transtentorial herniation by cranial computed tomography. *Radiology* 123:93–96, 1977.

37. Stovring J.: Contralateral temporal horn widening in unilateral supratentorial mass lesions: A diagnostic sign indicating tentorial herniation. *J. Comput. Assist. Tomogr.* 1:319–323, 1977.

38. Cordobes F., de la Fuenta M., Lobato R.D., et al.: Intraventricular hemorrhage in severe head injury. *J. Neurosurg.* 58:217–222, 1983.

39. Claussen C.D., Lohkamp F.W., Krastel A.: Computed tomography of trauma involving brain and facial skull (craniofacial injuries). *J. Comput. Assist. Tomogr.* 1:472–481, 1977.

40. Nelson W.E.: *Textbook of Pediatrics,* ed. 9. Philadelphia, W.B. Saunders Co., 1969, pp. 1–13.

41. Caffey J.: On the theory and practice of shaking infants. *Am. J. Dis. Child.* 124:161–169, 1972.

42. Caffey J.: The whiplash shaken infant syndrome: Manual shaking by the extremities with whiplash-induced intracranial and intraocular bleedings, linked with residual permanent brain damage and mental retardation. *Pediatrics* 54:396–403, 1974.

43. Tsai F.Y., Zee C.-S., Apthorp J.S., et al.: Computed tomography in child abuse head trauma. *Comput. Tomogr.* 4:277–286, 1980.

44. Ellison P.H., Tsai F.Y., Largent J.A.: Computed tomography in child abuse and cerebral contusion. *Pediatrics* 62:151–154, 1978.

45. Grunnet M.L., Shields W.D.: Cerebellar hemorrhage in the premature infant. *J. Pediatr.* 88:605–608, 1976.

46. Ravenel S.D.: Posterior fossa hemorrhage in the term newborn: Report of two cases. *Pediatrics* 64:39–42, 1979.

4

Nontraumatic Hemorrhage

JOSEPH A. HORTON, M.D.

ANEURYSMS

Most cerebral aneurysms result from a congenital defect in the arterial wall and are therefore referred to as congenital aneurysms.[1] This does not mean that the aneurysm is present at birth, only the abnormality of the arterial wall. Aneurysms presumably form as a result of pulsations on the defective arterial wall.[2] Most such aneurysms arise at or near the circle of Willis, the most common sites of origin being the anterior communicating artery (Figs 4–1 and 4–2), posterior communicating artery, and the middle cerebral artery trifurcation (Figs 4–3 to 4–5). Other common sites include the basilar apex (Figs 4–6 and 4–7), the intracavernous carotid artery (these are usually considered to be atherosclerotic rather than congenital), the carotid bifurcation, the supraclinoid internal carotid artery, and rarely at or along the course of the posterior inferior cerebellar artery (Fig 4–8). Aneurysms can occur almost anywhere, but these represent the vast bulk of the congenital ones. Noteworthy is the fact that if a patient has one aneurysm, he has about a 20% to 25% likelihood of having more than one (Fig 4–9).[1–3]

Congenital aneurysms are sometimes familial. Fox and Ko[4] have reported a family in which numerous siblings have harbored them. Those who were examined, even though asymptomatic, usually showed aneurysms. I have personally observed aneurysms in the same segment of the anterior cerebral artery on the same side in identical twin sisters, both of whom had subarachnoid hemorrhages. Mirror-image aneurysms are frequent, especially those near the midline, e.g., at the ophthalmic artery origins (Fig 4–10), and those involving the middle cerebral trifurcations.

Skull-base aneurysms may result from other etiologies, such as the abnormally high-flow states that one sees in vessels supplying arteriovenous malformations (AVM). Twenty-five percent of patients with an AVM have one or more aneurysms on the feeding vessel(s).[5]

Septic emboli can erode through an arterial wall, weaken it, and give rise to mycotic aneurysms.[6, 7] Patients especially prone to this are those with subacute bacterial endocarditis, those with extra- and intracardiac right-to-left shunts (thus missing the filtering effect of the pulmonary vascular bed), and intravenous drug abusers.[8] These aneurysms tend to be peripheral in location.

Other causes of peripheral aneurysms include tumor embolus, moyamoya syndrome, and trauma.[7, 9–11] In penetrating injuries, the mechanism of arterial trauma is obvious. In closed head injuries, the artery is assumed to be injured by massive brain motion in a manner not unlike that of shearing white matter injuries (see Chapter 3).

Most patients' aneurysms are discovered after a subarachnoid hemorrhage. They present with a severe headache, often focal, but the location is not diagnostic or informative of the location of the aneurysm. Loss of consciousness, localizing neurologic deficit, meningismus, and photophobia are also prominent features. A lumbar puncture reveals bloody CSF if it is performed acutely.

Occasionally, an aneurysm will present as a primary mass lesion.[12–16] A strategically located aneurysm may compress one or more cranial nerves, especially if it is within the cavernous sinus or adjacent to the brain stem. Giant or "tumorous" aneurysms may attain enormous size and even occupy a significant portion of, for example, the middle fossa, producing symptoms and signs of temporal lobe compression (Fig 4–11). These large aneurysms often have partially calcified walls and contain variable amounts of thrombus; occasionally, they are nearly or completely thrombosed. In most series,[12] giant aneurysms are considered to be safe lesions, i.e., unlikely to bleed, but one series[13] describes 13 patients with giant aneurysms, of whom 70% presented with subarachnoid hemorrhage.

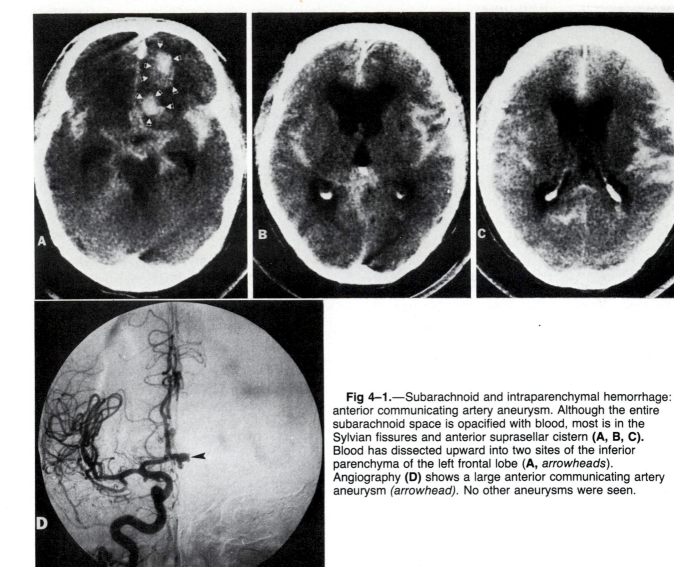

Fig 4–1.—Subarachnoid and intraparenchymal hemorrhage: anterior communicating artery aneurysm. Although the entire subarachnoid space is opacified with blood, most is in the Sylvian fissures and anterior suprasellar cistern **(A, B, C)**. Blood has dissected upward into two sites of the inferior parenchyma of the left frontal lobe **(A,** *arrowheads*). Angiography **(D)** shows a large anterior communicating artery aneurysm *(arrowhead)*. No other aneurysms were seen.

Transient ischemic attacks are an even rarer presenting complaint for patients with aneurysms[17] and seem to result from embolization of intra-aneurysmal thrombus.

CT Appearances

The Aneurysm

Small aneurysms are usually unresolvable on routine CT scans, because their size is similar to that of the parent vessel. Thus, an aneurysm and an artery in cross section appear identical. It has been suggested that aneurysms smaller than 2 cm are unreliably seen on CT.[18] Larger aneurysms, on the other hand, can often be visualized if they are sufficiently prominent and/or well separated from the skull base. Closely spaced thin sections and reformatted images may help in identifi-

cation of an aneurysm. While CT has not been traditionally used as the primary modality in the search for a bleeding source, 14 of 85 patients in one series had their aneurysms first diagnosed by CT.[19]

"Giant" aneurysms are readily seen, but can easily be confused with other types of mass lesions, especially neoplasms (see Figs 4–3, 4–5, 4–6, 4–8, 4–10, and 4–11). The clinical presentation depends upon the size and location. Calcium may outline none, part, or all of the wall,[20] and edema is rarely present.[21] Likewise, variable amounts of clot may fill the aneurysm.[17] This makes CT highly valuable in the preoperative work-up of an aneurysm patient. While angiography is very specific at identifying an aneurysm, it is only the lumen of the aneurysm that is shown. A partly thrombosed, broad-necked giant aneurysm may have the angio-

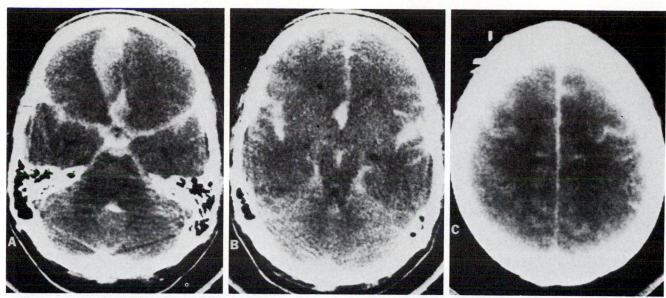

Fig 4–2.—Massive subarachnoid hemorrhage. A dramatic blood cisternogram (unenhanced scans **A, B,** and **C**) delineates the basal subarachnoid spaces. Most of the blood lies in the anterior interhemispheric fissure and within the parenchyma of the right frontal lobe, although extension into the ventricular system is shown by the presence of blood within the third **(B)** and fourth **(A)** ventricles. The patient did not survive to have an angiogram, but the picture is classic for rupture of an anterior communicating artery aneurysm.

graphic appearance of a small aneurysm with a distinct neck that is easily clippable. In such a case, CT more accurately defines the size of the lesion and therefore the probable neck size.

If an aneurysm is clotted entirely or in part, contrast enhancement is valuable. A mural thrombus may give the CT appearance of a crescentic zone of nonenhancement, while an almost completely thrombosed aneurysm may give a "target" or "bull's-eye" appearance, with the enhancing center of the "target" representing the persisting lumen. Occasionally, only the wall of a thrombosed aneurysm will enhance; surgical and pathologic observations suggest that this enhancement occurs because of the presence of vaso vasora in the wall of the aneurysm.

Because the static CT image of a giant aneurysm may resemble that of a tumor, diagnosis may be difficult. Rapid dynamic scanning during and immediately after injection can, in some cases, differentiate aneurysm from neoplasm. Time-density curves show a rapid opacification of the aneurysm with one of two washout patterns. If the aneurysm is higher than the supplying vessel, washout is rapid. On the other hand, if the aneurysm is in a dependent position, washout is slow, but a blood-contrast level may be present.

Subarachnoid Hemorrhage

ACUTE STAGE.—Once a subarachnoid hemorrhage occurs, the CT scan is usually abnormal.[22–24] Local he-

matoma and/or more generalized blood in the basal cisterns can be seen (see Figs 4–1, 4–2, 4–4, and 4–7). If the hematoma is localized, it may help localize the aneurysm.[25–27] For example, a clot confined to a Sylvian fissure suggests a middle cerebral artery aneurysm, especially if cisternal blood is absent. On the other hand, upward dissection of such a hematoma into the basal ganglia coupled with cisternal blood favors a posterior communicating artery location.

Localization based upon site of hematoma is not infallible, but can be of assistance in at least two ways. First, it directs angiography. The seriously ill patient who has had a subarachnoid hemorrhage is likely to have arterial spasm that may produce infarction. Each arterial injection may lead to further arterial irritability. Therefore, in the ill patient, CT localization of the probable aneurysm can lead to studying this vessel first (see Fig 4–4). If severe spasm is present and if an aneurysm is seen, the examination might be discontinued with the knowledge that the bleeding source has probably been found. Further angiographic work-up may await resolution of the arterial spasm.

The second advantage to the angiographer is the fact that a hematoma tends to surround or abut the aneurysm that bled; if several aneurysms are present, the one in or nearest to the hematoma is more likely the bleeder. Confronted angiographically with a large aneurysm and a small one, the large one is probably the one that bled, but if CT shows that the small one is within

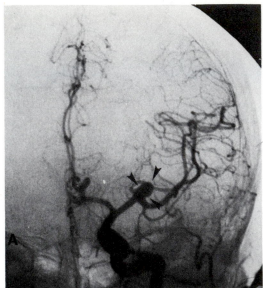

Fig 4–3.—Giant aneurysms: target sign. The angiogram in image **A** suggests that this middle cerebral artery aneurysm *(arrowheads)* is only about 1 cm in greatest diameter. **B, C,** the corresponding CT scan shows that, in reality, it is at least twice that size. The persistent lumen collects contrast material (**C,** *arrowheads*), and is surrounded by thrombus. The wall of the aneurysm enhances **(B),** secondary to vasa vasorum in the adventitia. In a second patient, a large, partially calcified giant aneurysm is clearly visible on the CT image **(D).** A target sign was present after constant enhancement (not shown). **E,** the smaller unclotted lumen of the aneurysm is seen at angiography. There is marked elevation of the A-1 segment of the right anterior cerebral artery, a reflection of the actual size of the aneurysm. Without CT, this would probably be interpreted as a subfrontal mass, such as a large hematoma, or a mass unrelated to the aneurysm.

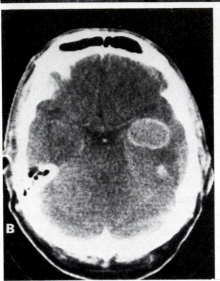

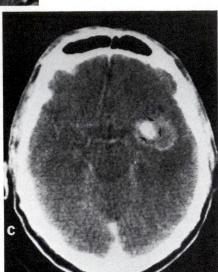

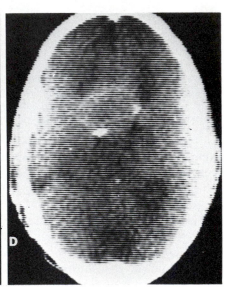

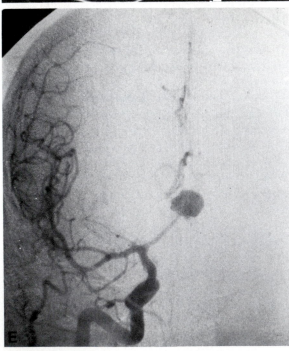

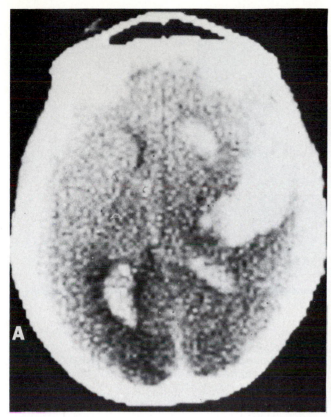

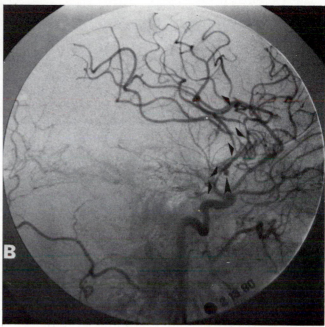

Fig 4–4.—Subarachnoid hemorrhage, middle cerebral artery trifurcation aneurysm. Acute hemorrhage opacifies the left Sylvian fissure and extends into the lateral ventricles **(A).** Anterior-superior displacement of the left trigone is present, indicating a large temporal mass effect. Left inter-nal carotid arteriogram, Haughton view **(B),** discloses the small middle cerebral artery aneurysm *(large arrowhead).* Note the marked spasm of the supraclinoid carotid artery as well as that of several middle cerebral arterial branches *(small arrowheads)* and the temporal lobe mass.

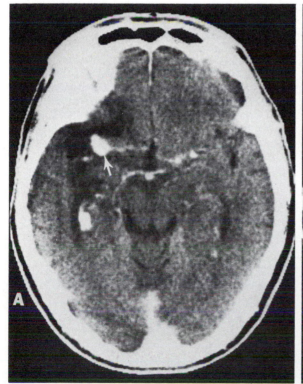

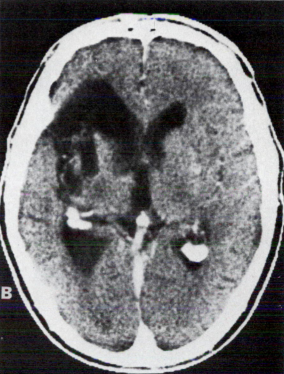

Fig 4–5.—Aneurysm with local infarction. Although this patient has never had a craniotomy or even angiography, it is possible to reconstruct the likely sequence of events leading to this CT appearance. A large right middle cerebral artery aneurysm **(A,** *arrow*) bled, producing both a local hematoma and considerable vasospasm. The spasm pro-duced an ischemic insult to the right temporal and frontal lobes while the local mass effect compromised the ipsilateral basal ganglia. This resulted in a persistent aneurysm, an enlarged Sylvian fissure, focal encephalomalacia, and local hydrocephalus *ex vacuo* producing dilatation of the frontal horn and trigone **(B).**

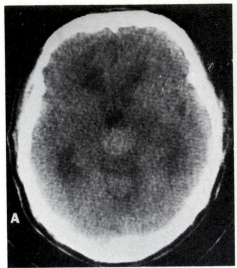

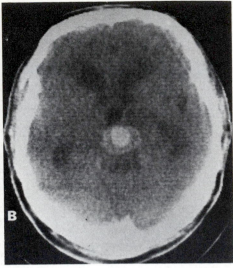

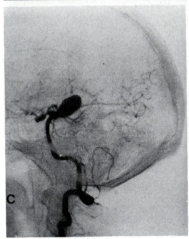

Fig 4–6.—Giant basilar apex aneurysm: target sign. This pair of studies illustrates the complementary values of CT scanning and angiography in the evaluation of large aneurysms. Angiography **(C)** shows the large basilar apex aneurysm, but CT **(A** and **B)** shows that only the central half of the lumen (linear measurement, therefore *one eighth the volume*) is opacified by contrast material. The angiogram underestimates the size of the aneurysm and can lull the unsuspecting neurosurgeon into believing that a readily approachable neck is present when, in fact, one is not. A large amount of mural thrombus within the aneurysm prevents complete opacification of the aneurysm at angiography, but the thrombus is dense enough to be resolved by CT. Compare the unenhanced **(A)** and enhanced **(B)** CT images to see opacification of the wall of the aneurysm; this is thought to occur through vasa vasora.

Fig 4–7.—Basilar artery aneurysm with mural thrombus. Gross subarachnoid hemorrhage has extended into the ventricular system and opacified both occipital horns **(A).** The aneurysm itself is easily seen on the unenhanced CT scan **(A,** midline density). Contrast administration **(B)** further opacifies the nonthrombosed part of the aneurysmal lumen; what does *not* enhance **(B,** between *arrowheads*) is clot.

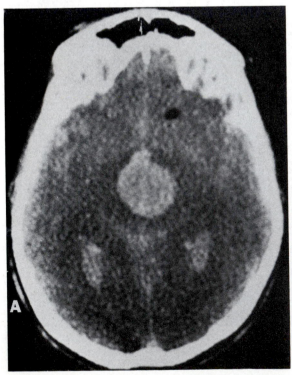

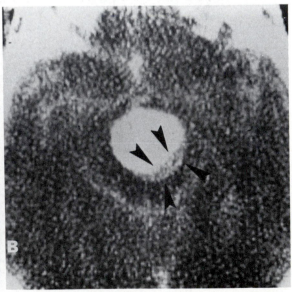

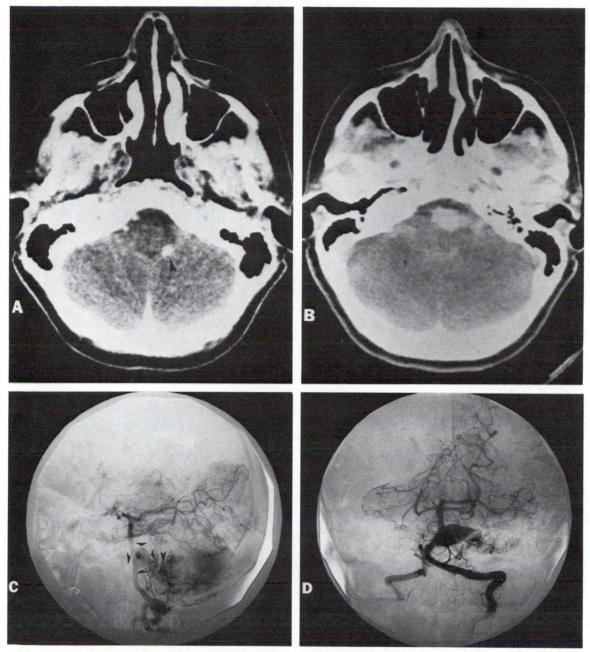

Fig 4–8.—Two posterior fossa aneurysms. The CT is somewhat confusing in that it is not readily apparent whether the smaller posterior density on the lower cut **(A,** *arrowhead)* is a part of or separate from the larger midline density on the higher cut **(B).** Angiography **(C** and **D)** shows a very large saccular aneurysm **(C,** *small arrowheads*) of the basilar artery, and a smaller posterior inferior cerebellar artery (PICA) aneurysm **(C,** *large arrowheads*). Thus, the smaller posterior CT density was the PICA aneurysm.

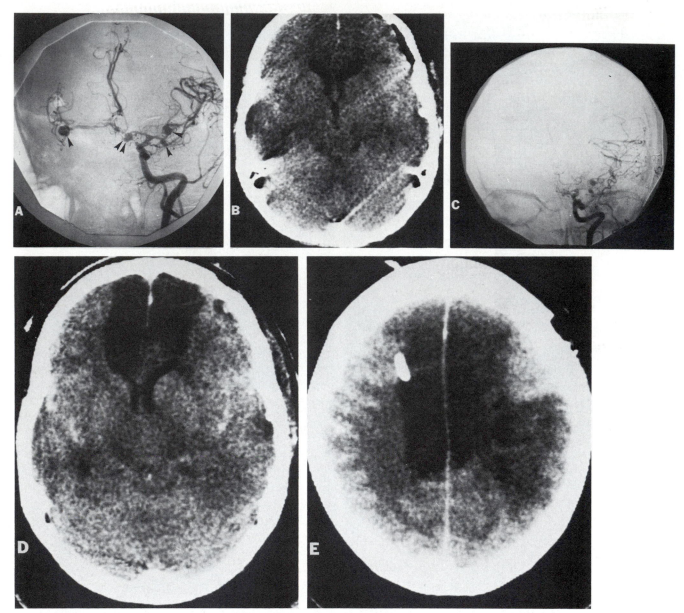

Fig 4–9.—Multiple aneurysms, infarction from vaso-spasm. **A,** angiography shows multiple aneurysms *(arrowheads)* and considerable spasm of the proximal anterior cerebral arteries. *Double arrowheads* point to the anterior communicating artery aneurysm, considered to have been the bleeder on clinical grounds as well as radiographic ones: vasospasm in its vicinity suggests the presence of blood. **B,** a CT scan done at approximately the same time suggests vague midline bifrontal lucencies (ischemia/infarc-tion). **C,** several days later, after clipping the anterior communicating artery aneurysm, the arterial spasm is extreme with no cross-filling and almost complete absence of opacification of the ipsilateral anterior cerebral artery. **D, E,** the classic "Mohican" appearance on CT confirms bilateral anterior cerebral distribution infarction. Note the interim development of mass effect with compression of the frontal horns.

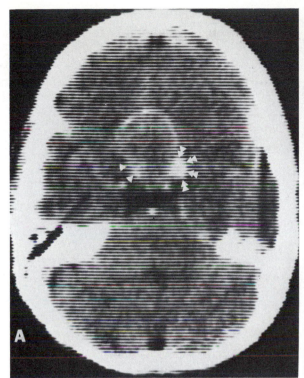

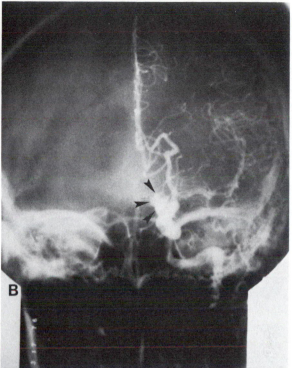

Fig 4–10.—Mirror image internal carotid artery aneurysms. Both CT **(A)** and angiography showed bilateral internal carotid artery aneurysms *(arrowheads),* but only one is a partially thrombosed giant aneurysm. Which one? The AP view of the left internal carotid artery injection **(B)** mirrors the right injection: both showed an aneurysm **(B,** *arrowheads),* but neither offered a clue as to which was the giant. On CT, it is evident that the opacifying aneurysmal lumen on the right **(A,** *single arrowhead)* is within the giant mass, but the left is outside. The density inside of the giant aneurysm is therefore its small unclotted lumen. Surgery confirmed a giant aneurysm on the right and a small aneurysm on the left. (From Latchaw R.E., Gold L.H.A., Tourje E.J.: Computerized tomography of intracranial tumors. *Minn. Med.* 60:554–559, 1977. Used by permission.

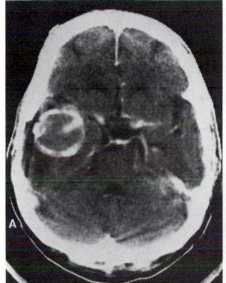

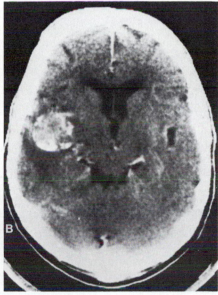

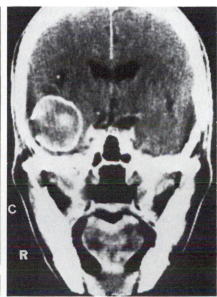

Fig 4–11.—Giant "tumoral" aneurysm. Temporal lobe seizures brought this patient to medical attention. Enhanced CT **(A, B, C)** showed a giant aneurysm with enhancement of a heavily calcified wall. The aneurysm was totally filled with clot, without a definite enhancing nodule to suggest a persisting lumen. The angiogram showed only an avascular mass in the right middle fossa. We presume that opacification of the aneurysm wall was by way of vasa vasora. These aneurysms are chronic and at low risk for hemorrhage. (R = patient's right.)

the hematoma while the large one is remote, the odds are reversed.

Hemorrhage from a ruptured aneurysm need not remain in the subarachnoid space. The hematoma, especially if loculated, can dissect into brain parenchyma (see Figs 4–1 and 4–4), the ventricular system (see Figs 4–4 and 4–7), or even the subdural space.[27] Anterior communicating artery aneurysms form anterior clots that, under pressure of continued arterial bleeding, can rupture the lamina terminalis and thereby gain entrance to the third ventricle. Blood from posterior communicating and middle cerebral artery aneurysms enter the choroidal fissure to reach the temporal horn. A basilar apex aneurysm may bleed through the floor of the posterior third ventricle. If blood has entered the ventricular system, the likelihood of an obstructive hydrocephalus is high: even a small clot may occlude the tiny aqueduct of Sylvius.

Free blood in the subarachnoid space causes a convexity block to normal flow and absorption of CSF, resulting in communicating hydrocephalus, which is more commonly encountered than obstructive hydrocephalus. Blood in the subdural space is usually a result of rupture of internal carotid bifurcation and middle cerebral artery trifurcation aneurysms (Fig 4–12).[28]

SUBACUTE STAGE.—Several changes characterize the subacute stage following subarachnoid hemorrhage. If an intra-axial hematoma is present, it becomes less dense over time, and will be surrounded by a lucent ring that occasionally enhances.[29] Positive mass effect may still be seen at this stage, but will be less marked than it is acutely. As resolution progresses, encephalomalacia occurs.

If obstructive hydrocephalus (see Fig 4–1) was not present initially, communicating hydrocephalus typically emerges at this time.[30–31] The degree may vary from mild to severe and is probably the result of increased CSF protein causing an increase in resistance to absorption of CSF. A mild hydrocephalus may resolve spontaneously, but if it is marked, decompressive shunting may be required.

Arterial spasm results from blood in CSF.[26, 31–35] Much work and speculation has centered on identifying the chemical(s) responsible. As of this writing, no definite entity has been proved,[36, 37] but there is reason to suspect serotonin to be at least one of the offending agents. Whatever the cause, ischemia from arterial spasm can be severe, so much so as to cause frank and even massive infarction (see Fig 4–9). Surgery performed in the face of such spasm carries a high risk; if CT demonstrates the low density of cerebral ischemia/infarction, the surgical risk is greater still.

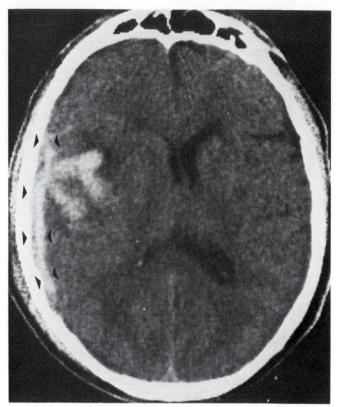

Fig 4–12.—Subarachnoid hemorrhage causing subdural hematoma. A right middle cerebral artery aneurysm bled into the Sylvian fissure. Continued bleeding, perhaps secondary to impaired coagulability, allowed blood to extend into the subdural space *(arrowheads)*. This is a rare finding.

LATE STAGE.—Communicating hydrocephalus may persist. Local-to-widespread encephalomalacia typically follows the hematoma if it is intra-axial. Significant ventricular asymmetry can result (see Fig 4–5), because the insulted hemisphere loses mass and the ventricle dilates as a local hydrocephalus *ex vacuo* (porencephaly).

Infantile Aneurysms and Diffuse Vascular Ectasia

Two types of aneurysms deserve special mention. Infantile and childhood aneurysms are rare and are an infrequent cause of subarachnoid hemorrhage, although they may bleed catastrophically. They are not necessarily related to underlying collagen or disseminated arterial disease, and they are unrelated to arteriosclerosis.

Fusiform dilatation and elongation of arteries may occur,[38, 39] especially of the vertebrobasilar system.[40, 41] This gives rise to megadolichobasilar artery (MDBA) or vertebrobasilar ectasia (Figs 4–13 and 4–14). The occurrence of MDBA can mimic a saccular aneurysm on CT, but must not be confused: the dilatation is the vertebral and/or basilar artery itself and therefore cannot

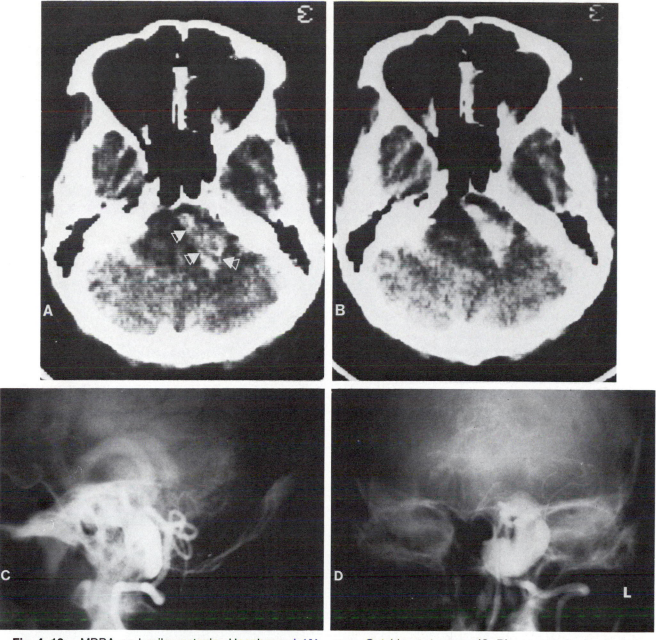

Fig 4–13.—MDBA or basilar ectasia. Unenhanced **(A)** and enhanced **(B)** CT sections show a wedge-shaped enhancing structure in the left side of the posterior fossa *(arrowheads).* The patient had presented with left tic doulou-reux. Outside angiograms **(C, D)** suggested a basilar artery aneurysm, but repeat angiography with a steep transfacial projection (not shown) showed massive basilar ectasia.

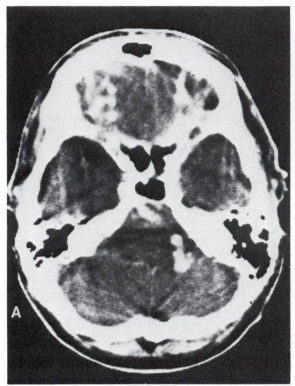

Fig 4–14.—MDBA. **A,** a large, densely enhancing serpiginous structure courses through the posterior fossa in this patient with trigeminal neuralgia. **B,** CT section through the circle of Willis shows marked ectasia of the carotid siphons *(arrowheads)* and enlargement of the distal basilar artery.

be safely isolated from the circulation. Most patients with this entity are hypertensive, but there have been reports of MDBA in normotensives. For this and other reasons, the potentially causal relation between hypertension and MDBA has been called into question. The condition is not associated with subarachnoid hemorrhage.

If symptomatic, MDBA usually presents as a cranial neuropathy,[42–47] either from direct vascular compression on the brain stem or cranial nerves or by traction on smaller vessels which, in turn, compress nerves. The trigeminal and facial nerves suffer most frequently.

Patients with MDBA often have hydrocephalus. Because of the proximity between the basilar artery and floor of the third ventricle, the hydrocephalus was once presumed to be obstructive in nature.[48, 49] More recent studies have shown that CSF pathways are not obstructed, but that hydrocephalus is instead secondary to transmission of large amplitude CSF pulsations ("water-hammer effect") throughout the ventricular system.[50–53]

HYPERTENSIVE HEMORRHAGE

Hypertensive cerebral hemorrhage[54, 55] is a catastrophic event, usually massive and generally involving the basal ganglia, particularly the putamen (Figs 4–15

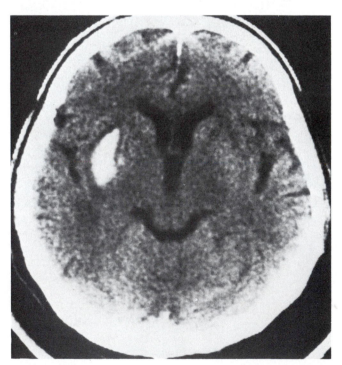

Fig 4–15.—Local basal ganglial hemorrhage. This right putaminal hemorrhage is isolated, produces little mass effect, and fails to reach either the ventricular system or the subarachnoid space. Chronic hypertension has probably played a causative role.

and 4–16). The thalamus may also be affected (Fig 4–17). Intraventricular extension is common, and death ensues rapidly if the hemorrhage is large (Figs 4–18 and 4–19). The classic CT appearance is that of a comma-shaped density near the midline and within the deep white matter of the brain.[56–59] It rarely extends to the subarachnoid space. Contrast enhancement about the rim can occur,[56] but in our experience is rare. Less commonly, there may be hemorrhage in the dentate nucleus of a cerebellar hemisphere.

If the patient survives the ictus, the course of resolution of the hematoma is the same as that for any

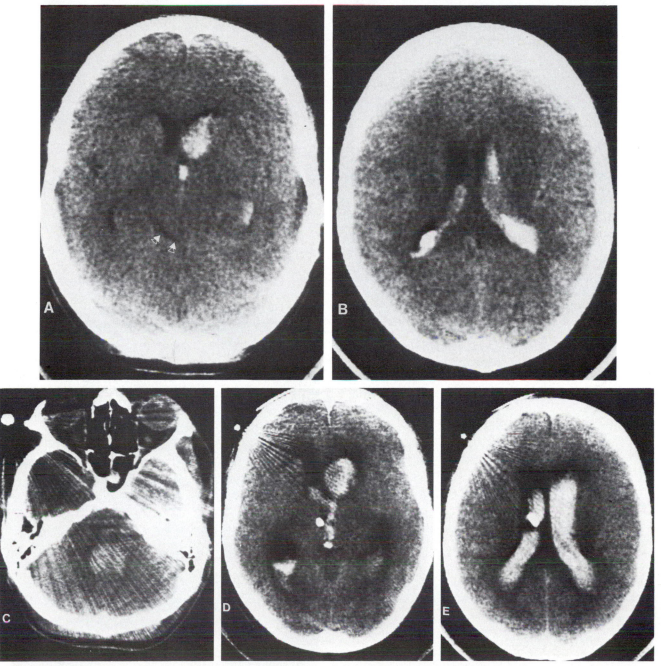

Fig 4–16.—Progressive hypertensive hemorrhage. **A, B,** at admission, the left caudate nuclear hemorrhage had already dissected into both lateral ventricles and into the third ventricle. Increased intracranial pressure is present, with compression of multiple cisterns. The right retrothalamic cistern (**A,** *arrowheads*) is still visible. **C, D, E,** by 72 hours, the degree of hemorrhage is considerably greater, a large amount of blood occupies the fourth ventricle **(C),** and despite shunting, the ventricular system is markedly dilated. Note the disappearance of the right retrothalamic cistern, indicating further pressure.

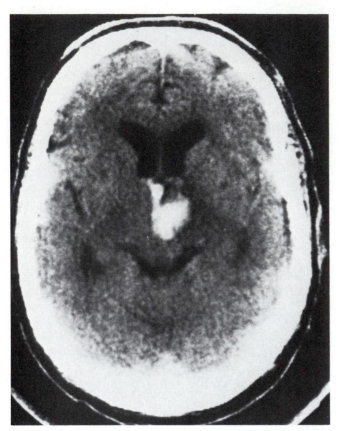

Fig 4–17.—Thalamic hemorrhage. Deep left thalamic hemorrhage has dissected into the third ventricle and across to the contralateral foramen of Monro. Obstructive hydrocephalus ensued, but responded well to shunting.

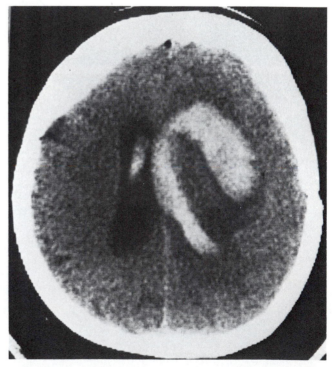

Fig 4–18.—Hypertensive hemorrhage. This white matter hemorrhage began above the level of the basal ganglia, dissected along the forceps minor into the ipsilateral frontal horn and ventricle, and across to the contralateral ventricle. Lower sections showed blood within the third ventricle.

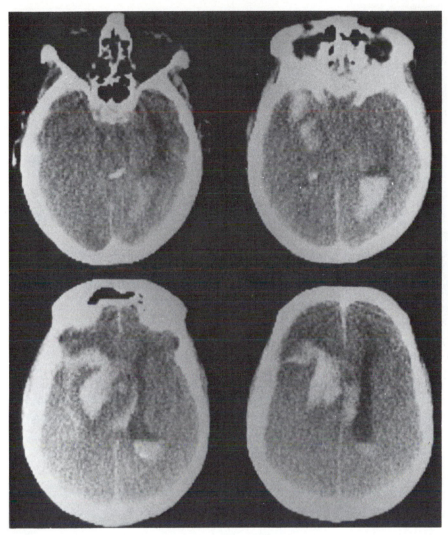

Fig 4–19.—Hypertensive hemorrhage. Hemorrhage into the right thalamus has produced an acute mass effect both by primary expansion and by rupture into the ventricular system, obstructing it. Some blood has dissected laterally and lies within the Sylvian fissure. This hemorrhage probably started in the right basal ganglia. Blood has ruptured into the ventricular system, producing obstructive hydrocephalus, and has dissected laterally to the right Sylvian fissure.

cause. Over time, the hematoma decreases in density, is surrounded by a zone of edema, and is replaced by malacic brain or porencephaly.[60]

GERMINAL MATRIX HEMORRHAGE

Prior to CT, intraventricular hemorrhage, particularly in the newborn, was considered to be fatal. The advent of CT scanning has permitted this hypothesis to be reexamined. In several prospective studies,[61–63] it has been shown that newborns with low birth weights (especially those of 1,500 gm or less) have a high incidence of germinal matrix hemorrhage (GMH) (Fig 4–20). Forty-four percent of one series of patients showed GMH, although in many it was asymptomatic. While low P_{O_2}, high P_{CO_2}, and prematurity are correlated with GMH,[64–68] the causal relations are not well documented. It appears that immaturity of the brain is probably the highest correlating factor.

The occurrence of GMH has been divided into four grades.[61] In Grade I, only the germinal matrix shows hemorrhage. In Grade II, there is extension into the ventricle, but without ventricular dilatation. Grade III shows intraventricular hemorrhage with dilatation. Grade IV is characterized by generalized hemorrhage into cerebral parenchyma as well. Predictably, the prognosis is directly related to grade of hemorrhage, patients with a Grade IV hemorrhage doing the worst.

Treatment consists of repeated lumbar punctures for decompression of the subarachnoid space. This does not seem to be associated with an increased incidence of herniation, even in the face of nearly ubiquitous ventricular dilatation. The progress of therapy is monitored by CT, but this may ultimately be replaced by diagnostic ultrasound through the patent anterior fontanel.

Long-term follow-up of these children sometimes shows prominence of the subarachnoid space and enlarged ventricles. In the face of an enlarging head, GMH may be the cause of so-called "benign subdural collections of infancy."

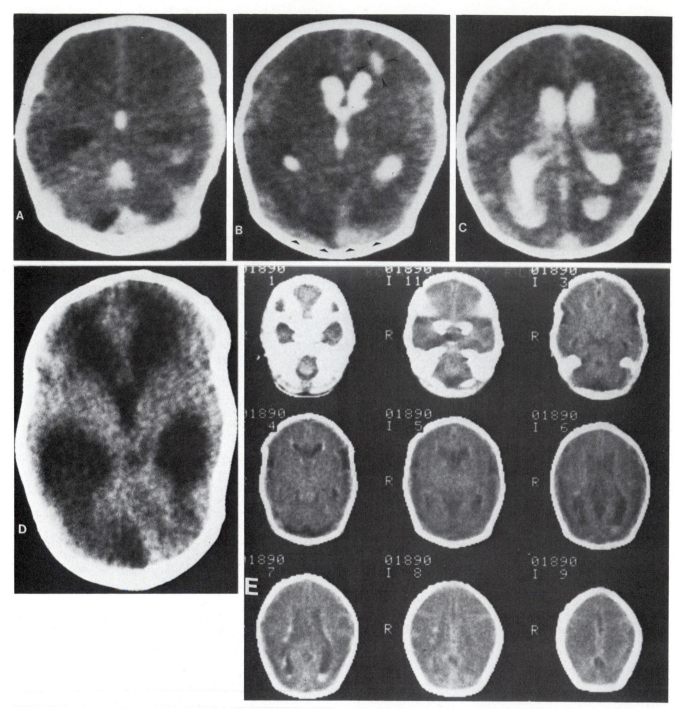

Fig 4–20.—Germinal matrix hemorrhages. **A, B, C,** the hemorrhage in this first patient began in the left germinal matrix and has extended into the ventricular system, the left frontal lobe parenchyma (**B,** *large arrowheads*), and the subarachnoid space (**B,** *small arrowheads*). This Grade IV germinal matrix hemorrhage patient was treated conservatively with repeated lumbar punctures. Five weeks later **(D),** the blood has resolved, but this is communicating hydrocephalus, a common sequela of germinal matrix hemorrhage. **E,** sequential cuts on a second patient show "sugar frosting" of the ventricles representing the germinal matrix hemorrhage with subependymal extension. Some blood has ruptured into the ventricular system, making this a Grade III hemorrhage.

ARTERIOVENOUS MALFORMATION

These lesions result from failure of the formation of a capillary bed between an artery or arteries and a vein or veins.[69, 70] Although they are considered to be congenital, they may enlarge over time[71, 72] or even disappear.[73] The dura, pia (Figs 4–21 to 4–23), or both may be sites of AVM, or they may arise from the ventricular ependymal surface (Figs 4–24 and 4–25). Less common is AVM of the choroid plexus. The term "pial AVM" tends to be misleading, because it suggests that these lesions are all peripheral or circumferential. However, these as well as the mixed pial-dural AVM may be massive and can occupy as much as an entire hemisphere.

Discovery of AVM may be incidental when a patient is examined for other reasons, such as trauma. Most

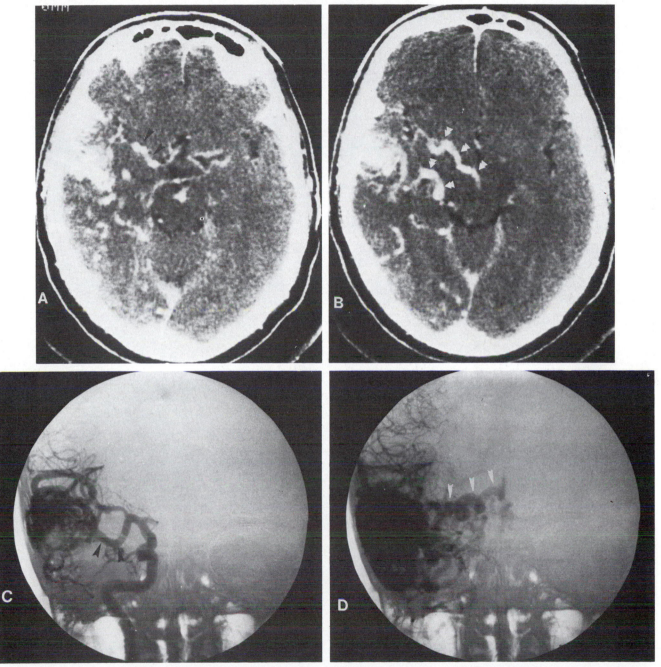

Fig 4–21.—AVM: Temporal lobe. **A, B,** CT shows a large right middle cerebral artery (**A,** *black arrowheads*) feeding the dense peripheral AVM. There are even larger, more ectatic veins draining it (**B,** *white arrowheads*). Correlation between CT and angiography is excellent: the arterial pedicle (**A, C,** *black arrowheads*), the nidus of the AVM, and its draining veins (**B, D,** *white arrowheads*) are clearly delineated on both.

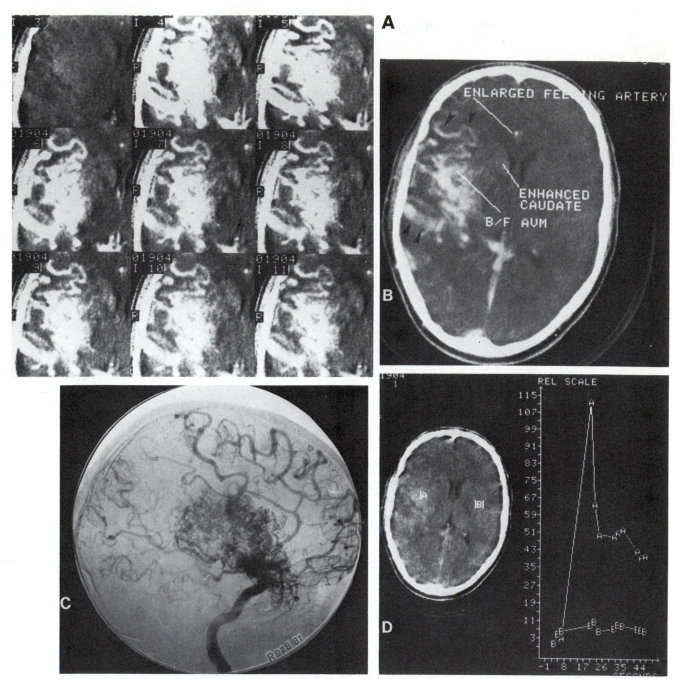

Fig 4–22.—A very large racemose pial AVM. This patient was originally studied for head trauma. Rapid-sequence segmented (every 3 seconds) **(A)** and static **(B)** CT images show the worm-like appearance of the malformation. Note that the draining veins (**B,** *arrowheads*) are much larger than the supplying arteries, a constant finding. **C,** corresponding right carotid angiography shows the network of small feeding arteries throughout the basal ganglia and the enlarged anterior and middle cerebral artery branches. **D,** speed of blood flow is illustrated graphically by plotting density of corresponding areas vs. time for the sequence shown in **A.** (*B/F AVM* in B = nidus of AVM)

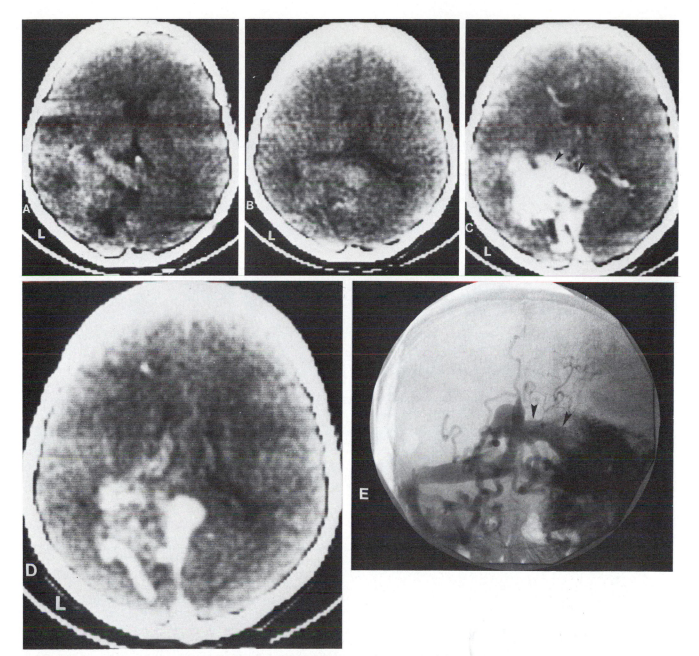

Fig 4–23.—Temporo-occipital AVM. A large AVM straddles the junction of the left temporal and occipital lobes (CT images reversed). Contrast enhancement densely opacifies the nidus and venous drainage routes; the smaller arterial supplies are obscured by venous structures. The value of scanning without **(A, B)** and with **(C, D)** contrast administration is well documented. An isolated enhanced scan would obscure calcification and hemorrhage, while an unenhanced scan would not define the nature of the abnormality. Note the increased density of the "blood pool" within the AVM on the unenhanced scan. A huge draining vein is seen on both angiography and CT **(C, E,** *arrowheads*). (L = patient's left.)

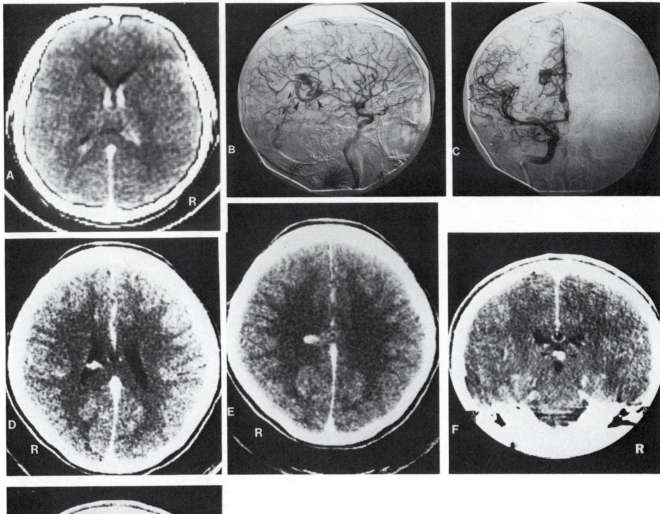

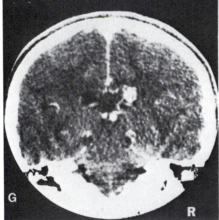

Fig 4–24.—Intraventricular hemorrhage: lateral ventricular AVM. This young patient presented with intraventricular hemorrhage **(A).** Right carotid angiography **(B, C)** disclosed an AVM, but whether midline pial (superficial) or ependymal (deep) is not certain. Note the dense opacification of the posterior portion of the right internal cerebral vein and vein of Galen (**B,** *large arrowheads*) as well as early filling of the straight sinus (**B,** *small arrowheads*). Enhanced CT scanning in axial **(D, E)** and coronal **(F, G)** projections shows the AVM to reside within the right lateral ventricle. Note the relative sizes of the two internal cerebral veins, the one ipsilateral to the AVM being much larger than its opposite normal counterpart (**F,** *arrowheads*). (*R* on CT scans = patient's right.)

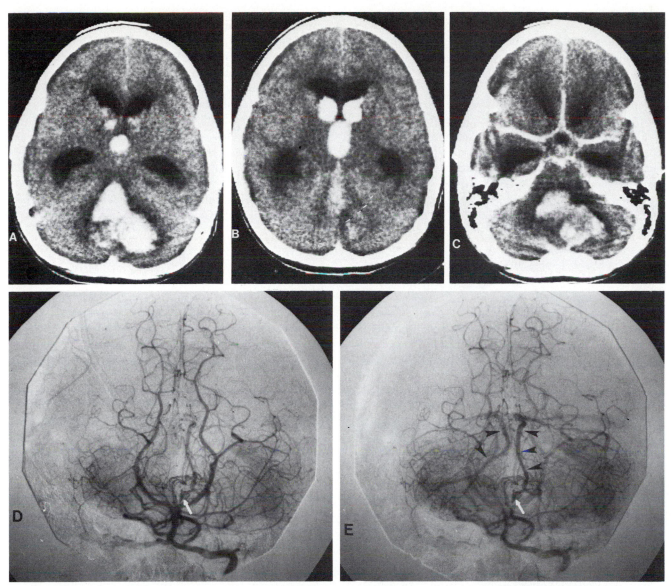

Fig 4–25.—Cryptic AVM: posterior fossa. **A, B, C,** extensive hemorrhage is confined to the ventricular system and left cerebellar hemisphere. **D, E,** vertebral angiography demonstrates a pair of draining veins (**E,** *arrowheads*) and a possible nidus (**D, E,** *white arrow*) along the left lateral aspect of the fourth ventricle. The extensive intraventricular hemorrhage is compatible with a location on the ependymal surface. Note the severe acute obstructive hydrocephalus.

patients present with symptoms of seizure, chronic neurologic deficit, or hemorrhage. Some patients with AVM harbor aneurysms of the feeding arteries, and these may be multiple. Whether the aneurysms are related to the increased flow through the supplying vessels, dysplasia of the vessels themselves, or both, is not clear.

If a pial or pial-dural AVM has bled, the hemorrhage is peripheral in location, and thus unusual for an aneurysm.[74–76] In addition, the enhanced CT appearance may be characterized by the presence of prominent vessels. While the arteries that supply AVM are enlarged, the veins that drain them are even larger and are the most likely vascular structures to be demonstrated on a contrast-enhanced scan.[77] The malformation itself may appear as an enhancing mass that may mimic a tumor,[75, 76] or even a cyst.[78] However, if a malformation is small ("cryptic"), only the draining vein may be identified. The aneurysms that are occasionally present may be demonstrated as well. If a cryptic AVM has obliterated itself either by bleeding or thrombosis of the artery or vein, it may be invisible on CT. If, on the other hand, the AVM is ependymal and therefore intraventricular, the hemorrhage may be either confined to the ventricular system or extend into the parenchyma adjacent to the site of the malformation.[79]

Because an AVM tends to divert blood away from normal brain, the brain surrounding an AVM may be dysplastic or atrophic. Ventricles adjacent to them may be small from mass effect, large from atrophic changes, or normal as a balance between these two opposing forces.

Venous angiomas are a type of vascular malformation. They are entirely venous in structure and represent local dysplasia of medullary veins and adjacent brain.[80] Generally, they drain to an aberrant central transparenchymal vein, which subsequently empties directly into a venous sinus (Fig 4–26).[81] Rarely, they may drain into deep vascular structures such as the thalamostriate vein (Fig 4–27). They occasionally bleed,[82] but are more commonly associated with headache or seizure. On the enhanced CT, there is a dense enhancing lesion, usually subcortical in location, and frequently serpiginous.[81] Overlying sulci may be generous, reflecting the locally dysplastic brain.

Other arteriovenous abnormalities can occur. In many cases, venous angiomata and cavernous angiomata are indistinguishable on CT scan. Carotid artery to cavernous sinus fistulae (Fig 4–28) can result from either rupture of an intracavernous carotid aneurysm or from traumatic laceration of an internal carotid artery within the cavernous sinus. An enlarged cavernous sinus may be seen, but a characteristic history coupled with demonstration of an enlarged superior ophthalmic vein makes the diagnosis.[83, 84] Proptosis and enlargement of intraorbital muscles, especially if unilateral, further suggest this diagnosis.

The term "aneurysm of the vein of Galen" (Fig 4–29) is a misnomer for a gigantic arteriovenous fistula of the vein of Galen. This usually does not produce a diagnostic problem. Most patients with this disease present in congestive heart failure at or shortly after birth. A loud bruit is held over the head. Scanning by CT reveals obstructive hydrocephalus and a large enhancing mass in the vicinity of the vein of Galen.[85, 86]

OTHER CAUSES OF HEMORRHAGE

Pituitary apoplexy[87] might be considered the prototype of intratumoral hemorrhage, but hemorrhage into other tumors has been described. Bleeding may occur in metastases, especially from melanoma and carcinoma of the lung, and in primary brain tumors, particularly gliomas.[88–90] A contrast-enhanced scan may demonstrate tumor surrounding the clot and thus suggest the correct diagnosis. Other tumor nodules may be seen on

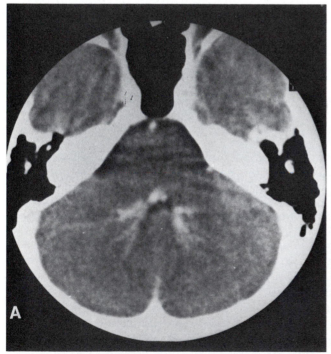
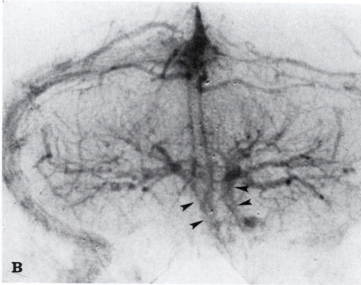

Fig 4–26.—Cerebellar venous angioma. Enhanced CT (**A**) shows bilateral stellate densities in the medial regions of both cerebellar hemispheres. A density in the anterior fourth ventricle represents confluence of the venous channels into a vein that crossed through the pons to the left cerebellopontine angle. The late venous phase of vertebral angiography demonstrates the bilateral venous angioma and the transpontine draining veins (**B,** *arrowheads*). (From Hacker D.A., Latchaw R.E., Chou S.N., et al.: Bilateral cerebellar venous angioma. *J. Comput Assist. Tomogr.* 5:424–426, 1981. Used by permission.)

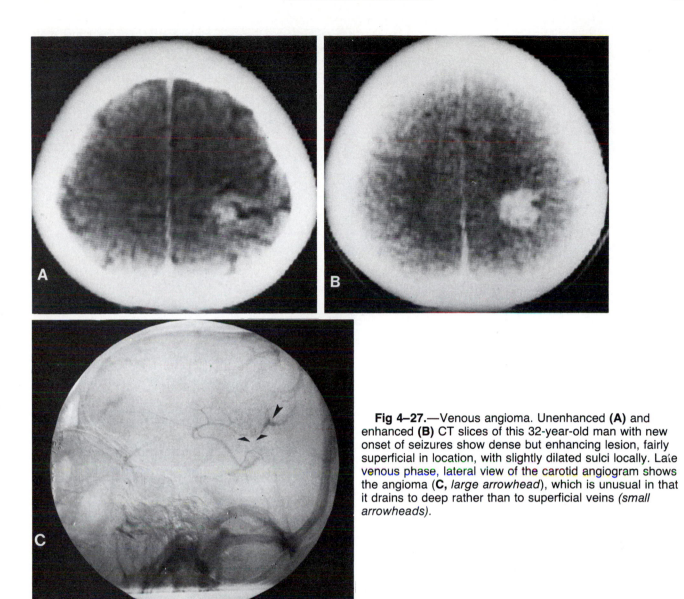

Fig 4–27.—Venous angioma. Unenhanced **(A)** and enhanced **(B)** CT slices of this 32-year-old man with new onset of seizures show dense but enhancing lesion, fairly superficial in location, with slightly dilated sulci locally. Late venous phase, lateral view of the carotid angiogram shows the angioma **(C,** *large arrowhead*), which is unusual in that it drains to deep rather than to superficial veins *(small arrowheads).*

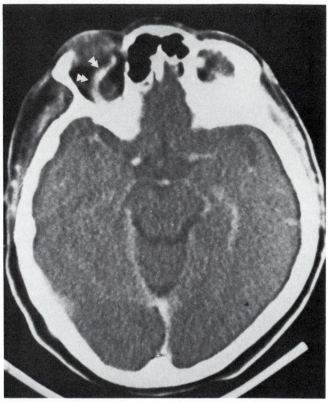

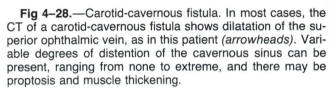

Fig 4–28.—Carotid-cavernous fistula. In most cases, the CT of a carotid-cavernous fistula shows dilatation of the superior ophthalmic vein, as in this patient *(arrowheads).* Variable degrees of distention of the cavernous sinus can be present, ranging from none to extreme, and there may be proptosis and muscle thickening.

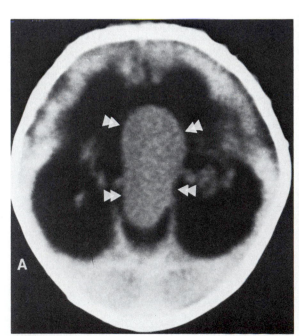

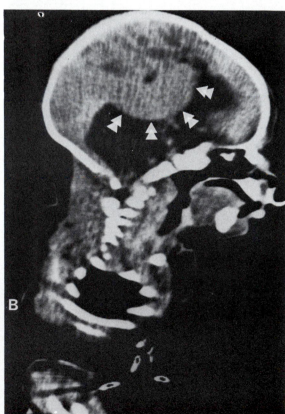

Fig 4–29.—Vein of Galen malformation. Axial **(A)** and direct sagittal **(B)** unenhanced scans demonstrate a large midline mass in the region of the vein of Galen *(arrowheads),* producing obstructive hydrocephalus. The patient presented with congestive heart failure and a loud cranial bruit.

the scan, suggesting metastases. In the case of hemorrhage into a glioma, unusual contrast enhancement or an unusual location for an intraparenchymal hemorrhage are appropriate clues. Other rarer causes of hemorrhage include coagulopathies,[91] amyloidosis,[92] and diseases with decreased platelet formation (Wiscott-Aldrich syndrome, etc.).

REFERENCES

1. Sekhar L.N., Heros R.B.: Origin, growth, and rupture of saccular aneurysms: A review. *Neurosurgery* 8:248–260, 1981.

2. Ferguson G.G.: Physical factors in the initiation, growth, and rupture of human intracranial saccular aneurysms. *J. Neurosurg.* 37:666–677, 1972.

3. Zacks D.J.: Multiple intracranial aneurysms. *A.J.R.* 130:180–182, 1978.

4. Fox J.L., Ko J.P.: Familial intracranial aneurysms: Six cases among 13 siblings. *J. Neurosurg.* 52:501–503, 1980.

5. Newton T.H., Troost B.T.: Arteriovenous malformations and fistulae, in Newton T.H., Potts D.G. (eds.): *Radiology of the Skull and Brain.* St. Louis, C.V. Mosby Co., 1974, vol. 2, book 4, p. 2512.

6. Frazee J.G., Cahan L.D., Winter J.: Bacterial intracranial aneurysms. *J. Neurosurg.* 53:633–641, 1980.

7. Olmsted W.W., McGee T.P.: The pathogenesis of peripheral aneurysms of the central nervous system: A subject review from the AFIP. *Radiology* 123:661–666, 1977.

8. Caplan L.R., Hier D.B., Banks G.: Current concepts of cerebrovascular disease—stroke: Stroke and drug abuse. *Stroke* 13:869–872, 1982.

9. Asari S., Nakamura S., Yamada O., et al.: Traumatic aneurysm of peripheral cerebral arteries: Report of two cases. *J. Neurosurg.* 46:795–803, 1977.

10. Miyazaki S., Fukushima H., Kamata K., et al.: False aneurysm with subdural hematoma and symptomatic vasospasm following head injury. *Surg. Neurol.* 16:443–447, 1981.

11. Bergstrom K., Hemmingsson A.: False cortical aneurysm in subdural haematoma following head injury without fracture. *Acta Radiol. Diag.* 14:657–661, 1973.

12. Sarwar M., Batnitzky S., Schechter M.M.: Tumorous aneurysms. *Neuroradiology* 12:79–97, 1976.

13. Sonntag V.K.H., Yuan R.H., Stein B.M.: Giant intracranial aneurysms: A review of 13 cases. *Surg. Neurol.* 8:81–84, 1977.

14. Pribram H.F.W., Hudson J.D., Joynt R.J.: Posterior fossa aneurysms presenting as mass lesions. *A.J.R.* 105:334–340, 1969.

15. Maxwell R.E., Chou S.N.: Aneurysmal tumors of the basifrontal region. *J. Neurosurg.* 46:438–445, 1977.

16. Cantore G.P., Ciappetta P., Vagnozzi R., et al.: Giant aneurysm of the anterior inferior cerebellar artery simulating cerebellopontine angle tumor. *Surg. Neurol.* 18:76–78, 1982.

17. Fukuoka S., Suematsu K., Nakamura J., et al.: Transient ischemic attacks caused by unruptured intracranial aneurysm. *Surg. Neurol.* 17:464–467, 1982.

18. Weisberg L.A.: Computed tomography in aneurysmal subarachnoid hemorrhage. *Neurology* 29:802–808, 1979.

19. Asari S., Satoh T., Sakurai M., et al.: Delineation of unruptured cerebral aneurysms by computerized angiotomography. *J. Neurosurg.* 57:527–534, 1982.

20. Lavyne M.H., Kleefield J., David K.R., et al.: Giant intracranial aneurysms of the anterior circulation: Clinical characteristics and diagnosis by computed tomography. *Neurosurgery* 3:356–363, 1978.

21. Ito H., Yamamoto S.: CT findings of tumorous aneurysms. *J. Comput. Assist. Tomogr.* 3:555, 1979.

22. Ghoshhajra K., Scotti L., Marasco J., et al.: CT detection of intracranial aneurysms in subarachnoid hemorrhage. *A.J.R.* 132:613–616, 1979.

23. Liliequist B., Lindqvist M., Valdimarsson E.: Computed tomography and subarachnoid hemorrhage. *Neuroradiology* 14:21–26, 1977.

24. Lim S.T., Sage D.J.: Detection of subarachnoid blood clot and other thin, flat structures by computed tomography. *Radiology* 123:79–84, 1977.

25. Kendall B.E., Lee B.C.P., Claveria E.: Computerized tomography and angiography in subarachnoid haemorrhage. *Br. J. Radiol.* 49:483–501, 1976.

26. Bryan R.N., Shah C.P., Hilal S.: Evaluation of subarachnoid hemorrhage and cerebral vasospasm by computed tomography. *Comput. Tomogr.* 3:144–153, 1979.

27. Scotti G., Ethier R., Melancon D., et al.: Computed tomography in the evaluation of intracranial aneurysms and subarachnoid hemorrhage. *Radiology* 123:85–90, 1977.

28. Handel S.F., Perpetuo F.O.L., Handel C.H.: Subdural hematomas due to ruptured cerebral aneurysms: Angiographic diagnosis and potential pitfalls for CT. *A.J.R.* 130:507–509, 1978.

29. Weisberg L.A.: Computerized tomography in intracranial hemorrhage. *Arch. Neurol.* 36:422–426, 1979.

30. Silver A.J., Pederson M.E. Jr., Ganti S.R., et al.: CT of subarachnoid hemorrhage due to ruptured aneurysm. *A.J.N.R.* 2:13–22, 1981.

31. Griffith H.B., Cummins B.H., Thomson J.L.G.: Cerebral arterial spasm and hydrocephalus in leaking arterial aneurysms. *Neuroradiology* 4:212–214, 1972.

32. Davis J.M., Davis K.R., Crowell R.M.: Subarachnoid hemorrhage secondary to ruptured intracranial aneurysm: Prognostic significance of cranial CT. *A.J.R.* 134:711–715, 1980.

33. Davis K.R., New P.F.J., Ojemann R.G., et al.: Computed tomographic evaluation of hemorrhage secondary to intracranial aneurysm. *A.J.R.* 127:143–153, 1976.

34. Allcock J.M., Drake C.G.: Ruptured intracranial aneurysms—the role of arterial spasm. *J. Neurosurg.* 22:21–29, 1965.

35. Wilkins R.H., Alexander J.A., Odom, G.L.: Intracranial arterial spasm: A clinical analysis. *J. Neurosurg.* 29:121–134, 1968.

36. Heros R.C., Zervas N.T., Negoro M.: Cerebral vasospasm. *Surg. Neurol.* 5:354–362, 1976.

37. Wellum G.R., Irvine T.W., Zervas N.T.: Cerebral vasoactivity of heme proteins in vitro: Some mechanistic considerations. *J. Neurosurg.* 56:777–783, 1982.

38. Bladin P.F., Donnan M.G.F.: Cerebral arterial ectasia. *Clin. Radiol.* 14:349–352, 1963.

39. Scotti G., DeGrandi C., Colombo A.: Ectasia of the intracranial arteries diagnosed by computed tomography. Megadolichobasilar artery: CT diagnosis. *Neuroradiology* 15:183–184, 1978.

40. Boeri R., Passerini A.: The megadolichobasilar anomaly. *J. Neurol. Sci.* 1:475–484, 1964.

41. Peterson N.T., Duchesneau P.M., Westbrook E.L., et al.: Basilar artery ectasia demonstrated by computed tomography. *Radiology* 122:713–715, 1977.

42. Deeb Z.L., Jannetta P.J., Rosenbaum A.E., et al.: Tortuous vertebrobasilar arteries causing cranial nerve syndromes: Screening by computed tomography. *J. Comput. Assist. Tomogr.* 3:774–778, 1979.

43. Carella A., Caruso G., Lamberti P.: Hemifacial spasm due to elongation and ectasia of the distal segment of the vertebral artery: Report of two cases. *Neuroradiology* 6:233–236, 1973.

44. Scott M., Stauffer H.M.: A case of aneurysmal malformation of the vertebral and basilar arteries causing cranial nerve involvement. *A.J.R.* 92:836–837, 1964.

45. Tridon P., Masingue M., Picard L., et al.: Hémispasme facial et mégadolichobasilaire à symptomatologie pseudotumorale. *Rev. Otoneuroophtalmol.* 43:279–286, 1971.

46. Kerber C.W., Margolis M.T., Newton T.H.: Tortuous vertebrobasilar system: A cause of cranial nerve signs. *Neuroradiology* 4:74–77, 1972.

47. Moseley I.F., Holland I.M.: Ectasia of the basilar artery: The breadth of the clinical spectrum and the diagnostic value of computed tomography. *Neuroradiology* 18:83–91, 1979.

48. Healy J.F., Wells M.V., Rosenkrantz H.: Computed tomographic demonstration of enlarged, ectatic basilar artery associated with obstruction of the anterior third ventricle. *Comput. Tomogr.* 5:239–245, 1981.

49. Rozario R.A., Levine H.L., Scott R.M.: Obstructive hydrocephalus secondary to an ectatic basilar artery. *Surg. Neurol.* 9:31–34, 1978.

50. Breig A., Ekbom K., Greitz T., et al.: Hydrocephalus due to elongated basilar artery: A new clinicoradiological syndrome. *Lancet* 1:874–875, 1967.

51. Greitz T., Ekbom K., Kugelberg E., et al.: Occult hydrocephalus due to ectasia of the basilar artery. *Acta Radiol. Diag.* 9:310–316, 1968.

52. Ekbom K., Greitz T., Kalmer M., et al.: Cerebrospinal fluid pulsations in occult hydrocephalus due to ectasia of basilar artery. *Acta Neurochir.* 20:1–8, 1969.

53. Tonali P., Laudisio A., Belloni G., et al.: Functional obstructive hydrocephalus. *Neuroradiology* 5:220–222, 1973.

54. Tanaka H., Ueda Y., Hayashi M., et al.: Risk factors for cerebral hemorrhage and cerebral infarction in a Japanese rural community. *Stroke* 13:62–73, 1982.

55. Caplan L.R., Mohr J.P.: Intracerebral hemorrhage: An update. *Geriatrics* 33:42–52, 1978.

56. Weisberg L.A.: Peripheral rim enhancement in supratentorial intracerebral hematoma. *Comput. Tomogr.* 4:145–154, 1980.

57. Kendall B.E., Radue E.W.: Computed tomography in spontaneous intracerebral haematomas. *Br. J. Radiol.* 51:563–573, 1978.

58. Wiggins W.S., Moody D.M., Toole J.F., et al.: Clinical and computerized tomographic study of hypertensive intracerebral hemorrhage. *Arch. Neurol.* 35:832–833, 1978.

59. Scott W.R., New P.F.J., Davis K.R., et al.: Computerized axial tomography of intracerebral and intraventricular hemorrhage. *Radiology* 112:73–80, 1974.

60. Messina A.V., Chernik N.L.: Computed tomography: The "resolving" intracerebral hemorrhage. *Radiology* 118:609–613, 1975.

61. Papile L.-A., Burstein J., Burstein R., et al.: Incidence and evolution of subependymal and intraventricular hemorrhage: A study of infants with birth weights less than 1,500 gm. *J. Pediatr.* 92:529–534, 1978.

62. Lee B.C.P., Grassi A.E., Schechner S., et al.: Neonatal intraventricular hemorrhage: A serial computed tomography study. *J. Comput. Assist. Tomogr.* 3:483–490, 1979.

63. Volpe J.J.: Intracranial hemorrhage in the newborn: Current understanding and dilemmas. *Neurology* 29:632–635, 1979.

64. Levene M.I., Fawer C.-L., Lamont R.F.: Risk factors in the development of intraventricular haemorrhage in the preterm neonate. *Arch. Dis. Child.* 57:410–417, 1982.

65. Deonna T., Payot M., Probst A., et al.: Neonatal intracranial hemorrhage in premature infants. *Pediatrics* 56:1056–1064, 1975.

66. Leech R.W., Kohnen P.: Subependymal and intraventricular hemorrhages in the newborn. *Am. J. Pathol.* 77:465–475, 1974.

67. Tsiantos A., Victorin L., Relier J.P., et al.: Intracranial hemorrhage in the prematurely born infant: Timing of clots and evaluation of clinical signs and symptoms. *J. Pediatr.* 85:854–859, 1974.

68. Friede R.L.: Acquired lesions in newborns and infants, in Friede R.L. (ed.): *Developmental Neuropathology.* New York, Springer-Verlag, 1975, pp. 1–37.

69. Newton T.H., Troost B.T.: Arteriovenous malformations and fistulae, in Newton T.H., Potts D.B. (eds.): *Radiology of the Skull and Brain.* St. Louis, C.V. Mosby Co., 1974, vol. 2, book 4, p. 2491.

70. Weisberg L.A., Nice C., Katz M.: Intracranial vascular malformations, in Weisberg L.A., Nice C., Katz M. (eds.): *Cerebral Computed Tomography.* Philadelphia, W.B. Saunders Co., 1978, pp. 94–104.

71. Peeters F.L.M.: Angiographically demonstrated large vascular malformation in a patient with a normal angiogram 23 years before. *Neuroradiology* 23:113–114, 1982.

72. Delitala A., Delfini R., Vagnozzi R., et al.: Increase in size of cerebral angiomas: Case report. *J. Neurosurg.* 57:556–558, 1982.

73. Conforti P.: Spontaneous disappearance of cerebral arteriovenous angioma: Case report. *J. Neurosurg.* 34:432–434, 1971.

74. Hayward R.D.: Intracranial arteriovenous malformations: Observations after experience with computerised tomog-

raphy. *J. Neurol. Neurosurg. Psychiatry* 39:1027–1033, 1976.

75. Bell B.A., Kendall B.E., Symon L.: Angiographically occult arteriovenous malformations of the brain. *J. Neurol. Neurosurg. Psychiatry* 41:1057–1064, 1978.

76. Kramer R.A., Wing S.D.: Computed tomography of angiographically occult cerebral vascular malformations. *Radiology* 123:649–652, 1977.

77. Terbrugge K., Scotti G., Ethier R., et al.: Computed tomography in intracranial arteriovenous malformations. *Radiology* 122:703–705, 1977.

78. Daniels D.L., Haughton V.M., Williams A.L., et al.: Arteriovenous malformation simulating a cyst on computed tomography. *Radiology* 133:393–394, 1979.

79. McCallum J.E., LoDolce D., Boehnke M.: CT scan in intraventricular hemorrhage: Correlation of clinical findings with computerized tomographic scans of the brain. *Neurosurgery* 3:22–25, 1978.

80. Senegor M., Dohrmann G.J., Wollmann R.L: Venous angiomas of the posterior fossa should be considered as anomalous venous drainage. *Surg. Neurol.* 19:26–32, 1983.

81. Michels L.G., Bentson J.R., Winter J.: Computed tomography of cerebral venous angiomas. *J. Comput. Assist. Tomogr.* 1:149–154, 1977.

82. Numaguchi Y., Kitamura K., Fukui M., et al.: Intracranial venous angiomas. *Surg. Neurol.* 18:193–202, 1982.

83. Weisberg L.A.: Computed tomographic findings in carotid-cavernous fistula. *Comput. Tomogr.* 5:31–36, 1981.

84. Merrick R., Latchaw R.E., Gold L.H.A.: Computerized tomography of the orbit in carotid-cavernous sinus fistulae. *Comput. Tomogr.* 4:127–132, 1980.

85. Spallone A.: Computed tomography in aneurysms of the vein of Galen. *J. Comput. Assist. Tomogr.* 3:779–782, 1979.

86. Martelli A., Scotti G., Harwood-Nash D.C., et al.: Aneurysms of the vein of Galen in children: CT and angiographic correlations. *Neuroradiology* 20:123–133, 1980.

87. Mohr G., Hardy J.: Hemorrhage, necrosis, and apoplexy in pituitary adenomas. *Surg. Neurol.* 18:181–189, 1982.

88. Wakai S., Yamakawa K., Manaka S., et al.: Spontaneous intracranial hemorrhage caused by brain tumor: Its incidence and clinical significance. *Neurosurgery* 10:437–444, 1982.

89. Zimmerman R.A., Bilaniuk L.T.: Computed tomography of acute intratumoral hemorrhage. *Radiology* 135:355–359, 1980.

90. Vincent F.M., Bartone J.R., Jones M.Z.: Cerebellar astrocytoma presenting as a cerebellar hemorrhage in a child. *Neurology* 30:91–93, 1980.

91. Ammirati M., Tomita T.: Spontaneous cerebellar hematoma in children: Report of two cases and review of the literature. *Neurosurgery* 11:426–429, 1982.

92. Tyler K.L., Poletti C.E., Heros R.C.: Cerebral amyloid angiopathy with multiple intracerebral hemorrhages: Case report. *J. Neurosurg.* 57:286–298, 1982.

5

Cerebral Infarction

JOSEPH A. HORTON, M.D.

CEREBRAL ISCHEMIA is a prevalent disease, affecting about 300,000 Americans annually. Half of these will develop fixed deficits from infarction of part of their brain. The other half will have transient ischemic attacks (TIA), the symptoms of which abate in less than 24 hours. *Any* transient neurologic deficit can be a manifestation of TIA, including amaurosis (fugax), paresis, apraxia, sensory deficit, and aphasia, but the first two are the most common presenting complaints.

Without doubt, atherosclerosis is the leading cause of cerebral vascular disease.[1, 2] Extracranial atheromata favor the carotid bifurcations, the posterior wall of the internal carotid artery origin being the most commonly affected. Lesions at this location produce signs and symptoms in three ways. First, atheromata reduce lumen size and thus decrease blood flow through the artery. While an intact circle of Willis can compensate for a single extracranial lesion (Fig 5–1), most patients with an atheroma in one vessel have more diffuse disease.

Ulceration of carotid atheromata causes the second problem, namely clot formation with distal embolization (Fig 5–2). It is common for endothelium to be absent over part or all of an atheroma, and the denuded segment may develop a crypt. But whether or not a crater is present, the locally absent endothelium serves as a nidus for clot formation. Once formed, the clot will either be lysed or detach and pass downstream to the eye and/or brain. Because the embolus so produced is flow-guided, it tends to strike the middle cerebral artery distribution more commonly than the anterior distribution, because flow in the middle exceeds that of the anterior cerebral artery.

The third and least common mechanism is distal embolization of the atheromatous material itself. Symptomatically, this is indistinguishable from thrombus embolization, but funduscopic examination may reveal the presence of Hollenhorst plaques (cholesterol emboli in the retinal vasculature). Even if such an atheroma does not produce a hemodynamically significant stenosis, it is not architecturally stable: fragmentation may occur, and surgery is indicated. Because the mechanism of embolization here is unrelated to clot formation, anticoagulation is insufficient.

Intracranial atherosclerosis may be isolated or coexist with cervical vascular disease. It most commonly affects the carotid siphon, but may involve the supraclinoid carotid as well as even small branches of an intracranial vessel. Even cerebellar arteries may be affected. As with cervical carotid disease, thrombus formation can ensue. Likewise, emboli from an extracranial origin can be trapped at the stenotic segment of the vessel.

Aseptic arteritides are rare causes of intracerebral arterial stenosis. Similar arteriopathies and atherosclerosis are responsible for lacunar infarction. In these, the vessels affected are primarily the lenticulostriate arteries.[3, 4]

Less common causes of cerebral arterial occlusion are septic emboli and hematogenously spread tumor. Septic and aseptic emboli are seen primarily in patients with subacute bacterial endocarditis or histories of intravenous drug abuse.[5] Patients with right-to-left shunts (intracardiac or extracardiac) lack normal filtering action of the pulmonary vascular bed, and they are thus at higher risk for both septic and tumoral embolization.

Thrombosis and embolization of the cerebral arterial system leads to cerebral ischemia. If collateral blood supply is available and vascular compromise is low, the patient might never have a symptom from the occlusion. If an embolus passes distally and/or collateral flow is absent or inadequate, symptoms of ischemia will result. If they resolve in less than 24 hours, the incident was a TIA. The longer that signs and symptoms continue without resolution, the more likely they are to evolve into a completed stroke.

Two other causes of cerebral ischemia and infarction deserve mention. Venous thrombosis, especially involving multiple and/or smaller cortical veins, produces in-

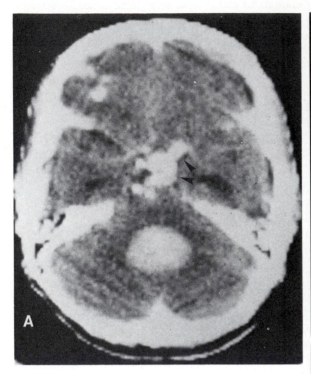

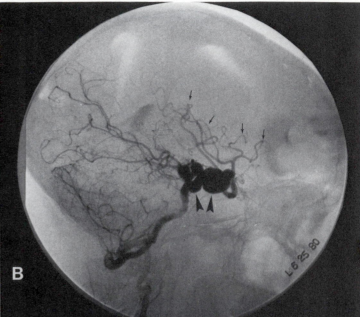

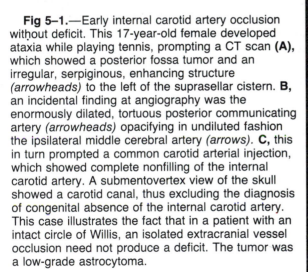

Fig 5–1.—Early internal carotid artery occlusion without deficit. This 17-year-old female developed ataxia while playing tennis, prompting a CT scan **(A)**, which showed a posterior fossa tumor and an irregular, serpiginous, enhancing structure *(arrowheads)* to the left of the suprasellar cistern. **B,** an incidental finding at angiography was the enormously dilated, tortuous posterior communicating artery *(arrowheads)* opacifying in undiluted fashion the ipsilateral middle cerebral artery *(arrows)*. **C,** this in turn prompted a common carotid arterial injection, which showed complete nonfilling of the internal carotid artery. A submentovertex view of the skull showed a carotid canal, thus excluding the diagnosis of congenital absence of the internal carotid artery. This case illustrates the fact that in a patient with an intact circle of Willis, an isolated extracranial vessel occlusion need not produce a deficit. The tumor was a low-grade astrocytoma.

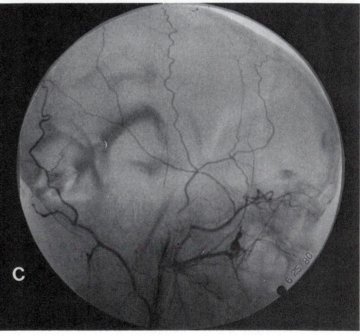

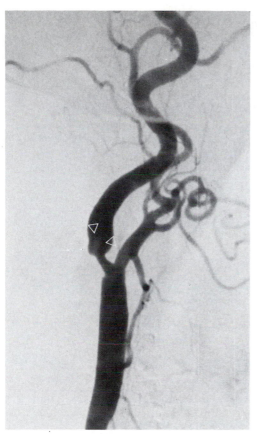

Fig 5–2.—Floating thrombus. Almost certainly related to the patient's TIA, the floating thrombus here seen as a filling defect *(arrowheads)* within the proximal internal carotid artery is barely attached to the wall. A cough, sneeze, massage of the neck, or selective catheterization is all that would be required to dislodge it.

creased venous back-pressure with consequent decreased perfusion. This can lead to so-called venous infarction. Thrombosis of a venous sinus is usually central so that numerous smaller collateral channels can open; in this setting infarction may be slightly less common than it is in isolated cerebral venous occlusions, because alternate venous pathways might open and prevent it. Low-flow states (hypotension, especially if superimposed upon arterial stenosis) can produce infarction in watershed* zones. Presumably, the tissue between two circulations is the first to suffer when blood pressure is decreased, because it is not central to either one.

Intracranial aneurysms can lead to infarction in either of two ways. First, if the aneurysm bleeds, subarachnoid hemorrhage can provoke arterial spasm se-

---

*Webster defines watershed as an area between two drainage zones. As used to describe infarction, it is the volume of brain between two perfusion zones.

vere enough to cause infarction. This is also discussed in Chapter 4. Secondly, clot formed within an aneurysm can leave it and pass into the cerebral circulation.[6]

CT APPEARANCES OF INFARCTION

For 12 hours after even the most massive ischemic insult, CT changes are at a minimum (Figs 5–3 and 5–4). Studies in baboons[7] correspond well to human experience and suggest that (1) no changes are usually seen for 12 to 24 hours, (2) the first changes are a decrease in density of the ischemic tissue and a concomitant increase in local ventricular size, and (3) animals in whom early changes are seen (within the 12- to 24-hour time period) have more extensive infarction than those in whom CT changes appear later.

Two inferences come to light from these findings. First, because there is an early local ventricular dilatation, it follows that the brain in the infarcted territory decreases in volume. Therefore, because blood is denser than brain tissue, the early lucency and brain shrinkage is almost certainly the result of a decrease in amount of blood within brain parenchyma. The second inference is that the almost uniformly negative study in TIA patients is predictable. In fact, by definition, the CT of TIA as an isolated event must be negative, because it resolves before CT changes can occur.

It is likely that the definitive acute CT evaluation of cerebral ischemia will revolve around imaging of cerebral blood flow. This topic is described in detail in Chapter 2.

Beyond 24 hours, lucency of the infarcted brain is a constant finding (Fig 5–5). It generally conforms to a vascular distribution (Fig 5–6). Delayed lucency differs partly in cause from acute changes. Dead tissue can excite considerable edema, and this pathology is reflected as local lucency.[8,9] Tissue necrosis further contributes to the density loss. Edema that follows can be extensive (Fig 5–7) and may exert mass effect severe enough to produce herniation, further vessel compromise, or even death.[10]

After several days to a week, so-called "luxury perfusion" allows dense enhancement of the affect area (Figs 5–8 and 5–9).[11-13] This enhancement occurs because of compromise of the blood-brain barrier at the interface of viable and nonviable brain or, in the case of cortical infarction, from a loss of autoregulation within leptomeningeal vessels. Enhancement of gyri is a constant finding if the infarction involves cortex (Figs 5–10 to 5–13). If only the periphery of a deep infarct enhances, a ring may be seen (Fig 5–14). Persistence of enhancement is variable, but may be as long as 8 to 10 weeks. Enhancement beyond this time is unusual for

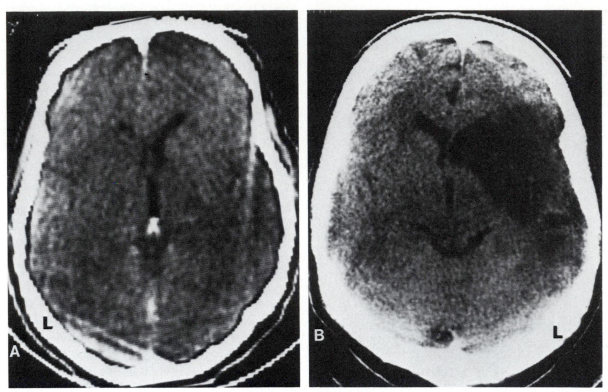

Fig 5–3.—Evolving infarct. **A,** about 6 hours after onset of this patient's right hemiplegia, the CT scan shows only effacement of the left frontal horn (patient's left *(L)* is on reader's left). **B,** seventy-two hours later, there is extreme lucency in the distribution of the left middle cerebral artery (patient's left *(L)* is on reader's right).

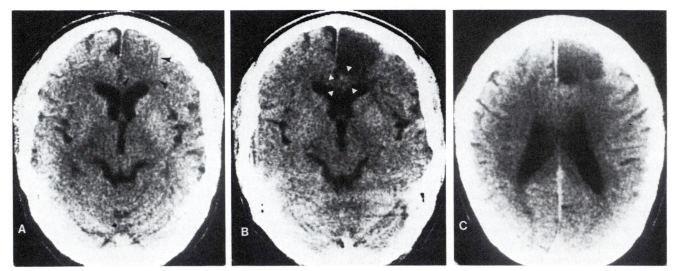

Fig 5–4.—Evolving anterior cerebral artery infarct. This 58-year-old woman presented with aphasia and right hemiparesis. **A,** the first CT scan is virtually normal. **B, C,** forty-eight hours later, marked lucency is seen in the distribution of the left anterior cerebral artery. In retrospect, a subtle lucency can be seen in this area on the first scan (**A,** *arrowheads*). Note that the corpus callosum itself is spared; its lack of lucency (**B,** *arrowheads*) shows it to remain preserved.

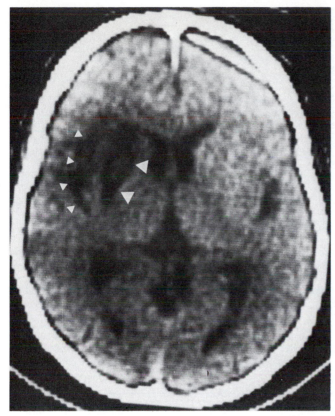

Fig 5–5.—Basal ganglion infarct. Lucency of the right lentiform nucleus *(large arrowheads)* marks this patient's infarct. Widening of the ipsilateral Sylvian fissure *(small arrowheads)* suggests some, but less, involvement of the middle cerebral artery distribution.

infarction. A more detailed description of contrast enhancement with infarction is found in Chapter 1.

Enhancement of brain parenchyma can occur without underlying *anatomical* abnormality, secondary to transient alteration of the blood-brain barrier. This is seen in the postictal state,[14] can conform to a vessel distribution, and have a CT appearance identical to that of an infarct. Over time, the CT scan returns to normal, the differentiating point (see Fig 5–13).

Delayed complications of infarction are not uncommon. Some seepage of blood through impaired endothelium can occur. If extensive, it may result in multiple petechial hemorrhages; this is by definition a hemorrhagic infarct. Contrasted with this is the more ominous gross hemorrhage into an infarct, which presents as an acute expanding intracranial mass and requires immediate decompression (Fig 5–15). Venous occlusion, with or without infarction, is associated with a higher likelihood of hemorrhage (Figs 5–16 and 5–17) than is arterial occlusion[15, 16] because of the transmitted back-pressure created by the venous occlusion.

Late CT changes consist of findings derivable from loss of brain: encephalomalacia, increase in sizes of subarachnoid space and ventricles, and, if the insult was massive, a displacement of normal tissue toward the area of encephalomalacia. This is typified by the Dyke-Davidoff syndrome,[17] in which intrauterine or neonatal carotid occlusion leads to hemispheric infarction in the growing skull (Fig 5–18). The radiographic syndrome comprises ventricular enlargement, elevation of the ipsilateral petrous bone and orbital roof, expansion of the frontal sinus on the affected side, and thickening of the skull over that hemisphere. Although unusual, dystrophic calcification can occur within an old infarct (Figs 5–18 and 5–19).

Patterns of infarction reflect the vascular territory involved.[18] As a rule, it is possible to determine the specific vessel(s) insulted. Thus, a wedge-shaped infarct results either from occlusion of several contiguous cortical arteries and is usually seen in the middle cerebral distribution (see Fig 5–3) or from hypotension and a watershed infarction. A "Mohican" appearance results from infarction of the anterior cerebral artery distribution (see Fig 5–4 and Chapter 4, Fig 4–9). This should be considered to be an axial view corresponding to the "Minnesota Vikings" sign, popularized for the lateral view of radionuclide brain scans. Basal ganglionic infarction may be isolated and result from fragmentation of a clot with immediate passage into the lenticulostriate arteries, or it may be associated with occlusion of the parent middle cerebral artery (see Figs 5–5 and 5–8). Other than with arteriopathy predisposing to the formation of lacunae, isolated thalamic infarction is rare, probably owing to the difficulty an embolus would have negotiating first the posterior communicating arteries and then the usually tiny thalamoperforate and thalamogeniculate arteries. Isolated posterior cerebral artery occlusion may cause lucency in the occipital and temporal lobes and in the thalamus, but if the vertebrobasilar system is more generally involved, the cerebellum and even brain stem may be affected (see Fig 5–6).

Infarction of the cerebellum is uncommon, reflecting rarity of embolization into the posterior circulation. Intracranial atherosclerosis, subclavian atheromata, aortic arch disease, or even intracardiac sources for emboli would be more likely than a primary vertebral artery source. Regardless of the cause, cerebellar infarction is a precarious state, because swelling can occur and may produce symptoms in at least three ways. First, the brain stem may be compressed. If a single hemisphere is involved, and this is the more common, the midbrain may be displaced against the *contra*lateral free edge of the tentorial incisura. Duret hemorrhages may further compromise function of the peduncle. In such a case, CT is invaluable, because the neurologic examination

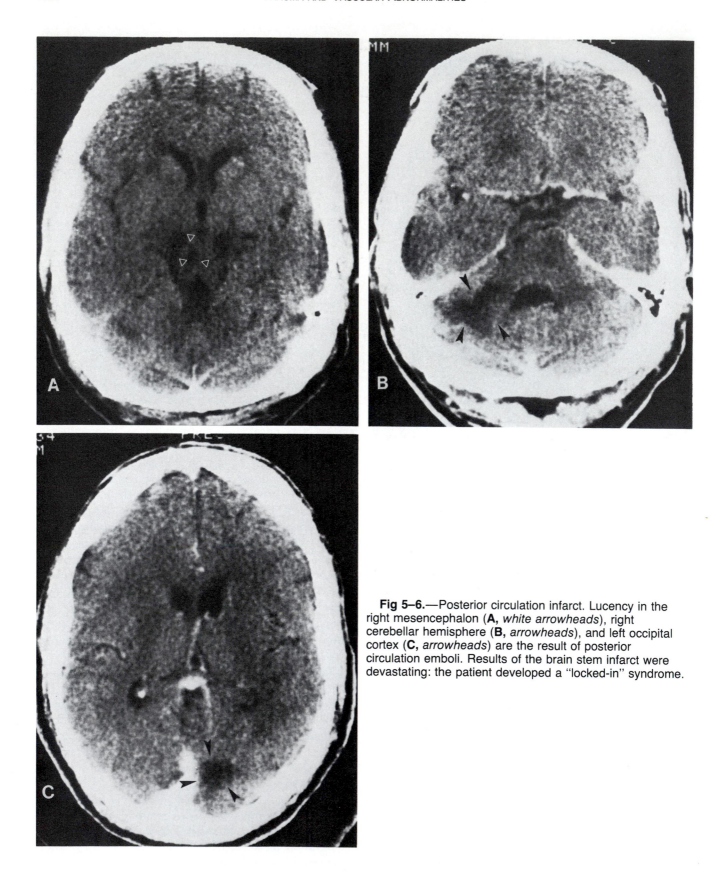

Fig 5–6.—Posterior circulation infarct. Lucency in the right mesencephalon (**A,** *white arrowheads*), right cerebellar hemisphere (**B,** *arrowheads*), and left occipital cortex (**C,** *arrowheads*) are the result of posterior circulation emboli. Results of the brain stem infarct were devastating: the patient developed a "locked-in" syndrome.

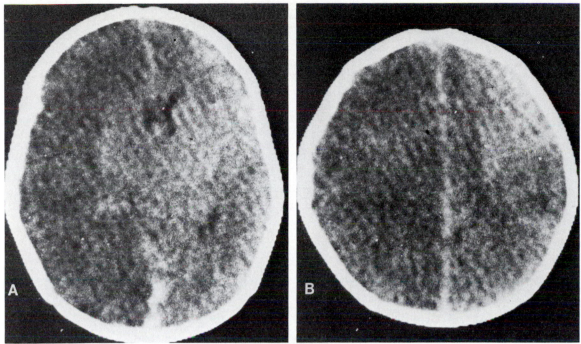

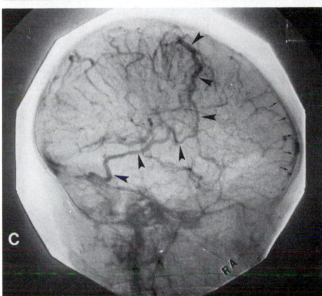

Fig 5–7.—Superior sagittal sinus thrombosis with extensive infarction. **A, B,** most of the right and the frontal pole of the left cerebral hemisphere are lucent and edematous from sagittal sinus thrombosis. **C,** lateral view, carotid angiography demonstrates some anterior opacification of the superior sagittal sinus *(arrows)*, but posteriorly it is unfilled. Large superficial collateral veins *(arrowheads)*—the vein of Trolard superiorly connecting to an ectatic vein of Labbé inferiorly—have replaced normal midline drainage.

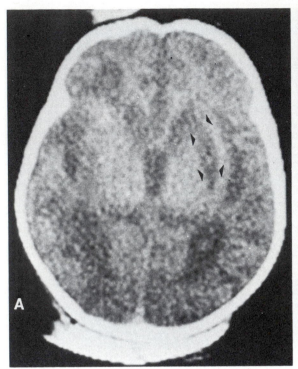

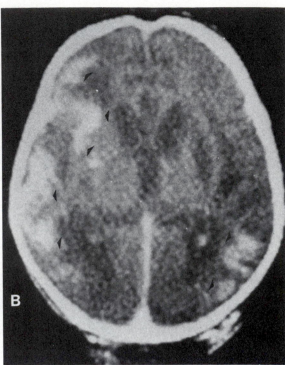

Fig 5–8.—Diffuse infarction following thoracic surgery. Multiple lucencies were noted on the scan of this patient, who had recently had correction of her great vessel transposition. Postoperatively, she had seizures and multiple confusing neurologic signs. **A,** the left lentiform nucleus *(arrowheads)* and numerous areas of cerebral cortex are lucent. **B,** contrast administration causes bilateral but patchy gyral enhancement *(arrowheads),* suggesting that these areas have been infarcted recently. Perhaps the other areas, e.g., the left lentiform nucleus, were involved preoperatively, probably as a result of the primary heart disease. Whether hypotension, a shower of emboli, or a combination of the two was responsible is uncertain.

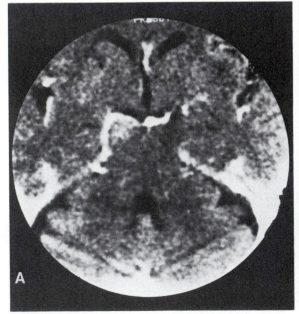

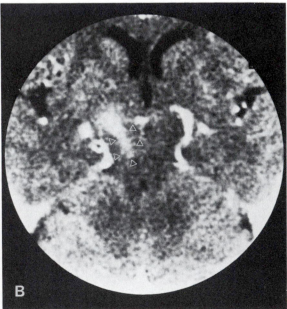

Fig 5–9.—Brain stem infarct: value of contrast enhancement. Infarction of the right cerebral peduncle **(A)** is seen with the use of contrast enhancement. Note how deeply the infarction penetrates the brain stem (**B,** *arrowheads*). The unenhanced study (not shown), even in retrospect, was normal.

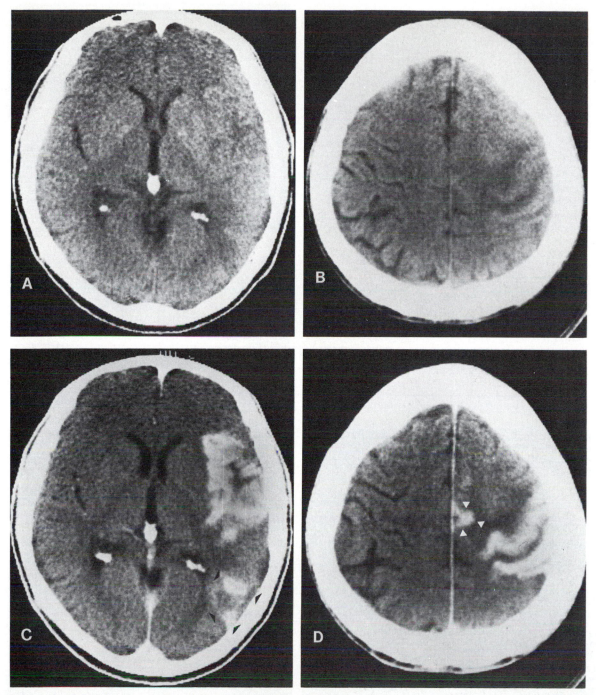

Fig 5–10.—Cortical infarction: value of contrast material. The lower unenhanced section **(A)** appears normal, while the higher one **(B)** demonstrates some effacement of cortical sulci, probably by gyral expansion. Contrast enhancement **(C, D)** of the posterior right frontal, temporal, and pa- rietal lobes to as high on the convexity as the midline shows the true extent of the infarct. Satellite areas of enhancement **(C, D,** *arrowheads*) suggest that the source was a shower of emboli.

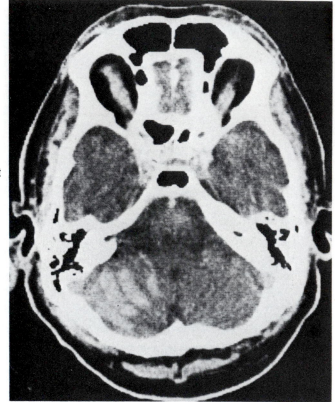

Fig 5–11.—Cerebellar infarction. Striate enhancement through the horizontal fissure of the right cerebellar hemisphere marks the infarcted tissue. The striated appearance of cerebellar infarction is analogous to the gyriform enhancement of cerebral cortical infarction.

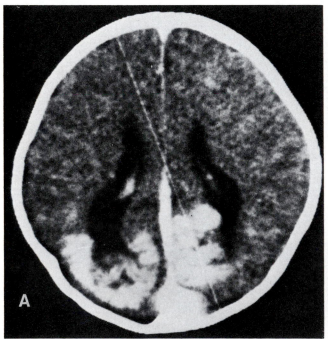

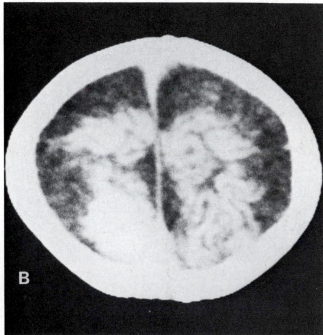

Fig 5–12.—Gyral enhancement with infarction. Extensive occipital **(A)** and parietal **(B)** infarction has resulted in enhancement of the involved cortex, enabling us to make the additional diagnosis of polymicrogyria in this child.

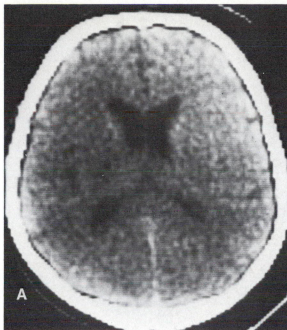 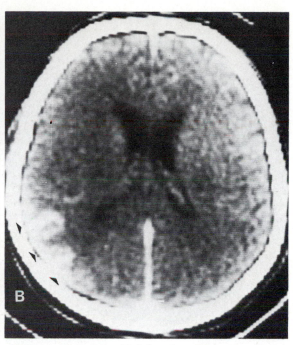

Fig 5–13.—Infarct-like enhancement with seizures. This patient had been having major motor seizures for 8 hours prior to the scan. Scans without **(A)** and with **(B)** contrast administration show cortical enhancement **(B,** *arrowheads*) similar to that seen with infarction. Clinical improvement with lack of deficit argued against a stroke. Follow-up studies were not required.

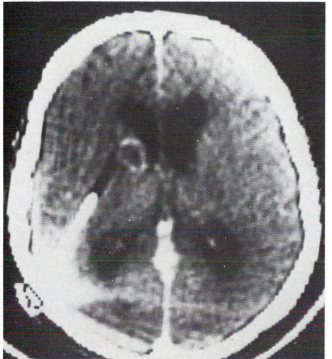

Fig 5–14.—Ring enhancement in infarct. The tract of a previous ventriculostomy catheter caused local encephalomalacia and infarction. Contrast administration has resulted in ring enhancement within the infarct.

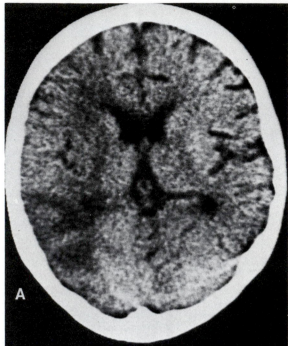 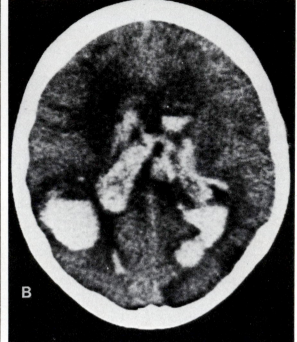

Fig 5–15.—Devastating hemorrhage into infarct. This heart transplant patient sustained a right temporo-occipital infarct. The first scan **(A)** shows a lucent lesion, and the patient was anticoagulated. Twenty-four hours later, there is massive intraparenchymal hemorrhage with extension into the ventricular system **(B).** Note the relaxed, generous subarachnoid space on the first study; intraventricular blood prevents normal CSF flow and produces an acute obstructive hydrocephalus. This expands the brain and effaces the subarachnoid space.

may give false localization. Secondly, downward herniation of the cerebellar tonsils and/or upward herniation of the upper pons and midbrain may occur. And third, compression of the aqueduct of Sylvius may cause an acute obstructive hydrocephalus.

If infarcts are multiple, and especially if they involve more than one hemisphere, an extracervical source should be sought (see Fig 5–8). Recall especially that hypotension and watershed infarction can also contribute to the pattern of multiple areas of involvement.

Differential diagnosis of infarction is not always simple. Acutely, an infarct is isodense, and an unenhanced CT scan will be normal. Thus, in the immediate state, a relative lack of normal contrast enhancement may be the only clue to the diagnosis. When blood flow measurements become more widespread and easier to perform, they will almost certainly make the diagnosis. One might expect nuclear magnetic resonance to be more sensitive than CT in the acute phase.

In the next phase, when the ischemic brain is lucent but does not yet contrast-enhance (see Figs 5–15,A, 5–4,B, and 5–4,C), differential diagnostic possibilities include low-grade tumor, especially astrocytoma, and demyelinating or other white matter disease processes. Because infarction usually involves cortex, also, cortical involvement favors infarct over tumor. If a mass effect

is present, the nontumorous possibilities can usually be excluded, but a neoplasm cannot. Again, even though low-grade tumor might not compromise the blood-brain barrier and become *denser* than normal brain after contrast infusion, it should change density by an amount similar to that of normal tissue, and over a similar time course.

Once contrast enhancement becomes a feature of infarction, inflammation must also be included as a CT diagnostic possibility (see Fig 5–14). Generally, contrast enhancement of infarcted brain is not associated with a positive mass effect and may even be seen with a negative one, corresponding to enlargement of ventricles and sulci. Conversely, an inflammatory process such as cerebritis with or without abscess formation tends to produce a positive mass effect, but occasionally produces none. A negative mass effect virtually excludes acute inflammation. In the enhancing phase, tumor may be even more difficult to discern from infarct unless the infarct is either wedge-shaped or cortical/gyral in distribution. Neither of these morphologies corresponds to any but the rarest of tumors. Here, even the time course of enhancement after infusion may be similar to that of a tumor; early venous drainage is angiographically consistent with both. Fortunately, during the enhancing phase, infarcts usually exert negative

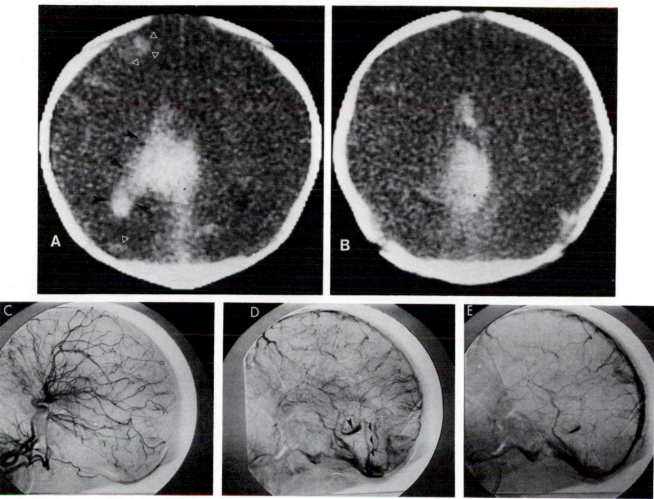

Fig 5–16.—Straight sinus and cortical venous thrombosis with resultant hemorrhage. **A, B,** CT shows intraventricular (**A,** *large arrowheads*), parenchymal, and subarachnoid hemorrhage. Additionally, small peripheral areas of hemorrhage (**A,** *small arrowheads*) probably result from multiple small cortical venous thromboses with local venous infarction and resultant hemorrhage. **C,** a single intracarotid metrizamide injection opacifies the entire intracranial circulation. **D,** while the deep venous system, including thalamostriate and internal cerebral veins, and particularly the vein of Galen *(large arrowhead)* are well opacified, only faint filling of the straight sinus (*small arrowheads*) is noted, and the basal veins of Rosenthal are not opacified, presumably secondary to increased venous back-pressure, itself caused by the partial straight sinus thrombosis. **E,** the late venous phase shows persistent opacification of the vein of Galen, but still only faint filling of the straight sinus; the vein of Galen cannot drain by any other route.

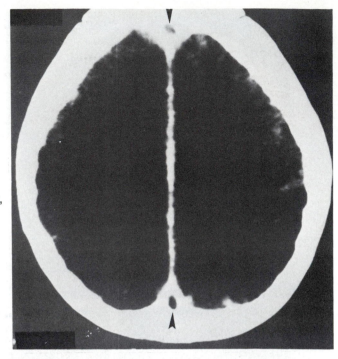

Fig 5–17.—Sagittal sinus thrombosis: delta sign. Normally, the enhanced sagittal sinus is homogeneously opaque. A thrombus within it usually appears as a filling defect, often triangular, and is referred to as a "delta" or "empty triangle" sign. Here, the thrombus is not triangular, but oval *(arrowheads)*.

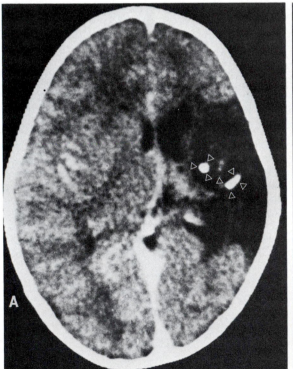

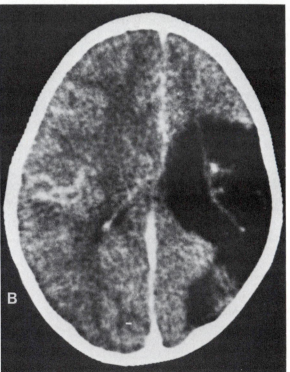

Fig 5–18.—Dystrophic calcification in old infarct. This patient's infarct occurred early in life, as can be inferred from the small hemicalvarium, large ventricle, and shift of midline structures to the small side of the skull. Dystrophic calcifications (**A,** *arrowheads*) lie within the malacic remains of the infarcted middle cerebral arterial territory (**A** and **B**).

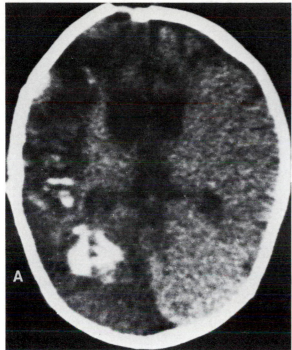 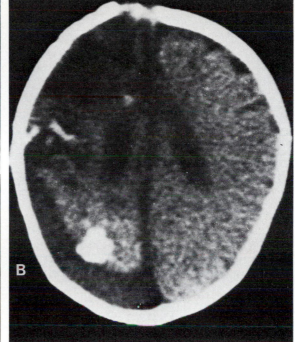

Fig 5–19.—Dystrophic calcification in infarct. Rarely reported, delayed changes of infarction can include parenchymal calcification as well as the common finding of loss of brain substance **(A, B).** Both are seen on this *un*enhanced study.

mass effects, and this generally supplies the needed clue. Persistence of enhancement for longer than 8 to 10 weeks strongly suggests tumor rather than infarction.

REFERENCES

1. Slager U.T.: Vascular disease, in Slager U.T. (ed.): *Basic Neuropathology.* Baltimore, Williams & Wilkins Co., 1970, pp. 45–66.
2. Schmidley J.W., Caronna J.J.: Transient cerebral ischemia: Pathophysiology. *Prog. Cardiovasc. Dis.* 22:325–342, 1980.
3. Mohr J.P.: Lacunes. *Stroke* 13:3–10, 1982.
4. Rascol A., Clanet M., Manelfe C., et al.: Pure motor hemiplegia: CT study of 30 cases. *Stroke* 13:11–17, 1982.
5. Caplan L.R., Hier D.B., Banks G.: Current concepts of cerebrovascular disease—stroke: Stroke and drug abuse. *Stroke* 13:869–872, 1982.
6. Duncan A.W., Rumbaugh C.L., Caplan L.: Cerebral embolic disease: A complication of carotid aneurysms. *Radiology* 133:379–384, 1979.
7. Drayer B.P., Dujovny M., Boehnke M., et al.: The capacity for computed tomography diagnosis of cerebral infarction. *Radiology* 125:393–402, 1977.
8. Hoff J.T., Nishimura M., Newfield P.: Pentobarbital protection from cerebral infarction without suppression of edema. *Stroke* 13:623–628, 1982.
9. Drayer B.P., Rosenbaum A.E.: Brain edema defined by cranial computed tomography. *J. Comput. Assist. Tomogr.* 3:317–323, 1979.
10. Kirshner H.S., Staller J., Webb W., et al.: Transtentorial herniation with posterior cerebral artery territory infarction. *Stroke* 13:243–246, 1982.
11. Skriver E.B., Olsen T.S.: Contrast enhancement of cerebral infarcts: Incidence and clinical value in different states of cerebral infarction. *Neuroradiology* 23:259–265, 1982.
12. Traupe H., Heiss W.-D., Hoeffken W., et al.: Hyperperfusion and enhancement in dynamic computed tomography of ischemic stroke patients. *J. Comput. Assist. Tomogr.* 3:627–632, 1979.
13. Caille J.M., Guibert F., Bidabe A.M., et al.: Enhancement of cerebral infarcts with CT. *Comput. Tomogr.* 4:73–77, 1980.
14. Rumack C.M., Guggenheim M.A., Fasules J.W., et al.: Transient positive postictal computed tomographic scan. *J. Pediatr.* 97:263–264, 1980.
15. Kingsley D.P.E., Kendall B.E., Moseley I.F.: Superior sagittal sinus thrombosis: An evaluation of the changes demonstrated on computed tomography. *J. Neurol. Neurosurg. Psychiatry* 41:1065–1068, 1978.
16. Matsuda M., Matsuda I., Sato M., et al.: Superior sagittal sinus thrombosis followed by subdural hematoma. *Surg. Neurol.* 18:206–211, 1982.
17. Dyke C.G., Davidoff L.M., Masson C.B.: Cerebral hemiatrophy with homolateral hypertrophy of the skull and sinuses. *Surg. Gynecol. Obstet.* 57:588–600, 1933.
18. Gado M.: CT correlative anatomy: The territories of the branches of anterior, middle, and posterior cerebral arteries. *J. Comput. Assist. Tomogr.* 3:553–554, 1979.

Infectious and Inflammatory Diseases of the Brain

6

Infectious Diseases of the Brain

ROBERT I. GROSSMAN, M.D.
ROBERT A. ZIMMERMAN, M.D.

THERE ARE a multitude of inflammatory and infectious diseases that affect the CNS. The brain responds to these in a limited fashion, so that a variety of pathologic processes result in similar radiographic pictures. Although these images are nonspecific with respect to the definitive organism, CT is exquisitely sensitive to its localization. With the clinical history, physical examination, and patient's age, the radiologist can more accurately interpret the CT images, and thus make a reasonable diagnosis.

There is no attempt in this chapter to consider all forms of infection and inflammation of the brain and its coverings. Special attention is devoted to pyogenic meningeal and parenchymal involvement. Specific nonpyogenic infectious and inflammatory diseases have been selected because of their importance and frequency. Tuberculosis and sarcoidosis are discussed as representative of granulomatous diseases. Coccidioidomycosis is an example of fungal infection; other fungal infections are discussed in Chapter 7. Cysticercosis is the most widespread parasitic cerebral infection in the world. Many viruses cause encephalitis, but herpes simplex encephalitis and subacute sclerosing panencephalitis secondary to postrubeola slow virus infection are two of the most important viruses affecting the brain.

EXTRAPARENCHYMAL INFECTION

Anatomy

There are three membranes that cover the brain. These are (from the outside inward) the dura mater, arachnoid, and pia mater. The dura mater is composed of two layers of very tough connective tissue. The outer layer is the skull's inner table periosteum. The inner layer is covered with mesothelium and lines the subdural space. The two layers separate to form the venous sinuses. The outer layer is adherent to the skull, espe-cially at the suture lines. The dura reflects and gives rise to the tentorium cerebelli, the falx cerebri, diaphragma sellae, and the falx cerebelli. The space between the inner table of the skull and the dura mater is the epidural space. The space between the outer dural covering and the arachnoid is the subdural space. This is a potential space containing bridging veins, which drain blood from the cortex into the venous sinuses, and outpouchings of the arachnoid (arachnoid villi), which project into the venous structures.

Beneath the subdural space are two layers of connective tissue, the pia and arachnoid, which together constitute the leptomeninges. The arachnoid is a delicate outer layer separated from the pia by the subarachnoid space, which contains the cerebrospinal fluid (CSF). The pia is closely applied to the brain and carries a vast network of blood vessels. Figure 6–1 illustrates this anatomy.

Locations and Forms of Infection

Leptomeningitis

The pathologic process of meningitis (leptomeningitis) involves inflammatory infiltration of the pia-arachnoid (Fig 6–2). The leptomeningeal inflammation most often occurs following hematogenous dissemination from a distant infectious focus. Direct extension from an infected site such as sinusitis or otitis media is much less common. Following septicemia, bacteria may lodge in venous sinuses and precipitate inflammatory changes, which in turn can interfere with CSF absorption. With stagnation of CSF absorption, bacteria are offered the opportunity of invading the meninges.[1]

Early in the course of infection, there is congestion of the pial vessels. Later, an exudate covers the brain, especially in the dependent sulci and basal cisterns. The leptomeninges become thickened.[2]

Clinical features are related to patient age (Table 6–1). Infants and particularly neonates may have a per-

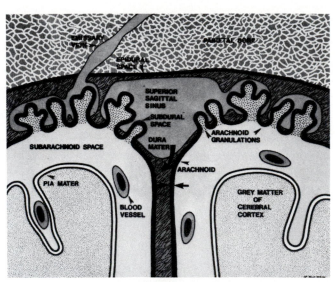

Fig 6–1.—Coronal section through sagittal sinus demonstrating the spaces around the brain and its coverings. The *curved arrow* is on the dura matter and the falx cerebri. The two *unmarked arrows* point to the dura and the arachnoid, with the potential subdural space between them.

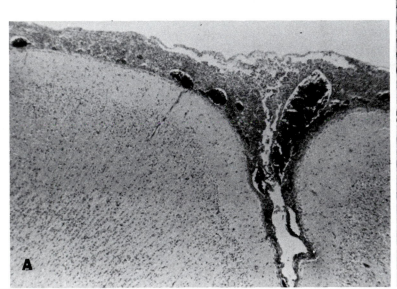 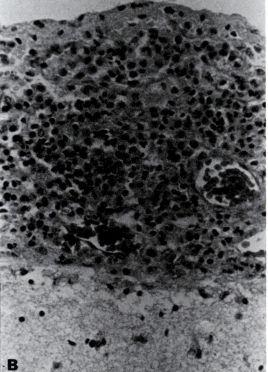

Fig 6–2.—Pathology of leptomeningitis: **A,** low-power view of thickened leptomeninges *(arrows)* in a patient with bacterial meningitis. **B,** high-power view of leptomeninges with dense polymorphonuclear infiltrate.

TABLE 6–1.—CLINICAL FEATURES
OF LEPTOMENINGITIS

INFANTS	ADULTS
Fever	Fever
Vomiting	Headache
Irritability	Photophobia
Anorexia	Pain and stiffness of neck
Constipation	Kernig's sign
Altered state of consciousness	
Seizures	
Bulging fontanel	
Kernig's sign	

plexing clinical picture, lacking signs that directly demonstrate meningeal irritation.

The CT findings in early as well as in successfully treated cases of meningitis are reported to be normal.[6] Exceptions to this in acute meningitis are (1) visualization of distended subarachnoid spaces (most easily recognized in children as abnormal, especially on sequential studies leading to recovery) (Fig 6–3) and (2) acute cerebral swelling (often leading to herniation and death). Communicating hydrocephalus with enlargement of the temporal horns and effacement of the basal cisterns may be visualized on the nonenhanced CT.

Within several days of the onset of meningitis, it is not uncommon to visualize marked contrast enhancement of the leptomeninges (Fig 6–4).[7, 8] This finding in itself does not appear to be of prognostic significance. Parenchymal abnormalities are primarily those of low-absorption areas, which may or may not enhance. These pathologically represent areas of infarction and subsequent necrosis secondary to focal vasculitis. Rarely, this represents cerebritis. The vasculitis may involve either arteries or veins; hence, the pattern of infarction will differ depending on the location, number, and type of vessels involved. Table 6–2 summarizes the spectrum of CT abnormalities in purulent meningitis.

Many complications occur as a result of inflammation involving the meninges. These sequelae are better imaged and characterized than are the manifestations of the meningitis itself. Communicating hydrocephalus occurs as both an early and late manifestation of leptomeningitis, not infrequently becoming symptomatic to the point of requiring ventricular shunting. The subacute CT findings of complicated leptomeningeal infection are those of atrophy, encephalomalacia (infarction), focal abscess, subdural empyema formation, and basilar loculations of CSF (Fig 6–5) (Table 6–3).[9]

Neonates represent a special case with respect to the cerebral sequelae of leptomeningitis. Gram-negative rods such as *Escherichia coli* are the chief offenders. The neonatal meningitides are believed to be acquired as a result of the delivery process. The lack of a developed immune system at birth makes the neonates susceptible to organisms that are normally not very virulent. These children frequently suffer severe parenchymal brain damage that ultimately produces a multi-

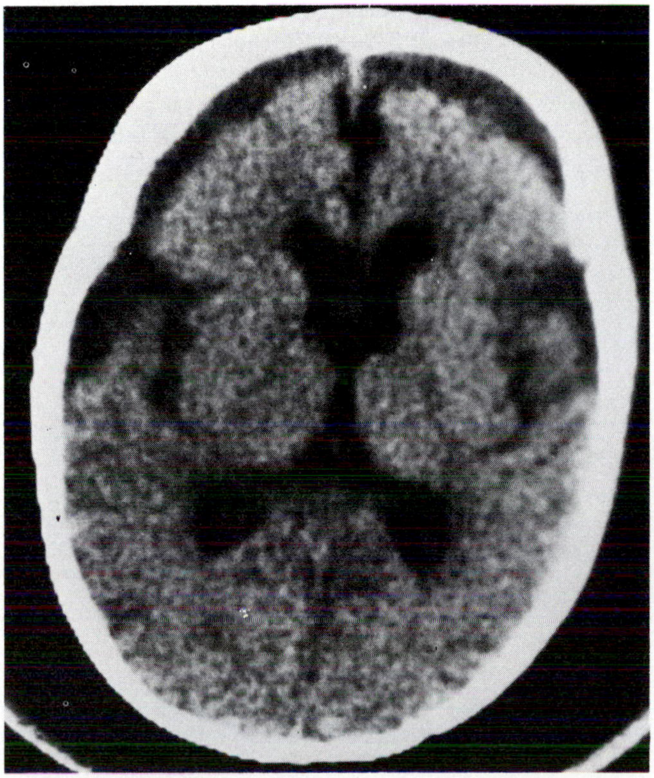

Fig 6–3.—Distended subarachnoid spaces in a child with *Hemophilus influenzae* meningitis.

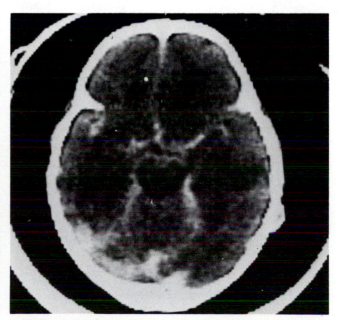

Fig 6–4.—Enhancement of the leptomeninges in bacterial meningitis.

TABLE 6–2.—SPECTRUM
OF CT FEATURES
OF LEPTOMENINGITIS

Normal scan
Enlargement of CSF spaces
Poor visualization of basal cisterns
Decreased parenchymal absorption
Focal parenchymal enhancement
General cerebral swelling
Diffuse meningeal enhancement
Communicating hydrocephalus
Subdural effusion

TABLE 6–3.—CT-DEMONSTRATED
COMPLICATIONS OF
LEPTOMENINGEAL INFECTION

Hydrocephalus
  A. Communicating
  B. Obstructive
Venous thrombosis
Arterial infarction
Atrophy
Encephalomalacia
Focal abscess formation
Basilar adhesions
Subdural empyema
Subdural hygroma
Epidural empyema

TABLE 6–4.—ETIOLOGIES
OF SUBDURAL EMPYEMA

Purulent bacterial meningitis
Postcraniotomy infection
Paranasal sinusitis
Otitis media
Osteomyelitis of the calvarium
Posttrauma
Hematogenous dissemination

cystic brain.[10] The CT findings are those of multifocal encephalomalacia leading to multiple distended intra- and paraventricular cysts (Fig 6–6).

Subdural Empyema

Disruption of the arachnoid meningeal barrier by infection leads to the formation of CSF collections within a potential compartment in the subdural space. These may present acutely or chronically, and they may be sterile or infected at time of presentation.

Empyema, rather than abscess, is the appropriate term for a purulent infection in this preformed space. Table 6–4 lists the etiologies of subdural empyema. Among the several possible mechanisms by which a subdural empyema is thought to form are (1) a distended arachnoid villus rupturing into the subdural space and infecting it; (2) phlebitic bridging veins (secondary to meningitis) infecting the subdural space; (3) the subdural space infected by direct hematogeneous dissemination, and (4) by direct extension through necrotic arachnoid membrane from the subarachnoid space.[11]

Clinical signs and symptoms in this group of patients include fever, vomiting, meningismus, seizures, and hemiparesis. The duration of symptoms prior to presentation ranges from 1 to 8 weeks. The mortality from subdural empyema has been reported to range from 25% to 40%. Prompt treatment with appropriate antibiotics and extensive craniotomy can result in a favorable outcome.[12–14]

Features in CT of subdural empyema are those of low-absorption extracerebral collections over the convex-

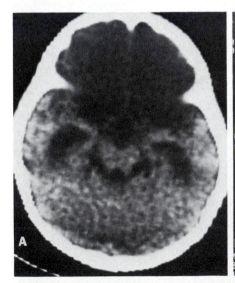
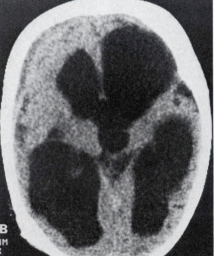
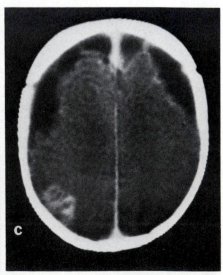

Fig 6–5.—Complications of leptomeningitis. **A,** frontal infarction following gram-negative leptomeningitis. **B,** same patient as in Figure 6–3, only 3 months later showing significant central parenchymal loss. **C,** subdural empyema and focal abscess after purulent leptomeningitis.

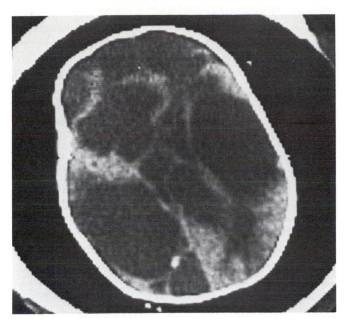

Fig 6–6.—Sequelae of neonatal leptomeningitis and ventriculitis: the polycystic brain.

ities and within the interhemispheric fissure (Fig 6–7). There may be effacement of the cortical sulci and mass effect on the ventricular system. After intravenous contrast, a rim of enhancement may be observed. This enhancement is predicated upon an adequate length of time for the development of granulation tissue. High-resolution coronal scanning following contrast is quite useful for confirming the diagnosis of an extracerebellar purulent collection. Depending upon the changes produced in the adjacent cerebral vessels, gyriform enhancement may also be demonstrated.

Epidural Abscess

Epidural abscess is most often the result of infection extending from the middle ear, paranasal sinuses, or cranium into the epidural space. Syphilis is one of the few causes of a primary epidural abscess (pachymeningitis externa).[15, 16] The CT findings of epidural abscess are those of a peripheral low-absorption area and mass effect. The epidural abscess can extend into the subgaleal space as well, a finding more frequent when the abscess occurs as a postoperative complication.[17]

Epidural abscesses can cross the midline, a finding that serves to distinguish the epidural abscess from the subdural empyema (Fig 6–8). A specific site of origin for the infection and its contiguous spread into the extracerebral space also helps to establish the diagnosis of epidural abscess.[18] Following intravenous contrast, an enhanced rim is frequently seen.

PARENCHYMAL PYOGENIC INFECTION

The advent of CT has radically altered both the diagnosis and management of pyogenic brain abscesses. Prior to CT, localization and detection of intracranial

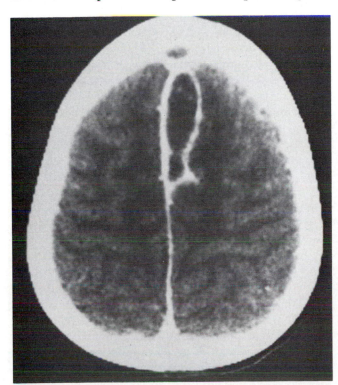

Fig 6–7.—Subdural empyema: contrast enhancement of subdural empyema with associated edema. Note that the empyema does not cross the midline and is dural based.

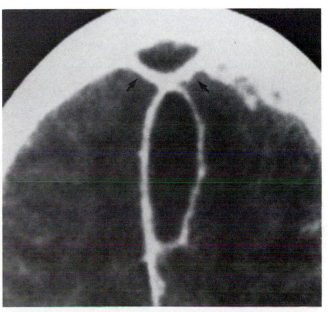

Fig 6–8.—Enhancing epidural abscess (arrows) in patients with subdural empyema. Patient had frontal sinus infection. Note that it straddles the midline and displaces the anterior attachment of the falx.

suppuration was highly dependent on clinical acumen. Headache, fever, vomiting, lethargy, focal neurologic deficit, and seizures are the most common presenting neurologic symptoms. Electroencephalographic slow-focus activity and radioisotope scanning were reasonably good localizing methods and were supplemented by ventriculography, angiography, and pneumoencephalography.[19] Mortality from cerebral abscess in the pre-CT era ranged between 30% to 60%. This has been drastically reduced in post-CT years, with some centers reporting no mortality with purulent abscess.[20, 21] This change has occurred because of CT's sensitivity in detection and its ability to localize lesions. Also, CT supplies a means whereby the results of surgery and antibiotics are readily monitored.

Cerebral abscess most often is the result of hematogenous dissemination from a primary infectious site. The various etiologies of cerebral abscess are listed in Table 6–5. The most frequent locations are the frontal and parietal lobes. Intracranial abscess affects predominantly the preadolescent and middle-age groups. This is related, in part, to the incidence of congenital heart disease, drug abuse, and to otitic and paranasal sinus infections (Fig 6–9). In all series, there is preponderance of males over females.[22] Abscesses may be unilocular or multilocular. They may be solitary or multiple. There are a variety of bacterial organisms commonly cultured from brain abscess (Table 6–6). In addition, there are numerous other pathogens that can infect the brain under the appropriate circumstances. Many of these latter conditions are covered in the chapter on the immunosuppressed host.

There have been several animal models of cerebral abscess. Wood and coworkers[23] used the monkey and embolized infected spheres via the internal carotid artery. He concluded that abscess formation was dependent upon stasis of bacteria as well as a focus of ischemic or necrotic brain. Enzmann and colleagues[24, 25] established brain abscesses in dogs by direct inoculation of bacteria into the brain parenchyma. He divided abscess formation into four stages: (1) early cerebritis (1 to 3 days), (2) late cerebritis (4 to 9 days), (3) early capsule formation (10 to 13 days), and (4) late capsule formation (14 days and later). The cerebritis phase of abscess formation consists of an inflammatory infiltrate of polymorphonuclear cells, lymphocytes, and plasma cells. By the third day, a necrotic center is forming. This deliquescent region is surrounded by inflammatory cells, new blood vessels, and hyperplastic fibroblasts. In the late cerebritis phase, extracellular edema and hyperplastic astrocytes are seen. Thus, the cerebritis phase of abscess formation starts as a suppurative focus, which breaks down and begins to become encapsulated by collagen at 10 to 13 days. This process continues with increasing capsule thickness.[24, 25]

The deposition of collagen is particularly important, because it directly limits the spread of the infection. Factors that affect collagen deposition include host resistance, duration of infection, characteristics of the organism, and drug therapy. Corticosteroids may decrease the formation of a fibrous capsule and may decrease the effectiveness of antibiotic therapy in the cerebritis phase, as well as reduce antibiotic penetration into the brain abscess.[26, 27] Brain abscesses that are hematogenously related usually occur at the junction of the gray and white matter. It is observed that collagen deposition is asymmetric with the side toward the white matter and ventricle having a thinner wall, resulting in a propensity for intraventricular rupture. Death from cerebral abscess is due to either its mass effect with herniation and/or the development of a ventricular empyema. In the late capsule phase, there is continued encapsulation and decreasing diameter of the necrotic center. Conservative therapy using antibiotics alone has been advocated in conjunction with close monitoring of the clinical and CT findings in patients with multiple abscesses, with those in sensitive locations, and with those who are poor surgical candidates.[28–30]

The characteristics of cerebral abscess depend upon the pathologic phase during which the abscess is being examined. In the cerebritis phase, CT demonstrates low-absorption abnormalities with appropriate mass effect. There is patchy or gyriform enhancement (Fig 6–10).[31] In the later cerebritis phase, ring enhancement may be present. Thus, the presence of ring enhancement should not unequivocally imply capsule formation.[24] Duration of symptoms is important in assessing

TABLE 6–5.—ETIOLOGIES
OF CEREBRAL ABSCESS

Hematogenous dissemination
  A. Pulmonary
  B. Cardiac
  C. Drug abuse
  D. Other
Direct extension
  A. Otitic
  B. Paranasal sinus
Trauma
  A. Penetrating injury
  B. Postsurgical

TABLE 6–6.—COMMON BACTERIA
CAUSING CEREBRAL ABSCESS

Aerobic bacteria	Anaerobic bacteria
Staphylococcus aureus	Streptococcus
Streptococcus viridans	Bacteroides
Hemolytic streptococcus	
Pneumococcus	
Gram-negative	
(E. coli, Proteus, Pseudomonas, H. influenzae)	

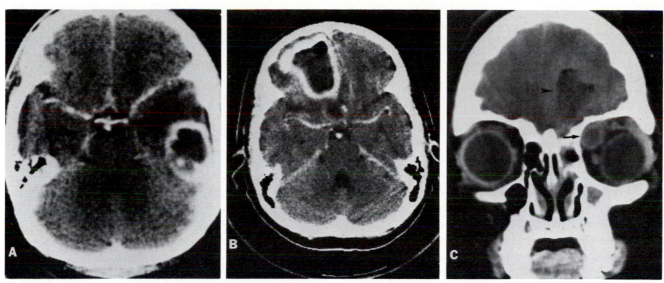

Fig 6–9.—A, intracranial abscess secondary to mastoiditis: ring-enhancing lesion in temporal lobe representing purulent bacterial abscess following mastoiditis. **B,** intracranial frontal abscess with gas-forming organism. **C,** coronal CT of patient **(B).** Note soft tissue in ethmoid sinuses, source of infection, which has produced an orbital abscess *(arrow).* Frontal abscess with gas is also demonstrable *(arrowhead).*

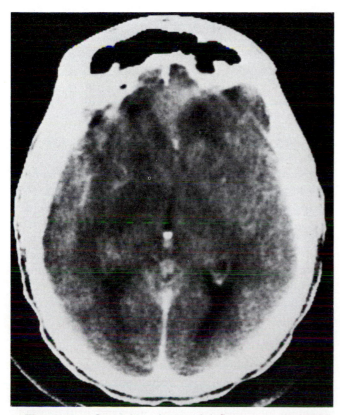

Fig 6–10.—Cerebritis phase of inflammatory reaction: patchy enhancement and mass effect in right frontotemporal region.

capsule formation. Britt and coworkers[25] suggest that the ring lesion of cerebritis may be distinguished from encapsulated abscess by delayed scanning. In the cerebritis phase, contrast was observed to have diffused into the necrotic center, while this did not occur in the well-formed brain abscess.

The encapsulated intracerebral abscess reveals a low-absorption center and usually has mass effect (see Fig 6–9,B). Very rarely does an abscess present as a high absorption on the plain scan[32] or as a homogeneous enhancing area on the postinjection study. With intravenous contrast, a uniform ring is most typical. The enhanced ring surrounds the central area of low absorption (necrotic center). A low density surrounds the enhanced ring and is due to edema fluid. It is a smooth, thin enhancing rim that suggests an abscess. Thickness, irregularity, and nodularity of the ring should raise the suspicion that one is dealing with a tumor (in most cases) or an unusual infection (fungus, etc.). However, many exceptions to this rule occur, and nodular, irregular pyogenic abscesses are not that infrequent.[33–35] Some of these represent subacute and chronic abscesses, while others are the result of adjacent daughter abscess formation. The ring-enhanced lesion should not be evaluated in a clinical vacuum. The appropriate history is essential for a specific diagnosis. Table 6–7 is a partial differential diagnosis of a ring-enhanced lesion. The treated brain abscess may enhance and show low absorption for long periods of time (over 8 months) in an otherwise asymptomatic patient.

TABLE 6–7.—Differential
Diagnosis of Ring Enhancement

Pyogenic brain abscess
Fungal infection
Infarction
Primary brain tumor
Metastatic brain tumor
Granuloma
Multiple sclerosis
Subacute hematoma

VENTRICULITIS

Infection of the ependyma of the ventricles may occur secondary to rupture of a parenchymal abscess into the ventricles, extension from a leptomeningeal infection, or following ventricular shunting. In neonates, ventriculitis may be the only manifestation of diffuse leptomeningitis. Chronic ventriculitis results in synechiae within the ventricles as well as obstruction of CSF egress. Small nodules on the ependymal surface are seen at autopsy on these patients.

Usually, CT reveals dilated ventricles with a thin rim of enhancement following the ependymal surface. Periventricular low absorption may also be seen (Fig 6–11).

NONPYOGENIC FORMS OF INFECTION AND INFLAMMATION

Tuberculosis

Although the incidence of intracranial tuberculosis has declined considerably in the past 40 years, it still remains a diagnostic dilemma. Intracranial tuberculosis has two related pathologic processes, tuberculous meningitis and the intracerebral tuberculoma. Tuberculous meningitis is seen in children associated with primary infection in geographic areas where tuberculosis is common. In the United States, tuberculous meningitis is noted among adults, particularly blacks and Asian immigrants.[36–39]

The pathophysiology of tuberculous meningitis begins with an initial focus that is usually pulmonic, but may occur in the abdomen or genitourinary tract. There is hematogenous dissemination of the bacilli to seed the leptomeninges and brain parenchyma. Often, granulomas are then formed. These granulomas may be dormant for years. The infection may completely resolve, or the granuloma may rupture into the subarachnoid space, discharging its necrotic debris and causing tuberculous meningitis. The granuloma is a small (1- to 3-mm diameter) nodule that may have a caseous center. There can be coalescence of these tubercles to form a large lesion. The basal cisterns are most affected by the exudative meningitis. Obstruction to the normal CSF flow results in hydrocephalus. Inflammatory changes in the blood vessels caused by this process leads to an ar-

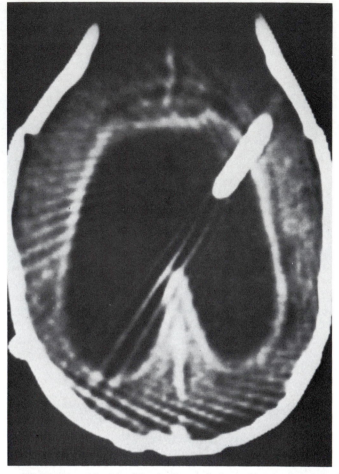

Fig 6–11.—Ventriculitis: hydrocephalus with shunt in left lateral ventricle and thin enhancement of ependyma of lateral ventricles.

teritis and infarction. Cranial nerve palsy occurs secondary to the basilar meningoneuritis.

Clinical features of tuberculous meningitis include confusion, headache, lethargy, and meningismus. This progresses in a subacute fashion with stupor, coma, decerebrate rigidity, cranial nerve palsy, and stroke possible. It is interesting to note that 19% of patients with tuberculous meningitis had *no* evidence of extrameningeal active disease at the time of diagnosis.[40, 41] Patients have low-grade fevers, with lumbar puncture revealing hypoglycorrhachia, increased protein, pleocytosis (predominantly lymphocytes), and negative smears.[42] The tuberculin skin test is often negative early in the disease.[43]

The intracerebral tuberculoma produces symptoms from mass effect and associated edema. These are related to the location of the lesion. Tuberculomas may be simple or multiple.[44] They can occur in the supra- and infratentorial regions. Features of CT depend upon the stage of the infection. In tuberculous meningitis, the basal and Sylvian cisterns are poorly visualized

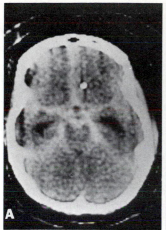
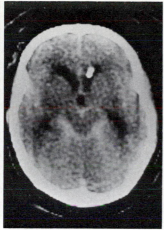
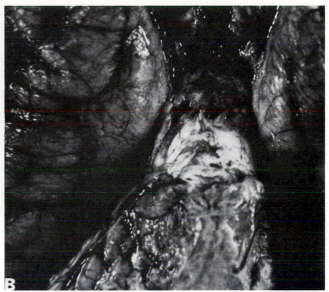

Fig 6–12.—Tuberculous meningitis. **A,** dense enhancement around basal *(left)* and perimesencephalic *(right)* cisterns with hydrocephalus. **B,** specimen in same patient. Note the purulent exudate around brain stem.

without contrast because of the dense exudate. They enhance uniformly and intensely (Fig 6–12).[45] Sequelae of the meningitis include hydrocephalus and low-absorption regions representing infarction secondary to the panarteritis.[46]

The intracerebral tuberculoma appears as a nodule that ranges from low to high absorption on plain scan. Calcification is reported in 1% to 6% of cases.[47, 48] The tuberculoma can cause hyperostosis, and as it enlarges it may adhere to dura, thus masquerading as a meningioma.[49] These nodules are associated with hydrocephalus and mass effect. They may be solitary or multiple. Contrast is necessary to demonstrate all the nodules. These lesions enhance, and some of them may show a characteristic punctate lucent center representing the central area of caseous necrosis.[50] The typical tuberculoma appears as an enhanced nodule with a small area of central low absorption (caseous necrosis) surrounded by a low-absorption region (edema) (Fig 6–13).

Intracerebral tuberculoma in cases of tuberculous meningitis is not necessarily revealed by CT, and obviously not all patients with intracerebral tuberculoma have meningeal enhancement.

Follow-up CT after appropriate antibiotic therapy reveals that the tuberculous nodules decrease in size and may show small areas of punctate calcifications at the tuberculoma site.[50] At times, the tuberculoma may be transformed into a calcified nodule that does not enhance. This calcified nodule may completely resorb.[51] In tuberculous meningitis, there is no demonstrable improvement in the degree of hydrocephalus.[52] This is secondary to the dense adhesions formed from the co-

pious exudate. The CT findings of CNS tuberculosis are summarized in Table 6–8.

Sarcoidosis

This systemic granulomatous disease of unknown etiology primarily occurs in the third and fourth de-

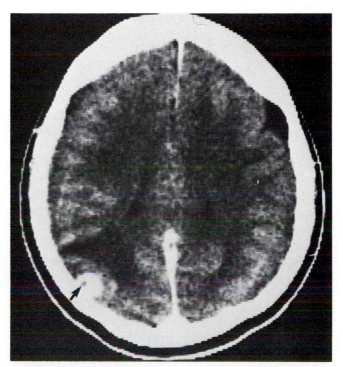

Fig 6–13.—Tuberculoma. Enhanced nodule with small central region of caseous necrosis *(arrow)* is surrounded by edema.

TABLE 6–8.—CT OF INTRACRANIAL TUBERCULOSIS

TUBERCULOMA NODULES (SOLITARY OR MULTIPLE)	MENINGITIS
Plain scan	Plain scan
Low-high absorption	Obliteration of basal and Sylvian cisterns
Mass effect	Calcification in basilar cisterns
Hydrocephalus	Hydrocephalus†
Calcification (1%–6%)*	Infarction
Hyperostosis (rare)	Contrast scan
Contrast scan	Uniform enhancement of leptomeninges
Uniform enhancement	Tuberculoma (occasionally)
Small lucent center	
Low absorption around nodule	
Meningeal enhancement	

*Nodules may decrease in size and show calcification following therapy.
†Ventricular dilatation usually remains in treated tuberculous meningitis.

cades, affecting the nervous system in approximately 5% of cases.[53] This figure includes involvement of peripheral nerves and myopathy. A very small percentage of patients have only the CNS disease without systemic manifestations.[54–56] Sarcoidosis of the CNS is an exclusionary diagnosis, because a positive biopsy only represents a nonspecific reaction to a variety of diseases.

Granulomatous intracranial disease has two patterns. The more common presentation is a chronic basilar leptomeningitis with involvement of the hypothalamus, pituitary gland, and optic chiasm. Patients may present with unilateral or bilateral cranial nerve (particularly VII) palsy and endocrine or electrolyte disturbances. These patients develop communicating hydrocephalus and may have signs of meningeal irritation. The granulomatous process frequently spreads from the leptomeninges to the Virchow-Robin spaces, invading and thrombosing affected blood vessels.[57, 58]

The second pattern is that of parenchymal sarcoid nodules. These granulomatous masses are usually associated with extensive arachnoiditis and microscopic granuloma throughout the brain parenchyma. They have been reported to cause obstructive hydrocephalus when located in the periaqueductal region.[59] These masses may be calcified and avascular. The sarcoid nodules produce signs and symptoms of an intracranial mass. The CSF abnormalities are those of elevated lymphocytes and protein with hypoglycorrhachia. These findings are quite nonspecific and not diagnostic for this disease.[60]

Unenhanced CT reveals hydrocephalus, either communicating or obstructive. Nodules may be calcified, of slightly increased absorption, or isodense and can occur throughout the brain parenchyma with a marked predilection for the base (pituitary, pons, hypothalamic) and periventricular regions. The nodules are not usually associated with edema.

Intravenous contrast produces homogeneous enhancement.[61] As opposed to tuberculoma nodules, sarcoid nodules do not develop lucent centers. The lepto-

meninges enhance when involved (Fig 6–14), and gyriform enhancement has also been reported.[62] Sarcoid has masqueraded as a brain tumor, pituitary lesion, meningioma, and even angiographically as a subdural hematoma.[60, 63–65] Dramatic response has been noted in some cases, with corticosteroid therapy producing a disappearance of the enhancing lesions.[53, 62] The CT picture clearly reflects the pathologic process, with hydrocephalus, homogeneously enhancing nodules, and leptomeninges as the hallmarks of intracranial sarcoid.

Herpes Simplex

Herpes simplex virus is the most common cause of fatal endemic encephalitis.[66] The survivors of this virus suffer severe memory and personality problems. Supposedly, early diagnosis and speedy therapy with antiviral agents can favorably affect the outcome.[67] Both the oral strain (Type 1) and the genital strain (Type 2) may produce encephalitis in man. Type 2 is responsible for infection in the neonatal period, presumably acquired either transplacentally or during birth from mothers with genital herpes.[68, 69] This strain may cause a variety

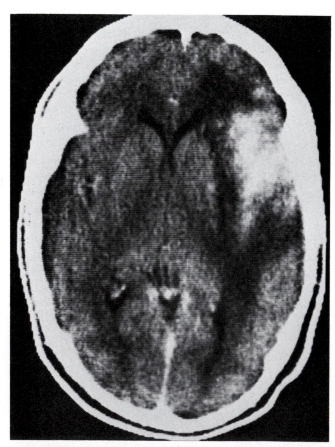

Fig 6–14.—Sarcoid: leptomeningeal enhancement in Sylvian cistern. (Courtesy of David Norman, M.D., University of California at San Francisco.)

of teratogenic problems, including intracranial calcifications, microcephaly, microphthalmia, and retinal dysplasia.[70] Sequelae from neonatal herpes also includes multicystic encephalomalacia, seizures, motor deficits, mental and motor retardation, and porencephaly.[71, 72]

The Type 1 virus produces the fulminant, necrotizing encephalitis seen in adults. The clinical picture is one of acute confusion and disorientation followed rapidly by stupor and coma. Seizures, viral prodrome, fever, and headache are also common presentations. Those patients with left temporal disease become symptomatic earlier because of their language impairment and thus may have more subtle CT findings at the time of presentation.

The pathologic findings are quite stereotyped. The virus asymmetrically attacks the temporal lobes, insula, orbitofrontal region, and cingulate gyrus. A possible explanation for the focality of herpes simplex Type 1 may depend on its known latency in the trigeminal ganglia. This latent virus under certain circumstances becomes reactivated and spreads along the trigeminal nerve fibers that innervate the meninges of the anterior and middle cranial fossae.[73] A diffuse meningoencephalitis with a predominant lymphocytic infiltration is seen. There is marked necrosis and hemorrhage with loss of all neural and glial elements. The end result, if the patient survives, is an atrophic cystic parenchyma. Laboratory diagnosis is dependent upon culturing the virus or on fluorescent antibody staining.[74, 75]

The CT features of intracranial neonatal herpes are quite different from those in adults and are summarized in Table 6–9.[76, 77] In adult Type 1 herpes encephalitis, CT findings within the first 5 days of the disease may be quite subtle.[78] The earliest abnormalities are low-absorption areas in the temporal lobe and insular cortex. These regions may be associated with mass effect and ventricular compression that progresses with time. Hemorrhage may be identified on unenhanced scans, although its incidence on CT varies depending on the reporting center.[78, 79] The areas of low absorption in the temporal lobe and insula abruptly end at the lateral putamen, which is characteristically spared. It is most unusual to have an isolated frontal or parietal involvement. The full extent of parenchymal damage is difficult to assess during the first 10 days of the disease.[78]

With intravenous contrast, linear, subarachnoid, or gyriform enhancement may be visualized. After 7 days,

TABLE 6–9.—CT FEATURES
OF NEONATAL HERPES SIMPLEX

Multiple cysts
Intracranial calcification (periventricular)
Hydrocephalus
Atrophy

almost all patients should have enhancement (Fig 6–15). Mass effect may persist for a considerable time period (39 days in one case).[80] Residual abnormalities include areas of low absorption and parenchymal loss at the site of involvement. Diffuse cortical calcification in an infant[79] (Fig 6–16) has also been described. Herpes simplex encephalitis is a potentially treatable encephalitis where outcome is dependent on early diagnosis, and CT remains of paramount importance in the diagnosis of this process.

Subacute Sclerosing Panencephalitis (SSPE)

This disease is a slow viral infection that occurs in children and young adolescents temporally following an innocent measles infection 3 to 9 years earlier. The infection progresses through stages. Initially, it starts with difficulty in language and behavioral changes.[81, 82] This is followed by intellectual deterioration, ataxia, chorea, dystonic rigidity, seizures, myoclonus, and ocular problems (optic atrophy, cortical blindness, chorioretinitis). In the final stages, the child is unresponsive, displaying severe autonomic dysfunction, and progresses to coma and death within months to years.[83, 84] The course occasionally is prolonged and associated with one or more remissions.

Supportive laboratory evidence of SSPE includes marked elevation of the CSF gamma globulin content. Electroencephalography is characterized by periodic high-voltage slow and sharp waves. Elevated levels of neutralizing antibody to measles (rubeola) virus are found in the CSF and serum[85, 86] It is rare to isolate rubeola from the brain tissue. Pathologic changes include eosinophilic intranuclear inclusions and demyelination of perivascular lymphocytic infiltration.

In patients with the rapidly progressive form of the disease, CT usually does not reveal significant abnormality; however, cerebral swelling with compression of the lateral ventricles has been reported early in SSPE.[87] Children with a prolonged course have extensive central and cortical parenchymal loss. In addition, areas of low absorption are seen in the subcortical and periventricular white matter. Low-absorption regions in the caudate nuclei have also been reported and may account for the movement problems (chorea, dystonia, rigidity) (Fig 6–17).[88] No demonstrable contrast enhancement has been reported. The effects of slow virus infection on the brain are reflected in CT of SSPE. These effects result ultimately in profound parenchymal loss.

Coccidioidomycosis

Most of the important CNS fungal diseases are considered in Chapter 7, which relates to the immunosuppressed host. Coccidioidomycosis is endemic in the

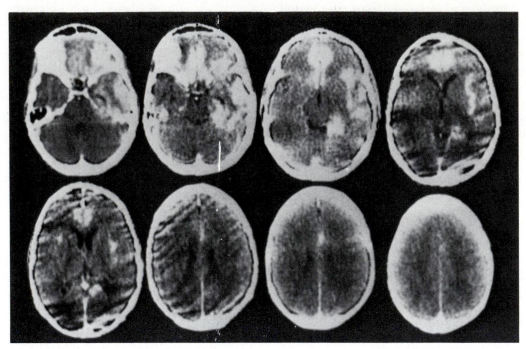

Fig 6–15.—Herpes simplex encephalitis: contrast enhancement bifrontally and left temporal region. (Courtesy of Kenneth Davis, M.D., Massachusetts General Hospital, Boston.)

southwestern United States and northern Mexico. The spore is inhaled, and a primary pulmonary focus develops. Hematogenous dissemination to the CNS occurs within a few weeks or months, but dissemination years later has been reported.[89] The intracranial infection may be manifested pathologically by a thick basilar meningitis with meningeal and parenchymal granulomas. The intra-axial granulomas have been reported to

have a propensity for the cerebellum.[90] Vasculitis producing occlusion has also been noted.[91] The disseminated cerebral form of coccidioidomycosis predominantly occurs in white males, and diagnosis is confirmed by CSF serology or culture.[90]

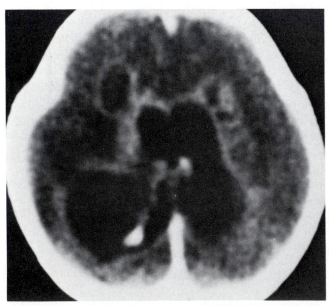

Fig 6–16.—Sequelae of neonatal herpes simplex type 2: polycystic brain with ependymal calcifications.

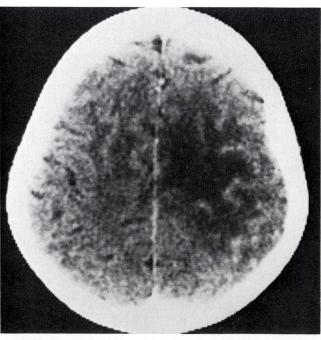

Fig 6–17.—SSPE: low absorption in white matter in child with SSPE. (Courtesy of Kenneth Davis, M.D., Massachusetts General Hospital, Boston.)

The CT picture is of basal arachnoiditis with obliteration and distortion of the cisterns. These may show increased absorption prior to contrast. Associated with this active arachnoiditis is communicating hydrocephalus. Contrasted scans reveal dense enhancement in the cisterns and sulci. When ependymitis is present, enhancement is noted around the ventricle. Focal low-absorption areas representing infarction secondary to vasculitis and enhancing nodules can occasionally be observed.

Cysticercosis

This parasite is endemic in parts of Latin America, Asia, Africa, and Europe. Man is the only known definitive host for the adult tapeworm (*Taenia solium*) as well as the intermediate host for the larval form (*Cysticercus cellulosae*), which prospers in the CNS.[92] The cestode is acquired by ingestion of insufficiently cooked pork containing the encysted larvae. The larva develops into the adult tapeworm in the human intestinal tract. The oncospheres (active embryo) released from ova of the adult tapeworm by gastric digestion burrow through the intestinal tract to reach the bloodstream, which carries them to the CNS and other regions where they form cysticerci. Man may also directly ingest the eggs (as an intermediate host) in contaminated food, via self-contamination by the anus-hand-mouth route, or by regurgitation of ova. Infestation of the CNS produces many neurologic problems (Table 6–10).[93-95] After several weeks, the embryo, which has lodged in the CNS, develops a cystic covering and a scolex. The interval

TABLE 6–10.—NEUROLOGIC
PROBLEMS ASSOCIATED WITH
CYSTICERCOSIS CEREBRI

Seizures
Hydrocephalus
   A. Communicating
   B. Obstructive
Headache
Dementia
Psychological disturbances
Vertigo
Paresthesias, paresis, paralysis
Visual disturbances

between the probable date of infection and the first distinctive symptom varies from less than 1 year to 30 years, the average being approximately 4.8 years.[94] The cysticerci vary in size from pinpoint to 6 cm in diameter.[96] They are located in the brain parenchyma, the meninges, and intraventricularly, or, rarely, intraspinally. Symptoms are related to the location of the parasites.

Classically, the plain skull radiographic features are of calcification in the brain parenchyma. These are quite characteristic with a slight off-center spherical calcification of 1 to 2 mm in diameter representing the scolex surrounded by a partially or totally calcified sphere (7 to 12 mm in diameter). The calcification only occurs in the dead larvae.[97] There are, however, a spectrum of CT findings associated with cysticercosis (Fig 6–18). The acute encephalitic phase of the infection is more common in children and is characterized by ei-

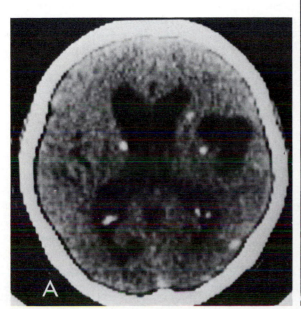 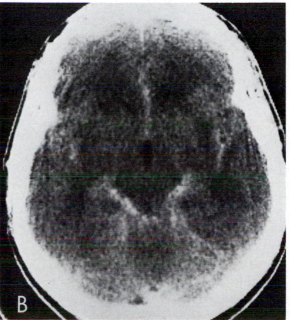

Fig 6–18.—Cysticercosis. **A,** multiple parenchymal calcifications as well as noncalcified cysts. **B,** eosinophilic meningitis in a patient with cysticercosis producing dense leptomeningeal enhancement.

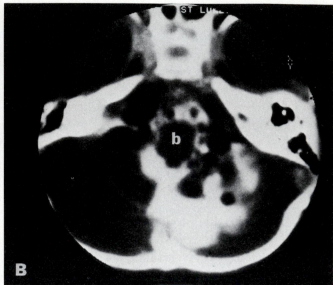

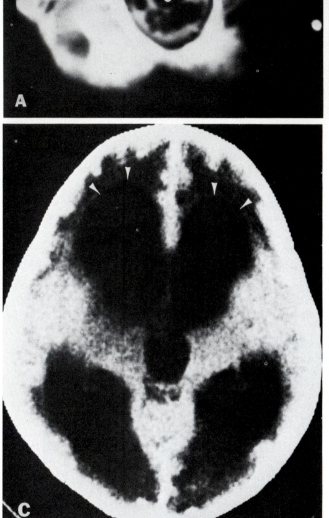

Fig 6–19.—Coenurosis. **A, B,** axial cuts at the level of the foramen magnum **(A)** and posterior fossa **(B)** following the intrathecal deposition of metrizamide demonstrate multiple cysts within the subarachnoid space. The cysts are of varying size and configuration and have densities between 20 and 35 Hounsfield units. (*c* = cervicomedullary junction; *b* = brain stem.) **C,** a supratentorial scan demonstrates pronounced dilatation of the third and lateral ventricles. It is difficult to distinguish between the ventricular margins *(arrowheads)* and the periventricular edema. The subarachnoid infection has produced a pronounced degree of communicating hydrocephalus. (Courtesy of G.A. Norris, M.D., St. Luke's Hospital, Duluth, Minn.)

ther multiple diffuse nodular lesions (85%) or localized lesions.[98] These foci are of low absorption and associated with edema. With intravenous contrast, the lesions uniformly enhance as dense nodules or small ring areas. The encephalitis phase of the disease lasts from 2 to 6 months, with edema persisting after enhancement disappears. Small calcifications may be detected by CT as early as 8 months after the acute phase.[98] These lesions occur in the white matter, cerebral cortex, and basal ganglia. Noncalcified nodules of increased absorption that enhance have also been reported.[99]

The brain parenchyma may concomitantly contain calcified dead larvae and low-absorption cysts. These low-absorption cysts may or may not enhance. These cysts may be found in the ventricles, where they have the same absorption as CSF. They may produce obstructive hydrocephalus and also cause a granular ependymitis by provoking an inflammatory reaction secondary to toxic substances released from the permeable cyst wall of the dead larvae.[100] Ventricular cysticercosis may be diagnosed with the aid of intraventricular metrizamide. The contrast material outlines the ventricular cysts and has also been reported to be taken up, after 5 hours, by the cyst.[101]

Hydrocephalus may also be secondary to meningeal involvement with basilar arachnoiditis. Cysticercosis has been reported on rare occasions to cause obstructive hydrocephalus by presenting as a mass at the foramen of Monro or as a cysticercotic cyst of the septum pellucidum.[102, 103] Larvae can have a racemose (grape-like clusters) form, which occurs in the subarachnoid spaces, and may simulate a low-absorption tumor in the sellar or cerebellopontine angle regions.[99, 104] The subarachnoid and intraventricular cysts do not calcify.[105]

Unusual neuroradiologic features of intracranial cysticercosis were described by Zee and coworkers[106] and include basal meningeal enhancement, positional cyst alteration, evidence of cortical enhancement with vasculitis, and mycotic aneurysm formation.[98]

Other Parasites

Other parasites may involve the CNS and present as lesions either within the parenchyma or the subarachnoid spaces. Such infestations include *Echinococcus* (hydatid cyst) and *Coenurus cerebralis*.[106] The latter is the larval cyst of the dog tapeworm, *Multiceps multiceps*, and infection usually occurs following ingestion of dog meat contaminated with the larvae.[106, 107] This unusual parasite infects the subarachnoid space and ventricular system, producing hydrocephalus (Fig 6–19).[107–109]

REFERENCES

1. Moxon E.R., Smith A.L., Averill D.R., et al.: Hemophilus influenzae meningitis in infant rats after intranasal inoculation. *J. Infect. Dis.* 129:154–162, 1974.
2. Adams R.D., Sidman R.L.: Meningeal infections, abscess and granulomas of the brain, in *Introduction to Neuropathology.* McGraw-Hill Book Co., New York, 1968.
3. Smith E.S.: Purulent meningitis in infants and children: A review of 409 cases. *J. Pediatr.* 45:425–436, 1954.
4. Dodge P.R., Swartz M.N.: Bacterial meningitis: A review of selected aspects. *N. Engl. J. Med.* 272:954–960, 1965.
5. Swartz M.N., Dodge P.R.: Bacterial meningitis: A review of selected aspects. *N. Engl. J. Med.* 272:725–731, 779–787, 842–848, 898–902, 954–960, 1003–1010, 1965.
6. Zimmerman R.A., Patel S., Bilaniuk L.: Demonstration of purulent bacterial intracranial infections by computed tomography. *A.J.R.* 127:155–165, 1976.
7. Bilaniuk L.T., Zimmerman R.A., Brown L., et al.: Computed tomography in meningitis. *Neuroradiology* 16:13–14, 1978.
8. Cockrill H.H. Jr., Dreisback J., Lowe B., et al.: Computed tomography in leptomeningeal infections. *A.J.R.* 130:511–515, 1978.
9. Feigin R.D., Dodge P.R.: Bacterial meningitis: Newer concepts of pathophysiology and neurologic sequelae. *Pediatr. Clin. North Am.* 23:541–556, 1976.
10. Packer R.J., Bilaniuk L.T., Zimmerman R.A.: CT parenchymal abnormalities in bacterial meningitis: Clinical significance. *J. Comput. Assist. Tomogr.* 6:1064–1068, 1982.
11. Rabe E.F.: Subdural effusions in infants. *Pediatr. Clin. North Am.* 14:831–850, 1976.
12. Hitchcock E., Andreadis A.: Subdural empyema: A review of 29 cases. *J. Neurol. Neurosurg. Psychiatry* 27:422–450, 1964.
13. Bannister G., Williams B., Smith S.: Treatment of subdural empyema. *J. Neurosurg.* 55:82–88, 1981.
14. Jacobson P.L., Farmer T.W.: Subdural empyema complicating meningitis in infants: Improved prognosis. *Neurology* 31:190–193, 1981.
15. Galbraith J.G., Barr V.W.: Epidural abscess and subdural empyema. *Adv. Neurol.* 6:257–267, 1974.
16. Segall H.D., Rumbaugh C.L., Bergeron R.T., et al.: Brain and meningeal infections in children: Radiological considerations. *Neuroradiology* 6:8–16, 1973.
17. Sandu V.K., Handel S.F., Pinto R.S., et al.: Neuroradiologic diagnosis of subdural empyema and CT limitations. *A.J.N.R.* 1:39–44, 1980.
18. Lott T., El Gammal T., Dasilva R., et al.: Evaluation of brain and epidural abscesses by computed tomography. *Radiology* 122:371–376, 1977.
19. Garfield J.: Management of supratentorial intracranial abscess: A review of 200 cases. *Br. Med. J.* 2:7–11, 1969.
20. Carey M.E., Chou S.N., French L.A.: Experience with brain abscesses. *J. Neurosurg.* 36:1–9, 1972.
21. Beller A.J., Sahar A., Praissi I.: Brain abscess: Review of 89 cases over a period of 30 years. *J. Neurol. Neurosurg. Psychiatry* 36:757–768, 1973.
22. Kerr F.W.L., King R.B., Meaghen J.N.: Brain abscess—a study of forty-seven consecutive cases. *J.A.M.A.* 168:868–872, 1958.
23. Wood J.H., Lightfoote W.E. II, Ommaya A.K.: Cerebral abscesses produced by bacterial implantation and septic embolisation in primates. *J. Neurol. Neurosurg. Psychiatry* 42:63–69, 1979.
24. Enzmann D.R., Britt R.H., Yeager A.S.: Experimental brain abscess evolution: Computed tomographic and neuropathologic correlation. *Radiology* 133:113–122, 1979.
25. Britt R.H., Enzmann D.R., Yeager A.S.: Neuropathological and computerized tomographic findings in experimental brain abscess. *J. Neurosurg.* 55:590–603, 1981.
26. Claman H.N.: Corticosteroids and lymphoid cells *N. Engl. J. Med.* 287:388–397, 1972.
27. Quartey G.R.C., Johnston J.A., Rozdilkey B.: Decadron

in the treatment of cerebral abscess. *J. Neurosurg.* 45:301–310, 1976.

28. Whelan M.A., Hillal S.K.: Computed tomography as a guide in the diagnosis and follow-up of brain abscesses. *Radiology* 135:663–671, 1980.

29. Rosenblum M.L., Hoff J.T., Norman D., et al.: Decreased mortality from brain abscesses since advent of computerized tomography. *J. Neurosurg.* 49:658–668, 1978.

30. Rosenblum M.L., Hoff J.T., Norman D., et al.: Nonoperative treatment of brain abscesses in selected high-risk patients. *J. Neurosurg.* 52:217–225, 1980.

31. Zimmerman R.A., Bilaniuk L.T., Shipkin P.M., et al.: Evolution of cerebral abscess: Correlation of clinical feature with computed tomography. *Neurology* 27:14–19, 1977.

32. Danziger A., Price H., Schechter M.M.: An analysis of 113 intracranial infections. *Neuroradiology* 19:31–34, 1980.

33. New P.F.J., David K.R., Ballantine H.T.: Computed tomography in cerebral abscess. *Radiology* 121:641–646, 1976.

34. Stevens T.A., Norman D., Kramer R.A., et al.: Computed tomographic brain scanning in intraparenchymal pyogenic abscesses. *A.J.R.* 130:111–114, 1978.

35. Joubert M.J., Stephanov S.: Computerized tomography and surgical treatment in intracranial suppuration. *J. Neurosurg.* 47:73–78, 1977.

36. Arseni C.: Two hundred and one cases of intracranial tuberculoma treated surgically. *J. Neurol. Neurosurg. Psychiatry* 21:308–311, 1958.

37. Ramamurthi B., Varodarajan M.G.: Diagnosis of tuberculomas of the brain: Clinical and radiological correlation. *J. Neurosurg.* 18:1–7, 1961.

38. Maurice-Williams R.S.: Tuberculomas of the brain in Britain. *Postgrad. Med. J.* 48:678–681, 1972.

39. Mayers M.M., Kaufman D.M., Miller M.H.: Recent cases of intracranial tuberculomas. *Neurology* 28:256–260, 1978.

40. Falk A.: U.S. Veterans Administration Armed Forces cooperative study on the chemotherapy of tuberculosis: XII. Tuberculous meningitis in adults, with special reference to survival, neurologic residuals, and work status. *Am. Rev. Resp. Dis.* 91:823–831, 1965.

41. Mayers M.M., Kaufman D.M., Miller, M.H.: Recent cases in intracranial tuberculomas. *Neurology* 28:256–260, 1978.

42. Kennedy D.H., Fallon R.J.: Tuberculous meningitis. *J.A.M.A.* 241:264–268, 1979.

43. Barrett-Connor E.: Tuberculous meningitis in adults. *South. Med. J.* 60:1061–1067, 1967.

44. Castio M., Lepe A.: Cerebral tuberculoma. *Acta Radiol. Diag.* 1:821–827, 1963.

45. Rovira M., Romero F., Torrent O., et al.: Study of tuberculous meningitis by CT. *Neuroradiology* 19:137–141, 1980.

46. Chu N.-S.: Tuberculous meningitis. *Arch. Neurol.* 37:458–460, 1980.

47. Dastur H.M.: Tuberculoma, in Vinken P.J., Bruyn G.W. (eds.): *Handbook of Clinical Neurology,* Amsterdam, North Holland Publishing Co., 1975, vol. 18, pp. 413–426.

48. Sibley W.A., O'Brien J.L.: Intracranial tuberculomas: A review of clinical features and treatment. *Neurology* 6:157–165, 1956.

49. Elisevich K., Arpin E.J.: Tuberculoma masquerading as a meningioma. *J. Neurosurg.* 56:435–438, 1982.

50. Whelan M.A., Stern J.: Intracranial tuberculoma. *Radiology* 138:75–81, 1981.

51. Peatfied R.C., Shawdon H.H.: Five cases of intracranial tuberculoma followed by serial computerized tomography. *J. Neurol. Neurosurg. Psychiatry* 42:373–379, 1979.

52. Price H.I., Danziger A.: Computed tomography in cranial tuberculosis. *A.J.R.* 130:769–771, 1978.

53. Delaney P.: Neurologic manifestations in sarcoidosis: Review of the literature with a report of 23 cases. *Ann. Intern. Med.* 87:336–345, 1977.

54. Wiederholt W.C., Siebert R.G.: Neurological manifestations of sarcoidosis. *Neurology* (Minneapolis) 15:1147–1154, 1965.

55. Silverstein A., Feuer M.M., Siltzback L.E.: Neurologic sarcoidosis. *Arch. Neurol.* 12:1–11, 1965.

56. Jefferson M.: Sarcoidosis of the nervous system. *Brain* 80:540–555, 1957.

57. Meyer J.S., Foley J.M., Compagna-Pinto D.: Granulomatous angiitis of the meninges in sarcoidosis. *Arch. Neurol. Psychiatry* 69:587–600, 1953.

58. Herring A.B., Urich H.: Sarcoidosis of the central nervous system. *J. Neurol. Sci.* 9:405–422, 1969.

59. Kumpe D.A., Rao C.V.G.K., Garcia J.H., et al.: Intracranial neurosarcoidosis. *J. Comput. Assist. Tomogr.* 3:324–330, 1979.

60. Cahill D.W., Saleman M.: Neurosarcoidosis: A review of the rarer manifestations. *Surg. Neurol.* 15:204–211, 1981.

61. Babu V.S., Eisen H., Pataki K.: Sarcoidosis of the central nervous system. *J. Comput. Assist. Tomogr.* 3:396–397, 1979.

62. Brooks J.J.R., Stuckland M.C., Williams J.P., et al.: Computed tomography changes in neurosarcoidosis clearing with steroid treatment. *J. Comput. Assist. Tomogr.* 3:398–399, 1979.

63. Decker R.E., Mardayat M., Mare J., et al.: Neurosarcoidosis with computerized tomographic visualization and transsphenoidal excision of a supra- and intrasellar granuloma. *J. Neurosurg.* 50:814–816, 1979.

64. Goodman S.S., Margulies M.E.: Boeck's sarcoid simulating a brain tumor. *A.M.A. Arch. Neurol. Psychiatry* 81:419–423, 1959.

65. deTribolet N., Zander E.: Intracranial sarcoidosis presenting angiographically as a subdural hematoma. *Surg. Neurol.* 9:169–171, 1978.

66. Meyer H.M. Jr., Johnson R.T., Crawford I.P., et al.: Central nervous system syndromes of "viral" etiology: A study of 713 cases. *Am. J. Med.* 29:334–347, 1960.

67. Whitley R.J., Soong S.J., Dolin R., et al.: Adenine arabinoside therapy of biopsy proven herpes simplex encephalitis. *N. Engl. J. Med.* 297:289–294, 1977.

68. South M.A., Tompkins W.A., Morris C.R., et al.: Congenital malformation of the central nervous system associated with genital type (type 2) herpes virus. *J. Pediatr.* 75:13–18, 1969.

69. Tuffli G.A., Mahmias A.J.: Neonatal herpetic infection: Report of two premature infants treated with systemic use of indoxuridine. *Am. J. Dis. Child.* 118:909–914, 1969.

70. Dublin A.B., Merten D.F.: Computed tomography in the evaluation of herpes simplex encephalitis. *Radiology* 125:133–134, 1977.

71. Haynes R.F., Amixi P.H., Cramblett G.H.: Fatal herpes virus hominis (herpes simplex virus) infections in children. *J.A.M.A.* 206:312–319, 1978.

72. Smith J.B., Groover R.V., Klass D.W., et al.: Multicystic cerebral degeneration in neonatal herpes simplex virus encephalitis. *Am. J. Dis. Child.* 131:568–572, 1977.

73. Davis L.E., Johnson R.T.: An explanation for the localization of herpes simplex encephalitis. *Ann. Neurol.* 5:2–5, 1979.

74. Taber L.H., Brasier F., Couch R.B., et al.: Diagnosis of herpes simplex virus infection by immunofluorescence. *J. Clin. Microbiol.* 3:309–312, 1976.

75. Tomlinson A.H., Chinn I.J., MacCallum F.O.: Immunofluorescence staining for the diagnosis of herpes encephalitis. *J. Clin. Pathol.* 27:495–499, 1974.

76. Sage M.R., Dubois P.J., Oakes J., et al.: Rapid development of cerebral atrophy due to perinatal herpes simplex encephalitis. *J. Comput. Assist. Tomogr.* 5:763–766, 1981.

77. Dublin A.B., Merten D.F.: Computed tomography in the evaluation of herpes simplex encephalitis. *Radiology* 125:133–134, 1977.

78. Zimmerman R.D., Russell E.J., Leeds N.E., et al.: CT in the early diagnosis of herpes simplex encephalitis. *A.J.R.* 134:61–66, 1980.

79. Enzmann D.R., Ranson B., Norman D., et al.: Computed tomography of herpes simplex encephalitis. *Radiology* 129:419–425, 1978.

80. Davis J.M., Davis K.R., Kleinman G.M., et al.: Computed tomography of herpes simplex encephalitis, with clinical pathological correlation. *Radiology* 129:409–417, 1978.

81. Measles—quick and slow. *Lancet* 2:27, 1971.

82. Rish W.S., Haddad F.S.: The variable natural history of subacute sclerosing panencephalitis. *Arch. Neurol.* 36:610–614, 1979.

83. Jabbour J.T., Garcia J.H., Lemmi H., et al.: SSPE: A multidisciplinary study of eight cases. *J.A.M.A.* 207:2248–2254, 1969.

84. Zeman W., Kolar O.: Reflections on the etiology and pathogenesis of subacute sclerosing panencephalitis. *Neurology* 18:1–7, 1968.

85. Sever J.L., Zeman W.: Serological studies of measles and subacute sclerosing panencephalitis. *Neurology* 18:95–97, 1968.

86. Connely J.H.: Additional data on measles virus antibody and antigen in subacute sclerosing panencephalitis. *Neurology* 18:87–89, 1968.

87. Pedersen H., Wulff C.H.: Computed tomographic findings of early subacute sclerosing panencephalitis. *Neuroradiology* 23:31–32, 1982.

88. Duda E.E., Huttenlocker P.R., Patronas N.J.: CT of subacute sclerosing panencephalitis. *A.J.N.R.* 1:35–38, 1980.

89. Einstein H.: Coccidioidomycosis of the central nervous system, in Thompson R.A., Green J.R. (eds.): *Advances in Neurology*. New York, Rosen, Richards, Press, Inc., 1974, vol. 6, pp. 101–105.

90. Dublin A.B., Phillips H.E.: Computed tomography of disseminated cerebral coccidioidomycosis. *Radiology* 135:361–368, 1980.

91. Ferris E.J.: Arteritis, in Newton T.H., Potts D.G. (eds.): *Radiology of the Skull and Brain*. St. Louis, C.V. Mosby Co., 1974, vol. 2, book 4, pp. 2566–2597.

92. Haining R.B., Haining R.G.: Cysticercosis cerebri. *J.A.M.A.* 172:2036–2039, 1960.

93. Simms N.M., Maxwell R.E., Christenson P.C., et al.: Internal hydrocephalus secondary to cysticercosis cerebri: Treatment with a ventriculoatrial shunt. *J. Neurosurg.* 30:305–309, 1969.

94. Dixon H.B.F., Lipscomb F.M.: Cysticercosis: An analysis and followup of 450 cases, in *Privy Council, Medical Research Council Special Report*, No. 229. London, Her Majesty's Stationery Office, 1961, pp. 1–59.

95. Stepien L.: Cerebral cysticercosis in Poland: Clinical symptoms and operative results in 132 cases. *J. Neurosurg.* 19:505–531, 1962.

96. Labato R.D., Lamas E., Portallo J.M.: Hydrocephalus in cerebral cysticercosis. *J. Neurosurg.* 55:786–793, 1981.

97. Santin G., Vargas J.: Roentgen study of cysticercosis of central nervous system. *Radiology* 86:520–527, 1966.

98. Rodriguez-Carbajal J., Salgado P., Gutierrez-Olvarado R., et al.: The acute encephalitic phase of neurocysticercosis: Computed tomographic manifestations. *A.J.N.R.* 4:51–55, 1983.

99. Carabajal J.S., Palacious E., Azar-Kia B., et al.: Radiology of cysticercosis of the central nervous system including computed tomography. *Radiology* 125:127–131, 1977.

100. Lobato R.D., Lamas E., Portillo J.M., et al.: Hydrocephalus in cerebral cysticercosis. *J. Neurosurg.* 55:786–793, 1981.

101. Zee C.S., Tsai F.Y., Segall H.D., et al.: Entrance of metrizamide into an intraventricular cysticercosis cyst. *A.J.N.R.* 2:189–191, 1981.

102. Dublin A.B., French B.N.: Cysticercotic cyst of the septum pellucidum. *A.J.N.R.* 1:205–206, 1980.

103. Jankowski R., Zimmerman R.D., Leeds N.E.: Cysticercosis presenting as a mass lesion at foramen of Monro. *J. Comput. Assist. Tomogr.* 3:694–696, 1979.

104. Stern W.E.: Neurosurgical considerations of cysticercosis of the central nervous system. *J. Neurosurg.* 55:382–389, 1981.

105. Bentson J.R., Wilson G.H., Helmer E., et al.: Computed tomography in intracranial cysticercosis. *J. Comput. Assist. Tomogr.* 1:464–471, 1977.

106. Zee C., Segall H.D., Miller C., et al.: Unusual neuroradiological features of intracranial cysticercosis. *Radiology* 137:397–407, 1980.

107. Danziger J., Bloch S.: Tapeworm cyst infestations of the brain. *Clin. Radiol.* 26:141–148, 1975.

108. Hoermos J.A., Healy G.R., Schultz M.G., et al.: Fatal human cerebral coenurosis. *J.A.M.A.* 213:1461–1464, 1970.

109. Schellhas K.S., Norris G.A., Loken T.: Disseminated subarachnoid coenurus (unpublished).

7

CNS Abnormalities in the Immunocompromised Host

ROBERT I. GROSSMAN, M.D.
ROBERT A. ZIMMERMAN, M.D.

THE COMPROMISED HOST (an unusual patient) represents a diagnostic dilemma to both the clinician and the radiologist, because he is not only susceptible to unusual infectious agents, but also to numerous other disorders as a result of his immunodeficient state. To add to this diagnostic dilemma are the difficulties encountered because (1) many of these different conditions have similar radiographic findings and (2) the circumstances that contribute to the immunosuppressed state frequently modify the classic CT characteristics of the pathologic process, i.e., corticosteroids decreasing contrast enhancement and mass effect.[1]

Table 7–1 enumerates some of the factors responsible for the immunosuppressed state. Explanation of the exact mechanism by which these processes alter the immune response is not possible in this chapter. Rather, we shall discuss those CT findings germane to the compromised host. The text is divided into two sections: (1) disorders that do not have a clear-cut infectious etiology (Table 7–2) and (2) a representative group of infectious diseases that affect the compromised host (Table 7–3).

TABLE 7–1.—FACTORS PRODUCING IMMUNOSUPPRESSED STATE

Postoperative
Posttraumatic
Foreign body in CNS
Host defense problems
  A. Humoral dysfunction
  B. Cell-mediated dysfunction
  C. Phagocytic dysfunction
Drug therapy
  A. Antibiotics
  B. Corticosteriods
  C. Chemotherapy
  D. Immunotherapy
Radiation therapy
Transplantation
Vascular dysfunction
  A. Diabetes mellitus
  B. Atherosclerosis
  C. Dehydration
Other
  A. Malnutrition
  B. Malignant disease
  C. Chronic alcoholism
  D. Metabolic disease

TABLE 7–2.—NONINFECTIOUS PROBLEMS ASSOCIATED WITH THE IMMUNOSUPPRESSED STATE

Dystrophic calcification
Disseminated necrotizing leukoencephalopathy
Radiation necrosis
Stroke
Leptomeningeal spread of tumor
Reticulum cell sarcoma

TABLE 7–3.—PATHOGENS IN PATIENTS WITH CELLULAR IMMUNE DEFICIENCY

Bacteria
  A. *Listeria*
Fungi
  B. *Nocardia*
  C. *Aspergillus*
  D. *Candida*
  E. *Cryptococcus*
  F. Mucormycosis
Protozoa
  G. *Toxoplasma*
Viruses
  H. Herpes zoster
  I. Papovavirus (PML)*

*Progressive multifocal leukoencephalopathy.

NONINFECTIOUS DISORDERS

Dystrophic Calcification

Calcification in the gray matter and basal ganglia may be demonstrated in patients who have received methotrexate and (or) irradiation months to years after cessation of therapy (Fig 7–1).[2–5] A microangiopathy is produced that is represented histologically by noninflammatory degeneration of small vessels associated with dystrophic calcification in adjacent gray matter. The most susceptible areas are the lentiform nucleus (putamen and globus pallidus), the vascular watersheds (anterior middle cerebral arteries, middle posterior cerebral arteries), and the cerebellar cortex.[6] Mineralizing angiopathy relates directly to length of survival from cessation of radiation therapy and the number of CNS relapses that occur.

The patients most commonly affected are children under age 10. These usually have been treated for acute lymphocytic leukemia. Subtle neurologic findings include memory loss, abnormal EEG, seizures, and personality changes.[7]

The CT findings include calcification that is usually symmetrically distributed in the areas previously described. Dilatation of the ventricles and subarachnoid spaces, as well as periventricular low absorption, are the other abnormalities that occur in this group of patients.[8]

Disseminated Necrotizing Leukoencephalopathy

Disseminated necrotizing leukoencephalopathy (DNL) is a syndrome that affects patients who have been treated with CNS radiation and chemotherapy, particularly intrathecal or intravenous methotrexate. Onset occurs shortly after completion of therapy. It is characterized clinically by a subacute course, the initial symptoms of which are confusion, ataxia, seizures, slurred speech, spasticity, dysphagia, and lethargy. This at times progresses to dementia, coma, and death.[9] Pathologic characteristics of this lesion include extensive areas of white matter demyelination and necrosis, astrocytosis, and a lack of inflammatory cellular response.[10]

The major CT finding in DNL is white matter low-absorption areas, symmetric and asymmetric (Fig 7–2).[11] The areas of white matter low absorption rarely exhibit contrast enhancement.[12] Direct instillation of methotrexate into the ventricle may also produce a necrotizing leukoencephalopathy with the finding of a focal low-absorption mass that may enhance with contrast material (Fig 7–3).[13]

Radiation therapy and chemotherapy are synergistic with respect to the CNS damage they elicit. Radiation disrupts the blood-brain barrier and increases the entry of chemotherapeutic drugs into the brain parenchyma, thus potentiating their effects. A case has been described in which periventricular low absorption without

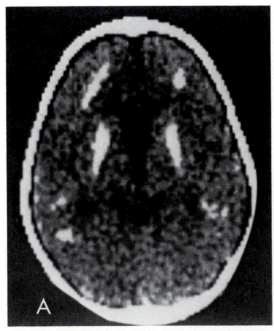
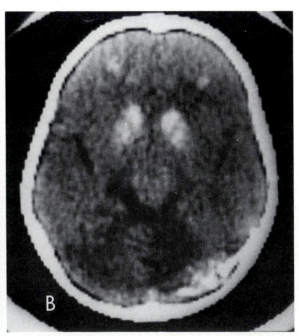

Fig 7–1.—**A,** dystrophic calcification in the lentiform nucleus and vascular watershed zones in a young leukemic patient treated with intrathecal methotrexate and irradiation. **B,** calcification in basal ganglia and parenchymal loss in cerebellum secondary to intrathecal methotrexate and radiation therapy for leukemia.

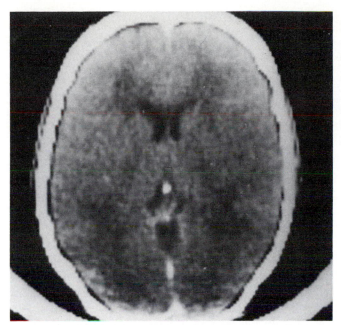

Fig 7–2.—DNL in 10-year-old patient with acute lymphocytic leukemia treated with irradiation and intravenous and intrathecal methotrexate. Note the low absorption in the periventricular white matter, which appeared just after cessation of therapy.

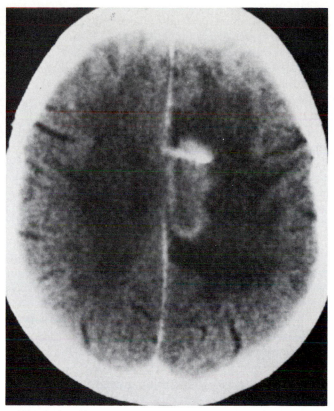

Fig 7–3.—Focal necrotizing leukoencephalopathy in a patient receiving intraventricular methotrexate. Note enhancing mass at the tip of the ventricular cannula. Also note absorption in white matter.

contrast enhancement, unassociated with the other characteristics, was noted within 2 months after CNS treatment (prophylaxis). As a result of this CT finding, therapy was stopped and treatment with corticosteroids instituted. Subsequent resolution of the low absorption in the white matter was documented on follow-up CT studies. The appearance of low-absorption abnormalities in this patient group may be the earliest manifestation of DNL.[14] In the spectrum of pathologic findings, the group of seemingly asymptomatic patients with periventricular low absorption fall somewhere between simple dystrophic calcification and the DNL syndrome.

Radiation Necrosis

Patients treated with radiation therapy for primary brain tumors, skull lesions, and intracranial metastasis have been noted by CT to frequently exhibit central and cortical parenchymal loss.[15, 16] The radiologist's dilemma, however, is in separating the findings of residual or recurrent tumor from radionecrosis. There are several factors that influence the development of radiation necrosis. These include total dose (6,000 rad), overall time of administration, size of each fraction of irradiation (200 rad/day), number of fractions per irradiation, and other radiomimetic influences such as chemotherapy and hypertension.[17] The signs and symptoms of radiation necrosis are nonspecific and do not differentiate it from recurrent tumor. The effects of ir-

radiation have been separated into those occurring early (within weeks) and late (4 months to many years later).[18] The former is transient and has no reported radiologic abnormality. The latter affects white matter to a much greater extent than gray matter and histologically involves vascular changes that include coagulative necrosis and hyalinization.[19] The usual time course during which symptoms evolve is about 2 years after therapy.

Unfortunately, it is exceedingly difficult on the basis of the CT scan to make the diagnosis of radiation necrosis, because CT may demonstrate a mass lesion that may or may not contrast enhance (just like a tumor!). The possibility of this diagnosis needs to be raised when a lesion is found in the appropriate temporal sequence to treatment. If the patient's symptoms are related to radiation necrosis, then removal of this necrotic tissue (if accessible) and therapy with corticosteroids are the treatment of choice and even at times curative.[20] The definitive diagnosis of radiation necrosis is made by surgical biopsy, but is suggested when the appropriate clinical information is correlated with the isodose reconstruction maps and the CT abnormalities.[21]

The radiologist may suggest the diagnosis of radiation necrosis with more certainty when bilateral symmetric lesions are visualized in a patient with an intact falx and a known unilateral tumor (Fig 7–4,A).[22] Another clinical setting that supports the diagnosis of radiation necrosis occurs when a patient with an irradiated extracranial neoplasm, without intracranial extension, presents with a purely intracranial mass (see Fig 7–4,B).[23]

Table 7–4 summarizes the CT abnormalities in intracranially irradiated individuals.

Stroke

In addition to the vasculopathy induced by radiotherapy,[24, 25] there are a number of other etiologies of stroke in the immunosuppressed patient (Table 7–5).[26–29] The compromised host presenting with CT evidence of stroke (infarction, hemorrhage, venous thrombosis) may have an unusual underlying problem. Coagulopathies are common in compromised patients, particularly in those patients with leukemia or when systemic infection has been superimposed on malignancy.[30] Small subcortical hemorrhage may be seen in disseminated intravascular coagulopathy (Fig 7–5). Chronic subdural hematoma has been described in one series in 10% of children with acute lymphocytic leukemia.[31]

TABLE 7–4.—CT ABNORMALITIES
IN IRRADIATED PATIENTS

Lesions of radiation necrosis:
  A. Low absorption
  B. Isodense   } ± Contrast enhancement
  C. High absorption
Strongly suggests radiation necrosis:
  A. Bilateral symmetric lesions in patients with intact falx and unilateral tumor
  B. Irradiated extracranial tumor without intracranial extension, and an intracranial mass
Stroke 2° to radiation-induced vasculopathy

Cerebral venous infarction is an important diagnosis that is easily overlooked as a diagnostic consideration, particularly if the physician is not attuned to the entity and its presenting CT characteristics. These include regions of low absorption, sometimes bilateral, in the parasagittal region or elsewhere, mass effect, hemorrhage, as well as gyriform contrast enhancement corresponding to a venous anatomical distribution. A thrombus can occasionally be seen in a cortical vein (cord sign), or following intravenous contrast material, in the superior sagittal sinus (empty triangle sign) (Fig 7–6).[32] Visualization of medullary veins has been reported following intravenous contrast.[33] High absorption on the unen-

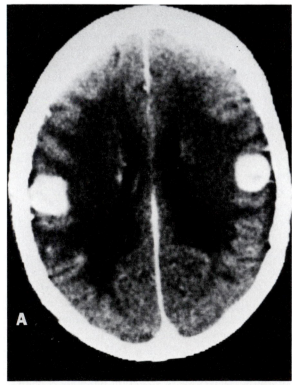
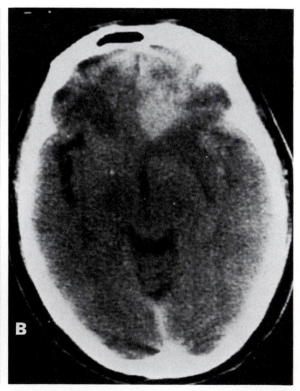

Fig 7–4.—A, radiation necrosis. Bilateral enhancing masses are present in a patient treated with opposing radiation ports (2 years prior to scan) for a temporal-lobe low-grade glioma. Low absorption is present in the white matter bilaterally. **B,** enhancing large frontal mass representing radiation necrosis in a patient treated with irradiation for a basal cell carcinoma of the forehead.

TABLE 7–5.—ETIOLOGY OF STROKE IN
IMMUNOSUPPRESSED PATIENTS

Nonbacterial thrombotic endocarditis
Bacterial endocarditis with mycotic aneurysm
Hyperviscosity syndromes
Hematologic dysfunction
    A. Disseminated intravascular coagulopathy
    B. Drug-induced thrombocytopenia and other coagulation
       disorders
Radiation-induced large vessel vasculopathy

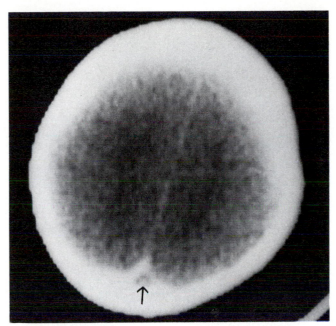

Fig 7–6.—Sagittal sinus thrombosis. Thrombus *(arrow)* within superior sagittal sinus is surrounded by contrast (empty triangle sign).

hanced scan, with dense enhancement on the contrasted images, has been observed in the tentorium in the case of sigmoid sinus thrombosis.[34] Although CT can strongly suggest the diagnosis, angiography or intravenous digital angiography is essential for confirmation. Table 7–6 lists some of the causes of venous thrombosis in this patient group.[35]

Leptomeningeal Spread of Tumor

When contrast enhancement is observed in the leptomeninges of cancer patients, the major clinical differential diagnosis involves infectious or granulomatous meningitis and leptomeningeal spread of tumor.[36] Certain malignancies (Table 7–7) produce a significant meningeal reaction with consequent leptomeningeal enhancement. Hematologic malignancies, however, do not evoke the reaction, and thus rarely show enhancement, despite the presence of leptomeningeal tumor.[37]

Lumbar puncture with cerebrospinal fluid (CSF) cytology is usually diagnostic when meningeal enhancement is noted and is a simple test for differentiating infection from tumor.[38]

The CT picture of leptomeningeal tumor spread includes obliteration of involved cisterns, leptomeningeal enhancement, and hydrocephalus with dilatation of the temporal horns (Fig 7–7). The differential diagnosis of these observations includes subarachnoid hemorrhage,

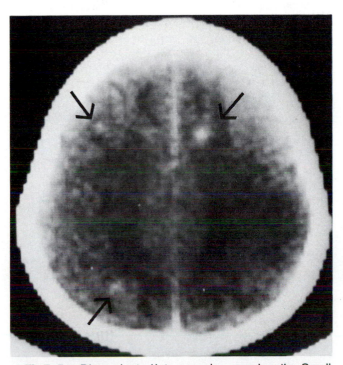

Fig 7–5.—Disseminated intravascular coagulopathy. Small cortical hemorrhages *(arrows)* are present in a patient with acute lymphocytic leukemia.

TABLE 7–6.—CAUSES OF VENOUS
THROMBOSIS IN IMMUNOSUPPRESSED PATIENTS

Tumors
    A. Compression or infiltration of venous structures
    B. Hypercoagulability
Infection
Dehydration
Inanition

TABLE 7–7.—TUMORS COMMONLY
PRODUCING LEPTOMENINGEAL
ENHANCEMENT

Primary brain tumor
    A. Pineal region tumors
    B. Medulloblastoma
    C. Ependymoma
    D. Glioma
Adenocarcinoma
Melanoma
Breast carcinoma
Squamous cell carcinoma

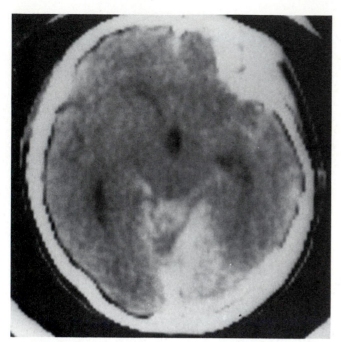

Fig 7–7.—Leptomeningeal spread of tumor. Enhancement of the leptomeninges and dilatation of the temporal horns are present in a patient with breast carcinoma.

pyogenic meningitis, granulomatous basal arachnoiditis, and metrizamide instillation.[39]

Reticulum Cell Sarcoma (RCS)

Primary RCS of the brain (microglioma, primary malignant lymphoma) has a predilection for immunosuppressed patients, particularly allograft recipients (cardiac, renal) and individuals with immunodeficiency states (Sjögren's syndrome).[40] This lesion's CT charac-

teristics include single or multiple areas of involvement with little mass effect relative to the tumor size. There is a marked predilection for the basal ganglion, cerebellar hemispheres, thalamus, brain stem, and corpus callosum. The tumor may be isodense or hyperdense on the preinfusion scan. It is unusual for this lesion to demonstrate central necrosis. Usually, RCS exhibits homogeneous enhancement following intravenous contrast (Fig 7–8).[41]

The RCS lesion is exquisitely sensitive to corticosteroids and radiation therapy. Prior therapy with corticosteroids may render the CT scan completely normal.[42]

INFECTIOUS COMPLICATIONS

Most of these CNS infections are related to defects in cell-mediated immunity secondary to either malignancy or drug therapy (corticosteroids, chemotherapy, etc.). Table 7–3 lists the pathogens we shall consider. In addition to those listed, the gram-negative bacilli, *Staphylococcus* and *Streptococcus*, produce meningitis and brain abscess in patients with neutropenia and impaired cellular immunity.[43]

Listerosis

This short gram-positive rod pathologically elicits meningitis, meningoencephalitis, and rarely brain abscess. *Listeria* does not present with a distinctive radiologic picture. The major problem lies in the difficulties encountered in laboratory diagnosis. Specimens from CSF often contain only a few *Listeria* organisms, which are easily mistaken for diphtheroids (gram-positive rods) and dismissed as a contaminant.[44] The diagnosis of *Listeria* infection should be considered in patients

Fig 7–8.—Reticulum cell sarcoma. *Top row,* unenhanced scan demonstrating high-absorption mass in parietal region. *Bottom row,* dense enhancement of mass following intravenous contrast.

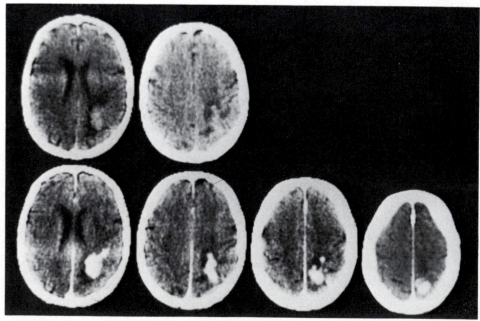

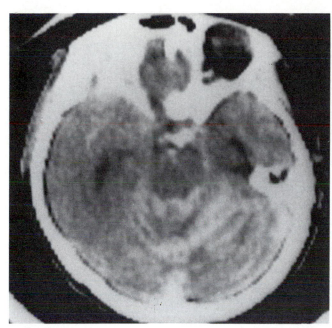

Fig 7–9.—*Listeria* meningitis. Note leptomeningeal enhancement.

with impaired cellular immunity, the suspicion of bacterial meningitis, and the CT findings of meningeal enhancement (or brain abscess) when the bacteriologic studies are negative (Fig 7–9).[45]

Nocardiosis

Nocardia, an aerobic fungus resembling *Actinomyces*, does not produce the sulfur granules seen with *Actinomyces*. Nocardia characteristically is associated with a state of compromised immunity, especially in the setting of corticosteroid therapy.[46] However, it may infect patients with normal immunity as well. *Nocardia* complicates a spectrum of diseases that includes pulmonary alveolar proteinosis, sarcoidosis, ulcerative colitis, and intestinal lipodystrophy.[47] Hematogenous dissemination occurs from a pulmonary focus into the CNS. This usually results in brain abscess formation, meningitis being rare. The onset of symptoms is often insidious.

Nocardial lesions on CT scans show an enhancing capsule commonly containing multiple loculations (Fig 7–10).[48] The diagnosis should be considered in the appropriate clinical setting, because *Nocardia* is quite sensitive to the sulfonamides.

Aspergillosis

In contradistinction to *Nocardia*, where a well-formed capsule is usually apparent, intracranial *Aspergillus* rarely presents with ring enhancement. This ubiquitous fungus primarily infects the compromised host. It may gain entry into the CNS by inoculation,

hematogenous dissemination, most often from a pulmonary focus, or by direct extension from the paranasal sinuses.

Pathologically, aspergillosis involves the brain in an aggressive form producing meningitis and meningoencephalitis with subsequent hemorrhagic infarction. Less malignant presentations include solitary cerebral abscess or isolated granulomas. In aggressive aspergillosis, histologically one visualizes invasion of blood vessels with secondary thrombosis and infarction.

Abnormalities on CT are subtle and include areas of low absorption with minimal mass effect, poor contrast enhancement, and usually no ring formation. In fact, the presence of true ring enhancement militates against the aggressive meningoencephalitic variety of aspergillosis. The relatively benign CT picture contrasts sharply with the consumptive nature of the infection (Fig 7–11). The lack of correlation between the radiographic and pathologic findings is related to the rapidity of the destructive process (inability to form an effective capsule) as well as suppression of enhancement by corticosteroid therapy. These CT findings, with the clinical setting of immunosuppression, corticosteroid therapy, fever, pulmonary infection, and neurologic findings (including a decreasing level of consciousness), suggest the aggressive form of intracranial aspergillosis, which implies an extremely poor prognosis.[49]

Candidiasis

Candida is the most common etiology of autopsy-proved cerebral mycosis. It has a propensity for neutro-

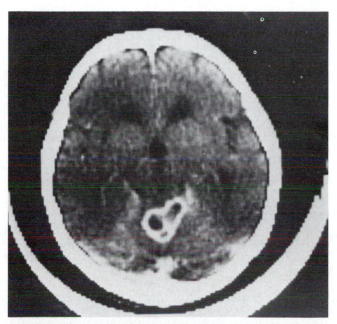

Fig 7–10.—*Nocardia* asteroides. Note multiloculated cerebellar abscess (enhanced scan) in a 79-year-old immunosuppressed patient with chronic lymphocytic leukemia.

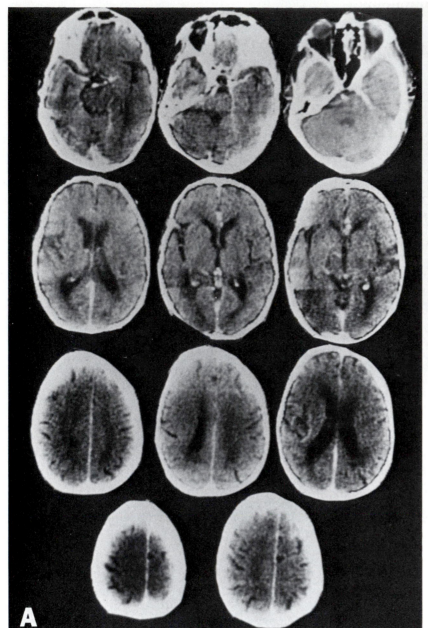

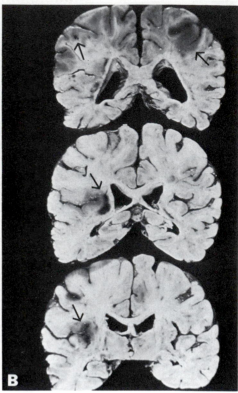

Fig 7–11.—A, intracranial aspergillosis. Enhanced scan is of a renal transplant patient with intracranial aspergillosis. Scan was performed the day patient expired and is quite unremarkable. **B,** pathologic specimen from same patient exhibiting multiple areas of septic infarction *(arrows).* The cerebellum was also involved.

penic patients who are receiving corticosteroids. *Candida* reaches the CNS by hematogenous dissemination via the respiratory or gastrointestinal tracts. Microscopic pathology includes vascular inflammation, thrombosis, infarction, or intraparenchymal microabscess formation, typically in the middle cerebral artery distribution. Noncaseating granulomas have also been observed.[50, 51] The gross pathologic findings induced by this yeast-like fungus include meningitis, pachymeningitis, septic infarction, abscess, or granuloma.[52, 53] These various pathologic presentations consequently generate different CT images, which include hydrocephalus (leptomeningeal disease), enhancing nodules with edema (granuloma), calcified granuloma, infarc-

tion, and abscess formation (Fig 7–12).[52, 54] The infectious presentation depends on the state of the host's natural defenses. The inability to mount an effective localizing cell-mediated immune response when challenged favors an aggressive infection rather than granuloma formation. Endophthalmitis is a complication of *Candida* septicemia.[55] This finding in the face of intracranial lesions in the suppressed host strongly supports the diagnosis of CNS candidiasis.

Cryptococcosis

Cryptococcus is a nonmycelial yeast with a polysaccharide capsule that distinctively stains with india ink. Sensitive immunologic diagnosis can also be made by

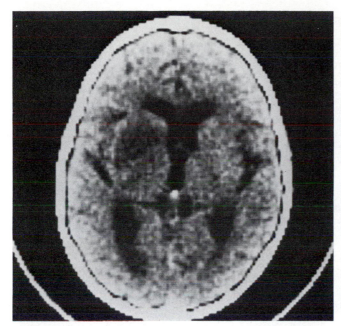

Fig 7–12.—*Candida* abscess. Large basal ganglionic abscess with minimal enhancement is noted in 15-year-old patient with acute lymphocytic leukemia and neutropenia. Patient had been treated with chemotherapy, corticosteroids, and radiation therapy.

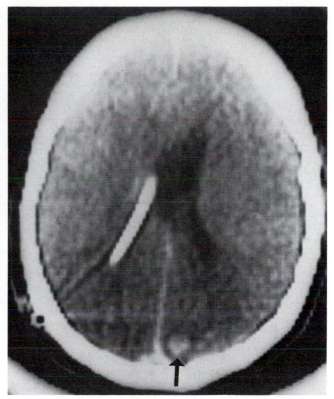

Fig 7–13.—Cryptococcosis. High-absorption nodule *(arrow)* on unenhanced CT enhances with intravenous contrast. Patient also had hydrocephalus secondary to cryptococcal meningitis.

detecting cryptococcal antigen or anticryptococcal antibody in the CSF or blood.[56] Pathologic findings include meningitis, meningoencephalitis, or granuloma formation.[57] Hematogenous dissemination from an inapparent pulmonary focus is the usual vector into the CNS. The surfaces of cerebral cortex, basal ganglia, and dorsal cerebellum are most frequently involved. The fungus seeds the meninges with subsequent rupture and secondary meningitis.[58] Its course is generally not as fulminant as *Aspergillus* or *Candida.*

Scanning with CT reveals hydrocephalus and leptomeningeal enhancement when the infection is meningeal in location. Plain scans will show a high-absorption nodule surrounded by edema that will enhance with intravenous contrast (Fig 7–13). While CT is not distinctive for *Cryptococcus,* the diagnosis may be suggested with positive laboratory results and appropriate scan abnormalities.

Mucormycosis

Mucormycosis affects patients with several problems related to abnormalities in host defenses, including altered cellular immunity. Particularly prone to this pathogen are diabetics in ketoacidosis or debilitated patients suffering from burns, uremia, or malnutrition.[59] The fungus is usually inhaled and rapidly destroys the nasal mucosa, forming black crusts. It may then spread into the paranasal sinuses, orbit, and the base of the skull or may extend through the cribriform plate, re-

sulting in involvement of the anterior cranial fossa.[60] Clinical symptoms include facial pain, bloody nasal discharge, dark swollen turbinates, chemosis, exophthalmus, cranial nerve palsy progressing rapidly to stroke, encephalitis, and death.[61]

Mucor has a striking tendency to proliferate along and through vascular structures, producing arteritis with aneurysm and pseudoaneurysm formation, as well as vascular occlusion and infarction.[62]

Features on CT of nasopharyngeal mucor include opacification and bony destruction of the paranasal sinuses, orbital extension from the ethmoid sinuses producing proptosis and chemosis, and obliteration of the nasopharyngeal tissue planes (Fig 7–14,A).[63] When this virulent fungus extends intracranially, low-absorption abnormalities are noted, particularly in the anterior cranial fossa, but may be in any part of the brain. These regions show mass effect and contrast enhancement.[64] Mucor may also cause large-vessel cerebral infarction with the appropriate CT abnormalities (see Fig 7–14,B).[65]

Toxoplasmosis

This ubiquitous protozoan parasite infects the CNS of adults with compromised cellular immunity (particu-

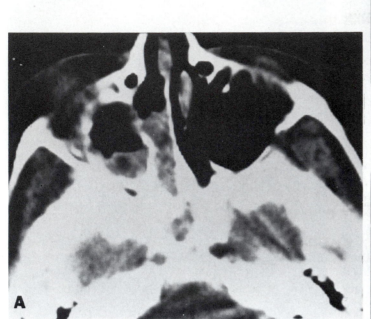
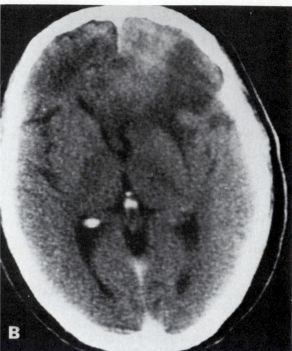

Fig 7–14.—A, mucor. Note involvement of nasal cavity and maxillary sinus in an immunosuppressed patient with chronic lymphocytic leukemia. **B,** same patient. Mucor has extended through the cribriform plate and produced a large frontal septic infarction.

larly defects in the lympocyte-monocyte system). Acute toxoplasmosis in compromised patients often occurs from reactivation of remotely acquired latent infection.[66] It can evoke an acute vascular thrombosis with infarction or be well localized in the form of granuloma at the corticomedullary junction or periventricular region.[66, 67] As opposed to congenital toxoplasmosis, calcification is not common.[68] Reported CT abnormalities have included areas of low absorption with little or no contrast enhancement, gyriform or ring contrast enhancement, and isodense nodules that enhance.[69, 70] Appropriate prompt antibiotic therapy may be curative after positive identification by serologic tests or the demonstration of *Toxoplasma* in the CSF.

Recently, *Toxoplasma* encephalitis has been associated with the acquired immune deficiency syndrome (AIDS) (Fig 7–15). These patients have multiple regions of involvement in the basal ganglia, thalamus, and corticomedullary junction. In most cases, CT shows low-absorption regions with progressive mass effect. Contrast enhancement is usually seen; however, the pattern of enhancement is not specific.[71]

Herpes Zoster

Herpes zoster is a DNA virus with a propensity for infecting immunosuppressed patients, particularly those individuals with lymphoma.[72, 73] These patients initially present with herpes zoster involvement of the eye and several weeks later develop contralateral hemiplegia. Pathology demonstrates an occlusive granulomatous vasculitis or meningoencephalitis.[72, 74] Cerebral angiography reveals multiple areas of segmental constriction usually involving proximal segments of the anterior and middle cerebral arteries without involvement of the extracranial vessels (Fig 7–16,A).[75]

This viral infection has CT features of low-absorption areas, mass effect, and gyriform contrast enhancement in the segmental distribution of the vasculitis (see Fig 7–16,B) or meningeal contrast enhancement in those cases with meningoencephalitis.[69]

There is some evidence that links herpes zoster with cerebral granulomatous angiitis.[76] Granulomatous angiitis has also been reported in immunosuppressed patients, particularly those with lymphoproliferative disorders.[77–79] There is diffuse infiltration, with lymphocytes, giant cells, and mononuclear cells, of small cerebral arteries and veins ($< 200 \mu$ in diameter).[80] Clinical manifestations include disorientation and impaired intellectual function, usually progressing to death within 1 year. Multiple low-absorption regions are shown on CT scans, which may or may not contrast enhance (Fig 7–17).[81, 82] These areas correspond to segmental abnormalities in the blood-brain barrier secondary to vasculitis. Thus, herpes zoster represents one

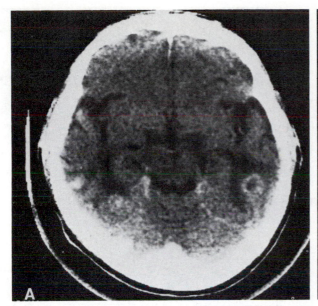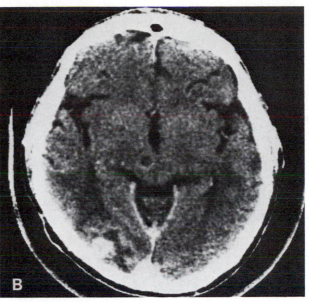

Fig 7–15.—Toxoplasmosis in a patient with AIDS. Enhanced scans demonstrate ring-enhancing lesions with surrounding low absorption at the corticomedullary junction of the left posterior temporal lobe (A) and within the right side of the midbrain (B). Nodules were also noted in the right-occipital and right-posterior temporal region.

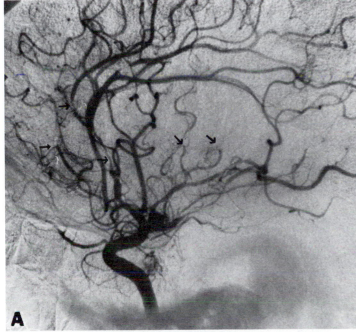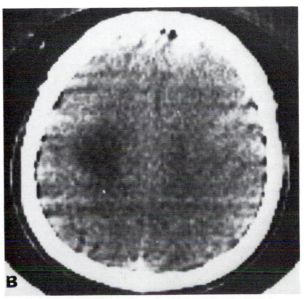

Fig 7–16.—Herpes zoster. A, a 60-year-old patient sustained a contralateral stroke 6 weeks after herpes zoster ophthalmicus. Cerebral angiography reveals multiple areas of vasculitis and occlusion (arrows). B, CT of same patient displaying low-absorption area (infarct) in middle cerebral "watershed" secondary to vasculitis.

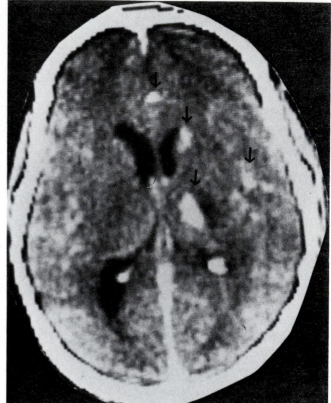

Fig 7–17.—Granulomatous angiitis. Enhanced CT shows multiple areas of involvement *(arrows)*. This patient had an acute change in personality.

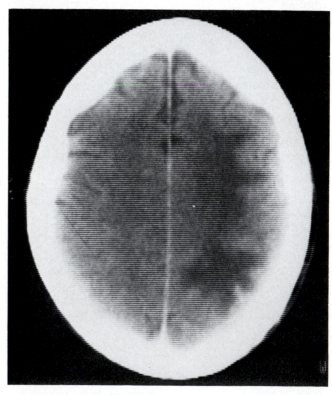

Fig 7–18.—PML in a 65-year-old man with chronic lymphocytic leukemia and a progressive 3-month history of mental deterioration. Scalloped areas of low absorption, without enhancement, are noted in the left central semiovale, particularly in the parieto-occipital region.

etiology with two unique manifestations (large-vessel infarction and cerebral granulomatous angiitis), each with discrete CT features.

Progressive Multifocal Leukoencephalopathy (PML)

Progressive multifocal leukoencephalopathy is a demyelinating disease that has been placed in the infectious section of this chapter because papovavirus (SV 40 virus) has been isolated from brains of patients with this disease.[83, 84] It most often affects the compromised host. Diseases associated with PML include lymphoma, leukemia, tuberculosis, sarcoid, systemic lupus erythematosus, and renal transplantation.[85] Recently, PML has been described in a young patient with AIDS.[86] Clinical symptoms depend upon the location of the involved white matter. Affected patients may present with ataxia, spasticity, or visual disturbances that progress inexorably to coma and death within 1 year.[87] The disease starts as focal areas of demyelination in the subcortical white matter and then coalesces into large areas, resulting in cystic atrophy.[88] There are no specific diagnostic tests for PML; however, CT is quite suggestive in the appropriate clinical circumstance.

The CT abnormalities observed in PML are scalloped low-absorption areas in the white matter, usually in the parieto-occipital region, that are not in a vascular distribution. These areas have no mass effect and may or may not contrast enhance (Fig 7–18).[89, 90] Late in the disease, there is parenchymal loss with ventricular dilatation. The differential diagnosis includes infarction, multiple sclerosis, infection, and tumor. Infarction is in a vascular distribution and associated with mass effect.

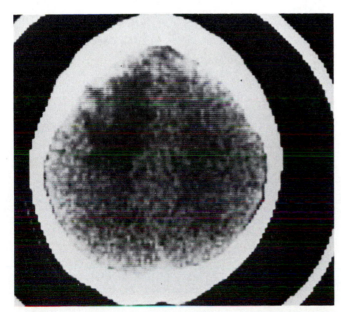

Fig 7–19.—Multiple sclerosis plaque. Large plaque with scalloped borders looks quite similar to those of PML.

Multiple sclerosis occurs most frequently in a periventricular location and in a patient population that is ostensibly immunologically competent. Large multiple sclerosis plaques could be quite similar to PML on CT (Fig 7–19). Tumor and infection have associated mass effect and do not respect the white matter.

Because of its viral etiology, PML may be potentially a treatable disease.[91] At this time, CT appears to be the most specific diagnostic modality available.

Acknowledgment

The authors wish to thank Kenneth R. Davis, M.D., of the Department of Radiology, Massachusetts General Hospital, Boston, for his contributions.

REFERENCES

1. Crocker E.F., Zimmerman R.A., Phelps M.E., et al.: The effect of steroids on the extravascular distribution of radiographic contrast material and technetium pertechnetate in brain tumors as determined by computed tomography. *Radiology* 119:471–474, 1976.
2. Flament-Durand J., Ketelbant-Balasse P., Maurus R., et al.: Intracerebral calcifications appearing during the course of acute lymphocytic leukemia treated with methotrexate and x-rays. *Cancer* 35:319–325,1975.
3. Lee K.I., Suh J.H.: CT evidence of gray matter calcification secondary to radiation therapy. *Comput. Tomogr.* 1:103–110, 1977.
4. McIntosh S., Fischer D.B., Rothman S.G., et al.: Intracranial calcifications in childhood leukemia. *J. Pediatr.* 91:909–913, 1977.
5. Numaguchi Y., Hoffman J.C., Sones P.J.: Basal ganglia calcification as a late radiation effect. *A.J.R.* 123:27–30, 1975.
6. Price R.A.: Pathology of central-nervous-system diseases in childhood leukemia, in Ongerboer de Visser B.W., Basch D.A., van Woerkrom, Eyhenboom W.M.H. (eds.): *Neuro-Oncology.* The Hague, Martinus Nijhoff Publishers, 1980, pp. 186–205.
7. Price R.A., Birdwell D.A.: The central nervous system in childhood leukemia. *Cancer* 42:717–728, 1978.
8. Peylan-Ramu N., Poplack D.G., Pizzo P.A., et al.: Abnormal CT scans of the brain in asymptomatic children with acute lymphocytic leukemia after prophylactic treatment of the central nervous system with radiation and intrathecal chemotherapy. *N. Engl. J. Med.* 298:815–818, 1978.
9. Rubinstein L.J., Herman M.M., Song T.F., et al.: Disseminated necrotizing leukoencephalopathy: A complication of treated central nervous system leukemia and lymphoma. *Cancer* 35:291–305, 1975.
10. Price R.A., Jamieson P.A.: The central nervous system in childhood leukemia. *Cancer* 35:306–318, 1975.
11. Lane B., Carroll B.A., Pedley T.A.: Computerized cranial tomography in cerebral diseases of white matter. *Neurology* 28:534–544, 1978.
12. Shalen P.R., Ostrow P.T., Glass P.J.: Enhancement of

the white matter following prophylactic therapy of the central nervous system for leukemia. *Radiology* 140:409–412, 1981.

13. Bjorgen J.E., Gold L.H.A.: Computed tomographic appearance of methotrexate-induced necrotizing leukoencephalopathy. *Radiology* 122:377–378, 1977.

14. Wendling L.R., Bleyer W.A., DiChiro G., et al.: Transient, severe periventricular hypodensity after leukemic prophylaxis with cranial irradiation and intrathecal methotrexate. *J. Comput. Assist. Tomogr.* 2:502–505, 1978.

15. Carella R.S., Pay N., Newall J., et al.: Computerized (axial) tomography in the serial study of cerebral tumors treated by radiation. *Cancer* 37:2719–2728, 1976.

16. Wilson G.H., Byfield J., Hanafee W.N.: Atrophy following radiation therapy for central nervous system neoplasms. *Acta Radiol. Ther. Phys. Biol.* 11:361–368, 1972.

17. Kramer S.: The hazard of therapeutic irradiation of the central nervous system. *Clin. Neurosurg.* 15:301–318, 1968.

18. Lampert P.W., Davis R.L.: Delayed effects of radiation on the human central nervous system: "Early and late" delayed reactions. *Neurology* 14:912–917, 1964.

19. Rottenberg D.A., Chernik N.K., Deck M.D.F., et al.: Cerebral necrosis following radiotherapy of extracranial neoplasms. *Ann. Neurol.* 1:339–357, 1977.

20. Mikhael M.A.: Radiation necrosis of the brain: Correlation between computed tomography, pathology, and dose distribution. *J. Comput. Assist. Tomogr.* 2:71–80, 1978.

21. Mikhael M.A.: Radiation necrosis of the brain: Correlation between patterns on computed tomography and dose of radiation. *J. Comput. Assist. Tomogr.* 3:241–249, 1979.

22. Brismar J., Roberson G.H., Davis K.R.: Radiation necrosis of the brain: Neuroradiological considerations with computed tomography. *Neuroradiology* 12:109–113, 1976.

23. Littman P., James H., Zimmerman R., et al.: Radionecrosis of the brain presenting as a mass lesion: A case report. *J. Neurol. Neurosurg. Psychiatry* 40:827–829, 1977.

24. Wright T.L., Bresnan M.J.: Radiation-induced cerebrovascular disease in children. *Neurology* 26:540–543, 1976.

25. Brant-Zawadzki M., Anderson M., DeArmond S.J., et al.: Radiation-induced large intracranial vessel occlusive vasculopathy. *A.J.R.* 134:51–55, 1978.

26. Bryan C.S.: Non-bacterial thrombotic endocarditis with malignant tumors. *Am. J. Med.* 46:787–793, 1969.

27. Gore R.M., Weinberg P.E., Anandappa E., et al.: Intracranial complications of pediatric hematologic disorders: Computer tomographic assessment. *Invest. Radiol.* 16:175–180, 1981.

28. Rosen P., Armstrong D.: Nonbacterial thrombotic endocarditis in patients with malignant neoplastic disease. *Am. J. Med.* 54:23–29, 1973.

29. Waldenström J.G.: Biological signs in the diagnosis of cancer, in *Paraneoplasia*. New York, John Wiley & Sons, 1978.

30. Coune A.: Coagulopathies in patients with tumors, in Klastersky J., Staquet M.J. (eds.): *Medical Complications in Cancer Patients*. New York, Raven Press, 1981.

31. Pitner S.E., Johnson W.W.: Chronic subdural hematoma in childhood acute leukemia. *Cancer* 32:185–190, 1973.

32. Buonanno F.S., Moody D.M., Ball M.R., et al.: Computed cranial tomographic findings in cerebral sinovenous occlusion. *J. Comput. Assist. Tomogr.* 2:281–290, 1978.

33. Banne M., Groves J.T.: Deep vascular congestion in dural venous thrombosis on computed tomography. *J. Comput. Assist. Tomogr.* 3:539–541, 1979.

34. Ingstrup H.M., Jorgensen P.S.: Tentorial changes in sigmoid sinus thrombosis. *J. Comput. Assist. Tomogr.* 5:760–762, 1981.

35. Sigsbee B., Deck M.D.F., Posner J.B.: Non-metastatic superior sagittal sinus thrombosis complicating systemic cancer. *Neurology* 29:139–146, 1979.

36. Little J.R., Dale A.J.D., Okazaki H.: Meningeal carcinomatosis. *Arch. Neurol.* 30:138–143, 1974.

37. Enzmann D.R., Krikorian J., Yorke C., et al.: Computed tomography in leptomeningeal spread of tumor. *J. Comput. Assist. Tomogr.* 2:448–455, 1978.

38. Morganroth J., Deisseroth A., Winokur S., et al.: Differentiation of carcinomatous and bacterial meningitis. *Neurology* 22:1240–1242, 1972.

39. Enzmann D.R., Norman D., Mani J., et al.: Computed tomography of granulomatous basal arachnoiditis. *Radiology* 120:341–344, 1976.

40. Williams R.S., Crowell R.M., Fisher C.M., et al.: Clinical and radiologic remission in reticulum cell sarcoma of the brain. *Arch. Neurol.* 36:206–210, 1979.

41. Enzmann D.R., Krikorian J., Norman D., et al.: Computed tomography in primary reticulum cell sarcoma of the brain. *Radiology* 130:165–170, 1979.

42. Case 49-1978: Case records of the Massachusetts General Hospital. *N. Engl. J. Med.* 299:1349–1359, 1978.

43. Hildebrand J.: Neurological disorders in cancer patients and their treatment, in Klostersky J., Staquet M.J., (eds.): *Medical Complications in Cancer Patients*. New York, Raven Press, 1981.

44. Buchner L.H., Schneierson S.S.: Clinical and laboratory aspects of Listeria monocytogenes infections. *Am. J. Med.* 45:904–921, 1968.

45. Lechtenberg R., Sierra M.F., Pringle G.F., et al.: Listeria monocytogenes: Brain abscess or meningoencephalitis. *Neurology* 29:86–90, 1979.

46. Smith P.W., Steinkraus G.E., Henricks B.W., et al.: CNS nocardiosis. *Arch. Neurol.* 37:729–730, 1980.

47. Case 20-1980: Case records of the Massachusetts General Hospital. *N. Engl. J. Med.* 302:1194–1199, 1980.

48. Tyson G.W., Welch J.E., Butler A.B., et al.: Primary cerebellar nocardiosis. *J. Neurosurg.* 51:408–414, 1979.

49. Grossman R.I., Davis K.R., Taveras J.M., et al.: Computed tomography of intracranial aspergillosis. *J. Comput. Assist. Tomogr.* 5:646–650, 1981.

50. Parker J.C., McCloskey J.J., Lee R.S.: The emergence of candidiasis: The dominant postmortem cerebral mycosis. *Am. J. Clin. Pathol.* 70:31–36, 1978.

51. Black J.T.: Cerebral candidiasis: Case report of brain abscess secondary to *Candida albicans*, and review of literature. *J. Neurol. Neurosurg. Psychiatry* 33:864–870, 1970.

52. Case 45-1981. Case records of the Massachusetts General Hospital. *N. Engl. J. Med.* 305:1135–1146, 1981.

53. Gorell J.M., Palutkas W.A., Chason J.L.: Candida pachymeningitis with multiple cranial nerve pareses. *Arch. Neurol.* 36:719–720, 1979.

54. Whelan M.A., Stern J., deNapoli R.A.: The computed tomographic spectrum of intracranial mycosis: Correlation with histopathology. *Radiology* 141:703–707, 1981.

55. Fishman L.S., Griffin J.R., Sapico F.L., et al.: Hematogenous Candida endophthalmitis—a complication of candidemia. *N. Engl. J. Med.* 286:675–681, 1972.

56. Bindschadler D.D., Bennett J.E.: Serology of human cryptococcosis. *Ann. Intern. Med.* 69:45–52, 1968.

57. Harper C.G., Wright D.M., Perry G., et al.: Cryptococcal granuloma presenting as an intracranial mass. *Surg. Neurol.* 11:425–429, 1979.

58. Everett B.A., Kusske J.A., Rush J.L., et al.: Cryptococcal infection of the central nervous system. *Surg. Neurol.* 9:157–163, 1978.

59. Blitzer A., Lawson W., Meyers B.R., et al.: Patient survival factors in paranasal sinus mucormycosis. *Laryngoscope* 90:635–648, 1980.

60. Long E.L., Weiss D.L.: Cerebral mucormycosis. *Am. J. Med.* 26:625–635, 1980.

61. Succar M.B., Nichols R.D., Burch K.H.: Rhinocerebral mucormycosis. *Arch. Otolaryngol.* 105:212–214, 1979.

62. Price D.L., Wolpow E.R., Richardson E.P. Sr.: Intracranial phycomycosis: A clinicopathological and radiological study. *J. Neurol. Sci.* 14:359–375, 1971.

63. Raji M.R., Agha F.P., Gabriele O.F.: Nasopharyngeal mucormycosis. *J. Comput. Assist. Tomogr.* 5:767–770, 1981.

64. Lazo A., Wilner H.I., Metes J.J.: Craniofacial mucormycosis: Computed tomographic and angiographic findings in two cases. *Radiology* 139:523–626, 1981.

65. Wilson W.B., Grotta J.C., Schold C., et al.: Cerebral mucormycosis: An unusual case. *Arch. Neurol.* 36:725–726, 1979.

66. Ruskin J., Remington J.S.: Toxoplasmosis in the compromised host. *Ann. Intern. Med.* 84:193–199, 1976.

67. Frenkel J.K., Nelson B.M., Ariss-Stella J.: Immunosuppressive and toxoplasmic encephalitis. *Hum. Pathol.* 6:97–111, 1975.

68. Carey R.M., Kimball A.C., Armstrong D., et al.: Toxoplasmosis: Clinical experiences in a cancer hospital. *Am. J. Med.* 54:30–38, 1973.

69. Enzmann D.R., Brant-Zawadzki M., Britt R.H.: CT of central nervous system infections in immunocompromised patients. *A.J.N.R.* 1:239–243, 1980.

70. Menges H.W., Fischer E., Valavanis A., et al.: Cerebral toxoplasmosis in the adult. *J. Comput. Assist. Tomogr.* 3:413–416, 1979.

71. Post M.J.D., Chan J.C., Hensley G.T., et al.: Toxoplasma encephalitis in Haitian adults with acquired immunodeficiency syndrome: A clinical-pathologic-CT correlation. *A.J.N.R.* 4:155–162, 1983.

72. Dolin R., Reichman R.C., Mazur M.H., et al.: Herpes-zoster-varicella infections in immunosuppressed patients. *Ann. Intern. Med.* 89:375–388, 1978.

73. Gallagher J.G., Merigan T.C.: Prolonged herpes-zoster infection associated with immunosuppressive therapy. *Ann. Intern. Med.* 91:842–846, 1979.

74. Hedges T.R. III, Albert D.M.: The progression of the ocular abnormalities of herpes zoster. *Ophthalmology* 39:165–177, 1982.

75. Mackenzie R.A., Forbes G.S., Karnes W.E.: Angiographic findings in herpes zoster arteritis. *Ann. Neurol.* 10:458–464, 1981.

76. Rosenblum W.I., Hadfield M.G.: Granulomatous angiitis of the nervous system in cases of herpes zoster and lymphosarcoma. *Neurology* 22:348–354, 1972.

77. Greco F.A., Kolins J., Rajjoub R.K., et al.: Hodgkin's disease and granulomatous angiitis of the central nervous system. *Cancer* 38:2027–2032, 1976.

78. Rosenblum W.I., Hadfield M.G.: Granulomatous angiitis of the nervous system in cases of herpes zoster and lymphosarcoma. *Neurology* 22:348–354, 1972.

79. Newcastle N.B., Tom N.I.: Noninfectious angiitis of the nervous system associated with Hodgkin's disease. *J. Neurol. Neurosurg. Psychiatry* 25:51–58, 1962.

80. Kolodny E.H., Rebeiz J.J., Caviness V.S., et al.: Granulomatous angiitis of the central nervous system. *Arch. Neurol.* 19:510–524, 1968.

81. Valavanis A., Friede R., Schubiger O., et al.: Cerebral granulomatous angiitis simulating brain tumor. *J. Comput. Assist. Tomogr.* 3:536–538, 1979.

82. Faer M.J., Mead J.H., Lynch R.D.: Cerebral granulomatous angiitis: Case report and literature. *A.J.R.* 129:463–467, 1977.

83. ZuRheim G.M., Chou S.M.: Particles resembling papovaviruses in human cerebral demyelinating disease. *Science* 148:1477–1479, 1965.

84. Weiner L.P., Herndon R.M., Narayon O.: Isolation of virus relation SV40 from patients with progressive multifocal leukoencephalopathy. *N. Engl. J. Med.* 286:385–390, 1972.

85. Legrain M., Graveleau J., Brion S., et al.: Progressive multifocal leukoencephalopathy after kidney transplantation. *Rev. Neurol.* 130:167–169, 1974.

86. Miller J.R., Barrett R.E., Britton C.B., et al.: Progressive multifocal leukoencephalopathy in a male homosexual with T-cell immune deficiency. *N. Engl. J. Med.* 307:1436–1437, 1982.

87. Lyon L.W., McCormick W.F., Schochet S.S., Jr.: Progressive multifocal leukoencephalopathy. *Arch. Intern. Med.* 128:420–426, 1971.

88. Richardson E.P., Jr.: Progressive multifocal leukoencephalopathy. *N. Engl. J. Med.* 265:815–823, 1961.

89. Heinz E.R., Drayer B.P., Haenggeli C.A., et al.: Computed tomography in white-matter disease. *Radiology* 130:371–378, 1979.

90. Carroll B.A., Lane B., Norman D., et al.: Diagnosis of progressive multifocal leukoencephalopathy by computed tomography. *Radiology* 122:137–141, 1977.

91. Marriott P.J., O'Brien M.D., Mackenzie I.C.: Progressive multifocal leukoencephalopathy: Remission with cytarabine. *J. Neurol. Neurosurg. Psychiatry* 38:205–209, 1975.

8

Diseases of the White Matter*

MEREDITH A. WEINSTEIN, M.D.
MICHAEL T. MODIC, M.D.
CHARLES K. KEYSER, M.D.

POSER[1] has divided the demyelinating diseases into two groups: the myelinoclastic (demyelinating) group, where myelin is normally formed and is subsequently injured or destroyed by either endogenous or exogenous agents or a combination of both; and the dysmyelinating diseases, in which some enzymatic disturbance interferes either with the formation of myelin or with its maintenance. The following classification of diseases of the white matter is primarily based on the classifications of Poser[1] and of Gilroy and Meyer.[2]

I. Myelinoclastic diseases
  A. Primary idiopathic (? acquired allergies and infections)
    1. Multiple sclerosis (MS)
    2. Diffuse sclerosis (Schilder, 1912)
    3. Optic neuromyelitis (Devic)
    4. Concentric sclerosis (Baló)
    5. Transitional sclerosis
  B. Acquired allergic and infectious diseases resulting in breakdown of myelin
    1. Postvaccinal encephalomyelitis
    2. Postinfectious encephalomyelitis (acute disseminated encephalomyelitis)
    3. Acute hemorrhagic leukoencephalitis
    4. Postinfectious polyneuritis (Landry-Guillain-Barré syndrome)
  C. Viral induced
    1. Subacute sclerosing panencephalitis (SSPE)
    2. Subacute rubella syndrome
    3. Progressive multifocal leukoencephalopathy (PML)
  D. Degenerative-toxic
    1. Central pontine myelinolysis (CPM)
    2. Marchiafava-Bignami disease
    3. Carbon monoxide encephalopathy
    4. Anoxic encephalopathy
  E. Vascular
    1. Binswanger's disease
    2. Maladie-de-Schilder-Foix
  F. Post-therapy
    1. Methotrexate leukoencephalopathy
    2. Disseminated necrotizing leukodystrophy (DNL)

II. Dysmyelinating diseases
  A. Leukodystrophies (genetically determined metabolic disorders with primary involvement of myelin)
    1. Metachromatic leukodystrophy
    2. Globoid cell leukodystrophy (Krabbe's disease)
    3. Spongy degeneration (Canavan's disease)
    4. Adrenoleukodystrophy
    5. Alexander's disease
    6. Pelizaeus-Merzbacher disease
  B. Lipid storage diseases with neuronal involvement (genetically determined metabolic disorders with secondary involvement of myelin)
    1. GM_2 gangliosidosis (Tay-Sachs disease)
    2. GM_1 gangliosidosis
    3. Ceroid lipofuscinoses
    4. Neimann-Pick (sphingomyelin lipidosis)
    5. Gaucher's disease (cerebroside lipoidosis)
    6. Cerebrotendinous xanthomatosis
    7. Fabry's disease
  C. Amino acidopathy

Brief synoposes of the clinical and CT findings of each of these diseases are given in Tables 8–1 and 8–2.

---

*Many of the illustrations in this chapter are reversed relative to others in this volume, with the patient's left on the reader's left. Those with the patient's left on the reader's right are indicated when significant.

TABLE 8–1.—MYELINOCLASTIC DISEASES

	AGE OF ONSET	ETIOLOGY	COMPUTERIZED TOMOGRAPHY

Multiple sclerosis	Any age
	Peak 15–45 yr
	Median 33 yr
		Unknown	Sharply marginated plaques 0.6–1.4 cm in diameter, predominantly periventricular, others elsewhere in white matter.
			  A. Decreased attenuation without contrast, increased with contrast (acute and subacute lesions).
			  B. Isodense without contrast, increased with contrast (acute and subacute lesions).
			  C. Decreased without and with contrast (chronic lesions).
			  D. Atrophy.
			  E. Mass effect (very rare).

Diffuse sclerosis	50% under 10 yr	Unknown. Same as multiple sclerosis?	Extensive bilateral areas of decreased attenuation with extensive enhancement in acute stage. Margins may be sharply or poorly defined.
Acute hemorrhagic leukoencephalitis	Young adults	Allergic response to virus	Decreased attenuation coefficients, focal or diffuse, unilateral or bilateral.
Subacute sclerosing panencephalitis	Most 5–15 yr	Measles	Rapidly progressive disease, normal-to-minimal abnormalities. Chronic course, decreased attenuation coefficients of white matter, caudate nuclei, or other basal ganglia without enhancement.
Subacute rubella syndrome	Congenital infection	German measles	Diffuse decreased attenuation white matter, basal ganglia, and centrum semiovale; may calcify.
Progressive multifocal leukoencephalopathy	See Chapter 7		
Central pontine myelinolysis	Any	Rapid increase in serum sodium	Variable-sized areas of decreased attenuation in pons. May have slight enhancement at periphery.
Marchiafava-Bignami	Adults	A. Alcholism B. Nutritional deficiency?	A. Acute, decreased attenuation corpus callosum. B. Subacute, enhancement corpus callosum. C. Chronic, atrophy corpus callosum and cortical atrophy, predominantly frontal.
Carbon monoxide and anoxic encephalopathy	All		Enlarged sulci and cortical atrophy, less commonly decreased attenuation of entire white matter, cerebral hemispheres.
Binswanger's disease	Elderly	Arteriosclerosis	Decreased attenuation of white matter without enhancement.
Methotrexate leukoencephalopathy	See Chapter 7		
Disseminated necrotizing leukodystrophy	See Chapter 7		

MYELIN

Abnormalities of the myelin sheath in the CNS are the subject of this chapter. All axons with a diameter greater than 1 μ in the central and peripheral nervous systems of vertebrates are surrounded by a myelin sheath.[3] The ratio of the diameter of the axon to the thickness of the myelin sheath varies from 5:1 to 25:1. Myelin is almost entirely absent in the cerebrum of the newborn, gradually increased during the first 3 months and more rapidly increases between the third and 13th month. From the 13th month to the age of 10 to 12 years, when the brain reaches its full adult size, there is a constant increase in myelin in relation to the lipids contained in the nerve cells and axons.[4] Five infant baboons were serially studied with CT during the first year of their lives to determine the rate and degree of normal white matter maturation in the frontal, occipital, and parietal areas. Frontal white matter was the most immature in the immediate postnatal period, but it became equal in attenuation to the other regions by 4 weeks of age.[5]

Myelin is a part of the cell wall membrane of the oligodendroglia in the CNS and of the Schwann cell in the peripheral nervous system. The formation and maintenance of myelin is dependent on both the oligodendroglia (or Schwann cell) and the axon; myelin is not formed by either axons grown alone or by oligoden-

TABLE 8–2.—DYSMYELINATING DISEASES (LEUKODYSTROPHIES)

	AGE OF ONSET	ETIOLOGY	COMPUTERIZED TOMOGRAPHY
Metachromatic leukodystrophy			Extensive, diffuse symmetric decreased attenuation coefficients of white matter without enhancement with mild-to-moderate ventricular dilatation.
A. Late infantile	12–18 mo	Decreased arylsulfatase A	
B. Juvenile	5–10 yr	Autosomal recessive	
C. Adult	Adulthood		
Globoid cell leukodystrophy (Krabbe's disease)	3–5 mo	Decreased galactocerebroside β-galactosidase Autosomal recessive	Ventricular or cortical atrophy. May have decreased attenuation of white matter.
Spongy degeneration (Canavan's disease)	2–3mo	Unknown Autosomal recessive	Megalencephaly, symmetric decreased attenuation of white matter.
Adrenoleukodystrophy	School-aged boys	Abnormal, long-chain fatty acid metabolism Sex-linked recessive	Type 1: Early phase: irregular areas decreased attenuation in occipital lobes; subsequent involvement of parietal, temporal, and frontal lobes. Enhancement along leading edge of lesion. Type 2: Enhancement of internal capsule, corona radiata, forceps major, and cerebral peduncles.
Alexander's disease	0–12 mo	Unknown Usually sporadic	Megalencephaly, decreased attenuation coefficient white matter, predominantly frontal lobes and anterior limbs internal capsule. May be decreased attenuation coefficient of basal ganglia, which may enhance.
Pelizaeus-Merzbacher disease	Early infancy	Unknown Sex-linked recessive	Decreased attenuation white matter.

droglia (or Schwann cells) grown alone in tissue culture. If an axon is interrupted, both the axon and its myelin sheath undergo degeneration even though the oligo-dendroglia is not injured. The process is known as Wallerian degeneration after Waller, who in 1850 cut the hypoglossal or glossopharyngeal nerves of frogs and showed degeneration of myelin.[6] To form and maintain myelin, an intact blood supply is also necessary.

Almost any injury or disease of the CNS can cause destruction of myelin. Trauma, infection, neoplasm, metabolic disease, and vascular lesions can cause demyelination associated with damage to neurons. Demyelinating disease is a condition in which there is an injury to myelin sheaths with relative preservation of axons, nerve cells, and supporting structures (periaxial degeneration). In most of the demyelinating diseases, degeneration of the axons and tissue necrosis may occur.[7]

MYELINOCLASTIC DISEASES

Primary Myelinoclastic Diseases

Multiple Sclerosis

HISTORY.—In 1838, Carswell[8] and, from 1839 to 1842, Cruveilhier[9] recognized and described the lesions of MS. In 1849, a German internist, Frerichs,[10] used the term "Hirnsklerose," and in 1866 a French neurologist, Vulpian,[11] described clinical and pathologic findings of patients with MS. In 1879, Charcot[12] recognized

the essential pathologic feature of MS, demyelination with relative preservation of axons.

EPIDEMIOLOGY.—The most common demyelinating disease, MS is relatively uncommon, with a prevalence rate of 58/100,000 in the United States (0.058%). On Jan. 1, 1976, there were 123,000 MS patients in the mainland United States. The age of the person at the first symptom was less than 20 in 13%, 20 to 29 in 30%, 30 to 39 in 28%, 40 to 49 in 14%, and 50-plus in 15%, for a median age of onset of 33 years. The average age of onset for females is 2 to 3 years earlier than for males. Females have a prevalence rate of 72/100,000, males of 42/100,000. Sixty-three percent of MS cases occur in females and 37% in males. Whites have a prevalence rate of 62/100,000; nonwhites have a rate of 31/100,000.[13]

There is ever-increasing evidence that MS is a disease acquired years before clinical onset. There is a marked variation in the incidence of MS that is related to latitude. Different races have markedly different susceptibilities to MS.

The compilation of nearly 200 studies has shown that MS is distributed throughout the world in three zones of high, medium, and low frequencies. The prevalence rates are over 30/100,000 in high-frequency areas, which include Europe between 45° and 65° latitude, southern Canada, northern United States, New Zealand, and southern Australia.[14]

Medium-frequency areas with prevalence rates of 5

to 25 (and mostly 10 to 15) per 100,000 are adjacent to high-frequency areas. and include southern Europe, southern United States, and most of Australia. In the United States, 37° latitude is the approximate border between the northern high-frequency areas and the southern medium-frequency regions. Incidence rates per 100,000 population (followed by latitude) for some representative United States and Canadian cities are Winnipeg, 40 (50°); Rochester, Minn., 64 (44°); Boston, 51 (42°); Denver, 37 (40°); San Francisco, 30 (37°); New Orleans, 12 (30°); Houston, 7 (30°); and Hawaii, 10 (20°).[15] Except for one white group in South Africa, all studied areas of Asia and Africa have low prevalence rates of MS (under 5/100,000).

White populations inhabit all the high- and medium-risk areas. In America, blacks, Orientals, and possibly Indians have much lower rates of MS than whites, but the incidence of each group parallels the geographic gradient found for whites.[14] Incidence of MS is very low in Japan, India, and Korea, with prevalence rates of 2/100,000 in Fukuoka (34° latitude), Sapporo (43°), Bombay (18°), and Seoul (38°).[15] No well-documented case of MS has been reported in African blacks.

While the etiology of MS is unknown, there is evidence suggesting an infectious (slow virus) etiology. Migration studies have shown that those migrating after age 15 retain the MS risk of their birthplace and that those migrating before 15 acquired the risk of their new residence.[14] In the Faroe Islands, a group of small islands between Norway and Iceland at latitude 62°, an epidemic of MS occurred. Between 1920 and 1977, 25 cases of MS occurred among native-born Faroese, excluding those with prolonged foreign residence. Twenty-four of these cases occurred between 1943 and 1960; one occurred in 1970. Before 1943, the prevalence rate was 0/100,000. After 1943, the prevalence rate was 87/100,000. All 14 early-onset cases (1943 to 1949) were in persons 11 to 45 years of age in 1940. All but two late-onset cases (1952 to 1960) were in persons up to 10 years of age in 1940. For 5 years beginning in April 1940, British troops occupied the Faroes in large numbers. All but three of the Faroese who had MS lived in locations where the British troops were stationed, and these three had direct contact with the British.[16] It is therefore probable that the British troops, or something brought along with the British troops such as dogs, caused an epidemic on the Faroes.

It is noteworthy that canine distemper was pandemic in the Islands during World War II. Canine distemper was absent before the British occupation, and since 1956 or 1957 there have been no further cases of canine distemper among dogs on the Faroe Islands. Other studies have shown an association between dogs with distemper and neurologic illnesses with symptoms of MS.[17–19]

In addition to the apparent association with dogs having distemper, other indications that MS may have an infectious etiology are similarities between the epidemiology of MS and poliomyelitis. A person has a 1.7 times greater chance of acquiring MS if he has had a tonsillectomy. This increased risk is similar to the increased risk of acquiring poliomyelitis after tonsillectomy.[20] Prior to immunization, the incidence of poliomyelitis had a variation with latitude that was similar to MS. It has been postulated that in equatorial regions where sanitation is poor, infection with the poliomyelitis virus and with the MS etiologic agent is universal early in life. It is further postulated that poliomyelitis does not cause paralytic disease, and the MS etiologic agent does not cause clinical manifestations of MS in this young age group. With improvement in the level of sanitation, there is a rising incidence in the level of paralytic poliomyelitis. There is an increased incidence of MS in people of a higher socioeconomic group who have grown up with a higher level of sanitation.[21] This was also true of paralytic poliomyelitis prior to immunization. It has therefore been postulated that MS may be an unusual manifestation of a common enteric virus in those people who have had less contact with this viral agent during early life and have failed to develop immunity by late childhood.[22]

The epidemiology of MS suggests a genetic or familial predisposition. Siblings of MS patients have a 20 times greater probability of acquiring MS, and children of MS patients have a 12 times greater probability of acquiring the disease.[23] Ten percent of patients with MS have a positive family history of MS. Identical twins of MS patients have a 20% to 25% chance of developing the disease, and fraternal twins have less than a 15% chance. The twin that is affected is more likely to have been exposed to tonsillectomies, infections, and animals.[24, 25]

Histocompatibility antigens (HLA) have been extensively studied because of their importance in organ transplantation. Several closely linked genes on chromosome no. 6 determine HLA types. The major human histocompatibility complex is called HLA, and several diseases are associated with particular HLA antigens. Among patients with MS, HLA-3 and HLA-7 have consistently been found to be increased in the range of 40%, compared with 25% in the normal population.[26] It is noteworthy that only one person in 100 infected with the virus of poliomyelitis develops a paralytic illness. It has been reported that there is an increase in HLA-3 and HLA-7 in patients with paralytic poliomyelitis.[27]

In summary, there is much evidence, but no proof, that MS is caused by a slow virus in a genetically susceptible group of people.[28, 29]

COMPUTERIZED TOMOGRAPHY.—Patients with clinically evident MS may have a normal CT scan. The abnormalities found with CT scanning in MS patients are plaques of decreased attenuation that do not enhance with contrast material in older lesions; plaques of decreased or isodense attenuation coefficients that enhance with contrast material in the acute phase; atrophy, both periventricular and cortical;[30] and much more rarely, large areas of decreased attenuation coefficients that enhance after the administration of contrast material and usually have mass effect.[31–33] Hemorrhagic complications of MS have also been rarely reported.[34]

Distribution of Lesions With Autopsy Correlation.— The distribution of MS lesions is highly variable. A case with extensive lesions in the spinal cord and optic nerves may show only a few small lesions in the cerebral hemispheres. In the brain, the lesions are roughly symmetric. Lesions are very commonly periventricular, in particular around the angles of the ventricles (frontal horns, atrium, posterior and temporal horns). These periventricular plaques may appear small in coronal sections, but they are often continuous from the tips of the occipital horns to the tips of the frontal and temporal horns.[35]

Myelin sheath stains show that lesions in the brain are frequently around the lateral and third ventricles. The lesions vary in size from that of a pinhole to almost an entire hemisphere. Varying size plaques may be found in the optic nerves, chiasm, or tracts. The lesions are most numerous in the white matter of the cerebrum, brain stem, cerebellum, and spinal cord. Lesions involving the gray matter of the brain and roots of the spinal and cranial nerves are unusual.[1]

Plaques numbering 1,594 were found on autopsy examinations of the brains of 22 patients with MS. Seventy-four percent of the plaques were in the white matter, 17% were in the junction of the cortex and white matter, 5% in the gray matter of the cortex, and 4% in the central gray matter. Forty percent of the lesions occurred in the periventricular regions. Large plaques were almost always periventricular, the largest occurring around the posterior and anterior horns. The gray matter cortical plaques were difficult to see microscopically. Almost all of the cortical plaques were found in only two of the 22 cases.[36]

Two cadaver brains from patients with MS were studied using a high-resolution CT scanner.[37] Plaques smaller than 0.6 cm were not detected with CT. Some larger plaques were misinterpreted as normal structures. In the first brain, 31 demyelinated plaques were found by pathologic examination. Five of these plaques, all larger than 1 cm, were detected with CT. Six additional lesions 1.6 to 3.2 cm in greatest diameter, located immediately adjacent to the lateral ventricles, were detected only after the anatomical specimens and CT images were compared. The remaining 20 lesions, ranging from 0.6 to 1.2 cm in diameter, were not detected prospectively or retrospectively. All lesions in this brain were periventricular.

Thirty-nine demyelinated plaques were found in the second brain. Only three of these plaques, 0.6 to 1.4 cm in greatest diameter, were detected with CT. The other 36 lesions, all less than 1 cm in diameter, were missed with CT both prospectively and retrospectively.

Although contrast enhancement may have aided in the detection of additional lesions, most of the small plaques undetected without contrast material would probably not have been detected after contrast enhancement. The incidence of low-attenuation areas visualized with CT has a very high correlation with autopsy series.

Plaques With Decreased Attenuation Coefficients.— Most of the plaques visualized with CT are periventricular, frequently near the anterior (Fig 8–1) and posterior horns, but the plaques are visualized in all parts of the white matter. Plaques of decreased attenuation coefficient have not been observed in the cortical gray matter. This correlates with the autopsy material, which showed cortical plaques were difficult to see microscopically. Most of the plaques seen with CT are 2 cm or less in size, although the low-attenuation coefficient areas in reported series vary in diameter from 0.3 to 7.2 cm.[38, 39]

The number of visualized plaques varies from one to eight per patient. The number of MS patients with visualization of plaques also varies in reported series from 18%[40] to 47%[41] of cases. In approximately 25% of the overall reported series, the plaques can be visualized using the CT image only (without an analysis of the CT number printout). The plaques have attenuation coefficients that vary from 10 to 27 Hounsfield units, with normal white matter having an average attenuation coefficient of 30 Hounsfield units.

Plaques visualized as areas of decreased attenuation coefficient in patients with an exacerbation of active disease may increase in size and number, may become isodense with the surrounding brain, or may remain stable (Figs 8–2 to 8–4).[30]

Although the CT visualization of MS plaques has been reported in the spinal cord,[42] brain stem, and optic nerves,[41] it is highly probable that some, if not most

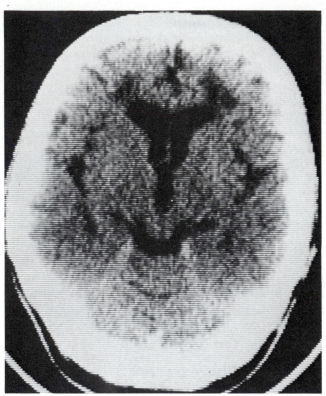

Fig 8–1.—MS in a 48-year-old woman. There are areas of decreased attenuation anterior to the frontal horns of both lateral ventricles on this enhanced scan. These lesions do not enhance. On another section, three other periventricular areas of decreased attenuation that did not enhance were seen. (From Weinstein M.A., Lederman R.J., Rothner A.D., et al.: *Radiology* 129:689–694, 1978. Used by permission.)

or all, of the reported lesions are artifacts and not true lesions. Many of these abnormalities were reported on early generation CT scanners, which produced a large number of artifactual densities.

Because MS plaques are small, more plaques should be detected in thin sections of the brain (approximately 4 or 5 mm) by minimizing overlap of plaque and normal brain tissue (partial volume effect). Because some plaques have almost the same attenuation coefficient as normal brain tissue, scanners with greater contrast resolution detect more of these plaques than earlier generation scanners.

Plaques With Contrast Enhancement.—In one report, 14 of 57 patients with moderate or severe signs and symptoms of an acute exacerbation of MS demonstrated a total of 48 well-delineated plaques on CT.[30] Twenty-two lesions were periventricular, and the remainder were elsewhere in the white matter. When they were first seen, 17 were decreased in attenuation coefficient both without and with contrast material, 16 were decreased in attenuation coefficient without con-

trast material and enhanced with it, and 15 could not be identified without contrast material and were seen well after enhancement (see Figs 8–2 to 8–4). Of the nine MS plaques that were not seen on the original nonenhanced CT scan, but were seen on a follow-up scan, eight showed contrast enhancement.

Over time, lesions that initially exhibited decreased attenuation coefficients without contrast material but showed contrast enhancement subsequently became decreased in attenuation coefficient both with and without contrast material. None of the lesions that failed to demonstrate contrast enhancement initially enhanced on follow-up scans. The lesions that did enhance initially showed decreased attenuation coefficients on both the preinfusion and postinfusion follow-up examinations. Some remained decreased in attenuation coefficient, and some became normal, both with and without contrast material. This data demonstrates that only acute MS lesions enhance with contrast material. It is likely that the enhancement usually clears after a period of weeks, but the enhancement may last or even increase over a period of several months, suggesting continuing active demyelination of the lesion (Figs 8–5 and 8–6).[31, 43]

Contrast enhancement in MS plaques represents a breakdown in the blood-brain barrier, which results in extravasation of contrast material.[44] Many substances that would readily enter other tissue and organs of the body are only selectively permeable to the vascular endothelium in the CNS. In general, the molecular size and polarity are inversely proportional to vascular permeability in the CNS. Liquids are highly permeable. Water, even though it is a dipolar substance, is highly permeable and follows the osmotic gradient. There are specific active transport mechanisms for certain sugars, biogenic amines, aminoacids, and ions. Outside the CNS, endothelial cells contain fenestrations and pinocytotic vesicles. The CNS endothelium does not contain these structures, but consists of continuous belts of tight junctions. The capillaries are completely enclosed by astrocytic perivascular foot processes, which are unique to the CNS. All of these features constitute the blood-brain barrier.[45] Compromise of the blood-brain barrier increases vascular permeability to the extravasation of plasma constituents into the extracellular space. The edema in MS is vasogenic, predominantly white matter edema. This is in distinction to cytotoxic edema, where the blood-brain barrier is intact and the edema due to influx of a plasma ultrafiltrate causing generalized intracellular overhydration; to ischemic edema, which affects both the white and gray matter and is secondary to infarction of the blood vessels; and to interstitial edema, which is secondary to hydrocephalus.

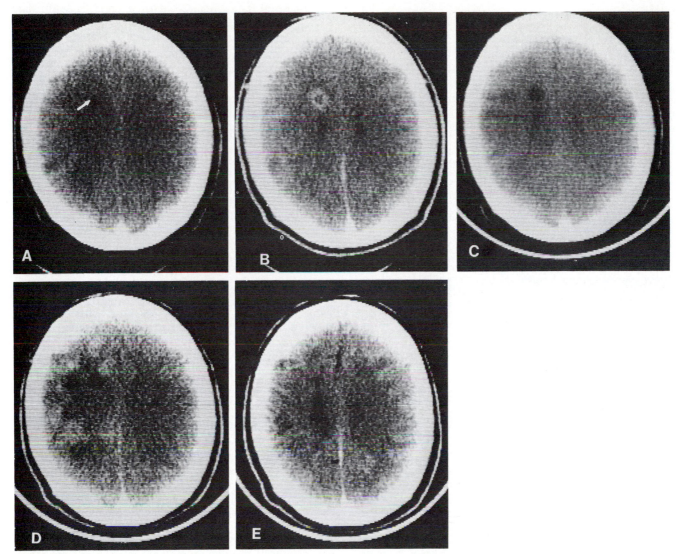

Fig 8–2.—MS in a 25-year-old man. **A,** nonenhanced scan shows an area of decreased attenuation *(arrow)* anterior to the body of the left lateral ventricle. **B,** scan same day with contrast material shows ring enhancement of the lesion. **C,** three weeks later (without contrast material), the area of decreased attenuation persists. In addition, a similar region not seen on the previous examination is visible lateral to the first lesion. **D,** same date as photo **C.** The previously observed lesions do not enhance. However, five discrete contrast-enhanced lesions, not seen on the unenhanced scans, are visible in the left hemisphere. **E,** five months later, the enhanced scan has returned to normal. (From Weinstein M.A., Lederman R.J., Rothner A.D., et al.: *Radiology* 129:689–694, 1978. Used by permission.)

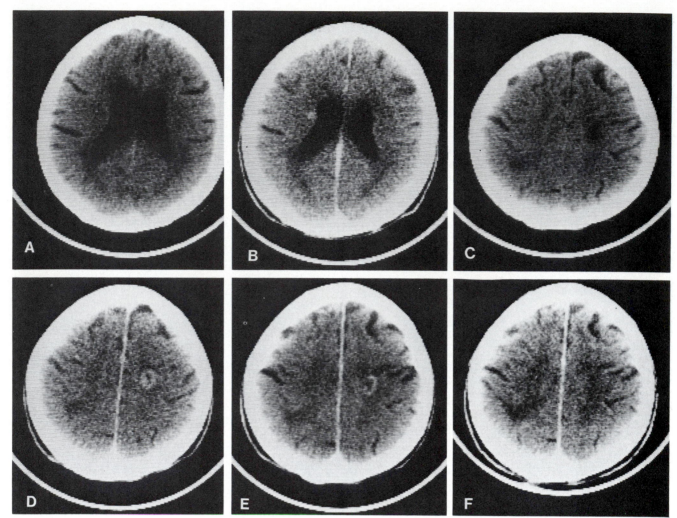

Fig 8–3.—MS in a 59-year-old man. Scans **A** through **E** were obtained on the same date. **A,** without contrast material. This scan and the scan taken at this level 7 months previously show mild dilatation of the sulci and ventricles. No lesions are seen. **B,** with contrast material. A periventricular lesion is shown on the left. On other sections, three other enhanced periventricular lesions were present, but were not seen on the unenhanced scans. CT scans with and without enhancement 8 days later showed no change. **C,** without contrast material. There is an area of decreased attenuation in each hemisphere. **D,** with contrast material. The lesion in the left hemisphere remains decreased in attenuation, while the one on the right exhibits ring enhancement. **E,** with contrast material. There is less enhancement of the ring lesion, but left lesion is unchanged. **F,** three months later (with contrast material), the left lesion remains unchanged. The right lesion can no longer be seen, either without or with contrast material. (From Weinstein M.A., Lederman R.J., Rothner A.D., et al.: *Radiology* 129:689–694, 1978. Used by permission.)

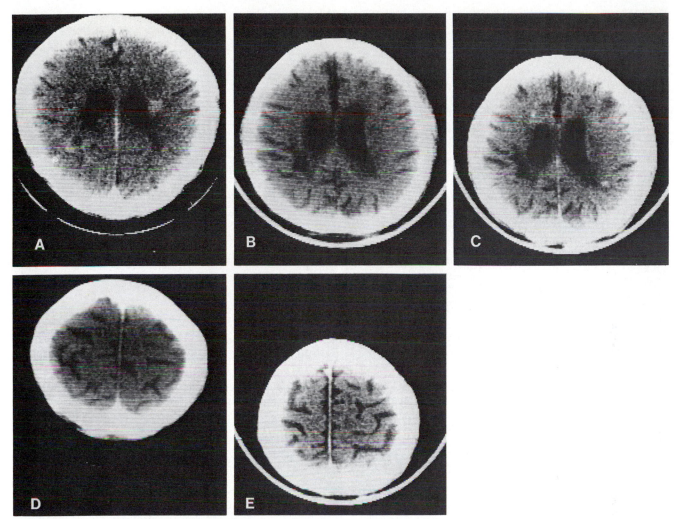

Fig 8–4.—MS in a 39-year-old woman. **A,** with contrast material. There is a lesion lateral to the body of the right lateral ventricle. A second lesion can be seen posterior to the body of the left lateral ventricle. On the unenhanced scan, the lesion on the right could not be seen, while the lesion on the left was decreased in attenuation. On another section, a periventricular lesion not visible without contrast material was seen on the enhanced scan. **B,** nineteen months later (without contrast material), the left lesion persists, while the right lesion is not visible. **C,** same date as photo **B,** with contrast material, the right lesion is now visible, while the left lesion does not enhance. Three additional enhanced periventricular lesions, not visible on the unenhanced scans, could be seen in the right and left hemispheres on different sections. **D,** same date as photo **A,** the sulci are normal in size. **E,** same date as photos **B** and **C,** the sulci are enlarged. (From Weinstein M.A., Lederman R.J., Rothner A.D., et al.: *Radiology* 129:689–694, 1978. Used by permission.)

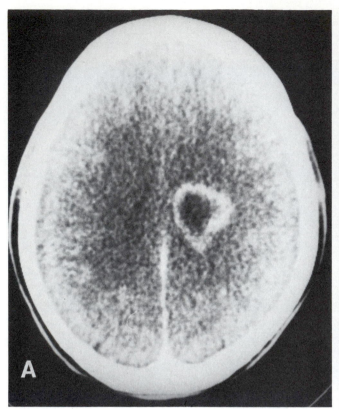

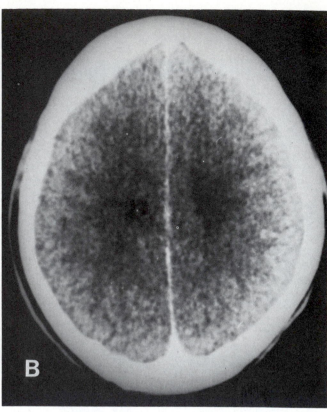

Fig 8–5.—MS. **A,** with contrast material. Scan obtained during acute clinical exacerbation of MS shows an enhancing ring lesion in the right parietal lobe. **B,** six weeks later (with contrast material). The previously visualized lesion is no longer enhanced, although a smaller area of decreased attenuation coefficient is again seen. (Courtesy of Lawrence H.A. Gold, M.D., University of Minnesota, Minneapolis.)

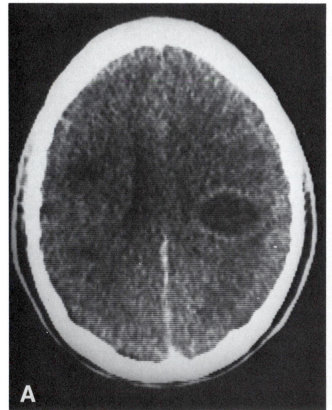

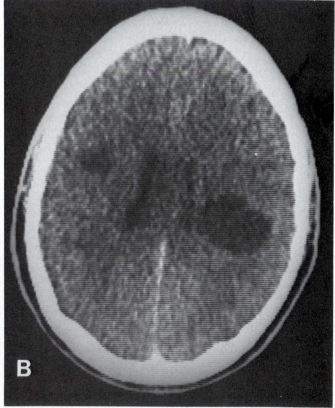

Fig 8–6.—MS. **A,** with contrast material. An area of ring enhancement with a central core of decreased attenuation coefficient is in the right parietal lobe. Mass effect is associated with this lesion. There is also a left frontal plaque. **B,** three weeks later (with contrast material), there is decreasing ring enhancement of the lesion. Mass effect persists. (Courtesy of Lawrence H.A. Gold, M.D., University of Minnesota, Minneapolis.)

Experience with radionuclide brain scans in MS is confirmatory that the enhancement of MS plaques is due to breakdown of the blood-brain barrier. In one reported series, five of 28 patients with a clinical diagnosis of MS had abnormal radionuclide images.[46] None of the 14 patients with inactive disease had an abnormal brain scan. In another series, three of 160 patients (1.8%) had abnormal radionuclide images representing a breakdown of the blood-brain barrier.[47] The radionuclide image will be abnormal only during the period when the CT scan shows contrast enhancement. Because smaller lesions can be better resolved with CT than with radionuclide imaging, and because plaques can be shown by CT but not by the radionuclide image when the blood-brain barrier is intact, more MS plaques are shown by CT than by radionuclide imaging.

Additional evidence that the enhancement of MS plaques is due to the breakdown of the blood-brain barrier is found in multiple reports that corticosteroids that reestablish the blood-brain barrier in vasogenic edema have been reported to suppress contrast enhancement of MS lesions.[45] Histologic and pathologic material, both in MS and in experimental allergic encephalomyelitis, also confirm the breakdown of the blood-brain barrier in MS.

Atrophy.—The incidence of atrophy in reported series ranges from 21% to 78%.[39, 48] The atrophy may be visualized as enlargement of the lateral ventricles, of the cortical sulci, of the basal cisterns, or of a combination of these. The atrophy is found both in patients with plaques and without plaques. Shrinkage of white matter secondary to sclerosis and tissue loss secondary to demyelination contribute to the atrophy found in MS. The longer the duration of MS signs and symptoms, the more likely is atrophy to be found. Patients with atrophy are more severely affected by dementia and diffuse hyperreflexia.[38, 39]

Mass Effect.—Very rarely, an MS plaque will present with mass effect.[31–33, 49] Most of the reported cases with mass effect have shown contrast enhancement. In the majority of these cases, the contrast enhancement has been around the periphery of the lesion, but in some cases the enhancement has occurred throughout the lesion. All of these lesions have been large in size. It has frequently been impossible to differentiate such lesions from primary and metastatic brain tumors on the original scan (Fig 8–7). Interval follow-up scans and clinical correlation may enable the correct diagnosis to be made in these cases, but several of these cases have been biopsied[31, 33] because they could not be differentiated from tumors. The results of the biopsies in these cases may be equivocal.

High Volume of Contrast Medium and Delayed Scanning.—In most CT examinations, 37 to 40 gm of iodine are used for contrast enhancement (100 ml of 76% methylglucamine diatrizoate equals 37 gm iodine). Studies have shown that if this dosage is doubled (74 to 82 gm iodine) and/or delayed scans (1 hour after contrast injection) are obtained, lesions may be seen that are not visualized on the regular contrast-enhanced scan: more metastases are visualized, areas of equivocal enhancement are more definitively defined, lesions are more distinct, the shape and size of the lesions are better seen, and macrocystic lesions can be differentiated from microcystic ones (Fig 8–8).[50–52]

Reports have shown that more MS plaques can be visualized with high doses and/or delayed scans.[53–55] Seventy consecutive patients with known MS or with signs and/or symptoms highly suspicious of acute or relapsing MS were studied in the largest of these reports.[55] The patients were examined before contrast medium infusion, immediately after 40 gm of iodine, and 1 hr after an additional rapid drip of 42 gm of iodine. The patients were divided into three groups: group 1, definite MS; group 2, suspected MS; group 3, MS eventually excluded. In the 39 cases in group 1, the conventional enhanced scan was positive in 25 cases and the high-volume delayed scan in 32 cases. The high-volume delayed scan added the following information in 23 of these 32 cases: (1) better visualization of equivocal areas in 17 cases, (2) enhancement of low-attenuation coefficient plaques not enhanced on the standard CT in 13 cases, (3) enhancement of isodense plaques not enhanced on the standard CT in 9 cases, and (4) visualization of low-attenuation plaques not seen on the standard CT in 4 cases. In 21 of the suspected MS cases, the conventional CT scan was positive in two cases and the high-volume delayed scan in 5 cases. Using a combination of high volumes of contrast media and 1-hour delayed scans, this study demonstrated previously unreported enhancing plaques in the cortical gray matter and in the gray/white matter junction areas.

CT: Clinical Correlation.—Patients with definite MS may have normal CT scans. Plaques may not be visualized because they are small, because they are isodense with the brain, because corticosteroids may mask the lesions, or because the lesions may be located in the brain stem, optic nerves, and spinal cord where they cannot be visualized because of CT artifacts from the surrounding bone.

Multiple reports have shown that in patients with abnormal CT scans, the location and activity of the clinically determined lesions may not correlate with the location and activity of the lesions as determined by the unenhanced and contrast-enhanced CT scans (Fig 8–

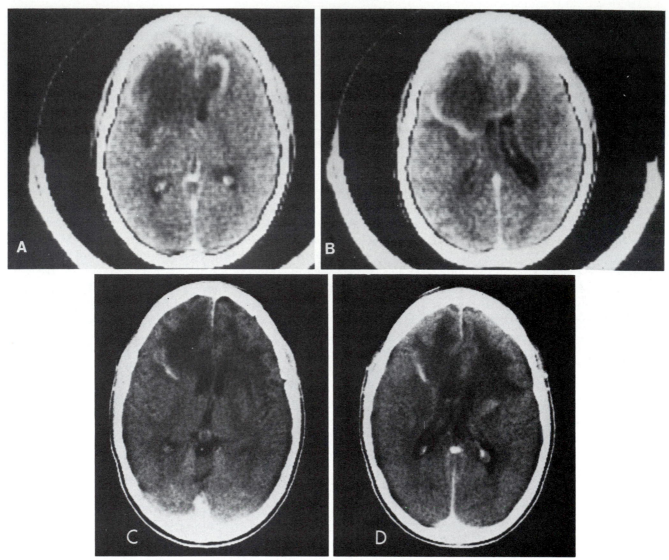

Fig 8–7.—A 23-year-old woman with a primary demyelinating disease (with contrast material). **A, B,** extensive areas of decreased attenuation coefficient present in both frontal lobes, greater on the left. There is compression of the frontal horns of the lateral ventricles and marked peripheral enhancement. The CT appearance is that of a "butterfly glioma" of the corpus callosum. **C, D,** six weeks later after corticosteroid therapy, scans show decreased mass effect and decreased enhancement. (From Rieth K.G., DiChiro G., Cromwell L.D., et al.: *J. Neurosurg.* 55:620–624, 1981. Used by permission.)

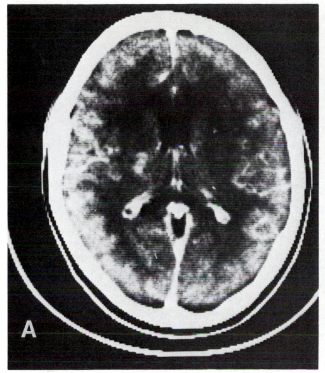
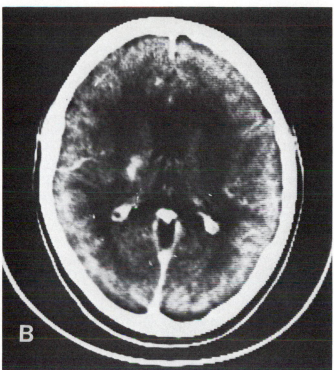

Fig 8–8.—A 35-year-old woman with MS (with contrast material, patient's left on reader's right). **A,** an area of enhancement is in the posterior portion of the right internal capsule of a scan obtained 20 minutes after the injection of 150 ml of contrast material. **B,** the area of enhancement is more apparent on a scan obtained 45 minutes after the injection of contrast material.

9).[30, 39, 44, 56, 57] One difficulty in relating the lesions to the clinical history is that there is no way to determine whether a demyelinated axon in a histologic or electron microscopic preparation was capable of transmitting nerve impulses during life. Total transverse demyelination can sometimes be observed in an optic nerve from a patient who was not blind in that eye and in the spinal cord from a patient who could walk. Therefore, some demyelinated axons must transmit impulses.[58] Clinical remission is most likely due to resumption of conduction in axons that were blocked at the time of acute demyelination. It is not known to what extent, if any, remyelination is related to remission. This indicates that conduction may occur through some of the plaques observed with CT and that CT does not detect other plaques that are present.

CT: Pathologic Correlation.—Plaques can be divided into active lesions (acute and subacute) and inactive (chronic) lesions. The early lesions are softer than the surrounding normal brain tissue and difficult to detect by microscopic examination in the first few days. Altered staining reactions and irregular bubbly expansion in the myelin sheaths, as well as microglial proliferation, can be seen in early lesions. During the next few weeks, the microglia become phagocytic and contain

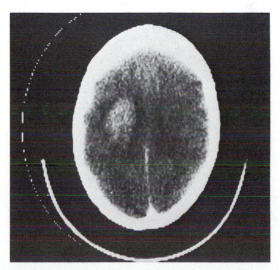

Fig 8–9.—A 30-year-old woman with MS (with contrast material). Typical contrast enhancement occurs in a pathologically and symptomatically regressing case of MS. Scan 2 weeks before did not show enhancement of this lesion. (From Marano G.D., Goodwin C.A., Ko J.P., et al.: *Arch. Neurol.* 37:523–524, 1980. Used by permission.)

fragments of myelin and globules of sudanophilic material. The bodies of nerve cells within the plaques appear normal, which differentiates the lesions from infarcts. After a few weeks, the well-differentiated plaques no longer stain for myelin. There is frequently lymphocytic cuffing of the small vessels within or around the lesion, but this cuffing is not prominent in the early stages and is often more conspicuous in older lesions.[58] These findings are consistent with macroscopic and histologic examination of the brains of MS patients who died shortly after enhancing lesions were visualized with CT[32, 58] and with biopsy specimens that were diagnostic of MS in patients with enhancing mass lesions.[31, 33]

The low attenuation in MS plaques is accounted for by a loss of myelin and increased water and not by accumulation of simple or complex lipids.[57] The etiology of the contrast enhancement is breakdown of the blood-brain barrier.

Regeneration of myelin was reported in five cases of MS.[59] The remyelinated fibers were present singly, in small clusters, and occasionally in large groups. In no instance did the number of fibrils exceed 10% of the number thought to be demyelinated in the affected plaque. This was thought to be peripheral myelin, which is usually produced by Schwann cells, as opposed to central myelin, which is produced by modified primitive mesenchymal cells, possibly microglial precursors.

In another plaque remyelination study in the brains of two patients, electron microscopy showed that remyelination by oligodendrocytes can occur in the adult CNS and that it is common in some cases of MS, although limited in its extent.[60]

Three inactive MS lesions were studied with an electron microscope. They demonstrated a very large extracellular space traversed by glial fibrils and normal-appearing axons running into or out of myelin sheaths, which retained their normal structures up to the abrupt terminations.[61] In old lesions, there is a dense network of glial fibers, explaining the increased consistency of these lesions. The name "multiple sclerosis" originates from these dense sclerotic lesions.

Diffuse Sclerosis

Diffuse sclerosis is also known as Schilder's disease (1912 type), diffuse myelinoclastic sclerosis, Schilder's cerebral sclerosis, and encephalitis periaxialis diffusa. This disease is a bilateral and relatively symmetric de-

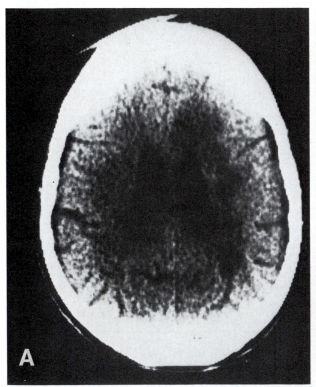 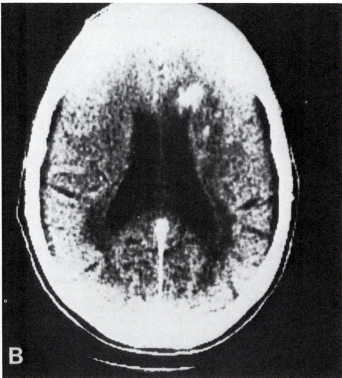

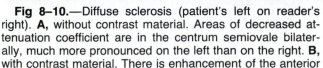

Fig 8–10.—Diffuse sclerosis (patient's left on reader's right). A, without contrast material. Areas of decreased attenuation coefficient are in the centrum semiovale bilaterally, much more pronounced on the left than on the right. B, with contrast material. There is enhancement of the anterior portion of the lesion on the left. This case shows a diffuse involvement of the white matter rather than just a focal plaque. (Courtesy of Lawrence H.A. Gold, M.D., University of Minnesota, Minneapolis.)

myelination of the centrum semiovale (cerebral hemispheric white matter that in sections superior to the corpus callosum has a semioval shape, mostly in the parieto-occipital lobes) (Figs 8–10 and 8–11). Demyelination of the centrum semiovale usually begins posteriorly and extends anteriorly (Figs 8–12 and 8–13). The U fibers (short-association fibers connecting adjacent gyri) are often uninvolved, but have a characteristic involvement if the lesions extend into the gray matter. Diffuse sclerosis usually has a continuous evolution compared with the episodic symptoms of MS.

Diffuse sclerosis occurs most frequently in children, with approximately one half of the cases starting before the age of 10 years. In children, MS is rare. Children probably rarely have MS, but rather the more virulent progressive disease that has been termed diffuse sclerosis.

In the past, children with many types of demyelinating diseases, including adrenoleukodystrophy and subacute sclerosing panencephalitis, were incorrectly said to have Schilder's disease. The term Schilder's disease causes confusion because it has been used for so many different disease processes, and its use should be avoided.

Optic Neuromyelitis (Devic's Disease)

This is a clinical syndrome of combined acute optic neuritis and transverse myelitis that is a variant of MS.

Concentric Sclerosis (Baló's Disease)

This is a histologic variant of both MS and diffuse sclerosis, with small or large areas of concentric, sharply demarcated bands of demyelination alternating with normally staining myelin, or with irregular blocks of demyelination. The disease frequently presents as a space-occupying lesion with an acute onset, short survival, and absence of remissions and exacerbations.

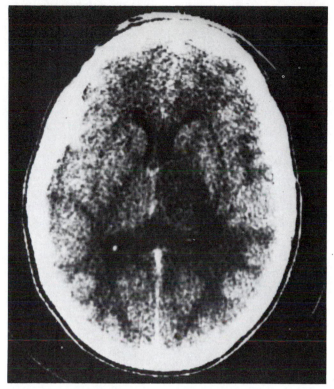

Fig 8–11.—Diffuse sclerosis in a 12-year-old (patient's left on reader's right). An extensive area of decreased attenuation coefficient is in the centrum semiovale on the left. This was best seen on a 3-hour delayed scan after a double dose of contrast material. (Courtesy of Trygve O. Gabrielson, M.D., University of Michigan, Ann Arbor.)

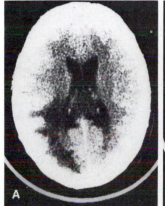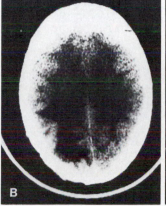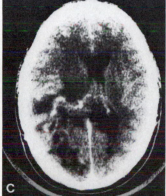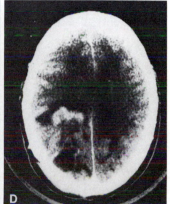

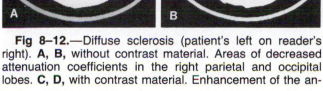

Fig 8–12.—Diffuse sclerosis (patient's left on reader's right). **A, B,** without contrast material. Areas of decreased attenuation coefficients in the right parietal and occipital lobes. **C, D,** with contrast material. Enhancement of the anterior portion of this lesion is visualized. (Courtesy of Lawrence H.A. Gold, M.D., University of Minnesota, Minneapolis.)

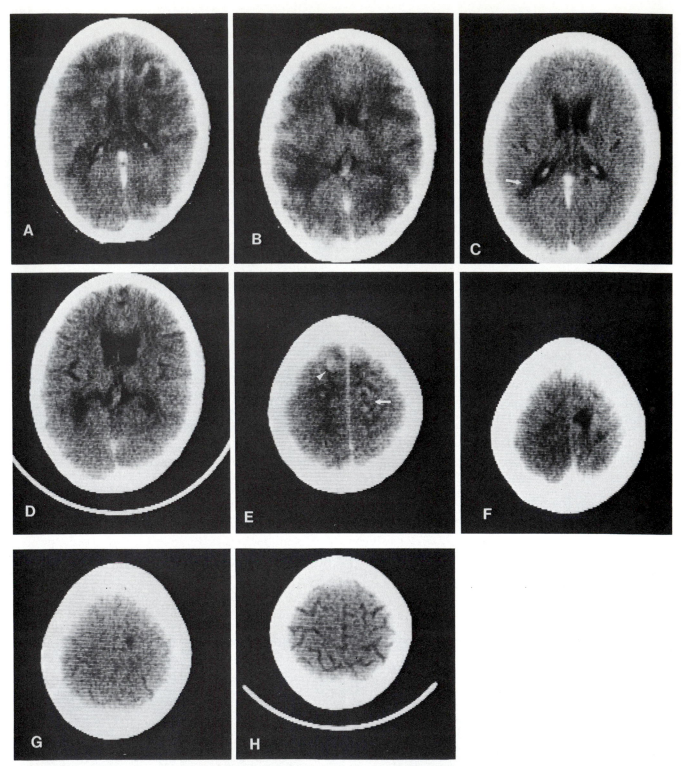

Fig 8–13.—Diffuse sclerosis in a 14-year-old girl. **A,** with contrast material. Diffuse, patchy areas of decreased attenuation can be seen in the white matter, together with focal areas of enhancement. **B,** six days later (with contrast material), the areas of decreased attenuation persist. There is no enhancement of the lesions. **C,** two months later (with contrast material), there is a residual area of decreased attenuation *(arrow)* lateral to the atrium of the left lateral ventricle. **D,** six months later (with contrast material), the scan has returned to normal. **E,** scan obtained at same time as photo **A** (with contrast material). There is a lesion *(arrow)* in the right parietal lobe. Without contrast material, it exhibited decreased attenuation. A second enhanced lesion *(arrowhead)* can be seen in the anterior part of the section on the left. **F,** scan obtained at the same time as photo **B** (with contrast material). The lesion on the right is no longer enhanced by contrast material. The lesion on the left cannot be seen. **G,** scan obtained at the same time as photo **C.** The lesion persists, but has decreased in size. **H,** scan obtained at the same time as photo **D.** The lesion can no longer be seen. The sulci have increased in size. (From Weinstein M.A., Lederman R.J., Rothner A.D., et al.: *Radiology* 129:689–694, 1978. Used by permission.)

Transitional Sclerosis
(Diffuse Disseminated Sclerosis)

Transitional sclerosis is a combination of Schilder's disease and MS. It has been used loosely in patients with at least one large area of demyelination and additional smaller areas of demyelination. The histopathology of transitional sclerosis is that of MS, but with large plaques in the subcortical white matter.

Acquired, Allergic, and Infectious Diseases Resulting in Myelin Breakdown

Postvaccinal Encephalomyelitis

The recommended schedule for childhood immunization is diphtheria, pertussis, tetanus, and trivalent polio vaccine at 2, 4, 6, and 15 months respectively, with measles, mumps, and rubella immunization at 15 months, and an additional diphtheria, pertussis, and tetanus immunization (DPT) at 48 months. Pertussis and possibly influenza, which are prepared from whole killed organisms, may cause allergic reactions producing encephalopathy. These reactions, occurring in less than one in 100,000 vaccine recipients, are characterized by acute demyelination occurring within 4 days of immunization. Recovery is usually complete. Guillain-Barré syndrome appears to have followed influenza immunization only after the 1976 swine flu immunizations.

Measles, mumps, rubella, and trivalent oral polio virus, which are prepared from live attenuated viruses, can cause symptomatic viral infections of the nervous system. Measles encephalitis occurs in one in 1,000,000 vaccine recipients; rubella neuritis occurs in less than one in 10,000 recipients; and paralytic poliomyelitis occurs in one in 3,000,000 vaccine recipients or close contacts of recipients.[62]

Until recently, rabies vaccine consisted of killed rabies virus produced in rabbit brain tissue. One in 750 patients receiving this vaccine developed encephalomyelitis, which was fatal 20% of the time. A duck embryo vaccine now used for rabies does not contain nerve tissue and causes fewer and less severe reactions.[63] After rabies, the most common postvaccinal encephalomyelitis had occurred after smallpox vaccination. The disease occurred in one in 4,000 vaccinations and about 20 times more frequently after primary vaccination than after revaccination.[63] Now that smallpox vaccinations have been eliminated, this common cause of postvaccinal encephalitis is no longer seen.

To our knowledge, there have been no reported cases of postvaccinal encephalitis with CT findings.

Postinfectious Encephalomyelitis

Neurologic complications used to occur most frequently after measles. One in 800 to one in 1,000 mea-sles patients developed encephalomyelitis with a 10% to 20% mortality rate and an equal rate of permanent neurologic damage.[63] With the widespread use of measles vaccination, measles encephalitis is becoming rarer. Encephalomyelitis occurs less frequently following chickenpox and rubella (German measles).

We are not able to report any cases of postinfectious encephalomyelitis with CT abnormalities.

Acute Hemorrhagic Leukoencephalitis

This is the most rapidly progressive demyelinating disease. It mainly affects young adults, but may also involve children. The disease appears to be an allergic response to a virus infection, with most of the cases preceded by approximately 10 days of an upper respiratory infection. The patient may present with headache, fever, stiff neck, hemiplegia, confusion, aphasia, and seizures. Invariably, peripheral leukocystosis is present, with counts ranging from 20,000 to 40,000 cells/mm. The cerebrospinal fluid is often under increased pressure, with polymorphonuclear pleocytosis up to 3,000 cells/mm. Most patients die within 2 to 4 days, but some patients have recovered with almost no residual symptoms.[63]

On CT, there are decreased attenuation coefficients of the white matter that may be focal and may be in one or both cerebral hemispheres (Fig 8–14). The margins of the lesions may be sharply or poorly defined. Rarely, there is enhancement of the lesions.[64, 65]

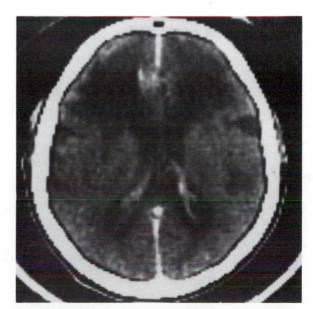

Fig 8–14.—Acute hemorrhagic leukoencephalitis. The white matter of both cerebral hemispheres shows decreased attenuation. The margins of the lesions are poorly defined. (From Adams R.D., Victor M. (eds.): *Principles of Neurology.* New York, McGraw-Hill, 1981, p. 662. Used by permission.)

Postinfectious Polyneuritis
(Landry-Guillain-Barré Syndrome)

This is a distinctive neuropathy characterized by inflammatory lesions scattered throughout the peripheral nervous system. The lesions consist of circumscribed areas in which myelin is lost, combined with an infiltrate of lymphocytes and macrophages.[66] Because this disease is predominantly one of the peripheral nervous system, it will not be discussed further in this chapter.

Viral-Induced Myelinoclastic Diseases

Subacute Sclerosing Panencephalitis

Subacute sclerosing panencephalitis is a slow-virus measles infection of the brain with an incidence of one in 1,000,000 in the United States. Acute measles encephalitis, which is a different, much more benign disease, occurs with approximately one in 800 to one in 1,000 measles patients. While SSPE is progressive and fatal, spontaneous remissions occur that may last for several years. One half of the patients have clinical measles after the age of 2 years. The latent period after the measles infection is approximately 6 years,[67] with most cases presenting between 5 and 15 years of age. One study demonstrated that SSPE patients lack antibodies to one of the viral proteins (M protein) despite high antibody titers to other viral proteins.[68]

The disease has been divided into four stages.[69] Stage 1 patients have decreased mental proficiency and behavioral abnormalities. In stage 2, there is progressive

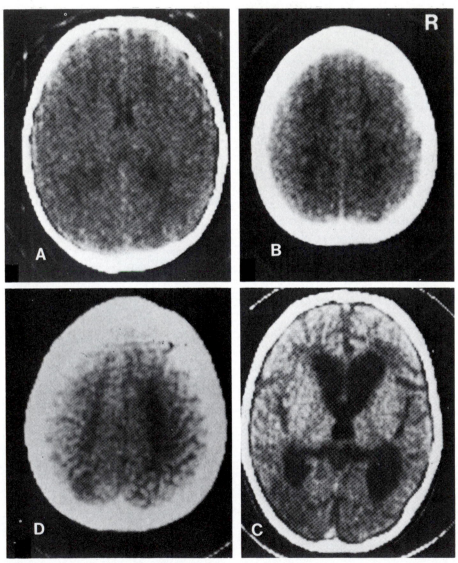

Fig 8–15.—SSPE in a 6-year-old boy. **A, B,** small lateral ventricles. Sulci and interhemispheric fissure are not visualized. **C, D,** seventeen months later, there is severe atrophy and decreased attenuation in both frontal lobes and in the left occipital region. (*R* = patient's right.) (From Pederson H., Wulff C.H.: *Neuroradiology* 23:31–32, 1982. Used by permission.)

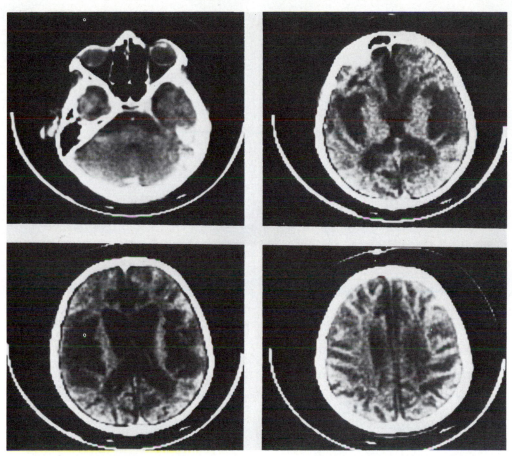

Fig 8–16.—SSPE in a 14-year-old boy. Note extensive atrophy affecting both white and gray matter of cerebral hemispheres, especially of temporal lobes. Pontine atrophy is visualized. (From Duda E.E., Huttenlocher P.R., Patronas N.J., et al.: *A.J.N.R.* 1:35–38, 1980. Used by permission.)

intellectual deterioration, myoclonic seizures, ataxia, and choreiform movements. One half of the patients have ocular signs, including cortical blindness, optic atrophy, and chorioretinitis. Coma, opisthotonos, and decerebrate rigidity occur in stage 3. Stage 4 patients have loss of cortical function. The disease is diagnosed by elevated titers of measles antibody in both the serum and cerebrospinal fluid and by EEG with characteristic synchronous periodic high-voltage complexes.

The cerebral cortex and white matter of both hemispheres and the brain stem are involved in SSPE. The cerebellum is usually spared. Patients with rapidly progressive clinical courses and in whom the pathologic changes are primarily cortical have normal or minimally abnormal CT scans. In patients with a chronic course, the CT shows diffuse and extensive atrophy, decreased attenuation in the white matter, and areas of decreased attenuation in the caudate nucleus or other basal ganglia (Figs 8–15 to 8–17). There is no contrast enhancement of the lesions.[70, 71]

Subacute Rubella Syndrome

Usually, the defects associated with congenital German measles are nonprogressive after the second or third year of life, although progression may occur after stable periods of 8 to 19 years. It appears that the German measles virus acquired in utero persists in the nervous system of these latter patients and may become active again, resembling SSPE.

The CT examination shows decreased attenuation coefficients of the white matter, which are believed to represent retardation of myelination (Fig 8–18). Calcifications may occur in the basal ganglia and centrum semiovale (Fig 8–19).[72]

Progressive Multifocal Leukoencephalopathy

See Chapter 7.

Degenerative-Toxic Myelinoclastic Diseases

Central Pontine Myelinolysis

This is a disease characterized by areas of demyelination of the pons, which may be only a few millimeters

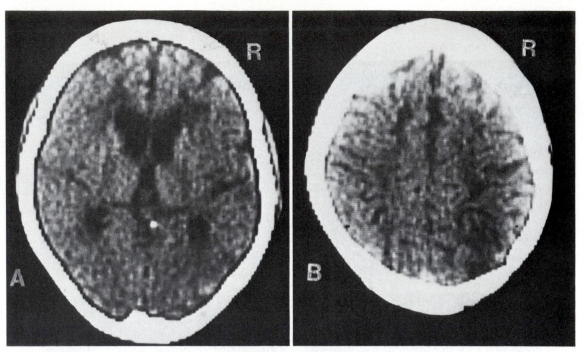

Fig 8–17.—SSPE in a 17-year-old girl who had symptoms for 86 months. **A, B,** focal areas of decreased attenuation in periventricular frontal white matter and in both gray and white matter of the right parietal lobe. Note diffuse cortical atrophy. (*R* = patient's right.) (From Duda E.E., Huttenlocher P.R., Patronas N.J., et al.: *A.J.N.R.* 1:35–38, 1980. Used by permission.)

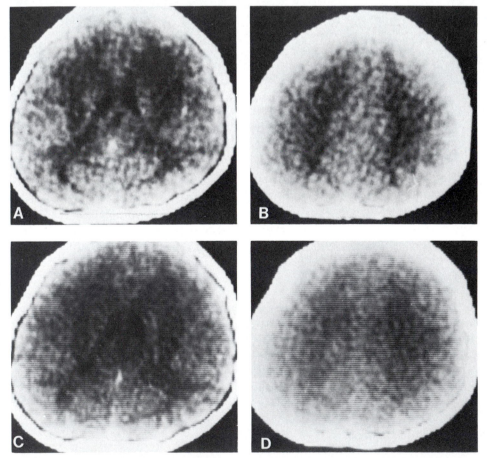

Fig 8–18.—Congenital rubella syndrome in a young female. **A, B,** scan at 19 months of age. **C, D,** scan at 3 years, 7 months of age. There is decreased attenuation of white matter in the earlier scan, somewhat improved in the later examination. (From Ishikawa A., Murayama T., Sakuma N., et al.: *Arch. Neurol.* 39:420–421, 1982. Used by permission.)

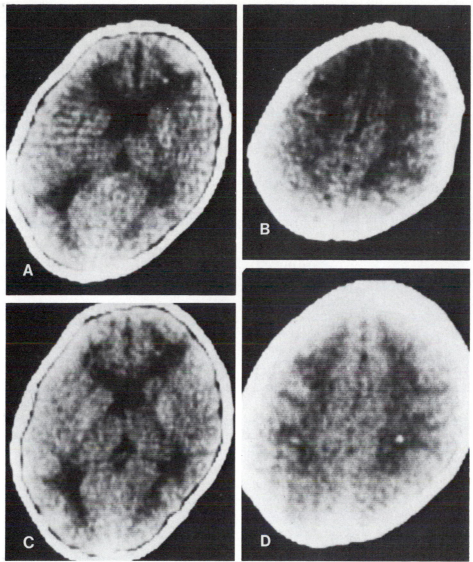

Fig 8–19.—Congenital rubella syndrome in a young male. **A, B,** scan at 19 months of age. **C, D,** scan at 3 years, 7 months of age. Both scans show decreased attenuation in the centrum semiovale (somewhat improved in the later scan). There are decreased attenuation white matter areas adjacent to the anterior and posterior horns of the lateral ventricles, increased attenuation of basal ganglia areas, and multiple calcified centrum semiovale nodules. (From Ishikawa A., Murayama T., Sakuma N., et. al.: *Arch. Neurol.* 39:420–421, 1982. Used by permission.)

in diameter or may occupy the entire pons. There is always a rim of intact myelin between the lesions and the surface of the pons. In extensive cases, the lesion may extend posteriorly into the medial lemnisci and rarely into the midbrain. Large lesions may be associated with demyelinating disease of the thalamus, internal capsule, lateral geniculate bodies, and cerebral cortex.[73]

The disease was originally considered to be secondary to chronic alcoholism, but subsequently has been found in children and other patients without a history of alcohol abuse. The disease is now thought to be associated with a rapid rise in the serum sodium (greater than 20 mEq/L in 1 to 3 days) in previously hyponatremic patients.[74] Almost always associated with some other severe, frequently life-threatening disease, CPM is difficult to diagnose during life, because the patients frequently are comatose from metabolic or other causes. The clinical syndrome of CPM is a sudden disturbance in mental status and flaccid quadriparesis occasionally associated with abnormal conjugate eye movements and pseudobulbar palsy.[73]

The CT in CPM shows a variable-sized area of decreased attenuation in the pons, which may have slight contrast enhancement at the periphery (Figs 8–20 and 8–21).[75, 76]

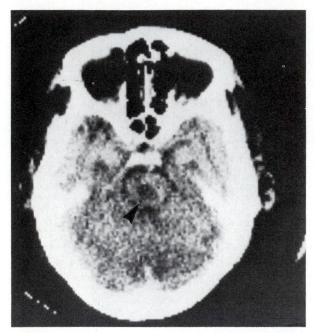

Fig 8–20.—A 53-year-old chronic alcoholic with CPM. Large area of decreased attenuation is in the pons *(arrow)*. This did not enhance when compared with preinfusion scan. (From Anderson T.L., Moore R.A., Grinnell V.S., et al.: *Neurology* 29:1527–1530, 1979. Used by permission.)

Marchiafava-Bignami Disease

This is a disease of necrosis of the corpus callosum in patients who usually have a long history of drinking red wines, but probably also occurs from ingesting other forms of alcohol. The disease has been reported in non-alcoholics and may represent a nutritional deficiency. The patients have clinical signs of acute and subacute

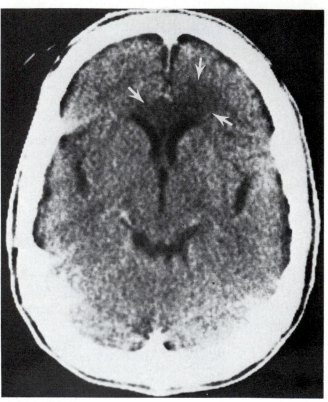

Fig 8–22.—Marchiafava-Bignami disease. Areas of decreased attenuation *(arrows)* are in the corpus callosum. (Courtesy of John C. Morris, M.D., Washington University, St. Louis.)

severe intellectual impairment, with callosal disconnection on psychometric testing. They may undergo spontaneous improvement to a more chronic stage.[73, 77]

During the acute stage, there is decreased attenuation of the corpus callosum (Fig 8–22). During the sub-

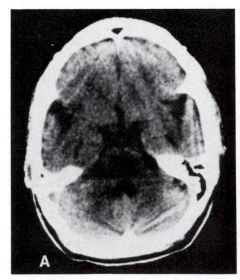
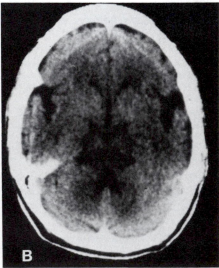

Fig 8–21.—A 51-year-old woman with CPM. **A, B,** areas of decreased attenuation coefficient are visualized in the pons. (From Telfer R.B., Miller E.M.: *Ann. Neurol.* 6:455–456, 1979. Used by permission.)

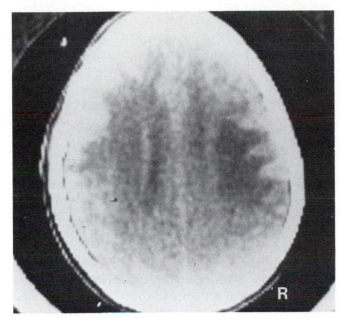

Fig 8–23.—Anoxic encephalopathy. There is decreased attenuation of the white matter of the cerebral hemispheres greater on the right than on the left. (R = patient's right.) (Courtesy of Robert I. Grossman, M.D., Hospital of the University of Pennsylvania, Philadelphia.)

acute stage, there may be contrast enhancement in the corpus callosum. In the chronic stage, there is atrophy of the corpus callosum and cortical atrophy, predominantly frontal.[77]

Carbon Monoxide and Anoxic Encephalopathies

Originally, it was thought that white matter changes occurred only as a delayed effect of hypoxia. It is now known that acute anoxic encephalopathy may affect the white matter.

The classic pathologic changes of anoxic encephalopathy are in the cortical and subcortical neurons, with relative sparing of the white matter. In both acute and chronic anoxic encephalopathy, the white matter may show demyelination.[78]

The most common CT findings of postanoxic encephalopathy are enlarged sulci from cortical atrophy. In some patients, there is decreased attenuation of the entire white matter of the cerebral hemispheres (Fig 8–23).[78]

Myelinoclastic Diseases of Vascular Etiology

Binswanger's Disease

Binswanger's disease, or subcortical arteriosclerotic encephalopathy, is a slowly progressive disorder caused by cerebral arteriosclerosis, in which the small arteries and arterioles of the white matter and basal ganglia are predominantly affected. The disease is clinically characterized by hypertension, dementia, spasticity, syncope, and seizures. Pathologically, there is diffuse demyelination or foci of necrosis.

The CT examination shows areas of decreased attenuation in the white matter without enhancement (Fig 8–24).[79, 80]

Maladie-de-Schilder-Foix Disease

This is a disease of nonprogressive demyelinating lesions of the white matter secondary to vascular disease.

Post-therapy Myelinoclastic Diseases

Methotrexate Leukoencephalopathy
See Chapter 7.

Disseminated Necrotizing Leukodystrophy
See Chapter 7.

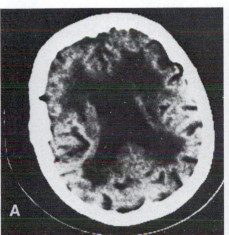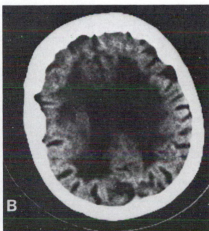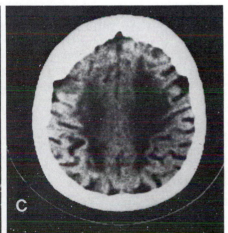

Fig 8–24.—Binswanger's disease (without contrast). **A, B, C,** there is extensive decreased attenuation of the white matter in the frontal, parietal, and temporal lobes.

DYSMYELINATING DISEASES

These are diseases in which an enzymatic disturbance interferes either with the formation of myelin or with its maintenance. The specific metabolic abnormalities remain unknown for some of these diseases.

Leukodystrophies

The leukodystrophies (leuko = white; dystrophy = defective nutrition) are a group of genetically determined metabolic disorders with primary involvement of myelin, but in which the metabolic abnormalities were originally unknown. Subsequently, some of the metabolic abnormalities of these diseases have been determined.

In the past, different classification systems of the leukodystrophies were based on histopathologic findings, staining properties, clinical findings, and age of onset. This has resulted in a large number of eponyms for the same disease and probably in different metabolic abnormalities being labeled as the same disease. Metachromatic and globoid cell leukodystrophy are now known to be lipid storage diseases; spongy sclerosis is found in many aminoacidopathies; and adrenoleukodystrophy is a fatty-acid metabolic defect.

The leukodystrophies will be discussed as a category of dysmyelinating disease because the term is widely used in the literature, with the realization that the term "leukodystrophy" should eventually be abandoned. The diseases currently classified as leukodystrophies should be recategorized by their metabolic abnormality when the enzymatic defect responsible for each disease becomes known. In some of the leukodystrophies, enzyme deficiencies result in defective catabolism of the lipid components of myelin. This leads to the accumulation of complex lipids that are weakly sudanophilic and of cholesterol esters that are strongly sudanophilic. Sudanophilic tissues are those readily stained with Sudan, which is a group of azo compounds used as stains for fats. The terms sudanophilic leukodystrophy or orthochromatic leukodystrophy (ortho = straight, normal, correct; orthochromatic = normally colored or stained) refer to a classification based upon histologic staining and include a heterogeneous group of diseases, including phenylketonuria, maple syrup urine disease, oasthouse urine disease, Cockayne's syndrome, adrenoleukodystrophy, and Pelizaeus-Merzbacher disease.[81] These staining classifications are differentiated from the metachromatic leukodystrophies. In metachromatic staining, different elements of a tissue take on different colors with the same dye.

Metachromatic Leukodystrophy

Metachromatic leukodystrophy, the most common leukodystrophy with at least 200 reported cases,[81] is due to a lack of the enzyme arylsulfatase A. The disease is diagnosed by low-to-absent arylsulfatase A in the urine, leukocytes, or cultured fibroblasts. There are three distinct forms of this disease: late infantile, juvenile, and adult. Each probably represents an independent autosomal recessive disorder.[2]

The most common type is the late infantile variety, in which symptoms develop between 12 and 18 months of age. The first symptom is clumsiness in walking as a result of weakness in the legs. Weakness and hypotonia of the lower extremities with reduction or absence of tendon reflexes are more common, but there may be spasticity. Upper limb involvement follows. There is progressive dementia, and 50% of those afflicted develop seizures. Death occurs between 2 and 10 years after the onset of the disease.[2, 81]

In the juvenile type, the age of onset is between 5 and 10 years, with progressive dementia and ataxia. The disease is more difficult to recognize in the adult and frequently presents as psychiatric illness with eventual progressive dementia.

The CT findings in all reported cases of metachromatic leukodystrophy are extensive, diffuse, symmetric decreased attenuation of the white matter without enhancement. There is mild-to-moderate ventricular enlargement (Fig 8–25).[82–84]

Globoid Cell Leukodystrophy (Krabbe's Disease)

This is an autosomal recessive disease with approximately 100 reported cases, secondary to a deficiency of galactocerebroside β-galactosidase. The disease is diagnosed by demonstrating a deficiency of this enzyme in serum, leukocytes, fibroblasts, or cultured amniotic

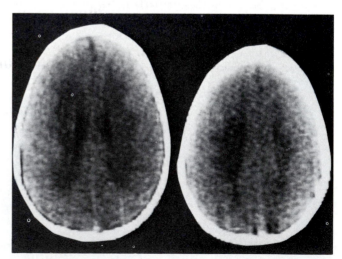

Fig 8–25.—Metachromatic leukodystrophy in late infant stage. There is extensive symmetric decreased attenuation of the white matter above *(right)* and at the level of bodies of the lateral ventricles *(left)*. (From Buonanno F.S., Ball M.R., Laster W., et al.: *Ann. Neurol.* 4:43–46, 1978. Used by permission.)

fluid. There are distended epithelioid (globoid) cells and collections of multinucleated bodies (globoid bodies) throughout the white matter. The brain is small with a diffuse loss of white matter.

The disease occurs almost entirely in infants of 3 to 5 months of age. Rarely, globoid cell leukodystrophy starts in the late infantile or juvenile period. The disease begins with increased irritability and crying and with extreme sensitivity to light and noise, which causes myoclonic jerks. The infant rapidly deteriorates and usually dies within 1 year of the onset of symptoms.[2, 81]

Descriptions of the CT findings in this disease are sparse. One case showed normal white matter and mild-to-moderate ventricular dilatation. Another case showed enlargement of the cortical sulci with questionable areas of decreased attenuation in the white matter.[84, 85]

Spongy Degeneration (Canavan's Disease)

This is an autosomal recessive disease of unknown etiology that occurs most often in Jewish families from eastern Europe. Approximately 90 cases of this disease have been reported. It begins in the first 2 or 3 months of life and usually leads to death within a few years. The infant develops flaccidity, apathy, blindness, and decorticate rigidity.[2, 81, 86]

Spongy degeneration of the brain has also been found in a number of inborn errors of amino acid metabolism, including maple syrup urine disease, homocystinuria, phenylketonuria, argininosuccinicaciduria, and nonke-

tonic hyperglycemia. It has also been seen in a case of 3-hydroxy-3-methylglutaryl-CoA-lyase deficiency, an extremely rare enzymatic defect of leucine metabolism.[87] Thus, spongy degeneration of the brain may be a nonspecific response of the brain to various abnormal metabolites.

Spongy degeneration and Alexander's disease are the only leukodystrophies that cause megalencephaly. Symmetric diffuse decrease in the attenuation of the white matter is demonstrated by CT (Figs 8–26 and 8–27).[86–89]

Adrenoleukodystrophy

This is a sex-linked recessive disease in which the exact inborn error of metabolism is unknown, but in which there is an abnormality of long-chain fatty-acid metabolism resulting in lipid storage. There is an accumulation of lipid-filled, p-aminosalicylic acid-positive inclusions within macrophages of the CNS, adrenal cortex, testes, and peripheral nerves. The adrenal glands are atrophic.

The disease occurs in school-age boys, with an insidious change in personality, mental deterioration, visual impairment, spasticity, and ataxia. The disease progresses rapidly, and most patients are demented, blind, deaf, and quadriparetic within several years.

Signs and symptoms of adrenal insufficiency usually precede the neurologic abnormalities. However, the adrenal insufficiency is variable in this disease, ranging from overt Addison's disease with abnormal skin pigmentation to normal adrenals by clinical and laboratory

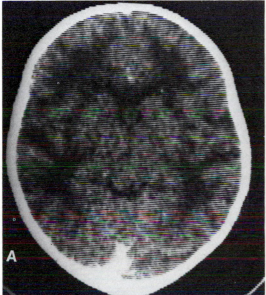
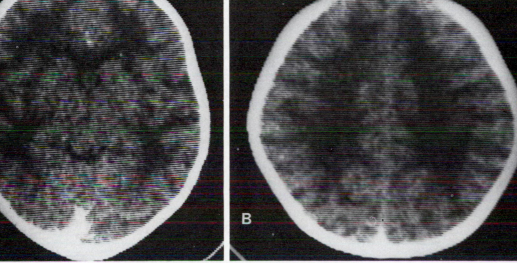

Fig 8–26.—Canavan's disease in a 7-month-old boy with increasing head circumference. **A,** there is decreased attenuation of the white matter with normal ventricles. **B,** a more cephalad section shows decreased attenuation of the centrum semiovale. (From Rushton A.R., Shaywitz B.A., Duncan C.C., et al.: *Ann. Neurol.* 10:57–60, 1981. Used by permission.)

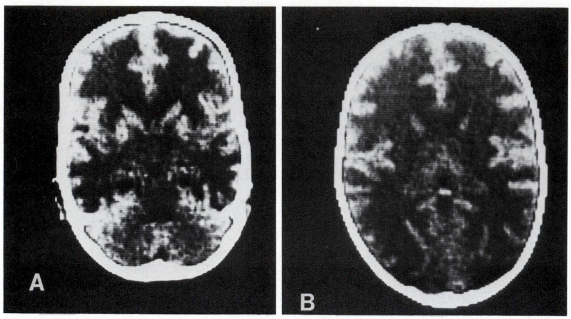

Fig 8–27.—Canavan's disease. **A, B,** there is a marked symmetric diffuse decrease in the attenuation of the white matter in this patient with megalencephaly. (Courtesy of David Weslowski, M.D., William Beaumont Hospital, Detroit.)

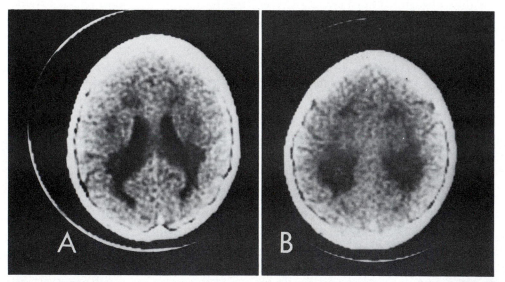

Fig 8–28.—Adrenoleukodystrophy, type 1, in an 11-year-old boy. **A, B,** areas of decreased attenuation coefficient are in the periventricular and posterior parietal regions. (From O'Neill B.P., Forbes G.S.: *Arch. Neurol.* 38:293–296, 1981. Used by permission.)

examination, but with a family history of Addison's disease. The diagnosis can be confirmed by finding elevated C_{26} fatty acid in cultured skin fibroblasts.[90]

Three histopathologic zones of destruction of the CNS white matter have been described in this disease, primarily in the parieto-occipital and posterior-temporal regions. Zone 1, along the leading edge of the lesion, shows myelin destruction with axonal sparing and little or no inflammatory response. Zone 2 shows increased demyelination with some axonal loss and many lipid-containing macrophages; there is a marked perivascular mononuclear inflammatory cell response. Zone 3 is inactive, central in location, and gliotic.[91]

The CT findings correlate with the histopathologic zones of destruction as described above. The earliest changes occur in the posterior cerebral regions (Fig 8–28). Irregular areas of decreased attenuation subsequently involve the parietal, temporal, and frontal lobes. These bilateral changes are not necessarily symmetric. Enhancement occurs along the leading edge of the lesion corresponding to zones 1 and 2. With progression of the disease, the areas of enhancement are located more anteriorly. Generalized central and cortical atrophy develop later as rim enhancement fades (Fig 8–29).[92–96]

There is another CT pattern in adrenoleukodystrophy that is called type 2 and is characterized by the absence of posterior periventricular areas of decreased attenuation. With contrast infusion, there is marked enhancement of various white matter tracts or fiber systems such as the internal capsule, corona radiata, forceps major, and cerebral peduncles (Fig 8–30). This pattern is believed to be specific for a phenotypic variant or an evolving stage of adrenoleukodystrophy.[97] Cases with both type 1 and type 2 findings and with calcification have been reported (Figs 8–31 and 8–32).[98, 99]

Alexander's Disease

This is the rarest of the leukodystrophies and is of uncertain pathogenesis. All proved cases have been sporadic except for one in which the family history strongly suggested that three siblings of an autopsy-proved case were affected. The brain is characterized by diffuse demyelination combined with Rosenthal fibers, which are believed to represent inert metabolic products from degeneration of astrocytes. The disease is usually manifest during the first year of life, with progressive retardation, symmetric spastic weakness, and convulsions in an infant with a rapidly enlarging head. Death occurs in months to years.

All cases have had megalencephaly. In one reported case, there were symmetric, well-demarcated lesions in the deep cerebral white matter on CT, sparing the subependymal regions and considerably more extensive in the frontal lobes than elsewhere. The lateral ventricles were moderately dilated. There was symmetric contrast enhancement of the caudate nuclei, the anterior columns of the fornices, the periventricular brain substance, the central portion of the forceps minor, and the region of the optic radiations (Fig 8–33). A second case in the same report showed symmetric decreased attenuation of the white matter of both frontal lobes, of the caudate and lenticular nuclei, and the anterior limbs of the internal capsules without abnormal enhancement (Fig 8–34).[100] A third case has been described with decreased attenuation of the white matter in the frontal lobes.[101]

Pelizaeus-Merzbacher Disease

This is an extremely rare condition with several rarer subtypes. The classic disease is sex-linked recessive and manifests in early infancy. There are characteristic areas

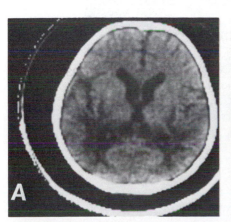
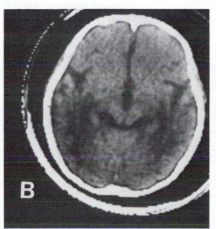
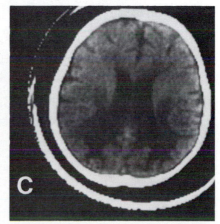

Fig 8–29.—Adrenoleukodystrophy, type 1, in a 6-year-old boy. **A, B, C,** areas of decreased attenuation coefficient are in the parietal and occipital regions. The lateral ventricles are enlarged. (From Furuse M., Obayashi T., Tsuji S., et al.: *Radiology* 126:707–710, 1978. Used by permission.)

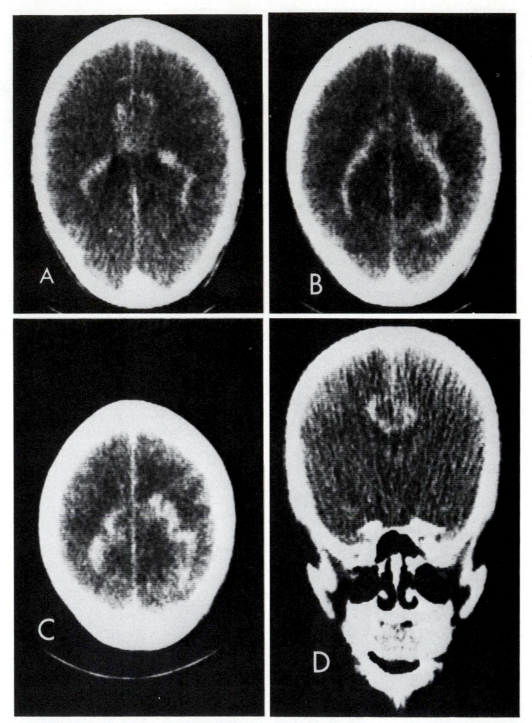

Fig 8–30.—An 11-year-old boy with adrenoleukodystrophy type 2 (with contrast). Axial **(A, B, C)** and coronal **(D)** scans show enhancement of the corpus callosum and corona radiata. (From DiChiro G., Eiben E.M., Manz H.J., et al.: *Radiology* 137:687–692, 1980. Used by permission.)

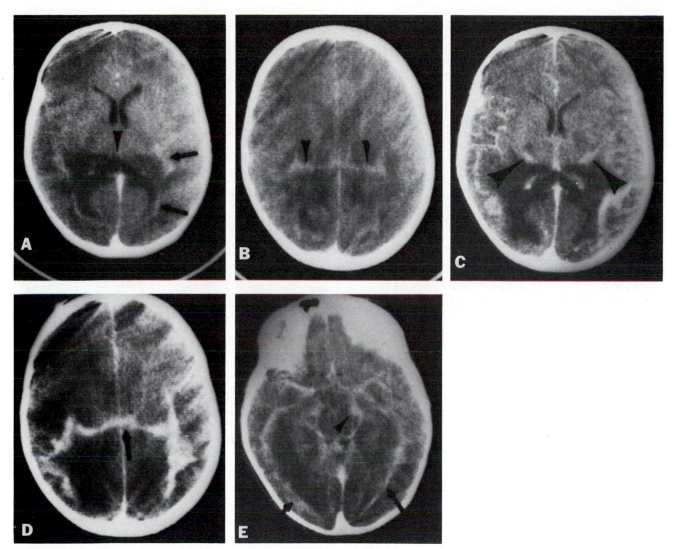

Fig 8–31.—An 8-year-old boy with adrenoleukodystrophy, combined types 1 and 2 (with contrast). **A,** enhancing lesions are adjacent to dilated occipital horns *(arrows).* Areas of decreased attenuation are in the splenium of the corpus callosum *(arrowhead).* **B,** a more superior section shows slight enhancement extending across the corpus callosum *(arrowheads).* **C, D,** scans obtained at the same level as photos **A** and **B** 7 months later show increase in the extent of low attenuation and postcontrast enhancement. New areas of enhancement are in the posterior limbs of the internal capsule *(arrowheads,* **C**). The *arrow* in photo **D** points to enhancement of the corpus callosum. **E,** enhancing lesions involve the inferior longitudinal fasciculi *(arrows).* Enhancement is also noted in the left cerebral peduncle *(arrowhead).* (From Brooks B.S., El Gammal T.: *J. Comput. Assist. Tomogr.* 6:385–388, 1982. Used by permission.)

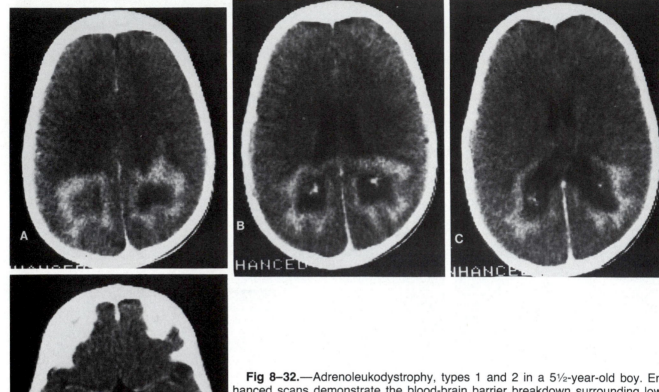

Fig 8–32.—Adrenoleukodystrophy, types 1 and 2 in a 5½-year-old boy. Enhanced scans demonstrate the blood-brain barrier breakdown surrounding low-attenuation areas **A, B, C,** and calcifications of the posterior centrum semiovale bilaterally **(B, C).** The enhancement involves the posterior limbs of the internal capsules and cerebral peduncles **(D).** Note the lack of gray matter involvement. (From Dubois P.J., Lewis F.D., Drayer B.P., et al.: *J. Comput. Assist. Tomogr.* 5:888–891, 1981. Used by permission.)

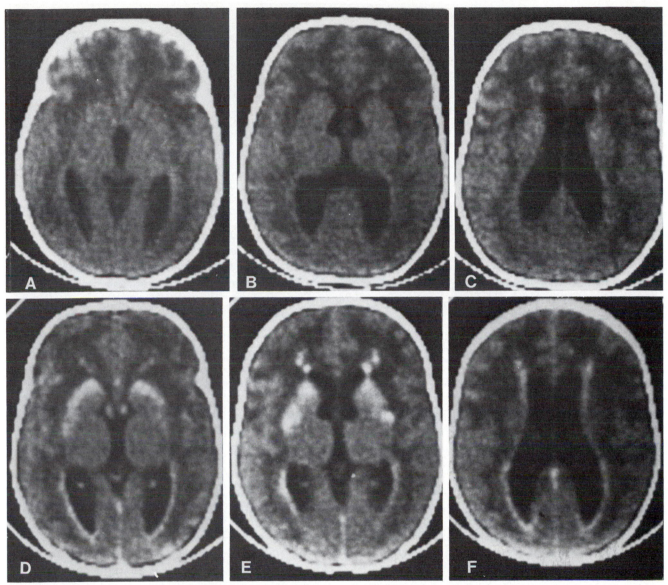

Fig 8–33.—Alexander's disease in a 7-month-old boy. **A, B, C,** unenhanced CT show symmetric low-attenuation areas in white matter. **D, E, F,** enhanced CT reveals increased attenuation in the caudate nuclei, the periventricu- lar areas, and the optic radiations. (From Holland I.M., Kendall B.E.: *Neuroradiology* 20:103–106, 1980. Used by permission.)

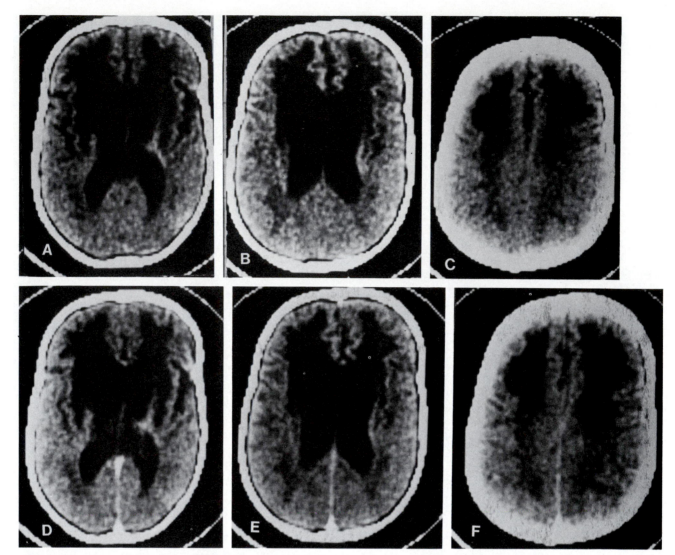

Fig 8–34.—Alexander's disease in a 6-year-old girl. **A, B, C,** unenhanced CT shows marked bilateral decreased attenuation of white matter in the frontal lobes, caudate nuclei, anterior limb of the internal capsules, and periependymal regions in parietal and occipital lobes. **D, E, F,** enhanced CT shows no unusual enhancement. (From Holland I.M., Kendall B.E.: *Neuroradiology* 20:103–106, 1980. Used by permission.)

of preserved myelin. There is a slow progression of the disease characterized by speech abnormalities, grimacing, ataxia, choreiform movements, spasticity, and mental deterioration. Pathologically, there is sclerosis of the white matter of the cerebrum and cerebellum.

In one 14-year-old patient with marked clinical symptoms, the CT was normal. However, CT examination of his 25-year-old uncle demonstrated cerebellar atrophy, periventricular areas of decreased absorption coefficients, and cortical atrophy (Fig 8–35).[102] A report of a 10-year-old patient with far-advanced disease discusses a subtle decrease in the attenuation of the frontal white matter.[84] A fourth reported case in an 18-month-old child described diffuse decrease in the attenuation of the white matter in the cerebrum and cerebellum.[83]

Lipid Storage Diseases With Neuronal Involvement

Mucopolysaccharidoses are inborn errors of metabolism in which mucopolysaccharides are not normally degraded. They collect in lysosomes, causing abnormality of metabolism of other large molecules.[103] Watts and colleagues[103] provide a good summary of the subject and associated CT findings.

While CT demonstrates gray matter abnormality, white matter often shows symmetric low-attenuation areas without specific association with hydrocephalus (Figs 8–36 to 8–38). Because they are not primarily demyelinating diseases, these diseases will not be discussed in this chapter.

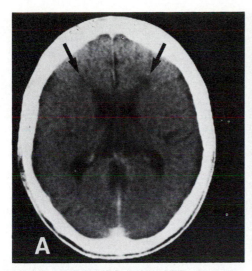
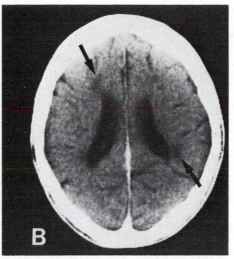

Fig 8–35.—Pelizaeus-Merzbacher disease in a 25-year-old man. **A, B,** with contrast. Low-attenuation areas are adjacent to the frontal horns and atria of the lateral ventricles (**A** and **B** arrows). Other scans showed a wide fourth ventricle, cerebellar atrophy, widened cortical sulci, and decreased attenuation of white matter of the upper centrum semiovale. (From Statz A., Boltshauer E., Schinzel A., et al.: Neuroradiology 22:103–105, 1981. Used by permission.

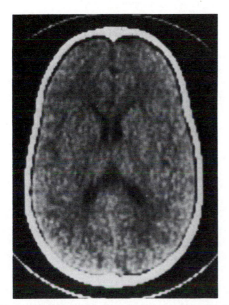
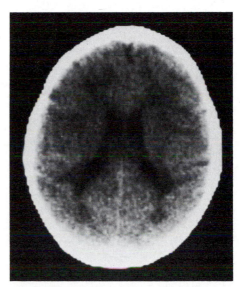

Fig 8–36.—Mucopolysaccharidosis I H/S in a 3-year, 9-month-old boy. Normal ventricles are present, with low attenuation in the parietal and frontal white matter. (From Watts R.W.E., Spellacy E., Kendall B.E., et al.: Neuroradiology 21:9–23, 1981. Used by permission.)

Fig 8–37.—Mucopolysaccharidosis II in a 4-year, 7-month-old boy. The scan shows abnormally low attenuation of deep parietal areas. (From Watts R.W.E., Spellacy E., Kendall B.E., et al.: Neuroradiology 9–23, 1981. Used by permission.)

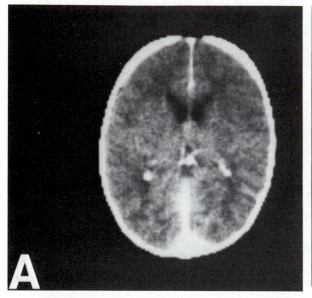 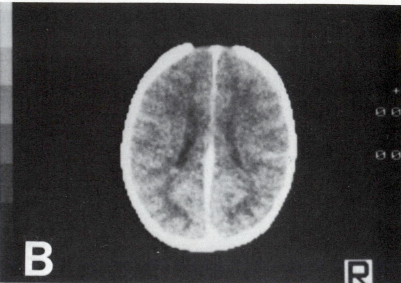

Fig 8–38.—Mucopolysaccharidosis in a 6-month-old girl. Enhanced scan shows below-normal attenuation in white matter of parietal lobes only. Ventricles are normal. Patient was clinically normal. (*R* = patient's right.) (From Watts R.W.E., Spellacy E., Kendall B.E., et al.: *Neuroradiology* 21:9–23, 1981. Used by permission.)

REFERENCES

1. Poser C.M.: Diseases of the myelin sheath, in Baker A.B. (ed.): *Clinical Neurology*. Philadelphia, Harper & Row, 1981, vol. 2, pp. 1–3, 7.
2. Gilroy J., Meyer J.S.: Demyelinating diseases of the nervous system, in Gilroy J., Meyer J.S. (eds.): *Medical Neurology*, ed. 3. New York, MacMillan Publishing Co., 1979, pp. 137–144.
3. Duncan D.: A relation between axone diameter and myelination determined by measurement of myelinated spinal root fibres. *J. Comp. Neurol.* 60:437–471, 1934.
4. Blackwood W.: Normal structure and general pathology of the nerve cell and neuroglia, in Blackwood W. (ed.): *Greenfield's Neuropathology*. Chicago, Year Book Medical Publishers, 1976, vol. 1, p. 10.
5. Quencer R.M.: Maturation of normal primate white matter: Computed tomographic correlation. *A.J.N.R.* 3:365–372, 1982.
6. Waller A.: Experiments on the section of the glossopharyngeal and hypoglossal nerves of the frog, and observations of the alterations produced thereby in the structure of their primitive fibres. *Philos. Trans. R. Soc. Lond. Biol.* 140:423–429, 1850.
7. Adams R.E., Kubic C.S.: The morbid anatomy of the demyelinative diseases. *Am. J. Med.* 12:510–546, 1952.
8. Carswell R.: Atrophy, in *Pathological Anatomy: Illustrations of the Elementary Forms of Disease*. London, Longman, 1838, plate 4.
9. Cruveilhier J.: *Anatomie Pathologique due Corps Humains*. Paris, Baillier, 1839–1842, vol. 2, part 52, plate 2.
10. Frerichs F.: Uber Hirnsklerose. *Haeser's Arch.* 10:334, 1849.
11. Vulpian E.: Notes sur la sclerose en plaque. *L'Union Med.* 30:475, 1866.
12. Charot J.M.: Lectures on the diseases of the nervous system. Delivered at La Salpetriere (translated from 2nd edition by G. Sigerson). Philadelphia, Lea & Febiger, 1879.
13. Baum H.M., Rothschild B.B.: The incidence and prevalence of reported multiple sclerosis. *Ann. Neurol.* 10:420–428, 1981.
14. Kurtzke J.F.: Epidemiologic contributions to multiple sclerosis: An overview. *Neurology* 30:61–79, 1980.
15. Alter M., Loewenson R., Harshe M.: The geographic distribution of multiple sclerosis: An examination of mathematical models. *J. Chronic Dis.* 26:755–767, 1973.
16. Kurtzke J.F., Hyllested K.: Multiple sclerosis in the Faroe Islands: I. Clinical and epidemiological features. *Ann. Neurol.* 5:6–31, 1979.
17. Chan W.W.C.: Multiple sclerosis and dogs. *Lancet* 1:487–488, 1977.
18. Cook S.D., Natelson B.H., Levine B.E., et al.: Further evidence of a possible association between house dogs and multiple sclerosis. *Ann. Neurol.* 3:141–143, 1978.
19. Cook S.D., Dowling P.C.: Distemper and multiple sclerosis in Sitka, Alaska. *Ann. Neurol.* 11:192–194, 1982.
20. Poskanzer D.C.: Tonsillectomy and multiple sclerosis. *Lancet* 2:1264, 1965.
21. Poskanzer D.C., Schapira K., Miller H.: Multiple sclerosis and poliomyelitis. *Lancet* 1:917, 1963.
22. Poskanzer D.C.: Etiology of multiple sclerosis: Analogy suggesting infection in early life, in Alter M., Kurtzke J.F. (eds.): *The Epidemiology of MS*. Springfield, Ill., Charles C. Thomas Publisher, 1968, pp. 62–74.
23. Berry R.J.: Genetical factors in the aetiology of multiple sclerosis. *Acta Neurol. Scand.* 45:459–483, 1969.

24. Schapira K., Poskanzer D.C., Miller H.: Familial and conjugal multiple sclerosis. *Brain* 86:315, 1963.

25. Kurtzke J.F., Bobowisk A.R., Brody J.A., et al.: Twin studies of multiple sclerosis: An epidemiologic inquiry. *Neurology* (Minneapolis) 27:341, 1977.

26. Naito S., Namerow N., Mickey M.R., et al.: Multiple sclerosis: Association with HL-A 3. *Tissue Antigens* 2:1–4, 1972.

27. Pietsch M.C., Morris P.J.: An association of HL-A 3 and HL-A 7 with paralytic poliomyelitis. *Tissue Antigens* 4:50–55, 1974.

28. Weiner H.L., Hauser S.L.: Neuroimmunology: I. Immunoregulation in neurological disease. *Ann. Neurol.* 11:437–449, 1982.

29. Lisak R.P.: Multiple sclerosis: Evidence for immunopathogenesis. *Neurology* 30:99–105, 1980.

30. Weinstein M.A., Lederman R.J., Rothner A.D., et al.: Interval computed tomography in multiple sclerosis. *Radiology* 129:689–694, 1978.

31. Rieth K.G., DiChiro G., Cromwell L.D., et al.: Primary demyelinating disease simulating glioma of the corpus callosum. *J. Neurosurg.* 55:620–624, 1981.

32. van der Velden M., Bots G.T.A.M., Endtz L.J.: Cranial CT in multiple sclerosis showing a mass effect. *Surg. Neurol.* 12:307–310, 1979.

33. Marano G.D., Goodwin C.A., Ko J.P.: Atypical contrast enhancement in computerized tomography of demyelinating disease. *Arch. Neurol.* 37:523–524, 1980.

34. Jankovic J., Derman H., Armstrong D.: Haemorrhagic complications of multiple sclerosis. *J. Neurol. Neurosurg. Psychiatry* 43:76–81, 1980.

35. Oppenheimer D.R.: Demyelinating diseases, in Blackwood W. (ed.): *Greenfield's Neuropathology.* Chicago, Year Book Medical Publishers, 1976, vol. 2, pp. 470–499.

36. Brownell B., Hughes J.T.: The distribution of plaques in the cerebrum in multiple sclerosis. *J. Neurol. Neurosurg. Psychiatry* 25:315–320, 1962.

37. Haughton V.M., Ho K.C., Williams A.L., et al.: CT detection of demyelinated plaques in multiple sclerosis. *A.J.R.* 132:213–215, 1979.

38. Aita J.F.: Cranial CT as an aid in diagnosis of multiple sclerosis. *Appl. Radiol.* 33–37, 1981.

39. Hershey L.A., Gado M.H., Trotter J.L.: Computerized tomography in the diagnostic evaluation of multiple sclerosis. *Ann. Neurol.* 5:32–39, 1979.

40. Jacobs L., Kinkel W.R.: Computerized axial transverse tomography in multiple sclerosis. *Neurology* 26:390–391, 1976.

41. Cala L.A., Mastaglia F.L., Black J.L.: Computerized tomography of brain and optic nerve in multiple sclerosis. *J. Neurol. Sci.* 36:411–426, 1978.

42. Coin C.G., Hucks-Folliss A.: Cervical computed tomography in multiple sclerosis with spinal cord involvement. *J. Comput. Assist. Tomogr.* 3:421–422, 1979.

43. Nelson M.J., Miller S.L., McLain W., et al.: Multiple sclerosis: Large plaque causing mass effect and ring sign. *J. Comput. Assist. Tomogr.* 5:892–894, 1981.

44. Aita J.F., Bennett D.R., Anderson R.E., et al.: Cranial CT appearance of acute multiple sclerosis. *Neurology* 28:251–255, 1978.

45. Sears E.S., Tindall R.S.A., Zarnow H.: Active multiple sclerosis. *Arch. Neurol.* 35:426–434, 1978.

46. Gize R.W., Mishkin F.S.: Brain scans in multiple sclerosis. *Radiology* 97:297–299, 1970.

47. Antunes J.L., Schlesinger E.B., Michelsen W.J.: The abnormal brain scan in demyelinating diseases. *Arch. Neurol.* 30:269–271, 1974.

48. Gyldensted C.: Computed tomography of the cerebrum in multiple sclerosis. *Neuroradiology* 12:33–42, 1976.

49. Weisberg L.: Contrast enhancement visualized by computerized tomography in acute multiple sclerosis. *Comput. Tomogr.* 5:293–300, 1981.

50. Davis J., Davis K.R., Newhouse J., et al.: Expanded high iodine dose in computed cranial tomography: A preliminary report. *Radiology* 131:373–380, 1979.

51. Raininko R., Majurin M.L., Virtama P., et al.: Value of high contrast medium dose in brain CT. *J. Comput. Assist. Tomogr.* 6:54–57, 1982.

52. Hayman L.A., Evans R.A., Hinck V.C.: Delayed high iodine dose contrast computed tomography. *Radiology* 136:677–684, 1980.

53. Morariu M.A., Wilkins D.E., Patel A.: Multiple sclerosis and serial computerized tomography: Delayed contrast enhancement of acute and early lesions. *Arch. Neurol.* 37:189–190, 1980.

54. Prendes J.L.: Contrast dose in CT scanning. *Arch. Neurol.* 38:67–68, 1981.

55. Vinuela F.V., Fox A.J., Debrun G.M., et al.: New perspectives in computed tomography of multiple sclerosis. *A.J.R.* 139:123–127, 1982.

56. Reisner T., Maida E.: Computerized tomography in multiple sclerosis. *Arch. Neurol.* 37:475–477, 1980.

57. Robertson W.C., Gomez M.R., Reese D.F., et al.: Computerized tomography in demyelinating disease of the young. *Neurology* 27:838–842, 1977.

58. Lebow S., Anderson D.C., Mastri A., et al.: Acute multiple sclerosis with contrast-enhancing plaques. *Arch. Neurol.* 35:435–439, 1978.

59. Feigin I., Popoff N.: Regeneration of myelin in multiple sclerosis. *Neurology* 16:364–372, 1966.

60. Prineas J.W., Connell F.: Remyelination in multiple sclerosis. *Ann. Neurol.* 5:22–31, 1979.

61. Perier O., Gregoire A.: Electron microscopic features of multiple sclerosis lesions. *Brain* 88:937–952, 1965.

62. Fenichel G.M.: Neurological complications of immunization. *Ann. Neurol.* 12:119–128, 1982.

63. Adams R.D., Victor M. (eds.): *Principles of Neurology,* ed. 2. New York, McGraw-Hill Book Co., 1981, pp. 658-662.

64. Valentine A.R., Kendall B.E., Harding B.N.: Computed tomography in acute haemorrhagic leukoencephalitis. *Neuroradiology* 22:215–219, 1982.

65. Reich H., Shu-Ren L., Goldblatt D.: Computerized tomography in acute leukoencephalopathy: A case report. *Neurology* 29:255–258, 1979.

66. Prineas J.W.: Pathology of the Guillain-Barré syndrome. *Ann. Neurol. Suppl.* 9:6–19, 1981.

67. Choppin P.W.: Measles virus and chronic neurological diseases. *Ann. Neurol.* 9:17–20, 1981.

68. Adams R.D., Victor M. (eds.): *Principles of Neurology*, ed. 2. New York, McGraw-Hill Book Co., 1981, p. 527.

69. Jabbour J.T., Garcia J.H., Lammi H., et al.: SSPE: A multidisciplinary study of eight cases. *J.A.M.A.* 207:2248–2254, 1969.

70. Duda E.E., Huttenlocher P.R., Patronas N.J.: CT of subacute sclerosing panencephalitis. *A.J.N.R.* 1:35–38, 1980.

71. Pederson H., Wulff C.H.: Computed tomographic findings of early subacute sclerosing panencephalitis. *Neuroradiology* 23:31–32, 1982.

72. Ishikawa A., Murayama T., Sakuma N., et al.: Computed cranial tomography in congenital rubella syndrome. *Arch. Neurol.* 39:420–421, 1982.

73. Adams R.D., Victor M. (eds.): *Principles of Neurology*, ed. 2. New York, McGraw-Hill Book Co., 1981, pp. 720–723.

74. Norenberg M.D., Leslie K.O., Robertson A.S.: Association between rise in serum sodium and central pontine myelinolysis. *Ann. Neurol.* 11:128–135, 1982.

75. Telfer R.B., Miller E.M.: Central pontine myelinolysis following hyponatremia, demonstrated by computerized tomography. *Ann. Neurol.* 6:455–456, 1979.

76. Anderson T.L., Moore R.A., Grinnell V.S., et al.: Computerized tomography in central pontine myelinolysis. *Neurology* 29:1527–1530, 1979.

77. Rancurel G., Gardeur D., Thibierge M., et al.: Computed tomography of Marchiafava-Bignami disease. Presented at the Twelfth Neuroradiologicum Symposium, Washington, D.C., Oct. 10–16, 1982.

78. Yagnik P., Gonzalez C.: White matter involvement in anoxic encephalopathy in adults. *J. Comput. Assist. Tomogr.* 4:788–790, 1980.

79. Rosenberg G.A., Kornfeld M., Stovring J., et al.: Subcortical arteriosclerotic encephalopathy (Binswanger): Computerized tomography. *Neurology* 29:1102–1106, 1979.

80. Rosenberg G.A., Kornfeld M., Stovring J., et al.: CT scan in subcortical arteriosclerotic encephalopathy. *Neurology* 30:791–792, 1980.

81. Poster C.M.: Diseases of the myelin sheath, in Baker A.B. (ed.): *Clinical Neurology*, revised ed., Philadelphia, Harper & Row, 1981, vol. 2, pp. 104–147.

82. Buonanno F.S., Ball M.R., Laster W., et al.: Computed tomography in late-infantile metachromatic leukodystrophy. *Ann. Neurol.* 4:43–46, 1978.

83. Robertson W.C., Gomez M.R., Reese D.F., et al.: Computerized tomography in demyelinating disease of the young. *Neurology* 27:838–842, 1977.

84. Heinz E.R., Drayer B.P., Haenggell C.A., et al.: Computed tomography in white-matter disease. *Radiology* 130:371–378, 1979.

85. Barnes D.M., Enzmann D.R.: The evolution of white matter disease as seen on computed tomography. *Radiology* 138:379–383, 1981.

86. Lane B., Carroll B.A., Pedley T.A.: Computerized cranial tomography in cerebral diseases of white matter. *Neurology* 28:534–544, 1978.

87. Lisson G., Leupold D., Bechinger D., et al.: CT findings in a case of deficiency of 3-hydroxy-3-methylglutaryl-CoA-lyase. *Neuroradiology* 22:99–101, 1981.

88. Rushton A.R., Shaywitz B.A., Duncan C.C., et al.: Computed tomography in the diagnosis of Canavan's disease. *Ann. Neurol.* 10:57–60, 1981.

89. Andriola M.R.: Computed tomography in the diagnosis of Canavan's disease. *Ann. Neurol.* 11:323, 1982.

90. O'Neill B.P., Moser H.W., Marmion L.C.: The adrenoleukomyeloneuropathy (ALMN) complex: Elevated C_{26} fatty acid in cultured skin fibroblasts and correlation with disease expression in three generations of a kindred, abstracted. *Neurology* 30:352, 1980.

91. Schaumburg H.H., Powers J.M., Raine C.S., et al.: Adrenoleukodystrophy: A clinical and pathological study of 17 cases. *Arch. Neurol.* 32:577–591, 1975.

92. Quisling R.G., Andriola M.R.: Computed tomographic evaluation of the early phase of adrenoleukodystrophy. *Neuroradiology* 17:285–288, 1979.

93. O'Neill B.P., Forbes G.S.: Computerized tomography and adrenoleukomyeloneuropathy: Differential appearance in disease subtypes. *Arch. Neurol.* 38:293–296, 1981.

94. Eiben R.M., DiChiro G.: Computer assisted tomography in adrenoleukodystrophy. *J. Comput. Assist. Tomogr.* 13:308–314, 1977.

95. Furuse M., Obayashi T., Tsuji S., et al.: Adrenoleukodystrophy. *Radiology* 126:707–710, 1978.

96. Duda E.E., Huttenlocher P.R.: Computed tomography in adrenoleukodystrophy: Correlation of radiological and histological findings. *Radiology* 120:349–350, 1976.

97. DiChiro G., Eiben E.M., Manz H.J., et al.: A new CT pattern in adrenoleukodystrophy. *Radiology* 137:687–692, 1980.

98. Dubois P.J., Lewis F.D., Drayer B.P., et al.: Atypical findings in adrenoleukodystrophy. *J. Comput. Assist. Tomogr.* 5:888–891, 1981.

99. Brooks B.S., El Gammal T.: An additional case of adrenoleukodystrophy with both type I and type II CT features. *J. Comput. Assist. Tomogr.* 6:385–388, 1982.

100. Holland I.M., Kendall B.E.: Computed tomography in Alexander's disease. *Neuroradiology* 20:103–106, 1980.

101. Boltshauser E., Spiess H., Isler W.: Computed tomography in neurodegenerative disorders in childhood. *Neuroradiology* 16:41–43, 1978.

102. Statz A., Boltshauser E., Schinzel A., et al.: Computed tomography in Pelizaeus-Merzbacher disease. *Neuroradiology* 22:103–105, 1981.

103. Watts R.W.E., Spellacy E., Kendall B.E., et al.: Computed tomography studies on patients with mucopolysaccharidoses. *Neuroradiology* 21:9–23, 1981.

Cranial and Intracranial Neoplasms

Introduction

Richard E. Latchaw, M.D.

There have been numerous attempts to classify the myriad of neoplasms involving the intracranial contents and their surrounding skull base and calvarium. In particular, the classification of the neuroectodermal tumors has been extremely controversial over many years, beginning with Baily and Cushing.[1] These authors studied the embryogenesis of the cellular components of CNS tumors and then attempted to classify these tumors according to the different morphological stages through which the cellular components pass in ontogenesis. In 1952, Kernohan and Sayre[2] produced a classification of glial tumors by assigning the numbers I through IV according to an increasing degree of malignancy. In their scheme, benign astrocytomas were Grade I, while glioblastoma multiforme represented Grade IV. Russell and Rubenstein[3] have classified neuroectodermal tumors according to their cell line, with categories including tumors of glial origin, those of the pineal parenchyma, those arising in the retina, and tumors of neuronal origin. More recently, Rorke[4] has suggested that neoplasms classified by Russell and Rubenstein in the group of tumors of neuronal origin, including medulloblastoma and neuroblastoma, and those of the group of pineal parenchymal tumors, be classified together as various forms of primitive neuroectodermal tumors. Finally, another attempt at the classification of all intracranial tumors has been made under the auspices of the World Health Organization.[5]

No one classification of intracranial tumors is agreeable to all parties concerned, nor can it satisfy all requirements made upon it. Any classification should have as its goal the organization of the components into a system that can be rationally considered at the time of differential diagnosis and that proves to be utilitarian for treatment and prognosis. For the purposes of this discussion of the radiologic appearances of the various cranial and intracranial neoplasms, the following classification will be utilized:

I. Neuroectodermal neoplasms
    A. Tumors of glial origin
        1. Astrocytoma
        2. Oligodendroglioma
        3. Tumors of ependymal origin
            a. Ependymoma
            b. Subependymoma
            c. Choroid plexus papilloma
            d. Colloid cyst
        4. Glioblastoma multiforme
    B. Primitive neuroectodermal tumors
        1. Medulloblastoma
        2. Neuroblastoma
        3. Pineal parenchymal tumors
    C. Tumors of ganglion cell origin
        1. Ganglioglioma
        2. Ganglioneuroma
II. Meningioma
III. Nerve sheath tumors
    A. Schwannoma
    B. Neurofibroma
IV. Congenital tumors
    A. Teratoma
    B. Germinoma
    C. Epidermoid
    D. Dermoid
    E. Lipoma
    F. Hamartoma
    G. Craniopharyngioma
V. Tumors of vascular origin
    A. Hemangioblastoma
    B. Hemangiopericytoma
    C. Chemodectoma
VI. Primary intracranial sarcomas
    A. Sarcomas of the meninges
    B. Sarcomas of the cerebral parenchyma
VII. Pituitary neoplasms
VIII. Metastatic tumors
IX. Tumors of the calvarium and skull base
    A. Calvarium
        1. Benign
            a. Epidermoid
            b. Hemangioma
        2. Aggressive and malignant
            a. Eosinophilic granuloma
            b. Sarcoma

B. Skull base
  1. Osteoma, osteochondroma, and osteogenic sarcoma
  2. Chondroma and chondrosarcoma
  3. Chordoma

Controversy exists regarding classification of the colloid cyst of the third ventricle. While some authors classify the colloid cyst with other nonneoplastic cystic lesions including arachnoid cyst, the colloid cyst is included with the other masses of ependymal origin in the classification by Russell and Rubenstein.[3] It is more convenient in this section to discuss colloid cysts with other intraventricular tumors representing differential diagnostic possibilities.

The clinical and radiologic diagnosis of a specific intracranial neoplasm depends upon many factors, one of which is location. Therefore, Chapter 9 will deal with tumors of the parenchyma, including the neuroectodermal tumors and primary sarcomas, while Chapter 10 will discuss extra-axial masses and tumors of the skull base and calvarium. Included in the extra-axial group are meningiomas, tumors of nerve sheath origin, and chemodectomas. Tumors of the skull base and calvarium include the tumors listed above under this category. The various congenital tumors, pineal parenchymal tumors, and tumors of blood vessel origin have multiple interrelationships and are therefore considered together in Chapter 11. The phakomatoses are those hereditary syndromes that include CNS neoplasms and hamartomas of a congenital origin and are therefore included in Chapter 11. Craniopharyngioma and pituitary tumors represent specific diagnostic problems and are therefore considered together elsewhere in this volume. Finally, a separate chapter in this section is devoted to the various manifestations of metastatic disease involving the cerebral parenchyma and meninges.

While a relatively short presentation could have been written that would be devoted to generalities on the typical appearances of the most common cranial and intracranial tumors, there is an attempt in this entire section to discuss in depth the CT scan appearances of many tumors. It has become apparent that the radiologist is frequently able to make a preoperative diagnosis of the type of neoplasm present in a large percentage of cases or to give a very accurate and short differential diagnosis. Such accuracy stems from the pattern of radiographic findings in any given neoplasm, including the site of occurrence, pattern of contrast enhancement, appearance of the tumor, margins and surrounding edema pattern, multiplicity, and a wealth of other radiographic findings. It is thus important to discuss the salient radiographic findings for both the more common cranial and intracranial neoplasms and the less common but significant differential diagnostic possibilities.

An effort has been made to discuss some of the more important neuropathologic concepts for a number of the tumor categories. An understanding of the pathology of these tumors is mandatory when attempting to explain the particular pattern of radiologic findings for any given neoplasm. Some physiologic concepts regarding contrast enhancement will also be discussed, although a more complete discussion of the mechanisms of enhancement will be found in Chapter 1 of this volume. Differential diagnosis is strongly emphasized throughout this section. Such differential diagnosis includes not only tumors that simulate the one under discussion, but nonneoplastic conditions as well. Chapter 13 of this section is devoted entirely to important points of differential diagnosis.

The techniques of radiographic evaluation are emphasized throughout these chapters. Contrast enhancement is vital in the evaluation of neoplastic conditions of the brain. Multiple projections such as sagittal and coronal views, in addition to the typical axial projection, are now easily available and are of great assistance in the evaluation of cranial and intracranial tumors. The role of delayed scanning following contrast infusion and the role of sequential studies over time are emphasized when evaluating difficult cases. Biopsy under CT control is no longer experimental, but a routine procedure in our institution, and is discussed throughout this section, particularly in Chapter 14. A much broader consideration of surgical diagnostic and therapeutic techniques is found in Chapter 34. Finally, there is an emphasis on new techniques that are either becoming available or are on the horizon for both the diagnosis and evaluation of intracranial tumors. Such techniques include CT numerical subtraction, dual energy analysis, three-dimensional imaging, and volumetric determination. A brief discussion of these new and exciting technical advances will be found in Chapter 14.

REFERENCES

1. Baily O., Cushing H.: *A Classification of Tumors of the Glioma Group.* Philadelphia, J.B. Lippincott, Co., 1926.
2. Kernohan J.W., Sayre G.P.: Tumors of the Central Nervous System. Atlas of Tumor Pathology, Armed Forces Institute of Pathology, 1952, section 10, fasc. 35.
3. Russell D.S., Rubenstein L.J.: *Pathology of Tumours of the Nervous System.* Baltimore, Williams & Wilkins Co., 1977.
4. Rorke L.B.: Cerebellar medulloblastoma and its relationship to primitive neuroectodermal neoplasms. *J. Neuropathol. Exp. Neurol.* 42:1–15, 1983.
5. Zulch K.J.: *Histological Typing of Tumors of the Central Nervous System.* Geneva, World Health Organization, 1979.

9

Primary Tumors of the Brain: Neuroectodermal Tumors and Sarcomas

RICHARD E. LATCHAW, M.D.

NEUROECTODERMAL TUMORS

The classification of neuroectodermal tumors listed in the Introduction to this section is appropriate for the pathologic evaluation and study of the behavior of neuroectodermal tumors. The classification is based upon cellular morphology, which is the particular province of the pathologist. Of greater import to the diagnostic radiologist is the macroscopic appearance of the tumor and the anatomical location of the mass, factors weighing heavily on the presurgical differential diagnosis of tissue type. Similar types of neuroectodermal tumors have a differing incidence within varying age groups, depending upon their anatomical location. Likewise, their macroscopic appearance on the CT scan differs to some degree according to the location of the neoplasm. For example, the cerebellar astrocytoma that is common in the pediatric age group frequently enhances markedly, even if it is pathologically benign, in contradistinction to the relatively sparse enhancement of the typical benign (low-grade) astrocytoma in the adult. Also, a brain stem astrocytoma may have a different radiographic appearance than either the cerebellar or cerebral astrocytoma, with little contrast enhancement even if the tumor is malignant. Therefore, it is more efficacious in the development of the appropriate differential diagnosis to divide neuroectodermal tumors according to their site of origin, utilizing the following outline:

A. Cerebral hemispheres
  1. Astrocytoma, benign and malignant
  2. Glioblastoma multiforme
  3. Oligodendroglioma
  4. Primitive neuroectodermal tumors, including primary intracranial neuroblastoma
  5. Ganglioglioma

B. Brain stem
  1. Astrocytoma, benign and malignant
  2. Glioblastoma multiforme
C. Cerebellum/fourth ventricle
  1. Astrocytoma, benign and malignant
  2. Glioblastoma multiforme
  3. Medulloblastoma
  4. Ependymoma
D. Intraventricular tumors
  1. Ependymoma; subependymoma
  2. Astrocytoma, benign and malignant
  3. Choroid plexus papilloma
  4. Colloid cyst
E. Pineal parenchymal tumors: pineocytoma and pineoblastoma

Neuroectodermal Tumors of the Cerebral Hemispheres

Astrocytoma and Glioblastoma Multiforme

The histologic characterization of glial tumors, which is based upon the predominating cell type and the grading of these glial tumors into benign and malignant forms relative to the degree of anaplasia, has undergone a great deal of change over the years, resulting in overlapping terms for the same neoplasm. In 1952, Kernohan and Sayre[1] divided astrocytic tumors into Grades I through IV, with Grade I being the most benign and Grade IV being the most malignant (glioblastoma multiforme). Today, such a grading system has been largely abandoned and replaced by a more simplified system based upon the degree of anaplasia present. The term "astrocytoma" (old astrocytoma I and II) refers to a neoplasm with a relatively benign appearance, having a homogeneous grouping of relatively typical cells with little atypicality or anaplasia. The term "malignant astrocytoma" (old astrocytoma III) refers to a neoplasm with a greater degree of anaplasia than the more benign form, but not containing all of the necessary malignant features to be called "glioblastoma." The term "glioblastoma multiforme" (old astrocytoma IV) is reserved for a malignant neoplasm having abundant glial pleomorphism, numerous mitotic figures and giant cells, pseudopalisading of cells, and vascular hyperplasia. The premortem classification of a particular astrocytic tumor is extremely difficult, with many neuropathologists emphasizing that true classification can only be made at autopsy. The actual grade or classification of such a neoplasm is based upon the most malignant portion present, and it is impossible to adequately sample a tumor at the time of either tumor resection or needle biopsy, particularly the latter. Therefore, many studies that have attempted to correlate the appearance of the tumor on the CT scan with the morphological characteristics and pathologic grade of the tumor have inherent error in the tumor sampling. Statements regarding the CT scan characteristics found with a particular degree of malignancy must be looked upon with some degree of skepticism.

On the unenhanced CT scan, the majority of astrocytomas present either with areas of decreased density (Fig 9–1) or with patchy areas of low density mixed with regions of isodensity (Fig 9–2). The rim so commonly seen with a malignant tumor on the enhanced scan may appear to be of slightly increased density relative to normal brain on the unenhanced views. This increased density may be more apparent than real because of the decreased density of the peritumoral edema combined with the low density of central necrosis or cyst formation (Fig 9–3). The borders of the lesion are usually poorly defined on the unenhanced scan, with those margins melding imperceptibly into areas of surrounding cerebral edema or into areas of more normal-appearing brain. Contrast enhancement is required for a better definition of the lesion and its margins. Various authors have suggested that if a brain tumor is suspected, there is little differential diagnostic value based on the nonenhanced CT scan.[2, 3] More importantly, some tumors that are isodense on the unenhanced scan would be missed if the radiographic findings on the preinfusion scan were to be used as the basis for administering contrast material.

The use of contrast material is vital in the evaluation of any cerebral neoplasm. The enhancement of an intracranial lesion with contrast material is a complex subject and is addressed more completely in Chapter 1 of

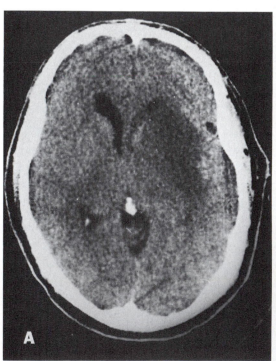 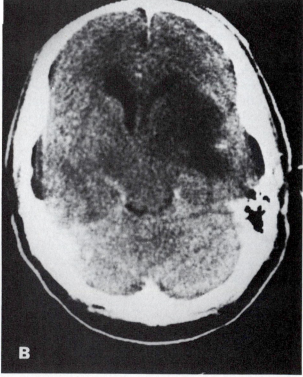

Fig 9–1.—Well-differentiated astrocytoma. Nonenhanced **(A)** and enhanced **(B)** scans demonstrated low density within the inferior left frontal and left temporal lobes. Only minimal enhancement along the lateral margin of the low density tumor is present **(B)**. Although the margins are relatively sharp and the neoplasm is quite low dense, no macroscopic or microscopic cysts were present.

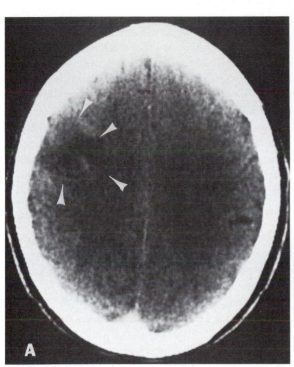

Fig 9–2.—Low-grade astrocytoma. The unenhanced scan **(A)** demonstrates patchy low density and isodensity in the high right frontoparietal junction *(arrowheads).* There is only minimal enhancement of the anterior portion **(B,** *anterior arrowhead)* of this low-grade glioma.

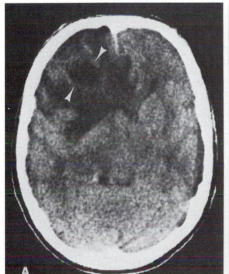
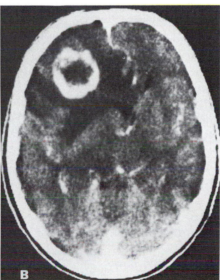
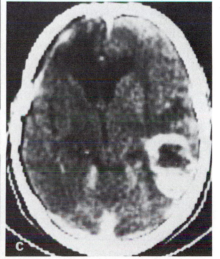

Fig 9–3.—Glioblastoma multiforme with intracranial metastasis via CSF. The unenhanced scan **(A)** demonstrates the rim of tumor tissue *(arrowheads)* surrounding a more central necrotic portion of the tumor. The ring is made more prominent by the central necrosis and surrounding peritumoral edema. The enhanced scan **(B)** demonstrates the shaggy ring of enhancing tumor. Note that there is no evidence of tumor in the left temporal region at this time. Five months later, following surgery and irradiation of the right frontal glioblastoma multiforme, the patient presents with a left posterior temporal enhancing centrally necrotic mass **(C).** The contiguity of the temporal mass to the surface of the brain suggests that this second lesion represents metastasis via the CSF pathways.

this book. In brief and simplified terms, enhancement depends upon either the presence of iodinated contrast material within the "blood pool" of a lesion or upon its passage across an abnormal blood-brain barrier to diffuse within the interstices of a lesion. In the former category are aneurysms, arteriovenous malformations, and certain extremely vascular neoplasms. In the latter category are cerebral infarcts, inflammatory lesions, and the majority of cerebral neoplasms. The degree of enhancement of a cerebral neoplasm depends primarily upon the degree of disruption of the blood-brain barrier and not upon the degree of vascularity within the lesion, whether angiographically or pathologically visualized. As seen with electron microscopy, malignant neoplasms produce a greater disruption of the blood-brain barrier than do more benign tumors. Therefore, malignant astrocytomas and glioblastomas generally enhance to a greater degree than do the more benign astrocytomas. This is a rough generalization, however, since some low-grade glial tumors are found to enhance more than might be expected for their degree of pathologic malignancy, and some malignant tumors demonstrate little enhancement. This subject of the "grading" of the degree of malignancy of glial tumors by the degree of contrast enhancement will be discussed later in greater detail.

The volume of contrast material that is used for contrast enhancement of intracranial lesions has steadily increased over the years. In our institution, 150 ml of a 60% iodinated contrast material is administered either as an infusion or by the combination of "IV push" of the first half of the contrast followed by infusion of the second half over approximately 5 minutes; both techniques result in the administration of 42 gm iodine to the patient. Some authors[4, 5] advocate a double dose of contrast material (84.6 gm iodine) administered over 10 to 15 minutes and followed by delayed scanning in 1 to 2 hours for the visualization of intracranial neoplasms. This delayed high-dose (DHD) technique produces high blood levels of iodine and allows for the time interval required for the movement of this contrast material across a relatively intact blood-brain barrier (see Fig 1–17). They, like other authors, gain little additional information from the nonenhanced scan, either for the diagnosis of a tumor or for the grading of a glioma. They have found this technique to be superior to either immediate scanning following a double dose of contrast material or to delayed scanning following a conventional dose.[4] Specifically, they found that the DHD technique allowed the visualization of single or multiple tumors not otherwise seen in 11.5% of cases in which the conventional dose was first utilized. No significant change in serum electrolyte values were

seen in patients who had normal renal function before the DHD scan.[4, 5]

In our institution, we have reserved this DHD technique for problem cases rather than for the routine case of suspected intracranial neoplasm. Such problem cases are generally those in which a mass effect is seen, but in which an area of definite enhancement cannot be visualized with the routine volume of contrast material. In some cases, before a definitive CT scan can be obtained, the patient has been placed on corticosteroids, which produce a relative "healing" of the blood-brain barrier; it may be difficult clinically to withdraw those corticosteroids in order to obtain a definitive CT scan. In such cases, the DHD technique has proven valuable in the diagnosis of neoplasia. One might also consider an attempt at osmotically breaking the blood-brain barrier with a drug such as mannitol. Disruption of the blood-brain barrier with intra-arterial mannitol has been performed for the perfusion of chemotherapy into malignant brain tumors (see Fig 1–19).[6]

Low-grade infiltrating astrocytomas generally have patchy areas of enhancement, slight to moderate in de-

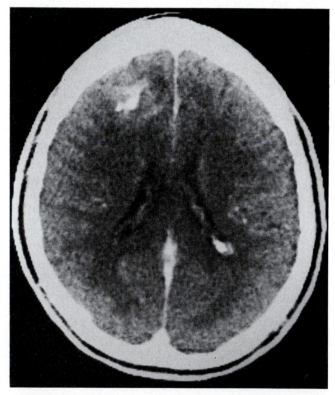

Fig 9–4.—Calcified anaplastic glioma. Forty-five-year-old man followed for a number of years with adult-onset seizure disorder and right frontal lobe calcific deposit. Scan now demonstrates slight enhancement around the calcification. This was most likely a low-grade astrocytoma or oligodendroglioma that underwent malignant degeneration.

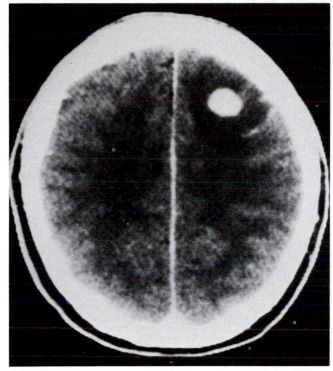

Fig 9–5.—Anaplastic astrocytoma having appearance of metastasis. This solid well-circumscribed neoplasm with abundant surrounding cerebral edema has an appearance more typical of solitary metastasis.

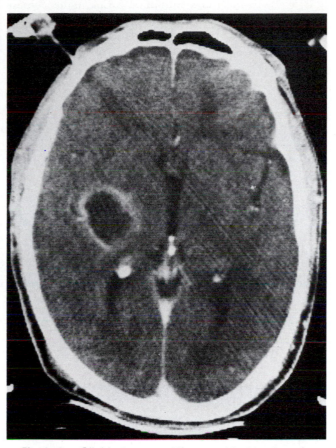

Fig 9–6.—Glioblastoma multiforme with thin ring of enhancement. Scan taken in stereotactic frame used for biopsy. Ring of enhancement of this malignant tumor is relatively thin.

gree (see Figs 9–1 and 9–2). The poorly enhancing margins blend with surrounding cerebral tissue, making marginal definition impossible. More malignant astrocytomas may have a similar infiltrative appearance (Fig 9–4) or may have much more circumscribed borders of enhancement, with marginal sharpness and homogeneity of enhancement more typically seen with benign lesions and metastases (Fig 9–5).

Glioblastoma multiforme commonly appears as a ring lesion caused by the rapid growth rate of the lesion beyond the capabilities of its blood supply to provide adequate nutrients, resulting in central necrosis. A thick shaggy rim is typically seen (see Fig 9–3), although a thin rim of enhancement may also be found (Fig 9–6). A variety of less common appearances have been seen with glioblastoma multiforme, including a relatively well-circumscribed lesion with little central necrosis (Fig 9–7), a combination of well-circumscribed nodules connected by or associated with diffusely infiltrating tumor (Figs 9–8 and 9–9), and a well-marginated lesion abutting the inner table of the skull and simulating a benign tumor such as meningioma (Fig 9–10). While the degree of contrast enhancement is moderate to marked in most malignant glial tumors, cases are seen

in which the degree of enhancement is minimal (Figs 9–4 and 9–11).

Low-density regions within astrocytic tumors may be due to one of three pathologic conditions. First, there may be central necrosis surrounded by a rim of more viable neoplasm. Stereotactic biopsy of both the rim and the central lucency[7] and many years of postmortem evaluation following CT scanning have established that the lucency within a rim is generally made up of necrotic tissue. However, the second reason for this low density is the presence of centrally located viable neoplasm that is slower to enhance than is the rim.[8] Histologic studies have suggested that although such low-density areas are made up in part of necrotic tissue, extensive areas of viable tissue may also be present.[9] Performance of DHD studies has demonstrated a progressive enhancement of the central portion of a ring lesion, not with a fluid-fluid level that would suggest the presence of a cystic component, but rather in a manner suggesting tissue that is slower to enhance.[5]

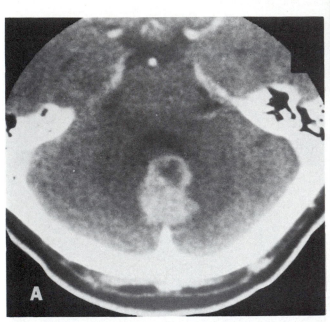

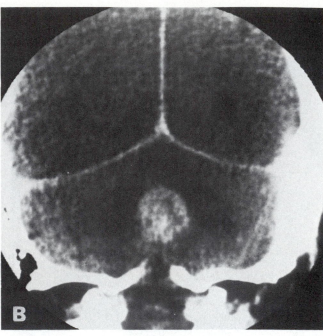

Fig 9–7.—Well-circumscribed glioblastoma multiforme with little surrounding edema or central necrosis. Glioblastoma of the cerebellar vermis, an unusual primary lesion, presents in this patient as a well-circumscribed enhancing mass lesion with little central necrosis or surrounding edema, as seen on the axial **(A)** and coronal **(B)** scans. This appearance is more typical of metastatic tumor.

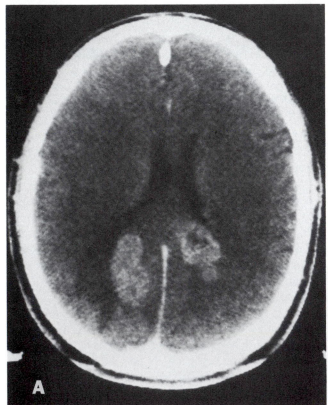

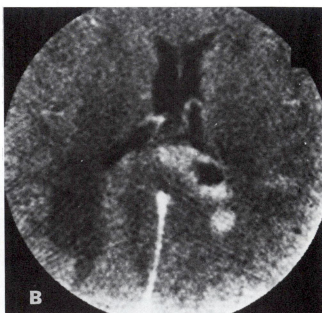

Fig 9–8.—Glioblastoma multiforme with extension through the splenium of the corpus callosum. The highest enhanced scan **(A)** demonstrates two well-circumscribed nodules of tumor in the medial portions of both parietal lobes. The slightly lower enhanced scan **(B)** shows connection of these tumor nodules through the splenium of the corpus callosum. This appearance is analogous to the more typical "butterfly glioma" of the frontal lobes with extension through the rostral corpus callosum.

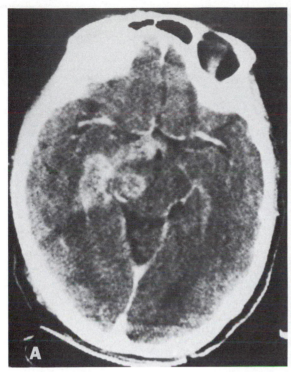

Fig 9–9.—Glioblastoma multiforme with both invasion of the brain stem and nodular fingers of tumor extension. A low-enhanced scan **(A)** demonstrates the malignant glioma within the right temporal lobe. Extension of tumor is into the brain stem and hypothalamus/optic chiasm. Fingers of tumor extended more superiorly, so that a higher cut **(B)** discloses separate nodules simulating hematogenous metastases.

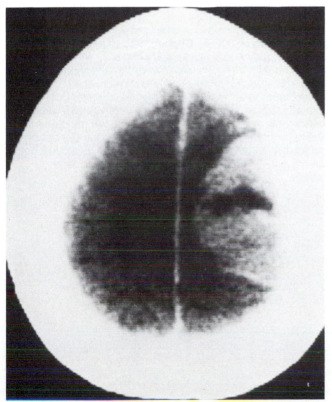

Fig 9–10.—Well-circumscribed high-convexity glioblastoma multiforme. The enhanced scan demonstrates a sharply marginated mass high over the left cerebral convexity and based along the inner table of the skull. Many of the features suggest a benign tumor such as meningioma. There is a central area of necrosis and/or cyst formation.

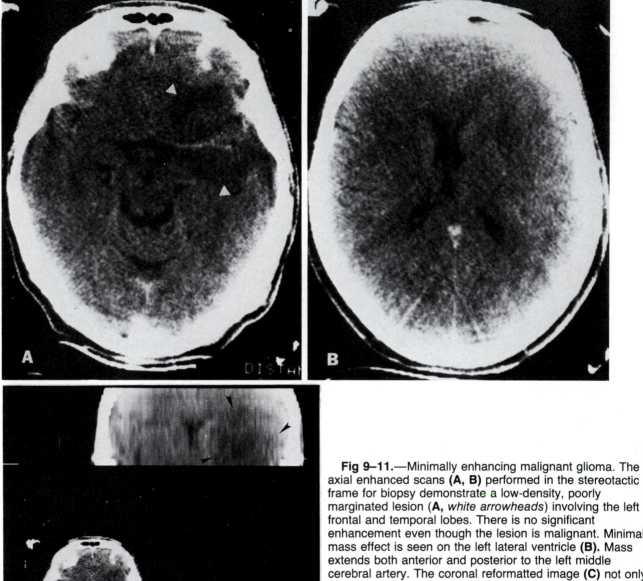

Fig 9–11.—Minimally enhancing malignant glioma. The axial enhanced scans **(A, B)** performed in the stereotactic frame for biopsy demonstrate a low-density, poorly marginated lesion (**A,** *white arrowheads*) involving the left frontal and temporal lobes. There is no significant enhancement even though the lesion is malignant. Minimal mass effect is seen on the left lateral ventricle **(B).** Mass extends both anterior and posterior to the left middle cerebral artery. The coronal reformatted image **(C)** not only demonstrates the tumor *(black arrowheads)* as well or better than the axial views, but the mass effect is easier to visualize.

Lastly, there may be a true cyst within the neoplasm, with tumor tissue present either as a nodule (Fig 9–12) or located more diffusely around the rim of the cyst (Fig 9–13). The diagnosis of a cyst within a neoplasm can be surgically important, because the mass effect of the tumor can be markedly decreased by drainage of the cystic component (see Fig 9–13). The diagnosis of a cyst rather than a central area of necrosis demands the presence of smooth inner margins; attenuation coefficients alone are generally of little value.[10] In addition, contrast material that penetrates the blood-brain barrier in such a cystic tumor may form a fluid-fluid level (see Fig 12–7)[11] generally not present with necrotic tumors.[10]

When the enhanced CT scan demonstrates a mass lesion with ring enhancement, a malignant primary cerebral neoplasm must be a major consideration. The biopsy diagnosis of a lower-grade tumor must be viewed with suspicion, because there is the possibility that the site of biopsy was in an area of lesser-grade astrocytoma. However, other lesions may be present with such an appearance, as will be discussed in Chapter 13. Briefly, metastatic tumors (see Fig 12–4) and resolving hematomas may present with an irregularly marginated rim and may therefore be impossible to distinguish from a malignant primary cerebral neoplasm. An intracerebral abscess generally has a smoother margin (see

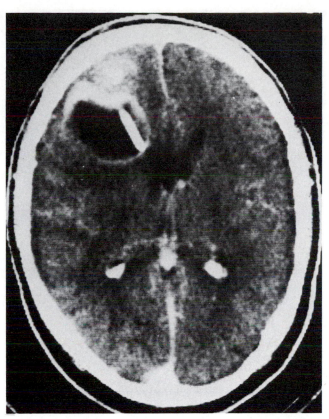

Fig 9–13.—Cystic astrocytoma with shunt. The right frontal lobe neoplasm is cystic as indicated by the sharp margins of the internal lucency. A shunt has been placed into the cyst cavity for decompression.

Fig 13–2), although it can be difficult, if not impossible, to distinguish the two on the basis of CT appearance alone. The ring of a resolving cerebral infarct (see Fig 5–14) is generally partial or incomplete.

Some astrocytomas present as low-density lesions without evidence of contrast enhancement (Fig 9–14) and with absorption coefficients that may be as low as that for cerebrospinal fluid (CSF). Such an appearance suggests a cystic tumor or possibly a nonneoplastic process such as porencephaly, arachnoid cyst, or infarct. It has been well demonstrated that such tumors may vary in histologic grade from benign to malignant.[12-14] The margins of such a low-density tumor are usually not as sharp and smooth as a grossly cystic lesion, and the low density is accounted for either by the presence of interstitial or intracellular microcysts, or by a relatively high water content.[12] It must be emphasized that a CT diagnosis of neoplasia in such a case does not rest on the presence of contrast enhancement, nor on the level of absorption coefficients, but on the gross morphological characteristics such as the margins of the lesion.

Occasionally, we may see a low-density, nonenhancing peripheral mass that is sharply demarcated and

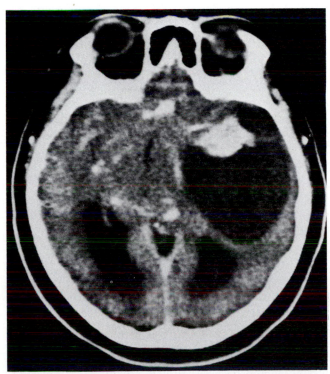

Fig 9–12.—Cystic astrocytoma. The left temporal cystic astrocytoma contains a densely enhancing solid nodule anteriorly. The sharp internal margination of the lucency is indicative of a true cyst.

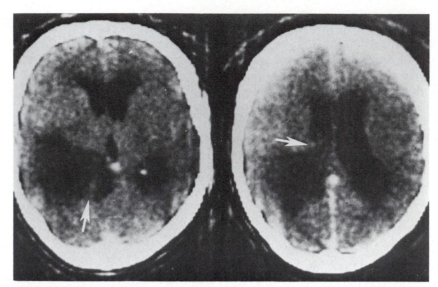

Fig 9–14.—High-grade astrocytoma with microcystic components. A large low-density parietal lobe mass is present with absorption coefficients close to that of the CSF within the ventricular system. The mass does not represent a dilated ventricular atrium, but is separated from the lateral ventricle *(arrows)*, which is compressed and distorted. A grossly solid lesion was found at the time of surgery, not a grossly cystic lesion, although intracellular microcysts were found on pathologic examination, accounting for the low density of this lesion. (From Latchaw R.E., Gold H.L.A., Moore J.S., et al.: *Radiology* 125:141–144, 1977. Used by permission.)

smoothly marginated in all projections (Fig 9–15). The lack of marginal irregularity in at least one projection would tend to exclude the usual noncystic low-density glial tumor, while the lack of a rim or nodule of enhancement as in Figures 9–12 and 9–13 would exclude a typical cystic glioma. The most likely diagnoses would appear to be arachnoid or epidermoid cysts, although a purely cystic astrocytoma cannot be excluded. In such a case, a radionuclide scan may be of value. While cerebral radionuclide studies have been infrequently used since the advent of CT scanning, they can occasionally give valuable information not derived from CT alone. In the case shown in Figure 9–15, the radionuclide scan was positive in the area of abnormality, indicating a diagnosis of neoplasm, because a nonneoplastic cyst would not be expected to take up isotope.

The low density that is seen surrounding the enhancing portion of a tumor is called cerebral edema. Postmortem pathologic studies generally demonstrate a variable amount of cerebral edema surrounding a neoplasm. However, to attribute that low density surrounding an enhancing lesion simply to cerebral edema is to misunderstand the nature of the pathologic process. Lilja and coworkers[9] have studied a group of high-grade gliomas undergoing CT scanning immediately before patient death, followed by extensive postmortem sectioning and radiologic-pathologic correlation. They have found that areas of little or no enhancement that are either isodense or of low density contain fingers of viable neoplasm throughout the entire region. Areas of nonenhancing low-density tumor with histologic characteristics of malignancy have a CT appearance similar to that of edematous areas. Certainly, the areas of enhancement, particularly the borders of a ring lesion, do not represent the true margins of the neoplasm.

With the assumption that some of the surrounding low density represents edema, the amount of this surrounding edema is variable in tumors of the astrocytic series. Generally, the more malignant lesions produce a greater degree of disruption of the blood-brain barrier and therefore more surrounding cerebral edema (see Figs 9–3 and 9–5). Many infiltrative neoplasms have little in the way of surrounding edema (see Figs 9–2 and 9–4). However, these statements are generalizations, with the amount of edema variable and not always dependent upon histologic grade only, as seen with the relatively sparse edema around the malignant astrocytomas of Figures 9–6 through 9–9.

The cerebral edema surrounding an astrocytoma/glioblastoma involves only the white matter, presenting "fingers" of edema (Figs 9–3 and 9–16) as the edema spreads along white matter tracts in a similar fashion to the spread of tumor along these same fiber tracts.[15] Infarcts, on the other hand, involve gray matter in 98% of cases, with both gray and white matter involvement in over two thirds of cases.[15]

The amount of mass effect in any given tumor is dependent to a large degree upon the amount of surrounding "edema." Infiltrating neoplasms with little surrounding edema may produce little or no apparent

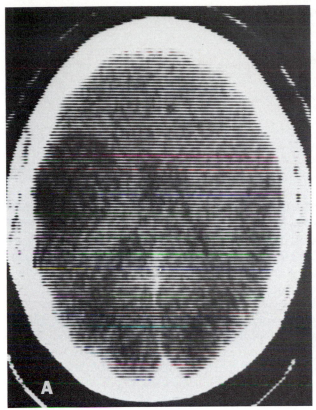

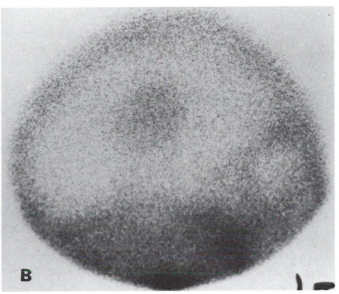

Fig 9–15.—Low-grade cystic astrocytoma with positive radionuclide scan. The enhanced axial scan **(A)** demonstrates a sharply marginated low-density mass within the posterior frontal and temporal lobes. No enhancement could be visualized on multiple slices. The sharp margination on all slices suggested an arachnoid cyst, although a cystic neoplasm in this adolescent male could not be excluded. A radionuclide scan **(B)** demonstrates an area of isotope uptake. Arachnoid cysts are not generally positive on radionuclide studies. Surgery revealed a low-grade cystic astrocytoma. (From Latchaw R.E., Gold L.H.A., Moore J.S., et al.: *Radiology* 125:141–144, 1977. Used by permission.)

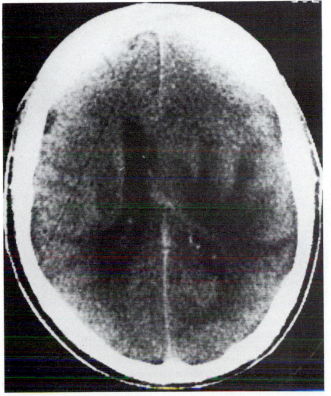

Fig 9–16.—"Fingers of edema." This nonenhanced scan at a level above a left temporal lobe glioblastoma multiforme demonstrates extensions of edema along white matter tracts and between gray matter structures, thereby simulating the fingers of a hand.

mass effect on the ventricular system (see Figs 9–4 and 9–6), the structure upon which mass effect is most apparent. A lack of apparent mass effect does not exclude a diagnosis of neoplasm. Temporal and occipital lobe masses and high-convexity tumors may produce little distortion of the distant ventricular system, although effacement of cortical sulci may be present with high convexity masses (see Figs 9–5 and 9–10). It must be stressed that the axial view of a CT scan is only one projection that is used in evaluating the brain; sagittal and coronal views may be of value in detecting mass effect if present (see Fig 9–11).

Hemorrhage into an astrocytoma/glioblastoma is more common with the higher grades of malignancy, although hemorrhage into lower-grade gliomas does occur (Fig 9–17). Such hemorrhage generally results as the tumor outgrows its blood supply, producing areas of necrosis and secondary hemorrhage. Hemorrhage may also occur because tumor vessels have relatively weak walls that rupture easily, or because of growth of the neoplasm into normal cerebral vessels.[16] Hemorrhage may be the initial neurologic event in a patient without known cerebral tumor. The diagnosis of tumorous over nontumorous hemorrhage depends upon a high degree of suspicion with a hemorrhage in an unusual location, with a dispersed distribution of the blood unlike the usual consolidated traumatic hematoma, or with an unusual history such as progressive neurologic deficit accompanied by a sudden catastrophic event (see Fig 9–17). In such a case, contrast enhancement may be present at the periphery of the hemorrhage, suggesting underlying neoplasm. It must be remembered that a resolving hematoma will have an abnormal blood-brain barrier after a number of days to weeks, with marginal enhancement occurring at that time.

Calcification within an astrocytoma (see Fig 9–4) is indicative of its long-standing presence and slow growth and is therefore indicative of a relatively low-grade astrocytoma. However, such a tumor may undergo malignant degeneration so that calcified low-grade tumor is seen contiguous to more malignant tumor.

Astrocytoma/glioblastoma infiltrates into the surrounding parenchyma by coursing along white matter tracts. Infiltration into the corpus callosum (see Fig 9–8) or the anterior or posterior commissures allows spread to the opposite hemisphere. Infiltration into the brain stem may also occur (see Fig 9–9), allowing extension into the posterior fossa. Infiltration into subependymal tissues produces a periventricular mode of spread (Fig 9–18). This is generally an ominous sign for

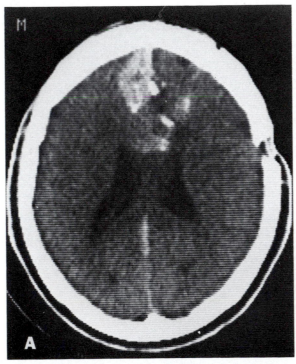
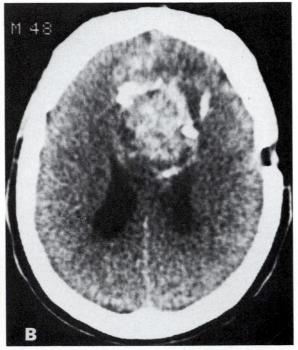

Fig 9–17.—Calcified oligodendroglioma with hemorrhage. The enhanced CT scan **(A)** demonstrates a calcified neoplasm originating in the anteromedial right frontal lobe, extending posteriorly into the corpus callosum, and into the medial left frontal lobe. The patient had had a previous left frontal craniotomy for biopsy. Repeat nonenhanced scanning **(B)** was performed 5 months later following the sudden and catastrophic onset of stupor leading to coma. The scan demonstrates diffuse and mottled hemorrhage within the neoplasm. (Courtesy of Lawrence H.A. Gold, M.D., University of Minnesota, Minneapolis.)

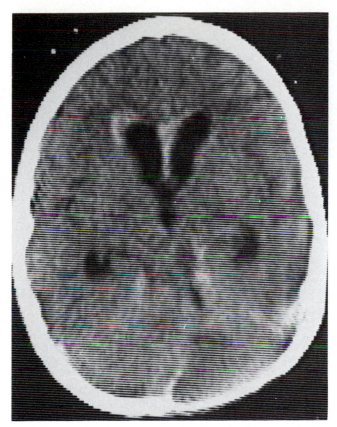

Fig 9–18.—Periventricular spread of glioma. Six-year-old child with previous partial resection of cerebellar grade II astrocytoma. Spread by CSF pathways had led 1 year later to diffuse periventricular extension of neoplasm, a very ominous prognostic sign.

the patient's prognosis; even when the neurologic condition appears stable, periventricular spread is usually indicative of a rapid downhill course.[17]

The extension of neoplasm to a ventricular or cortical surface allows seeding of tumor cells via CSF pathways. This may occur with many intracranial neoplasms, but is most common with malignant astrocytoma/glioblastoma (see Fig 9–3), medulloblastoma (see Figs 9–32 to 9–36), and germinoma. Occasionally, one sees multiple foci of malignant gliomas that represent separate sites of primary tumor (multifocal glioma) rather than metastases via CSF pathways. The necessary pathologic criteria for a diagnosis of multifocal glioma include the lack of linkage between the tumor masses along white matter tracts and the lack of contiguity of the tumor to cortical or ependymal surfaces.[18] If both lesions presented simultaneously, the probable CT scan diagnosis would be metastases rather than multifocal glioma, and there would be no way to make the distinction without biopsy.

Astrocytoma/glioblastoma may grow into the dural coverings of the brain, but does not completely pene-

trate the dural structures. Dural invasion is usually an imperceptible finding on CT scan, although it is well known angiographically, with tumor vessels to the glioma being supplied by the meningeal vascular system. Rather than penetration of the falx, infiltration of the opposite hemisphere usually requires parenchymal extension such as through the corpus callosum or seeding of tumor cells via CSF pathways.

Numerous authors have attempted to grade the degree of malignancy of astrocytic tumors using radiographic criteria on the CT scan. In general, the non-enhanced scan has not been helpful in differentiation, with both benign and malignant tumors presenting with an admixture of low density and isodensity.[3, 12, 19, 20] The amount of surrounding cerebral edema has proved to be somewhat more useful, with the more malignant astrocytomas tending to have a greater amount of surrounding cerebral edema than their benign counterparts.[19, 21] Most authors have tended to grade the tumor by the degree and character of contrast enhancement. In general, malignant astrocytomas and glioblastomas have been found to enhance markedly in 95% to 100% of cases; low-grade astrocytomas have been found to enhance in a range between only a few percentage of cases to as high as 40%, with that enhancement generally being spotty and nonhomogeneous when present; and intermediate-grade astrocytomas enhance between 60% and 90% of the time. According to these authors, if no enhancement is present, a low-grade glioma can be inferred, while marked enhancement is extremely unusual with low-grade tumors. The enhancement of a malignant astrocytoma/glioblastoma is generally nonhomogeneous, and a ring of enhancement is common.[19–23]

While these generalizations can be trusted in the majority of cases, numerous examples have been seen that rail against the use of such simplification. Pure low-density tumors as seen in Figure 9–14 may be benign or malignant, with neither the degree of contrast enhancement or the level of attenuation coefficients corresponding to the grade of malignancy.[12–14] Malignant astrocytomas may have little enhancement and be quite infiltrating in nature, as in Figures 9–4 and 9–11. Marked enhancement in low-grade tumors may also be seen (Fig 9–19). In addition, one source has found that the generalizations cited above are helpful for supratentorial tumors, but that the correlation of enhancement and tumor grade is not consistent in posterior fossa astrocytomas.[22]

Potential errors in the correlation of the CT scan appearance and the pathologic grading at the time of biopsy may be produced by the site of biopsy, as discussed earlier in this chapter. The grade of the tumor is the most malignant portion, but the biopsy may be

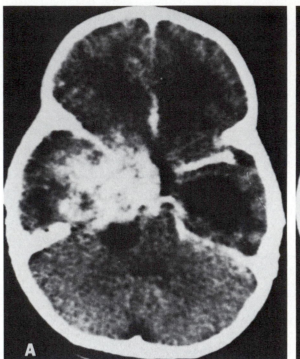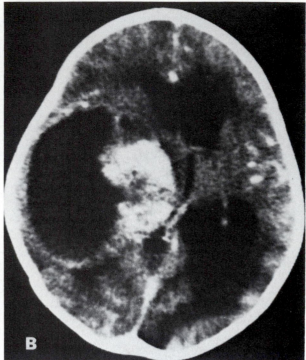

Fig 9–19.—Cystic grade II astrocytoma with marked enhancement. This 14-month-old child presented with increasing head size. Enhanced scans demonstrate a huge cystic neoplasm of the right cerebral hemisphere with a solid component medially and inferiorly **(A)** that markedly enhances, even though histologically this was a low-grade glioma. The tumor invades deeply into the thalamus and brain stem. There is a true cyst as denoted by the sharp margination of the lucent component **(B)**.

from a more benign portion of the tumor. Tumors behave differently in various intracranial locations, as indicated in the difference in enhancement patterns between supratentorial and infratentorial tumors of similar histologic types. The degree of enhancement of any neoplasm is dependent upon the degree of breakdown of the blood-brain barrier, the amount of contrast material utilized, and the timing of the scan following contrast infusion. Many tumors that obviously would not enhance with a conventional dose of contrast material are visualized with a high dose of contrast media,[4, 5] and tumors that appear centrally necrotic may fill in over time.[5] These factors are indicative of differences between tumors of similar grades in the alteration of the blood-brain barrier. Whether this difference in alteration among tumors of similar grade is significant for prognosis is conjectural. Silverman and Marks[24] followed 22 low-grade tumors over 4 years, dividing the group into enhancing and nonenhancing astrocytomas. There was no apparent difference in survival between the two groups, although it is admitted that the patient numbers may be too small or the 4 years too short a period of observation.

All too few studies concerned with the CT appearances of varying types and grades of gliomas have had precise pathologic-radiologic correlation. Such correlation is absolutely essential when attempting to make any prediction of histology from radiographic appearances. Two good studies are of interest in this discussion. Butler and coworkers[22] found that the degree of enhancement in malignant supratentorial gliomas correlated with increased tumor vascularity and necrosis. However, this relationship was not linear, so that once the threshold of enhancement was reached, there was no increasing enhancement with increased necrosis and tumor vascularity. Rather, increasing enhancement did not appear to depend upon microscopic findings, but rather upon functional parameters; the authors inferred a greater degree of abnormality of the blood-brain barrier with increasing malignancy. A similar correlation was not found with posterior fossa astrocytomas as previously discussed. Lilja and associates[9] attempted to correlate pathologic sections of eight malignant supratentorial gliomas with their immediate premorten CT scans. They found that the differences in enhancement patterns did not correlate with any specific histologic changes of malignancy, in contradistinction to the study of Butler and colleagues.[22] Multiple areas of high-grade tumor extended into the parenchyma surrounding areas of enhancement, but these areas of tumor extension did not show any enhancement and were frequently of low-attenuation value, mimicking the surrounding cerebral edema. Tumor extensions were frequently of isodensity and therefore not discernible by CT. The ring of neoplasm certainly did not define the limits of the tumor. These authors believed that the degree of enhancement correlated with the degree of abnormality of the blood-brain barrier, but not necessarily with any histologic changes of malignancy. They believed that the correlation between malignancy and intense enhancement was not constant and that there were definite limitations of the CT scan, both to the grading and to the delineation of the boundaries of a glioma.[9]

Further pathologic-radiologic studies with precise technique are needed for a more complete understanding of the anatomical and functional factors that lead to CT scan appearances, not only of intracranial neoplasms, but of all lesions visualized by CT scan. The CT scan characteristics for the more typical benign and malignant astrocytomas are useful, but must be viewed as generalizations at best. Errors will be made when attempting to rely upon only CT scan criteria for the definition and histologic characterization of an intracranial neoplasm. Biopsy of multiple areas of the glioma, as will be described in Chapter 34, is necessary for the appropriate characterization of the tumor.

Oligodendroglioma

Many of the statements made for astrocytomas can be made equally for oligodendrogliomas. An oligodendroglioma may be indistinguishable from an astrocytoma on the CT scan, with this distinction being made only at pathologic examination. However, there are two radiographic features that may give a presurgical indication of oligodendroglioma. The first is that of rather abundant calcification (Fig 9–20). While an astrocytoma may also calcify, an oligodendroglioma appears to have a propensity for rather extensive calcification. This calcification may be either peripheral or central, and while the curvilinear appearance as seen on skull films has been described as typical for oligodendroglioma, a nodular appearance is more common on the CT scan.[25]

The second feature is the relatively frequent appearance of a purely low-density tumor, with little if any enhancement (Fig 9–21).[13] The attenuation coefficients may be very low, simulating a nonneoplastic cyst or an area of encephalomalacia. Such a low density may not be associated with a true cyst, but a relatively high interstitial water content or microcystic change may be present to account for the low density. The presence of irregular margins on at least one projection rules out the diagnosis of arachnoid cyst, which should be smoothly marginated in all projections. The coronal

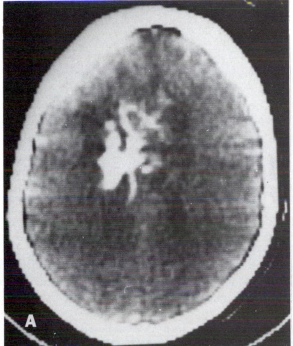

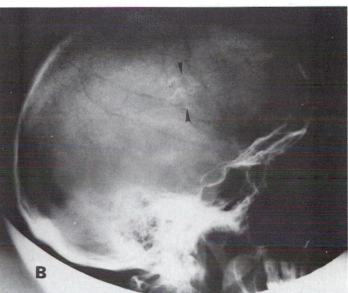

Fig 9–20.—Oligodendroglioma with curvilinear calcifications. The axial CT scan (A) demonstrates clumpy, confluent, and curvilinear calcifications involving the medial right frontal and parietal lobes and adjoining corpus callosum. An enhanced scan (not shown) demonstrated extensive enhancing neoplasm throughout the same regions. The curvilinear calcifications (arrowheads) as seen on the lateral skull film (B) are characteristic of oligodendroglioma.

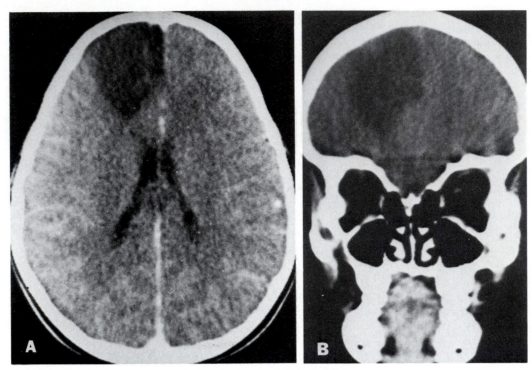

Fig 9–21.—Low-dense, nonenhancing oligodendroglioma. The axial enhanced scan **(A)** demonstrates a low-density lesion in the right frontal tip without definite mass effect and with sharp margination, suggesting the possibility of a long-standing cyst or other nonneoplastic process. The coronal scan **(B)** better demonstrates the irregular margination of the lesion, indicative of neoplasm. At surgery, this was a noncystic low-grade glioma. (From Varma R.R., Crumrine P.K., Bergman I., et al.: *Neurology* 33:806–808, 1983. Used by permission.)

projection (see Fig 9–21,B) may be a necessary addition to the axial projection in order to visualize the irregular margination. Oligodendroglioma may undergo malignant degeneration, with the CT scan demonstrating a combination of heavily calcified tumor contiguous to infiltrating and/or obvious necrotic and rapidly growing neoplasm.

Primitive Neuroectodermal Tumor (PNET)

The group of PNET encompasses various subtypes of malignant cerebral neoplasms that occur in children and that appear to have both similar histologic characteristics and similar course and prognosis. Rorke[26] has attempted to subclassify these tumors according to the line of cellular differentiation in any given tumor. Five subtypes are recognized, including the following categories: glial, ependymal, neuronal, bipotential, and unspecified. The neuronal subtype includes primary intracranial neuroblastoma. Medulloblastoma represents differentiation along neuronal lines by a tumor originating in the cerebellum. The pineal parenchymal tumors, pineoblastoma and pineocytoma, also are in this spectrum. Such a classification would explain the occasional diagnosis of "cerebral medulloblastoma," which simply would be a neuronal subtype of primitive neuroectodermal tumor located in the supratentorial compartment.[26]

Primary intracranial neuroblastoma represents the differentiation of primitive cells into more mature ganglion-like cells that in the better differentiated varieties form Homer-Wright rosettes as in extracranial neuroblastoma. The less well-differentiated varieties may require electron microscopy to identify dendritic processes characteristic of the neoplasm to separate it from the other forms of PNET.[27] This rare neoplasm has probably been called ependymoma or oligodendroglioma in the past.[28] The malignant tumor may invade venous structures, leading to extracranial metastases.[29] Metastases via the CSF pathways are also common. Primary intracranial neuroblastoma is to be differentiated from metastatic neuroblastoma from an extracranial site, in which metastases are generally to the calvarium, base of the skull, and orbits, while metastases to intracranial structures from an extracranial site are extremely rare.[30]

The CT scan findings are nonspecific and consist of a diffusely enhancing mass lesion (Fig 9–22) with a variable amount of surrounding cerebral edema, simulating

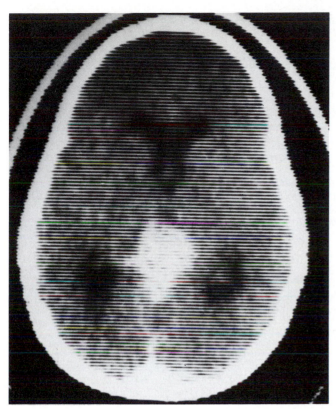

Fig 9–22.—Primary intracranial neuroblastoma. A diffusely enhancing neoplasm behind and above the third ventricle was found in this 6-year-old child. Biopsy revealed neuroblastoma, and there was no site of origin of extracranial neuroblastoma. Metastatic extracranial neuroblastoma rarely involves the cerebral parenchyma. (From Latchaw R.E., L'Heureux P.R., Young G., et al.: *A.J.N.R.* 3:623–630, 1982. Used by permission.)

any type of glial tumor.[30] However, three radiographic findings singly or in combination may suggest the appropriate diagnosis. First, there is a relatively high incidence of hemorrhage within the neoplasm.[31, 32] In one series, two out of three primary intracranial neuroblastomas demonstrated intratumoral hemorrhage.[32] Intratumoral hemorrhage in other types of neoplasms in the pediatric age group is uncommon. Second, cyst formation within the tumor is a common finding, with six out of 11 cases in one series demonstrating intratumoral cyst formation.[31] Third, neuroblastomas are frequently vascular at angiography.[30]

Ganglioglioma

This uncommon benign neoplasm may be found in a wide range of age groups, from the young to middle age. It is made up of a combination of ganglion and glial cells,[33, 34] and the lesion appears to grow very slowly as denoted by the frequent presence of calcification and

contoural changes in the skull.[25] True cyst formation is common (Fig 9–23).[33, 34] Enhancement is moderate to marked, even though the lesion has a benign histologic character. This enhancement may either be diffuse and homogeneous (Fig 9–24),[34] or peripheral about the margins of the cyst (see Fig 9–23).

Brain Stem Tumors

Brain stem expansions most commonly occur in children, with two out of three patients being children in a study of 41 brain stem expansions. In the same series, three out of four brain stem tumors were gliomas, so that 80% of brain stem gliomas occurred in the childhood age group.[35] Histologic evidence of malignancy (malignant astrocytoma, glioblastoma) is common even in brain stem gliomas occurring in childhood, with close to 50% having pathologic evidence or a clinical course of malignancy.[35]

The appearance of the unenhanced CT scan is that of a diffuse expansion of low density, isodensity, or an admixture of densities. It produces mass effect on the fourth ventricle with anterolateral bulging of the belly of the pons (Figs 9–25 to 9–28). Hemorrhage into the

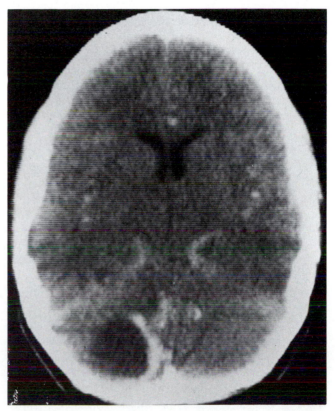

Fig 9–23.—Cerebellar ganglioglioma. The enhanced scan demonstrates a cystic neoplasm involving the right cerebellar hemisphere with a medial rim of enhancing solid tumor. A cystic component is common with ganglioglioma.

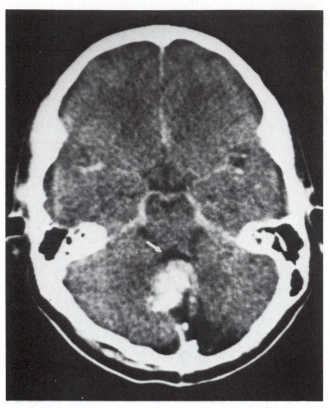

Fig 9–24.—Cerebellar ganglioglioma. Ten-year-old child presenting with an enhancing mass in the inferior vermis of the cerebellum, compressing and displacing the fourth ventricle *(arrow)* anteriorly. A portion of the dense mass is calcification as seen on the preinfusion scan (not shown).

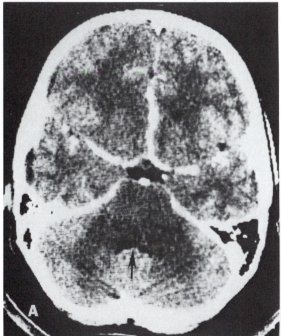

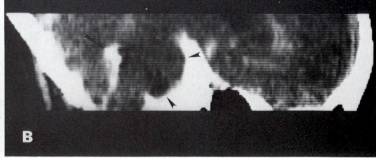

Fig 9–25.—Nonenhancing brain stem glioma. Enhanced axial scan **(A)** demonstrates diffuse low density throughout the pons, compressing the anterior portion of the fourth ventricle *(arrow)*. There is diffuse spread of nonenhancing neoplasm through the cerebellar peduncles into both cerebellar hemispheres. A reformatted sagittal view **(B)** performed during Amipaque cisternography demonstrates the diffuse bulging of the pons *(arrowheads)* and posterior displacement of the fourth ventricle *(arrow)*.

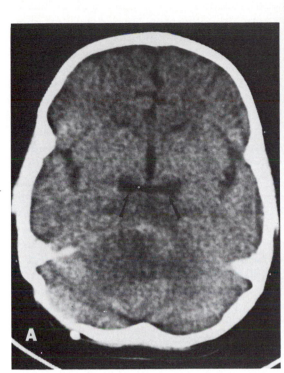

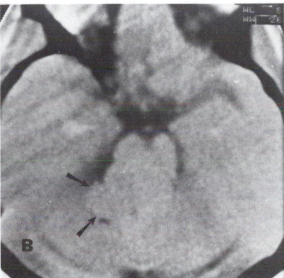

Fig 9–26.—Malignant brain stem glioma. Previous biopsy of a purely low-dense brain stem neoplasm in a 6-year-old child revealed a low-grade glioma. Seven months later, tumor has spread superiorly into the upper brain stem to compress the quadrigeminal and ambient cisterns (**A,** *arrows*). The enhanced scan (**B**) demonstrates intense enhancement involving the right lateral aspect of the pons extending to the cerebellopontine angle.

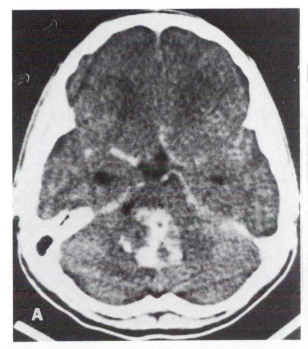

Fig 9–27.—Brain stem glioma with exophytic component. The enhanced axial scan (**A**) demonstrates an irregularly enhancing neoplasm involving the posterior portion of the pons and contiguous cerebellum. A reversed view of an Amipaque cisternogram (**B**) demonstrates an eccentric nodular component *(arrows)* extending from the right lateral aspect of the brain stem, distorting the ambient cistern. A grade I astrocytoma of the brain stem was found at surgery.

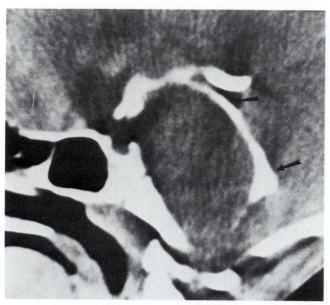

Fig 9–28.—Brain stem glioma demonstrated by Amipaque ventriculogram. A direct sagittal view following the placement of Amipaque through an intraventricular shunt demonstrates contrast material within the third and fourth ventricles and aqueduct. There is pronounced posterior displacement of both the aqueduct and fourth ventricle *(arrows)* by the diffuse brain stem expansion.

lesion is uncommon, as is calcification, while cystic or necrotic changes are relatively common.[35] Contrast enhancement varies from no enhancement (see Fig 9–25) to pronounced enhancement (see Fig 9–26). The enhancement pattern does not correlate well with the histologic grade of malignancy. Pathologic findings or a clinical course of malignancy are common with brain stem tumors and may be present with nonenhancing purely low-density tumors. In addition, low-grade tumors may enhance (see Fig 9–27), again pointing to the difficulty of attempting to grade the histologic degree of malignancy on the basis of the CT scan alone.

While the typical brain stem glioma is rather symmetric in location, producing bilateral neurologic findings, there may be an exophytic component to the tumor, with extension anteriorly into the prepontine subarachnoid cisterns or laterally towards the cerebellopontine angle (see Figs 9–26 and 9–27). This exophytic component may show a greater degree of contrast enhancement than the typical glioma confined to the brain stem and therefore may mimic an extra-axial mass lesion.[35] Spread of tumor occurs through the cerebellar peduncles into the cerebellum (see Fig 9–25), inferiorly into the medulla and spinal cord (see Fig 9–28), or superiorly through the upper brain stem into the cerebral hemispheres.

Metrizamide cisternography may be of great help in the evaluation of a brain stem neoplasm by filling the fourth ventricle, prepontine, and perimesencephalic cisterns to outline the brain stem. Not only may the routine axial and positional coronal projections be obtained, but a sagittal view of the brain stem may be obtained either by reformatting the axial slices (see Fig 9–25) or by obtaining a true sagittal view, performed by placing the child's head and one arm through the hole in the gantry (see Fig 9–28). The multiple views with metrizamide outlining the brain stem help in demonstrating both a subtle brain stem expansion and the deformation of contiguous structures indicative of spread of neoplasm. Metrizamide cisternography has also found use in our institution for the presurgical evaluation of a biopsy site. Our surgeons generally insist on a biopsy for the definitive diagnosis of a brain stem lesion, but wish to biopsy the lesion in a site that is easily accessible and not productive of significant neurologic deficit. In such cases, when an obvious exophytic component has not been seen on the routine CT scan, we have employed metrizamide cisternography with axial, coronal, and sagittal views, so that an area of relative bulging may be seen and selected as the biopsy site (see Figs 9–25, 9–27, and 9–28).[36]

Tumors of the Cerebellum and Fourth Ventricle

Primary neoplasms involving the cerebellum and fourth ventricle are far more common in children than adults. The differential diagnosis of these primary neoplasms include astrocytoma, medulloblastoma, ependymoma, and choroid plexus papilloma of the fourth ventricle. Hemangioblastoma is more commonly found in the adult, with the other tumors in this age group being primary astrocytoma/glioblastoma and primary lymphoma, all of which are relatively rare. A solitary cerebellar mass lesion in an adult is more typically a metastatic tumor or an hemangioblastoma. Cerebellar astrocytoma, medulloblastoma, and ependymoma are discussed here, while choroid plexus papilloma and primary lymphoma are covered later in this chapter. Hemangioblastoma will be discussed in Chapter 11.

Astrocytoma

Three out of four cerebellar astrocytomas originate within the cerebellar hemisphere, while the rest begin within the cerebellar vermis.[37] The typical appearances are either a solid lesion (Figs 9–29 and 9–30) or a cystic tumor (Fig 9–31), with an equal division between the cystic and solid types.[38]

On the unenhanced CT scan, a variety of appearances may be present, including slight increased density (see Fig 9–29), isodensity (see Fig 9–30), or mixed high and low density.[38] Enhancement may be homogeneous in character (see Figs 9–29 and 9–30) or inho-

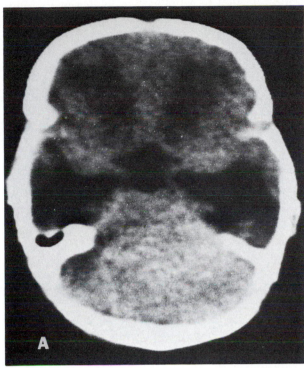
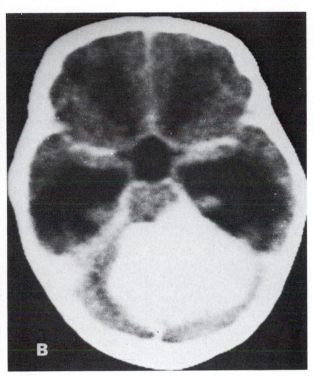

Fig 9–29.—Low-grade solid cerebellar astrocytoma. The unenhanced scan **(A)** in this child demonstrates diffuse increased density throughout much of the posterior fossa. The enhanced scan **(B)** demonstrates a sharply marginated neoplasm that enhances intensely and homogeneously. A relatively low-grade astrocytoma was found at the time of surgical excision.

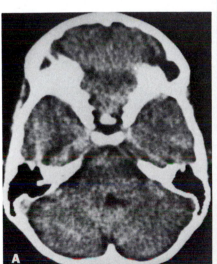
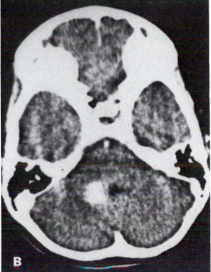
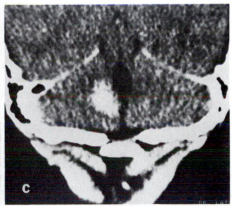

Fig 9–30.—Low-grade cerebellar astrocytoma. The non-enhanced axial scan **(A)** demonstrates amputation of the right lateral recess of the fourth ventricle. There is minimal low and high density in the region of abnormality. The enhanced scan **(B)** shows diffuse homogeneous enhancement of a small lesion in the periventricular region. Direct coronal scanning **(C)** demonstrates extension of the neoplasm into the right cerebellar tonsil and the relationship of the mass to the fourth ventricle and vallecula.

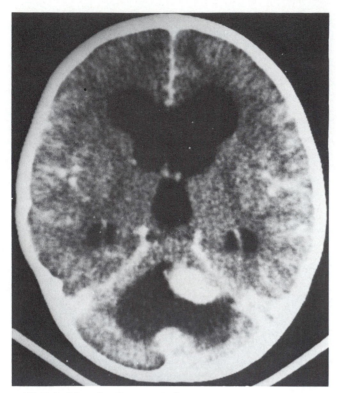

Fig 9–31.—Cystic cerebellar astrocytoma. Axial enhanced scan demonstrates a large cystic neoplasm of the cerebellum with a densely enhancing solid nodule anteriorly.

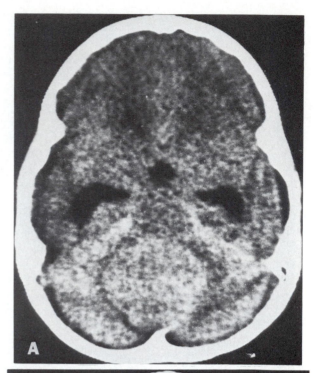

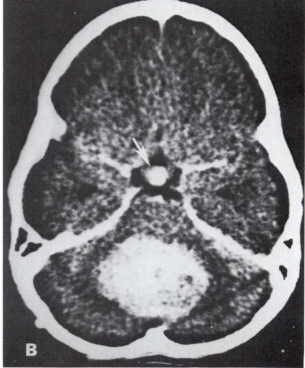

mogeneous, with the cystic tumors having either a solid nodule (see Fig 9–31) or a rim of enhancement. The degree of enhancement does not correlate with the degree of malignancy, with marked enhancement being seen in relatively benign tumors.[22, 39] Extension into the brain stem and spinal cord is a common occurrence.

Medulloblastoma

Medulloblastoma ranks close to the incidence of astrocytoma in pediatric cerebellar masses. When presenting in childhood, medulloblastoma usually originates in the cerebellar vermis along the roof of the fourth ventricle.[40, 41] However, a variant of the medulloblastoma occurs in the adolescent and young adult age groups, originating laterally within a cerebellar hemisphere. These latter tumors are frequently desmoplastic and have been called cerebellar sarcomas.

The usual vermian medulloblastoma has a characteristic CT scan appearance. There is a centrally located mass lesion of slight-to-moderate increased density without contrast material, compressing the fourth ventricle and producing obstructive hydrocephalus (Fig 9–32). The mass characteristically enhances markedly and homogeneously, with the margins sharply demarcated from the surrounding brain (Figs 9–32 and 9–33).

Fig 9–32.—Medulloblastoma. The unenhanced scan **(A)** demonstrates a sharply circumscribed mass of moderate increased density occupying the cerebellar vermis and medial hemispheres. There is obstructive hydrocephalus. The enhanced scan **(B)** demonstrates diffuse homogeneous enhancement of this lesion, typically seen with medulloblastoma. There is seeding of tumor via CSF pathways, with a suprasellar neoplastic nodule *(white arrow)*.

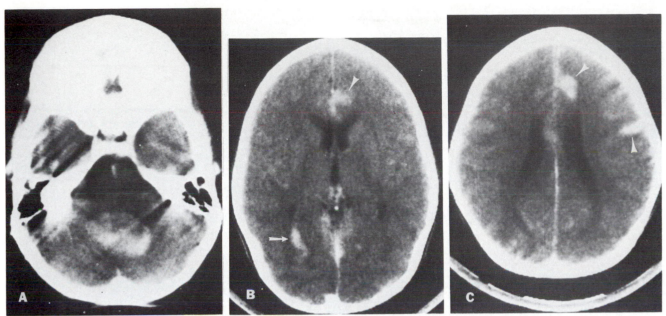

Fig 9–33.—Medulloblastoma with diffuse subarachnoid and intraventricular seeding. The enhanced scan in the posterior fossa **(A)** demonstrates a well marginated midline enhancing neoplasm typical of medulloblastoma. The quality of the scan is marred by motion artifact. Higher enhanced cuts **(B, C)** demonstrate multiple tumor deposits in cerebral sulci *(arrowheads)* and intraventricular spread producing a deposit with the right occipital horn **(B,** *arrow).*

There is usually no evidence of cyst formation or calcification, findings that are more typical of astrocytoma and ependymoma, respectively. Occasionally, however, less common features will be present, including small cysts (Fig 9–34), areas of calcification, or hemorrhage.[42] The combination of increased density on the preinfusion scan and the marked and homogeneous enhancement in a midline tumor strongly suggests the diagnosis of medulloblastoma, although astrocytoma may have a similar appearance (see Fig 9–29).

The more laterally originating medulloblastoma in the older age group may simulate astrocytoma. In our limited experience with such lesions, the degree of contrast enhancement has not been as florid as that with the midline childhood medulloblastomas (Fig 9–35). This is certainly in keeping with the histologic finding of an extensive amount of dense fibrous tissue within the lesion.

Medulloblastoma may invade contiguous parenchymal structures, including the brain stem and spinal cord (see Fig 9–35). These tumors commonly metastasize via CSF pathways to produce a suprasellar mass (see Figs 9–32 and 9–34), multiple enhancing masses on the surface of the brain (see Fig 9–33), ependymal implants along the ventricular surface (see Fig 9–33), or "dropped metastases" along the outer surface of the spinal cord (see Fig 9–35). The contrast-enhanced scan demonstrating diffuse cisternal enhancement (Fig 9–36) is indicative of widespread implants throughout the

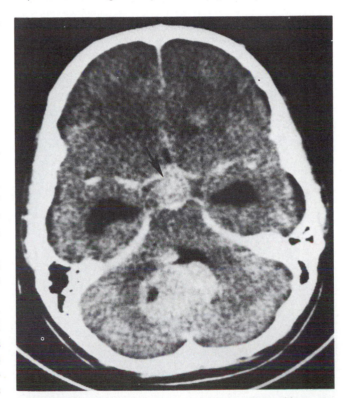

Fig 9–34.—Partially cystic medulloblastoma with suprasellar metastasis. The enhanced scan demonstrates a well-marginated neoplasm of the cerebellar vermis compressing and distorting the fourth ventricle. There is a small cyst in the right lateral aspect of the tumor. CSF seeding has occurred, with a large suprasellar metastasis *(arrow).*

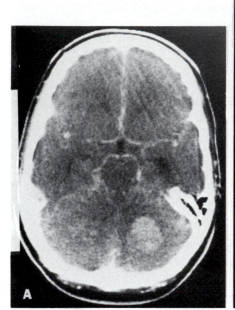
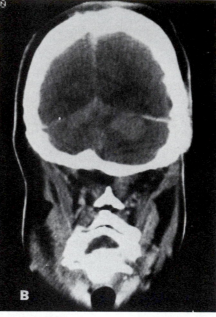
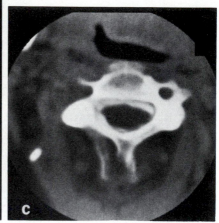

Fig 9–35.—Cerebellar hemispheric medulloblastoma in an adult. The axial enhanced scan **(A)** demonstrates a well-circumscribed homogeneous mass within the left cerebellar hemisphere. The degree of enhancement is only moderate, which appears to be typical with adult medulloblastoma. The coronal view **(B)** not only demonstrates the primary tumor focus within the superior portion of the left cerebellar hemi-sphere, just below the tentorium, but diffuse subtentorial tumor extension and invasion into the vermis. Postoperative Amipaque myelography **(C)** demonstrates enlargement of the cervical spinal cord, which has an irregular margin. At the time of posterior fossa craniotomy for excisional biopsy of the cerebellar mass, diffuse infiltration both into the cervical spinal cord and along its outer margins was found.

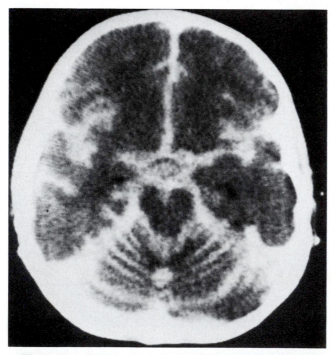

Fig 9–36.—Diffuse meningeal enhancement produced by seeding of medulloblastoma. Diffuse CSF seeding with medulloblastoma has produced such intense enhancement with the intravenous contrast agent that the scan simulates an Amipaque cisternogram.

subarachnoid spaces. Spread of medulloblastoma may be present relatively early, and all patients in our institution undergo myelography following initial surgery to detect spinal cord involvement.

Ependymoma

Three of four ependymomas occur in the posterior fossa, with the rest occurring supratentorially, arising either within a ventricle or within the cerebral parenchyma itself.[43] While the majority of ependymomas occur in childhood, between 23% and 46% will occur in patients greater than 18 years of age.[43–45] Of the pediatric posterior fossa masses, ependymoma is much less common than either medulloblastoma or astrocytoma.

Posterior fossa ependymomas generally originate from the floor of the fourth ventricle. While they are frequently isodense on the precontrast scan, 50% of the lesions are calcified (Fig 9–37).[43] Enhancement of a patchy or nonhomogeneous character (see Fig 9–37) is more common than homogeneous enhancement. The characteristics of calcification and nonhomogeneous enhancement distinguish these lesions from typical posterior fossa astrocytomas and medulloblastomas. Seeding along CSF pathways is similar to medulloblastoma.

Supratentorial ependymomas may originate either

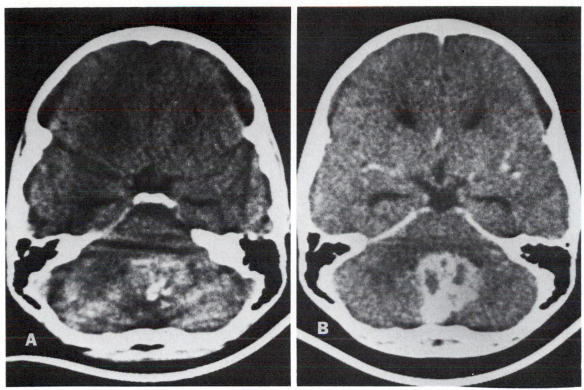

Fig 9–37.—Fourth ventricular ependymoma. The unenhanced scan **(A)** demonstrates a calcified mass lesion in the midline of the cerebellum in the region of the fourth ventricle, which is not visualized. The enhanced scan **(B)** shows nonhomogeneous enhancement of the mass lesion, which has multiple cystic areas. The combination of calcification and nonhomogeneous enhancement is typical of ependymoma.

along the ependymal lining of a ventricle or within the white matter of a cerebral hemisphere. In the latter situation, it is theorized that the ependymoma originates from ependymal rest cells, which are far from the ventricular lining, but are connected to the ventricle by a band of ependymal tissue.[43] These parenchymal ependymomas are frequently large at the time of presentation and commonly contain true cysts (Fig 9–38). The differential diagnosis of supratentorial hemispheric ependymoma includes ganglioglioma, which is a slower-growing, relatively benign lesion; oligodendroglioma; astrocytoma; and primitive neuroectodermal tumor. The ependymoma presenting within a lateral ventricle is typically of large size at the time of diagnosis as a result of its decompression into the ventricular system, with parenchymal mass effect and obstructive hydrocephalus occurring late.

Intraventricular Neuroectodermal Tumors

The differential diagnosis of lesions originating or presenting primarily within a ventricle include ependymoma, subependymoma (subependymal astrocytoma), choroid plexus papilloma, colloid cyst, and meningioma. Ependymomas arising within a ventricle or within the cerebral parenchyma have been discussed above. Meningiomas will be considered in greater detail in Chapter 10.

Subependymoma (Subependymal Astrocytoma)

The subependymoma is a variant of ependymoma in which there is a proliferation of subependymal astrocytes.[46] The majority of these tumors occur within the fourth ventricle, although 27% may be supratentorial, located along the walls of the lateral ventricle.[47] The majority of these tumors are asymptomatic, without evidence of active growth nor obstruction to the outflow of CSF, and are incidental findings at autopsy in elderly males.[46, 47] However, the symptomatic tumors are either strategically located to produce blockage of the CSF flow or are large at the time of presentation, with their intraventricular placement allowing for a large size before symptoms are produced. The septum pellucidum is a common supratentorial intraventricular location;[46] the centripetal growth produces a well-circumscribed mass lesion within the frontal horns (Fig 9–39).

A variant of the subependymal astrocytoma is the subependymal giant-cell astrocytoma that is seen in tuberous sclerosis. These tumors most frequently occur in the region of the foramen of Monro, producing obstruction to CSF flow, and are associated with the periven-

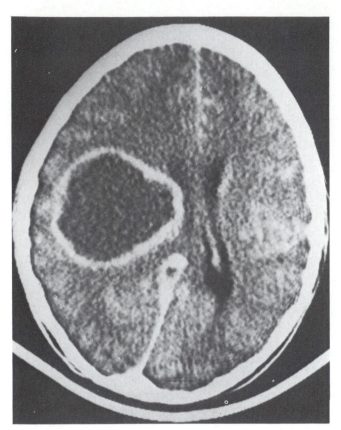

Fig 9–38.—Parietal ependymoma. This 13-year-old child presented with a large mass lesion of the right parietal lobe, compressing the right lateral ventricle. The lesion may have originated from either the ventricular ependyma or from ependymal rest cells within the hemisphere. The lesion is primarily cystic, with a densely enhancing rim.

tricular calcifications classically seen in tuberous sclerosis (Fig 9–40). While benign tubers may undergo calcification, the neoplasm occurring from degeneration of a tuber may be isodense on the preinfusion scan. It is therefore extremely important to perform an enhanced scan on all patients with tuberous sclerosis in order to detect an underlying neoplasm. This entity will be described more fully in Chapter 11.

Choroid Plexus Papilloma

Choroid plexus papilloma is a rare benign neoplasm, amounting to 0.5% of all intracranial tumors.[46] The most common point of origin is within the trigone of the lateral ventricle, although third and fourth ventricular papillomas have been reported.[48, 49] While choroid plexus papillomas have been most frequently seen during childhood, they may present at any age.[49] The CT scan appearance is that of a well-margined lesion with increased density before contrast enhancement (Figs 9–41 and 9–42),[49] and calcification is frequent. The lesion enhances markedly (see Figs 9–41 and 9–42), with ei-

ther a homogeneous or nonhomogeneous texture.[49, 50] Intraventricular meningioma has a similar appearance, although this tumor is extremely unusual in the pediatric age group.

Hydrocephalus is typically present with these tumors. While hemorrhage from this vascular tumor, producing adhesions and secondary obstruction to CSF flow, has been suggested as an etiology of the hydrocephalus,[51] the more widely accepted explanation is that of overproduction of CSF. Gudeman and coworkers[52] have nicely documented the decrease of CSF production following the removal of a choroid plexus papilloma and a secondary decrease in ventricular size without ventricular shunting. Thus, as illustrated in Figure 9–42, hydrocephalus associated with a lesion that could not produce ventricular obstruction by its position alone is further evidence for the preoperative diagnosis of choroid plexus papilloma.

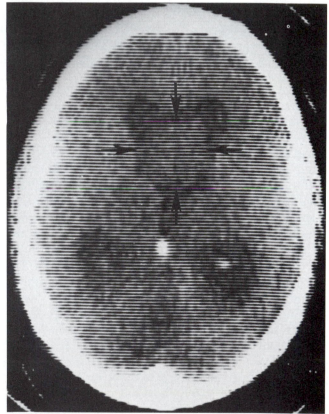

Fig 9–39.—Intraventricular glioma arising from the septum pellucidum. There is a sharply marginated round lesion (arrows) that is relatively isodense to the rest of the brain and has its epicenter in the septum pellucidum. The mass obstructs the foramina of Monro, producing dilatation of both frontal horns. Surgery revealed a well-circumscribed low-grade glioma that could be removed in its entirety. (From Latchaw R.E., Gold L.H.A., Tourje E.J.: *Minnesota Medicine* 60:554–559, 1977. Used by permission.)

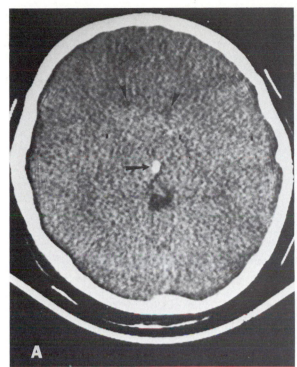

Fig 9–40.—Tuberous sclerosis with subependymal astro-cytoma in a child. The unenhanced scan **(A)** demonstrates a focus of calcification *(arrow)* near the third ventricle. There is a mass lesion of slightly greater than normal brain density compressing both frontal horns *(arrowheads).* The en-hanced scan **(B)** demonstrates the diffuse enhancement of this subependymal astrocytoma. A contrast scan is critical in differentiating a neoplasm from a tuber.

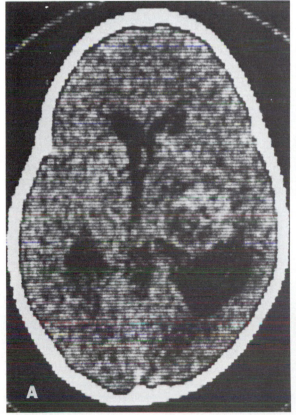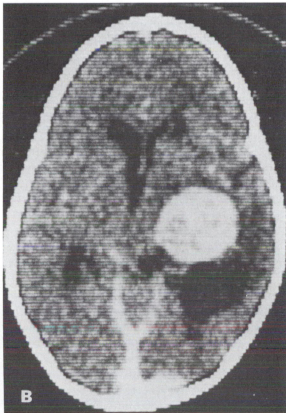

Fig 9–41.—Choroid plexus papilloma. The unenhanced scan **(A)** demonstrates a well-circumscribed mass of mod-erately increased density within the left temporal horn, pro-ducing dilatation of the left ventricular atrium. The enhanced scan **(B)** demonstrates diffuse and homogeneous enhance-ment of this neoplasm.

219

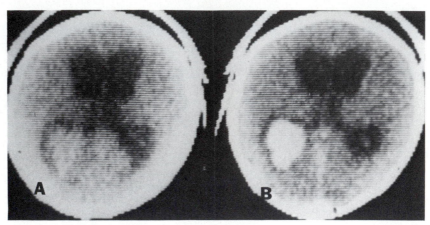

Fig 9–42.—Choroid plexus papilloma producing hydrocephalus. The unenhanced scan **(A)** demonstrates the high-dense mass within the atrium of the right lateral ventricle. There is intense and homogeneous enhancement of the lesion **(B)** in this 6-month-old child. The appropriate diagnosis can be made on this scan, because the lesion is not strategically situated to produce the hydrocephalus present. An increased production of CSF by the neoplasm accounts for the hydrocephalus.

Colloid Cyst

Colloid cyst is included in this chapter because of its neuroepithelial origin,[46, 53] although it could also be included under congenital tumors of maldevelopmental origin.[54] The lesion arises from the roof of the third ventricle, just behind the foramen of Monro. Although this lesion is probably present from birth, its very slow growth means that it does not generally present until adulthood.[54]

The CT scan appearance is classically that of a lesion located at the foramen of Monro, having a moderate-to-marked density without the use of contrast enhancement (Figs 9–43 and 9–44). This density is secondary to a combination of desquamated material within the cyst, hemosiderin, and calcium.[53] The lesion obstructs the foramina of Monro, leading to dilatation of the lateral ventricles and a small or normal-sized third ventricle (Figs 9–43 to 9–45). Occasionally, the lesion may be of an isodense nature (see Fig 9–45),[53] making its diagnosis much more difficult. Because the foramina of Monro are only a few millimeters in width, a small isodense lesion strategically located at the foramen may produce a marked degree of hydrocephalus, yet be difficult to visualize because of the marked enlargement of the lateral ventricles. Colloid cysts occasionally enhance with contrast material, which may be secondary to blood vessels on the wall of the cyst with leakage of contrast into the cyst cavity.[53] The enhanced scan may also show separation of the veins at the foramina of Monro by the cyst (see Fig 9–44).

The major differential diagnostic consideration of a mass in this region is an astrocytoma. Typically, such a glioma is evident on the contrast-enhanced scan (Fig 9–46) and has irregular margins in contradistinction to the

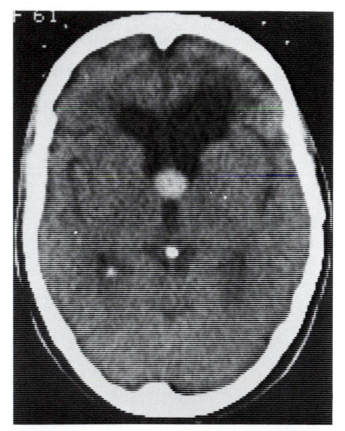

Fig 9–43.—Hyperdense colloid cyst. This nonenhanced scan demonstrates the classic appearance of a colloid cyst of the third ventricle. The mass is of a high density and is located at the foramina of Monro, producing moderate dilatation of the frontal horns, but a normal-sized third ventricle. (Courtesy of Lawrence H.A. Gold, M.D., University of Minnesota, Minneapolis.)

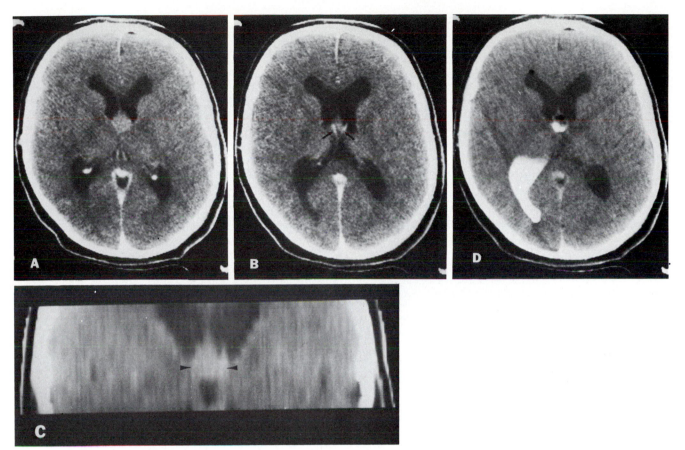

Fig 9–44.—Classic colloid cyst of the third ventricle, with stereotactic aspiration. The enhanced axial scans **(A, B)** demonstrate the classic appearance of a hyperdense mass located at the foramen of Monro. There is separation of the internal cerebral veins **(B,** *arrows*) by the mass. The coronal reformatted image **(C)** demonstrates the relationship of the hyperdense mass *(arrowheads)* to the lateral and third ven-tricles. Image **D** was performed with the patient in the ste-reotactic frame following placement of a needle into the cyst and aspiration of the cyst contents. A small amount of air within the cyst cavity and right frontal horn persists from the procedure. Amipaque has been introduced to evaluate com-munication between the lateral and third ventricles. Some of the contrast agent has run into the cyst cavity.

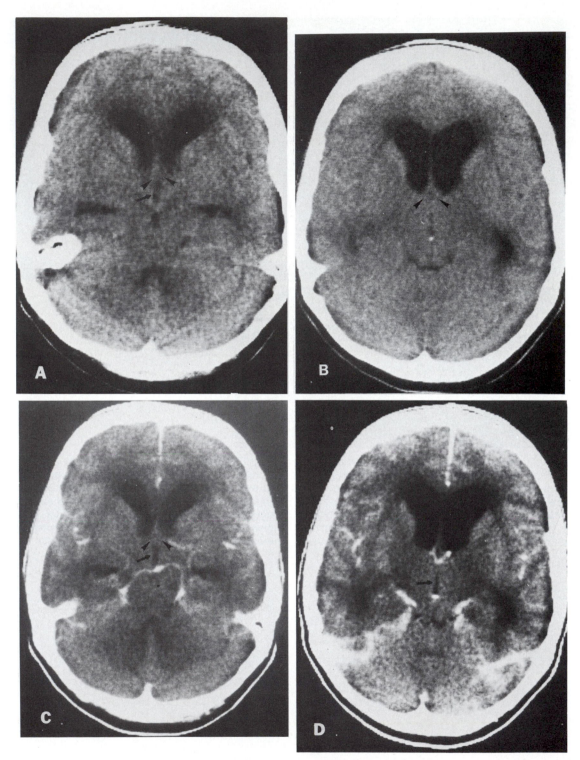

Fig 9–45.—Isodense colloid cyst. The nonenhanced scans **(A, B)** demonstrate moderate enlargement of the lateral ventricles, but a small third ventricle **(A,** *arrow*). There is an isodense mass *(arrowheads)* located at the foramina of Monro to produce this lateral ventricular obstruction. The enhanced views **(C, D)** again demonstrate the small third ventricle *(arrows),* the isodense mass **(C,** *arrowheads*) at the foramina of Monro, and slight separation of the internal cerebral veins **(D).** There is a cap-like impression on the anterior portion of the third ventricle **(C).** A colloid cyst may rarely be isodense, with its presence suspected by the differential size of the third and lateral ventricles.

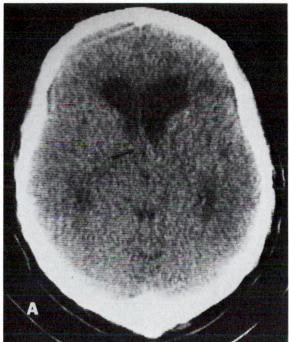
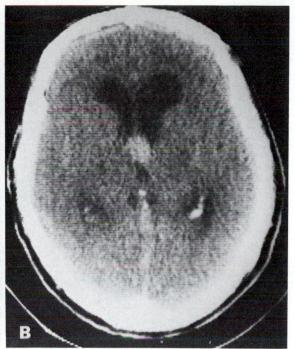

Fig 9–46.—Third ventricular glioma simulating colloid cyst. The unenhanced scan **(A)** demonstrates an isodense mass *(arrow)* in the region of the foramina of Monro. This is similar to the isodense colloid cyst in Figure 9–45. However, the enhanced scan **(B)** demonstrates an enhancing, slightly irregular mass at the junction of the third and lateral ventri- cles, which was surgically proved to be an astrocytoma. Colloid cysts only rarely enhance; the appearance in this case is more compatible with a glioma. (Courtesy of Lawrence H.A. Gold, M.D., University of Minnesota, Minneapolis.)

sharp margins of the typical colloid cyst. However, some irregularity of margins of a colloid cyst has also been seen (Fig 9–47) caused by contiguous choroid plexus.

It has been the policy in the author's institution that patients who present with lateral ventricular dilatation and a small third ventricle, without an obvious obstructing mass lesion of the foramen of Monro, are studied with metrizamide ventriculography. Such a ventriculogram performed after therapeutic decompressive shunting of the lateral ventricles has revealed a subtle colloid cyst in a few cases (see Fig 9–47). This cyst may also be stereotactically punctured under CT control, with the aspiration of mucoid material and secondary decompression of the ventricular system (see Fig 9–44). The growth rate of these cysts is so slow that decompression without complete removal may be sufficient to alleviate symptoms.

Pineal Parenchymal Tumors

The pineal parenchymal tumors, pineocytoma and pineoblastoma, are tumors of neuroectodermal origin. However, they are relatively rare compared with other tumors originating in the pineal region, particularly germinoma and teratoma, which are tumors of congen-ital origin. The entire group of pineal region tumors will therefore be discussed in Chapter 11.

SARCOMAS

A number of primary sarcomas of the CNS have been described, including primary diffuse sarcoma of the meninges;[55, 56] focal meningosarcoma, which will be discussed in Chapter 10; sarcoma following irradiation, particularly parasellar fibrosarcoma following radiation therapy for pituitary tumor;[57, 58] and primary reticulum cell sarcoma of the brain (histiocytic lymphoma, microglioma). While the term "histiocytic lymphoma" is a commonly used term today for this latter entity, there is disagreement as to the cell of origin which may be the β-lymphocyte rather than the histiocyte.[59] As such, some authors favor the term "primary malignant lymphoma of the brain." This tumor has become of greater interest today because of its appearance in patients receiving long-term immunosuppressant drugs, particularly for transplantation (Fig 9–48).[5, 60]

Up to one half of the patients with primary malignant lymphoma have multiple cerebral lesions, which are generally located deep within the hemisphere in areas such as the basal ganglia, thalamus, and corpus cal-

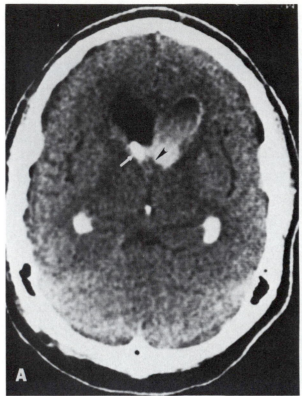

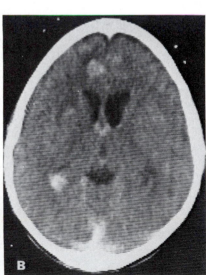

Fig 9–47.—Irregularly marginated isodense colloid cyst, demonstrated with Amipaque ventriculography. Axial scans with and without intravenous contrast enhancement (not shown) demonstrated an isodense mass in the region of the foramina of Monro, producing dilatation of the lateral ventricles, but a small third ventricle, similar to the case in Figure 9–45. A shunt was placed into the right lateral ventricle (*white arrow,* **A**), through which Amipaque was introduced with subsequent scanning. The axial scan **(A)** demonstrates an irregularly marginated lesion in the region of the foramina of Monro *(black arrowhead),* with a small third ventricle that is compressed anteriorly. The direct coronal view **(B)** also demonstrates a midline mass lesion, which produces a cap-like impression on the third ventricle *(black arrow).* At surgery, a colloid cyst was found; the irregularity of the margins of the lesion was due to contiguous choroid plexus.

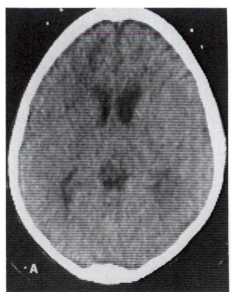

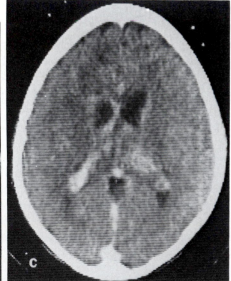

Fig 9–48.—Post-transplant primary lymphoma of the brain. Progressive somnolence occurred while this patient was on immunosuppressive therapy a number of months following renal transplantation. This led to a CT scan. The unenhanced scan **(A)** demonstrates some patchy low density within both frontal lobes and distortion of the frontal horns. The enhanced scans **(B, C)** demonstrate multiple ho-mogeneously enhancing nodular densities within the parenchyma and diffuse periventricular enhancement producing distortion of the ventricular contour. Infection was considered, but there was little improvement with antibiotics and antifungal agents. At autopsy, diffuse primary lymphoma of the brain was found.

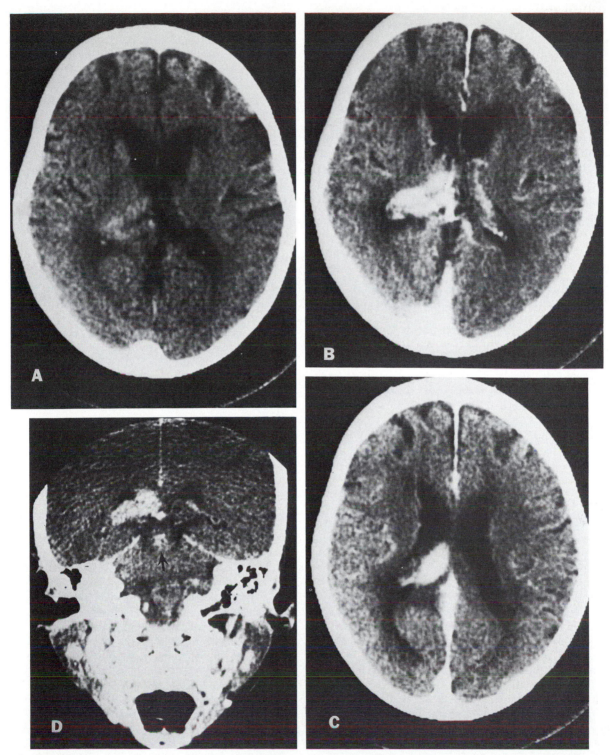

Fig 9–49.—Primary histiocytic lymphoma of the brain. Headache prompted a CT scan, with an unenhanced view **(A)** demonstrating a neoplasm of moderate increased density compressing and distorting the body and atrium of the right lateral ventricle. The enhanced axial views **(B, C)** dem- onstrate diffuse, homogeneously enhancing tumor infiltrating around and through the right lateral ventricle and contiguous parenchyma. The coronal view **(D)** demonstrates the relationship of the neoplasm to the ventricular system and infiltration into the quadrigeminal plate *(arrow).*

losum (Figs 9–48 and 9–49).[59, 60] On the preinfusion scan, the tumor has been described as varying from low to high density, with the isodense and hyperdense appearances being more common.[59–61] The increased density is most likely due to the dense packing of the cells, similar to medulloblastoma.[61] There is generally homogeneous enhancement, with the lesions being well circumscribed (Figs 9–48 and 9–49).[60, 62] There is usually little edema, and periventricular spread is common (see Fig 9–48).[60]

The diagnosis of malignant lymphoma of the brain may be suggested on the basis of the homogeneous enhancement of multiple deep lesions. Typically, glial tumors have patchy or mixed enhancement patterns,[62] and hematogenous metastases present with sharper margins and more surrounding edema than the typical lesions of primary malignant lymphoma.

REFERENCES

1. Kernohan J.W., Sayre G.P.: *Tumors of the Central Nervous System.* Atlas of Tumor Pathology, Armed Forces Institute of Pathology, 1952, section 10, fasc. 35.
2. Latchaw R.E., Gold L.H.A., Tourje E.J.: A protocol for the use of contrast enhancement in cranial computed tomography. *Radiology* 126:681–687, 1978.
3. Butler A.R., Kricheff I.I.: Non-contrast CT scanning: Limited value in suspected brain tumor. *Radiology* 126:689–693, 1978.
4. Hayman L.A., Evans R.A., Hinch V.C.: Delayed high iodine dose contrast computed tomography: Cranial neoplasms. *Radiology* 136:677–684, 1980.
5. Shalen P.R., Hayman L.A., Wallace S., et al.: Protocol for delayed contrast enhancement in computed tomography of cerebral neoplasia. *Radiology* 139:397–402, 1981.
6. Neuwelt E.A., Frenkel E.P., Diehl J., et al.: Reversible osmotic blood-brain barrier disruption in humans: Implications for the chemotherapy of malignant brain tumors. *Neurosurgery* 7:44–52, 1980.
7. Boethius J., Collins V.P., Edner G., et al.: Stereotactic biopsies and computer tomography in gliomas. *Acta Neurochir.* 40:223–232, 1978.
8. Norman D., Enzmann D.E., Levin V.A., et al.: Computed tomography in the evaluation of malignant glioma before and after therapy. *Radiology* 121:85–88, 1976.
9. Lilja A., Bergstrom K., Spansare B., et al.: Reliability of computed tomography in assessing histopathological features of malignant supratentorial gliomas. *J. Comput. Assist. Tomogr.* 5:625–636, 1981.
10. Afra D., Norman D., Levin V.A.: Cysts in malignant gliomas: Identification by computerized tomography. *J. Neurosurg.* 53:821–825, 1980.
11. Messina A.V., Potts D.G., Rottenburg D., et al.: Computed tomography: Demonstration of contrast medium within cystic tumors. *Radiology* 120:345–347, 1976.
12. Latchaw R.E., Gold L.H.A., Moore J.S., et al.: The nonspecificity of absorption coefficients in the differentiation of solid tumors and cystic lesions. *Radiology* 125:141–144, 1977.
13. Varma R.R., Crumrine P.K., Bergman I., et al.: Childhood oligodendrogliomas presenting with seizure and low density lesion on CT scan. *Neurology* 33:806–808, 1983.
14. Handa J., Nakaro Y., Handa H.: Computed tomography in the differential diagnosis of low-density intracranial lesions. *Surg. Neurol.* 10:179–185, 1978.
15. Monajati A., Heggeness L.: Patterns of edema in tumors vs. infarcts: Visualization of white matter pathways. *A.J.N.R.* 3:251–255, 1982.
16. Zimmerman R.A., Bilaniuk L.T.: Computed tomography of acute intratumoral hemorrhage. *Radiology* 135:355–359, 1980.
17. McGeachie R.E., Gold L.H.A., Latchaw R.E.: Periventricular spread of tumor demonstrated by computed tomography. *Radiology* 125:407–410, 1977.
18. Kieffer S.A., Salibi N.A., Kim R.C., et al.: Multifocal glioblastoma: Diagnostic implications. *Radiology* 143:709–710, 1982.
19. Joyce P., Bentson J., Takehashin M., et al.: The accuracy of predicting histologic grades of supratentorial astrocytomas on the basis of computerized tomography and cerebral angiography. *Neuroradiology* 16:346–348, 1978.
20. Marks T.E., Gado M.: Serial computed tomography of primary brain tumors following surgery, irradiation and chemotherapy. *Radiology* 125:119–125, 1977.
21. Tchang S., Scotti G., Terbrugge K., et al.: Computerized tomography as a possible aid to histological grading of supratentorial gliomas. *J. Neurosurg.* 46:735–739, 1977.
22. Butler A.R., Horii S.C., Kricheff I.I., et al.: Computed tomography in astrocytomas: A statistical analysis of the parameters of malignancy and the positive contrast enhanced CT scan. *Radiology* 129:433–439, 1978.
23. Steinbhoff H., Lanksch W., Kazner E., et al.: Computed tomography in the diagnosis and differential diagnosis of glioblastomas: A qualitative study of 295 cases. *Neuroradiology* 14:193–200, 1977.
24. Silverman C., Marks J.E.: Prognostic significance of contrast enhancement in low-grade astrocytomas of the adult cerebrum. *Radiology* 139:211–213, 1981.
25. Vonofakos D., Barcu H., Hacker H.: Oligodendrogliomas: CT patterns and emphasis on features indicating malignancy. *J. Comput. Assist. Tomogr.* 3:783–788, 1979.
26. Rorke L.B.: Cerebellar medulloblastoma and its relationship to primitive neuroectodermal neoplasms. *J. Neuropathol. Exp. Neurol.* 42:1–15, 1983.
27. Priest J., Dehner L.P., Sung J.H., et al.: Primitive neuroectodermal tumors (embryonal gliomas) of childhood: A clinicopathologic study of 12 cases, in Humphrey G.B., Bennett G. (eds.): *Pediatric Oncology.* The Hague, Boston, London, Martinua Nijhoff Publishers, 1981, pp. 247–264.
28. Horten B.C., Rubinstein L.J.: Primary cerebral neuroblastoma: A clinicopathological study of 35 cases. *Brain* 99:735–756, 1976.
29. Sakaki S., Mori Y., Motozaki T., et al.: A cerebral neuroblastoma with extracranial metastases. *Surg. Neurol.* 16:53–59, 1981.

30. Latchaw R.E., L'Heureux P.R., Young G., et al.: Neuroblastoma presenting as central nervous system disease. *A.J.N.R.* 3:623–630, 1982.

31. Chambers E.F., Turski P.A., Sobel D., et al.: Radiologic characteristics of primary cerebral neuroblastomas. *Radiology* 139:101–104, 1981.

32. Zimmerman R.A., Bilaniuk L.T.: CT of primary and secondary craniocerebral neuroblastoma. *A.J.N.R.* 1:431–434, 1980.

33. Zimmerman R.A., Bilaniuk L.T.: Computed tomography of intracranial ganglioglioma. *J. Comput. Tomogr.* 3:24–30, 1979.

34. Nass R., Whelan M.A.: Gangliogliomas. *Neuroradiology* 22:67–71, 1981.

35. Bilaniuk L.T., Zimmerman R.A., Littman P., et al.: Computed tomography of brainstem gliomas in children. *Radiology* 34:89–95, 1980.

36. Latchaw R.E., Vries J.: Metrizamide CT scanning in the evaluation of a biopsy site for brainstem expansions (unpublished).

37. Naidich T.P., Lin J.P., Leeds N.E., et al.: Primary tumors and other masses of the cerebellum and fourth ventricle: Differential diagnosis by computed tomography. *Neuroradiology* 14:153–174, 1977.

38. Zimmerman R.A., Bilaniuk L.T., Bruno L., et al.: Computed tomography of cerebellar astrocytoma. *A.J.R.* 130:929–933, 1978.

39. Tadmor R., Harwood-Nash D.C.F., et al.: Brain tumors in the first two years of life: CT diagnosis. *A.J.N.R.* 1:411–417, 1980.

40. Zimmerman R.A., Bilaniuk L.T., Pahlajani H.: Spectrum of medulloblastoma demonstrated by computed tomography. *Radiology* 126:137–141, 1978.

41. Enzmann D.R., Domar D., Levin V., et al.: Computed tomography in the follow-up of medulloblastomas and ependymomas. *Radiology* 128:57–63, 1978.

42. Zee C.-S., Segall H.D., Miller C., et al.: Less common CT features of medulloblastoma. *Radiology* 144:92–102, 1982.

43. Swartz J.D., Zimmerman R.A., Bilaniuk L.T.: Computed tomography of intracranial ependymomas. *Radiology* 143:97–101, 1982.

44. Kricheff I.I., Becker M., Schneck S.A., et al.: Intracranial ependymomas: Factors influencing prognosis. *J. Neurosurg.* 21:7–14, 1964.

45. Dohrmann G.J., Farwell J.R., Flannery J.T.: Ependymomas and ependymoblastomas in children. *J. Neurosurg.* 45:273–283, 1976.

46. Russell D.S., Rubinstein L.J.: Primary tumors of neuroectodermal origin, in *Pathology of Tumors of the Nervous System.* Baltimore, Williams & Wilkins Co., 1977, pp. 146–282.

47. Sheithauer B.W.: Symptomatic subependymoma: Report of 21 cases with review of the literature. *J. Neurosurg.* 29:689–696, 1978.

48. Tomasello F., Albanese V., Beinini F., et al.: Choroid plexus papilloma of the third ventricle. *Surg. Neurol.* 16:69–71, 1981.

49. Hawkins J.C. III: Treatment of choroid plexus papilloma in children: A brief analysis of twenty years' experience. *Neurosurgery* 6:380–384, 1980.

50. Coin C.G., Coin J.W., Glover M.B.: Vascular tumors of the choroid plexus: Diagnosis by computed tomography. *J. Comput. Assist. Tomogr.* 1:146–148, 1977.

51. Milhorat T.H.: Choroid plexus and cerebrospinal fluid production. *Science* 166:1514–1516, 1969.

52. Gudeman S.K., Sullivan H.G., Rosver M.J., et al.: Surgical removal of bilateral papillomas of the choroid plexus of the lateral ventricles with resolution of hydrocephalus: Case report. *J. Neurosurg.* 50:677–681, 1979.

53. Ganti S.R., Antunes J.L., Louis K.M., et al.: Computed tomography in the diagnosis of colloid cysts of the third ventricle. *Radiology* 138:388–391, 1981.

54. Wilson C.B., Moossy J., Boldrey E.B., et al.: Pathology of intracranial tumors, in Newton T.H., Potts G.D. (eds.): *Radiology of the Skull and Brain.* St. Louis, C.V. Mosby Co., 1977, vol. 3, pp. 3016–3018.

55. Russell D.S., Rubinstein L.J.: Tumors of meninges and of related soft tissues, in *Pathology of Tumors of the Nervous System.* Baltimore, Williams & Wilkins Co., 1977, pp. 65–100.

56. Latchaw R.E., Gabrielsen T.O., Seeger J.F.: Cerebral angiography in meningeal sarcomatosis and carcinomatosis. *Neuroradiology* 8:131–139, 1974.

57. Kingsley D.P.E., Kendall B.E.: CT of the adverse effects of therapeutic radiation of the central nervous system. *A.J.N.R.* 2:453–460, 1981.

58. Martin W.H., Cail W.S., Morris J.L., et al.: Fibrosarcoma after high energy radiation therapy for pituitary adenoma. *A.J.N.R.* 1:469–472, 1980.

59. Tadmor R., Davis K.R., Roberson G.H., et al.: Computed tomography in primary malignant lymphoma of the brain. *J. Comput. Assist. Tomogr.* 2:135–140, 1978.

60. Enzmann D.R., Kirkorian J., Norman D., et al.: Computed tomography in primary reticulum cell sarcoma of brain. *Radiology* 130:165–170, 1979.

61. Kasner E., Wilske J., Steinhoff H., et al.: Computer assisted tomography in primary malignant lymphomas of the brain. *J. Comput. Assist. Tomogr.* 2:125–134, 1978.

62. Ralvany J., Levine H.: Computed tomography in the diagnosis of primary lymphoma of the central nervous system. *J. Comput. Assist. Tomogr.* 2:215–217, 1978.

10

Primary Tumors of the Brain: Extra-Axial Tumors

RICHARD E. LATCHAW, M.D.

THIS CHAPTER is devoted to tumors that arise from the meninges and extra-axial soft tissues, including nerve sheaths and chemoreceptor tissue at the base of the brain, and to tumors arising in the bones of the calvarium and base of the skull. An extensive discussion of tumors involving the petrous bone and contiguous cerebellopontine angle, particularly the acoustic schwannoma and glomus jugulare tumor, will be found in Chapter 23.

TUMORS OF THE MENINGES

Meningioma

Meningiomas constitute approximately 15% of all intracranial neoplasms, second in incidence only to neuroectodermal tumors. The most common site is high over the convexity, with the majority in this location adjoining the superior sagittal sinus. Most favor the middle third of the sinus, with the anterior third the next most common.[1] Other common locations for meningioma include the meninges near the lateral sinuses and torcula, the pterion, the sphenoid ridges, tuberculum sellae and planum sphenoidale, olfactory grooves, the parasellar region, the posterior aspect of the petrous bone, the clivus and margin of the foramen magnum, the falx, and the tentorium. Intraventricular meningioma is rare and is thought to be secondary to an infolding of meningeal tissue during formation of the stroma of the choroid plexus.[1] Meningioma in the pineal and third ventricular region most commonly is attached to the falx-tentorial junction ("carrefour falcotentorial meningioma"), but may also arise from the meningeal tissue within the velum interpositum.[2] Finally, meningioma may arise from the sheath of a cranial nerve, particularly the optic nerve, to give a meningioma located at the optic foramen or within the orbit.

The CT scan characteristics of meningiomas in these various locations are essentially the same, and all the lesions will be considered together. Meningiomas have been divided into numerous histologic varieties, ranging from meningothelial to the angioblastic. Again, the CT scan characteristics of these histologic varieties are essentially the same; the rapidity of growth and propensity to recur may differ among the various types, but the radiologic appearances are indistinguishable.

The nonenhanced CT scan usually demonstrates a homogeneous mass that is isodense or of slightly increased density relative to normal brain (Fig 10–1). The presence of calcification is extremely variable and may be nodular or very fine and punctate (psammomatous) (Fig 10–2). Occasionally, the entire meningioma will be densely calcified with no enhancement visible through the calcification (Fig 10–3).

Because meningiomas are located along the margins of the brain, away from anatomical structures that denote mass effect such as the ventricular system, it may be extremely difficult to visualize these tumors without the use of contrast material. Characteristically, there is intense enhancement of a homogeneous nature, and the margins are sharply demarcated in all projections (Figs 10–1, 10–2, 10–4, and 10–5). A meningioma is typically broad-based upon a bony or dural margin; coronal views are very helpful in evaluating the relationship to the bony and dural structures and to the brain (Figs 10–4 and 10–5).

The amount of cerebral edema surrounding a meningioma is quite variable. While there is frequently little, if any, edema surrounding the slow-growing benign lesions (see Figs 10–2, 10–4, and 10–5), moderate-to-marked edema may be present in up to 42% of meningiomas (Figs 10–1 and 10–6).[3] The presence of abundant edema may falsely suggest the presence of a parenchymal lesion such as a metastatic tumor (see Fig

229

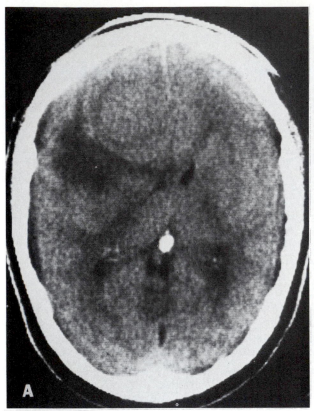
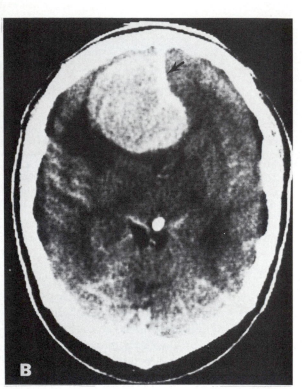

Fig 10–1.—Falx meningioma. The unenhanced scan **(A)** demonstrates a large mass lesion of slight increased density relative to the normal brain, located in the right frontal region. There is a moderate amount of surrounding edema and compression of the frontal horns. The enhanced scan

(B) demonstrates intense homogeneous enhancement of this lesion with sharp margination. The mass is based along the falx *(arrow)* and has all the characteristics of a falx meningioma.

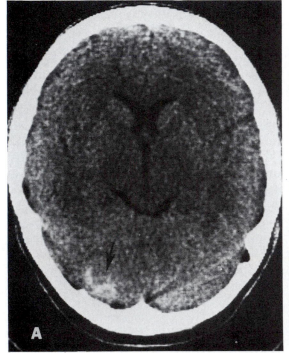
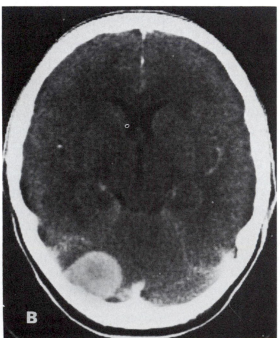

Fig 10–2.—Meningioma with psammomatous calcification. The unenhanced scan **(A)** shows punctate calcification in the right occipital region *(arrow)*. The enhanced scan **(B)** demonstrates homogeneous enhancement of the calcified

mass, with sharp margination. The mass is based along the inner table of the right occipital bone and has all the characteristics of a meningioma containing psammomatous calcification.

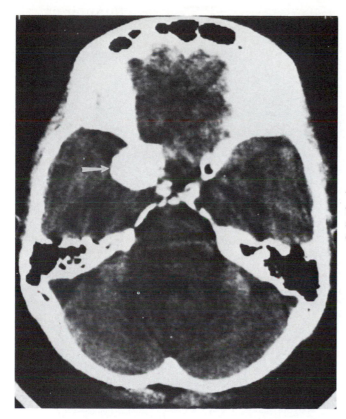

Fig 10–3.—Heavily calcified sphenoid meningioma. There is a large rounded calcific mass *(arrow)* attached to the right anterior clinoid process and the lesser wing of the sphenoid. This heavily calcified meningioma did not enhance.

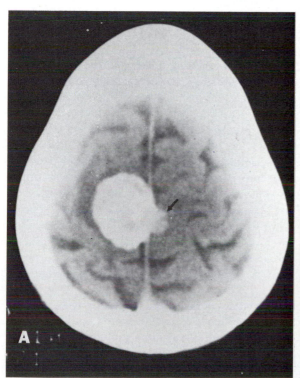

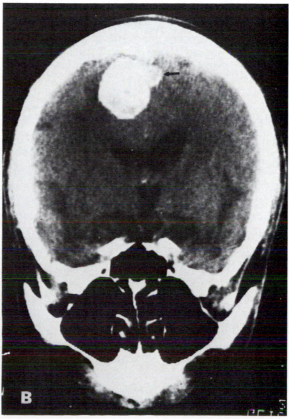

Fig 10–4.—Heavily calcified parafalcine meningioma with extension through the falx. Nonenhanced axial **(A)** and coronal **(B)** scans demonstrate a heavily calcified parafalcine meningioma with extension of calcified tumor through the falx *(arrows)*.

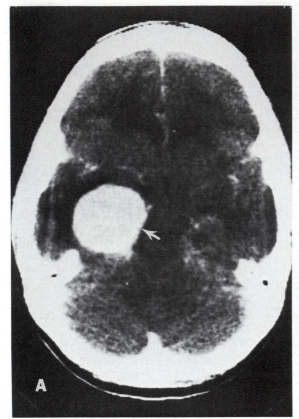
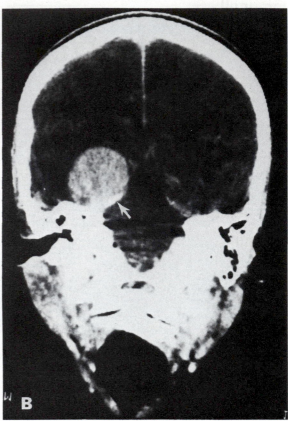

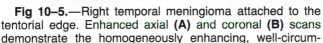

Fig 10–5.—Right temporal meningioma attached to the tentorial edge. Enhanced axial **(A)** and coronal **(B)** scans demonstrate the homogeneously enhancing, well-circum- scribed mass located within the right temporal fossa. The medial portion of the tumor is attached to the free edge of the tentorium *(arrows).*

10–6). The amount of cerebral edema is not proportional to the size of the tumor, nor to the location, type of meningioma, presence of bony invasion, or evidence of malignant degeneration. There is also no correlation between the amount of edema and the presence of obstruction of cerebral veins and dural sinuses.[3, 4]

Benign meningiomas may invade the surrounding tissues, including the dura (see Fig 10–4) and contiguous bony structures. Bony invasion frequently produces an osteoblastic response, with hyperostosis seen in up to 27% of meningioma cases, especially those located in the planum sphenoidale/parasellar regions (Fig 10–7).[3] The tumor may completely penetrate the calvarium to invade the scalp. Rarely, there is extension through and destruction of the bones at the base of the skull, with spread of meningioma into the parapharyngeal and facial regions (Fig 10–8). Such extensive invasion and spread is not necessarily indicative of malignant degeneration. Intracranial tumors may spread along the optic nerve to be both intracranial and intraorbital,[5] and primary intraorbital meningiomas may spread posteriorly to produce an intracranial component.

In a recent study, Russell and colleagues[6] found that 15% of the meningiomas reviewed had atypical features. Necrosis and scarring produce irregularity of the tumor margins and nonhomogeneous enhancement (Fig 10–9), occasionally resulting in a "ring sign." The necrosis was present in up to 14% of the cases and was thought to be due to rapid growth with secondary tumor ischemia. Focal high-density areas were found to be due to acute hemorrhage within the tumor. Such tumors were not necessarily of the angioblastic variety, but the hemorrhage was considered secondary to rupture of thin tumor vessels. Old hemorrhage produced areas of low density, as did regions of lipomatous degeneration. Finally, low-density zones contiguous to typical meningiomas represented trapped cerebrospinal fluid (CSF) within arachnoid cysts. All of the posterior fossa meningiomas in their series were typical in appearance; if cystic changes were found in posterior fossa mass, the lesion was not a meningioma. However, this author has occasionally seen necrotic or cystic change in large posterior fossa meningiomas.

The majority of meningiomas are easily recognized, and there is usually only a limited differential diagnosis. A primary glioma originating in the high convexity may

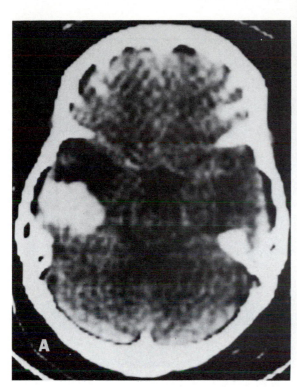

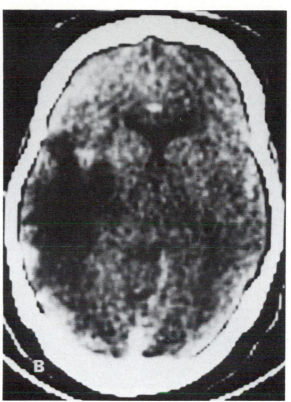

Fig 10–6.—Right temporal meningioma with extensive parenchymal edema. An axial slice through the midtemporal fossae (A) demonstrates a homogeneously enhancing, well-marginated mass that appears to be within the right temporal lobe. There is extensive edema anterior to the lesion. A higher cut (B) demonstrates extensive edema throughout the right temporal, frontal, and parietal lobes. While the position of the lesion and the amount of edema are consistent with a nonmeningiomatous lesion such as a solitary metastasis, the homogeneity of enhancement and the sharp marginations are consistent with meningioma. The extensive edema may be seen with meningioma and is not a reflection of malignancy or venous obstruction. At surgery, the mass was found to be attached to the junction of the squamous portion of the right temporal bone and petrous bone.

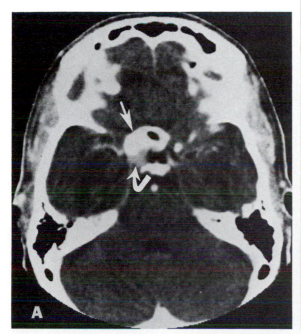

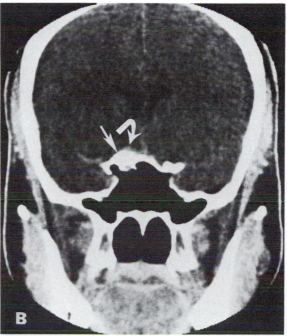

Fig 10–7.—Tuberculum sellae meningioma. The axial (A) and coronal (B) scans demonstrate hyperostosis of the right lateral margin of the tuberculum sellae (straight arrows). The homogeneously enhancing soft-tissue mass (curved arrows) is seen contiguous to the hyperostosis.

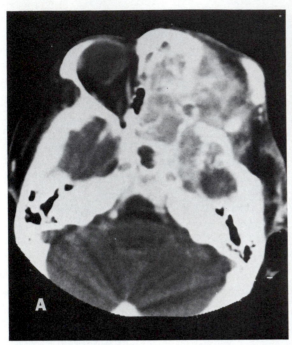 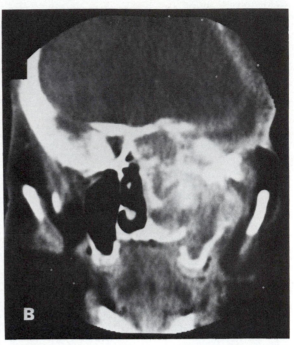

Fig 10–8.—Meningioma with extension into the face. The axial **(A)** and coronal **(B)** scans demonstrate a massive, enhancing neoplasm involving the left temporal fossa, sphenoid, left orbit and nose, left maxillary antrum, and contiguous facial structures. Histologically, this was a benign meningioma. Long-standing meningiomas of the temporal fossae and/or orbit may invade the facial structures and produce extensive bony destruction, mimicking a malignant neoplasm. Such extensive spread is not necessarily indicative of malignant degeneration of the meningioma.

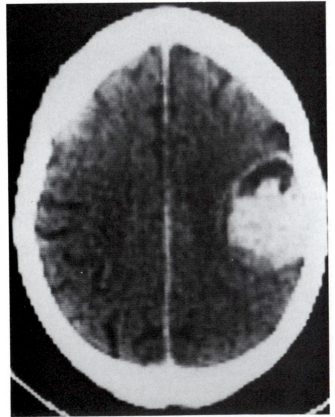

Fig 10–9.—Partially cystic/necrotic meningioma. There is a well-marginated mass based along the inner table of the skull of the high left cerebral convexity. While the majority of this mass enhances in a homogeneous fashion typical of meningioma, there is cystic and/or necrotic component anteriorly. Histologically, this was a typical meningioma. Fourteen percent of meningiomas have atypical features such as necrosis and cyst formation.

appear to be based along the inner table of the skull, simulating meningioma (see Fig 9–10). Occasionally, a large exophytic mass originating within the bony calvarium may project into the brain; if the mass is sharply marginated and enhances homogeneously as can be seen with many metastatic tumors such as carcinoma of the prostate, the appearance may simulate meningioma (see Fig 12–9). It may be difficult to distinguish between an intra-axial and extra-axial mass lesion, particularly if there is a large amount of surrounding cerebral edema (see Fig 10–6). While a peripheral intra-axial mass may destroy the gray matter/white matter junction (Fig 10–10), an extra-axial benign mass typically leaves this junction intact, but displaces the cortex from the inner table of the skull and buckles the underlying white matter.[7] It may be impossible to distinguish between schwannoma and meningioma, particularly in the parasellar region (see Figs 10–17 and 10–18). Both typically have a homogeneous enhancement pattern and sharp margination. Clinical symptomatology such as facial pain will suggest the presence of schwannoma rather than a meningioma. The distinction between schwannoma and meningioma may also be difficult when the lesion is located in the cerebellopontine angle. The findings of increased density on the preinfusion scan, calcification, a broad-base against the petrous bone, an eccentric relationship to the internal auditory canal, and the lack of necrosis and cyst formation all favor meningioma. The meningioma may extend through the tentorial notch to the middle cranial fossa, producing a "comma" shape (Fig 10–11); we have rarely seen this configuration with acoustic schwannoma.

Multiple Meningiomas and Meningosarcoma

Multiple meningiomas (Fig 10–12) may occur in neurofibromatosis, in which there are not only meningiomas, but also schwannomas, neurofibromas, and various gliomas. Multiple meningiomas may also occur without the syndrome. Malignant meningiomas not only invade neighboring tissues, as do benign meningiomas, but also infiltrate the CNS.[8] While a malignant meningioma can have a similar CT scan appearance to that of a benign lesion, the diagnosis of malignancy may be suggested in a patient with an extensively spreading meningioma that quickly recurs (Fig 10–13).

Other lesions of the meninges include diffuse pri-

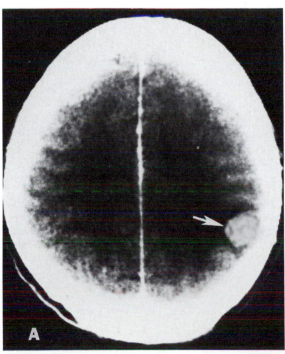
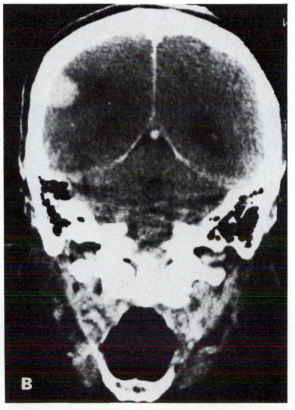

Fig 10–10.—Right parietal metastasis simulating meningioma. The axial (A) and coronal (B) projections demonstrate a solitary metastatic lesion (A, arrow) from carcinoma of the lung. The metastasis was to the corticomedullary junction, destroying the interface between the gray and white matter. This latter characteristic confirms the intraparenchymal location of the lesion, even though the extension of the mass to the inner table of the skull suggests a diagnosis such as meningioma.

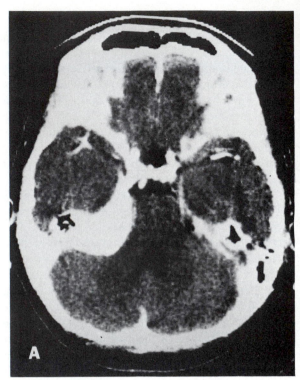

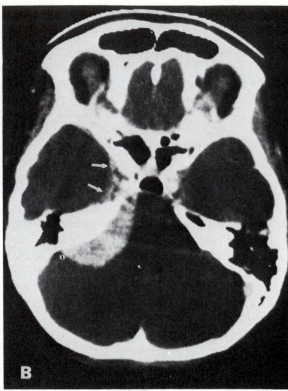

Fig 10–11.—Cerebellopontine meningioma extending into the middle cranial fossa. The enhanced axial scans demonstrate a large homogeneously enhancing, well-marginated tumor involving the right cerebellopontine angle and producing mild compression of the lateral aspect of the fourth ventricle **(A).** The lesion is centered along the ridge of the right petrous bone, typical of meningioma and unusual for acoustic schwannoma. Image **B** was taken with a wide window (bone window) to allow separation of the enhancing tumor from the underlying petrous bone. There is extension of tumor into the medial aspect of the right middle cranial fossa, producing displacement of the lateral margin of the right cavernous sinus *(arrows).* Extension into the middle cranial fossa to produce a "comma shape" is characteristic for meningioma.

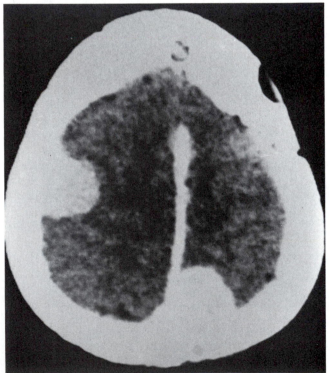

Fig 10–12.—Multiple meningiomas in neurofibromatosis. This enhanced scan demonstrates two homogeneously enhancing, well-circumscribed meningiomas based along the inner table of the skull. There is also diffuse spread of meningioma in the interhemispheric fissure.

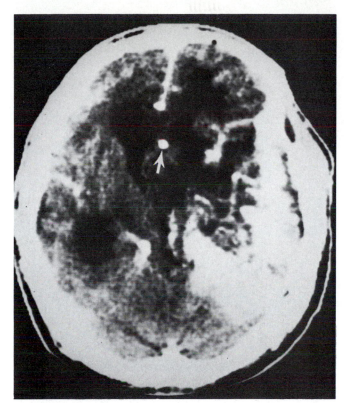

Fig 10–13.—Meningosarcoma. There is extensive homogeneously enhancing neoplasm along the inner table of the left frontal, temporal, and parietal bones, with extension medially along the left side of the tentorium. The patient has undergone previous left-sided craniotomy for attempted resection. There is a shunt *(arrow)* within the compressed and displaced left frontal horn. The mass quickly recurred and spread along the meninges within a 6-month period of time, consistent with the histologic diagnosis of meningosarcoma.

mary meningeal sarcomatosis,[8, 9] primary leptomeningeal melanoma,[10] and neurocutaneous melanosis, which is a malignant condition closely related to the other phakomatoses, particularly neurofibromatosis, with the presence of café-au-lait spots.[11, 12]

SOFT-TISSUE TUMORS AT THE BASE OF THE SKULL

Schwannoma and Neurofibroma

Tumors originating from cranial nerve roots are either schwannomas or neurofibromas. The term schwannoma refers to the origin of the neoplasm from the Schwann cell, the cell that lines the axon beyond the pia. "Neuroma," "neurinoma," and "neurilemmoma" are all terms that do not refer to true anatomical structures and therefore should be discarded.[13] Neurofibromas are also tumors that originate from cranial nerve roots similar to schwannomas, but are found in patients with neurofibromatosis (von Recklinghausen's disease).

While a neurofibroma may be difficult, if not impossible, to distinguish pathologically from a schwannoma, it frequently has a looser texture than a schwannoma.[13]

The most common schwannoma is that of the eighth cranial nerve ("acoustic neuroma"). The second-most-common nerve of origin is the fifth cranial nerve ("trigeminal neuroma"), originating anywhere along the course of that nerve, including the exit of the nerve from the pons, at its point of dural penetration at Meckel's cave, within the cavernous sinus, or at the points of exit from the skull by the three components of the nerve, including the superior orbital fissure, foramen rotundum, and foramen ovale. Rarely, a schwannoma may originate from cranial nerves IX, X, or XI as it passes through the jugular foramen, or from the twelfth cranial nerve.[14–16]

The CT scan appearance of the schwannoma and the neurofibroma are essentially similar and will be considered together. The radiographic diagnosis of a neurofibroma rather than a schwannoma depends upon the clinical knowledge of the presence of neurofibromatosis or on the radiographic appearance of bilateral eighth nerve tumors, which is presumptive evidence of neurofibromatosis, or upon the presence of multiple intracranial tumors, including eighth nerve tumors, gliomas, and meningiomas, again indicative of neurofibromatosis. The CT scan appearance of schwannoma/neurofibroma is essentially similar, whatever the location, and therefore a discussion of the typical CT appearances can be condensed. Because of the frequency of eighth nerve schwannomas and the extensive and varied radiographic work-up of this tumor, it will be discussed more extensively in Chapter 23.

Typically, schwannomas are of low density or isodensity before the administration of contrast material. The degree of contrast enhancement is moderate to marked and may be homogeneous (Fig 10–14) or nonhomogeneous in character as a result of cystic change (Fig 10–15). A schwannoma of cranial nerves IX, X, or XI has a similar appearance to an eighth nerve schwannoma, with the only difference being the location of the lesion; a schwannoma of cranial nerves IX, X, or XI produces erosion of the jugular foramen (Fig 10–16), while an eighth nerve tumor produces erosion of the internal auditory canal (see Fig 10–14).

A major differential diagnostic consideration of an enhancing mass in the cerebellopontine angle is meningioma. A meningioma is almost always homogeneous in its contrast enhancement, frequently has a broad-base of attachment to the petrous bone, is somewhat eccentric from the internal auditory canal, and may extend in "comma" fashion through the tentorial incisura to lie partially within the middle cranial fossa (see Fig 10–11), a finding this author has only rarely seen with an acous-

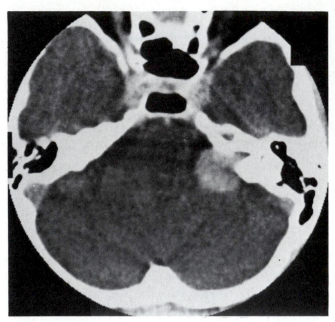

Fig 10–14.—Classic acoustic schwannoma. The neoplasm in the left cerebellopontine angle enhances homogeneously, and there is extension of tumor into an enlarged left internal auditory canal. These are classic findings of an eighth nerve schwannoma.

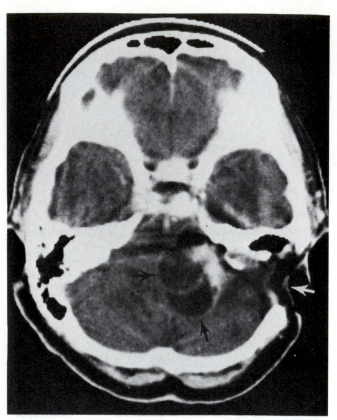

Fig 10–15.—Cystic acoustic schwannoma mimicking intracerebellar tumor. There is a large neoplasm *(black arrows)* with both cystic and solid components involving the left cerebellopontine angle and cerebellar hemisphere with extension to the midline. The patient has had a previous retromastoid craniotomy *(white arrow)*. The combination of solid and cystic components is common with schwannomas. The deep invagination into the cerebellar hemisphere mimics a primary intracerebellar tumor such as cystic astrocytoma.

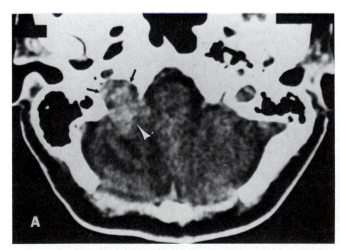

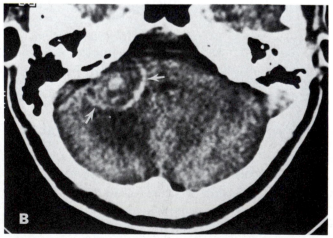

Fig 10–16.—Schwannoma originating in the jugular fossa. The enhanced axial scan seen in photo **A** demonstrates an enhancing neoplasm *(white arrowhead)* within and extending beyond an enlarged right jugular fossa *(black arrows)*. A slightly higher cut **(B)** demonstrates the more superior portion of the tumor, which has the appearance of a "target." There is a peripheral rim of enhancement *(white arrows)* with a central collection of enhancement and non-enhancing, partially necrotic tumor between the areas of enhancement. An acoustic schwannoma may have an identical appearance to that seen in photo **B.** The enlargement of the jugular fossa by tumor is evidence for the origin of the schwannoma from a cranial nerve within the fossa. At the time of surgery, it was believed that the schwannoma originated from the right eleventh cranial nerve.

tic schwannoma. Acoustic schwannoma, on the other hand, is generally located at or in the internal auditory canal and produces erosion of that structure, is frequently inhomogeneous or cystic in its enhancement pattern, and stays below the tentorium. Occasionally, it can be difficult to distinguish an extra-axial posterior fossa lesion from an intra-axial lesion of the cerebellar hemisphere.[17] A slow-growing extra-axial mass may invaginate into the cerebellar parenchyma, simulating a cerebellar mass lesion (see Fig 10–15), and likewise a cerebellar mass may have an exophytic component projecting into the cerebellopontine angle.

A trigeminal schwannoma located at the petrous apex may have an identical appearance to an acoustic schwannoma, with the only difference being presentation of pain in the fifth nerve distribution and the relatively high position of the lesion on the CT scan relative to the cerebellopontine angle. A schwannoma located in the middle cranial fossa presents as an enhancing mass lesion with either a homogeneous or inhomogeneous character,[18] producing erosion of the lateral wall of the sella and the base of the skull; coronal sections are of great value in defining the extent of the mass and involvement of the cavernous sinus and contiguous sella (Fig 10–17). The major differential diagnostic considerations for a parasellar mass are meningioma (Fig 10–18) and carotid artery aneurysm. This differentiation may be extremely difficult on the CT scan alone. Meningiomas may produce hyperostosis of the surrounding bony structures (see Fig 10–7), and a trigeminal schwannoma classically presents with facial pain. Dynamic CT scanning with rapid filling of an aneurysm would aid in distinguishing this entity. Trigeminal schwannoma may occasionally erode the base of the skull and extend deeply into the parapharyngeal and facial structures (Fig 10–19) in a manner similar to meningioma (see Fig 10–8).

Chemodectoma

The chemodectoma (paraganglioma) arises from chemoreceptor tissue located in the middle ear (glomus tympanicum tumor), jugular foramen (glomus jugulare tumor), upper neck at the level of the second cervical segment (vagus body tumor), or in the midneck at the level of the carotid bifurcation (carotid body tumor). All of these tumors are very vascular, with the classic an-

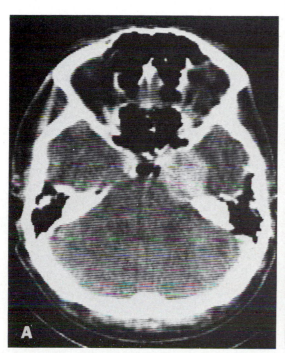
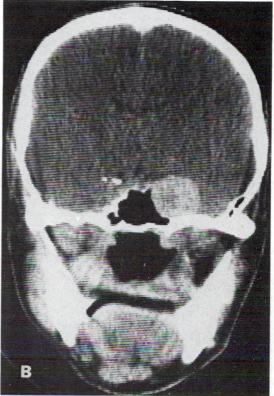

Fig 10–17.—Trigeminal schwannoma. The enhanced axial **(A)** and coronal **(B)** scans demonstrate a homogeneously enhancing, round, well-marginated mass in the medial aspect of the middle cranial fossa. The long-standing presence of this tumor is denoted by the concave deformity of the lateral wall of the sphenoid sinus. Differential diagnosis includes aneurysm, schwannoma, and meningioma. No hyperostosis can be seen to suggest meningioma, and the patient presented with facial pain. Left carotid angiography demonstrated a subtle stain.

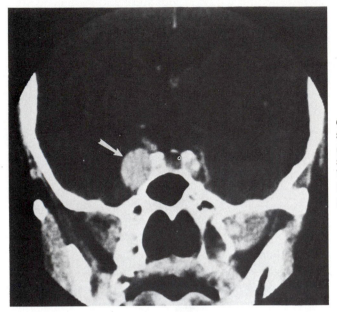

Fig 10–18.—Parasellar meningioma. This enhanced coronal scan demonstrates a homogeneously enhancing, sharply marginated mass in the right parasellar region *(arrow),* having a similar appearance to the schwannoma seen in Figure 10–17. However, this was a meningioma. Without contiguous bony hyperostosis, it may be impossible to distingish between parasellar meningioma and schwannoma on routine scan.

giographic findings of hypervascularity and a prolonged stain. The CT findings of a glomus jugulare tumor include enlargement of a jugular foramen with local bone erosion (Fig 10–20); enlargement alone is not a sufficient criterion for the presence of a mass, because

asymmetry in the size of the jugular foramina is a common and normal variant. A dense mass is seen within the jugular foramen following contrast administration (see Fig 10–20). Extension may occur either inferiorly into the upper neck (see Fig 10–20) or superiorly into

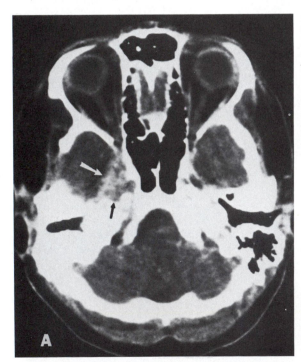

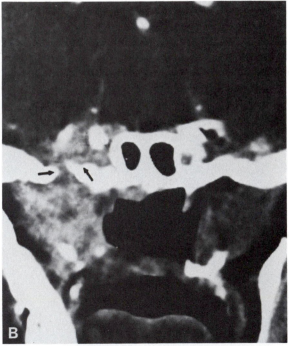

Fig 10–19.—Trigeminal schwannoma extending into the parapharyngeal soft tissues. The axial scan **(A)** demonstrates an inhomogeneously enhancing mass *(white arrow)* within the right cavernous sinus and parasphenoidal region, producing bone erosion and destruction of the apex of the right petrous bone *(black arrow).* The patient has had a previous right temporal craniotomy for biopsy. The coronal

scan **(B)** demonstrates the bone erosion and destruction at the base of the skull *(black arrows),* with extension of the right parasphenoidal tumor inferiorly into the parapharyngeal soft tissues. This appearance is similar to that of meningioma extending into the face, seen in Figure 10–8. (Courtesy of Drs. Modesti and Cacayorin, Upstate Medical Center, State University of New York, Syracuse.)

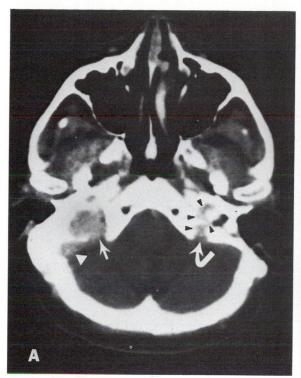
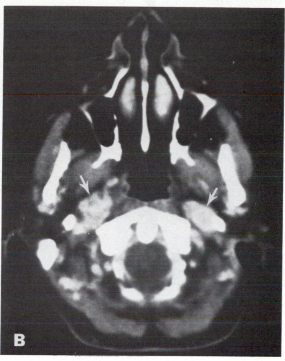
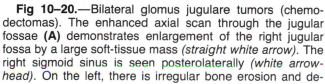

Fig 10–20.—Bilateral glomus jugulare tumors (chemodectomas). The enhanced axial scan through the jugular fossae **(A)** demonstrates enlargement of the right jugular fossa by a large soft-tissue mass *(straight white arrow)*. The right sigmoid sinus is seen posterolaterally *(white arrowhead)*. On the left, there is irregular bone erosion and de-struction *(black arrowheads)* of the jugular fossa by an enhancing soft-tissue mass *(curved white arrow)*. The axial scan at the level of C-1 **(B)** demonstrates homogeneously enhancing, well-marginated tumors in the region of the jugular veins bilaterally *(white arrows)*. These represent extension of the bilateral chemodectomas into the upper neck.

the cerebellopontine angle (Fig 10–21).[19] While a glomus jugulare tumor is histologically benign, the tumor may produce a marked degree of bone erosion and extension into the posterior and middle cranial fossae, spinal canal, and cervical soft tissues (see Fig 10–21). Approximately 10% of patients have bilateral glomus jugulare tumors (see Fig 10–20).

Any mass lesion seen in the region of the jugular foramen should have angiography for preoperative confirmation of a chemodectoma, possibly followed by embolization. Other masses may originate in the region of the jugular foramen, including a schwannoma of cranial nerves IX, X, or XI (see Fig 10–16) and occasionally meningioma. These lesions may be slightly vascular on angiography, but do not have the extreme degree of hypervascularity and staining as the chemodectoma.

PRIMARY TUMORS OF THE CALVARIUM AND BASE OF THE SKULL

Tumors of the Calvarium

Primary tumors of the calvarium range from the benign epidermoid and hemangioma to the more aggres-sive eosinophilic granuloma and finally to the sarcomas. Bone erosion is best defined by using the bone window on the CT scanner. The degree of bony irregularity suggests the benign or malignant nature of the lesion (Fig 10–22). Variable degrees of mass affecting the extradural space and scalp are present with the different tumors, and distinguishing the various lesions on the basis of CT alone is difficult. Early localized Paget's disease of the calvarium (osteoporosis circumscriptus cranii) may have a similar appearance to metastatic disease, although in advanced cases, marked thickening of the diploic space is evident, supporting the diagnosis of Paget's disease (Fig 10–23).

Tumors of the Base of the Skull

Chordoma

The chordoma originates from notochordal remnants and therefore may be found anywhere along the craniospinal axis from the sphenoid bone to the sacrum, with the two ends favored in location.[1, 20] The most common intracranial locations are the body of the sphenoid bone and the clivus. The chordoma is a slow-

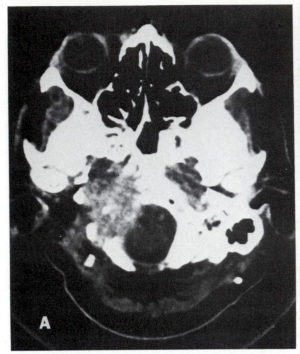
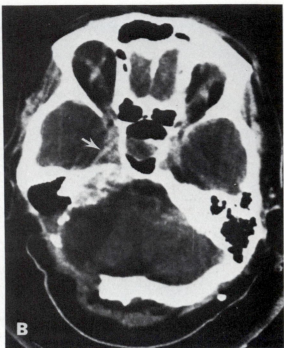

Fig 10–21.—Glomus jugulare tumor with extension into the spinal canal and middle cranial fossa. There is extensive bone destruction on the right from both the tumor itself and previous surgery in this patient with a huge recurrent glomus jugulare tumor. The lower enhanced scan **(A)** demonstrates extensive neoplasm eroding the edge of the foramen magnum and extending into the right side of the spinal canal. There is erosion of the right petrous bone **(B)** with extension of enhancing neoplasm into the right cavernous sinus, producing lateral displacement of the sinus margin *(arrow)*. Right internal carotid angiography (not shown) demonstrated supply to the tumor from the petrous and cavernous portions of the artery, with encasement of that vessel.

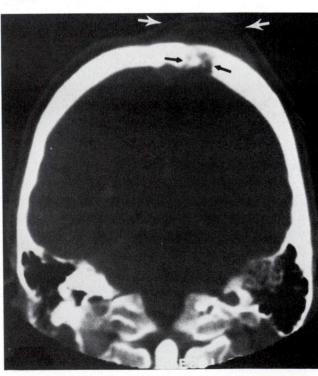

Fig 10–22.—Metastatic chondrosarcoma to the calvarium in Maffucci's syndrome (multiple enchondromatosis with soft-tissue hemangiomas). The direct enhanced coronal scan demonstrates irregular bony destruction of the high convexity of the left parietal bone near the midline *(black arrows)*, with an overlying soft-tissue mass of the scalp *(white arrows)*. The irregular margination of the bone destruction involves the inner and outer tables and intervening diploic space, giving evidence for the presence of an aggressive and destructive lesion.

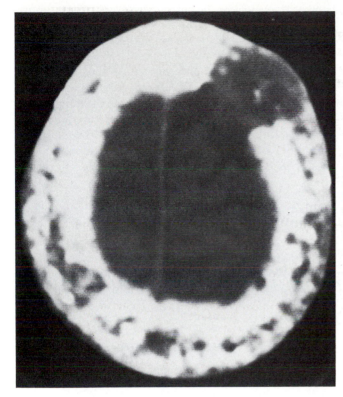

Fig 10–23.—Paget's disease of the skull. There is extensive thickening of the calvarium characteristic of Paget's disease. There are both osteolytic and osteoblastic areas, with some of the osteoblastic areas being nodular ("cotton wool" appearance typical of Paget's disease). In the left frontoparietal region, there is a large confluent lytic area more typical of stage 1 of this disease (osteoporosis circumscripta cranii). The rest of the skull has the appearance of stage 2, the combined phase.

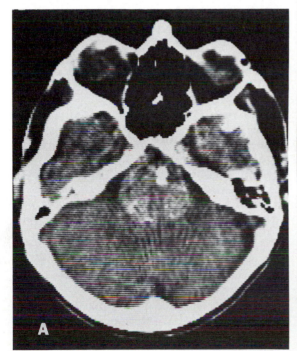

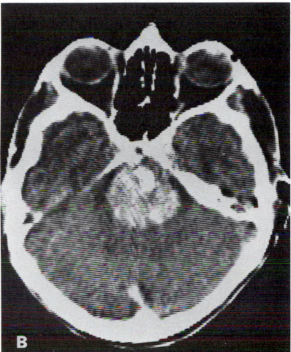

Fig 10–24.—Clival chordoma. The unenhanced scan **(A)** demonstrates a large well-circumscribed mass containing central calcification, located in the usual region of the brain stem. The brain stem is markedly compressed and dis- placed posterior to this lesion. There is erosion and destruc- tion of the clivus anterior to the mass. The enhanced scan **(B)** demonstrates a mild degree of diffuse but patchy en- hancement of this slow-growing tumor.

growing neoplasm with a long latent period, but is locally invasive and tends to recur following any but the most radical of surgical procedures.

The CT scan characteristics include that of a mass of increased density on the preinfusion scan, frequently with multiple areas of calcification, on a moderate-to-marked degree of contrast enhancement (Fig 10–24).[21] The clival chordoma generally produces compression and posterior displacement of the contiguous brain stem and may penetrate the dura and cause multiple cranial nerve palsies.[1] Extension into the sphenoid sinus and nasopharynx is common.

A neoplasm with a similar appearance on a CT scan is a clival meningioma. Like the chordoma, the meningioma may enhance markedly and contain calcium.

However, evaluation of bony structures with appropriate windows commonly demonstrates clival destruction with the chordoma, whereas meningioma generally produces a scalloped and deformed clivus rather than bone destruction. The presence of calcification and irregular bone destruction helps to distinguish a chordoma of the body of the sphenoid from a benign intrasellar-parasellar neoplasm such as a pituitary adenoma. It may be difficult to distinguish a sphenoidal chordoma from other primary calcifying malignant tumors in this region, such as chondrosarcoma (Fig 10–25).

Others

Other tumors of the bones of the skull base include osteoma, osteochondroma, chondroma, and chondrosarcoma, among others.[22] Benign osteoma is heavily calcified, while there is variable calcification within the chondroma and osteochondroma. Chondrosarcoma is a rare lesion that may present with a rim of enhancement in addition to calcification and/or bone destruction (see Fig 10–25).

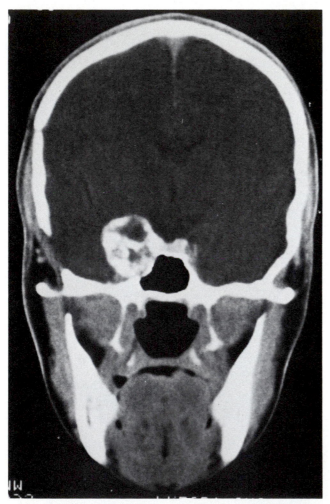

Fig 10–25.—Parasellar embryonal chondrosarcoma. This coronal enhanced scan was imaged at a wide window width (bone window). The patient has had a previous right temporal craniotomy for biopsy. The right parasellar mass contains multiple nodular areas of calcification, multiple areas of cyst formation, and rim-like enhancement. The long-standing presence of the mass is denoted by the deformed right lateral wall of the sphenoid sinus.

REFERENCES

1. Wilson C.B., Moossy J., Boldrey E.B., et al.: Pathology of intracranial tumors, in Newton T.H., Potts D.G. (eds.): *Radiology of the Skull and Brain.* St. Louis, C.V. Mosby Co., 1977, vol. 3, pp. 3016–3048.
2. Rozario R., Adedman L., Prager R.J., et al.: Meningiomas of the pineal region and third ventricle. *Neurosurgery* 5:489–495, 1979.
3. New P.F.J., Aronow S., Hesselink J.R.: National Cancer Institute study: Evaluation of computed tomography in the diagnosis of intracranial neoplasms: IV. Meningiomas. *Radiology* 136:665–675, 1980.
4. Smith H.P., Cahha V.R., Moody D.M., et al.: Biological features of meningiomas that determine the production of cerebral edema. *Neurosurgery* 8:428–433, 1981.
5. Nakagawa H., Lusino O.: Biplane computed tomography of intracranial meningioma with extracranial extension. *J. Comput. Assist. Tomogr.* 4:478–483, 1980.
6. Russell E.J., George A.E., Kricheff I.I., et al.: Atypical computed tomographic features of intracranial meningioma: Radiological-pathological correlation in a series of 131 consecutive cases. *Radiology* 135:673–682, 1980.
7. George A.E., Russell E.J., Kricheff I.I.: White matter buckling: CT sign of extra-axial intracranial mass. *A.J.N.R.* 1:425–430, 1980.
8. Russell D.S., Rubenstein L.J.: Tumours of meninges and of related tissues, in *Pathology of Tumours of the Nervous System.* Baltimore, Williams & Wilkins Co., 1977, pp. 65–100.
9. Latchaw R.E., Gabrielsen T.O., Seeger J.F.: Cerebral angiography in meningeal sarcomatosis and carcinomatosis. *Neuroradiology* 8:131–139, 1974.
10. Tamura M., Kanafuchi J., Nagaya T., et al.: Primary leptomeningeal melanoma with epipharyngeal invasion. *Acta Neurochir.* 58:59–66, 1981.

11. Lamas E., Lobato R.D., Sotelo T., et al.: Neurocutaneous melanomas. *Acta Neurochir.* 36:93–105, 1977.

12. Russell D.S., Rubenstein L.J.: Congenital tumours of maldevelopmental origin, in *Pathology of Tumours of the Nervous System.* Baltimore, Williams & Wilkins Co., 1977, pp. 24–64.

13. Russell D.S., Rubenstein L.J.: Tumours of the nerve roots and peripheral nerves, in *Pathology of Tumours of the Nervous System.* Baltimore, Williams & Wilkins Co., 1977, pp. 372–401.

14. Latchaw R.E., Gold L.H.A.: The diagnosis of schwannomas involving the jugular foramen (unpublished).

15. Ulso C., Sebested P., Overgaard J.: Intracranial hypoglossal neurinoma: Diagnosis and post-operative care. *Surg. Neurol.* 16:65–68, 1981.

16. Dolan E.J., Tacher W.S., Rotenberg D., et al.: Intracranial hypoglossal schwannoma as an unusual cause of facial nerve palsy. *J. Neurosurg.* 56:420–423, 1982.

17. Miller E.M., Newton T.H.: Extra-axial posterior fossa lesions simulating intra-axial lesions on computed tomography. *Radiology* 127:675–679, 1978.

18. Goldberg R., Byrd S., Winter J., et al.: Varied appearance of trigeminal neuroma on CT. *A.J.R.* 134:57–60, 1980.

19. Marsman J.W.P.: Tumors of the glomus jugulare complex (chemodectoma) demonstrated by cranial computed tomography. *J. Comput. Assist. Tomogr.* 3:795–799, 1979.

20. Russell D.S., Rubenstein L.J.: Secondary neoplasms of the nervous system, in *Pathology of Tumours of the Nervous System.* Baltimore, Williams & Wilkins Co., 1977, pp. 348–360.

21. Kendall B.E., Lee B.C.P.: Cranial chordomas. *Br. J. Radiol.* 50:687–698, 1977.

22. Matz S.H., Iraeli Y., Shalit M.N., et al.: Computed tomography in intracranial supratentorial osteochondroma. *J. Comput. Assist. Tomogr.* 5:109–115, 1981.

11

Primary Tumors of the Brain: Tumors of Congenital, Pineal, and Blood Vessel Origin, and the Phakomatoses

RICHARD E. LATCHAW, M.D.

CONGENITAL TUMORS, pineal tumors, tumors of blood vessels, and the syndromes of the phakomatoses are all considered together in this chapter because of their multiple interrelationships. The congenital tumors include the teratoma, germinoma (atypical teratoma), dermoid, epidermoid, lipoma, hamartoma, and craniopharyngioma. A teratoma is derived from all three germ cell layers (ectoderm, mesoderm, and endoderm), and therefore many different tissues may be found in such a lesion. A dermoid is a teratomatous lesion that is derived from two germ cell layers (ectoderm and mesoderm), while an epidermoid is derived from the single germ cell layer (ectoderm). A germinoma represents a form of teratoma in which a single but multipotential tissue predominates, the germ cell itself. The lipoma frequently accompanies other congenital anomalies, such as agenesis of the corpus callosum, and is thought to result from abnormalities of the closure of the neural tube. A hamartoma is a mass made up of normal and mature cells, but arranged in a disorganized fashion. Of particular import in this discussion is the hamartoma of the tuber cinereum that is associated with precocious puberty. Malformations of the blood vessels, including arteriovenous malformation and capillary, venous, and cavernous angiomas, are all hamartomatous lesions involving the blood vessels. While the first three entities are discussed in Chapter 4 of Section II, cavernous angiomas typically present as a mass and will therefore be discussed with tumors of blood vessel origin. Finally, craniopharyngioma is thought to arise from a remnant of Rathke's pouch and is therefore of a congenital origin. This entity will be discussed more fully in Chapter 16, which deals with intrasellar and suprasellar abnormalities.

One of the most common locations for the intracranial teratoma is the pineal region. The most common pineal tumor is the germinoma, and dermoid, epidermoid, and lipoma are all seen in that area. Therefore, a discussion of pineal region tumors must not only include these teratomatous lesions, but also the neuroectodermal tumors, pineocytoma and pineoblastoma.

The tumors of blood vessel origin include the hemangioblastoma and hemangiopericytoma. Hemangioblastoma is a component of one of the phakomatoses, the von Hippel-Lindau syndrome. The phakomatoses are those hereditary syndromes that are associated with neoplasms and/or hamartomas of the CNS. Not only is the hemangioblastoma a component of one of the phakomatoses, but the tuber of tuberous sclerosis is a form of hamartoma, and the angiomatous lesions of the Sturge-Weber syndrome are hamartomas of blood vessel origin.

CONGENITAL TUMORS

Teratoma

Intracranial teratoma, like any teratoma elsewhere in the body, is derived from all three germ cell layers. Therefore, these tumors may contain a variety of tissue types, including ectodermal elements such as epidermis and nervous tissue; mesodermal elements such as fat, muscle, cartilage, and bone; and endodermal elements such as mucosa and secretory glands. Any of these tissue types may undergo malignant degeneration. Cyst formation is also typical. The most common location for these tumors is in the pineal gland, with the intrasellar/suprasellar region and the posterior fossa less common sites of origin.[1]

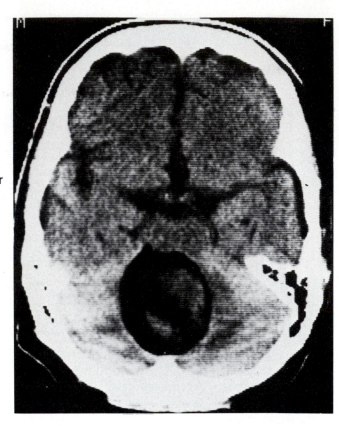

Fig 11–1.—Teratoma (lipomyocele). The nonenhanced scan demonstrates a large cystic lesion within the posterior fossa, containing a solid component centrally and low-density fat peripherally. The central solid component was primarily muscle tissue, but there were also collagenous elements and hamartomatous groups of blood vessels present, along with a minor contribution from tissues of endodermal origin.

The CT scan appearance of these lesions varies considerably according to the tissue type present. Figure 11–1 shows the CT of a lipomyocele of the cerebellar vermis. The lesion was primarily cystic, contained a great deal of fat with a large central core of muscle fibers, and had a peripheral nodule of abnormal vascularity representing a hamartomatous collection of blood vessels.

Dermoid

The lining of the dermoid cyst is squamous epithelium, and in addition dermal elements are present, including hair follicles and sebaceous and sweat glands.[2] The sebaceous secretions produce very low-attenuation coefficients, with the hair and desquamated epithelial debris producing higher numbers (Fig 11–2). The attenuation coefficients, therefore, range from 16 HU (Hounsfield units) down through −100 HU.[2, 3] Calcification of the wall may occur (Fig 11–3), or there may be more chunk-like calcifications representing either vestigial or well-formed teeth (Figs 11–2 and 11–3).[4] There is no enhancement of these low-density lesions.

Dermoid cysts are almost always located in or near the midline, giving support to the theory of their development from an abnormality of the closure of the neural tube, and therefore there may be associated midline abnormalities. For example, a dermoid of the posterior fossa may have an underlying dermal sinus connecting the cyst to the skin.[1] There may also be coloboma of the iris and retina[5] or other midline abnormalities.

Patients with intracranial dermoid present in a variety of fashions, including seizure disorder, hydrocephalus, or symptoms related to compression of contiguous neurologic structures.[4, 5] Rupture of a dermoid allows the sebaceous material to spread throughout the subarachnoid and/or ventricular spaces, producing a granulomatous meningitis that may be rapidly fatal.[1, 5, 6] The CT findings in such a case are those of the primary tumor along with fatty density in the subarachnoid spaces[5] or a fat-cerebrospinal fluid (CSF) level in the ventricular system (Fig 11–4).[6]

Epidermoid

The epidermoid is derived from ectoderm and has a lining of simple stratified squamous epithelium. There is progressive desquamation of keratinized material, which breaks down to form a thick waxy material rich in cholesterol.[1]

While these lesions may occasionally present in the midline, such as within the fourth ventricle[7] or within the suprasellar cisterns, they are generally eccentric in location, as opposed to the dermoid cyst. The most common locations are the cerebellopontine angle, the middle cranial fossa, the suprasellar cisterns, the diploic

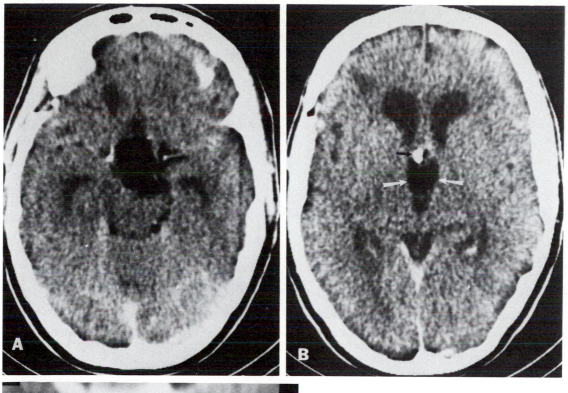

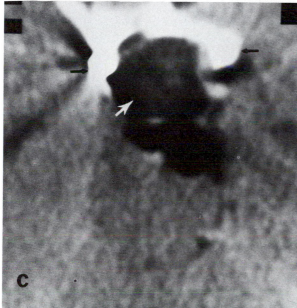

Fig 11–2.—Suprasellar dermoid tumor containing hair, fat, and calcium. The enhanced axial scan at the level of the suprasellar space and brain stem **(A)** demonstrates a large low-density expansion, having attenuation coefficients equal to fat. There is extension posteriorly against the anterior aspect of the brain stem. A higher cut **(B)** demonstrates protrusion of the fatty mass into the lower portion of the third ventricle *(white arrows),* and a focal nodule of calcification *(black arrow)* just below the right foramen of Monro. A magnified view **(C)** at the level of the anterior clinoid processes *(black arrows)* demonstrates a solid component *(white arrow)* within the fat-containing mass. This solid component was made up primarily of hair and collagenous elements. (Courtesy of Lawrence Gold, M.D., University of Minnesota, Minneapolis.)

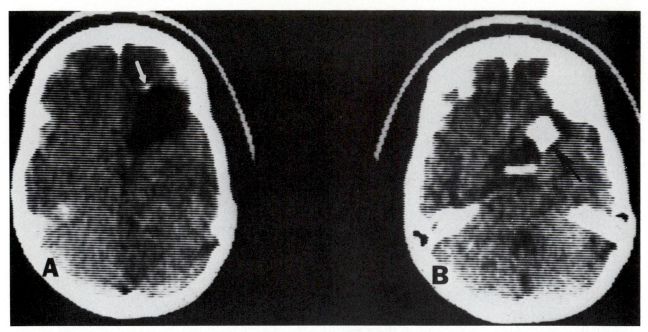

Fig 11–3.—Calcified left frontal dermoid tumor. Two non-enhancing views demonstrate a large fat-containing mass projecting into the left frontal lobe. There is rim calcification *(white arrow)* on the higher cut **(A)**, while the lower cut **(B)** demonstrates a large nodule of calcification *(black arrow).*

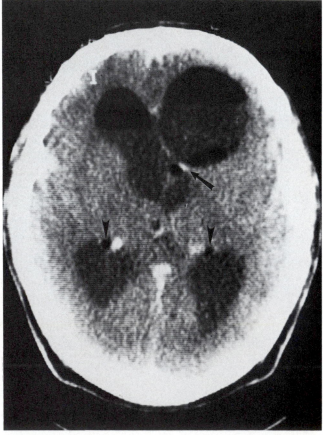

Fig 11–4.—Left frontal dermoid with rupture giving intraventricular fat. There is a large fat-containing mass in the left frontal lobe with rim calcification *(arrow).* Communication of the fat with the CSF of the ventricular system produces fat-CSF levels. Small globules of fat are present near the rim of calcification and in both ventricular atria *(arrowheads).* (Courtesy of A. Norris, M.D., Duluth, Minn.)

space of the calvarium, the fourth ventricle, the intraspinal subarachnoid spaces, and within a lateral ventricle such as the body or temporal horn.[1, 8]

The combination of desquamated epithelium and cholesterol produces attenuation coefficients close to that of CSF, with a range from approximately −5 to +20 HU.[4, 8, 9] The attenuation coefficients usually do not reach the low levels of the dermoid, although there is a considerable range of densities that may be present. Mural calcifications may be present as with the dermoid (Fig 11–5),[4, 8, 9] along with bony deformities reflecting the congenital nature of the lesion.

Symptoms are usually related to local compression of neurologic structures, and there is no invasion of brain. Because the mass is so slow growing, the epidermoid is usually large at the time of its discovery.[7] Malignant change with local invasion of brain is rare[10] and is secondary to malignant degeneration of squamous epithelium to produce squamous cell carcinoma.

The major differential diagnosis is that of arachnoid cyst, which usually has more regular margins than does the epidermoid and does not have mural calcification (see Figs 22–54 to 22–59). The marginal irregularity of the epidermoid is secondary either to growth of the lesion into crevices[9] or to visualization of the concentric lamellae within the cyst following capsular rupture. A "frond-like" appearance is classically seen during pneumoencephalography because of coating by air of the internal architecture of the cyst following such capsular rupture. The same appearance may be seen with the use of metrizamide cisternography and CT scanning.

Lipoma

The lipoma is almost always located in the midline, giving support to its theorized origin from an abnormality of the closure of the neural tube. The most common locations are the genu of the corpus callosum (Fig 11–6); the region of the pineal gland, splenium of the corpus callosum, quadrigeminal plate cistern, and velum interpositum (Fig 11–7); and the intraspinal subarachnoid spaces.[11–13] Midline dysraphism is very common with these congenital tumors, including an absent septum pellucidum, partial or complete agenesis of the corpus callosum, agenesis of the cerebellar vermis, encephalocoele, myelomeningocele, and spina bifida.[11–13] The majority of the lipomas are clinically silent,[4, 14] with the patient's symptoms generally related to the associated dysraphic state.

These tumors are purely of fat density, without associated hair or keratinized tissue to give areas of density higher than fat. Calcification at the periphery is a common finding, particularly with lipomas of the rostral corpus callosum (see Fig 11–6).[12] The midline lipoma may also be associated with extensions of lipomata into the choroid plexus of the lateral ventricle. Change of head position may show a change of position of the choroidal lipomata as they float on the denser CSF.[13]

Hamartoma

The hamartoma is a focus of mature but disorganized or ectopic tissue. Two groups of hamartomatous lesions are of particular interest in this chapter. The first is the

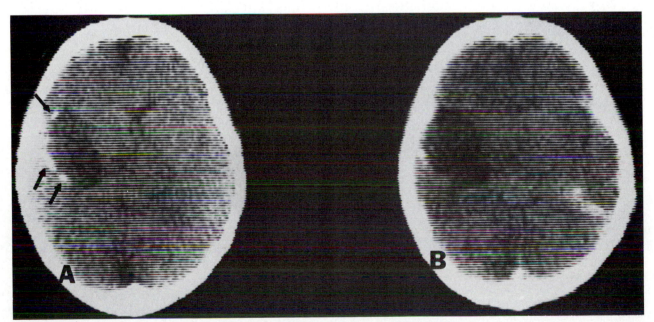

Fig 11–5.—Intracranial epidermoid tumor. **A, B,** two nonenhanced scans demonstrate a large extracerebral mass that projects into the right frontotemporal parenchyma. The higher cut **(A)** demonstrates rim calcification *(arrows)*. The lesion is not as low in its attenuation coefficients as the dermoid tumors of Figures 11–2 through 11–4.

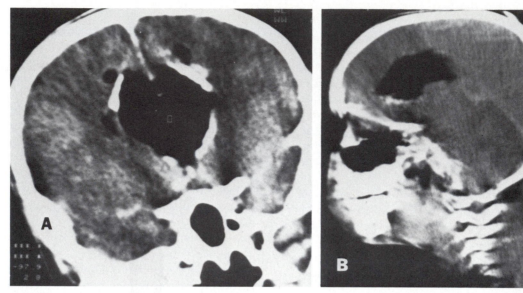

Fig 11–6.—Agenesis of the corpus callosum with lipoma. Coronal **(A)** and direct sagittal **(B)** enhanced scans demonstrate a large fat-containing mass in the region of the rostral portion of the corpus callosum. The mass measured −98 HU, typical of fat. There is peripheral calcification.

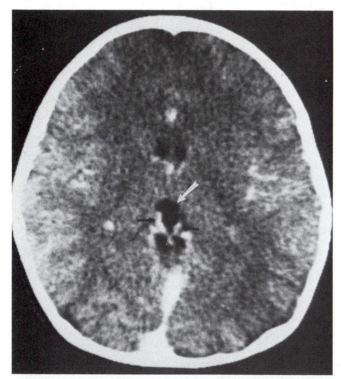

Fig 11–7.—Lipoma involving the velum interpositum. A small lipoma *(white arrow)* involves the subarachnoid space above the third ventricle (velum interpositum) and probably the contiguous corpus callosum. The small benign, probably insignificant mass produces bilateral displacement of the internal cerebral veins *(black arrows)* running within the velum interpositum.

hamartoma that is generally attached by a thick stalk to the tuber cinereum or mammillary bodies.[1] This lesion more commonly occurs in the male and produces precocious puberty. It is a nonenhancing or minimally enhancing lesion that may be difficult to define on a routine CT scan. Metrizamide cisternography is of great value in defining this mass (Fig 11–8), which may be removed in its entirety.

The second group of hamartomas of interest here are those of the phakomatoses. These will be discussed later in this chapter.

PINEAL TUMORS

The term "pinealoma" refers to a group of neoplasms occurring in the pineal region, not to a single neoplasm. Included in this tumor category are neoplasms of germ cell origin, including the teratoma, germinoma (atypical teratoma, which is the most common tumor in this region), epidermoid and dermoid, embryonal cell carcinoma with its variant the endodermal sinus tumor, and choriocarcinoma; tumors of pineal cell origin, the pineocytoma and pineoblastoma; glial tumors, particularly astrocytoma; and lipoma.[4, 14]

A number of pineal region tumors have distinctive clinical or radiologic findings. For example, the pineal region is the most common location for the intracranial teratoma, which has an admixture of tissue types including fatty elements, muscle, and other soft tissues, calcification, and teeth (Fig 11–9). Lipomas occur in the pineal gland or in the region of the quadrigeminal cis-

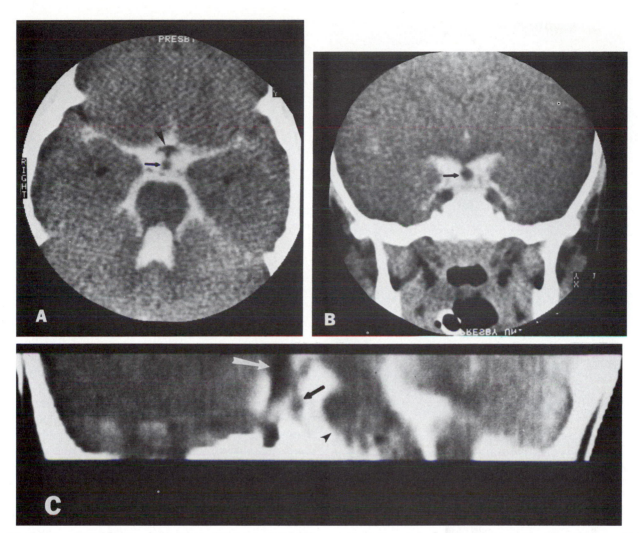

Fig 11–8.—Hamartoma of the tuber cinereum. Axial **(A)** and direct coronal **(B)** scans were performed during Amipaque cisternography. The sagittal view **(C)** is a reformatted image. There is a small mass (*black arrow,* **A, B, C**) that appears on the axial scan to be attached by a stalk to the posterior margin of the optic chiasm (*large arrowhead,* **A**). The sagittal image shows to good advantage the attach- ment of the stalk to the tissue behind the third ventricle (tuber cinereum). The third ventricle is indicated in photo **C** by the *white arrow,* with the *small arrowhead* denoting the pons. Multiple views with Amipaque allow for a complete evaluation of the relationships of the small mass to contiguous structures.

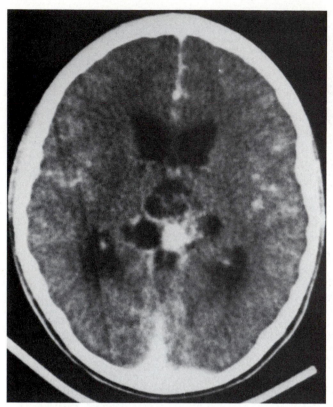

Fig 11–9.—Pineal teratoma. The enhanced scan demonstrates a multicompartmental lesion in the region of the pineal gland and velum interpositum. There is a solid component posteriorly and multiple cystic areas anteriorly and laterally with enhancing margins. Histologically, the mass was made up of multiple tissue elements including muscle, connective tissue, and glandular elements from digestive tract precursors.

tern, velum interpositum, and splenium of the corpus callosum and project into the pineal area (see Fig 11–7); these lesions are denoted by their uniformly low-attenuation coefficients. Epidermoid tumors frequently have mural calcification and are closer to CSF density. Germinomas account for over 50% of pineal tumors,[15] while the neoplasm of pineal cell origin (pineoblastoma and pineocytoma) account for less than 20%. Teratomatous tumors including teratoma, germinoma, and embryonal cell carcinoma almost always present in males, while tumors of pineal cell origin are more commonly present in females.[15]

Calcification of pineal tumors is a frequent but nonspecific finding. In one series, 75% of all pineal region tumors contained calcification, including two thirds of germinomas and 80% of pineal cell neoplasms.[16] Because the majority of pineal region tumors occur during childhood, the age limit for pineal calcification has been evaluated on both plain skull films and CT scans, which are more sensitive to the presence of small amounts of calcification. Small specks of normal pineal calcification can be seen in children as young as 6 years, with normal pineal calcification rarely visualized as early as 2 years of age. In general, pineal calcification below the age of 6 years suggests the possibility of a pineal region tumor;[17] other authors utilize 10 years of age as the cutoff, with the upper limits of size being 1 cm.[16]

Germinomas typically have a slight increase in their density on the preinfusion CT scan, with marked homogeneous enhancement.[18] The margins may be relatively sharp, or they may be irregular, indicative of infiltration into surrounding tissues. Embryonal cell carcinoma (Fig 11–10) and tumors of pineal cell origin (Fig 11–11) have a similar CT appearance to germinoma.[15] Glial tumors may originate in the pineal gland or in the thalamus, hypothalamus, or mesencephalic tectum. These tumors are generally of a low density before contrast and enhance to a moderate degree, generally with an inhomogeneous character so typical of glial tumors.[15]

In summary, the presence of calcification and the density on the pre- and postcontrast scans are of little help in distinguishing the most common varieties of pineal region tumors, which are the germinoma, embryonal cell carcinoma, and pineal cell neoplasms. The relative densities of the tumors may be of value in distinguishing the teratoma, lipoma, dermoid and epidermoid, and glial tumors. If the patient is female, a pineal cell origin is more likely. Finally, choriocarcinoma of the pineal gland is frequently hemorrhagic, typical of choriocarcinoma present elsewhere in the brain.[19]

Confusion has arisen with the term "ectopic pinealoma," which refers to a germinoma present in the suprasellar region, thought to represent a metastatic extension of a pineal region tumor. Some patients with suprasellar germinomas do indeed have pineal region tumors, and germinomas are known to seed throughout the neural axis via CSF pathways. However, suprasellar germinoma may occur independently of a pineal region germinoma, and germinomas are known to occur in other midline locations such as the mediastinum. With an abnormality of the closure of the neural tube, it is quite possible that germinomas and other teratomatous lesions will form in the pineal or suprasellar regions or both.[14, 15] Germinomas may also occur in a paramedian location, including the basal ganglia and thalamus.[20]

Controversy has long existed as to the role of surgery vs. radiation therapy without biopsy for treatment of pineal region tumors. The surgical approach to this region is difficult and may produce a relatively high degree of morbidity/mortality. In addition, many of the "pinealomas" are quite radiosensitive, including the most common variety, the germinoma, as well as pineal cell neoplasms and embryonal cell carcinoma.[15, 21] In

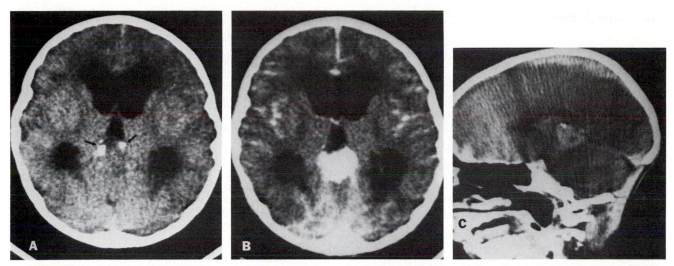

Fig 11–10.—Embryonal cell carcinoma of the pineal region. The unenhanced scan **(A)** demonstrates an isodense mass containing calcium *(arrows)* projecting into the posterior portion of the third ventricle and producing obstructive hydrocephalus. The enhanced study **(B)** demonstrates in-tense enhancement of this malignant pineal region tumor. A direct sagittal scan **(C)** demonstrates the relationship of the calcified and enhancing mass to the posterior portion of the ventricular system and corpus callosum and to the posterior fossa.

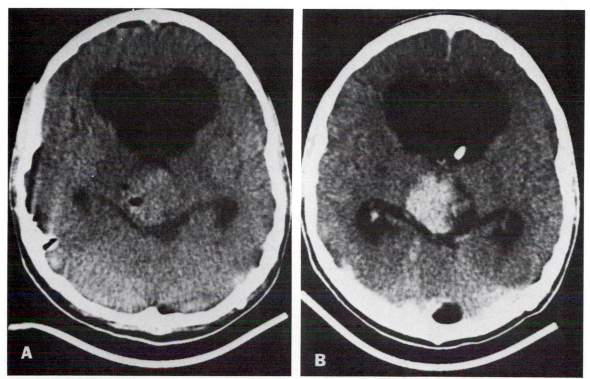

Fig 11–11.—Pineoblastoma with stereotactic biopsy. The unenhanced scan **(A)** was taken following a stereotactic biopsy, which left a small amount of air within the lesion at the biopsy site. The mass is relatively well circumscribed and greater than brain density on the preinfusion study. The enhanced scan **(B)** was performed a few days before **A** and demonstrates diffuse and homogeneous enhancement of the lesion. The tip of an intraventricular shunt is seen, but the ventricles remain markedly dilated.

our institution, we have found that CT-guided stereotactic biopsy (see Fig 11–11) has given the histologic
diagnosis with extremely low morbidity; this diagnostic
procedure is followed by radiation therapy for the sensitive histologic types.

TUMORS OF BLOOD VESSEL ORIGIN

Hemangioblastoma

Hemangioblastoma is the most common primary cerebellar neoplasm in the adult and comprises 7% to 12%
of all adult posterior fossa tumors when considering
both primary and metastatic neoplasms.[22] While this
tumor is associated with von Hippel-Lindau syndrome,
only approximately 25% of patients presenting with hemangioblastoma have the other manifestations of the
syndrome, which include angioma of the retina (von
Hippel's disease), nonneoplastic cysts of the pancreas
and kidney, neoplasms of the kidney (in particular hypernephroma) and adrenal glands (especially pheochromocytoma), and hemangioblastomas of the spinal
cord.[14, 23] While supratentorial hemangioblastoma has
been described,[24] the majority of such cases have probably been angioblastic meningiomas.[14] Occasionally,
one may see hemangioblastomas in both the infratentorial and supratentorial compartments, with this multiplicity indicative of the von Hippel-Lindau syndrome
(Fig 11–12).[24, 25]

Hemangioblastoma presents in three forms on the
CT scan. The most common, accounting for approximately 50% of cases,[26] is that of a large cystic lesion
with a small mural nodule (Fig 11–13), simulating a
cystic astrocytoma of childhood. The nodule generally
enhances homogeneously to a marked degree. The nodule may be quite small in comparison to the large cystic
component, requiring multiple overlapping cuts and
close scrutiny for identification of the enhancing nodule. The other 50% of tumors are split between a diffusely enhancing mass containing cystic areas (Figs 11–
12 and 11–14) and a totally solid homogeneous lesion
without cyst formation (Fig 11–15).

Whichever mode of presentation occurs, the lesion is
well circumscribed, and there is generally little, if any,
surrounding cerebral edema. The mass effect, which is
frequently due to the large cystic component, may produce obstructive hydrocephalus. Classically, there is intense staining of the nodular component of the tumor
at angiography.

Spinal cord CT scans reveal a similar appearance to
the cystic lesion with a mural nodule seen in Figure
11–13. All patients with hemangioblastoma require ex-
cretory urography to exclude hypernephroma.

Hemangiopericytoma

Hemangiopericytoma arises from the capillary peri-
cyte and generally has its intracranial site of origin in
the meninges.[14, 27] This tumor was originally thought to
be an angioblastic meningioma, although reticulin
staining demonstrates its relationship to vascular channels.[14] The tumor has a high recurrence rate and may
metastasize to extracranial locations.

Typically, the tumor is of isodensity or increased
density on the preinfusion scan and enhances homogeneously in a similar fashion to a meningioma (Figs 11–
16 and 11–17).[27] Bone changes such as sclerosis and
calcification are not seen as in some meningiomas. A
peripherally located lesion based along the inner table
of the skull may be indistinguishable from a meningioma on the CT scan alone (see Fig 11–16). The angiographic demonstration of meningeal blood supply and a
persisting homogeneous stain (see Fig 11–17) likewise
makes distinction from meningioma difficult or impossible. The appropriate diagnosis may be suggested by
the presence of such a lesion in a location not common
for meningioma and with a history of rapid recurrence
after previous surgery or by the presence of metastases
(see Fig 11–17).

Cavernous Hemangioma

Cavernous hemangioma is a type of blood vessel hamartoma and is therefore related to arteriovenous malformation and the capillary and venous angiomas. This entire group of lesions is discussed more completely in
Chapter 5. Cavernous hemangioma is included in this
chapter because of its frequent CT presentation as a
tumor mass.

Cavernous hemangioma is a relatively rare lesion,
and its CT scan appearance has been infrequently described.[28–30] The lesion generally is dense without the
use of contrast material (Fig 11–18,A) because of the
"blood pool" that is present, although the presence of
hemorrhage, fibrosis, and calcification may also play a
role in this increased density. The degree of contrast
enhancement varies from none to marked (see Fig 11–
18,B) in the few cases that have been described, and
the amount of mass effect is generally minimal or none.
This hamartomatous lesion generally has a rounded
configuration, and some authors have frankly stated that
they are unable to distinguish this lesion preoperatively
from meningioma, glioma, or simple intracerebral
hemorrhage.[28] The possibility could be suggested by a
combination of an intraparenchymal location, sharply
defined borders, increased density before enhancement, and an unchanged appearance on sequential
scans.

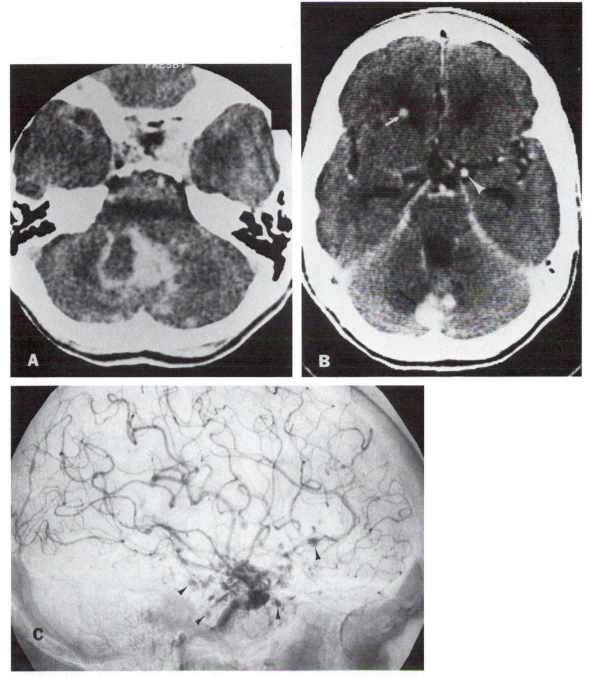

Fig 11–12.—Cerebellar hemangioblastoma with multiple supratentorial hemangioblastomas. The scan through the midportion of the cerebellum **(A)** demonstrates a large intensely enhancing mass lesion located within the cerebellar vermis and right cerebellar hemisphere. The mass is primarily solid, with an internal cyst. A higher cut **(B)** demonstrates the superior portion of the cerebellar hemangioblastoma *(black arrow)* located in the posterior portion of the cerebellar vermis. There are multiple enhancing nodules supratentorially, located in the subarachnoid cisterns *(white arrowhead)* and right frontal horn *(white arrow)*. There may also be other nodules in the Sylvian fissures simulating vascular structures. A right carotid angiogram **(C)** demonstrates multiple staining nodules within the basal portions of the brain and subarachnoid cisterns, some of which are marked by *black arrowheads.*

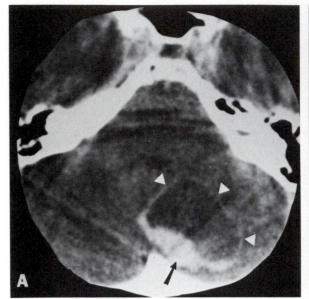

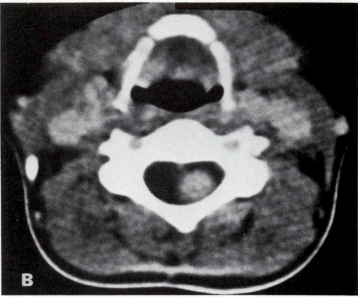

Fig 11–13.—Cerebellar and spinal cord cystic hemangioblastomas in von Hippel-Lindau syndrome. The enhanced axial scan of the posterior fossa **(A)** demonstrates a large cystic mass *(white arrowheads)* with a small mural nodule *(black arrow)* that stains intensely, located within the cerebellar vermis and left cerebellar hemisphere. A scan through the upper cervical spinal canal **(B)** following intravenous contrast enhancement demonstrates a large cystic expansion within the spinal canal with an intensely staining nodule to the left of the midline.

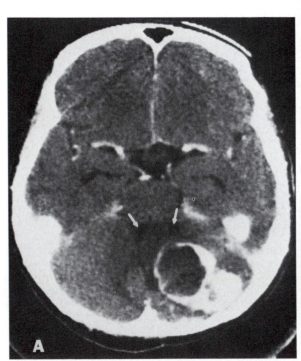

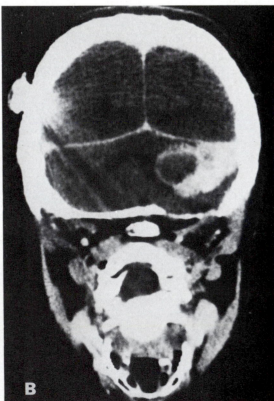

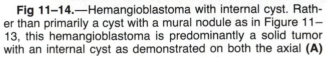

Fig 11–14.—Hemangioblastoma with internal cyst. Rather than primarily a cyst with a mural nodule as in Figure 11–13, this hemangioblastoma is predominantly a solid tumor with an internal cyst as demonstrated on both the axial **(A)** and coronal **(B)** projections. There is compression of the fourth ventricle *(arrows, A)* and extension of the mass to the underside of the tentorium.

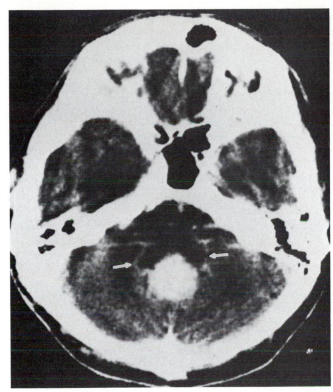

Fig 11–15.—Solid hemangioblastoma. There is a solid well-circumscribed mass in the region of the fourth ventricle. The enhancement is intense and homogeneous, and there are contiguous vascular structures *(arrows).* Angiographically and histologically, this was a classic hemangioblastoma. (Courtesy of Louis Scotti, M.D., St. Francis General Hospital, Pittsburgh.)

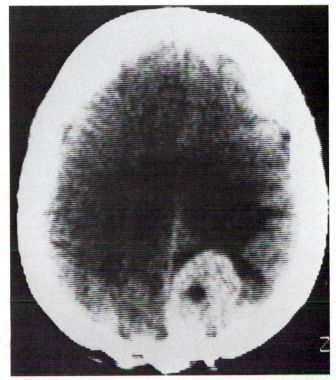

Fig 11–16.—Hemangiopericytoma. This well-circumscribed, intensely enhancing mass based along the inner table of the skull has an appearance similar to many meningiomas. The internal area of cyst formation or necrosis can be seen with some meningiomas, as can edema as extensive as in this case. (Courtesy of Richard Kasdan, M.D., CT Scan Associates, Inc., Pittsburgh.)

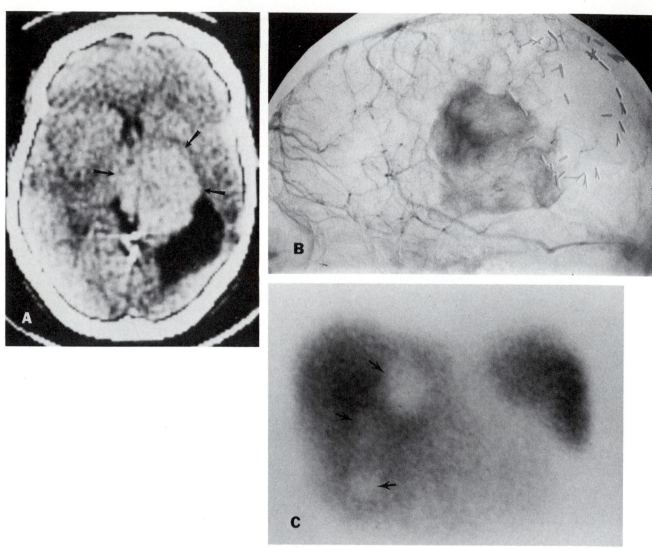

Fig 11–17.—Metastatic hemangiopericytoma. The axial enhanced CT scan **(A)** demonstrates a large, homogeneously enhancing and relatively well-circumscribed mass lesion located deep within the left cerebral hemisphere and midline *(arrows)*. The patient has had previous surgery, as denoted by metallic clips posterior to the lesion in the midline, with the diagnosis of hemangiopericytoma. The lateral view of the left carotid angiogram **(B)** showed persistence of the intense stain of the well-demarcated lesion into the venous phase. Metastases have occurred, as denoted on the anteroposterior view of the liver/spleen radionuclide scan **(C)**, with multiple metastatic lesions in the right lobe of the liver *(arrows)*.

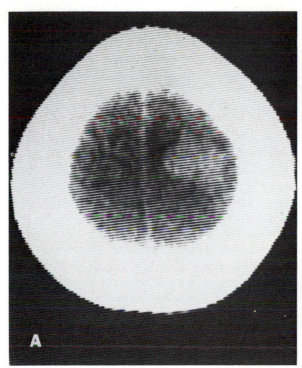

Fig 11–18.—Cavernous hemangioma. This 12-year-old child with a seizure disorder has a mass lesion in the high left cerebral convexity. The mass has greater-than-normal brain density on the unenhanced scan, **(A)** and has intense enhancement on the postinfusion study **(B).** Angiographically, the mass was avascular. Neoplasm was suspected, and surgery revealed a well-circumscribed cavernous hemangioma, which was totally removed.

PHAKOMATOSES (DYSGENETIC SYNDROMES)

The diseases herein considered are all associated with neoplasms and/or hamartomas of the CNS and have a hereditary basis. There is overlap among the various phakomatoses, such as café-au-lait spots of the skin occurring in both neurofibromatosis and tuberous sclerosis. There are a number of recorded cases with other forms of clinical and pathologic overlap indicative of the close relationship of these syndromes.[31] The neoplasms and/or hamartomas of these syndromes are emphasized in this section; discussion of the hereditary patterns and extracranial manifestations of the phakomatoses is not possible within the limitations of this book.

Neurofibromatosis (von Recklinghausen's Disease)

Neurofibromatosis is a neuroectodermal dysplasia that presents with a myriad of intracranial, intraspinal, osseous, cutaneous, and vascular abnormalities. These lesions include the following: arterial occlusive disease involving the renal, brachiocephalic, and intracranial vasculature; café-au-lait spots and cutaneous neurofibromas; focal bone erosion from overlying neurofibromas or bony abnormalities not related to local tumor, such as pseudarthrosis of a bone of an extremity; spinal abnormalities including scoliosis (which frequently involves a short segment and is angular in configuration), dural ectasia, and multiple intraspinal tumors such as multiple neurofibromas, meningioma, and nerve root enlargement without focal neoplasms; and finally, the intracranial tumors that have been found in association with neurofibromatosis, including almost all categories of neoplasms. The most common tumors associated with this syndrome are neurofibromas and schwannomas involving cranial nerves, particularly the eighth cranial nerves; meningiomas; optic nerve gliomas; and tumors of glial origin, whatever the location. The CT scan appearance of each of these lesions is dealt with separately throughout this section or in other portions of the book. Even without the more common cutaneous and osseous abnormalities found in this syndrome, neurofibromatosis may be suggested when there is a multiplicity of intracranial and/or intraspinal tumors, such as bilateral acoustic tumors or a combination of optic nerve glioma and acoustic tumor.

Tuberous Sclerosis (Bourneville's Disease)

Tuberous sclerosis is characterized by seizures and mental retardation; cutaneous lesions including adenoma sebaceum, café-au-lait spots, and shagreen patches; osseous lesions including cystic areas in the phalanges and flame-shaped cortical densities in periarticular locations; and the presence of tubers of the brain. A tuber, a form of hamartoma, contains both neurons and astrocytes, with many of the latter being of giant size,[1] and most commonly occurs in a subependymal location.

The subependymal tubers frequently calcify (Fig 11–19), and the appearance of multiple subependymal calcifications is classic for tuberous sclerosis and diagnostic even with a lack of more typical features of this syndrome. Multiple subependymal calcifications may also occur with one of the intrauterine inflammatory conditions such as toxoplasmosis or cytomegalic inclusion disease (Chapter 22), but the inflammatory process generally produces other cerebral abnormalities such as hydrocephalus, microcephaly, areas of encephalomalacia, etc. Calcifications may also be present in other portions of the brain with tuberous sclerosis.

A common location for a tuber is near the foramen of Monro (see Figs 9–40 and 11–19), and this lesion may produce obstruction to the outflow of one or both lateral ventricles. A tuber may undergo degeneration to the so-called giant cell astrocytoma,[1] and it is therefore extremely important to perform CT scanning in patients with tuberous sclerosis, both with and without contrast material. While the unenhanced scan will demonstrate the classic subependymal calcifications (see Fig 11–19,A), the neoplasm may not contain calcification and may be relatively isodense on the unenhanced scan (see Fig 11–19,B). The enhanced scan will demonstrate this lesion (see Fig 11–19,C) as the contrast material passes the abnormal blood-brain barrier of the neoplasm, indicating that the mass is neoplastic and not a simple tuber with an intact blood-brain barrier.

von Hippel-Lindau Syndrome

The von Hippel-Lindau syndrome has been previously discussed in this chapter under Hemangioblastoma. The syndrome consists of hemangioblastomas of the cerebellum, spinal cord, and rarely of the supratentorial structures (see Figs 11–12 to 11–15); retinal angiomas (von Hippel's disease); and various cysts and neoplasms of the abdominal viscera, most notably hypernephroma of the kidney and pheochromocytoma of the adrenal gland. Only approximately 25% of patients with hemangioblastoma are part of this diffuse syndrome. As previously discussed, hemangioblastoma presents with three CT scan appearances, including a mural nodule within a cystic lesion, a solid enhancing neoplasm, and an enhancing tumor containing multiple cystic areas (Figs 11–12 to 11–15).

Sturge-Weber Syndrome (Encephalotrigeminal Angiomatosis)

Sturge-Weber syndrome consists of blood vessel hamartoma formation involving the face and ipsilateral ce-

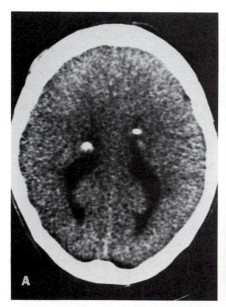 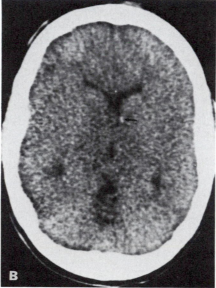 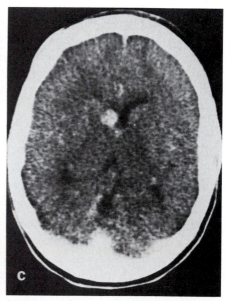

Fig 11–19.—Tuberous sclerosis with subependymal giant cell astrocytoma. The unenhanced scans **(A, B)** demonstrate calcification within multiple subependymal tubers. Image **B** demonstrates a subtle tuberous calcification on the left *(arrow)* and slight mass effect on the right frontal horn. The enhanced scan **(C)** demonstrates a well-circumscribed enhancing subependymal neoplasm in this right caudate region. Pathology revealed a typical giant cell astrocytoma. Contrast enhancement is vital in evaluating patients with tuberous sclerosis, because many of the neoplasms are isodense, and degeneration of a tuber into a neoplasm cannot be adequately assessed without an enhanced study.

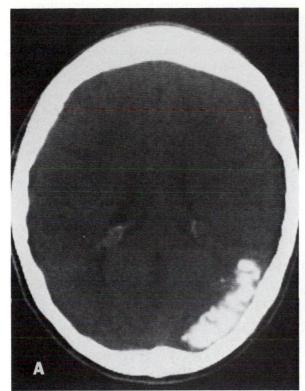
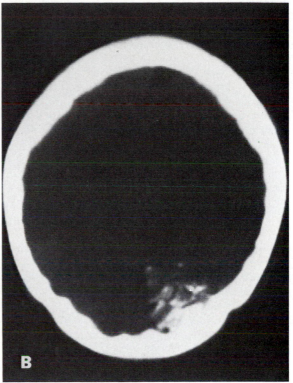

Fig 11–20.—Calcifications in the Sturge-Weber syndrome. **A, B,** unenhanced scans taken at wide window widths (bone window) demonstrate gyriform calcifications in the left parieto-occipital region characteristic of the Sturge-Weber syndrome.

rebral hemisphere. The cutaneous abnormality is most frequently a port-wine stain, typically involving the cutaneous distribution of the ophthalmic division of the trigeminal nerve. Congenital buphthalmus and glaucoma may also be present.[23] The intracranial abnormality is a capillary-venous malformation involving the pia and underlying cerebral cortex, typically in the parieto-occipital region. Calcifications in the deep layers of the cortex occur in the region of the malformation, producing parallel and wavy densities ("tram-line") on skull films.

The CT scan findings are that of extensive calcification, which has the same wavy appearance as seen on the plain skull films (Fig 11–20), and focal or hemispheric atrophy. Occasionally, one may also see a subtle area of contrast enhancement representing the pial vascular malformation.

Neurocutaneous Melanosis

The predominant feature of this rare disease is the presence of an increased number of melanin-containing cells within areas of the skin and meninges.[1] Melanoma of the meninges may occur, having an appearance on the CT scan of a homogeneously enhancing extra-axial tumor and simulating meningioma.[32, 33]

REFERENCES

1. Russell D.S., Rubenstein L.J.: Congenital tumours of maldevelopmental origin, in *Pathology of Tumours of the Nervous System.* Baltimore, Williams & Wilkins Co., 1977, pp. 24–64.
2. Mikhael M.A., Mattar A.G.: Intracranial pearly tumors: The roles of computed tomography, angiography and pneumoencephalography. *J. Comput. Assist. Tomogr.* 2:421–429, 1978.
3. Lee S.H., Delgado T.E., Ruchheit W.A.: Intracranial dermoid tumor: Diagnosis by computed tomography: A case report. *Neurosurgery* 1:281–283, 1977.
4. Zimmerman R.A., Bilaniuk L.T., Dolinhas C.: Cranial computed tomography of epidermoid and congenital fatty tumors of maldevelopmental origin. *J. Comput. Tomogr.* 3:40–50, 1979.
5. Murphy M.J., Risk W.S., Van Geldes J.C.: Intracranial dermoid cyst in Goldenbar's syndrome. *J. Neurosurg.* 53:408–410, 1980.
6. Healy J.F., Brahme F.J., Rosenkrantz H.: Dermoid cysts and their complications as manifested by computed cranial tomography. *Comput. Tomogr.* 4:111–115, 1980.
7. Rosario M., Becker D.H., Conley F.K.: Epidermoid tumors involving the fourth ventricle. *Neurosurgery* 9:9–13, 1981.
8. Chambers A.A., Lubin R.R., Tomsick T.A.: Cranial epi-

dermoid tumors: Diagnosis by computed tomography. *Neurosurgery* 1:276–279, 1977.

9. Davis K.R., Roberson G.H., Taveras J.M.: Diagnosis of epidermoid tumors by computed tomography. *Radiology* 119:347–353, 1976.

10. Dubois P.J., Sage M., Luther J.S., et al.: Malignant change in an intracranial epidermoid cyst. *J. Comput. Assist. Tomogr.* 5:443–435, 1981.

11. Faerber E.N., Wolpert S.M.: The value of computed tomography in the diagnosis of intracranial lipomata. *J. Comput. Assist. Tomogr.* 2:297–299, 1978.

12. Zee C.-S., McComb J.G., et al.: Lipoma of the corpus callosum associated with frontal dysraphism. *J. Comput. Assist. Tomogr.* 5:201–205, 1981.

13. Yock D.H.: Choroid plexus lipomas associated with lipoma of the corpus callosum. *J. Comput. Assist. Tomogr.* 4:678–682, 1980.

14. Russell D.S., Rubenstein L.J.: Pineal neoplasms, in *Pathology of Tumours of the Nervous System.* Baltimore, Williams & Wilkins Co., 1977, pp. 283–298.

15. Zimmerman R.A., Bilaniuk L.T., Wood J.H., et al.: Computed tomography of pineal, parapineal, and histologically related tumors. *Radiology* 137:669–677, 1980.

16. Lin S.R., Crane M.D., Lin Z.S., et al.: Characteristics of calcification in tumors of the pineal gland. *Radiology* 126:721–726, 1978.

17. Zimmerman R.A., Bilaniuk L.T.: Age-related incidence of pineal calcification detected by computed tomography. *Radiology* 142:659–662, 1982.

18. Futrell N.N., Osborn A.G., Cleson B.D.: Pineal region tumors: Computed tomographic-pathologic spectrum. *A.J.N.R.* 2:415–420, 1981.

19. Kawakami Y., Kamada O., Tabuci K., et al.: Primary intracranial choriocarcinoma. *J. Neurosurg.* 53:369–374, 1980.

20. Kobayashi T., Kageyama N., Kida Y., et al.: Unilateral germinomas involving the basal ganglia and thalamus. *J. Neurosurg.* 55:55–62, 1981.

21. Inoue Y., Takeuchi T., Tamaki M., et al.: Sequential CT observations of irradiated intracranial germinomas. *A.J.R.* 132:361–365, 1979.

22. Seeger J.F., Burke D.P., Knake J.E., et al.: Computed tomographic and angiographic evaluation of hemangioblastomas. *Radiology* 138:65–73, 1981.

23. Russell D.S., Rubenstein L.J.: Tumours and hamartomas of the blood vessels, in *Pathology of Tumours of the Nervous System.* Baltimore, Williams & Wilkins Co., 1977, pp. 116–145.

24. Tomasello F., Albanese V., Iannotti F., et al.: Supratentorial hemangioblastoma in a child: Case report. *J. Neurosurg.* 52:578–583, 1980.

25. Diehl P.R., Simon L.: Supratentorial intraventricular hemangioblastoma: Case report and review of the literature. *Surg. Neurol.* 15:435–443, 1981.

26. Naidich T.P., Lin J.P., Leeds N.E., et al.: Primary tumors and other masses of the cerebellum and fourth ventricle: Differential diagnosis by computed tomography. *Neuroradiology* 14:153–174, 1977.

27. Osborne D.R., Dubois P.R., Drayer B.P., et al.: Primary intracranial meningeal and spinal hemangiopericytoma: Radiologic manifestations. *A.J.N.R.* 2:69–74, 1981.

28. Ishikawa M., Handa H., Moritake K., et al.: Computed tomography of cerebral cavernous hemangiomas. *J. Comput. Assist. Tomogr.* 4:587–591, 1980.

29. Pozzati E., Padorani R., Morrone B., et al.: Cerebral cavernous angiomas in children. *J. Neurosurg.* 53:826–836, 1980.

30. Bartlett J.E., Koshore P.R.S.: Intracranial cavernous angioma. *A.J.R.* 128:653–656, 1977.

31. Vouge M., Pasquini V., Salvalini U.: CT findings of atypical forms of phakomatosis. *Neuroradiology* 20:99–101, 1980.

32. Tamura M., Kanafuchi J., Nagaya T., et al.: Primary leptomeningeal melanoma with epipharyngeal invasion. *Acta Neurochir.* 58:59–66, 1981.

33. Lamas E., Lobato R.D., Sotelo T., et al.: Neurocutaneous melanomas. *Acta Neurochir.* 36:93–105, 1977.

MDBA –

mega dolicho basilar artery
or vertebro basilar ectasia

May simulate a saccular
aneurysm – often associated
c̄ hydrocephalus – non
obstructive (third ventricle)
so called water hammer
effect of CSF pulsations –

GMH –

Germinal Matrix
Hemorrhage – usually in
newborn c̄ low birth wts
(under 1500 gm or less)
Immaturety of brain
is highest correlating factor
Communicating hydrocephalus
common sequelae

12

Metastases

RICHARD E. LATCHAW, M.D.

METASTATIC INVOLVEMENT of the brain takes many forms, ranging from hematogenous metastases to the brain and meninges, direct spread to the brain and meninges from tumors of the face and neck, or intracranial dissemination of primary and secondary brain tumors via cerebrospinal fluid (CSF) pathways. Likewise, metastases may primarily involve the calvarium or skull base.

This chapter will be broken into four sections, beginning with hematogenous metastases to the brain and meninges. The involvement of the brain and meninges by systemic lymphoma and leukemia warrants a separate section, because there is a characteristic pattern of initial meningeal involvement followed by infiltration into the contiguous parenchyma. Bony involvement is divided into metastatic lesions involving the calvarium and metastases to the base of the skull. Finally, dissemination of primary and secondary CNS tumors to other portions of the brain will be discussed.

HEMATOGENOUS METASTASES TO THE BRAIN AND MENINGES

The most common sites of origin for metastases to the CNS are the lung, breast, kidney, colon and rectum, skin (particularly melanoma), and paranasal sinuses.[1] While the majority of hematogenous metastases occur at the gray matter/white matter junction (Figs 10–10, 12–1, and 12–2)[1] metastatic involvement of the deeper parenchymal structures is frequent. Metastasis to the brain stem (see Fig 12–2) is less common,[2] while metastasis to the choroid plexus of a ventricle is rare.[3]

The findings on the unenhanced CT scan are extremely variable. Areas of low density have been seen, particularly with metastases from the lung, breast, and kidney, and with lymphoma and melanoma.[1, 4] Metastases with increased attenuation coefficients have been seen with lung, kidney, colon, melanoma, choriocarcinoma, and various sarcomas, particularly osteogenic

sarcoma. All of these latter lesions are known to be frequently hemorrhagic or contain calcium, which may account for their increased density (Fig 12–3).[1, 5] However, hemorrhage or calcification has not always been found pathologically in metastases of increased density (Figs 12–1 and 12–4),[4, 6] with the increased density probably on the basis of the cellular compactness.

In many cases, the decreased density seen with metastatic lesions is probably a reflection of the amount of surrounding cerebral edema. Many metastatic tumors are isodense on the unenhanced scan, without much surrounding edema (Figs 12–5 and 12–6). These lesions may be extremely difficult to detect without the use of contrast material. Multiple lesions may be present and "balance" each other so that there is no detectable mass effect. A contrast-enhanced scan is therefore imperative when evaluating the presence of metastatic tumor, not only to better visualize a lesion with obvious mass effect, but to look for occult metastases not detectable on the unenhanced scan and to determine if multiple lesions are present when there is only one obvious area of abnormality, confirming the diagnosis of metastatic tumor (Fig 12–7). While most hematogenous metastases enhance to a moderate or marked degree, occasionally some metastases are difficult to define with a single dose of contrast material. Some authors advocate performing a high-dose delayed contrast-enhanced scan, with the administration of over 80 gm of iodine and scanning 1 to 2 hours after infusion, whenever there is a question of metastatic disease. In such cases, lesions difficult to define may become evident, and multiple lesions not previously detected with a single dose of contrast material may be seen.[7, 8] In one series, 44% of patients undergoing this delayed high-dose technique had additional lesions seen with more information provided by this technique than on the conventional enhanced scan in two thirds of the cases; 11.5% of the cases were false-negative until the delayed high-dose technique was utilized.[8]

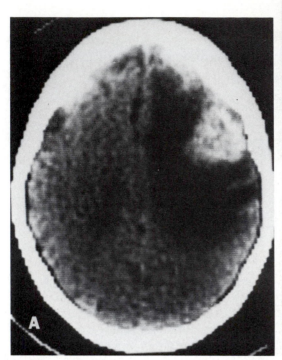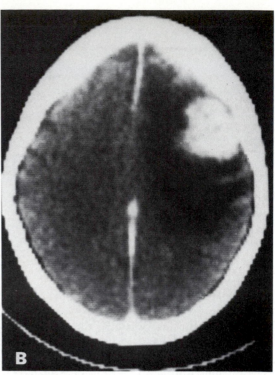

Fig 12–1.—Dense solitary metastasis. The unenhanced scan **(A)** demonstrates a dense mass centered at the corticomedullary junction of the left frontal and parietal lobes. There is extensive cerebral edema. The enhanced scan **(B)** demonstrates intense enhancement. Histologically, this was a metastasis from adenocarcinoma of the colon, and there was no evidence of intratumoral hemorrhage. Punctate areas of calcification in mucinous adenocarcinomas of the colon can be responsible for increased density on the unenhanced scan, but such was not true in this case.

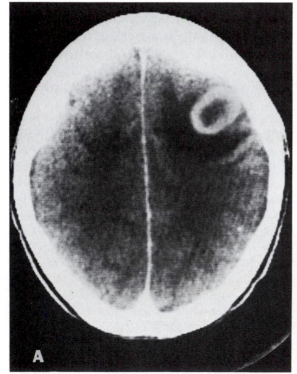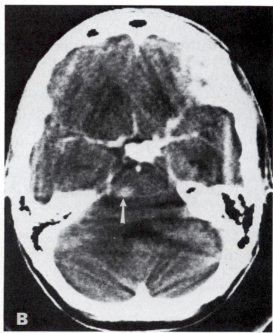

Fig 12–2.—Metastasis with thick ring of enhancement in frontal lobe, with second lesion in the pons. The enhanced axial scan above the ventricular system **(A)** demonstrates a tumor in the posterior left frontal lobe having a thick ring of enhancement, a central area of necrosis, and peripheral edema of moderate amount. A scan through the upper pons **(B)** demonstrates a second lesion *(arrow)* within the right side of the brain stem. This 38-year-old female had adenocarcinoma metastases throughout the body, of unknown origin.

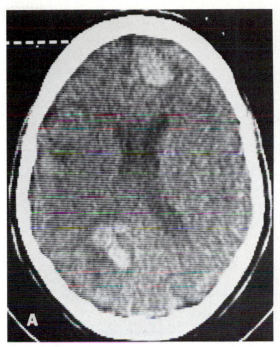
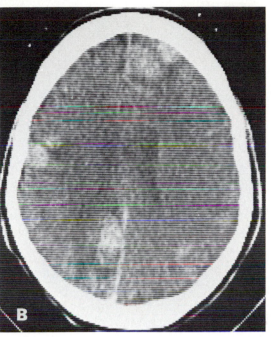

Fig 12–3.—Metastatic melanoma with multiple dense hemorrhagic metastases. The unenhanced scan **(A)** demonstrates multiple dense masses, while the enhanced study **(B)** at a slightly different level demonstrates more metastatic lesions that enhance. Many of these metastatic nodules contained hemorrhage, typical of metastatic melanoma. (Courtesy of Lawrence Gold, M.D., University of Minnesota, Minneapolis.)

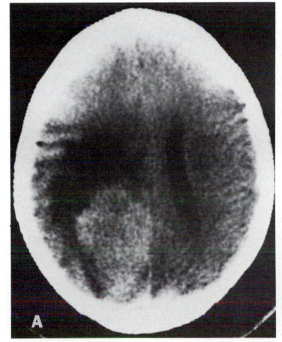
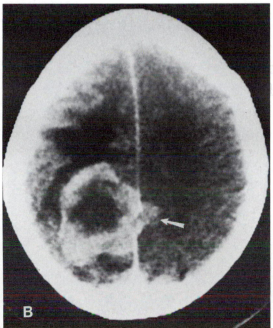

Fig 12–4.—Metastatic oat cell carcinoma penetrating the falx. The unenhanced scan **(A)** demonstrates a relatively dense large metastasis of oat cell carcinoma, with abundant surrounding cerebral edema. The enhanced study **(B)** demonstrates intense enhancement with central necrosis. The aggressive nature of the lesion is demonstrated by growth of tumor through the falx into the opposite cerebral hemisphere (*arrow,* **B**) in this 35-year-old woman with rapid deterioration.

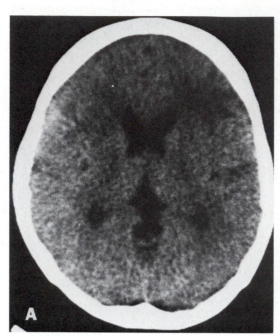
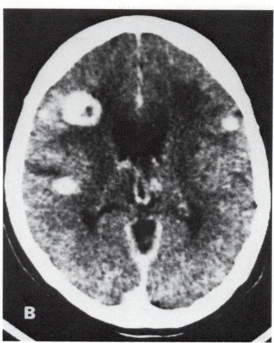

Fig 12–5.—Enhancement of multiple isodense metastases. This 38-year-old woman with metastatic melanoma has an unenhanced CT scan **(A)** with left frontal lobe edema and some patchy edema in the left temporal and right frontal regions. The enhanced scan **(B),** however, demonstrates intense enhancement of multiple metastatic nodules not seen on the unenhanced scan.

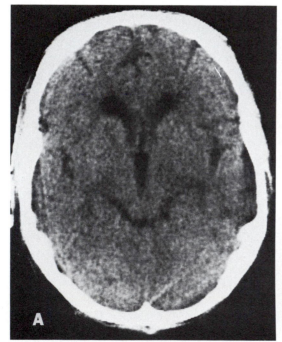
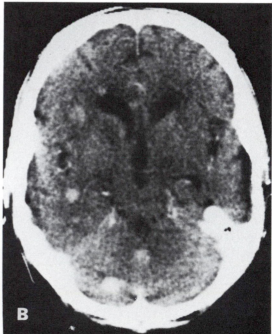

Fig 12–6.—Enhancement of multiple occult metastases. The unenhanced scan **(A)** is unremarkable in this patient with known metastatic oat cell carcinoma. The enhanced scan **(B)** at a very slightly different angle demonstrates multiple enhancing cerebral and cerebellar nodules. None of these nodules could be identified on the preinfusion study, nor was there evidence of edema or mass effect to suggest multiple tumor deposits.

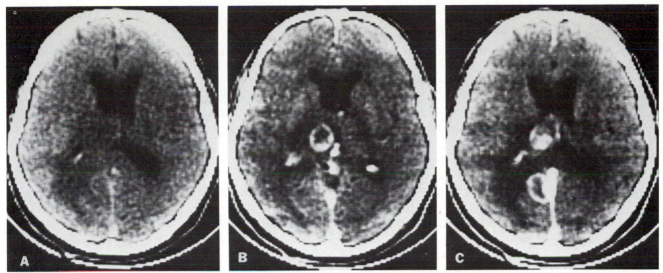

Fig 12–7.—Metastatic large cell carcinoma of the lung with contrast-fluid level. The unenhanced scan **(A)** demonstrates compression of the body and atrium of the right lateral ventricle, with diffuse low density throughout the right thalamus and contiguous structures. The enhanced study **(B, C)** demonstrates a metastatic lesion with a ring of enhancement in the right thalamus. The straight inferior margin of enhancement is indicative of a contrast-fluid level within the centrally necrotic tumor. A high cut **(C)** demonstrates the dome of the right thalamic tumor nodule and a second "ring" of metastasis in the medial right parietal lobe.

While many metastatic lesions have a round, homogeneously enhancing appearance on the enhanced scan (see Figs 12–1, 12–3, 12–5, and 12–6), the "ring sign" is also a frequent finding (see Figs 12–2, 12–4, and 12–7). The appearance of rim enhancement is nonspecific and may occur with either primary or secondary tumors, abscesses, resolving hematomas, and occasionally infarcts. The lucent area within the metastatic tumor represents necrosis as the tumor outgrows its blood supply. Extracellular fluid or blood accumulation within the cavity may produce a fluid level;[9] contrast material may also leak into the cavity to produce a fluid-fluid level on the enhanced scan (see Fig 12–7). Metastases may be truly cystic, and there may be both a solid and a cystic component with the solid portion appearing like a mural nodule, suggesting cystic astrocytoma or hemangioblastoma.[10] Absorption coefficients do not separate a true cyst from necrosis; a true cyst is differentiated from necrosis when the margins of the lucency within the ring of enhancement are sharp. The diagnosis of a cystic component can be surgically important, because drainage of the cyst without complete tumor removal may give temporary palliation of the mass effect.

The amount of edema surrounding a metastatic lesion is variable, but is generally moderate to marked (see Figs 12–1, 12–2, 12–4, and 12–7).[1] However, only minimal edema may be present (see Figs 12–3, 12–5, and 12–6), and when associated with an isodense mass on a precontrast scan, the metastasis may be difficult or impossible to detect without the use of contrast material (see Figs 12–5 and 12–6).

Certain metastatic tumors have a high propensity to bleed, and acute intracranial hemorrhage or a stroke-like clinical picture may be the initial neurologic presentation.[11] The most common metastases presenting with hemorrhage are metastatic choriocarcinoma, melanoma (see Fig 12–3), lung, and kidney.[11–13] The important differential diagnostic features from simple hemorrhage include an atypical location of the hemorrhage relative to that expected from aneurysm, arteriovenous malformation, or hypertension; contrast enhancement in the area of hemorrhage, particularly during the acute phase when delayed enhancement around a resolving hematoma would not be expected; and the multiplicity of lesions as seen on the enhanced scan (see Fig 12–3).[12]

Unless specific features such as hemorrhage are present that might help in defining a particular subgroup of metastatic lesions, it appears to be impossible to differentiate one source of metastatic tumor from another. This is true not only on the unenhanced scan, but on the contrast-enhanced study as well.[1] Likewise, it may be difficult to distinguish a solitary metastasis from a primary brain tumor. In one series, only 40% of single melanoma metastases had the characteristics most commonly associated with hematogenously disseminated tumor, including a round enhancing mass and moderate-to-marked edema. Many of the lesions had an appearance more typically associated with primary brain tumor, including less enhancement and edema than typically seen with metastatic tumor.[14] It may be difficult to distinguish a solitary metastasis from a meningioma, particularly if the metastatic tumor is based along the falx or if axial cuts through the high convexity show the mass is based along the inner table of the skull (Fig 12–8). Coronal cuts in such a case may be of value. Finally, differentiation of a solitary metastasis with a ring of enhancement from other lesions such as primary brain tumor, abscess, or a resolving hematoma may be impossible. For example, while it has been said that abscesses typically have a thin wall while tumors have a thicker, more irregular wall, metastatic tumors with a ring of enhancement have been seen having either a thick rim of enhancement (see Figs 12–2 and 12–4), or a thin rim (Fig 12–9) mimicking abscess. The differentiation in any given case may be extremely difficult or impossible. This subject will be discussed further in Chapter 13.

Metastatic tumors generally respect dural boundaries as they grow, similar to primary CNS parenchymal tumors. While a tumor may invade a dural structure, actual growth through that structure into contiguous parenchyma is rare. For example, the spread of metastatic tumor from one hemisphere to another does not usually occur through the falx, but requires passage through the corpus callosum. Rarely, a very aggressive metastatic neoplasm may grow through the falx to invade the contralateral hemisphere (see Fig 12–4). Periventricular spread of metastatic tumor may also occur, as with primary CNS tumors (see Fig 9–18).[15]

There is variable visualization of tumor metastases to the meninges to produce meningeal carcinomatosis without evidence of parenchymal metastases, depending upon the tumor type. In one series, 44% of patients with metastatic carcinoma had pathologic enhancement of the meninges; 100% of patients with metastatic melanoma had visualization; but there was visualization in only 3% of patients with proved meningeal involvement by leukemia and lymphoma.[16] Our experience has been that while meningeal thickening and enhancement *may* be seen in meningeal carcinomatosis, visualization of a CT abnormality is frequently indefinite, requiring cytologic evaluation of the CSF for diagnosis.

LYMPHOMA/LEUKEMIA

Cerebral involvement by systemic lymphoma usually is of the leptomeninges rather than the parenchyma, while primary malignant lymphoma of the brain (also

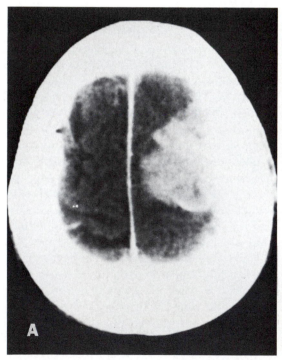
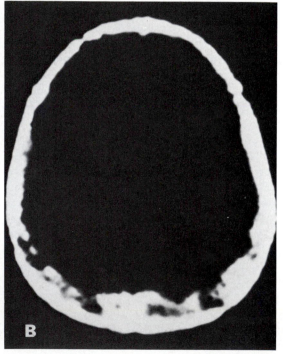

Fig 12–8.—Metastatic carcinoma of the prostate projecting into the cerebral parenchyma, simulating meningioma. The enhanced scan high over the convexity **(A)** demonstrates a well-circumscribed, homogeneously enhancing mass bordered along the inner table of the skull. The appearance could well represent meningioma. However, visualization of the calvarium with a wide window (bone window) as seen in **B** demonstrates multiple irregularities of the calvarium indicative of the multiple metastases to the skull by this carcinoma of the prostate. It may be difficult to differentiate a mass originating intracranially from one originating in the bone and projecting intracranially. Evaluation of the bony structures allows such differentiation.

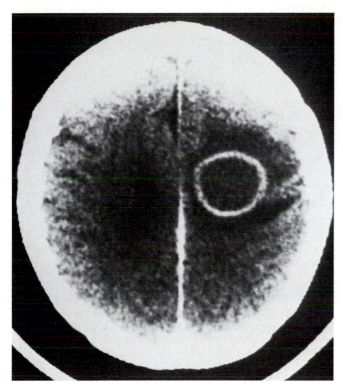

Fig 12–9.—Solitary metastasis with thin ring of enhancement from carcinoma of the lung. While many tumors have a thick, shaggy ring and while the thin ring is said to be typical of abscess, both primary and metastatic neoplasm may have a relatively thin ring.

called reticulum cell sarcoma or histiocytic lymphoma) is more common in the parenchyma, as discussed in Chapter 9.[17] Lymphoma, like leukemia, spreads along the leptomeninges, dipping into the Virchow-Robin spaces with the pial vasculature.[18] Occasionally, tumor may spread into the contiguous gray matter to form a parenchymal mass.[19] Movement of tumor cells via the CSF into the ventricular system will allow growth in subependymal locations and periventricular spread.[20]

Identification by CT scan of lymphomatous involvement of only the meninges, without parenchymal tumor, is unusual.[16, 18, 19] This is true even if a double dose of contrast material is utilized.[18] The parenchymal extensions of tumor are generally isodense or mildly hyperdense, relative to the surrounding brain on the precontrast scan, and enhance homogeneously (Figs 12–10 and 12–11).[18–20] The parenchymal masses are frequently multifocal with minimal surrounding edema (see Fig 12–10). This appearance of multiple lesions with minimal edema and margins that are less sharp than hematogenous metastases is different from that usually seen with hematogenous metastatic tumor and may suggest the appropriate diagnosis.

Leukemic involvement of the brain, like lymphoma, generally involves the leptomeninges with spread along the Virchow-Robin spaces, with only the occasional penetration into contiguous brain to form a focal leukemic mass ("chloroma"). With spread via CSF into the ventricular system, a chloroma may be present within the deep periventricular parenchyma (Fig 12–12).

Parenchymal leukemic deposits are generally isodense or of slight increased density on the nonenhanced scan and enhance homogeneously (Figs 12–12 and 12–13).[18, 21, 22] The borders of the enhancing mass may be relatively sharp,[21] but infiltration into surrounding parenchyma with irregular margination may also be present (Figs 12–12 to 12–14). Such irregular margination may allow differentiation of a solitary focus of leukemia (see Fig 12–14) from a solitary hematogenous metastasis (see Fig 12–2) when there is inadequate history of the type of systemic tumor.

The CT appearance of parenchymal involvement by lymphoma and leukemia is important to recognize relative to other pathologic conditions that occur in patients with these diseases, particularly cerebritis/abscess, hemorrhage, and infarction. Infarction is generally of low density on the precontrast scan, while the enhanced study shows peripheral enhancement, involvement of both gray and white matter, and a wedge-shaped configuration in a vascular distribution. Acute hemorrhage is dense without the use of contrast material, cerebritis is generally patchy in its enhancement pattern, and abscess usually is seen as a ring of enhancement. All of these CT appearances are different from the appearance of parenchymal involvement by either leukemia or lymphoma, and, in most cases, parenchymal involvement by tumor should be readily distinguished from these other complications.

METASTASES TO THE SKULL

Metastases to the bones of the skull in the adult age group may occur from a wide variety of tumors, with metastases from carcinoma of the breast, the prostate, and multiple myeloma being particularly common offenders.[23] The dural boundary is almost always respected by metastatic lesions, even when there is extensive bony involvement (Fig 12–15). Rarely, aggressive metastases may break through the dura to invade the brain (Fig 12–16). Carcinoma of the prostate frequently involves the calvarium and produces either a mixed lytic and blastic appearance (see Figs 12–8 and 12–16) or may produce an osteoblastic response that mimics the hyperostosis of meningioma.

Bone involvement in the pediatric age group is generally from neuroblastoma (Fig 12–17), lymphoma, leukemia, or any of the sarcomas.[23–25] Deposits of neuro-

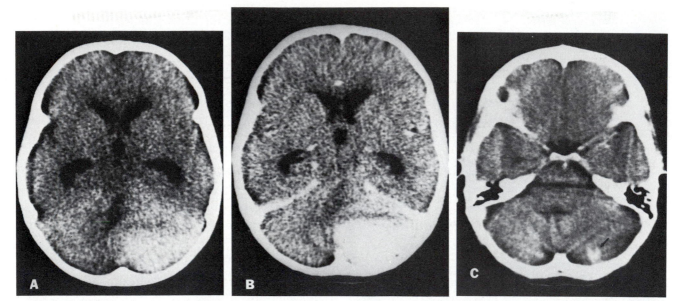

Fig 12–10.—Non-Hodgkin's lymphoma of the cerebellar hemisphere. The unenhanced scan **(A)** demonstrates a high-dense mass within the left cerebellar hemisphere, contiguous to the inner table of the left occipital bone, producing compression of the fourth ventricle and obstructive hydrocephalus. There is intense enhancement of the postinfusion study **(B).** Although of a high density on the unenhanced scan, the appearance is not typical of hemorrhage, because the mass was not as high dense as the typical hematoma, nor were the margins as sharp, and enhancement occurred, which is characteristic of neoplasm. This child had a history of diffuse systemic involvement with lymphoma, and the intracranial mass undoubtedly began in the meninges with spread into the contiguous cerebellum. Following radiation therapy, there has been a rapid diminution in the size of the cerebellar mass in only 10 days **(C),** with only a small tumor nodule remaining *(arrow).*

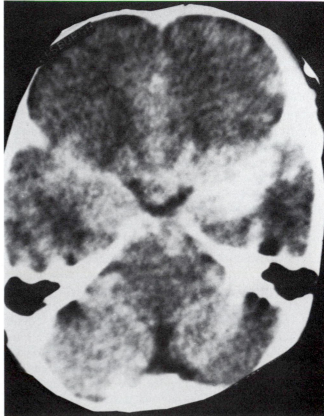

Fig 12–11.—Leptomeningeal lymphoma with spread into contiguous parenchyma. The enhanced scan at the base of the brain demonstrates extensive enhancing leptomeningeal deposits of lymphoma, which are spreading into the contiguous cerebral and cerebellar parenchyma.

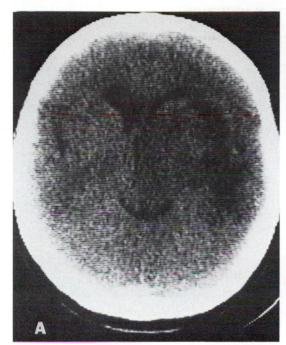
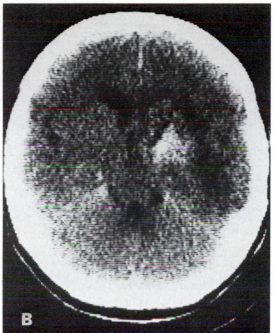

Fig 12–12.—Cerebral involvement with leukemia. This patient with a long history of leukemia presented with progressive right hemiparesis. The unenhanced CT scan **(A)** demonstrates edema in the medial left temporal lobe and basal ganglia, an isodense mass in the left basal ganglia, and mass effect on the left frontal horn and third ventricle. The enhanced scan **(B)** demonstrates homogeneous enhancement of the irregularly marginated deposit of leukemia.

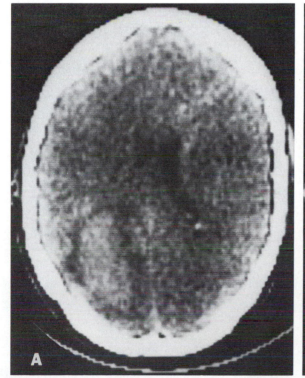
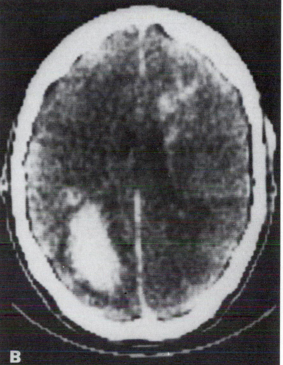

Fig 12–13.—Leukemic involvment of the brain (chloroma). The unenhanced scan **(A)** demonstrates a mass of moderate high density within the right parietal and occipital lobes, producing compression of the right lateral ventricle. There is also patchy density within the left frontal lobe. The enhanced scan **(B)** shows marked homogeneous enhancement of the right parieto-occipital leukemic deposit and enhancement of the patchy and infiltrating left frontal lobe deposit. There is also periventricular extension along the body of the left lateral ventricle.

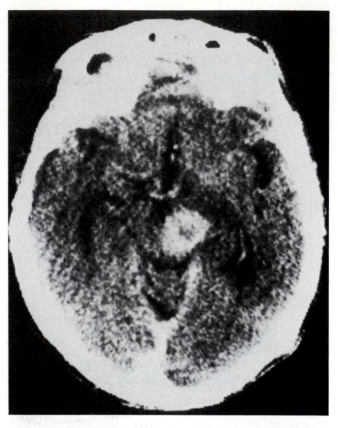

Fig 12–14.—Solitary leukemic deposit within the brain stem. A 70-year-old woman presented with progressive right-sided weakness, and the CT scan appearance of an enhancing mass within the left side of the upper brain stem. The irregular margination was not typical for a hematogenous metastasis to the brain stem, as in Figure 12–2, and systemic leukemia was subsequently discovered. The central lucency within this mass was not typical for a leukemic deposit, suggesting the possibility of an abscess. Stereotactic biopsy confirmed the diagnosis of a leukemic mass.

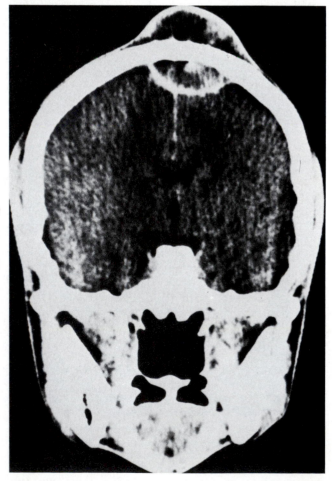

Fig 12–15.—Ewing's sarcoma metastasis to the calvarium with epidural deposit. The enhanced scan in the coronal projection demonstrates a mass in the left frontal bone, producing elevation of the scalp. There is extension of neoplasm into the epidural space with inferior displacement of the enhancing dura. The epidural location is denoted by intracranial tumor crossing the midline.

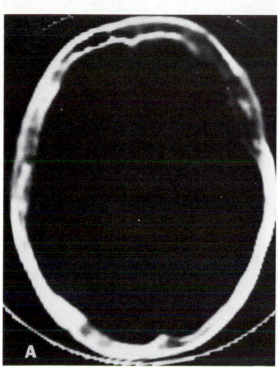

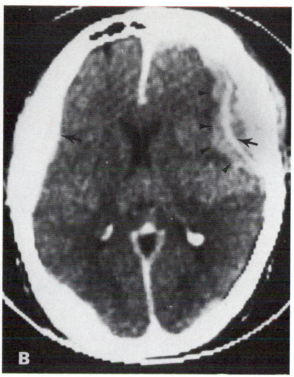

Fig 12–16.—Metastatic carcinoma of the prostate to the calvarium, with dural penetration. The axial scan with a wide window (bone window) **(A)** demonstrates multiple areas of bone destruction involving the calvarium, most prominent in the frontal regions bilaterally. The enhanced scan of the head with windowing for the cerebral parenchyma **(B)** shows elevation of the dura (arrows) in the regions of the bone destruction, indicative of epidural extension of tumor. This aggressive neoplasm has penetrated the dura on the left, with spread into the contiguous cerebral parenchyma (arrowheads).

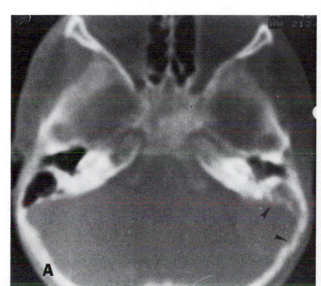

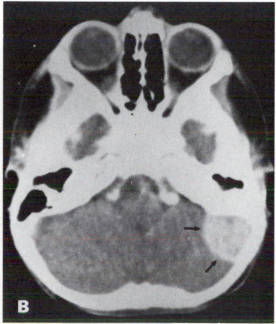

Fig 12–17.—Metastatic neuroblastoma to the left petrous and occipital bones. Neuroblastoma has metastasized to the left petrous and occipital bones (arrowheads, **A**), best seen on an image with wide window. The epidural mass projects into the region of the left cerebellar hemisphere as seen on the enhanced scan **(B)**, displacing the dura (arrows) ahead of it.

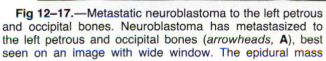

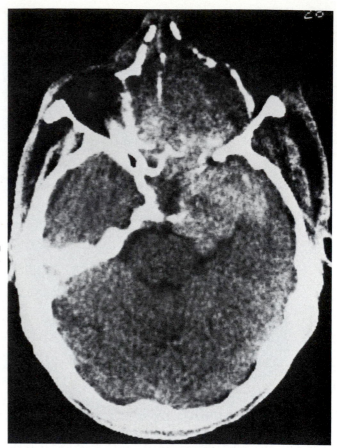

Fig 12–18.—Carcinoma of the palate with extensive intracranial extension. This nonenhanced scan demonstrates extensive neoplasm producing bone destruction in the face. There is destruction of the anterior portion of the base of the skull, with extension of dense tumor into the left middle cranial fossa. There is destruction of the left lateral wall of the sphenoid sinus and growth of tumor as far posteriorly as the brain stem.

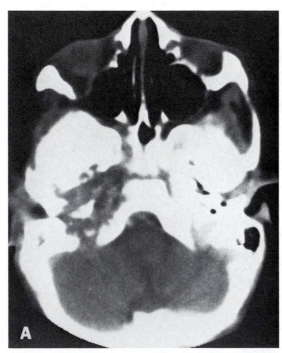
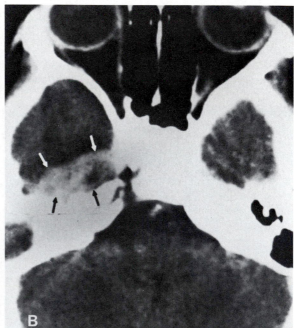

Fig 12–19.—Rhabdomyoscarcoma of the nasopharynx with extension into the middle and posterior cranial fossae. This 3-year-old child with previous treatment for rhabdomyosarcoma of the nasopharynx presented with palsies of the right fifth through twelfth cranial nerves. The scan at the base of the skull **(A)** demonstrates extensive bone destruction involving the base of the skull on the right, right petrous and temporal bones, and the right side of the body of the sphenoid bone. The enhanced intracranial scan **(B)** demonstrates a large focal tumor within the inferior and posterior portion of the right temporal fossa *(arrows)*. There was undoubtedly parameningeal extension of tumor, as well, to produce the lower cranial nerve palsies.

276

blastoma may spread along the epidural spaces to the cranial sutures, producing focal erosions of those sutures that simulate the split sutures of increased intracranial pressure.[24, 25]

Certain tumors that begin in the soft tissues of the upper neck and face have a propensity to extend through the neural foramina or directly through the bony base of the skull to produce intracranial deposits (Fig 12–18). Metastases to the base of the skull from more distant sources may likewise produce epidural deposits of tumor displacing neural structures. In the child, extracranial rhabdomyosarcoma, neuroblastoma, lymphoma, and histiocytosis X may produce bone destruction and an enhancing intracranial mass (Fig 12–19); in general, the various tumors cannot be distinguished on CT scan alone.[26] In our institution, any patient who presents with a tumor of the upper neck or face requires CT scanning of the head to evaluate the possibility of parameningeal involvement. Such in-

volvement will alter the therapeutic regimen, with the addition of radiation therapy to the cranial cavity or intrathecal chemotherapy.

Benign tumors may also extend intracranially if they erode the bones of the base of the skull. For example, angiofibroma of the nasopharynx frequently extends laterally into the subtemporal fossa or into the sphenoid sinus. Erosion of the lateral walls of the sphenoid sinus or of the bony margins of the temporal fossa will allow tumor to extend into the middle cranial fossa (Fig 12–20).

SPREAD OF NEOPLASM THROUGH CSF PATHWAYS

Many primary and secondary tumors involving the cerebral parenchyma may be seeded to other portions of the brain via CSF pathways. Any tumor that extends to a cortical or ventricular surface will have access to

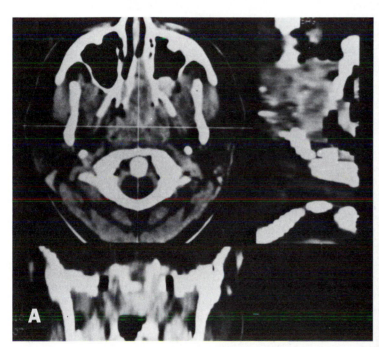

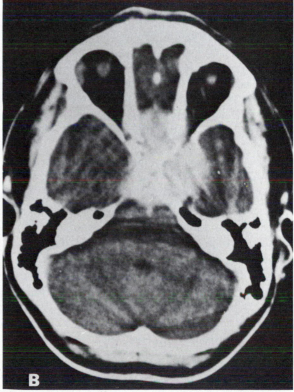

Fig 12–20.—Angiofibroma of the nasopharynx with intracranial extension. Photo **A** is a composite figure, with the axial scan through the nasopharynx located in the top left of the figure, the coronal reformatted image located below this, and the sagittal reformation located to the right. The sagittal image has been turned 90°, so that the face is toward the top of the page. The figure demonstrates a large nasopharyngeal mass extending into the left nasal cavity. There is extensive destruction of the sphenoid bone and planum sphenoidale, with a large component of tumor intracranially.

The axial enhanced scan **(B)** shows the extensive enhancing angiofibroma within the sphenoid body and region of the sella, both temporal fossae, and extension below the frontal lobes. The mass also extends as far posteriorly as the basilar artery. A combined extracranial and intracranial approach allowed displacement of tumor into the nasopharyngeal wound with complete removal of this benign neoplasm. (Courtesy of Daniel Bursick, M.D., Mercy Hospital, Pittsburgh.)

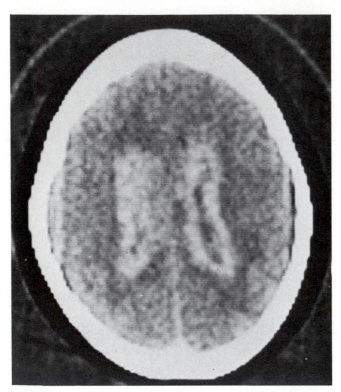

Fig 12–21.—Pineal region germinoma with periventricular spread of tumor. There is extensive enhancement of periventricular tumor in this patient with previous therapy for pineal region germinoma.

the CSF, with the potential for seeding of tumor cells. Malignant tumors based around the ventricular system have a greater propensity to produce such internal metastases. Of the primary CNS tumors, medulloblastoma, ependymoma, and glioblastoma frequently produce meningeal seeding as denoted by meningeal enhancement on the contrast-enhanced CT scan (see Fig 9–36). There may be extension of this leptomeningeal tumor through the cortical surface to produce a focal parenchymal mass. Multiple foci of glioblastoma may result from seeding of this type (see Fig 9–3), although multiple focal masses can result from the spread of fingers of tumor through the parenchyma (see Figs 9–8 and 9–9). Occasionally, primary multifocal glioblastoma occurs. The distinction of this entity from spread of a single tumor requires pathologic confirmation of separate lesions not connected by fingers of tumor and the placement of the second tumor away from the cortical surface, where spread via CSF pathways would have placed the lesion.[27]

Metastatic tumors may also spread via CSF pathways. Penetration of the leptomeninges may produce a focal parenchymal mass, as previously demonstrated with lymphoma and leukemia (see Figs 12–10 to 12–14).

Periventricular spread of tumor occurs with many malignant primary and metastatic tumors (Figs 9–18 and 12–21). Tumor invades the brain to reach the subependymal tissues, with spread of tumor along the ventricular margins. Scanning by CT demonstrates a dense rim of enhancement around the ventricles (see Figs 9–18 and 12–21) and may also demonstrate the focal mass or masses of the primary or hematogeneously disseminated metastatic tumor. The major differential consideration is ventriculitis, with an easy clinical distinction between these two entities in most cases. Periventricular spread of tumor is generally an ominous sign, even when the patient appears to be unchanged neurologically.[15]

REFERENCES

1. Potts D.G., Albott G.F., von Sneidern J.V.: National Cancer Institute study: Evaluation of computed tomography in the diagnosis of intracranial neoplasms: III. Metastatic tumors. *Radiology* 136:657–664, 1980.
2. Weiss H.D., Richardson E.P.: Solitary brainstem metastasis. *Neurology* 28:562–566, 1978.
3. Healy J.F., Rosenkrantz H.: Intraventricular metastases demonstrated by cranial computed tomography. *Radiology* 136:124, 1980.
4. Deck M.D.F., Messina A.V., Sackett J.F.: Computed tomography in metastatic disease of the brain. *Radiology* 119:115–120, 1976.
5. Danzinger J., Wallace S., Handel S.F., et al.: Metastatic osteogenic sarcoma to the brain. *Cancer* 43:707–710, 1979.
6. Gouliamos A.D., Jimenez J.P., Goree G.A.: Computed tomography and skull radiology in the diagnosis of calcified brain tumor. *A.J.R.* 130:761–764, 1978.
7. Hayman L.A., Evans R.A., Hinch V.C.: Delayed high iodine dose contrast computed tomography: Cranial neoplasms. *Radiology* 136:677–684, 1980.
8. Shalen P.R., Hayman L.A., Wallace S., et al.: Protocol for delayed contrast enhancement in computed tomography of cerebral neoplasia. *Radiology* 139:397–402, 1981.
9. Dublin A.B., Norman D.: Fluid-fluid level in cystic cerebral metastatic melanoma. *J. Comput. Assist. Tomogr.* 3:650–652, 1979.
10. Whelan M.A., Ascherl G.F., Schlesinger E.B.: Cerebellar metastases from ovarian carcinoma. *J. Comput. Assist. Tomogr.* 5:583–585, 1981.
11. Mandybur T.I.: Intracranial hemorrhage caused by metastatic tumors. *Neurology* 27:650–655, 1977.
12. Gildersleeve N. Jr., Koo A.H., McDonald C.J.: Metastatic tumor presenting as intracerebral hemorrhage. *Radiology* 124:109–112, 1977.
13. Ginoldi S., Wallace S., Shalen P., et al.: Cranial computed tomography of malignant melanoma. *A.J.N.R.* 1:531–535, 1980.
14. Enzmann D.R., Kramer R., Norman D., et al.: Malignant melanoma metastatic to the central nervous system. *Radiology* 127:177–180, 1978.

15. McGeachie R.E., Gold L.H.A., Latchaw R.E.: Periventricular spread of tumor demonstrated by computed tomography. *Radiology* 125:407–411, 1977.
16. Enzmann D.R., Krikorian J., Yoke C., et al.: Computed tomography in leptomeningeal spread of tumor. *J. Comput. Assist. Tomogr.* 2:448–455, 1978.
17. Enzmann D.R., Krikorian J., Norman D., et al.: Computed tomography in primary reticulum cell sarcoma of brain. *Radiology* 130:165–170, 1979.
18. Pagani J.J., Libshitz H.I., Wallace S., et al.: Central nervous system leukemia and lymphoma: Computed tomographic manifestations. *A.J.N.R.* 2:397–403, 1981.
19. Brandt-Zawadzki M., Enzmann D.R.: Computed tomographic brain scanning in patients with lymphoma. *Radiology* 129:67–71, 1978.
20. Dubois P.J., Martinez A.J., Myerowitz R.L., et al.: Subependymal and leptomeningeal spread of systemic malignant lymphoma demonstrated by cranial computed tomography. *J. Comput. Assist. Tomogr.* 2:217–221, 1978.
21. Wendling L.R., Cromwell L.D., Latchaw R.E.: Computed tomography of intracerebral leukemic masses. *A.J.R.* 132:217–220, 1979.
22. Sauers J.J., Moody D.M., Naidich T.P., et al.: Radiographic features of granulocytic sarcoma (chloroma). *J. Comput. Assist. Tomogr.* 3:226–233, 1979.
23. Healy J.F., Marshall W.H., Brahme P.J., et al.: CT of intracranial metastases with skull and scalp involvement. *A.J.N.R.* 2:335–338, 1981.
24. Latchaw R.E., L'Heureux P.R., Young G., et al.: Neuroblastoma presenting as central nervous system disease. *A.J.N.R.* 3:623–630, 1982.
25. Chirathivat S., Post M.J.D.: CT demonstration of dural metastases in neuroblastoma. *J. Comput. Assist. Tomogr.* 4:316–319, 1980.
26. Scotti G., Harwood-Nash D.C.: Computed tomography of rhabdomyosarcoma of the skull base in children. *J. Comput. Assist. Tomogr.* 6:33–39, 1982.
27. Kieffer S.A., Salibi N.A., Kim R.E., et al.: Multifocal glioblastoma: Diagnostic implications. *Radiology* 143:709–710, 1982.

13

Differential Diagnosis of Intracranial Tumors

RICHARD E. LATCHAW, M.D.

TWO ASPECTS of the differential diagnosis of cerebral neoplasms utilizing CT scan characteristics will be emphasized in this chapter: first, those characteristics that help in distinguishing one type of tumor from another; second, those characteristics that are of value in distinguishing a neoplasm from a nonneoplastic process. No one CT scan characteristic can be utilized in differentiating one type of tumor from another, nor in separating neoplastic from nonneoplastic processes. However, a combination of findings will generally give a high probability in the diagnosis of a particular neoplasm. While biopsy will always be necessary to insure the appropriate diagnosis, the prediction of neoplasm, and usually a specific type of tumor, can be made preoperatively in the majority of cases.

CT SCAN CHARACTERISTICS FOR DIFFERENTIATING TUMOR TYPES

The four most common tumor types have been selected for analysis and evaluation according to their CT scan characteristics. The tumors compared and contrasted are the benign astrocytoma, malignant astrocytoma/glioblastoma multiforme, meningioma, and hematogenous metastasis. The CT scan characteristics include the density before contrast enhancement, the degree and homogeneity of enhancement, the speed of that enhancement and the sharpness of the tumor margins following enhancement, and the degree of peritumoral edema and mass effect (Table 13–1). The characteristics for any one specific tumor are obviously generalizations, and exceptions will always be found. In addition, each generalization concerns the usual supratentorial tumor in an adult. For example, a low-grade astrocytoma of the cerebellum in a child may enhance to a rather marked degree and be homogeneous in appearance, whereas most low-grade supratentorial astrocytomas in the adult enhance only to a slight degree, with that enhancement patchy in nature. In addition,

there is a subset of astrocytomas that are of a purely decreased density without evidence of enhancement, but are varied in degree of histologic malignancy. These tumors likewise are exceptions to the generalizations in this chapter. Of all the neuroectodermal tumors, only the benign and malignant astrocytomas are considered in this evaluation. Other neuroectodermal tumors such as oligodendroglioma, medulloblastoma, ependymoma, ganglioglioma, and primary intracranial neuroblastoma have CT scan characteristics that are sufficiently different from the generalizations given that they cannot be included in this discussion. The specific appearances of these latter tumors are described more fully in Chapter 9. The congenital tumors and associated neoplasms discussed in Chapter 11 are sufficiently uncommon and have specific radiographic or clinical findings (age, position of the tumor, fatty density, associated clinical manifestations) so that they usually do not enter into the differential diagnosis of the four major classes of neoplasms to be herein compared and contrasted. Finally, lymphoma or leukemic deposits in the brain may have an appearance identical to neuroectodermal or metastatic tumors, and it may be impossible to distinguish them without further clinical data or without biopsy. In summary, this evaluation of the differential diagnostic features emphasizes the four most common types of neoplasms seen in the adult, with an emphasis on their most typical appearance on the CT scan. The generalization for each CT scan characteristic is listed in Table 13–1; only brief additional comments are given below.

Density Before Contrast Enhancement

Distinction must be made between the actual tumor itself and the peritumoral edema surrounding the lesion. It is admitted that the low density surrounding an actual tumor mass is called "edema," whereas it most likely represents a combination of actual edema and infiltrating tumor in many cases (see Chapter 9). Never-

TABLE 13–1.—DIFFERENTIAL DIAGNOSTIC FEATURES OF CEREBRAL NEOPLASMS

CHARACTERISTIC	SUPRATENTORIAL ASTROCYTOMA	MALIGNANT ASTROCYTOMA/ GLIOBLASTOMA	MENINGIOMA	HEMATOGENOUS METASTASIS
Density without contrast	Decreased to isodense, mixed	Variable: decreased to increased, mixed	*Isodense to increased, homogeneous	Variable: decreased to increased
Calcification	Common	Uncommon, unless malignant degeneration of benign astrocytoma	Frequent	Uncommon
Hemorrhage	Rare	Common	Rare	Common in certain metastases
Degree of enhancement	*None to moderate	Moderate to marked	Marked	Moderate to marked
Homogeneity of enhancement	Usually patchy	Patchy, ring	Homogeneous	Homogeneous or ring
Enhancement over time	*Slow	Moderate to rapid, ring may fill in	Rapid	Moderate to rapid, ring may fill in
Tumor margins after contrast	Irregular, poorly defined	Mixed: sharp, irregular	Sharp	Sharp
Edema	Minimal	Abundant	Minimal	Abundant
Mass effect	Variable: none to moderate	Moderate to marked	Variable: slight to moderate	Frequently marked

*Denotes significant differential characteristic.

theless, when describing the CT scan characteristics of a lesion, it is helpful to make the distinction between a relatively well-circumscribed mass, which itself may be either homogeneous or patchy in its density, and the surrounding low density, which will be called edema.

The precontrast scan may be helpful in differential diagnosis if a tumor of isodensity to hyperdensity is seen. As seen in Table 13–1, benign and malignant astrocytomas and hematogenous metastases are variable in density on the precontrast scan, whereas meningiomas tend to be isodense to hyperdense; in particular, the meningioma has a homogeneous appearance (see Fig 10–1). If there is a large amount of edema surrounding the meningioma, the appearance may be similar to a hematogenous metastasis, which may also have a relatively homogeneous tumor nodule on the preinfusion scan (see Fig 12–1) and a large amount of surrounding edema. The presence of diffuse low density tends to exclude the diagnosis of meningioma.

Calcification

Calcification is a rather nonspecific finding and may be seen with many neuroectodermal tumors, even the more malignant varieties such as in long-standing astrocytomas that undergo malignant degeneration. Calcification is also common in meningiomas. Calcification is uncommon in most metastases, although certain metastatic tumors such as osteogenic sarcoma and adenocarcinoma of the gastrointestinal tract may have well-defined foci of calcification. In addition, the increased density in some metastatic tumors is said to be on the basis of either hemorrhage or punctate, microscopic calcification.

Hemorrhage

Hemorrhage is distinctly rare in meningioma or benign astrocytoma, but is relatively common in malignant neoplasms as they rapidly outgrow their blood supply (see Figs 9–17 and 12–3). The presence of hemorrhage tends to exclude a diagnosis of either benign astrocytoma or meningioma.

Degree of Enhancement

Malignant astrocytoma/glioblastoma (see Fig 9–3), meningioma (see Fig 10–1), and many metastatic tumors (see Fig 12–5) enhance to a marked degree. On the other hand, benign astrocytoma tends to have a relatively intact blood-brain barrier, and therefore there is a degree of enhancement that varies from none to minimal in a large number of cases (see Figs 9–1 and 9–2), with moderate enhancement in a few of the cases. Again, one must realize that many low-grade astrocytomas, particularly those in children, may have a moderate-to-marked degree of enhancement (see Figs 9–19 and 9–29).

Homogeneity of Enhancement

The texture of enhancement is frequently a helpful finding in distinguishing the four types of tumors. Benign astrocytomas tend to be patchy in their enhancement pattern (see Figs 9–1 and 9–2), whereas malignant astrocytomas and glioblastomas vary from a patchy appearance (Fig 9–4) to a relatively well-circumscribed although irregular appearance (see Figs 9–8 and 9–9). The ring of enhancement is common with glioblastoma (see Fig 9–3), with irregular margins of the ring being characteristic. Meningiomas are almost always homogeneous in their enhancement pattern (see Fig 10–1), although up to 14% of meningiomas may have unusual appearances such as hemorrhage, cyst formation, or irregular margins.[1] Hematogenous metastatases usually have either a homogeneous (see Fig 12–1) or a ring type of enhancement (see Fig 12–2).

It should also be stressed that the homogeneity of enhancement may be in part time-dependent. A ring lesion may partially fill in over time, and this has been seen with both primary gliomas and metastatic lesions.[2–4]

In summary, the heterogeneity of enhancement excludes meningioma; the presence of a ring of enhancement tends to exclude benign astrocytoma; and patchy enhancement tends to exclude most hematogenous metastases and meningioma.

Evaluation Over Time

This CT scan characteristic depends upon the serial observations of the neoplasm over time, with an evaluation of the changing attenuation coefficients. Early studies by Hatam and coworkers[5] suggested that tumor diagnosis may be facilitated by such serial observation. Graphic representation of the enhancement pattern of various tumors demonstrated that relatively vascular meningiomas and metastases enhance quickly, while gliomas tend to enhance over a slower period of time. Unfortunately, these early studies relied upon relatively slow scanners. Follow-up studies to this early work have been uncommon.[6] With the advent of dynamic scanning, there is again a chance for the study of the dynamics of tumor enhancement, which may prove helpful in the differential diagnosis of the various classes of tumors.

In general, benign astrocytomas tend to enhance relatively slower over time than their more malignant counterparts. The enhancement of a metastatic lesion depends upon the degree of alteration of the blood-brain barrier, which is variable with different metastatic tumors. The rings of both malignant astrocytomas and hematogenous metastases may fill in over time as previously indicated. Finally, extra-axial tumors such as meningiomas, schwannomas, and pituitary tumors all appear to lack a blood-brain barrier, but all enhance rapidly with the movement of contrast material across the blood-tissue interface. Meningiomas tend to have a relatively rapid clearance of that enhancement, while the clearance may be slower in schwannomas.[6]

Tumor Margins

Most hematogenous metastases tend to be sharply demarcated on the enhanced scan, with a sharp margin separating the actual tumor nodule from the peritumoral edema (see Fig 12–2). The same is true of meningiomas (see Fig 10–1). Malignant astrocytomas and glioblastomas may have either an irregular enhancing margin (see Fig 9–4) or a relatively sharp margin (see Fig 9–7), particularly when a ring of enhancement is present (see Fig 9–3). That ring is generally irregular in contour, as opposed to nonneoplastic rings of enhancement such as is found in abscess. Finally, benign astrocytomas generally have poorly defined, irregular margins, as the tumor blends imperceptibly into the surrounding parenchyma (see Figs 9–1 and 9–2).

Edema

It must be stressed again that the low density surrounding a tumor mass is referred to as "edema," while it must be recognized from pathologic studies[7] that the low densities surrounding a more malignant tumor usually represent a combination of edema and poorly enhancing malignant fingers of tumor. In general, however, most benign astrocytomas have minimal surrounding edema because of the relatively intact blood-brain barrier, whereas there is usually abundant edema surrounding the malignant glial tumor. Likewise, the edema surrounding metastatic tumors is generally abundant. Peritumoral edema surrounding meningioma is extremely variable. The "classic" appearance is that of minimal edema (see Fig 10–2), whereas up to 47% of meningiomas may have a moderate or occasionally even marked degree of peritumoral edema (see Fig 10–6).[8]

Mass Effect

The amount of mass effect from the malignant tumors, whether of a primary glial or metastatic origin, tends to be moderate to marked, secondary to the amount of peritumoral edema that is present. Benign astrocytomas may have a mass effect that varies from none to moderate, depending upon the amount of associated edema and the size of the lesion. Relatively infiltrating astrocytomas may have no mass effect and only patchy enhancement (see Figs 9–1 and 9–2) and may therefore represent a major diagnostic problem. Meningiomas grow very slowly, frequently indenting the brain and causing little diffuse mass effect, even when a very large tumor is present. Peritumoral edema may be moderate to marked, however, with that edema occurring very quickly in some cases. The reason for this rapid accumulation of edema fluid with meningioma is unknown, but may produce a marked degree of mass effect and rapid neurologic change (see Chapter 10).

Summary

It can be seen from Table 13–1 and the generalizations described that no one feature of the CT scan appearances of these four major classes of intracranial tumors is sufficient for distinguishing the tumor type.

Rather, it is generally a combination of features that points to the correct diagnosis. The salient features for each tumor type can be listed as follows:

1. *Benign astrocytoma:* Hypodense or isodense lesion with inhomogeneous and patchy texture before enhancement; may be calcified, but no evidence of hemorrhage; slight-to-moderate enhancement occurring slowly and giving a nonhomogeneous appearance with poor visualization of the margins; slight or no edema and mild mass effect.

2. *Malignant astrocytoma/glioblastoma:* Inhomogeneously low-to-isodense lesion without calcification, but possibly hemorrhagic on the unenhanced scan; moderate-to-marked enhancement occurring in a moderate period of time, but producing an inhomogeneous texture and frequently a ring of enhancement; margins are frequently sharply defined, particularly when a ring is present, although margins are ragged in contour; moderate surrounding edema and mass effect.

3. *Meningioma:* Homogeneously isodense-to-slightly-hyperdense lesion on the nonenhanced scan, frequently containing calcifications, but no blood; rapid, marked, and homogeneous enhancement; sharp margination with little-to-mild surrounding edema and mass effect.

4. *Hematogenous metastasis:* Variable density before contrast; may have hemorrhage, but no focal calcification; enhancement in a moderate period of time, and to a moderate or marked degree; texture is usually either homogeneous or a ring, with sharp margination and abundant surrounding edema.

CT SCAN CHARACTERISTICS DIFFERENTIATING NEOPLASTIC FROM NONNEOPLASTIC LESIONS

The major disease categories to be differentiated from cerebral neoplasm are infarction; inflammatory lesions including infection, noninfectious granulomatous disease such as sarcoidosis, and demyelinating disease; aneurysm and arteriovenous malformation (AVM); radiation necrosis; and nonneoplastic mass such as arachnoid cyst. The specific CT scan features of infarction, inflammatory lesions, and aneurysms/AVM are presented elsewhere in this volume. Radiation necrosis is discussed more fully in this chapter, while arachnoid cyst has been extensively discussed in Chapter 22. The emphasis in this section is on those features that are helpful in distinguishing neoplastic from nonneoplastic lesions.

Infarction

Neoplasms are included in the differential diagnosis of lesions producing cerebrovascular symptoms. While the rapid onset of symptoms in a particular vascular distribution generally suggests thrombosis, embolism, or hemorrhage, a mass lesion such as neoplasm or subdural hematoma may occasionally produce a sudden change in neurologic status and therefore mimic a vascular lesion.[9] In such a case, the appearance of the lesion on the CT scan will generally distinguish neoplasm from infarction.

Infarction involves the gray matter in almost all cases, and a combination of gray and white matter in two thirds of cases.[10] Gliomas and hematogenous metastases involve the deep gray matter, white matter, or gray/white interface, with relative sparing of the cortex itself. Meningiomas may indent the cortex, but do not destroy superficial gray matter, and the appearance is distinctly different from that of infarct.

Infarcts are classically wedge shaped, in a vascular distribution, and have peripheral and nonhomogeneous enhancement. This enhancement is at the margin of viable tissue where there is still a blood-brain barrier, albeit damaged, whereas the central portion of the infarct has undergone necrosis. Both primary and secondary neoplasms may have a rim of enhancement (see Figs 9–3, 9–6, and 12–4), and at times the peripheral enhancement of an infarct (see Fig 5–14) may simulate the ring enhancement of a neoplasm. However, the peripheral enhancement of an infarct is generally an incomplete ring, and this finding in combination with the position of the lesion in a vascular distribution and the clinical history will differentiate infarction from neoplasm in the overwhelming majority of cases.

Inflammatory Lesions

Within the broad category of inflammatory lesions are included infection by viral, bacterial, and mycobacterial agents; noninfectious granulomatous disease such as sarcoidosis; and demyelinating disease such as multiple sclerosis.

Infection

When discussing infection, a distinction must be made between cerebritis and abscess. Cerebritis is a diffuse encephalitic process with poor margins and irregular enhancement (Fig 13–1) that may go on to frank abscess formation with relatively sharp margins and the appearance of a ring lesion (Fig 13–2). It may be extremely difficult to distinguish cerebritis from a diffuse infiltrating neoplasm. In both, irregular borders and heterogeneous density, both with and without contrast enhancement, may be present. The distinction between cerebritis and infarction may likewise be extremely difficult, and the correct distinction between infiltrating neoplasm, cerebritis, and infarction may depend upon the patient's history, clinical findings, and the progression of the lesion. Biopsy may be mandatory in early stages for appropriate diagnosis.

Likewise, it may be impossible to distinguish abscess

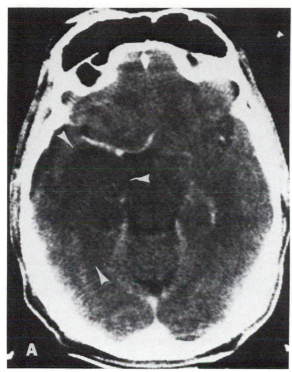 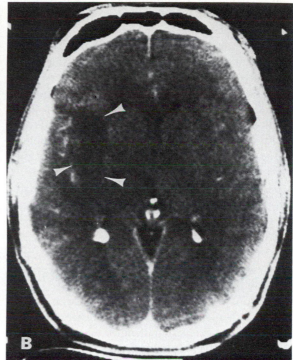

Fig 13–1.—Herpes encephalitis of the right temporal lobe. The lower enhanced axial scan **(A)** demonstrates a poorly marginated area of moderate decreased density and no enhancement *(white arrowheads)* involving the inferior portion of the right temporal lobe. There is some anterior displacement of the middle cerebral artery. A higher cut **(B)** demonstrates a more sharply circumscribed area of low density *(arrowheads)* within the superior right temporal lobe. Intracellular inclusion bodies typical of herpes simplex encephalitis were found by stereotactic biopsy (scans performed in stereotactic frame).

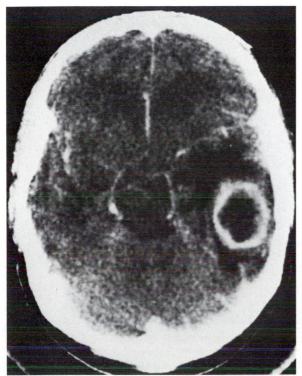

Fig 13–2.—Left temporal lobe abscess. The enhanced axial scan demonstrates the classic ring of enhancement within this left temporal lobe abscess. There is abundant surrounding edema and a moderately irregular and shaggy rim.

with its ring formation from either primary malignant glioma or metastatic tumor. Many abscesses have sharp inner margins to the ring of enhancement, while the inner margin of a necrotic tumor is frequently shaggy. However, utilization of the appearance of the ring alone frequently leads to a wrong diagnosis. Abscesses may be seen to have relatively shaggy margins (see Fig 13–2), while both primary and secondary neoplasms may have sharply marginated rings (see Figs 9–6 and 12–9). The appearance of the ring of an abscess is time dependent, with a more shaggy margination occurring in the early stages of abscess formation. The sharp margination of the ring of a neoplasm is indicative of its cystic nature. In any given case, the distinction between abscess and tumor may be impossible. The clinical history, including the rapidity of progression and the presence of extracranial infection, may be necessary for appropriate diagnosis. Biopsy and drainage under CT control may be both diagnostic and therapeutic.

Tuberculous involvement of the cerebral parenchyma varies from the ring enhancement of an abscess to the solid nodule of a tuberculoma. In addition, there may be a diffuse meningitis, particularly at the base of the brain, characterized by meningeal enhancement. It is said that a tuberculous abscess frequently has thick, irregular walls, and is multilocular, whereas bacterial abscesses classically have thinner walls;[11] in such a case, distinguishing tuberculous abscess from primary or metastatic tumor would probably be impossible on the CT scan alone. Tuberculomas may be isodense before contrast enhancement, with either a homogeneous or a ring appearance produced on the postinfusion scan.[12] Calcification may or may not be present to help in distinguishing such a nodule from metastatic tumor.

Sarcoid

Up to 14% of patients with systemic sarcoidosis will have meningeal or parenchymal deposits of sarcoid. Meningeal involvement is more common, with parenchymal involvement usually being peripheral as a result of spread of the lesion through the meninges. The CT scan appearance will therefore vary from only meningeal enhancement similar to meningitis or meningeal carcinomatosis of any form to a peripheral parenchymal mass lesion that enhances homogeneously and mimics many other types of neoplasms.[13–16] Multiple deposits may be present (Fig 13–3), simulating diffuse metastatic disease.[15] The combination of meningeal and peripheral parenchymal involvement of a homogeneous nature is also found in lymphoma and leukemia (see Figs 12–10 to 12–14), and distinction from sarcoid probably cannot be made without a history of the particular systemic disease or biopsy.

Demyelinating Disease

The most common demyelinating disease is multiple sclerosis, which is usually characterized by a long history of waxing and waning of neurologic symptoms, in-

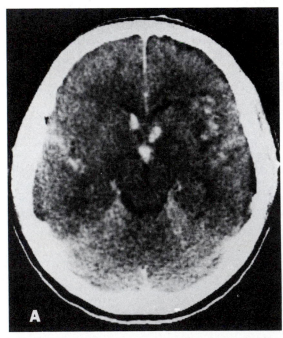 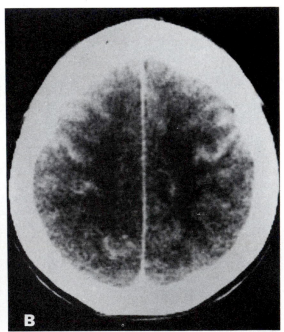

Fig 13–3.—Meningeal and parenchymal sarcoid. The lower cut **(A)** demonstrates multiple nodular deposits of sarcoid in the region of the left hypothalamus, right caudate nucleus, and third ventricle. There is a propensity for sarcoid involvement of the hypothalamus, pituitary, and basal ganglia. There are also further deposits of sarcoid in the temporal lobes bilaterally. A higher scan **(B)** demonstrates multiple areas of gyral enhancement, similar to the appearance of leptomeningeal neoplasm or pyogenic meningitis.

cluding blurred vision, ataxia, incoordination, and slurred speech. The presence of periventricular lucencies on the CT scan (see Fig 8–1) and enlargement of sulci are typical of such a classic presentation. Some of these plaques may enhance with contrast material during an acute exacerbation, representing a transient breakdown of the blood-brain barrier (see Figs 8–3 and 8–4). Enhancement of multiple nodules may suggest a diagnosis of metastases in a case without the typical clinical history, although the location of the periventricular nodular enhancement is so typical of multiple sclerosis that this diagnosis should be entertained.

Occasionally, a previously normal patient will present with a solitary enhancing lesion on the CT scan, accompanying the acute onset of neurologic symptoms. That lesion may have heterogeneous enhancement with irregular borders, thereby simulating either a primary neoplasm or a solitary metastases (see Fig 8–5). In such a case, the correct diagnosis at the time of initial scan may be impossible. High gamma globulin levels in the CSF or subtle historical points such as transient visual blurring may give a hint to the correct diagnosis. Serial CT scans will show a change in the appearance of the lesion as it undergoes remission. Corticosteroids may hasten that remission, and although the amount of edema and the degree of enhancement of a neoplasm will decrease with the use of corticosteroids, discontinuing the corticosteroids will allow visualization of the neoplasm in time, whereas the lesion of multiple sclerosis may go into remission. Therefore, in suggestive cases, a trial of corticosteroids may be of benefit before undertaking biopsy.

Other forms of demyelinating disease may present with acute symptomatology and enhancing lesions that simulate neoplasms (see Fig 8–7). Bilateral frontal lobe lesions with involvement of the corpus callosum may be present, simulating a "butterfly glioma."[17] While some of these lesions may be part of the spectrum found in adrenoleukodystrophy or progressive multifocal leukoencephalopathy, the history and pathologic findings may be insufficient for any diagnosis other than nonspecific demyelinating disease.

Aneurysm and AVM

A giant aneurysm presents as a mass, with a well-circumscribed, homogeneously enhancing density (see Figs 4–7 and 4–8). The presence of the lesion in the distribution of one of the major cerebral blood vessels may arouse suspicion for the presence of an aneurysm. Laminated clot may be present within the aneurysm so that there is only peripheral enhancement, representing relative vascularity of the wall of the aneurysm, or a central nodule of enhancement, representing the persistent patent lumen of the aneurysm surrounded by laminated clot (see Figs 4–3 and 4–6). Calcification of

the wall of the aneurysm may also be present (see Figs 4–10 and 4–11). A parasellar aneurysm that is dense before the administration of contrast material because of the presence of the "blood pool," which does not have calcification in the wall and which enhances homogeneously, will simulate a meningioma or trigeminal schwannoma (see Figs 10–17 and 10–18). In such cases, a dynamic CT scan may be of help, demonstrating rapid opacification of the aneurysm as opposed to slower opacification even in such vascular neoplasms as meningioma and schwannoma.

The classic AVM has large serpiginous and curvilinear densities representing the feeding arteries and draining veins (see Fig 4–21). The classic appearance is unlike any typical neoplasm, allowing distinction between AVM and neoplasm to be made. Unfortunately, some cases of AVM present primarily as irregular, nonhomogeneous but relatively confluent densities on the enhanced scan, thereby simulating neoplasm. The presence of increased density on the preinfusion scan may suggest an increased "blood pool." Hemorrhage in the vicinity may strongly suggest a vascular lesion such as

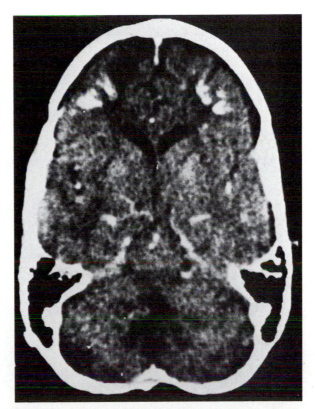

Fig 13–4.—Frontal lobe calcifications following methotrexate and cranial irradiation for medulloblastoma. This single enhanced axial view demonstrates midline encephalomalacia within the posterior fossa following previous resection, chemotherapy, and irradiation for medulloblastoma. There are areas of frontal lobe encephalomalacia bilaterally, associated with multiple nodular calcifications in both frontal lobes.

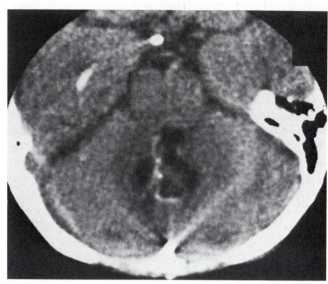

Fig 13–5.—Radiation necrosis of the cerebellar vermis. This axial enhanced scan through the posterior fossa demonstrates that a previous midline posterior fossa craniotomy has been performed for ependymoma in this adolescent female. There is curvilinear enhancement just to the right of the midline. The patient had symptoms of progressive ataxia and midline cerebellar dysfunction, prompting surgical exploration for possible recurrent ependymoma. Surgery and pathologic examination revealed only radiation necrosis.

AVM, although hemorrhage into a tumor is not uncommon. Fortunately, cases of AVM do not typically present with a history suggestive of progressive mass effect, but rather with that of seizure or hemorrhage, and clinical suspicion is raised as to the possibility of vascular malformation on clinical grounds alone. Angiography provides the definitive diagnosis.

While venous angiomas tend not to bleed because of their low intravascular pressure, they may do so. In addition, they frequently present on the CT scan as an enhancing lesion simulating tumor (see Fig 4–27). A high-resolution scan may show the classic appearance of a venous angioma, with the radiating venules converging into a nidus, from which exits a large transcerebral

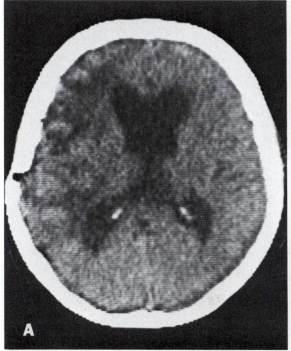

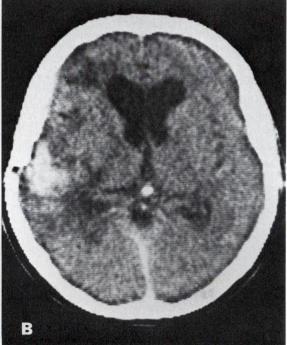

Fig 13–6.—Right frontotemporal radiation necrosis. The patient had multiple previous craniotomies for attempted removal of a right sphenoid wing meningioma. Radiation therapy was administered in an attempt to prevent recurrence. The unenhanced scan **(A)** demonstrates multiple patchy high- and low-density areas within the right frontal and temporal lobes. The enhanced scan **(B)** shows a confluent and homogeneously enhancing focus in the right parietotemporal region. The enhancing focus simulates neoplasm. Surgery revealed radiation necrosis only. (Courtesy of Lawrence Gold, M.D., University of Minnesota, Minneapolis.)

vein (see Fig 4–26).[18] This classic appearance should not be confused with any type of neoplasm.

Finally, a ring of enhancement may be present with a resolving hematoma. If no history of previous hemorrhage is available, this ring may be thought to represent abscess, primary glioma, or metastatic neoplasm, without any distinguishing characteristics to differentiate these pathologic processes. The ring represents the abnormality of the blood-brain barrier surrounding the resolving hematoma, with the more central low density being the liquifying portion of the clot. A history of previous acute neurologic symptoms or sequential CT scans demonstrating the progressive resolution of the lesion will aid in appropriate diagnosis.

Radiation Necrosis

Irradiation to the head has been reported to produce numerous findings, including osteoradionecrosis of the calvarium;[19] radiation-induced sarcoma, particularly fibrosarcoma in the parasellar region following pituitary irradiation;[20–22] parenchymal calcification with areas of white matter hypodensity and atrophy (Fig 13–4) following the combined use of radiation and chemotherapy for intracranial leukemia, lymphoma, and other neoplasms;[23, 24] or the appearance of either patchy or well-circumscribed contrast enhancement with or without mass effect, representing necrosis from radiation alone.[25–28] The production of parenchymal necrosis from radiation alone has a latent period of 1 month to 14 years and generally occurs with doses of 6,000 rad or greater.[25]

An area of radiation necrosis may appear on the enhanced CT scan as an irregular region of enhancement without mass effect (Fig 13–5),[25] a solid area of enhancement with or without mass effect (Fig 13–6),[27] or a ring lesion simulating malignant primary brain tumor, metastatic tumor, recurrent or persistent tumor, or abscess (Fig 13–7).[25–27] While it has been suggested that radiation dose curves can be compared to the zones of CT scan abnormality, with areas of enhancement below 5,500 rad of irradiation probably representing recurrent tumor and not radiation necrosis,[29] in the majority of cases it is probably impossible to definitely distinguish areas of radiation necrosis from recurrent tumor.[28] This has certainly been our experience, with the varieties of presentation of radiation necrosis and the similarities of its appearance with that typically seen with aggressive neoplasms precluding appropriate diagnosis on a single

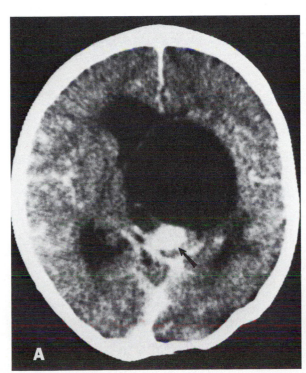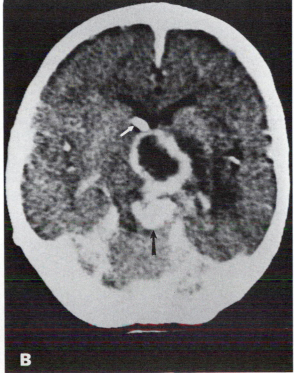

Fig 13–7.—Radiation necrosis following interstitial irradiation. Enhanced CT scan **(A)** demonstrates a large recurrent thalamic glioma with both a cystic component anteriorly and a solid component posteriorly *(arrow)*. The patient went to Stockholm, Sweden, for the placement of yttrium into the cyst cavity in an attempt to decrease the mass effect and the rate of recurrence. Follow-up scanning 6 months later **(B)** shows a nodular component *(black arrow)* more posteriorly, a shunt within the right lateral ventricle *(white arrow)* decompressing the ventricular system, but an area of ring enhancement in the midline. Fearing further tumor recurrence, surgery was performed, which revealed extensive radiation necrosis without evidence of tumor, thereby accounting for the ring of enhancement.

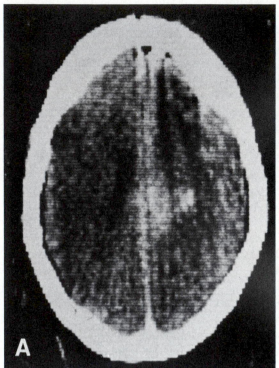
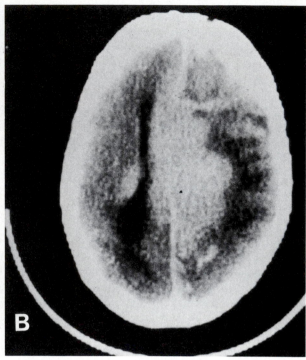

Fig 13–8.—Radiation necrosis simulating recurrent neoplasm. The initial enhanced scan **(A)** demonstrates an enhancing mass in the region of the posterior portion of the corpus callosum. Unfortunately, the scan is marred by artifact. Biopsy revealed malignant astrocytoma, and the patient underwent radiation therapy. Four months later, the patient became markedly somnolent, and CT scanning revealed a massive area of enhancement involving the medial portions of both cerebral hemispheres **(B)**. Autopsy revealed that the majority of the enhancing mass represented radiation necrosis, with only a small amount of tumor present. (Courtesy of Robert Selker, M.D., Montefiore Hospital, Pittsburgh.)

CT scan (Figs 13–7 and 13–8). Either biopsy or sequential CT scans, particularly following the administration of corticosteroids,[26] may be helpful in determining the correct diagnosis.

Nonneoplastic Cysts

A nonneoplastic cyst such as an arachnoid cyst does not enhance, is located in an extra-axial position, and mimics a nonenhancing mass such as an epidermoid cyst. Arachnoid cysts are discussed extensively in Chapter 22.

REFERENCES

1. Russell E.J., George A.E., Kricheff I.I., et al.: Atypical computed tomographic features of intracranial meningioma: Radiological-pathological correlation in a series of 131 consecutive cases. *Radiology* 135:673–682, 1980.
2. Norman D., Enzmann D.E., Levin V.A., et al.: Computed tomography in the evaluation of malignant glioma before and after therapy. *Radiology* 121:85–88, 1976.
3. Messina A.V., Potts D.G., Rottenburg D., et al.: Computed tomography: Demonstration of contrast medium within cystic tumors. *Radiology* 120:345–347, 1976.
4. Shalen P.R., Hayman L.A., Wallace S., et al.: Protocol for delayed contrast enhancement in computed tomography of cerebral neoplasia. *Radiology* 139:397–402, 1981.
5. Hatam A., Bupvall U., Lewander R., et al.: Contrast medium enhancement with time in computer tomography: Differential diagnosis of intracranial lesions. *Acta Radiol. Suppl.* 346:63–81, 1975.
6. Takeda N., Tanaka R., Nakai I., et al.: Dynamics of contrast enhancement in delayed computed tomography of brain tumors: Tissue-blood ratio and differential diagnosis. *Radiology* 142:663–668, 1982.
7. Lilja A., Bergstrom K., Spansare B., et al.: Reliability of computer tomography in assessing histopathological features of malignant supratentorial gliomas. *J. Comput. Assist. Tomogr.* 5:625–636, 1981.
8. New P.F.J., Aronow S., Hesselink J.R.: National Cancer Institute study: Evaluation of computed tomography in the diagnosis of intracranial neoplasms: IV. Meningiomas. *Radiology* 136:665–675, 1980.
9. Weisberg L.A., Nice C.M.: Intracranial tumors simulating the presentation of cerebrovascular syndromes: Early detection with cerebral computed tomography (CCT). *Am. J. Med.* 63:517–524, 1977.
10. Monajati A., Heggeness L.: Patterns of edema in tumors vs. infarcts: Visualization of white matter pathways. *A.J.N.R.* 3:251–255, 1982.

11. Reichenthal E., Cohen M.L., Schujman E., et al.: Tuberculum brain abscess and its appearance on computerized tomography. *J. Neurosurg.* 56:597–600, 1982.

12. Price H.I., Danzinger A.: Computed tomography in cranial tuberculosis. *A.J.R.* 130:769–771, 1978.

13. Kendall B.E., Tatler G.L.V.: Radiological findings in neurosarcoidosis. *Br. J. Radiol.* 51:81–92, 1978.

14. Cahill D.W., Salamon M.: Neurosarcoidosis: A review of the rarer manifestations. *Surg. Neurol.* 15:204–211, 1981.

15. Kempe D.A., Ras C.V.G.K., Garcia J.H., et al.: Intracranial neurosarcoidosis. *J. Comput. Assist. Tomogr.* 3:324–330, 1979.

16. Brooks J., Steckland M.C., Williams J.P., et al.: Computed tomography changes in neurosarcoidosis, clearing with steroid treatment. *J. Comput. Assist. Tomogr.* 3:398–399, 1979.

17. Reith K.G., DiChiro G., Cromwell L.D., et al.: Primary demyelinating disease simulating glioma of the corpus callosum. *J. Neurosurg.* 55:620–624, 1981.

18. Hacker D.A., Latchaw R.E., Chou S.N., et al.: Bilateral cerebellar venous angioma. *J. Comput. Assist. Tomogr.* 5:424–426, 1981.

19. Latchaw R.E., Gabrielsen T.O.: Osteoradionecrosis of the skull. *Univ. Mich. Med. Center J.* 39:166–169, 1973.

20. Kingsley D.P.E., Kendall B.E.: CT of the adverse effects of therapeutic radiation of the central nervous system. *A.J.N.R.* 2:453–460, 1981.

21. Robinson R.G.: A second brain tumor and irradiation. *J. Neurol. Neurosurg. Psychiatry* 41:1005–1012, 1978.

22. Martin W.H., Cail W.S., Morris J.L., et al.: Fibrosarcoma after high energy radiation therapy for pituitary adenoma. *A.J.N.R.* 1:469–472, 1980.

23. Shalen P.R., Ostrow P.T., Glass P.J.: Enhancement of the white matter following prophylactic therapy of the central nervous system for leukemia: Radiation effects and methotrexate leukoencephalopathy. *Radiology* 140:409–412, 1981.

24. Peylan-Ramu N., Poplack D.G., Pizzo P.A., et al.: Abnormal CT scans of the brain in asymptomatic children with acute lymphatic leukemia after prophylactic treatment of the central nervous system with radiation and intrathecal chemotherapy. *N. Engl. J. Med.* 298:815–823, 1978.

25. Mikhael M.A.: Radiation necrosis of the brain: Correlation between patterns on computed tomography and dose of radiation. *J. Comput. Assist. Tomogr.* 3:241–249, 1979.

26. Baron S.H.: Brain radiation necrosis following treatment of an esthesioneuroblastoma olfactory neurocytoma. *Laryngoscope* 89:214–223, 1979.

27. Sundersen N., Galicich J.H., Deck M.D.F., et al.: Radiation necrosis after treatment of solitary intracranial metastases. *Neurosurgery* 8:329–333, 1981.

28. Deck M.D.F.: Imaging techniques in the diagnosis of radiation damage to the central nervous system, in Gilbert H.A., Kagan A.R. (eds.): *Radiation Damage to the Nervous System.* New York, Raven Press, 1980.

29. Mikhael M.A.: Radiation necrosis of the brain: Correlation between computed tomography, pathology, and dose distribution. *J. Comput. Assist. Tomogr.* 2:71–80, 1978.

14

New Concepts for the CT Scan Diagnosis and Therapy of Intracranial Tumors and Other Abnormalities

RICHARD E. LATCHAW, M.D.

SOME RECENT and imminent developments in CT scanning make the diagnosis and therapy of certain intracranial processes far easier and more efficacious than in the past. Such changes include improvements in CT resolution, manipulation of images to allow stereoscopic and three-dimensional viewing, as well as techniques for biopsy and placement of radioactive seeds into a neoplasm under CT control.

INCREASED LOW-CONTRAST RESOLUTION

New developments in CT scanners have steadily improved their spatial resolution of high-contrast objects. The newest high-resolution scanners allow a spatial resolution of high-contrast objects as close as 0.25 mm. While such spatial resolution is extremely important in the evaluation of fine bony detail, in the separation of the sharp margins of a high-contrast object such as an enhancing neoplasm from contiguous bone and tissue, and in the precise placement of a therapeutic device such as a biopsy probe, the early detection of a subtle neoplasm such as a low-grade astrocytoma requires excellent *low-contrast* resolution. The newest CT scanners allow for low-contrast resolution of 0.3%, and even better resolution may be on the horizon. A trade-off of spatial and contrast resolution has always been necessary in CT scanning, and while a large increase in the photon flux delivered to the patient has been required in the past for improved low-contrast resolution, such resolution is possible on the newer machines with no increase in radiation dose and without loss of spatial resolution. Hopefully, improvements in low-contrast resolution will aid in the detection of subtle abnormalities such as diffuse infiltrating neoplasms that leave the blood-brain barrier intact, subtle areas of infarction, poorly defined regions of cerebritis, and early changes of demyelinating disease.

HISTOGRAMS AND THE "SIGMA SCAN"

In the early years of CT, it was hoped that a singular value of attenuation coefficient might be found for each pathologic process or type of neoplasm. It rapidly became obvious that many diseases had identical attenuation coefficients and CT numbers, and that morphological anatomy of the lesion proved more helpful in diagnosis than any particular CT-derived number. A slightly different approach has been the production of a histogram of densities found throughout a lesion. A graph of the frequency of CT numbers in a lesion may be produced and correlated with pathology. To date, such histographic analysis has not proved to be any more diagnostic than visualizing the radiographic position and characteristics of the lesion.

Another technique that emphasizes the homogeneity of a lesion is the Sigma scan.[1] People are able to perceive slight differences in brightness between adjacent objects, but the variations in density within an object are often slight and difficult to perceive. The Sigma scan is an image of the variance of density that occurs within an object or lesion. Density variations are slight within a meningioma and rather marked in glioblastoma multiforme. This technique attempts to quantitate this variation and correlate it with pathology.

DUAL kVp/EFFECTIVE ATOMIC NUMBER DETERMINATION

A number of years ago, we demonstrated the ability of dual kVp scanning to define the effective atomic number of a neoplasm and to differentiate three classes of intracranial neoplasms (glial tumors, metastatic lesions, and meningiomas) to a very high degree of statistical significance.[2, 3] The old technique for such dual kVp scanning involved sequential scanning at a particular level, first at one kVp and then at a second energy level. In such a system, when motion occurred between slices, artifact produced significant error. Current research efforts are aimed at allowing a rapid change in kVp so that two images of a single slice are acquired during a single x-ray tube rotation, each at a different energy level. Manipulation of the two values for each pixel obtained at the two energy levels produces a single image corresponding to the effective atomic number at each pixel location (the so-called Z-scan).[4] While the electronic engineering of a dual kVp system is not simple, requiring both a rapid kVp switching device and different software filter functions for each energy, Z-scans may prove important to tumor identification and differentiation. It will also be important in the quantification of the amount of a high atomic-numbered material (high Z) present in a slice, such as calcium or iodinated contrast material.

CT SUBTRACTION

A method called CT subtraction determines precisely the amount of contrast enhancement that occurs for each pixel in a slice. The technique requires scanning a level first without enhancement and then with enhancement. Digital subtraction of the attenuation coefficients allows the production of a perfectly "subtracted" image. This technique may improve our ability to detect subtle enhancement in a low-grade neoplasm, early infarction and infection, and diffuse demyelinating disease. Unfortunately, the technique has been associated with a large error, because the patient must be absolutely motionless between the preinfusion and postinfusion scans. While rapid scanning of 2 to 3 seconds is now common and of great benefit for such a technique, the error associated with interscan motion during the administration of contrast material may make the method without value.

ELECTRONIC RADIOGRAPHY FOR LOCALIZATION

Utilizing the x-ray tube of the CT scanner, a low x-ray dose of approximately 50 millirads is used to produce an electronic radiograph. For example, movement of the supine patient's head past the x-ray tube within the CT scan gantry produces a lateral view of the skull. While this image is not of the same quality as a plain radiograph utilizing a film/screen combination, it is today a routine technique to localize the level of a partic-

ular subsequently performed scan of the intracranial contents. The level of the slice is superimposed on the electronic image of the skull (Fig 14–1). Therefore, the level of the slice of interest, such as through the midportion of an intracranial neoplasm, can be directly related to the skull, allowing the surgeon to determine the optimal site for craniotomy. By knowing the anteroposterior relationships of the tumor to the rest of the intracranial contents while the entire plane of the scan is visualized, the location of the tumor can be determined. Alternatively, scanning in both the axial and coronal projections may be performed, with the patient's head marked at the level of each slice through the area of pathology (see Fig 14–1). The crossing of the axial and coronal planes, as marked on the skin of the patient, indicates the appropriate site for craniotomy.

A future software upgrade for the General Electric CT/T scanning systems will be the superimposition of an entire area of interest onto the lateral view of the head ("CORRELATE" and "LOCATE" programs). For example, the margins of an intracranial tumor seen on multiple slices may be defined, with this area of interest directly superimposed on the lateral electronic radiograph. The surgeon or the radiation therapist may then relate the entire tumoral margin to external landmarks.

THREE-DIMENSIONAL IMAGING

Scanning and/or reformation in the sagittal and coronal planes, in addition to axial imaging, have been major advances in visualizing intracranial lesions in three dimensions. These techniques replace what the viewer normally does, namely the tedious mental reconstruction and transference of a series of two-dimensional images—the collection of CT scan slices—into the three-dimensional patient. While radiologists have traditionally been trained to perform this mental task, it is one that is difficult, because it is not an intrinsically natural process for the brain to perform. The fact that it requires years to be able to do this well means that those not intensively trained in this process do it only with great difficulty. Helpful as it is to have multiple projections available, the next major step is the actual production of a three-dimensional or stereoscopic image, giving the perception of depth to an intracranial lesion and its relation to other intracranial structures. This is extremely helpful for all, but especially for the surgeon, allowing him to preoperatively visualize the relationship of a lesion to contiguous structures and to plan an appropriate surgical approach.

One method of three-dimensional visualization of a tumor is the reformation of the lesion within a "wire-

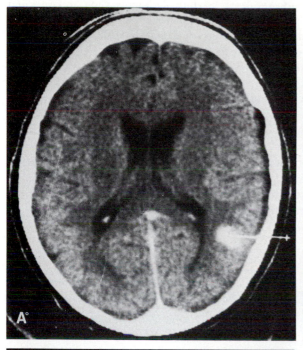

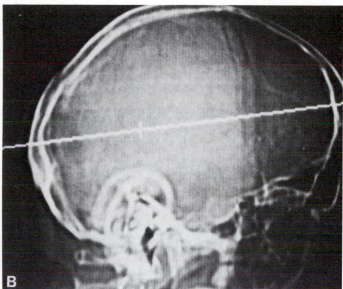

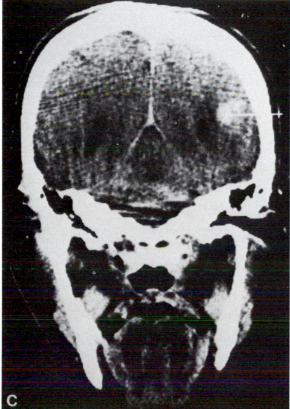

Fig 14–1.—Electronic radiography for localization. The axial enhanced scan **(A)** demonstrates a metastatic neoplasm at the left inferior parietal corticomedullary junction. The linear line that extends from the tumor beyond the skull has been drawn on the imaging console. A direct measurement from the center of the tumor to the skull may be made to determine the depth of the biopsy. The plane of this scan may be directly superimposed on an electronic lateral image of the skull **(B),** so that the plane of the abnormality may be directly related to bony contours. A direct coronal image **(C)** can be used to visualize the neoplasm, similar to **A.** The plane of the scan through the tumor in **C** may likewise be related to the skull. The intersection of the laser light beams of the axial and coronal planes, as seen and marked on the patient's skin, indicates the exact point of the intracranial neoplasm.

frame" contoural depiction of the skull (Fig 14–2).[5, 6] This technique requires 16 or more contiguous 5-mm or thinner slices through the entire lesion. At the present time, only the surface of a lesion may be related to the contour maps of the skull; reformation of contiguous anatomical structures is not part of the software program.

Reformation of a series of slices may be performed with a portion "removed" to reveal internal anatomy. This is similar to viewing a pie at an angle, with a slice removed to reveal the pieces of apple within. We have used this technique in the evaluation of regional cerebral blood flow as determined by CT scanning during stable xenon inhalation (see Chapter 2).

General Electric currently has an experimental program in which high-contrast objects such as bone may be visualized in three dimensions. The technique depends upon assigning darker gray-scale values to areas at increasing depth from the surface, thereby producing a three-dimensional effect. The entire object, e.g., the skull or spine, may be rotated around a number of axes to evaluate all aspects. The goal is to be able to manipulate any part of the image and change its relationship to the whole. This would allow preoperative reconstructive "surgery" to be performed on the spine or face before actual surgery. At the present time, such reformatting techniques require the scanning of high-density tissues such as bone to produce adequate edges in the reformatted image.

Finally, recent work has centered on coupling one of

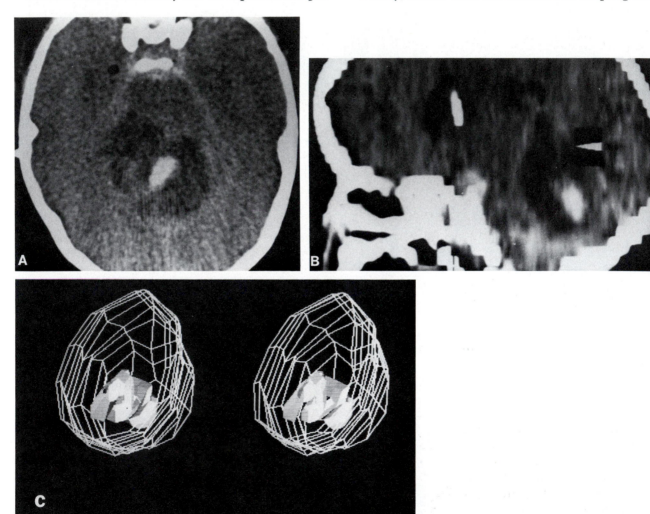

Fig 14–2.—Three-dimensional imaging utilizing a computer reproduction of an intracranial neoplasm relative to a wire-frame model of the skull. The axial CT scan following the deposition of metrizamide into the intracranial subarachnoid cisterns **(A)** demonstrates a large low-density neoplasm within the cerebellar vermis. There is a central collection of high density. The reformatted sagittal view **(B)** shows the relationship of this neoplasm to contiguous structures. There is a shunt within a lateral ventricle. Figure **C** is a computer-generated three-dimensional image of the neoplasm and its relationship to the wire-frame model of the skull, which is projected obliquely as if the patient were looking up and to the right. (From Vries J.K.: *Concepts Pediatr. Neurosurg.* 4:1–11, 1983. Used by permission.)

two series of reconstructed images of the same lesion to each of two eyepieces in a stereoscopic headpiece.[7] Viewing the lesion through the stereoscope (or crossing one's eyes in the traditional manner for stereoscopic viewing) gives a sense of depth to the CT image and a perception of the relationship of the lesion to contiguous structures (Fig 14–3).

VOLUMETRIC DETERMINATION

A number of new high-resolution CT scanners allow for the volumetric determination of any three-dimensional region of interest. The region is defined either by hand-drawing with the cursor around the margin of the particular region of interest over a series of scans or by selecting a range of attenuation coefficients within an area encompassing the region of interest (Fig 14–4). Either procedure allows the determination of the volume of any particular intracranial structure or lesion. For example, a volumetric determination of the cerebral ventricles may be made to evaluate ventricular enlargement in patients with dementia (see Fig 14–4).[8, 9] Calculation of the volume of a neoplasm, such as a cystic craniopharyngioma (Fig 14–5), helps in the determination of the appropriate amount of radioactive isotope to be instilled into the cystic tumor for its treatment. The implantation of radioactive seeds for interstitial irradiation of a neoplasm (Fig 14–6) is greatly facilitated by volumetric determination of the neoplasm so that the appropriate isodose curves can be computed.

CT-GUIDED STEREOTACTIC NEUROSURGERY

The role of the CT scanner in determining the coordinates of an intracranial area of interest in relation to a stereotactic frame is covered in far greater detail in Chapter 34. In brief, a special Leksell stereotactic frame has been devised that is density-compatible with the CT scanner, so that few artifacts are produced while scanning the patient within the frame. The coordinates taken from the CT scan are directly transferable to the frame. Not only are appropriate coordinates for the site of biopsy or probe placement determined on the CT scanner, but the therapeutic procedure is actually performed under CT control. This allows for the visualization of the exact site of probe placement and the determination of any intraoperative or postoperative complications such as hemorrhage.

The neurosurgical procedures performed under CT control may be divided into functional and morphological stereotaxis. Functional procedures include thalamotomy for movement and pain disorders and electrode placement for EEG recording and subsequent chronic seizure therapy. All functional stereotactic procedures have relied on deep brain markers such as the anterior and posterior commissures and the intercommissural (IC) line as reference points to determine the position of a specified thalamic nucleus. Although CT now allows direct visualization of the thalamus and contiguous structures such as the internal capsule, scanning in a plane parallel to the important IC line has not been possible. Recently, however, we have devised a technique for generating coronal oblique reformatted images that are parallel to the IC line. Briefly, the diencephalon is scanned with contiguous 1.5-mm cuts, the anterior commissure is located on one slice and the posterior commissure on another. Because two points determine a plane, a reformatted axial image may be generated that is at a cephalocaudad angle to the original slices and parallel to the important IC line. Measurements to specific targets may be made from this coronal oblique image or from images above or below this plane.[10] This technique of generating coronal oblique planes and images in other surgically useful planes has aided CT scanning in revolutionizing stereotactic procedures for functional neurosurgery.

Morphological stereotactic procedures under CT control include the biopsy of tumors, drainage of cysts and abscesses, and placement of radioactive seeds into a neoplasm. The biopsy of tumors and areas of infection such as herpes encephalitis is an important diagnostic procedure that spares the patient a craniotomy. This procedure represents a large volume of the stereotactic work performed and is discussed thoroughly in Chapter 34. The drainage of a cyst such as a colloid cyst (see Fig 9–44) may be the only therapy that is necessary, because the colloid is so slow to accumulate. A cystic craniopharyngioma that cannot be removed surgically without producing damage to surrounding vital structures may be punctured under CT guidance for the instillation of radioactive phosphorus (see Fig 14–5). The cyst of an inoperable neoplasm may be decompressed for symptomatic relief. Radioactive seeds may be accurately placed into an inoperable tumor (see Fig 14–6) following the computer generation of isodose curves, aided by a volumetric evaluation of the neoplasm.

The applications of CT-guided neurosurgery continue to grow. Cerebral blood flow determinations will be made in the future during occlusive vascular procedures (see Chapter 2). Brain and cerebrovascular surgery may be performed directly on the scanner to monitor results. The applications of CT-guided surgery have proved so successful, and the future possibilities appear so limitless, that we have installed a scanner in an operating room to facilitate CT-guided interventional pro-

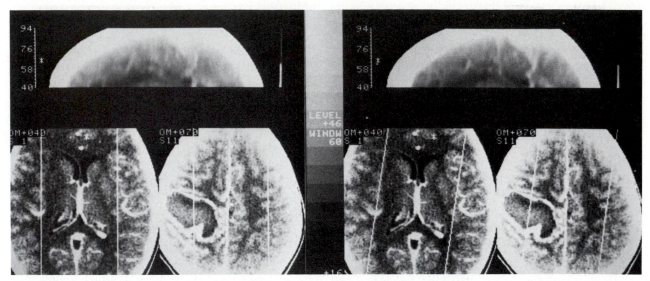

Fig 14–3.—Three-dimensional imaging utilizing stereo-scopic views. Two reformatted sagittal images have been produced from the two axial scans seen in the *bottom row* of this figure. There is a "ring" of enhancement of a neo-plasm in the high right parietal lobe. The sagittal image on the *left* was produced in a plane parallel to the long axis of the head, while the image on the *right* is at a small angle from the long axis. By crossing one's eyes while looking at the sagittal reformatted images of this figure, one can obtain a three-dimensional view of the enhancing margin of this neoplasm and relate it to contiguous neural structures such as the underlying ventricle.

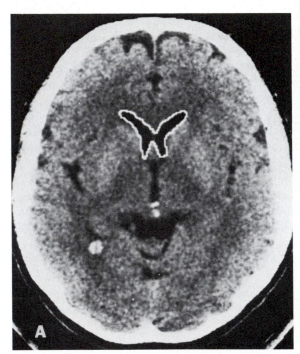
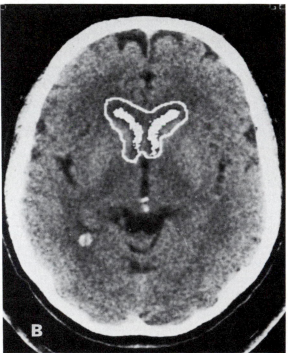

Fig 14–4.—Volumetric determination of the cerebral ven-tricles. The area of any intracranial structure may be deter-mined on a single slice in two ways. The contours of the structure may be drawn by hand **(A),** utilizing the "track-ball" of the scanner console. Alternatively, the general out-line of the structures to be evaluated may be encircled **(B),** with the range of attenuation coefficients specified within that general area of interest. Each pixel within that range is added to the area measurement **(B).** A volumetric determi-nation may be made on one slice by knowing the slice thick-ness or by summation on contiguous slices through a larger volume.

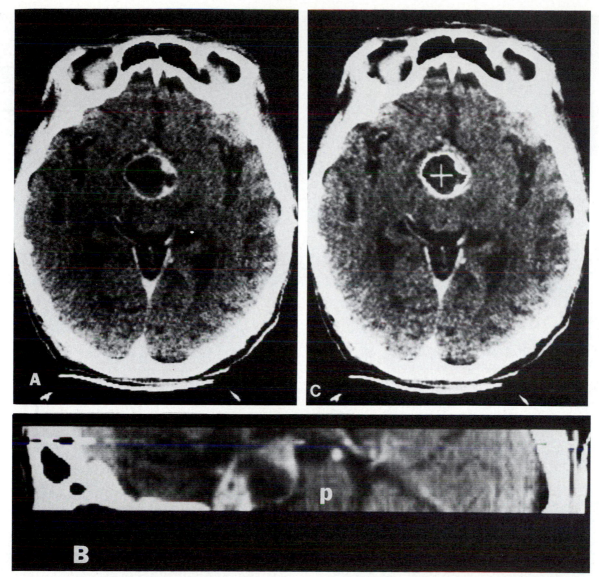

Fig 14–5.—Volumetric determination of a cystic neoplasm. The craniopharyngioma demonstrated on the enhanced axial **(A)** and reformatted sagittal **(B)** images can be evaluated volumetrically. (In **B,** *p* denotes the pons.) A line may be drawn with the track-ball of the computer console along the inner margins of the craniopharyngioma cyst **(C)** and the area of the cyst determined. By knowing the thickness of each slice, a volume per slice may be calculated. Summation of the cyst volume in each slice gives the total cyst volume. Thin slices are required to reduce error.

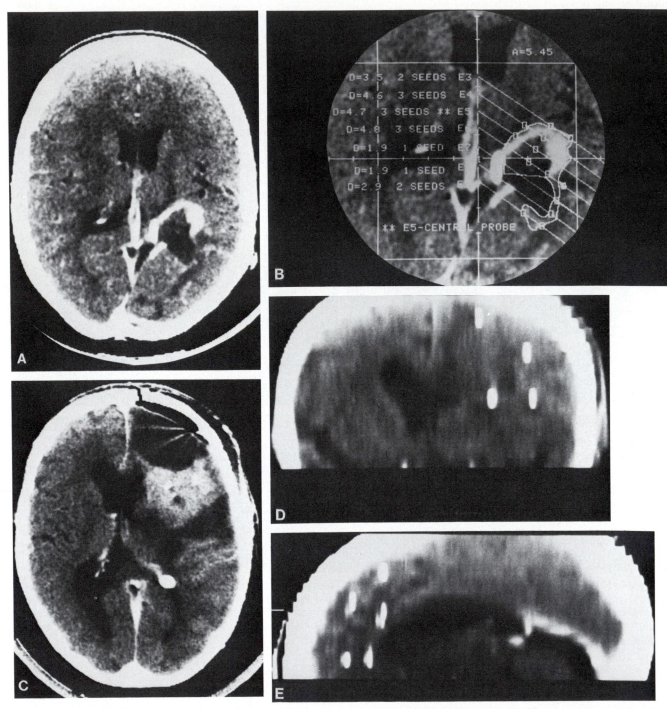

Fig 14–6.—Utilization of volumetric determination for interstitial irradiation. There is a neoplasm in the left parietal lobe, near the atrium of the left lateral ventricle, with an anterior ring of enhancement **(A).** This was histologically proved to be glioblastoma multiforme. Volumetric determination of the tumor was performed over multiple contiguous scans, which allowed the production of isodose curves for the implantation of seeds containing ^{125}I. The number and location of those seeds for appropriate irradiation of the entire tumor bed is indicated in **B.** Those seeds are then implanted under CT-guided stereotactic control. **C,D,E,** a different patient than **A** and **B** is seen to have a large partially cystic and partially solid left frontal lobe tumor **(C).** Following volumetric analysis of the tumor and the plotting of appropriate isodose curves, seeds containing ^{125}I have been placed with CT-guided stereotactic control. The coronal **(D)** and sagittal **(E)** reformatted images show the position of some of the seeds.

cedures. The fields of neuroradiology and neurosurgery move ever closer.

REFERENCES

1. Horton J.A., Kerber C.W.: The grain in the stone: A computer search for hidden CT patterns. *Radiology* 129:427–431, 1978.
2. Latchaw R.E., Payne J.T., Gold L.H.A.: Effective atomic number and electron density as measured with a computed tomography scanner: Computation and correlation with brain tumor histology. *J. Comput. Assist. Tomogr.* 2:199–208, 1978.
3. Latchaw R.E., Payne J.T., Loewenson R.B.: Predicting brain tumor histology: Change of effective atomic number with contrast enhancement. *A.J.N.R.* 1:289–294, 1980.
4. Marshall W.H., Alvarez R.E., Macovski A.: Initial results with prereconstructive dual-energy computed tomography (PREDECT). *Radiology* 140:421–430, 1981.
5. Batnitzky S., Price H.I., Cook P.N., et al.: Three-dimensional computer reconstruction from surface contours for head CT examinations. *J. Comput. Assist. Tomogr.* 5:60–67, 1981.
6. Vries J.K.: REX: A comprehensive information management system for neurosurgical practice. *Concepts Pediatr. Neurosurg.* 4:1–11, 1983.
7. Horton J.A., Kennedy W.H., Rhodes M., et al.: Stereoscopic reformatting and display of CT images. Presented at the Twenty-first Annual Meeting of the American Society of Neuroradiology, San Francisco, June 1983.
8. George A.E., de Leon M.J., Rosenbloom S., et al.: The relationship of CT ventricular volume to cognitive deficit. *Radiology* 149:493–498, 1983.
9. Gado M.H., Hughes C.P., Danzinger W., et al.: Volumetric measurements of the cerebrospinal fluid spaces in demented subjects and controls. *Radiology* 144:535, 1982.
10. Latchaw R.E., Lunsford L.D., Kennedy W.H.: Reformatted imaging to define the intercommissural line for CT-guided stereotactic functional neurosurgery. *A.J.N.R.*, to be published.

The Sellar and Parasellar Regions

15

Normal Intrasellar and Parasellar Anatomy and Techniques of Examination

HELEN M.N. ROPPOLO, M.D.

ROUTINE CT TECHNIQUES

Sellar Region

Lesions of the pituitary gland and sella turcica are optimally evaluated with 1.5-mm thick contiguous CT sections. The use of thin sections prevents overlooking small lesions, which could be obscured on thicker sections by partial volume averaging.

Coronal CT scanning is preferable to axial scanning for demonstrating abnormalities within the sella. During coronal scanning, maximum hyperextension of the head is necessary in order to avoid artifacts from teeth; this is most effectively achieved in the prone position. However, accurate positioning (i.e., absence of even the slightest head rotation), which is critical for an accurate evaluation based on normal coronal anatomy, is most effectively achieved when positioning the patient while supine. Therefore, it is difficult to unequivocally recommend the prone or the supine technique. However, in the older age population or in patients with relatively short and/or thick necks where hyperextension is most difficult to achieve, the prone position is recommended. In either the supine or prone positions, complete immobilization of the head is necessary in order to avoid inadvertent head movement. Head movement is a source of unwanted motion artifacts; it may also result in a failure to scan through some portions of the gland.

In addition to coronal sections, 1.5-mm thick contiguous axial CT sections may be performed. However, axial scanning is necessary only if teeth artifacts obscure detail on the direct coronal scans. The axial scans should be performed at a $-10°$ to $-20°$ angulation to the orbitomeatal line. This angulation is necessary to avoid low-attenuation streak artifacts between the orbital and petrous ridges.[1] Coronal reconstructions of these axial scans, if available, should be obtained.

Nonenhanced scans are not performed for the routine evaluation of the pituitary gland. However, because acidophilic tumors may be relatively dense on CT compared to adjacent tissue both before and after contrast infusion,[2-4] nonenhanced scans may be helpful for their detection and delineation.

Following contrast infusion, the concentration of contrast within the vascular space rapidly declines,[5] and the density difference between the very vascular normal pituitary tissue and the often less-vascular pituitary lesions also declines. Therefore, it is desirable to establish a high initial vascular concentration of contrast and maintain this level throughout scanning. This can be achieved with the rapid infusion of 75 ml of 60% iodinated contrast solution prior to scanning, followed by a drip infusion of 75 ml during scanning.

A technique of 120 kV and at least 1,180 milliampere seconds (mAs) is recommended for the evaluation of the pituitary gland and sella turcica. The use of a lower mAs may be satisfactory for large lesions, but it may interfere with the detection of small microadenomas.

The optimal window width for filming the coronal sections is 250, with window widths of 150 or 300 sometimes having supplemental value. Filming at a 2.5- to 3-times magnification factor is recommended. Either simple or computerized magnification appears to be adequate.

Parasellar Regions

Techniques used for the routine evaluation of the cavernous sinuses and parasellar regions are similar to those used for the evaluation of the pituitary gland and sella turcica. However, in addition to enhanced coronal sections, enhanced axial sections are also routinely obtained. Either the routine axial projection ($+20°$ to the orbitomeatal line) or the modified axial projection used for the sellar region ($-10°$ to $-20°$ to the orbitomeatal line) may be used. For most lesions, 1.5-mm thick sections are recommended. However, if a large lesion is suspected, 5-mm thick sections are more appropriate. In addition, in the parasellar regions, the knowledge of the nonenhanced CT density of a lesion and of the presence or absence of calcification or hemorrhage may be helpful in establishing the diagnosis. Therefore, nonenhanced contiguous 5- or 10-mm thick sections in either the coronal or axial projections may also be obtained.

SPECIAL CT TECHNIQUES

Metrizamide Cisternography

Indications for metrizamide cisternography include the following: (1) the evaluation of the pituitary gland surface for a subtle superior convexity that could indicate an underlying mass; (2) the differentiation of an empty sella from a large cystic lesion when routine intravenous-enhanced CT is indeterminate; (3) the determination of the existence of a questionable parasellar lesion; and (4) the evaluation of the extent of large parasellar masses.

This procedure is usually performed via a lumbar puncture using a 22-gm needle. Approximately 5 ml of metrizamide at a concentration of 170 to 190 mg iodine/ml are instilled. The needle is removed, and for sellar and parasellar lesions the prone patient is tilted 60° (Trendelenburg's position) for 45 to 60 seconds. The patient is then returned to the horizontal position and scanned prone in both the coronal and modified axial (−10° to −20° to the orbitomeatal line) projections. Contiguous sections of 1.5-mm thickness are obtained for small lesions, and 5-mm thick contiguous or overlapping sections are obtained for larger lesions.[6, 7]

Dynamic CT Scanning

Dynamic CT scanning may be performed for the evaluation of the internal carotid arteries and their branches. This technique can differentiate a vascular from a soft-tissue lesion; it can also evaluate lateral extension of a pituitary infiltrative process by demonstrating vascular displacement and/or vascular encasement. Dynamic CT scanning may be a potential alternative technique to arteriography in the presurgical evaluation of pituitary adenomas.[8]

In dynamic CT scanning, coronal scans are usually obtained initially. The patient is placed either prone or supine with the head hyperextended. Contiguous baseline scans may be performed from the tuberculum anteriorly to the dorsum sellae posteriorly. These nonenhanced scans may be helpful subsequently when attempting to differentiate arterial structures from bone, cavernous sinus, or tumor.[8] Contrast agent such as Renografin 76 is then injected into a large antecubital vein through an 18-gm angiocatheter. This may either

be performed manually by injecting 50 ml over 10 seconds or mechanically by injecting 40 ml over 4 to 5 seconds.[8] Arm-to-brain transit time is about 8 seconds. The scan sequence is initiated so that the first scan coincides with the arrival of contrast in the cavernous internal carotid. Thus, if rotor preparation time is 2 seconds and scan time is 4.8 seconds (GE 8800), the midpoint of the first scan will occur 4.4 seconds after initiation of the scan sequence. In order to cause the midpoint of the first scan to coincide with the arrival of contrast in the cavernous carotid, contrast infusion should begin 3.6 seconds prior to the onset of scanning, assuming arm-to-brain transit time is 8 seconds.

If a graphic analysis plotting change in contrast over time is desired, a single section is selected. A preinjection baseline scan is obtained, and the region of interest cursor is centered over the appropriate structure. Continuous scans for 15 to 30 seconds followed by single scans having gradually increasing time intervals between them are obtained. Although the most meaningful scans are acquired within the first 2 minutes postinfusion, additional scans obtained during the next 20 to 30 minutes may be helpful.[9] Following dynamic coronal scanning, the same technique may be applied for dynamic axial scanning.

NORMAL ROUTINE CT EVALUATION

The Normal Pituitary Gland and Sella Turcica

Intraglandular Architecture

On gross examination of the pituitary gland, the anterior lobe partially envelopes the posterior lobe (Fig

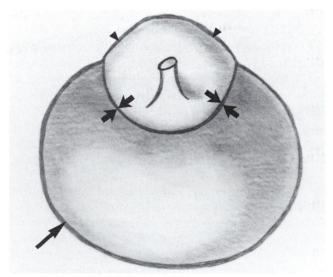

Fig 15–1.—Pituitary gland seen from above depicts the gross anatomical interrelationships of the anterior lobe *(large arrow)*, pars intermedia *(small thick arrows)*, and posterior lobe *(arrowheads)*.

15–1). The region of the pars intermedia is interposed between them (see Fig 15–1).[10]

On microscopic examination, the anterior lobe consists of three glandular cell types: chromophobic, acidophilic, and basophilic. These cell types may be intermingled with each other or found separately. Their distribution forms distinct areas within the anterior lobe. Those areas that are composed of cells with prominent cellular granularity and/or of tissue having a significant degree of tissue compactness correspond to areas of increased CT density on nonenhanced and usually also on enhanced CT sections.[2]

The pars intermedia is a thin structure extending the height of the gland, which contains colloid cysts.[11] When these cysts are numerous and/or large, they are detectable on CT examination as lucent areas; they do not increase in density with contrast infusion.[2]

On microscopic examination, the posterior lobe consists of bundles of neurohypophyseal tissue with varying degrees of compactness and vascularity. The more compact and/or vascular the tissue, the more dense it is on CT examination.[2]

On contiguous 1.5-mm coronal CT sections through the gland, CT patterns may be present. These patterns are similar in both the nonenhanced and enhanced glands. They result from the gross anatomical interrelationships of the anterior lobe, pars intermedia, and posterior lobe to each other (see Fig 15–1) as well as from the histologic architecture within the anterior and posterior lobes.[2, 10]

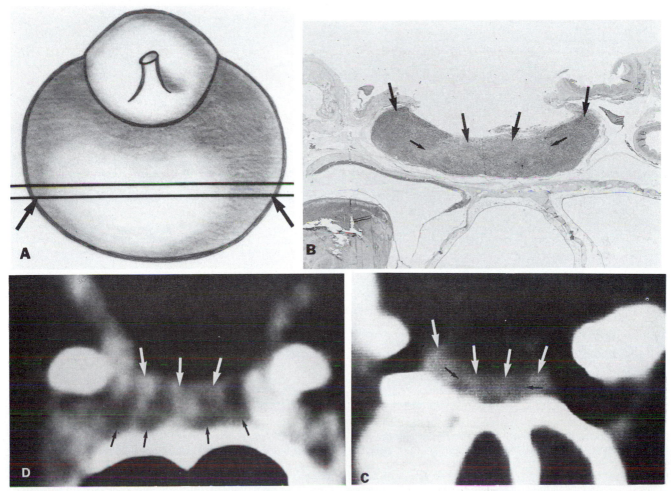

Fig 15–2.—A, schematic representation of the location of a coronal section through the anterior portion of the anterior lobe (large arrows). B, coronal histologic section (hematoxylin-eosin) through this section. C, closely corresponding specimen CT section. Strongly staining areas in B (large black arrows) consist of tightly compacted tissue with heavily granulated acidophilic cells; they correspond to CT-dense areas in C (large white arrows). Weakly staining areas in B (small black arrows) consist of loosely compacted tissue with chromophobic and/or mildly-to-moderately granulated basophilic cells; they correspond to CT-lucent areas in C (small black arrows). D, contrast-enhanced section from a normal patient through this region demonstrating similar CT-dense (large white arrows) and CT-lucent (small black arrows) areas. Sections similar to B–D may also be found more posteriorly within the anterior lobe, as diagrammatically represented in Figure 15–3, A.

When a coronal CT section is taken through the anterior portion of the anterior lobe (Fig 15–2,A), CT-lucent and CT-dense areas of similar configuration often alternate with each other from one side of the gland to the other, creating a repetitive type of pattern (see Fig 15–2,C and D). The CT-lucent areas usually correspond to areas of loosely compacted tissue with chromophobic and/or mildly-to-moderately granulated basophilic cells; the CT-dense areas usually correspond to areas of tightly compacted tissue with heavily granulated acidophilic cells (see Fig 15–2,B).[2]

When a coronal CT section is taken through the midportion of the anterior lobe (Fig 15–3,A), an identical CT pattern to that described above is frequently seen. However, in this region, as well as occasionally more anteriorly, laterally located CT-dense areas may be present with CT-lucent areas concentrated more medially (see Fig 15–3,C and D). Histologically, these CT-

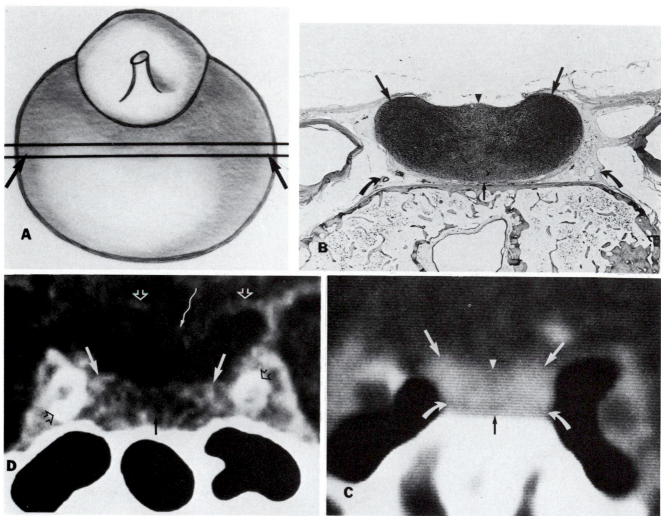

Fig 15–3.—A, schematic representation of the location of a coronal section through the midportion of the anterior lobe *(large arrows).* **B,** coronal histologic section (hematoxylin-eosin) through this region. **C,** closely corresponding specimen CT section. Strongly staining areas in **B** *(large black arrows)* consist of tightly compacted tissue with heavily granulated acidophilic cells; they correspond to CT-dense areas in **C** *(large white arrows).* Weakly staining areas in **B** *(small black arrow)* consist of loosely compacted tissue with chromophobic and/or mildly-to-moderately granulated basophilic cells; they correspond to CT-lucent areas in **C** *(small black arrow).* Weakly staining areas along the superior surface of the gland (**B,** *black arrowhead*) consist primarily of loosely compacted fibrous tissue with only a few intermingled glandular cells; they correspond to CT-lucent areas in **C** *(white arrowhead).* Weakly staining areas in **B** *(curved black arrows)* consist of extraglandular adipose and fibrous tissue and correspond to CT-lucent areas in **C** *(curved white arrows).* **D,** contrast-enhanced CT section from a normal patient through this region demonstrating similar CT-dense *(large white arrows)* and CT-lucent *(small black arrow)* areas. Also note bilateral carotid calcification *(open black arrows),* the A-1 segments of the anterior cerebral arteries *(open white arrows),* and the optic chiasm *(wavy arrow)* in the suprasellar cistern. Sections similar to **B–D** could also be located more anteriorly within the gland, as diagrammatically represented in Figure 15–2, A.

lucent and CT-dense areas are similar to those seen in the repetitive pattern (see Figs 15–2,B and 15–3,B). In addition, especially in nonenhanced glands in this region, CT-lucent areas are often present along the superior border (see Fig 15–3,C). Histologically, these areas are composed predominantly of loosely compacted and often very vascular fibrous tissue; a few acidophilic, chromophobic, and/or basophilic cells are interspersed throughout. These regions are contiguous posteriorly with similar areas at the base of the infundibulum. They are not usually identifiable in enhanced glands, presumably because of their frequent very vascular nature.

The CT sections of anterior and midportions of the anterior lobe do not always contain interspersed CT-lucent and CT-dense areas; their CT pattern may be relatively homogeneous. Histologically in these instances, there is usually a relatively uniform degree of tissue compactness. Chromophobic, mildly-to-moderately granulated basophilic cells and moderately or heavily granulated acidophilic cells are interspersed either diffusely with each other or as scattered small foci of the individual cell types.[2]

Within the anterior lobe on both sides of the gland, compact bands of dense connective tissue and vessels course in an anteroposterior direction; they are referred to as fibrous cores (Fig 15–4).[12] These fibrous cores are surrounded by loosely compacted glandular tissue, from which they cannot be differentiated on nonenhanced CT examination. Although the vessels in the fibrous cores are larger than those in the adjacent tissue, the relative vascularity-per-unit volume of these two tissues is usually similar. This helps to explain why in contrast-enhanced patients, these fibrous cores are unable to be discerned as identifiable CT-dense areas.[2]

Between the anterior lobe and cavernous sinus, CT-lucent areas are sometimes present (Figs 15–3,C and 15–5,D) that are not part of the normal anterior lobe tissue. These CT-lucent areas have been shown frequently to correspond histologically to adipose and/or connective tissue (see Fig 15–3,B).[2] However, it is also possible that some of them represent loculations of cerebrospinal fluid (CSF).

When a coronal CT section is taken further posteriorly in the gland (Fig 15–5,A), the posterior portions of the anterior lobe are located laterally, and the anterior portion of the pars intermedia is located centrally. Histologically, the posterior portions of the anterior lobe consist primarily of heavily granulated and densely compacted acidophilic cells embedded in a vascular stroma (see Fig 15–5,B and E); these areas tend to be CT-dense on both nonenhanced and enhanced CT sections (see Fig 15–5,C, D, F, and G). The centrally located pars intermedia may contain colloid cysts. When

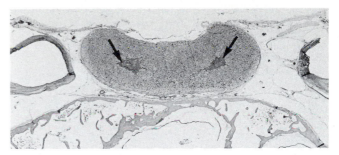

Fig 15–4.—Coronal histologic section through the anterior lobe of an autopsy specimen demonstrating symmetric fibrous cores (arrows).

present, these cysts are identifiable on CT either as small, round, midline, CT-lucent areas (see Fig 15–5,C and D) or as elongated, midline, CT-lucent areas extending from the inferior to the superior border of the gland and often having a rectangular or wedge-shaped configuration (see Fig 15–5,F and G). Because of their cystic nature, the CT-lucent areas of the pars intermedia possess better margination than most other CT-lucent areas in the pituitary gland. Unlike most of the other CT-lucent areas, those in the pars intermedia do not enhance; this causes them to be relatively more CT-lucent than the others on postinfusion scans.[2]

When a coronal CT section is taken further posteriorly in the gland (Fig 15–6,A), the central region corresponds to the anterior portion of the posterior lobe. Histologically, this portion often consists of very vascular and compact neurohypophyseal tissue (see Fig 15–6,B). It is usually the most vascular portion of the posterior lobe, receiving vessels directly from superior and inferior vascular networks located on the surface of the gland.[12] This portion of the posterior lobe tends to be relatively homogeneous and dense on CT (see Fig 15–6,C–E). Immediately adjacent to the posterior lobe on either side is the diverging pars intermedia. When colloid cysts are large and/or abundant in the pars (see Fig 15–6,B), the CT appearance will usually be that of two elongated lucent areas extending the entire height of the gland. They slant medially as they extend from the inferior to the superior border of the pituitary gland, producing a tent-like configuration (see Fig 15–6,C and D). Lateral to the pars, on either side of the gland, are the most posterior portions of the anterior lobe. Histologically, they usually consist of the most densely compacted and heavily granulated acidophilic cells in the anterior lobe (see Fig 15–6,B); they are often the most CT-dense portions of this lobe both before and after enhancement (see Fig 15–6,C–E). Following enhancement, however, they are usually less dense than the centrally located posterior lobe. Like the posterior lobe, these laterally located portions of the anterior

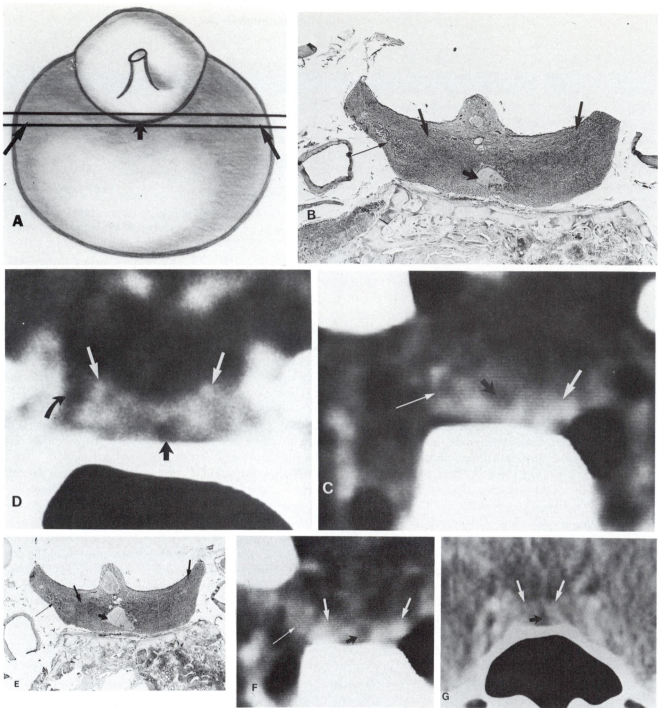

Fig 15–5.—A, schematic representation of the location of a coronal section through the anterior portion of the pars intermedia *(small thick arrow)* and the posterior portions of the anterior lobe *(large arrows).* **B,** specimen coronal histologic section (hematoxylin-eosin) demonstrates a colloid cyst *(short thick arrow)* situated centrally, densely compacted acidophilic tissue *(long thick arrows)* situated laterally, and an unsuspected loosely compacted chromophobic microadenoma *(long thin arrow)* with the acidophilic tissue on the right. **C,** closely corresponding specimen CT section demonstrates a central CT-lucent area *(short thick arrow)* corresponding to the colloid cyst. The lateral CT-dense areas *(long thick arrow)* correspond to the densely compacted acidophilic tissue. The right lateral CT-lucent area *(long thin arrow)* corresponds to the region of the microadenoma. **D,** contrast-enhanced CT section from a normal patient demonstrates similar CT-dense *(long thick arrows)* and

CT-lucent *(short thick arrow)* areas, except that the CT-dense areas *(long thick arrows)* are now symmetric. In this instance, the right lateral CT-lucent area *(curved arrow)* appears extraglandular and probably corresponds to extraglandular fat and/or connective tissue. **E,** specimen coronal histologic section (hematoxylin-eosin) slightly posterior to **B** demonstrates the central colloid cyst *(short thick arrow),* which at this point extends almost the entire height of the gland. The appearances of the microadenoma *(long thin arrow)* and of the densely compacted acidophilic tissue *(long thick arrows)* are unchanged. **F,** closely corresponding specimen CT section demonstrates the elongated central CT-lucent cyst *(short thick arrow),* the CT-lucent microadenoma *(long thin arrow),* and the CT-dense acidophilic tissue *(long thick arrows).* **G,** contrast-enhanced CT section from a normal patient demonstrates similar CT-lucent *(short thick arrow)* and CT-dense *(long thick arrows)* areas.

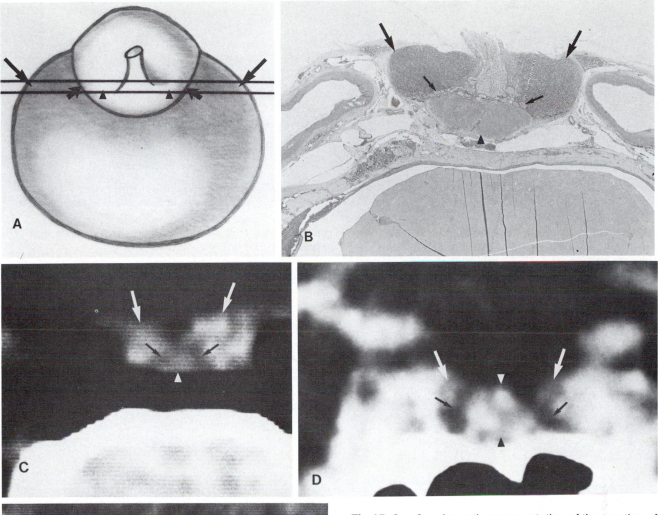

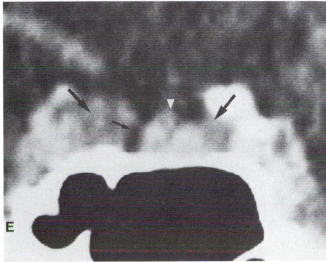

Fig 15–6.—A, schematic representation of the location of a coronal section through the midregion of the pituitary gland involving the anterior portion of the posterior lobe *(arrowheads),* the lateral portions of the pars intermedia *(small thick arrows),* and the posterior portions of the anterior lobe *(large arrows).* **B,** coronal histologic section (hematoxylin-eosin) through this region. **C,** closely corresponding specimen CT section. Strongly staining posterior portions of the anterior lobe in **B** *(large arrows)* consist of tightly compacted tissue with heavily granulated acidophilic cells; they correspond to CT-dense areas in **C** *(large arrows).* Weakly staining anterior portion of the posterior lobe in **B** *(arrowhead)* consists of compact and very vascular neurohypophyseal tissue; it corresponds to the central CT-dense area in **C** *(arrowhead).* Portions of the colloid cyst-containing pars intermedia in **B** *(small arrows)* correspond to CT-lucent areas in **C** *(small arrows).* **D, E,** contrast-enhanced patient CT sections demonstrate less enhancement of the posterior portions of the anterior lobe *(large arrows)* than of the more vascular anterior portion of the posterior lobe *(arrowheads).* The pars intermedia is CT-lucent bilaterally in **D** and unilaterally in **E** *(small arrows).* There is a slight superior convexity to the posterior lobe *(white arrowhead)* near the region of the insertion of the infundibulum in both **D** and **E.**

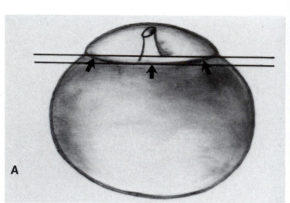

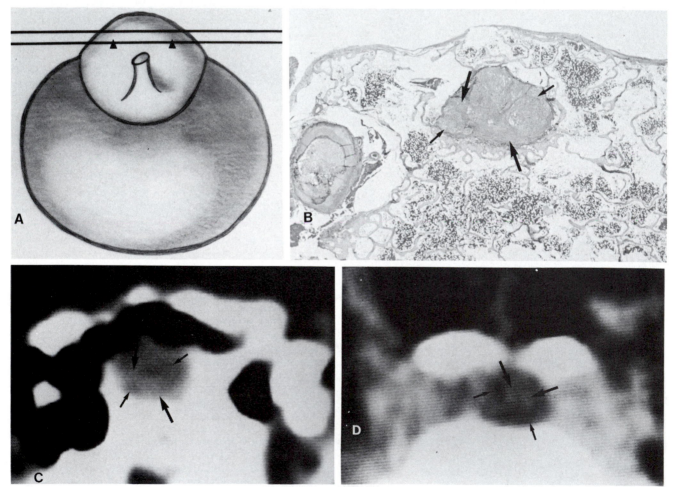

Fig 15–7.—A, schematic representation of the location of a coronal section through the midregion of a pituitary gland in which the pars intermedia *(arrows)* is transversely orientated. **B,** enhanced coronal CT section demonstrates a transversely sectioned CT-lucent pars intermedia *(arrows)* on both sides of the centrally positioned posterior lobe *(arrowhead).*

Fig 15–8.—A, schematic representation of the location of a coronal section *(arrowheads)* through the posterior lobe. **B,** coronal histologic section (hematoxylin-eosin) through the region. **C,** closely corresponding specimen CT section. Bundles of neurohypophyseal tissue in **B** consist of areas of greater *(large arrows)* and lesser *(small arrows)* degree of compactness; these areas correspond in **C** to CT-dense *(large arrows)* and CT-lucent *(small arrows)* areas respectively. **D,** contrast-enhanced normal patient with similar CT-dense *(large arrows)* and CT-lucent *(small arrows)* areas.

312

lobe tend to be relatively homogeneous on CT. A CT section through this region often includes the base of the pituitary infundibulum, which frequently gives the surface of the gland a very slight central superior convexity. The area of infundibular insertion is very CT-dense following enhancement, presumably because of its very vascular nature (see Fig 15–6,D and E).[2]

An alternative pattern is frequently seen in this midportion of the gland, presumably resulting from a more transversely positioned pars intermedia (Fig 15–7,A). The relatively lucent inferolateral regions are thought to correspond to partially volume-averaged colloid cysts in the more transversely sectioned pars intermedia. The more dense central region corresponds to the anterior portion of the posterior lobe (see Fig 15–7,B).

More posterior coronal CT slices (Fig 15–8,A) pass through the posterior lobe (see Fig 15–8,B). In this region, the posterior lobe is often inhomogeneous on CT, sometimes having a "cystic" appearance (see Fig 15–8,C and D). However, true cysts are not present. On histologic examination, bundles of neurohypophyseal tissue of differing degrees of vascularity and compactness are present. The more lucent areas on CT examination correspond to the less compact and/or less vascular bundles on histologic examination. This region of the posterior lobe may also be homogeneous on CT, in which instance it has a relatively uniform histologic

composition.[2] The most posterior portion of the posterior lobe is often embedded in a cupped dorsum sellae (Fig 15–9,A and B). The posterior lobe may also be embedded in a cupped posteroinferior sellar floor (see Fig 15–9,C).[2]

The above description of contiguous CT slices is summarized in Figure 15–10. It is dependent on strict adherence to proper technique. Head rotation must be conscientiously avoided. Coronal CT slices must be perpendicular or nearly perpendicular to the floor of the sella. Suboptimal head extension or suboptimal tube or gantry angulation will result in oblique CT slices having a superiorly positioned posterior lobe and an inferiorly positioned anterior lobe.[2]

Gland Height

Measurements of the heights of normal pituitary glands demonstrate a slightly greater mean gland height for females as compared with that of males. Syvertsen and associates[13] report a mean gland height of 4.8 ± 1.3 mm for females, with a range of 2.7 to 6.7 mm; they report a mean gland height of 3.5 ± 1.5 mm for males, with a range of 1.4 to 5.9 mm. Roppolo and coworkers,[10] performing midline measurements in the region of the anterior lobe, report a mean gland height of 4.2 ± 1.42 mm for females, with a range of 2.7 to 6.1 mm and mean gland height of 3.5 ± 0.96 mm for males,

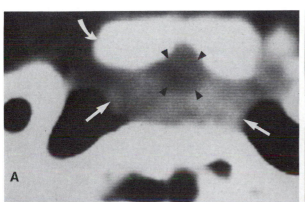

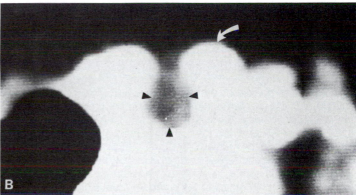

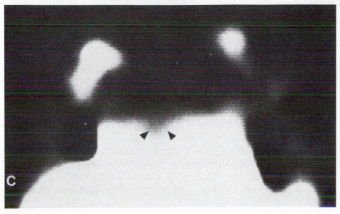

Fig 15–9.—A, axial CT section of autopsy sphenoid bone and pituitary gland specimen demonstrates a cupped dorsum sellae *(curved white arrow),* which partially envelopes a normal posterior lobe *(arrowheads).* The anterior lobe *(white arrows)* is also depicted. **B,** coronal CT section of the same cupped dorsum sellae *(curved white arrow)* as seen in **A** with its normal posterior lobe *(arrowheads).* **C,** coronal section of another autopsy specimen demonstrates cupping *(arrowheads)* in the floor of the sella turcica posteriorly and immediately adjacent to the dorsum; this cup also contains normal posterior lobe tissue.

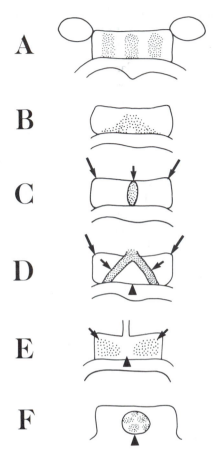

Fig 15–10.—Diagrammatic representation of frequent CT patterns formed by CT-lucent *(stippled)* and CT-dense *(solid white)* areas. Diagrams **A** and **B** correspond to sections through the anterior lobe only; diagrams **C** and **D** correspond to sections through the midregion of the gland. Diagram **C** corresponds to sections through the posterior portions of the anterior lobe *(long arrows)* and through the anterior-most portion of the pars intermedia *(small arrow)*. Diagram **D** depicts the posterior-most portions of the anterior lobe *(large arrows)*, diverging portions of the pars intermedia *(small arrows)*, and the anterior-most portions of the posterior lobe *(arrowhead)*. Diagram **E** corresponds to sections through the midregion of a gland in which the diverging pars intermedia *(small arrows)* is transversely orientated. The anterior-most portion of the posterior lobe is central *(arrowhead)*. Diagram **F** corresponds to sections through the posterior lobe *(arrowhead)* where it is embedded in the dorsum sellae.

with a range of 1.9 to 4.5 mm. Peyster and colleagues[14] report gland heights of up to 9 mm in both normal females and males between the ages of 12 and 21. Swartz and coworkers[15] have found normal-appearing glands up to 9.6 mm in height in normal females of childbearing age. Preliminary results[10] indicate a lesser gland height in two age groups, namely in the prepubertal age group and in the age group over 60. The decreased gland height in the prepubertal age group presumably correlates with the lesser degree of pituitary function in

that population. Possible etiologies for the decreased gland height in the age group over 60 include regression of the pituitary tissue from decreasing function, progressive compression of the pituitary gland from prolonged and persistent CSF pressure over time through an incompetent diaphragma sellae, and/or volume loss from ischemic changes in the anterior lobe. The anterior lobe is more prone to ischemia than the posterior lobe, presumably due to the different source and nature of its major blood supply. The anterior lobe is supplied predominantly by portal vessels originating from the superior hypophyseal arteries, which in turn arise from the supratentorial segments of the internal carotid arteries, whereas the posterior lobe receives its blood supply directly from the inferior hypophyseal arteries.[12, 16]

Cisternal Herniation

Intrasellar cisternal herniation may be defined as the invagination of the suprasellar cistern into the sella turcica (Fig 15–11). The superior border of the sella turcica corresponds to a line drawn between the points of juncture of the cavernous sinuses bilaterally with the diphragma sellae (see Fig 15–11,A). When these points of juncture are not obvious on coronal CT, they may be

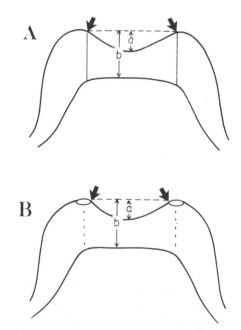

Fig 15–11.—Diagrammatic representations of cisternal herniation. **A,** the level of the superior border of the sella turcica is represented by a line *(dotted line)* drawn between the points of juncture of the cavernous sinuses bilaterally with the diaphragma sellae *(arrows)*. The percent of cisternal herniation = a/b × 100. **B,** when these points of juncture are not discernible, the level of the superior border of the sella may be empirically estimated to correspond to a line *(dotted line)* drawn between the tips of the anterior clinoid processes *(arrows)*.

empirically estimated to correspond to the tips of the anterior clinoid processes (see Fig 15–11,B). The degree of cisternal herniation may be calculated and then graded on a scale of 1 to 4 (Table 15–1).[10]

The *diaphragma sellae* borders the pituitary gland superiorly and is often concave in configuration in glands associated with cisternal herniation. In these instances, the more central portions of the diaphragma project into the confines of the sella turcica (Fig 15–12,A and B).[17] However, when the diaphragma sellae is incomplete centrally, cisternal herniation may occur through the incompetent central portion; the lateral competent portions may remain relatively flat (see Fig 15–12,C).[18] When cisternal herniation occurs in normal patients, it may be caused by persistent normal CSF pulsations on the diaphragma sellae and/or on the pituitary gland. Also, because cisternal herniation has been reported[10] in 84% of a combined normal patient and autopsy specimen population over the age of 34, and in only 16% in those younger than the age of 34, an additional normal cause for cisternal herniation may

be decreasing glandular function and therefore size with age. Pathologic causes for cisternal herniation will be discussed in Chapter 16.

Superior Glandular Surface Configuration

Roppolo and coworkers[10] report that in their combined normal patient and autopsy specimen population, the superior surface of the *anterior lobe* was flat in 56% of cases and concave in 42%. In the remaining 2%, it had a scalloped configuration consisting of a superior biconvexity with a central depression (Fig 15–13,A). This scalloped type of configuration was more frequently seen on sections of glands containing portions of the pars intermedia (see Fig 15–13,B) than on sections containing only anterior lobe tissue. In the former instances, the pars itself was the source of the central depression (see Fig 15–13,B).[10] In addition, the superior surface of the *anterior lobe* may normally have a convex configuration. This has been observed in both normal males and females between the ages of 12 and 21[14] as well as in normal females between 18 and 35.[15]

The superior surface of the *posterior lobe* may be flat, slightly concave, or even convex. Convexity is usually present when the CT section is through the posterior lobe at the point of infundibular insertion (see Fig 15–6) or through the posterior lobe where it is embedded in the dorsum sellae (see Fig 15–8).[10]

The superior surface of the *anterior lobe* of a gland

TABLE 15–1.—DEGREE OF CISTERNAL HERNIATION

Grade	1	2	3	4
$\dfrac{\text{Ht* sella} - \text{ht gland}}{\text{Ht sella}} \times 100 = \%$	1–25	26–50	51–75	76–100

*Height.

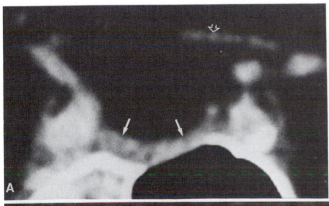

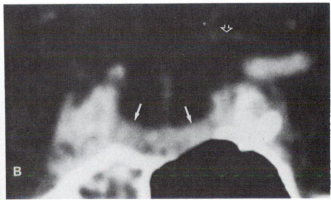

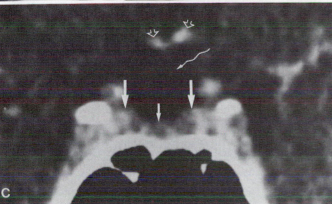

Fig 15–12.—Enhanced coronal CT sections demonstrating cisternal herniation. **A,** concave superior surface anteriorly (**A,** *small arrows*) and posteriorly (**B,** *small arrows*) is present in a gland associated with an apparent competent diaphragma sellae. A concave superior surface centrally (**C,** *small arrow*) with a flat superior surface laterally (**C,** *large arrows*) is present in a gland associated with an incompetent diaphragma sellae. Note the A-1 segments of the anterior cerebral arteries (**A, B,** and **C,** *open white arrows*) and the optic chiasm (**C,** *wavy arrow*) in the suprasellar cistern.

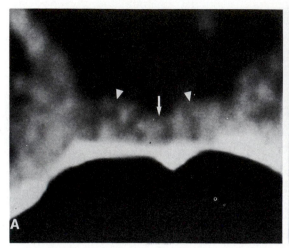
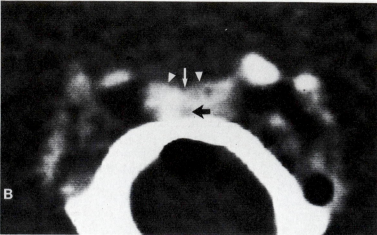

Fig 15–13.—Coronal CT. **A,** section of a patient's pituitary gland demonstrates a biconvexly scalloped superior surface *(arrowheads)* with a central depression *(large arrow)* in the region of the *anterior lobe.* **B,** section of an au-topsy specimen pituitary gland demonstrates a biconvexly scalloped superior surface *(arrowheads)* with a central depression *(small arrow)* in the region of the *pars interme-dia.* Lucent area *(large arrow)* corresponds to a colloid cyst.

associated with cisternal herniation usually has a concave configuration. Rarely, this superior surface may be scalloped with a superior biconvexity and a central depression as described previously (see Fig 15–13,A). Unless a patient is prepubertal, however, it is unusual for the superior surface of the *anterior lobe* of a gland associated with cisternal herniation to be flat.

The superior surface of the *posterior lobe* of a gland *affected by* cisternal herniation is also usually concave, but tends to have a lesser degree of concavity than the superior surface of its anterior lobe.[10]

Infundibular Displacement

While infundibular displacement often indicates the presence of a mass,[4, 13] slight displacement may occur normally.[13] This latter finding can result from the presence of a slightly eccentrically positioned posterior lobe into whose midline region the infundibulum normally inserts.[10]

Caution must be exercised to avoid mistaking tortuous anterior cerebral arteries for a displaced infundibulum. This potential error can be avoided by carefully following the course of the infundibulum from the infundibular recess of the third ventricle to the superior surface of the gland. This course may extend over several coronal CT sections. Also, because the infundibulum is generally not seen on the anterior sections of the pituitary gland where the anterior cerebral arteries characteristically reside, determining the position of the involved CT section in the gland is helpful.[10]

Bone Changes

In CT scanning, alterations of window level can easily produce areas of apparent bone thinning, simulating bone erosion (Fig 15–14). These areas range from per-pendicular or slanting linear bony defects from less than 1 mm to several millimeters in width (see Fig 15–14). Particularly when symmetric, these changes in the floor of the sella should be ignored. Although focal inferior cupping in the bony sellar floor suggests abnormality, this finding may be normal when present immediately adjacent to the dorsum sellae (see Fig 15–9,C). In addition, focal areas of anterior cupping of the dorsum sellae are almost invariably normal (see Fig 15–9,A and B). In each of the above instances, this cupping contains normal posterior lobe.[10]

Potential Problems

Because microadenomas may present with subtle or no mass effect and as CT-lucent areas, care must be taken not to mistake a lucent pars intermedia containing discernible colloid cysts for a small lucent microadenoma. This error is particularly likely when evaluating a CT section through the anterior-most portion of the pars intermedia. If the pars intermedia contains large and/or numerous colloid cysts in this section, a central lucency will be seen (see Fig 15–5,C, D, F, and G). When contiguous 1.5-mm sections are performed, this central lucency should not pose too great a diagnostic problem, because the adjacent posterior section will usually demonstrate a dense, centrally located posterior lobe with the diverging lucent pars on either side (see Fig 15–6,C–E). The presence of this latter section indicates the location of the previous section within the gland. When lucent, the diverging pars itself can be differentiated from an abnormality by its typical elongated configuration and by its tendency to slant medially as it progresses superiorly in the gland (see Fig 15–6,C–E). In addition, the sides of these normal pars lu-

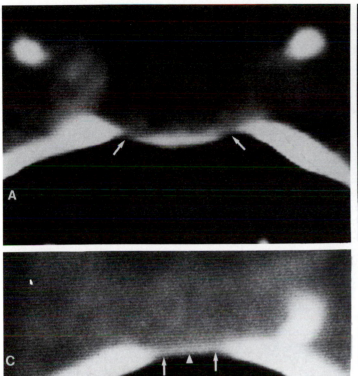

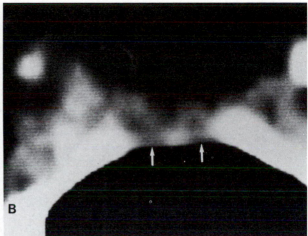

Fig 15–14.—Normal bone thinning. **A,** bilaterally symmetric oblique thinning *(arrows).* **B,** focal areas of perpendicular thinning *(arrows).* **C,** generalized thinning *(arrowhead)* with bilaterally symmetric areas of focal perpendicular thinning *(arrows).*

cencies are often parallel, a finding that would be unexpected in an expanding mass lesion.[10]

On the same section in which we see the diverging pars intermedia, another potential source for diagnostic error exists. The central, often dense and homogeneous posterior lobe, especially when flanked on either side by a lucent pars, may have the appearance of an enhancing mass lesion (see Fig 15–6,D and E). This error is particularly likely if the infundibulum inserts into the superior surface of the posterior lobe on this CT section, producing the appearance of a superior convexity at its point of insertion (see Fig 15–6,D and E).[10]

Another potential problem on anterior CT sections of the pituitary gland can result from faint visualization of the tuberculum sellae as a result of partial volume averaging (Fig 15–15). In such an instance, the gland may also appear to have an abnormal superior convexity and therefore to possess mass effect. Comparing the involved CT section with its anterior and posterior contiguous sections will help to clarify whether the source of this convexity is the extraglandular tuberculum sellae or an abnormal intraglandular mass.[10]

The Normal Suprasellar Cistern

In the routine axial projection, i.e., +20° to the orbitomeatal line, the normal suprasellar cistern has a star-shaped configuration.[19] This star is five-pointed when the pons forms its posterior border, but six-pointed when the cerebral peduncles with their interpeduncular cistern (the sixth point) are present posteriorly (Fig 15–16). The posterolateral points of the star bilaterally are formed by the portions of the perimesencephalic cisterns interposed between the lateral margins of the pons or cerebral peduncles and the medial margins of the temporal lobes. The anterolateral points of the star are interposed between the anteromedial margins of the temporal lobes and the posterolateral margins of frontal lobes. The anterior point is interposed between the medial margins of both frontal lobes and is continuous with the interhemispheric fissure anteriorly. The optic nerves and chiasm are present within the anterior portion of the suprasellar cistern, often forming a V-shaped configuration. The vascular structures comprising the circle of Willis outline its perimeter (see Fig 15–16).

The modified axial projection, i.e., −10° to −20° to the orbitomeatal line, used primarily for evaluating of the contents of the sella turcica in order to avoid low-attenuation streak artifacts, may also be used for evaluation of the suprasellar cistern. In this projection, the optic nerves, chiasm, infundibulum, and vessels of the circle of Willis are identifiable, and the free edge of the tentorial margin is seen to excellent advantage (Fig 15–17). The average transverse diameter of the optic

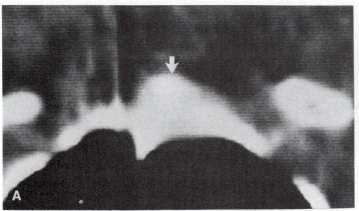

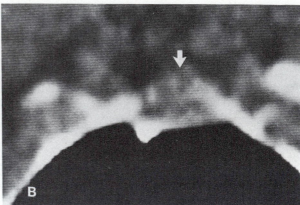

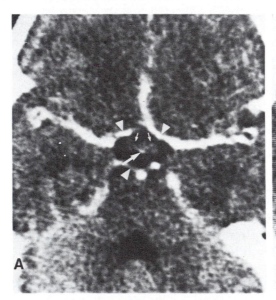

Fig 15–15.—**A,** coronal section immediately anterior to the first CT section through glandular tissue. Note the superiorly convex appearance to the bony tuberculum sellae *(arrow).* **B,** on the next contiguous section, partial volume averaging gives a similar superiorly convex configuration to the superior surface of the gland *(arrow).* **C,** on the next contiguous section, the normal flat superior border of the gland is seen *(arrow).*)

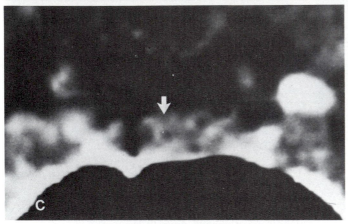

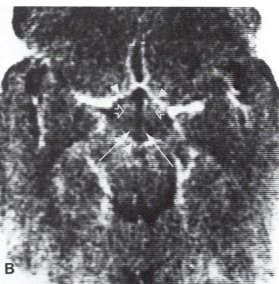

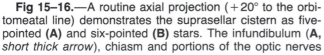

Fig 15–16.—A routine axial projection (+20° to the orbitomeatal line) demonstrates the suprasellar cistern as five-pointed (**A**) and six-pointed (**B**) stars. The infundibulum (**A,** *short thick arrow*), chiasm and portions of the optic nerves (**A,** *short thin arrows*), tuber cinereum (**B,** *open arrows*), and mammillary bodies (**B,** *long thin arrows*) are identifiable. Vessels of the circle of Willis border the periphery (**A** and **B,** *arrowheads*).

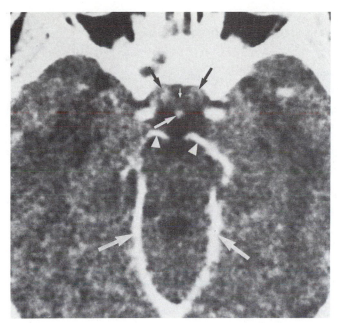

Fig 15–17.—Modified axial projection (−20° to the orbitomeatal line), which also demonstrates the infundibulum *(short thick white arrow)*, optic chiasm *(short thin white arrow)*, optic nerves *(short thick black arrows)*, and vessels of the circle of Willis *(white arrowheads)*. The tentorial margins are well seen *(large white arrows)*.

chiasm determined from axial CT sections performed at 0° to −10° to the orbitomeatal line is 1.8 cm, with a range of 1.2 to 2.7 cm.[20]

In the coronal projection, the anterior cerebral arteries and optic chiasm are located in the anterior portion of the suprasellar cistern (see Figs 15–3,D and 15–12). The average transverse diameter of the optic chiasm in this projection is 1.5 cm, with a range of 0.9 to 1.8 cm, and the average vertical diameter is 0.4 cm, with a range of 0.3 to 0.6 cm.[20] Posteriorly, the infundibulum courses from the infundibular recess of the third ventricle to the superior border of the pituitary gland in the midline (see Fig 15–12,B). The entire infundibulum may be seen on one CT section, or adjacent portions may be visible over several sections.

The Normal Cavernous Sinus

Anatomy

The superior and lateral walls of the cavernous sinus are composed of a thick layer of dura, continuous inferolaterally with the dural floor of the middle cranial fossa (Fig 15–18) and superomedially with a dural bridge between the tuberculum sellae and posterior clinoid processes (Fig 15–19,A).[21] The medial and inferior walls consist of much thinner fibrous layers, which blend with the thicker dural layers of the superior and lateral

walls (see Fig 15–18).[21] The third and fourth cranial nerves and the first and sometimes the second divisions of the fifth cranial nerve all reside within the thick lateral dural wall of the cavernous sinus (see Fig 15–18).[21–23]

The third cranial nerve pierces the dural roof of the cavernous sinus anterolateral to the posterior clinoids (see Fig 15–19). It descends slightly as it courses anteriorly along the superolateral wall of the cavernous sinus toward the superior oribtal fissure (see Figs 15–18 and 15–19,B–D).[22, 23]

The fourth cranial nerve pierces the dura slightly posterolateral to the third cranial nerve and courses inferior to it through most of the cavernous sinus (see Fig 15–19). However, just posterior to the superior orbital fissure, the fourth cranial nerve assumes a position superior to the third.[24] Within the cavernous sinus, these two nerves lie in close proximity to each other, often separated by only their thin dural coverings (see Figs 15–18 and 15–19,B–D). The fourth cranial nerve is significantly smaller than the third and often indistinguishable from it on CT.[22–24]

The fifth nerve ganglion (trigeminal ganglion) is embedded in two folds of dura, i.e., Meckel's cave, situated on the anterior aspect of the petrous apex just posterior to the cavernous sinus (see Fig 15–19,B–D). The third division of the fifth cranial nerve exits inferiorly from the ganglion toward the foramen ovale without ever entering the cavernous sinus (see Fig 15–19,B–D). The second division of the fifth cranial nerve exists anteroinferiorly from the ganglion toward the foramen rotundum (see Fig 15–19,B–D).[26] There is considerable debate as to whether this second division ever courses within the cavernous sinus.[24–26] The first division of the fifth cranial nerve enters the cavernous sinus inferiorly, courses anterosuperiorly within its lateral

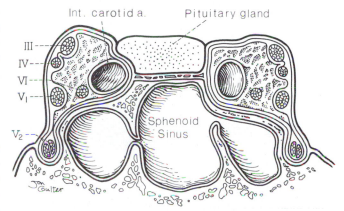

Fig 15–18.—Diagrammatic representation of a coronal section through the midcavernous sinus. (*III, IV,* and *VI* = cranial nerves; *V₁* and *V₂* = first and second divisions of fifth cranial nerve.)

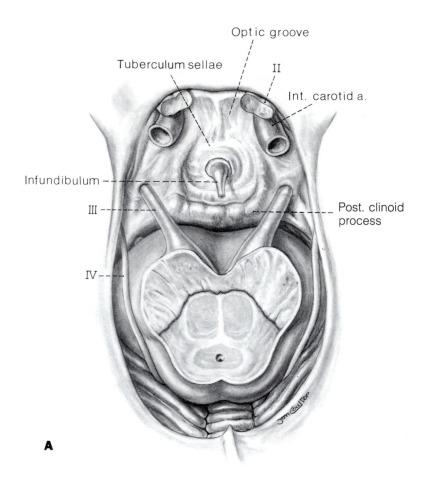

A

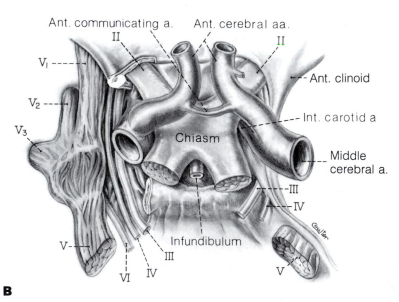

B

Fig 15–19.—A, anatomical illustration of the midbrain and sella turcica as viewed from above, depicting dural connections between the tuberculum sellae anteriorly and the posterior clinoids posteriorly. These connections define the superolateral margins of the sella turcica and the superomedial margins of the cavernous sinuses. Also depicted are the medial margins of the tentorium, which define the superolateral borders of the cavernous sinuses. (*II, III,* and *IV* = cranial nerves.) **B,** anatomical illustration of cavernous sinuses and suprasellar cistern as viewed from above. The dural coverings of the left cavernous sinus have been excised. (*II, III, IV, V,* and *VI* = cranial nerves; *V₁, V₂,* and *V₃* = divisions of the fifth cranial nerve.)

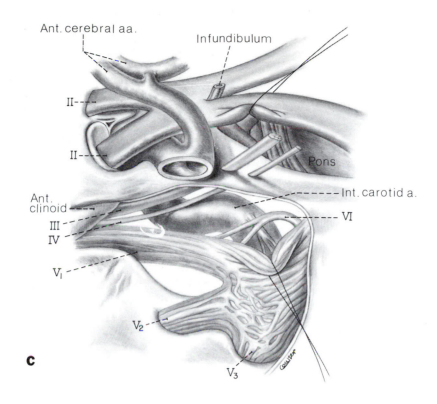

Ant. cerebral aa.

Infundibulum

II

II

Pons

Int. carotid a.

Ant. clinoid

III
IV

VI

V₁

V₂

V₃

C

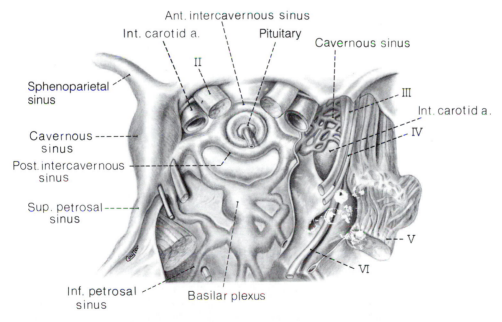

Ant. intercavernous sinus

Int. carotid a.   Pituitary

Cavernous sinus

II

Sphenoparietal sinus

III

Int. carotid a.

Cavernous sinus

IV

Post. intercavernous sinus

Sup. petrosal sinus

V

VI

Inf. petrosal sinus   Basilar plexus

D

Fig 15–19, cont.—C, anatomical illustration of cavernous sinus and suprasellar cistern as viewed from the side. The lateral dural wall of the cavernous sinus has been excised. (*II, III, IV,* and *VI* = cranial nerves; *V₁, V₂,* and *V₃* = divisions of fifth cranial nerve.) **D,** anatomical illustration of the sella turcica and cavernous sinuses as viewed from above, depicting venous connections to and from the cavernous sinuses (*center* and *left*) as well as the venous anatomy within the cavernous sinus (*right,* dural covering excised). (*II, III, IV,* and *V* = cranial nerves.)

wall, and exits at the superior orbital fissure (see Figs 15–18 and 15–19,B–D).[23, 24]

The sixth cranial nerve enters the cavernous sinus posteriorly, approximately 2 cm beneath the posterior clinoid process (see Fig 15–19,B–D).[24] It courses anteriorly frequently as multiple rootlets[23] on the inferolateral wall of the cavernous carotid artery and deep to the first division of the fifth cranial nerve (see Figs 15–18 and 15–19,B–D). It exits the sinus anteriorly through the superior orbital fissure.

The plexus of venous channels within the cavernous sinus is predominantly situated in its central and superior portions and may be partially embedded in adipose tissue (see Figs 15–18 and 15–19,D).[21] This plexus most commonly receives venous drainage anteriorly via the superior and inferior ophthalmic veins, the central retinal vein, and sometimes from the sphenoparietal sinus. It drains posteriorly primarily into the superior and inferior petrosal sinuses and inferiorly into the pterygoid plexus through the foramen lacerum, the foramen ovale, and the foramen of Vesalius (see Fig 15–19,D).[23, 27, 28] The cavernous sinuses interconnect with each other through anterior and posterior intrasellar intercavernous sinuses, usually located on the superior surface of the gland, and also through sinuses located posteriorly on the dorsum sellae (see Fig 15–19,D).[21, 23, 28]

The internal carotid artery, measuring approximately 2 cm in length, is located inferomedially within the cavernous sinus, generally deep to the venous channels and usually embedded in adipose tissue (see Figs 15–18 and 15–19,B–D). Its inferomedial border often lies within a bony groove on the lateral aspect of the sphenoid bone. Its superomedial border may abut against the pituitary gland or be separated from it by adipose tissue or more rarely by venous channels.[29] Because the cavernous carotid is anchored in position only at its point of entrance into and at its exit from the cavernous sinus, arterial tortuosity within the sinus may develop. This results in indentation of the lateral aspect of the pituitary gland by the carotid (see Fig 15–18), which is seen in 28% of glands. This indentation may be associated with a tongue-like projection of anterior lobe tissue over the carotid artery (Fig 15–20). The mean separation between the pituitary gland and carotid is 2.3 mm, with a maximum separation of 7 mm.[23]

CT Appearance

The cavernous sinus is best evaluated with enhanced 1.5-mm thick coronal CT sections performed as described previously in this chapter under Routine CT Techniques. The coronal projection is superior to the axial projection for evaluating the contents and bound-

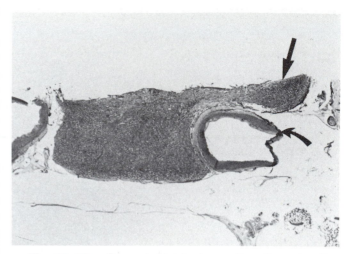

Fig 15–20.—Coronal histologic section (hematoxylin-eosin) through the pituitary gland of a normal autopsy specimen. Note indentation of its anterior lobe by the cavernous carotid artery *(curved arrow)* associated with a tongue-like extension of the anterior lobe over the carotid *(straight arrow).*

aries of the cavernous sinus, although the latter may provide supplementary information.

Normal cavernous sinuses are relatively symmetric bilaterally and have well-defined boundaries (Figs 15–21 and 15–22). They have a mediolateral diameter of 5 to 7 mm, a vertical diameter of 5 to 8 mm, and an anteroposterior diameter of 10 to 15 mm.[22] Following contrast enhancement, the carotid arteries are indistinguishable from venous structures unless they are encased by tumor, give rise to partially thrombosed aneurysms, and/or are calcified (see Fig 15–3,D). Cranial nerves, however, are frequently identifiable within the enhanced cavernous sinuses as small focal lucent areas (Figs 15–21 and 15–22).[24]

On enhanced coronal CT, the third cranial nerve is frequently able to be visualized as a small lucent area superolaterally, located immediately beneath the anterior clinoid process anteriorly and lateral to the posterior clinoid process posteriorly (see Fig 15–21,A). The fourth cranial nerve is usually not visualized as a separate entity from the third, both because of its small size and its close proximity to the third nerve. The first division of the fifth cranial nerve is present inferiorly (see Fig 15–21,A). The second division can sometimes be identified inferolaterally.[24] The fifth nerve ganglion can be discerned posteriorly adjacent to the dorsum sellae (see Fig 15–21,B). Usually, the third division of the fifth cranial nerve can be identified coursing from it toward the foramen ovale (see Fig 15–21,B).

In the axial projection, 1.5-mm thick sections through the inferior portion of the cavernous sinus may

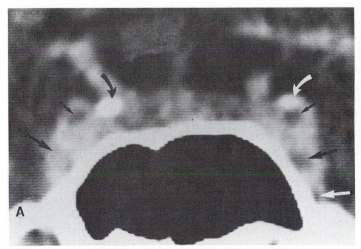

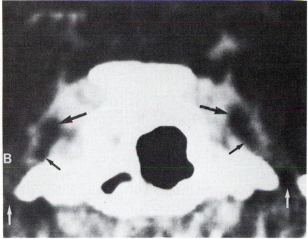

Fig 15–21.—A, enhanced coronal CT section through the midcavernous sinus. Note cranial nerve III *(small black arrows)* immediately inferior to the anterior clinoid process *(curved white arrow)* on the left and lateral to the posterior clinoid process *(curved black arrow)* on the right. The first division of the cranial nerve V *(large black arrows)* is visualized bilaterally inferior to cranial nerve III. Also demonstrated is the second division of the cranial nerve V *(large white arrow)* adjacent to or possibly within the inferior portion of the cavernous sinus. **B,** enhanced coronal CT section in the region of the dorsum sellae demonstrates the trigeminal ganglion *(large black arrows)* with the third division of cranial nerve V *(small black arrows)* coursing from it toward the foramen ovale *(small white arrows).*

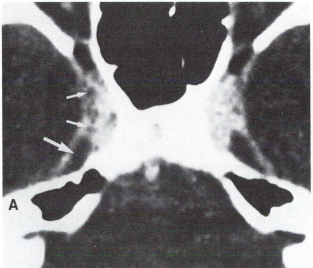

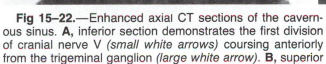

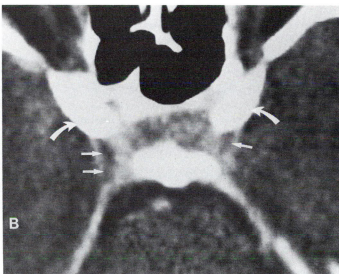

Fig 15–22.—Enhanced axial CT sections of the cavernous sinus. **A,** inferior section demonstrates the first division of cranial nerve V *(small white arrows)* coursing anteriorly from the trigeminal ganglion *(large white arrow).* **B,** superior section demonstrates cranial nerve III *(small white arrows)* coursing anteriorly, disappearing beneath the anterior clinoid processes *(curved arrows).*

demonstrate the first division of the fifth cranial nerve coursing anteriorly from the fifth nerve ganglion (see Fig 15–22,A). More superior sections may demonstrate the third cranial nerve with a similar course (see Fig 15–22,B).

NORMAL CT EVALUATION WITH METRIZAMIDE CISTERNOGRAPHY

Metrizamide CT cisternography is employed to further evaluate areas that appear suspicious on routine CT examination. It can clarify the existence of subtle convexities on the surface of the gland and differentiate intrasellar cystic lesions of CSF density from intrasellar cisternal herniation.

In the coronal projection, the superior surface of the gland is normally flat, concave, biconvexly scalloped with a central depression, or, as previously discussed, occasionally convex. The supraclinoid segments of the internal carotid arteries appear as filling defects in the metrizamide and are located medial to the anterior clinoids and superior to the cavernous sinuses (Fig 15–23,A). They divide into the middle and anterior cerebral arteries, the latter of which course anteromedially, superior to the optic chiasm (see Fig 15–23,A). If the vessels are tortuous and if cisternal herniation is present, the anterior cerebral arteries may dip into the sella turcica immediately anterior to the optic chiasm. The infundibulum is identifiable on one or several contiguous CT sections as it extends inferiorly from the infundibular recess of the third ventricle to the superior surface of the posterior half of the gland in the midline (see

Fig 15–23,B). If cisternal herniation is present posteriorly, the infundibulum will insert into the gland beneath the level of the posterior clinoids (see Fig 15–23,B).[30]

In the axial projection, the sellar and parasellar regions are best evaluated with metrizamide, with the CT sections performed at −10° to −20° to the orbitomeatal line. Because the diaphragma bridges the tuberculum sellae anteriorly with the posterior clinoids posteriorly, CT sections obtained beneath these two structures can be used for the diagnosis of cisternal herniation. However, care must be exercised not to use the section immediately at the tuberculum level, because a false impression of herniation may be deduced as a result of partial volume averaging. When cisternal herniation is present posteriorly, the infundibulum is surrounded by metrizamide below the level of the diaphragma sellae (Fig 15–24,A).[30] In the suprasellar cistern, the vessels of the circle of Willis are identifiable as curved linear filling defects located peripherally (see Fig 15–24,C). The optic nerves course posteromedially from the optic foramina toward the optic chiasm (see Fig 15–24,C); the optic tracts course posterolaterally from the chiasm toward the medial aspects of the temporal lobes (see Fig 15–24,D). The infundibulum and infundibular recess of the third ventricle are situated immediately posterior to the optic chiasm (see Fig 15–24,C and D). Mammillary bodies are identifiable between the infundibular recess of the third ventricle and the cerebral peduncles (see Fig 15–24,D), immediately inferior to the main substance of the hypothalamus. Occasionally, cranial nerves are discernible in the postclival region (see Fig 15–24,B).

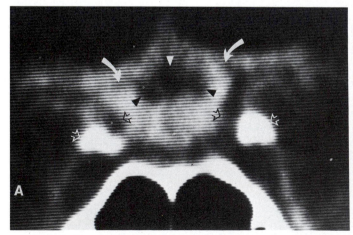

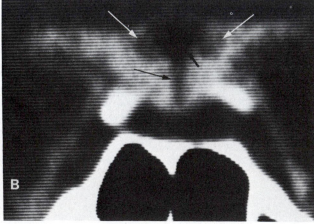

Fig 15–23.—Metrizamide cisternogram in the coronal projection. **A,** anterior CT section demonstrates the internal carotid arteries *(open black arrows)* entering the suprasellar space as they exit the cavernous sinuses just medial to the anterior clinoid processes *(open white arrows).* The A-1 segments of the anterior cerebral arteries *(curved white arrows)* course superior to the optic nerves *(black arrow-* *heads).* Note the optic recess *(white arrowhead)* situated between the optic nerves. **B,** posterior section demonstrates the infundibulum *(thin black arrow)* coursing from the infundibular recess to the third ventricle *(small black arrow)* to the pituitary gland. Note the optic tracts *(thin white arrows)* adjacent to the infundibular recess.

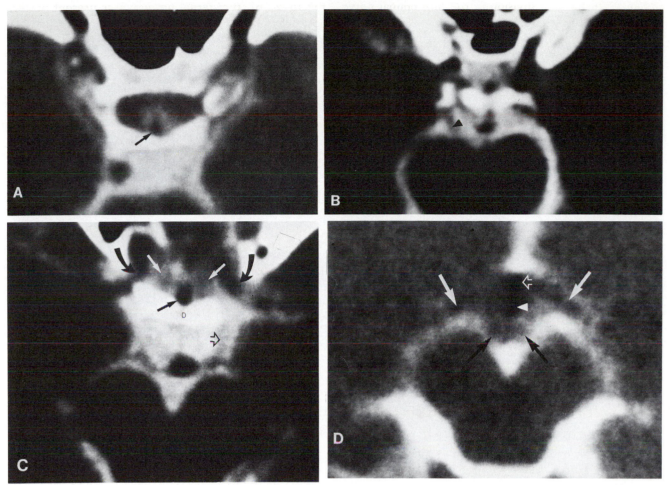

Fig 15–24.—Metrizamide cisternogram in the axial projection. **A,** cisternal herniation is demonstrated by the presence of metrizamide within the sellae, outlining the infundibulum *(small black arrow).* **B,** section slightly superior to **A** demonstrates cranial nerve III *(black arrowhead)* coursing anteriorly from the cerebral peduncle to the cavernous sinus. **C,** section slightly superior to **B** demonstrates the optic nerves *(small white arrows).* The suprasellar segments of the internal carotid arteries *(curved black arrows)* are lateral to the infundibulum *(small black arrow)* and anterior to the posterior communicating artery *(open black arrow).* (D = dorsum sellae.) **D,** section slightly superior to **C** demonstrates the optic tracts *(large white arrows),* infundibular recess *(white arrowhead),* mammillary bodies *(large black arrows),* and optic recess *(open white arrow).*

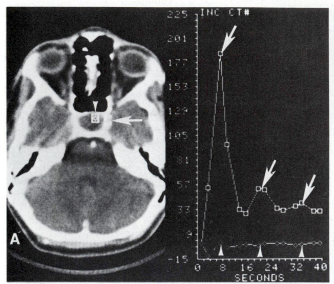

Fig 15–25.—Dynamic CT scanning demonstrates a sharp initial rise and fall in CT density followed by a small recirculation rise in both the carotid (**A,** *large arrows*) and basilar (**B,** *large arrows*) arteries. A nonenhancing area within the sella demonstrates essentially no change in CT density (**A,** *arrowheads*). An enhancing area within the sella demonstrates a gradual rise in CT density to form a plateau (**B,** *small arrows*). (Courtesy of Wendy A. Cohen, M.D., New York University Medical Center, New York.)

NORMAL CT EVALUATION WITH DYNAMIC SCANNING

On routine CT examination, the cavernous segment of the internal carotid artery is usually indistinguishable from venous channels within the cavernous sinus and may also be indistinguishable from adjacent isodense portions of the normal pituitary gland or isodense microadenomas. Dynamic CT scanning allows the cavernous segment of the internal carotid to be visualized as a separate entity (Fig 15–25). It also provides good visualization of its suprasellar segment and its branches. In addition, primary arterial structures can also be differentiated from normal pituitary gland and from tumors by means of graphic analysis of the rates of contrast accumulation. Primary arterial structures demonstrate a rapid, sharp rise and fall in CT density over the first 15 to 20 seconds; a small recirculation rise occurs during the next 15 to 20 seconds (see Fig 15–25). By contrast, normal pituitary gland and enhancing portions of tumors demonstrate a gradual rather than sharp increase in CT density during the first 30 seconds; a plateau is then reached that extends into the recirculation phase (see Fig 15–25,B).[8, 9] Nonenhancing areas such as cysts have a relatively flat curve throughout (see Fig 15–25,A).[8, 9]

REFERENCES

1. Ernest F., McCullough E.C., Frank D.A.: Fact or artifact: An analysis of artifact in high resolution computed tomographic scanning of the sella. *Radiology* 140:109, 1981.
2. Roppolo H.M.N., Latchaw R.E.: The normal pituitary gland: II. Microscopic anatomy—CT correlation. *A.J.N.R.* 4:937–944, 1983.
3. Sakoda K., Mukada K., Yonezawa M., et al.: CT scan of pituitary adenoma. *Neuroradiology* 20:249, 1981.
4. Gardeur D., Naidich T.P., Metzger J.: CT analysis of intrasellar pituitary adenomas with emphasis on patterns of contrast enhancement. *Neuroradiology* 20:241, 1981.
5. Leppick I.E., Thompson G.J., Ethier R., et al.: Diatrizoate in computed cranial tomography: A quantitative study. *Invest. Radiol.* 12:22, 1977.
6. Rosenbaum A.R., Drayer B.P.: CT cisternography with metrizamide. *Acta Radiol. Suppl.* 355:323, 1977.
7. Drayer B.P., Rosenbaum A.E., Kennerdell J.S., et al.: Computed tomographic diagnosis of suprasellar masses by intrathecal enhancement. *Radiology* 123:339, 1977.
8. Cohen W.A., Pinto R.S., Kricheff I.I.: Dynamic CT scanning for visualizing parasellar carotid arteries. *A.J.N.R.* 3:185, 1982.
9. Wing D.S., Anderson R.E., Osborn A.G.: Dynamic cranial computed tomography: Preliminary results. *A.J.N.R.* 1:135, 1980.
10. Roppolo H.M.N., Latchaw R.E., Meyer J.D., et al.: The normal pituitary gland: I. Macroscopic anatomy—CT correlation. *A.J.N.R.* 4:927–935, 1983.
11. Chambers E.F., Turski P.A., LaMasters D., et al.: Regions of low density in the contrast-enhanced pituitary gland: Normal and pathological processes. *Radiology* 144:109, 1982.
12. Stanfield J.P.: The blood supply of the human pituitary gland. *J. Anat.* 94:257, 1960.

13. Syvertsen A., Haughton V., Williams A.L., et al.: The computed tomographic appearance of the normal pituitary gland and pituitary microadenomas. *Radiology* 133:385, 1979.

14. Peyster R.G., Hoover E.D., Viscarello R.R., et al.: CT appearance of the adolescent and pre-adolescent pituitary gland. *A.J.N.R.* 4:411, 1983.

15. Swartz J.D., Russell K., Basile B.A., et al.: The high resolution CT appearance of the intrasellar contents in women of childbearing age. *Radiology* 147:115, 1983.

16. Sheehan H.L., Stanfield J.P.: The pathogenesis of postpartum necrosis of the anterior lobe of the pituitary gland. *Acta Endocrinol.* 37:479, 1961.

17. Rhoton A.L., Hardy D.G., Chambers S.M.: Microsurgical anatomy and dissection of the sphenoid bone, cavernous sinus and sellar region. *Surg. Neurol.* 12:63, 1979.

18. Kaufman B.: The "empty" sella turcica—a manifestation of intrasellar subarachnoid space. *Radiology* 90:931, 1968.

19. Naidich T.P., Pinto R.S., Kushner M.J., et al.: Evaluation of sellar and parasellar masses by computed tomography. *Radiology* 120:91, 1978.

20. Daniels D.L., Haughton V.M., Williams A.L., et al.: Computed tomography of the optic chiasm. *Radiology* 137:123, 1980.

21. Parkinson D.: Anatomy of the cavernous sinus, in Smith J.L. (ed.): *Neuro-ophthalmology Symposium of the University of Miami and the Bascom Palmer Eye Institute.* St. Louis, C.V. Mosby Co., 1972, pp. 73–101.

22. Hasso A.N., Pop P.M., Thompson J.R., et al.: High resolution thin-section computed tomography of the cavernous sinus. *RadioGraphics* 2:83, 1982.

23. Harris F.S., Rhoton A.L.: Anatomy of the cavernous sinus: A microsurgical study. *J. Neurosurg.* 45:169, 1976.

24. Kline L.B., Acker J.D., Post M.J.D., et al.: The cavernous sinus: A computed tomographic study. *A.J.N.R.* 2:229, 1981.

25. Williams P.L., Warwick R.: *Gray's Anatomy,* ed. 36. Philadelphia, W.B. Saunders Co., 1980, p. 746.

26. Henderson W.R.: A note on the relationship of the human maxillary nerve to the cavernous sinus and to an emissary sinus passing through the foramen ovale. *J. Anat.* 100:905, 1966.

27. Hasso A.N., Bentson J.R., Wilson G.H., et al.: Neuroradiology of the sphenoid region. *Radiology* 114:619, 1975.

28. Doyle D.L., Aton-Rosa D.S., Ramee A.: Orbital veins and cavernous sinus, in Newton T.H., Potts D.G. (eds.): *Radiology of the Skull and Brain: Angiography.* St. Louis, C.V. Mosby Co., 1974, vol. 2, pp. 2225–2227.

29. Fujii K., Chambers S.M., Rhoton A.L.: Neurovascular relationships of the sphenoid sinus: A microsurgical study. *J. Neurosurg.* 50:31, 1979.

30. Haughton V.M., Rosenbaum A.E., Williams A.L., et al.: Recognizing the empty sella by CT: The infundibulum sign. *A.J.N.R.* 1:527, 1980.

16

Intrasellar and Parasellar Abnormalities

HELEN M.N. ROPPOLO, M.D.

ABNORMALITIES in the sellar and parasellar regions may be caused by local mass-producing lesions, such as tumors or arachnoid cysts, or may result from more remote pathology, such as primary endocrine gland failure or generalized increased intracranial pressure.

Clinically, these abnormalities may be associated with hypo- or hypersecretion of pituitary hormones. Visual disturbances may develop from compression of the optic chiasm, nerves, and/or tracts; other cranial nerve dysfunctions may result from involvement of the cavernous sinuses.

In the following paragraphs, the CT appearances of sellar and parasellar abnormalities will be described. An attempt will be made to correlate these appearances with underlying histopathologic features.

CISTERNAL HERNIATION: "EMPTY SELLA"

Intrasellar herniation of the suprasellar cistern may occur in association with either a *competent* or an *incompetent* diaphragma sellae. The term "empty sella" classically refers to a sella into which the suprasellar cistern has herniated through an *incompetent* diaphragma[1,2] and usually implies associated expansion and remodelling of the bony sellar floor (Fig 16–1).[3]

Cisternal herniation can be a normal finding, as discussed in Chapter 15. In these instances, it is usually the result of persistent normal CSF pulsations directly on the pituitary gland or diaphragma sellae. However, cisternal herniation may also result from disease processes that cause a prolonged increase in intracranial pressure, such as benign increased intracranial pressure in the pickwickian syndrome.[2] In addition, it may occur in association with a loss of intraglandular and/or intratumoral volume secondary to pituitary infarction,[4] spontaneous tumor necrosis,[5] tumor resection, or tumor treatment with bromocriptine or radiation therapy.[6-8]

Cisternal herniation with or without an incompetent diaphragma is usually greatest in the anterior portion of the sella, resulting in a posteroinferior compression of the gland.[2,3] Factors that encourage anterior herniation include the following: (1) superior anchoring of the posterior lobe by the infundibulum as a result of direct continuity of their tissues; (2) greater vulnerability of the anterior lobe to ischemia;[4,9] and (3) greater frequency of tumors in the anterior lobe. Herniations that are primarily posterior in location have been reported in patients with diabetes insipidus, a condition associated with decreased posterior lobe function.[10]

Sellar enlargement with bony remodelling frequently accompanies an "empty sella." In the absence of coexisting tumor, five types of bony sellar configurations, as viewed sagittally, may result: cup-like, quadrangular, omega-shaped, balloon-like, and deep.[3] In the presence of tumor, areas of thinning and/or slanting of the sellar floor with or without focal inferior bony concavities may be present.

As discussed in Chapter 15, cisternal herniation with or without an incompetent diaphragma can be diagnosed on coronal CT following intravenous contrast infusion or the intrathecal instillation of metrizamide. Cisternal herniation can be differentiated from a mass lesion of CSF density in the sella, such as a cystic tumor or an arachnoid cyst, if the infundibulum can be identified below the level of the posterior clinoids (see Fig 16–1,B).[11] In difficult cases, metrizamide cisternography will establish the position of the infundibulum and outline the superior surface of the gland.[11] In addition to cisternal herniation, metrizamide cisternography can also detect slight convexities on the superior surface that can suggest the presence of an underlying microadenoma or other mass-producing abnormality.

PITUITARY GLAND HYPERPLASIA

Pituitary hyperplasia is caused either by excessive stimulation of the pituitary gland or by obstruction of

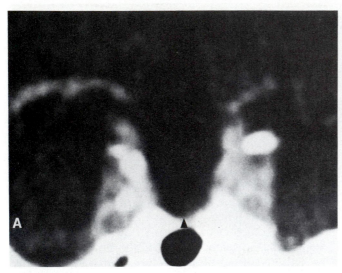

Fig 16–1.—Empty sella. **A,** enhanced coronal CT section through the anterior portion of the sella demonstrates marked cisternal herniation with remodelling of the bony floor *(arrowhead)*. **B,** posterior section demonstrates the infundibulum *(arrow)* extending deeply into the sella below the level of the posterior clinoid processes.

the normal pathways of pituitary inhibition. Excessive stimulation may result from primary end-organ failure, such as primary hypothyroidism or primary hypogonadism.[12–15] These conditions are also associated with the development of focal pituitary adenomas.[15] Obstruction of pathways of normal inhibition may result from the use of dopamine antagonists. Physiologically, dopamine is released by the hypothalamus and acts directly on the pituitary gland to inhibit the secretion of certain hormones. Also, the hypothalamic release of dopamine itself is mediated by dopamine receptors. Therefore, dopamine antagonists obstruct both the release of dopamine at the hypothalamic level and its direct inhibitory effect on the pituitary gland.[14, 16]

Hyperplastic glands tend to have an increased overall size. Their surfaces are usually superiorly convex, and their adjacent sellar floors often demonstrate bone erosion. Hyperplastic glands in the absence of focal adenomas have not as yet been implicated in causing abnormal-appearing areas within the gland on CT. However, different regions of the pituitary gland contain different concentrations of various cell types (see Chapter 15).[17] Because in hyperplasia only specific cell types may be stimulated, certain selective regions may significantly alter their degree of cellular granularity, tissue compactness, and/or tissue vascularity. Therefore, it is possible that focal CT-dense or CT-lucent areas may result in simulating adenomas.

RATHKE'S CLEFT CYST

Colloid cysts are normally present in the pars intermedia, originating from remnants of Rathke's cleft. They are lined by epithelial cells, which are cuboidal to columnar in configuration and which may or may not be ciliated. Mucin-secreting goblet cells may also be present.[18]

Occasionally, these Rathke's cleft cysts become abnormally large and produce considerable mass effect. The major portions of their central cystic areas are hypodense or isodense to brain tissue on nonenhanced CT and do not enhance following contrast infusion.[19] However, the rims and occasionally septations emanating from the rims of these cysts contain fibrous connective tissue that routinely enhances with contrast infusion (Fig 16–2) and may develop foci of nodular calcification.

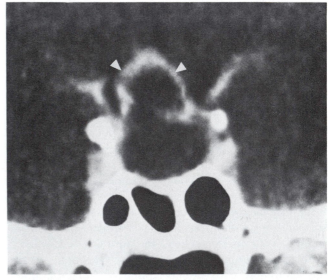

Fig 16–2.—Rathke's cleft cyst. Contrast-enhanced coronal CT section demonstrates an enhancing rim of tissue *(arrowheads)* surrounding a central low-dense cystic area. An enhancing septation is present within the cyst.

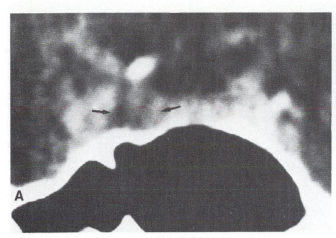

Fig 16–3.—PRL-secreting microadenomas. **A,** enhanced coronal CT section demonstrates a predominantly low-dense inhomogeneous microadenoma (arrows). At surgery, a cavity of liquified neoplastic material was encountered. Pathologic examination of solid elements of tumor demonstrated a chromophobic microadenoma. **B,** enhanced coronal CT section demonstrates focal erosion of the anteroinferior floor of the sella from a low-dense microadenoma (arrow). Pathologic examination of the surgical specimen demonstrated a chromophobic microadenoma.

PITUITARY ADENOMAS

Pituitary adenomas originate from the adenohypophyseal tissue of the anterior lobe of the pituitary gland. Clinically, they are usually identified by the hormone or hormones they secrete. By light microscopy, they are classified as chromophobic, acidophilic, basophilic, or as a mixed cell type. Most prolactin (PRL)-secreting adenomas are composed of chromophobic cells by light microscopy, although some contain acidophilic cells or a mixture of both. Growth hormone (GH)-secreting adenomas usually consist of acidophilic cells, although chromophobic cells may also be present. Adrenocorticotrophic hormone (ACTH)-secreting adenomas usually consist of both basophilic and chromophobic cells. Most nonfunctioning adenomas consist predominantly of chromophobic cells, although acidophilic cells may also be present.[20]

Adenomas Less Than 10 mm in Diameter

Microadenomas are defined as adenomas less than 10 mm in maximum diameter. They are confined to the region of the sella turcica and are best evaluated with enhanced coronal CT. Because microadenomas often possess an ill-defined shape, they can be difficult to separate from the remainder of the gland (Fig 16–3,A). Among the various types of microadenomas, GH-secreting tumors in younger patients tend to have the best margination.[19]

Microadenomas usually present with some evidence of mass effect, namely a superior convexity to the surface of the gland, infundibular displacement, bone erosion, and/or distortion of normal structural patterns within the gland (Figs 16–3 to 16–8).

In their nonenhanced state, microadenomas are usually hypodense or isodense to the most dense regions in the normal portions of the gland. Microadenomas that are GH-secreting tend to be the most CT-dense (see Fig 16–7).[19] This is at least partially due to the presence of numerous acidophilic granules within their cytoplasm.[17, 21] Microadenomas only rarely contain discernible calcification.

Microadenomas are best evaluated following contrast infusion. As in their nonenhanced state, GH-secreting tumors tend to be more CT-dense than other microadenomas following enhancement. However, PRL-secret-

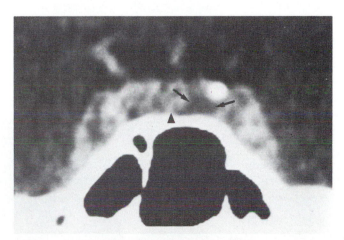

Fig 16–4.—ACTH-secreting microadenoma. Enhanced coronal CT section demonstrates a low-dense microadenoma (arrows) located in the posterolateral portion of the anterior lobe immediately adjacent to the posterior lobe (arrowhead). At surgery, this microadenoma consisted of soft tannish-pink tissue containing basophilic ACTH-positive cells.

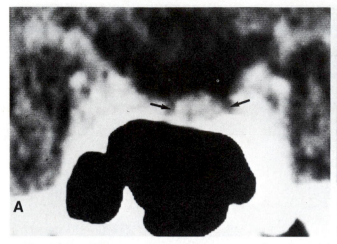

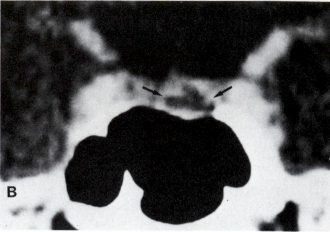

Fig 16–5.—PRL-secreting microadenoma. **A,** enhanced coronal CT section performed prior to treatment demonstrates a microadenoma (between *arrows*), which is predominantly homogeneous and isodense. **B,** on bromocriptine therapy, the microadenoma *(arrows)* became predominantly hypodense.

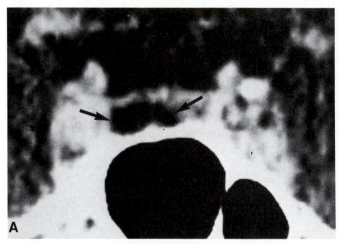

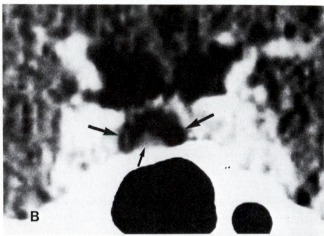

Fig 16–6.—Bromocriptine-treated, PRL-secreting microadenoma. Enhanced coronal CT sections demonstrate an abnormal low-dense area on the anterior section (**A,** *large arrows*) and both a low-dense area (**B,** *large arrows*) and a high-dense area (**B,** *small arrow*) on the posterior section. At surgery, the tumor consisted of a separate cystic portion containing yellow fluid and a solid portion containing chromophobic cells and concentric laminated calcospherites.

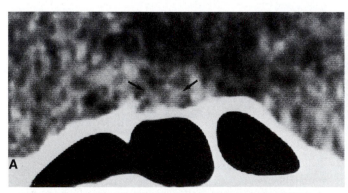

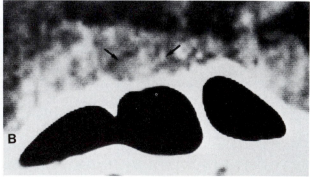

Fig 16–7.—GH-secreting microadenoma. Nonenhanced coronal CT section **(A)** demonstrates a CT-dense microadenoma (**A,** *arrows*), which enhances (**B,** *arrows*) following contrast infusion.

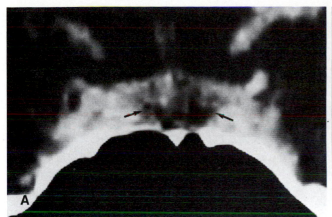
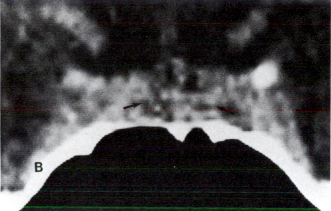

Fig 16–8.—PRL-secreting microadenoma with delayed concentration. Enhanced coronal CT sections immediately **(A)** and 30 minutes **(B)** following contrast infusion demonstrate a microadenoma, which is predominantly lucent on the immediate postinfusion scan (**A,** *arrows*), but which demonstrates an accumulation of contrast on the delayed scan (**B,** *arrows*). (Courtesy of V.M. Haughton, M.D., Milwaukee County Medical Complex, Milwaukee.)

ing tumors tend to exhibit the greatest change in CT density.[19]

At least initially following contrast infusion, the degree of microadenoma enhancement appears to depend predominantly on its degree of vascularity.[17, 19] This suggests that low-dense microadenomas or low-dense areas within microadenomas may correspond to sheets of poorly vascularized tumor cells, areas of intratumoral necrosis or cyst formation, abscesses, and/or liquified hematomas.[19, 21] Delayed enhancement may occur in at least some of these low-dense areas (see Fig 16–8).[22]

Following contrast infusion, microadenomas demonstrate one of four patterns of enhancement: (1) pattern 1: homogeneous and dense (see Figs 16–5 and 16–7); (2) pattern 2: homogeneous and hypodense to gland (see Figs 16–3,B and 16–4); (3) pattern 3: heterogeneous (see Figs 16–3,A, 16–6, and 16–8); and (4) pattern 4: pattern not discernible because of significant cisternal herniation, i.e., grade 3 or grade 4 cisternal herniation.

In the series of Gardeur and coworkers,[21] approximately one third of *PRL-secreting* microadenomas presented as dense homogeneous areas (pattern 1), one fifth as hypodense homogeneous areas (pattern 2), and approximately one third as heterogeneous areas (pattern 3). Findings of others,[6, 17, 23, 24] suggest that pattern 2, homogeneous and hypodense, is the most common presentation for PRL-secreting microadenomas, at least initially following contrast infusion.[22] Quite frequently, different CT enhancement patterns are present on different CT sections through a single PRL-secreting microadenoma (see Fig 16–6).

In the series of Gardeur and colleagues,[21] half of *nonfunctioning* chromophobic adenomas presented as dense homogeneous areas (pattern 1). One fourth were heterogeneous (pattern 3) and one fifth were relatively hypodense (pattern 2). Nonfunctioning chromophobic tumors tend to be holosellar in extent at the time of presentation, as compared with the PRL-secreting microadenomas, which are often more focal. This reflects the nonfunctioning nature of these chromophobic tumors, which often delays their detection until they become large and produce a mass effect.

Also in the series of Gardeur and coworkers,[21] none of the *GH-secreting* tumors presented as homogeneous and dense (pattern 1) or as homogeneous and hypodense (pattern 2). One fourth were heterogeneous (pattern 3) and half presented with an empty sella. In one fourth, no pathologic enhancement was discernible. Results of others[19] indicate a high frequency of homogeneous and dense tumors (pattern 1) in this group (see Fig 16–7).

Tumors that secrete *ACTH* have been reported to be predominantly hypodense (pattern 2) (see Fig 16–3,B) or to be associated with a significant degree of cisternal herniation (pattern 4).[12, 19] However, only a very few cases have been reported to date.

Adenomas Greater Than 10 mm in Diameter

If clinical symptoms resulting from hormones secreted by microadenomas go unnoticed or if the microadenomas are hormonally inactive, they may continue to enlarge, eventually extending beyond the confines of the sella turcica. Significant symmetric or asymmetric intrasphenoidal extension of tumor may result (Figs 16–9 to 16–11).[24, 25] Extension of tumor superiorly into the suprasellar cistern may also occur (Figs 16–9 to 16–12). In these latter instances, two thirds of the tumors will be positioned symmetrically above the sella, with one third growing asymmetrically.[25] Within

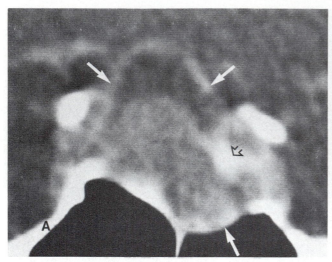

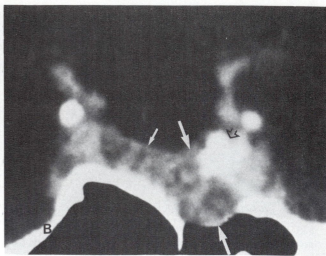

Fig 16–9.—Effects of bromocriptine on a PRL-secreting adenoma. Contrast-enhanced CT sections prior to **(A)** and following **(B)** bromocriptine therapy demonstrate a marked decrease in tumor size (**A, B,** *large arrows*). Note the different appearance of the normal glandular tissue (**B,** *small ar-* *row*) with a pattern of alternating lucent and dense areas that can be seen normally, as compared with the residual tumor tissue, which appears inhomogeneous (**B,** *large arrows*). Tumor calcification is present (**A, B,** *open arrow*).

the suprasellar cistern, pituitary adenomas extend predominantly anteriorly, superiorly, and laterally, causing symptomatology as a result of compression on the optic chiasm and/or optic nerves. Their margins are rounded, lobulated, or irregular (see Figs 16–9 to 16–12).[25] When these tumors extend above the suprasellar cistern, they cause an upward displacement of the third ventricle (see Fig 16–11,A).[24, 25] Obstruction of the foramen of Monro with subsequent hydrocephalus occurs in 12% of suprasellar adenomas.[24] Extension into one of the frontal fossae[25] with asymmetric compression of one of the lateral ventricles[24] may result from further growth. When suprasellar pituitary adenomas extend posteriorly, they cause backwards displacement of the brain stem, dilating the interpeduncular and prepontine cisterns, and/or splaying the cerebral peduncles.[25]

On nonenhanced CT, suprasellar components of pituitary adenomas have a CT density greater than brain tissue in 74% of cases, are isodense in 9%, and contain single or multiple low-dense zones in at least 17%.[25] As with their intrasellar counterparts, the solid components of suprasellar GH-secreting tumors tend to be more CT-dense than the solid components of other pituitary adenomas, a feature that is at least partially the

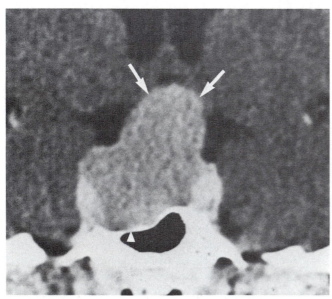

Fig 16–10.—Nonfunctioning chromophobic adenoma. Contrast-enhanced coronal CT section demonstrates sellar enlargement *(arrowhead)*, suprasellar extension *(arrows)*, and homogeneous enhancement.

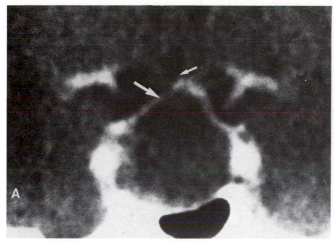
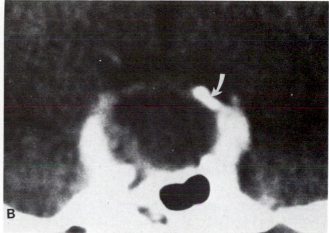

Fig 16–11.—Nonfunctioning chromophobic adenoma 6 years postradiation treatment. **A,** enhanced coronal CT section demonstrates suprasellar extension of a predominantly low-dense tumor *(large arrow)* with impingement on the third ventricle *(small arrow).* **B,** a more posterior section demonstrates capsular calcification *(curved arrow).* At surgery, approximately 8 cc of darkened old blood was aspirated, indicating a previous apoplectic episode.

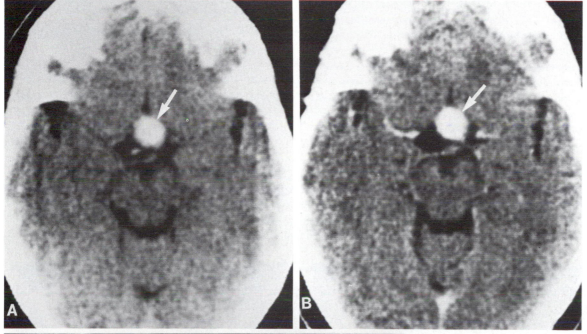

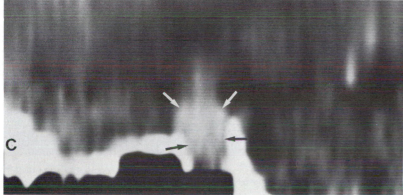

Fig 16–12.—Pituitary apoplexy. Nonenhanced **(A)** and enhanced **(B)** axial CT sections demonstrate a nonenhancing hyperdense mass *(arrow)* in the suprasellar cistern corresponding to acute hemorrhage within a chromophobic adenoma. Enhanced sagittal reconstruction **(C)** demonstrates both the intrasellar *(black arrows)* and suprasellar *(white arrows)* portions of this hemorrhagic adenoma.

result of their heavy granulation and their tendency to be densely compacted.[17, 19] When acute tumoral enlargement (pituitary apoplexy) occurs as a result of intratumoral hemorrhage, the CT density of an acute blood clot is present (see Fig 16–12). In such an instance, the area of acute hemorrhage is usually surrounded by viable tumor tissue that enhances following contrast infusion.[26] Approximately 50% of the low-dense zones in pituitary adenomas correspond to necrotic tissue, 36% to fluid, and 14% to a combination of both necrotic tissue and fluid.[27] Occasionally, a low-dense zone may represent an old blood clot (see Fig 16–11).[19]

Calcification occurs in 2% to 12% of suprasellar adenomas; the calcifications may have a rim-like or nodular appearance. The rim-like calcifications may surround a solid enhancing mass or be present in the wall of cystic structure (see Fig 16–11,B). The nodular calcifications may be distributed as scattered small foci or form a large conglomerate mass within the tumor (Fig 16–13); they may be confused with the calcifications of craniopharyngiomas.[25, 26] Pituitary adenoma calcification occurs more commonly following radiation or operative treatment than prior to therapy.

Suprasellar extensions of pituitary adenomas can enhance significantly. This enhancement is homogeneous in 44% to 51% of cases (see Fig 16–10).[21, 27] It is heterogeneous in the remaining 49% to 56%, where it consists of separate low- and high-dense zones (see Fig 16–9). Of these, 14% to 28% are almost exclusively low-dense, demonstrating only rim enhancement (see Fig 16–11).

Invasive Adenomas

Pituitary adenomas may become invasive, reflecting a malignant transformation. This may occur secondary to radiation therapy. The clinical hallmark of this malignant transformation is a rapid progression of symptoms.[28]

These adenomas may invade the sphenoid bone, the cavernous sinuses, and the trigeminal ganglia (Fig 16–14). They may also invade the dorsum posteriorly and extend directly into the brain stem cisterns of the immediate postsellar region.

Effects of Bromocriptine Therapy

The hypothalamus has a predominantly inhibitory effect on the pituitary gland with respect to its release of prolactin. This effect is mediated through dopamine, which normally acts directly upon the hypothalamus as well as directly upon the pituitary gland to effect a decrease in prolactin secretion.[14, 16] Bromocriptine is a dopamine agonist that, like dopamine, inhibits prolactin secretion. In PRL-secreting adenomas, bromocriptine usually reduces serum prolactin levels. In some patients with GH-secreting adenomas, bromocriptine can reduce serum GH levels.[29] On CT examination, Bonneville and colleagues[6] report a modification in size or density of PRL-secreting pituitary microadenomas in 75% of patients while on bromocriptine therapy. Large tumors may decrease more than 50% in size (see Fig 16–9). Small tumors may decrease in size to the point where they become indistinguishable from the normal gland. Reduction of tumor size is often rapid, occurring within the first month of therapy.[7] A more delayed reduction may occur in some patients 4 to 8 months after initiation of therapy.[7] The mechanism of decrease in tumor size is unknown, but may relate to a decrease in intracellular volume because of decreased function, to cellular necrosis, and/or to resorption of necrotic or cystic components.

During bromocriptine therapy, the CT density of

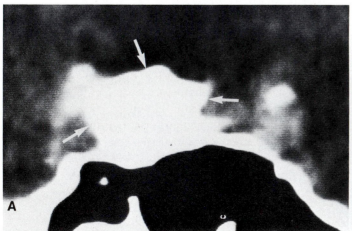
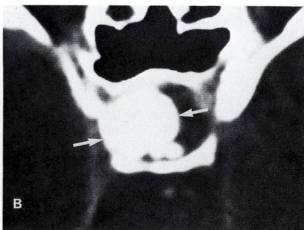

Fig 16–13.—Pituitary calculus. Enhanced coronal (A) and axial (B) CT sections demonstrate intrasellar calcification (arrows) in a patient who has undergone subtotal resection of a PRL-secreting adenoma by the subfrontal approach and who is currently on bromocriptine therapy.

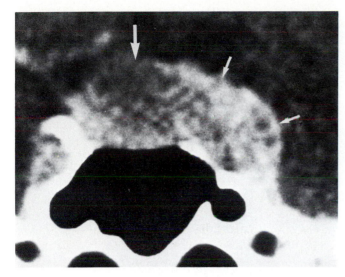

Fig 16–14.—Invasive pituitary adenoma. Enhanced coronal CT section demonstrates invasion and resultant enlargement of the cavernous sinus *(small arrows)* from a pituitary adenoma *(large arrow)*.

PRL-secreting adenomas may decrease, approaching cerebrospinal fluid (CSF) density (see Fig 16–5). Those tumors or tumor areas that reach CSF density have probably undergone necrotic cyst formation.[6] The CT density of PRL-secreting adenomas may also increase during bromocriptine therapy, approaching the CT density of the normal gland.[6, 30] Occasionally, these adenomas may change in density without any change in size.[6] Whether of high or low density, PRL-secreting adenomas generally tend to become more homogeneous during bromocriptine therapy.[30]

Evidence to date indicates that upon discontinuance of bromocriptine therapy, a rapid resurgence of tumor growth and/or function usually occurs.[29] Serum prolactin levels tend to become elevated within 1 month following termination of therapy.[29] However, in large PRL-secreting adenomas, prolactin levels may remain considerably below pretreatment levels for at least several months.[31] In small adenomas, prolactin levels that have returned to normal during therapy may, on rare occasions, remain normal for an extended period of time following discontinuance.

MENINGIOMAS

Parasellar meningiomas most frequently arise from the tuberculum sellae. In these instances, they are centered over the tuberculum in the midline (Fig 16–15) or slightly off the midline. This centering is slightly anterior to that of most suprasellar extensions of pituitary adenomas, reflecting their more anterior site of origin (see Fig 16–15,A and B).[26] Other meningiomas in the parasellar region include those originating from the planum sphenoidale, the sphenoid wings, the clinoid processes (Figs 16–16 and 16–17), the diaphragma sella, and the cavernous sinuses (Fig 16–18). Hyperos-

tosis of adjacent bone is a frequent occurrence in meningiomas (see Figs 16–15,C–E, 16–16,A, and 16–17). However, this feature is often difficult to evaluate on CT in the sellar area because of the normal presence of very dense bone in this region.

On CT examination, meningiomas usually appear rounded or slightly lobulated with sharply defined margins (see Figs 16–15,A,B, and E, 16–16, and 16–17).[24, 26] Prior to contrast infusion, they are generally more dense than adjacent brain tissue (see Fig 16–15,A).[24, 26] They may possess scattered calcifications, and a few are densely calcified (see Fig 16–16).[24] Unlike some meningiomas in other locations, suprasellar meningiomas are not usually associated with a decreased density in the adjacent brain tissue.[25] Following contrast infusion, suprasellar meningiomas, like meningiomas in other locations, usually demonstrate a dense homogeneous enhancement (see Figs 16–15,B and E and 16–16 to 16–18).[32]

CRANIOPHARYNGIOMAS

Craniopharyngiomas arise from epithelial remnants of Rathke's pouch.[33] Histologically, they are composed of nests of epithelial cells or of cysts lined by epithelial cells embedded in loose connective tissue or glial stroma.[34, 35] Twenty percent originate in the sella turcica (Fig 16–19).[34, 36] The remaining 80% originate in the suprasellar cistern or very rarely in the third ventricle.[25, 35] At the time of presentation, approximately 86% occupy primarily the suprasellar cistern.[32] Within the suprasellar cistern, craniopharyngiomas tend to be situated more posteriorly than suprasellar extensions of pituitary adenomas (Fig 16–20).[7] Approximately 60% of all craniopharyngiomas cause obstruction of the foramen of Monro (see Fig 16–19),[25, 35] compared with 12%

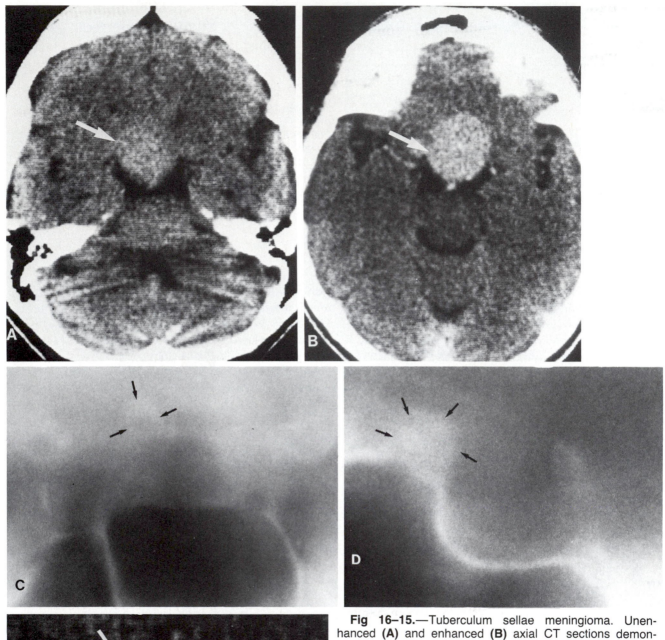

Fig 16–15.—Tuberculum sellae meningioma. Unenhanced **(A)** and enhanced **(B)** axial CT sections demonstrate the meningioma **(A, B,** *arrow*) centered in the anterior portion of the suprasellar cistern over the tuberculum sellae with no evidence of adjacent edema. The meningioma is of greater-than-brain-tissue density in its unenhanced state **(A,** *arrow*) and enhances homogeneously **(B,** *arrow*) following contrast infusion. Anteroposterior **(C)** and lateral **(D)** polytomograms demonstrate "blistering" of bone **(C, D,** *arrows*) caused by the meningioma. Enhanced coronal CT **(E)** demonstrates the corresponding CT appearance of "blistering" **(E,** *small arrow*) beneath the enhancing meningioma **(E,** *large arrow*).

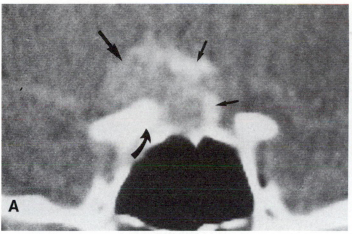

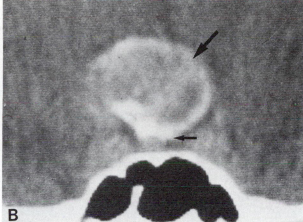

Fig 16–16.—Anterior clinoid process meningioma. **A,** enhanced coronal CT section demonstrates an enhancing meningioma *(large arrow),* which possesses peripheral calcifications *(small arrows)* and which is associated with hyperostosis of the anterior clinoid process *(curved arrow).* **B,** a more posterior CT section demonstrates the meningioma *(large arrow)* with peripheral calcifications *(small arrow)* at its junction with the pituitary gland.

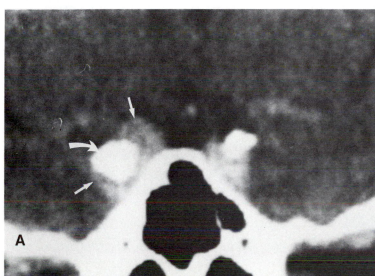

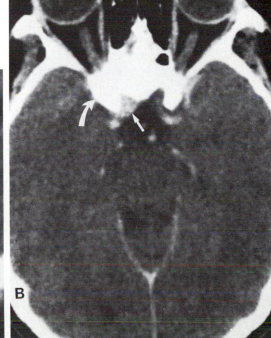

Fig 16–17.—Anterior clinoid process meningioma. Enhanced coronal **(A)** and axial **(B)** CT sections demonstrate hyperostosis of the anterior clinoid process **(A, B,** *curved* *arrow)* associated with an enhancing meningioma **(A, B,** *straight arrows).*

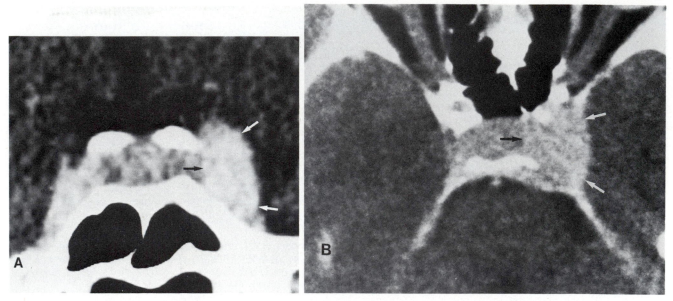

Fig 16–18.—Cavernous sinus meningioma. Enhanced coronal **(A)** and axial **(B)** CT sections demonstrate diffuse enlargement of the left cavernous sinus (**A, B,** *arrows*).

of suprasellar pituitary adenomas.[24] Craniopharyngiomas, particularly their cystic components, may extend into the frontal, temporal, and posterior fossae (Fig 16–21). Their margins may be rounded, lobulated, or irregular. Calcification is present in 58% to 77% of all cases on CT.[24, 26, 27, 32, 35] It occurs more frequently in children than adults, i.e., in 70% to 90% of children compared with 34% to 50% of adults.[24, 36]

Sixty percent of all craniopharyngiomas are primarily cystic.[34] Eighty four percent demonstrate at least some degree of cyst formation pathologically.[34] Cyst formation in craniopharyngiomas is thought to result from three possible mechanisms: (1) degenerative changes in the center of nests of adamantinomatous cells, giving rise to microcysts; (2) degenerative changes in the glial stroma; and (3) maturation and desquamation of squamous epithelium. All of these mechanisms of cyst formation may give rise to varying and sometimes high concentrations of protein within the cysts. These high protein concentrations may also be due to the presence of fenestrated capillaries, which may allow passage of protein from the vessels into the cysts.[35, 37] Craniopharyngioma cysts may also have a high cholesterol content resulting from the desquamation of cholesterol-containing squamous epithelium into them. Pathologically, 50% of these cysts have a "motor oil" consistency, 14% appear clear, and the remainder consist of a material that has a pasty, grumous, or blood-stained appearance.[34]

On nonenhanced CT examination, there is a wide variation in CT density among these cysts, ranging from near CSF density (see Figs 16–19 to 16–21,A) to a den-

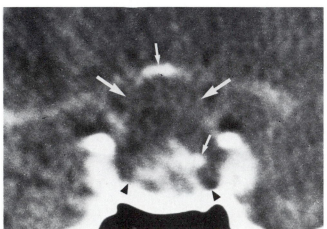

Fig 16–19.—Primary intrasellar craniopharyngioma. Coronal enhanced CT section demonstrates an intrasellar craniopharyngioma of mixed densities, including calcium *(small arrows)*. Sellar enlargement *(arrowheads)* and suprasellar extension *(large arrows)* are present.

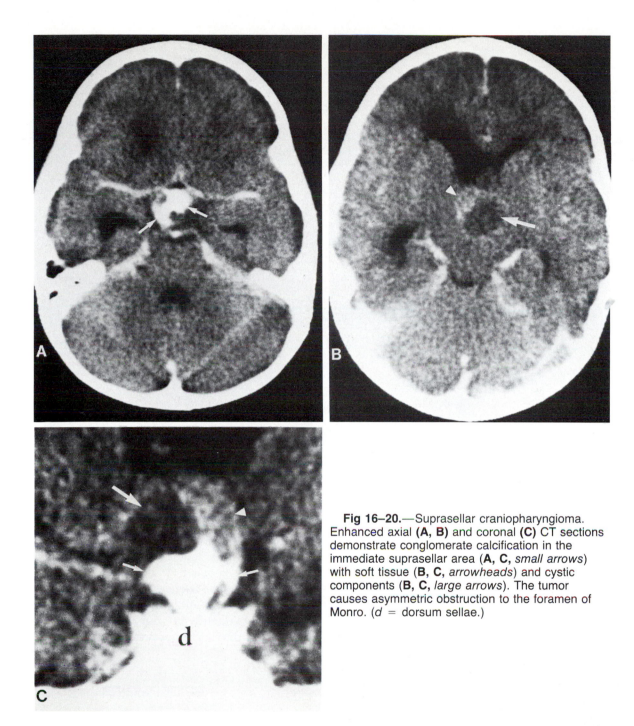

Fig 16–20.—Suprasellar craniopharyngioma. Enhanced axial **(A, B)** and coronal **(C)** CT sections demonstrate conglomerate calcification in the immediate suprasellar area **(A, C,** *small arrows*) with soft tissue **(B, C,** *arrowheads*) and cystic components **(B, C,** *large arrows*). The tumor causes asymmetric obstruction to the foramen of Monro. (*d* = dorsum sellae.)

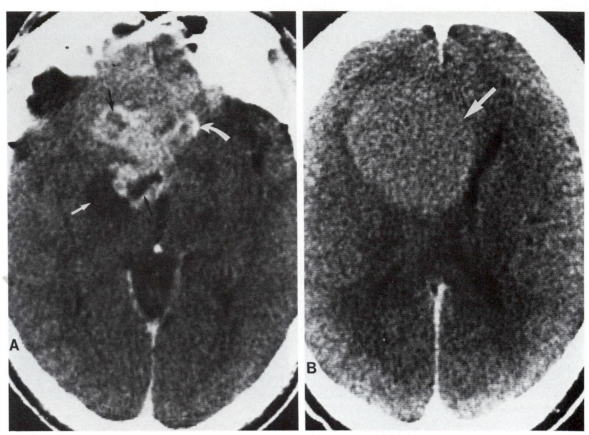

Fig 16–21.—Suprasellar craniopharyngioma. **A,** enhanced axial CT section demonstrates a cyst with a nonenhancing rim *(small white arrow)* as well as cysts with enhancing rim *(small black arrows).* Rim calcification *(curved arrow)* is present. **B,** a more superior CT section demonstrates a high-density cyst extending into the right frontal fossa *(large white arrow).*

sity greater than brain tissue (see Fig 16–21,B).[37] Low density is probably due to a high cholesterol content,[26, 38] whereas high density is the result of a high protein concentration.[37] The CT-density cannot indicate whether a cyst is composed of solid necrotic material or is of fluid consistency. Daniels and associates[27] report six cases in which cysts were isodense with CSF, three of which represented necrotic tumor and three of which corresponded to fluid.

On CT examination, calcification in craniopharyngiomas are usually conglomerate in nature. These conglomerate calcifications are most often located in the immediate suprasellar areas (see Figs 16–19 and 16–20,A and C). However, the calcifications may also be rim-like, forming discontinuous rims around the cysts (see Figs 16–21,A). In these instances, they are thought to result from degeneration of the cysts' outer epithelial lining cells.[36]

Predominantly cystic craniopharyngiomas may show no change in density with contrast infusion. Those that are predominantly soft tissue in nature or have discernible soft-tissue rims surrounding their cystic compo-

nents may demonstrate significant enhancement (see Figs 16–20,B and C, and 16–21,A). Their degree of enhancement is similar to that seen in suprasellar extensions of pituitary adenomas.[39] Enhancing soft-tissue areas, cystic areas, and areas of conglomerate calcification are all frequently present adjacent to each other on CT sections through the suprasellar region (see Fig 16–20,C).

EPIDERMOIDS

Epidermoid tumors within the cranium originate from ectoderm that is ectopically located as a result of its incomplete cleavage from the neural tube at the time of closure.[33] Epidermoids consist solely of squamous epithelium, which, through progressive maturation and desquamation, forms a central tumor core of proteinaceous material and cholesterol crystals. These tumors grow in a linear fashion similar to all epithelial tissue.

Epidermoids can be intradural or extradural in location. They arise either in the midline or slightly off the midline, as compared with dermoids, which are characteristically only midline in origin.[38] When they arise in the sella or in the suprasellar cistern, they are difficult to differentiate from craniopharyngiomas; indeed, in these regions the two entities may be synonymous.[24, 26, 34] Above the suprasellar cistern, epidermoids may also arise within the third ventricle. In addition, they may originate within the middle cranial fossa and from there extend medially, compressing the cavernous sinus and remodelling the sphenoid bone.[40] Posteriorly, they may arise extradurally, especially in the paratrigeminal region, where they can cause erosion and decalcification of the petrous apex.[40] Epidermoids have irregular, nodular, or rounded margins. Nodular margins are present in the portions of intradural tumors that insinuate into crevices around the brain.[38]

On nonenhanced CT examination, epidermoids are usually near or slightly below CSF in density (see Chapter 11, Fig 11–5). Rarely, however, they may approach the density of brain tissue. Their CT density range results from their varying cholesterol and protein concentrations.[24, 26, 36, 41] Rim-like capsular calcification may occur.[42] With contrast infusion, epidermoids typically fail to enhance, a finding reflecting their "cystic" centers and their thin hypovascular "cyst" walls.

DERMOIDS

Dermoids possess elements of the ectodermal and mesodermal germ cell layers. Although these tumors are characteristically midline in location, they only rarely arise in the suprasellar region. Like epidermoids, they contain squamous epithelium. In addition, they also contain sebaceous glands, sweat glands, and/or hair follicles.[33, 38] The capsules of dermoids are thicker and more frequently contain calcification than the capsules of epidermoids (see Chapter 11, Fig 11–2). This calcification is rim-like[38] or conglomerate in nature.[36, 41] Like most epidermoids, the "cystic" components of dermoids are low-dense, and the soft-tissue components demonstrate little if any enhancement (Fig 16–22). In dermoids, fat density may be present (see Chapter 11, Fig 11–3).

TERATOMAS

Teratomas may contain elements of all three germ cells layers.[38] Occasionally, they possess mixed malignant elements including germinomas, carcinomas, and choriocarcinomas.[42] They usually occur in the midline. Seventeen percent arise in the suprasellar region. They

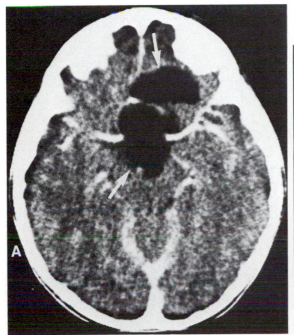
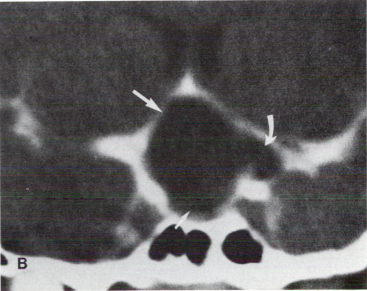

Fig 16–22.—Suprasellar dermoid cyst. **A,** enhanced axial CT section demonstrates a nonenhancing dermoid cyst *(arrows)* of CSF density extending from the suprasellar cistern into the left frontal fossa beneath A-1 segment of the left anterior cerebral artery. Histologically, it was composed of keratinizing epithelium keratin debris and pilosebaceous material. **B,** coronal CT section from a metrizamide cisternogram demonstrates insinuation of the dermoid cyst *(curved arrow)* between the basal ganglia and temporal lobe. A line of demarcation *(small arrow)* between the dermoid cyst *(large straight* and *curved arrows)* and the pituitary gland is identifiable.

are seen more frequently only in the pineal region, where they occur 70% of the time.[42]

On CT examination, the margins of teratomas are usually slightly irregular.[41] These tumors may contain very dense globules of calcification or ossification (see Chapter 11, Fig 11–9). The calcification may be central, a feature that helps to differentiate them from dermoids and epidermoids.[35] Fat density may be present, reflecting the adipose nature of some of the tissues (see Chapter 11, Figs 11–1 and 11–9). They often enhance inhomogeneously.[41]

GERMINOMAS

Suprasellar germinomas, also referred to as atypical teratomas or ectopic pinealomas, arise from primitive germ cells prior to their differentiation into germ cell layers. These tumors may be mass-like, compressing adjacent structures, and/or invasive, extending into them. When mass-like, their margins are well demarcated and lobulated (Fig 16–23); when invasive, their margins are ill defined. Invasive germinomas infiltrate structures of the suprasellar cistern, including the infundibulum and the optic chiasm, nerves, and tracts,

eventually obliterating the entire space. They can extend superiorly and posteriorly, invading the periventricular regions around the third and lateral ventricles.[42] Whether invasive and/or mass-like, bony changes including erosion of the posterior clinoids and ballooning of the sella turcica may occur.[42]

On nonenhanced scans, germinomas are either equal or slightly higher in density than in normal brain tissue (see Fig 16–23,A).[25, 42] They do not exhibit calcification. With contrast infusion, they characteristically demonstrate intense enhancement (see Fig 16–23,B).[25]

MESENCHYMAL CHONDROSARCOMAS

Parasellar mesenchymal chondrosarcomas (chondromyxoid fibromas) are embryonic in origin, arising from cartilaginous differentiation of mesenchymal cells in the meninges.[43] They usually originate in the region of the petrous apex and adjacent sphenoid bone, where they may cause destructive and/or sclerotic changes. They tend to grow anteriorly into the middle cranial fossa, displacing the cavernous sinus in the process. The lateral wall of the cavernous sinus and presumably the cranial nerves that course through it are displaced lat-

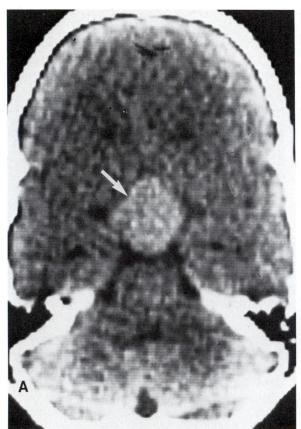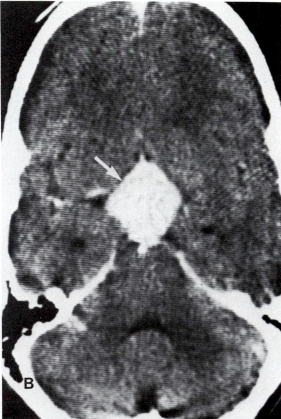

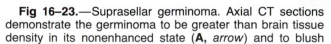

Fig 16–23.—Suprasellar germinoma. Axial CT sections demonstrate the germinoma to be greater than brain tissue density in its nonenhanced state (**A,** arrow) and to blush intensely following contrast infusion (**B,** arrow). Margins are well demarcated and lobulated.

erally. The cavernous carotid artery is displaced inferiorly and anteriorly.

Parasellar mesenchymal chondrosarcomas may possess dense nodular central calcifications and may have a heavily calcified peripheral rim (Fig 16–24). Low-dense areas are interspersed between the calcific regions. These tumors, however, may also demonstrate no evidence of calcification and present only as low-dense regions on nonenhanced scans.[44]

Following contrast infusion, rim enhancement may be discernible in portions adjacent to the lateral dural wall of the cavernous sinus (Fig 16–25). Part or all of this enhancement may represent enhancing dura and/or laterally displaced and partially compressed venous portions of cavernous sinus. In the low-dense portions of these tumors, mild patchy enhancement may be present (see Figs 16–24 and 16–25).

CHORDOMAS

Chordomas arise from notochordal remnants. Histologically, they consist of lobules of mucoid tissue surrounded by fibrous septae. These lobules are contained within well-defined capsules. They are composed of sheets or cords of cells possessing varying amounts of intracellular mucin; the cells are embedded in a background of extracellular mucin. Osseous sequestra and dystrophic calcification may be present.[45] These tumors present as bulky, lobulated masses, which are soft or firm depending upon their degree of calcification.[36]

Intracranial chordomas may arise on the dorsal surface of the clivus or dorsum sellae.[45] Erosion of the clivus occurs in 53% to 62%,[45–47] of the dorsum sellae in

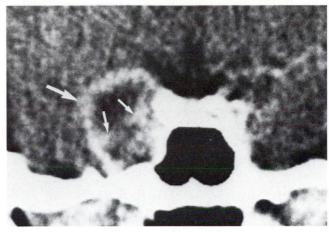

Fig 16–25.—Mesenchymal chondrosarcoma. Enhanced coronal CT section demonstrates peripheral rim enhancement (large arrow), at least a portion of which represents enhancing dura. Patchy central areas of enhancement (small arrows) are also present.

34% to 69%,[45–47] of the petrous bone in 30% to 50%,[46, 47] of the orbital fissure in 20% to 25%,[46–48] and of the foramen ovale in 23%.[46–48] After eroding either the clivus or dorsum sellae, chordomas may invade the retropharyngeal airspace, the sphenoid sinus, and the sella turcica.[47] Sclerosis of bone occurs in 5% of cases.[48]

Tumor calcification is present in 34% to 86%.[47, 48] Lindgren and DiChiro[49] have classified these calcifications in the following way: (1) reticular, resembling fine lace work; (2) solid nodular; (3) scattered flecks measuring 1 to 2 mm; (4) cystic rim; and (5) combination of nodular and rim.

On CT scans, the margins of chordomas may be regular or irregular. Prior to contrast infusion, their soft-tissue components may be of low or intermediate density. Their actual CT density most likely reflects their ratio of cellular-to-mucoid elements, with the cellular elements possessing the greater CT density. When chordomas contain calcifications, the amount is variable; sometimes they are densely calcified (see Chapter 10, Fig 10–24).

Following contrast infusion, large low-dense chordomas do not enhance. Intermediate-density tumors may enhance, but the degree of enhancement is less than that of meningiomas.[26, 47, 48] Densely calcified tumors may demonstrate no enhancement or show only rim enhancement;[46] the rim enhancement may represent only enhancing dura.

HAMARTOMAS

A hamartoma is a congenital maldevelopment of tissue consisting of an area of focal overgrowth. A favorite site of origin for this type of tumor in the nervous sys-

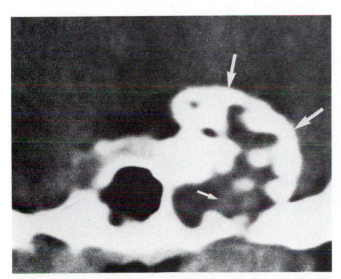

Fig 16–24.—Mesenchymal chondrosarcoma. Enhanced coronal CT section demonstrates thick rim calcification (large arrows) and more central nodular calcifications interspersed with patchy areas of enhanced tissue (small arrow).

tem is the hypothalamus. Hypothalamic hamartomas usually originate in the tuber cinereum, which is located in the floor of the third ventricle. From there, they grow into the interpeduncular and suprasellar cisterns; they frequently remain attached to the tuber cinereum by only a stalk. Clinically, these tumors present with precocious puberty, seizures, and/or laughing spells. On nonenhanced and enhanced CT examinations, hamartomas show the same CT density as normal brain tissue (Fig 16–26). Their margins are slightly lobulated and/or irregular.[50]

SCHWANNOMAS

Schwannomas (neurofibromas, neurinomas, neurilemmomas) are nerve sheath tumors that may arise in the parasellar region in association with cranial nerves II to VI. When associated with cranial nerve II, they can arise in the suprasellar cistern, optic canal, and/or orbit. When associated with cranial nerves III to VI, they may involve the cavernous sinus. Schwannomas of the trigeminal ganglion arise in the region of the Meckel's cave, immediately posterior to the cavernous sinus. Bone erosion and destruction may be associated with schwannomas (see Chapter 10, Fig 10–17). Following contrast enhancement, they tend to be isodense with

the cavernous sinus either in their entirety or in their peripheral portions.[44]

GLIOMAS

Gliomas originating within the suprasellar cistern may be derived from the optic chiasm, nerves, or tracts. They can infiltrate superiorly into the hypothalamus, laterally into the temporal lobes, or anteriorly into the orbital canals. When present within the orbital canals, they may be associated with bone erosion. Primary suprasellar gliomas tend to be better marginated and less malignant than primary hypothalamic gliomas.[24, 36] Except for their cystic or necrotic portions, they can enhance mildly or intensely (Figs 16–27 and 16–28). When they are confined to the region of the optic chiasm, nerves, and/or tracts, they tend to enhance poorly (see Fig 16–27). When large (see Fig 16–28), they tend to enhance intensely and are difficult to differentiate from primary hypothalamic gliomas. A vertical diameter of the optic chiasm greater than 6 mm suggests a chiasmal tumor.[51]

METASTASES

Metastases to the sellar and parasellar regions commonly occur. They may spread from distant sites or be

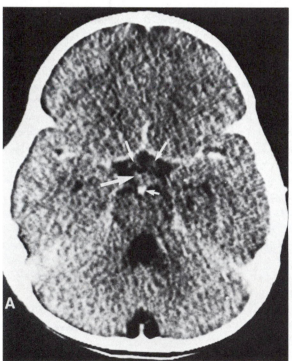

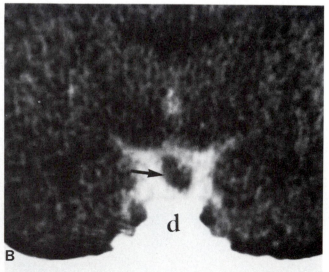

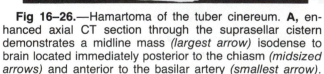

Fig 16–26.—Hamartoma of the tuber cinereum. **A,** enhanced axial CT section through the suprasellar cistern demonstrates a midline mass *(largest arrow)* isodense to brain located immediately posterior to the chiasm *(midsized arrows)* and anterior to the basilar artery *(smallest arrow).*

B, coronal section of metrizamide cisternogram demonstrates the hamartoma *(arrow)* located immediately above the dorsum *(d).* The thin residual connection with the hypothalamus was unable to be identified on CT.

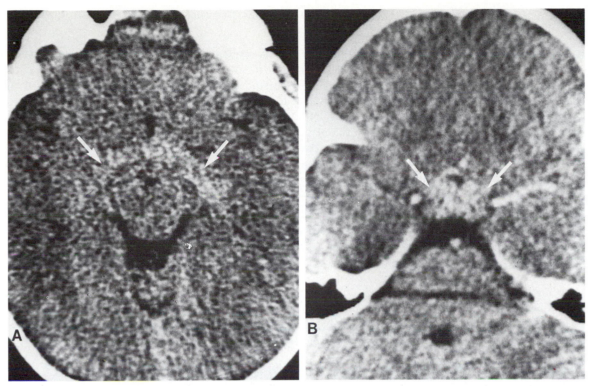

Fig 16–27.—Chiasmal glioma. **A,** nonenhanced axial CT section demonstrates a slightly hyperdense chiasmal glioma invading the optic tracts *(arrows)*. **B,** the enhanced axial CT section through the suprasellar cistern demonstrates a bilobulated configuration to the chiasmal glioma in this region *(arrow)*. Only minimal enhancement is present.

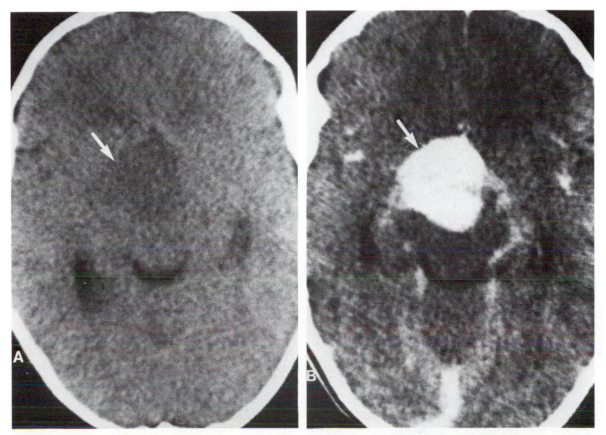

Fig 16–28.—Optic nerve glioma. Nonenhanced **(A)** and enhanced **(B)** axial CT sections demonstrate a glioma that is low-dense **(A,** *arrow)* prior to contrast infusion and enhances intensely **(B,** *arrow)* postinfusion.

the result of direct extension from adjacent structures. A common form of direct extension is from the orbit to the cavernous sinus. Metastases sometimes spread between the sellar and suprasellar regions via the infundibulum. When this occurs, a mass with a dumbbell-shaped configuration can result; one portion of the mass is confined to the sella turcica beneath a bulging diaphragma, and the other portion is situated within the suprasellar cistern. With contrast infusion, metastatic tumors usually enhance; their most dense regions are frequently isodense with the cavernous sinus (Fig 16–29). These metastatic tumors, especially in the suprasellar region, may become cystic and demonstrate rim enhancement.

ARACHNOID CYSTS

Arachnoid cysts may be congenital, post-traumatic, or post-inflammatory in origin. Congenital arachnoid cysts originate as a result of entrapment of CSF during the development of the leptomeninges; post-traumatic and post-inflammatory arachnoid cysts result from arachnoidal adhesions.

Arachnoid cysts may be divided into two types. The first is the true arachnoid cyst, in which there is no communication between the cyst and the subarachnoid space. The second is more properly called an arachnoid pouch, because communication between the two does exist (Fig 16–30). A ball-valve phenomenon may be operative in these cases to allow entrapment of CSF.[52]

Arachnoid cysts may rarely originate within the sella turcica.[53] More commonly, however, they arise in the suprasellar cistern. From here, they can extend inferiorly into the intrasellar region or superiorly, displacing the third ventricle upwards and ultimately causing obstruction at the foramen of Monro (see Fig 16–30,C). Arachnoid cysts may also originate from or extend into the lateral parasellar regions (see Fig 16–30), where

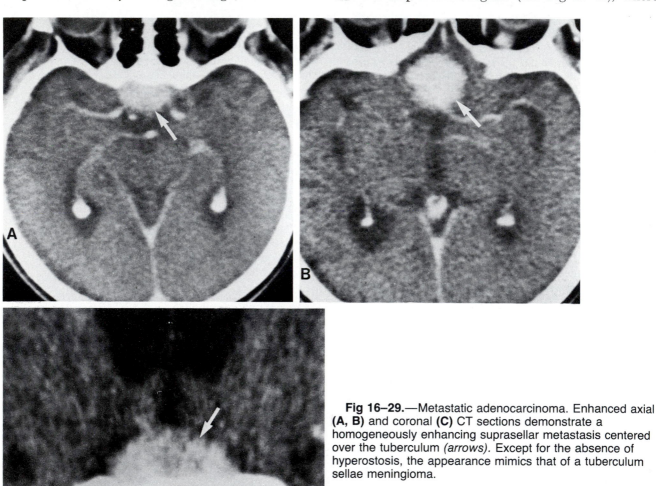

Fig 16–29.—Metastatic adenocarcinoma. Enhanced axial **(A, B)** and coronal **(C)** CT sections demonstrate a homogeneously enhancing suprasellar metastasis centered over the tuberculum *(arrows)*. Except for the absence of hyperostosis, the appearance mimics that of a tuberculum sellae meningioma.

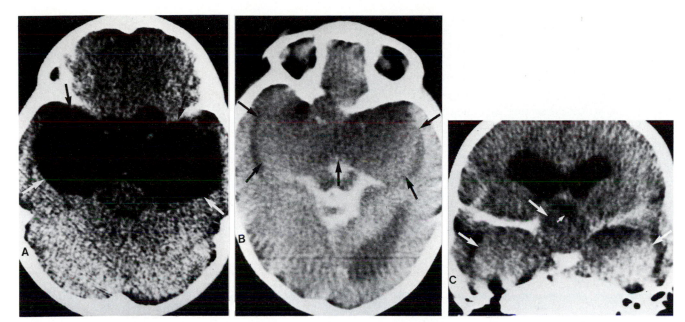

Fig 16–30.—Arachnoid cyst. **A,** nonenhanced axial CT section demonstrates a large arachnoid cyst *(large arrows)* extending laterally from the suprasellar cistern into both temporal fossae. **B,** axial cisternogram CT section demonstrates immediate filling of the arachnoid cyst *(large arrows)* with metrizamide, indicating communication between the subarachnoid space and the cyst. **C,** coronal cisternogram CT section demonstrates superior displacement and invagination of the third ventricle *(small arrow)* by the arachnoid cyst *(large arrows)*.

they may cause expansion of the temporal fossa, particularly in children.

On CT examination, the margins of arachnoid cysts are sharply defined; they may be round, straight, biconvex, semicircular, or even concave, often molding to the structures with which they come into contact (see Fig 16–30). They are of CSF density and do not calcify. They do not demonstrate central or rim enhancement following contrast infusion.

Arachnoid cysts can be differentiated from large CSF-containing cisterns when they result in a displacement of brain tissue or vascular structures or cause bony remodelling. They may be indistinguishable on CT from neuroepithelial (ependymal) cysts, which occasionally occur in this region (Fig 16–31). Noncommunicating arachnoid or neuroepithelial cysts can be differentiated from communicating arachnoid cysts by metrizamide cisternography (see Figs 16–30 and 16–31). However, because even noncommunicating cysts may accumulate contrast material late by absorption through their walls, it is necessary to scan the patient immediately after the instillation of metrizamide to establish the presence of communication. A suprasellar cyst can be differentiated from an enlarged third ventricle that has herniated into the suprasellar cistern and sella turcica when continuity between the herniated and nonherniated portions of the third ventricle can be identified on coronal CT (Fig 16–32).

VASCULAR PROCESSES

Aneurysms of the sellar and parasellar regions originate from cavernous (Fig 16–33) and suprasellar (Fig 16–34) portions of the internal carotid arteries and from the anterior communicating artery.[53] With enlargement, aneurysms from the cavernous and immediate supraclinoid segments of the internal carotid may extend laterally into the middle cranial fossa or medially into the sella turcica. Extension into the sella may be associated with remodelling of the sphenoid bone, which tends to be more asymmetric than seen with most pituitary adenomas (see Fig 16–33,A).[27, 54] Erosion of the clinoid processes may also occur.[44]

Prior to contrast infusion, the central portions of aneurysms are usually isodense or hyperdense to adjacent brain.[24] Their margins are round or fusiform. Approximately two thirds contain rim calcification (see Figs 16–33,A and 16–34).[27, 44] Occasionally, underlying thrombus is also calcified.[44] With contrast infusion, rim enhancement occurs in many instances (see Fig 16–34). Homogeneous enhancement of the entire lesion occurs in approximately 55% of cases[55] and indicates absence of significant thrombus formation (see Fig 16–33). When thrombus is present, only partial enhancement of the aneurysm will occur. This results in the formation of a target lesion, with the enhancing central or eccentric target area representing the patent lumen (see Fig 16–34).[44, 55] When there is complete thrombo-

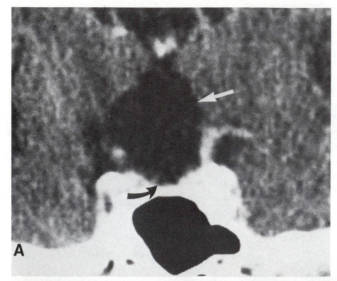

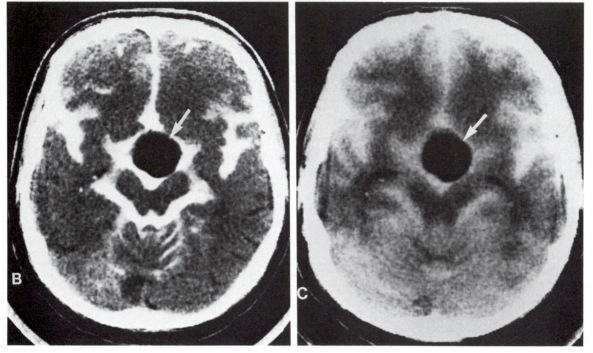

Fig 16–31.—Neuroepithelial cyst. **A,** enhanced coronal CT section demonstrates a CSF-density cyst situated predominantly in the suprasellar cistern (**A,** *large arrow*) and extending into the sella turcica (**A,** *curved arrow*). Axial CT sections immediately (**B**) and several hours following (**C**) the intrathecal instillation of metrizamide demonstrate absence of communication of the cyst (**B, C,** *large arrow*) with the subarachnoid space.

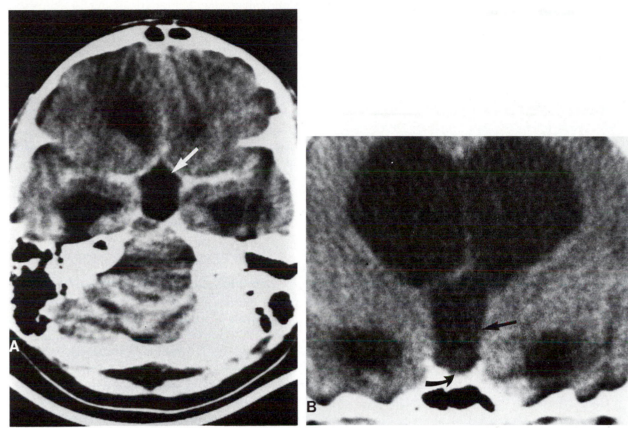

Fig 16–32.—Intrasellar herniation of third ventricle secondary to obstructive hydrocephalus. **A,** contrast-enhanced axial CT section demonstrates ahexagonal configuration to the circle of Willis caused by the herniated third ventricle *(arrow).* **B,** contrast-enhanced coronal CT section demonstrates contiguity of the intrasellar *(curved arrow)* and suprasellar *(straight arrow)* components of the third ventricle, which has a less rounded configuration than most cysts.

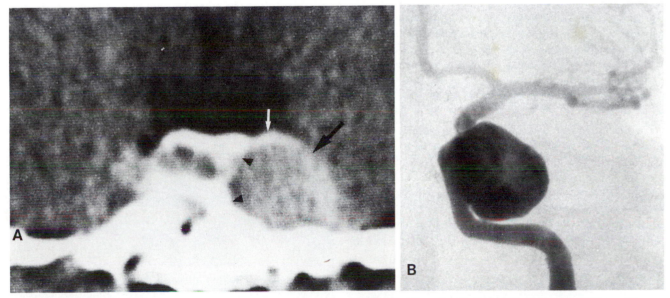

Fig 16–33.—Cavernous carotid aneurysm. **A,** enhanced coronal CT scan demonstrates a homogeneously enhancing cavernous carotid aneurysm *(large arrow)* possessing rim calcification *(small arrow),* but having no evidence of thrombus formation. Bony remodelling of the dorsum sellae *(arrowheads)* is present. **B,** corresponding angiogram.

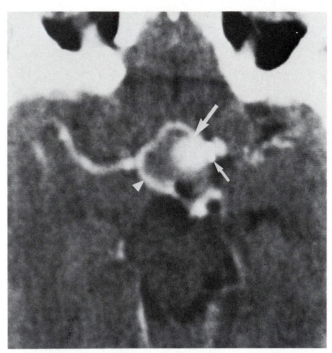

Fig 16–34.—Suprasellar carotid aneurysm. Enhanced axial CT section demonstrates an enhancing eccentric aneurysmal lumen *(large arrow)*, aneurysmal rim enhancement *(arrowhead)*, and rim calcification *(small arrow)*.

sis or when a portion of the patent lumen is not included in a particular CT section, only rim enhancement will be identifiable.[55] Occasionally, the parent vessel of an aneurysm will be visible in continuity with it, demonstrating the aneurysmal neck.[24] If aneurysms are scanned 10 to 15 minutes postinfusion, they may have a mottled appearance for uncertain reasons.[24, 25] In these instances, the aneurysm may be difficult to differentiate from neoplastic disease.

Carotid-cavernous fistulas and arteriovenous malformations in the region of the cavernous sinus usually cause enlargement of the sinus and often of the superior ophthalmic vein (see Chapter 17, Fig 17–49).[4]

Tortuosity of the cavernous carotid artery without aneurysmal dilatation can cause lateral sellar erosion with asymmetric sellar enlargement.[56] This phenomenon may be bilateral.

Dynamic CT scanning is helpful in differentiating primary vascular abnormalities, such as aneurysms, carotid-cavernous fistulas, or arteriovenous malformations, from other lesions by their earlier filling and by the characteristic enhancement curves they produce (see Chapter 15).

INFLAMMATORY PROCESSES

Sellar and parasellar infectious processes may result in the formation of abscesses with low-dense centers

and rim enhancement (Figs 16–35 and 16–36). Erosive bone changes may be present. When the granulomas of tuberculosis[57] or of sarcoidosis are present in the suprasellar region,[58] they may form well-demarcated, homogeneously enhancing mass lesions (Fig 16–37). The tuberculomas may calcify. Involvement of the parasellar meninges by cysticercosis can result in the formation of nonenhancing cysts of CSF density indistinguishable from arachnoid cysts.[59] Lymphoid adenohypophysitis, an infiltrative inflammatory process of the pituitary gland, can result in an enlarged homogeneously enhancing gland that often extends into the suprasellar space.[60] This abnormality is usually seen in young women with rapidly developing hypopituitarism and is thought to be autoimmune in origin.

DIFFERENTIAL DIAGNOSIS

Intrasellar Abnormalities

Abnormalities *confined to the sella* that can be *predominantly low-dense* on CT include pituitary adenomas (see Figs 16–3,B, 16–4, and 16–5,B), Rathke's cleft cysts (see Fig 16–2), craniopharyngiomas, metastases, epidermoids, and arachnoid cysts. Intrasellar abnormalities that may *enhance inhomogeneously* include pituitary adenomas (see Figs 16–3,A, 16–6, and 16–8), craniopharyngiomas (see Fig 16–21,A), metastases, and abscess (see Figs 16–35 and 16–36). Those abnormalities that can enhance homogeneously include pituitary adenomas (see Figs 16–5,A and 16–7), metastases (see Fig 16–29), pituitary glandular hyperplasia, and lymphocytic adenohypophysitis. Intrasellar lesions that can calcify include craniopharyngiomas (see Fig 16–19) and pituitary adenomas (see Fig 16–13), the latter cal-

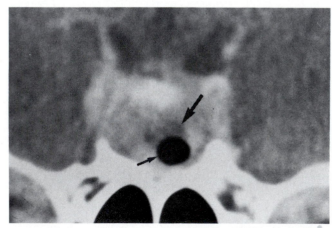

Fig 16–35.—Pituitary abscess. A low-dense center *(large arrow)* with gas *(small arrow)* is present within an abscess developing 3 years after resection of a chromophobic adenoma. Because a nongas-forming organism was cultured, the gas presumably indicates the existence of a communication between the enlarged sella and nasopharynx.

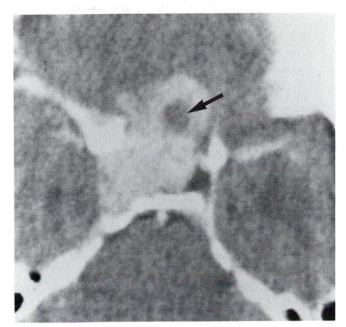

Fig 16–36.—Pituitary abscess. Abscess developing within an adenoma demonstrates a low-dense center *(arrow)* with an enhancing rim of tissue.

cifying most frequently following radiation treatment or surgical intervention.

Primary Intrasellar vs. Primary Suprasellar Abnormalities

Abnormalities that are intrasellar in origin, but extend into the suprasellar space, can usually be differentiated from primary suprasellar abnormalities extending secondarily into the sella. This differentiation is possible when continuity of the suprasellar and intrasellar tissues is evident on coronal CT (see Figs 16–2 and 16–9 to 16–11). In addition, primary intrasellar lesions frequently cause the lateral walls of the sella to be *convex* laterally (see Figs 16–2, 16–11, and 16–19). In secondary lesions, the lateral walls are usually funnel-shaped in configuration (see Figs 16–1,A and 16–32,B). Also, although both primary and secondary intrasellar abnormalities may result in sellar enlargement with remodelling of the bony floor (see Figs 16–1 to 16–3, 16–5 to 16–11, 16–13,A, 16–14, and 16–35), the degree of sellar enlargement in secondary lesions is less than would be expected from similarly sized primary intrasellar abnormalities.

Parasellar Abnormalities: Primary and Secondary

Nonenhancing Low-Dense Regions

Parasellar abnormalities, whether primary or secondary, frequently possess nonenhancing low-dense regions representing cysts, necrotic material, or poorly vascularized low-dense tissue. The nonenhancing areas

of craniopharyngiomas range in density from near *CSF to greater-than-brain-tissue density;* the *rims of these areas may enhance* and *calcify* (see Figs 16–19 to 16–21). Gliomas and rarely meningiomas may also possess nonenhancing low-dense areas; although their *rims may enhance, they only rarely calcify.* Suprasellar extensions of pituitary adenomas and Rathke's cleft cysts may possess low-dense areas with *rim enhancement* (see Figs 16–2, 16–9,A, and 16–11). The low-dense areas of adenomas may rarely possess *rim calcification* (see Fig 16–11,B); those of Rathke's cleft cysts may occasionally possess peripheral *focal nodular calcification.* The *rims* of low-dense areas of parasellar metastases and abscesses also *enhance,* but these *do not calcify.* The *rims* of nonenhancing low-dense areas of dermoids and epidermoids *rarely enhance* but may *calcify* (see Fig 16–22). In the case of extradural epidermoids, however, the presence of enhancing dura on one side of the lesion and of the bone on the other may mimic rim enhancement. The CT density of the nonenhancing low-

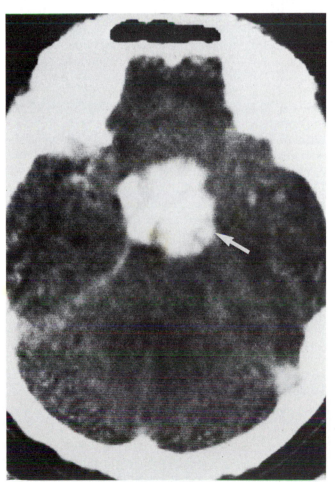

Fig 16–37.—Suprasellar tuberculoma. Enhanced axial CT section demonstrates a markedly enhancing mass lesion *(arrow),* which demonstrated greater-than-brain-tissue density on the nonenhanced scan.

dense areas of epidermoids and dermoids is usually *near CSF density* (see Fig 16–22). In epidermoids, however, this density may rarely approach that of brain tissue, and in dermoids, fat density may be present. When a nonenhancing low-dense area does not demonstrate rim enhancement or calcification, it must be differentiated from an arachnoid cyst (see Fig 16–30), a neuroepithelial cyst (see Fig 16–31), a cyst of cysticercosis, or an enlarged third ventricle that has herniated into suprasellar cistern (see Fig 16–32).

Poorly Enhancing Regions

Hamartomas (see Fig 16–26) and early optic chiasm gliomas (see Fig 16–27) enhance poorly following contrast infusion, appearing nearly isodense to brain tissue. Both lesions occur most frequently in childhood.

Homogeneously Enhancing Regions

Solid abnormalities originating within or extending into the parasellar spaces and that possess homogeneously enhancing areas include meningiomas (see Figs 16–15,B and E, and 16–16 to 16–18), chiasmal (see Fig 16–27,B), optic nerve (see Fig 16–28,B), optic tract and hypothalamic gliomas, craniopharyngiomas (see Figs 16–20,B and C, and 16–21,A), germinomas (see Fig 16–23,B), embryonal cell carcinomas, teratomas, schwannomas, metastases (see Fig 16–29), granulomas (see Fig 16–37), aneurysms (see Figs 16–33,A and 16–34), pituitary adenomas (see Fig 16–10), hyperplastic pituitary glands, histiocytic lymphomas, lymphocytic adenohypophysitis, and hypothalamic histiocytosis. Rim calcification in association with dense homogeneous enhancement usually indicates the presence of an aneurysm (see Fig 16–33,A), although meningiomas (see Fig 16–16) and pituitary adenomas may mimic this appearance.

Central Nodular Calcification

Parasellar lesions that may possess central nodular calcification include craniopharyngiomas (see Figs 16–19 and 16–20,A and C), meningiomas, pituitary adenomas (usually post-treatment) (see Fig 16–13), mesenchymal chondrosarcomas (see Fig 16–24), and chordomas. Pituitary apoplexy may also cause central increased CT density as a result of acute intratumoral hemorrhage (see Fig 16–12).

REFERENCES

1. Kaufman B., Chamberlain W.B. Jr.: The ubiquitous "empty sella" turcica. *Acta Radiol.* 13:413, 1973.
2. Kaufman B.: The "empty" sella turcica—a manifestation of intrasellar subarachnoid space. *Radiology* 90:931, 1968.
3. Bajraktari X.: Skull changes with intrasellar cisternal herniation. *Neuroradiology* 13:89, 1977.
4. Plaut A.: Pituitary necrosis in routine necropsies. *Am. J. Pathol.* 28:883, 1952.
5. Smaltino F., Bernini F.P., Muras I.: Computed tomography for diagnosis of empty sella associated with enhancing pituitary microadenoma. *J. Comput. Assist. Tomogr.* 4:592, 1980.
6. Bonneville J.E., Poulignot D., Cattin E., et al.: Computed tomographic demonstration of the effects of bromocriptine on pituitary microadenoma size. *Radiology* 143:451, 1982.
7. Scotti G., Scialfa G., Pieralli S., et al.: Macroprolactinomas: CT evaluation of reduction of tumor size after medical treatment. *Neuroradiology* 23:132, 1982.
8. Lee W.M., Adams J.E.: The empty sella syndrome. *J. Neurosurg.* 28:351, 1968.
9. Stanfield J.P.: The blood supply of the human pituitary gland. *J. Anat.* 94:257, 1960.
10. Marano G.D., Horton J.A., Vazquez A.M.: Computed tomography in diabetes insipidus: Posterior empty sella. *Br. J. Radiol.* 54:263, 1981.
11. Haughton V.M., Rosenbaum A.E., Williams A.L., et al.: Recognizing the empty sella by CT: The infundibulum sign. *A.J.N.R.* 1:527, 1980.
12. Okuno T., Sado M., Momoi T., et al.: Pituitary hyperplasia due to hypothyroidism. *J. Comput. Assist. Tomogr.* 5:600, 1980.
13. Lawrence A.M., Wilber J.F., Hagen T.C.: The pituitary and primary hypothyroidism: Enlargement and unusual growth hormone secretory responses. *Arch. Intern. Med.* 132:327, 1973.
14. Murad E., Haynes R.C.: Hormones and hormone antagonists, in Gilman A.G., Goodman L.S., Gilman A. (eds.): *The Pharmacological Basis of Therapeutics.* New York, Macmillan Publishing Co., 1980, pp. 1380–1383.
15. Danzinger J., Wallace S., Handel S., et al.: The sella turcica in primary end organ failure. *Radiology* 131:111, 1979.
16. Frantz A.G.: Prolactin. *Phys. Med. Biol.* 298:201, 1978.
17. Roppolo H.M.N., Latchaw R.E.: The normal pituitary gland. Part II: Microscopic anatomy—CT correlation. *A.J.N.R.* 4:937, 1983.
18. Shanklin W.M.: The incidence and distribution of cilia in the human pituitary with a description of micro-follicular cysts derived from Rathke's cleft. *Acta Anat.* 11:24, 1951.
19. Sakoda K., Mukada K., Yonezawa M., et al.: CT scan of pituitary adenomas. *Neuroradiology* 20:240, 1981.
20. Martinez A.J., Lee A., Moossy J., et al.: Pituitary adenomas: Clinicopathological and immunohistochemical study. *Ann. Neurol.* 7:24, 1980.
21. Gardeur D., Naidich T.P., Metzger J.: CT analysis of intrasellar pituitary adenomas with emphasis on patterns of contrast enhancement. *Neuroradiology* 20:241, 1981.
22. Hemminghytt S., Kalkoff R., Daniels D.L., et al.: Computed tomographic study of hormone-secreting microadenomas. *Radiology* 146:65, 1983.
23. Syvertsen A., Haughton V.M., Williams A.L., et al.: The computed tomographic appearance of the normal pituitary gland and pituitary microadenomas. *Radiology* 133:385, 1979.
24. Naidich T.P., Pinto R.S., Kushner M.J., et al.: Evaluation of sellar and parasellar masses by computed tomography. *Radiology* 120:91, 1976.

25. Leeds N.E., Naidich T.P.: Computerized tomography in the diagnosis of sellar and parasellar lesions. *Semin. Roentgenol.* 12:121, 1977.

26. Fahlbusch R., Grumme T.H., Aulich A., et al.: Suprasellar tumors in the CT scan, in Lanksch W., Kazner E. (eds.): *Cranial Computerized Tomography.* Berlin, Heidelberg, New York, Springer Publishing Co., 1976, pp. 114–127.

27. Daniels D.L., Williams A.L., Thornton R.S., et al.: Differential diagnosis of intrasellar tumors by computed tomography. *Radiology* 141:697, 1981.

28. Salvolini U., Menichelli F., Pasquini U.: Sellar region: Normal and pathological conditions, in Baert A., Jeanmart L., Wackenheim A. (eds.): *Clinical Computed Tomography.* Berlin, Heidelberg, New York, Springer Publishing Co., 1978, pp. 14–37.

29. Luboshitzky R., Barzilai D.: Bromocriptine for an acromegalic patient: Improvement in cardiac function and carpal tunnel syndrome. *J.A.M.A.* 244:1825, 1980.

30. Roppolo H.M.N., Meyer J.D., Latchaw R.E., et al.: High resolution computerized tomographic evaluation and comparison of the normal pituitary gland and prolactin secretion adenomas. Presented at the 19th Annual Meeting of the American Society of Neuroradiology, Chicago, April 4–9, 1981.

31. Eversman T., Fahlbusch R., Rjosk K.H., et al.: Persisting suppression of prolactin secretion after long term treatment with bromocriptine in patients with prolactinomas. *Acta Endocrinol.* 92:413, 1979.

32. Numaguchi Y., Kishikawa T., Ikeda J., et al.: Neuroradiological manifestations of suprasellar pituitary adenomas, meningiomas, and craniopharyngiomas. *Neuroradiology* 21:67, 1981.

33. Toglia J.U., Netsky M.G., Alexander E.: Epithelial (epidermoid) tumors of the cranium: Their common nature and pathogenesis. *J. Neurosurg.* 23:384, 1965.

34. Petito C.K., DeGirolami U., Earle K.: Craniopharyngiomas: A clinical and pathological review. *Cancer* 37:1944, 1976.

35. Fitz C.R., Wortzman G., Harwood-Nash D.C., et al.: Computed tomography in craniopharyngiomas. *Radiology* 127:687, 1978.

36. Weisberg L.A., Nice C., Katz M.: The juxtasellar region–visual, endocrine or radiographic abnormalities, in Weisberg L.A., Nice C., Katz M. (eds.): *Cerebral Computed Tomography: A Text-Atlas.* Philadelphia, W.B. Saunders Co., 1978, pp. 162–191.

37. Braun I.F., Pinto R.S., Epstein F.: Dense cystic craniopharyngiomas. *A.J.N.R.* 3:139, 1982.

38. Davis K.R., Roberson G.H., Taveras J.M., et al.: Diagnosis of epidermoid tumor by computed tomography: Analysis and evaluation of findings. *Radiology* 119:347, 1976.

39. Hatam A., Bergstrom M., Greitz T.: Diagnosis of sellar and parasellar lesion computed tomography. *Neuroradiology* 18:249, 1979.

40. Kline L.B., Acker J., Post M.J.D., et al.: The cavernous sinus: A computed tomographic study. *A.J.N.R.* 2:299, 1981.

41. Gonzalez C.F., Grossman C.B., Palacios E.: Neoplastic Disease, in Gonzalez C.F., Grossman C.B., Palacios E. (eds.): *Computed Brain and Orbital Tomography.* New York, John Wiley & Sons, 1976, pp. 57–149.

42. Tekeuchi J., Morik K., Moritake K., et al.: Teratomas in the suprasellar region: Report of five cases. *Surg. Neurol.* 3:247, 1975.

43. Rollo J.L., Green W.R., Kahn L.B.: Primary meningeal mesenchymal chondrosarcoma. *Arch. Pathol. Lab. Med.* 103:239, 1979.

44. Hasso A.N., Pop P.M., Thompson J.R., et al.: High resolution thin section computed tomography of the cavernous sinus. *Radio Graphics* 2:83, 1982.

45. Utne J., Pugh D.G.: The roentgenologic aspect of chordoma. *A.J.R.* 74:59, 1955.

46. Tan W.S., Spigos D., Khine N.: Case report: Chordoma of the sellar region. *J. Comput. Assist. Tomogr.* 6:154, 1982.

47. Schechter M.M., Liebeskind A.L., Azar Kia B.: Intracranial chordomas. *Neuroradiology* 8:67, 1974.

48. Kendall B.E., Lee B.C.P.: Cranial chordomas. *Br. J. Radiol.* 50:687, 1977.

49. Lindgren E., DiChiro G.: Suprasellar tumors with calcification. *Acta Radiol.* 36:173, 1951.

50. Mori K., Handa H., Takeuchi J., et al.: Hypothalamic hamartoma. *J. Comput. Assist. Tomogr.* 5:519, 1981.

51. Daniels D.L., Haughton V.M., Williams A.L., et al.: Computed tomography of the optic chiasm. *Radiology* 137:123, 1980.

52. Banna M.: Arachnoid cysts on computed tomography. *A.J.R.* 127:979, 1976.

53. Ring B.A., Waddington M.: Primary arachnoid cysts of the sella turcica. *A.J.R.* 98:611, 1966.

54. Raymond L.A., Tew J.: Large suprasellar aneurysms imitating pituitary tumour. *J. Neurol. Neurosurg. Psychiatry* 41:83, 1978.

55. O'Neill M., Hope T., Thompson G.: Giant intracranial aneurysms: Diagnosis with special reference to computerized tomography. *Clin. Radiol.* 31:27, 1980.

56. Anderson R.D.: Tortuosity of the cavernous carotid arteries causing sellar expansion simulating pituitary adenoma. *A.J.R.* 126:1203, 1976.

57. Whelan M.A., Stern J.: Intracranial tuberculoma. *Radiology* 138:75, 1981.

58. Brooks B.S., Gammal T.E., Hungerford G.D., et al.: Radiological evaluation of neurosarcoidosis: Role of computed tomography. *A.J.N.R.* 3:513, 1982.

59. Bentson J.R., Wilson G.H., Helmer E., et al.: Computed tomography in intracranial cysticercosis. *J. Comput. Assist. Tomogr.* 1:464, 1977.

60. Hungerford G.D., Biggs P.J., Levine J.H., et al.: Lymphoid adenohypophysitis with radiological and clinical findings resembling a pituitary tumor. *A.J.N.R.* 3:444, 1982.

The Orbit

Introduction

WILLIAM E. ROTHFUS, M.D.

Computed tomography has unquestionably changed the diagnostic approach to pathology of the orbit. Conventional tomography, venography, and arteriography are no longer used with regularity, their usefulness being limited to specific clinical situations. With its ability to distinguish grades of soft-tissue density, to image small objects, and to obtain and display information in multiple projections, CT has rapidly displaced these older methods as the examination of choice in complicated orbital cases. Versatile and easily performed, it has proved useful in a wide variety of clinical settings.

Because of its superb ability to define the anatomy of the orbit, the primary role of orbital CT scanning has been anatomical. That is, it has been used mainly to locate orbital lesions, determine their size, and elucidate the extent of involvement of other orbital or periorbital structures. Orbital trauma serves as an example. A penetrating metallic foreign body can be precisely located, as can associated bony fractures. In addition, soft-tissue injury of the globe, optic nerve, or muscle along the path of the foreign body can be seen and quantitated. So too, orbital infection can be described by primary location of involvement and the degree of spread through the orbital soft tissue.

Other orbital processes, like neoplasm, noninfectious inflammatory masses, and vascular abnormalities, can be characterized by more than an anatomical description. Surely CT is critical in delineating the location and extent of these lesions, but other characteristics, like texture, density before and after contrast, method of spread, and shape can give insight into the specific nature of the pathologic process. Indeed, in many instances, the CT characteristics may be specific enough to suggest the correct histology of the process. Few articles in the literature have addressed this aspect, differential diagnosis, as it relates to CT scanning of the orbit.

The purpose of this section, therefore, is twofold. Firstly, it is to emphasize the utility of high-resolution orbital scanning in a variety of clinical contexts, all of which require precise anatomical information. Secondly, it is to provide some structure for the analysis of this anatomical information. Thus, the section is divided into chapters representing problems that present commonly on CT scans of the orbit. Some of these problems, e.g., infection or trauma, simply require an orderly anatomical approach to solve. Other problems, e.g., tumors or enlarged optic nerve sheath, are more difficult. They have a variety of differential diagnostic possibilities that must be considered. The more frequent differentials are discussed in the appropriate chapters.

It is emphasized that exact histologic diagnosis is often not possible on the basis of the CT scan alone. As in any radiologic approach to differential diagnosis, different diseases may present similarly. Being in the right "ballpark," however, is frequently as important as getting the exact diagnosis, because it affects the course of further diagnostic studies and therapeutic measures.

In this regard, CT may, in fact, contribute even more to the acquisition of information about a particular orbital process than anatomical localization and differential diagnosis. Using CT guidance, fine-needle aspiration biopsy can obtain tissue samples. Direct histologic information is gained, with which appropriate and definitive clinical decisions can be made.

17

Normal Orbital Anatomy and CT Scanning Techniques

WILLIAM E. ROTHFUS, M.D.

NORMAL ANATOMY

The bony orbit forms a cavity that is shaped like a four-sided pyramid, the apex of which is the optic foramen. Its roof, which slopes inferiorly from anterior to posterior, is made up mostly of the orbital portion of the frontal bone, with a posterior component from the lesser wing of sphenoid. The medial wall, which is oriented in the sagittal plane, is composed of the nasal process of the maxilla, lacrimal bone, lamina papyracea of the ethmoid, and part of the greater wing of the sphenoid. The floor, which slants upward, is formed by the zygomatic bone and orbital processes of the maxilla and palatine bones. The lateral wall is angled about 45° from the sagittal plane and does not extend anteriorly as far as the medial wall. It is formed by the zygomatic bone anteriorly and greater sphenoidal wing posteriorly. The bones are covered by a layer of periosteum called the periorbita. This periorbita is loosely attached, except at suture lines and foramina. Periosteal reflections (orbital septa) extend from the orbital margins and insert at the tarsal plates.[1] Thus, the orbital contents are enveloped by a protective "sock" of periosteum.

The orbital boundaries are very thin along the floor and medial wall. These areas of thinning are important sites of potential weakness in trauma, infection, and neoplasm. Actual dehiscences occur in the lamina papyracea, forming a direct (though small) connection between the ethmoids and the orbit.

When the bony walls are scanned by CT, account must be taken of their varying degrees of angulation from the true axial, coronal, and sagittal planes. The medial wall, oriented in the sagittal plane, is most easily evaluated in the usual axial (−10° from the orbitomeatal baseline) and coronal sections. The other walls diverge from these planes, and are therefore scanned obliquely. Complete evaluation of the walls, e.g., in a complex fracture of the orbits, must take this into account. Use of reconstruction techniques, especially off-axis sagittal and coronal planes, is often needed to gain adequate three-dimensional information about the walls.

The bony margins of the orbit have variable thickness on CT. Natural areas of thinning, mentioned previously, may be so thin that the bone cannot be resolved. Instead, the air of the sinus appears to abut directly against extraconal fat. Besides the floor and medial wall, the roof and lateral walls may have such areas of thinning (Figs 17–1,A and B, and 17–2,A and B). Knowledge of these areas is essential to avoid misdiagnosing wall destruction by inflammatory or neoplastic disease.

Normal foramina present as bony defects with smooth, corticated margins. Familiarization with the major foramina is important, because they serve as important neurovascular conduits for the orbital extension of extraorbital disease. The superior orbital fissure is a triangular-shaped orifice extending between the superior and lateral walls and running from the cranial cavity to the orbit.[1] Best delineated in axial section, it is shown on sequential scans just anterior to the cavernous sinus (see Fig 17–1,C). The inferior orbital fissure is between the lateral and inferior walls anterior to the superior orbital fissure. It connects the inferior orbit with the pterygopalatine fossa posteriorly and the infratemporal fossa anteriorly.[1] It is best appreciated in axial or coronal sections (see Figs 17–1,A and 17–2,B). The optic canal projects anteriorly, laterally, and inferiorly from the cranial cavity to the orbital apex. Just superior to the superior orbital fissure, it is evaluated well in axial scans, particularly if performed in a plane −40° to the orbitomeatal baseline.[2] With less severe angulation, portions of the canal are seen sequentially (see Fig 17–1,D). The nasolacrimal canal runs coronally from the

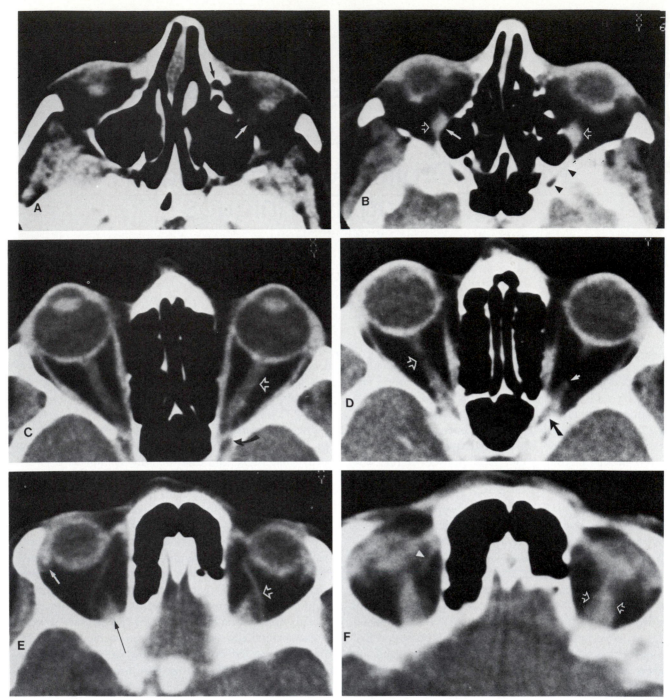

Fig 17–1.—A, normal orbit, inferior level, axial section. The lateral maxillary wall *(white arrow)* is quite thin, looking as though it is nonexistent. The nasolacrimal duct *(black arrow)* is a well-defined foramen running coronally from the anteromedial orbit to the nasal cavity. **B,** normal orbit, inferior level, axial section. The lateral wall of the ethmoid sinus *(closed arrow)* is so thin that it appears to be absent. The inferior orbital fissure *(arrowheads)* is seen posteriorly behind the inferior rectus muscle *(open arrows).* **C,** normal orbit, midlevel, axial section. The superior orbital fissure *(curved arrow)* provides communication between the orbit and cavernous sinus. Its walls are well defined. The globe is divided into anterior and posterior chambers by the lens. The medial and lateral recti are thin fusiform structures inserting into the posterior globe. The left optic nerve sheath *(open arrow)* is uniform in caliber, having been sectioned directly down its axis. **D,** normal orbit, midlevel, axial section. The posterior portion of the intraorbital optic nerve is seen entering the anterior aspect of the optic canal *(black

arrow).* The optic nerve sheath is sectioned above its "knee." Partial volume averaging causes apparent caliber and density change *(open arrow).* Portions of the ophthalmic artery *(white arrow)* are seen coursing over the optic nerve. **E,** normal orbit, superior level, axial section. The lacrimal gland *(white arrow)* is a small soft-tissue structure just lateral and superior to the globe. Posteriorly, it is outlined by fat. Only the posterior aspect of the superior rectus/superior levator palpebrae muscle complex *(long arrow)* is seen, because of scan angle. The midportion of the superior ophthalmic vein is easily identified *(open arrow).* **F,** normal orbit, superior level, axial section. The superior rectus/superior levator palpebrae muscle complex *(open arrows)* is seen as a rectangular density extending toward the posterosuperior globe. The most anterior part of the superior ophthalmic vein *(arrowhead)* lies just medial to the superior globe. Just anterior to this is a portion of the superior oblique muscle, draped over the globe.

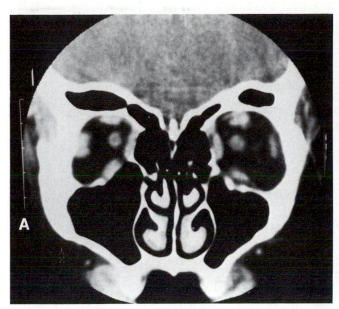

Fig 17–2.—A, normal orbit, direct coronal section. Midorbital sections behind the globe project the optic nerves in the medial half of the orbit. The rectus muscles are clearly seen. The superior oblique can be distinguished just above the medial rectus, and the levator palpebrae superioris can be identified just above the superior rectus in the orbit to the reader's right. **B,** normal orbit, direct coronal section. This section is taken just posterior to photo **A**. The orbits have changed shape from round to triangular. Because the patient's head is slightly oblique, a portion of the inferior orbital fissure is seen on the left *(arrows),* but not on the right.

anteromedial portion of the orbital floor to the nasal cavity and can be seen on axial or coronal scan (see Fig 17–1,A).

The Globe and Lacrimal Gland

The globe dominates the structures of the anterior orbit. Roughly spherical in shape, it lies slightly closer to the lateral wall than the medial wall and closer to the roof than the floor.[3] It is made up of two chambers, separated by the lens. The anterior chamber is volumetrically much smaller than the posterior. It is covered by cornea, while the posterior chamber is covered by retina, choroid, sclera, and Tenon's capsule. These walls and their enclosed chambers are well defined by CT. The walls are uniform in width and density, except for a slight protuberance and change in density at the insertion of the optic nerve posteriorly (papilla). The various layers of the walls cannot be distinguished by CT. The aqueous and vitreous chambers have uniformly low density, while the lens stands out as a higher density structure in the anterior globe (see Fig 17–1,C).

Various methods to evaluate globe proptosis have evolved with CT. One easy method is to project a line from one zygomatic process to the other on a well-positioned midorbital axial scan. Normally, about one third of the globe should project behind this line. Less than one third suggests significant exophthalmos.[4]

The lacrimal gland resides in the superolateral aspect of the anterior orbit, just medial to the zygomatic process of the frontal bone. It is most commonly seen on axial scans. A well-defined oval or bean-shaped structure, it has a homogeneous density roughly equal to that of muscle. Its posterior aspect is the most easily distinguished, by virtue of being outlined by the extraconal fat (see Fig 17–1,E).

The Extraocular Muscles

The recti muscles arise from a common tendinous ring at the orbital apex. This ring, the annulus of Zinn, surrounds the medial portion of the superior orbital fissure and the optic foramen.[5] It therefore has a critical relationship to important nervous and vascular structures. From the annulus, the muscles extend anteriorly, gradually diverging as they parallel the orbital walls, thus forming the well-known muscle cone. At their most anterior portions, the muscles have fairly dense tendinous sheaths, which insert into different quadrants of Tenon's capsule. This capsule surrounds the posterior globe, attaches the sclera and optic nerve, and forms the base of the cone. Two major surgical spaces are defined by the muscle cone—the intraconal space and the extraconal space. Although an intermuscular fascial membrane has been described, further separating the intraconal and extraconal spaces,[6] recent anatomical work has raised doubt about the existence of such a structure.[7]

The superior oblique muscle also originates at the

apex. It courses close to the superomedial wall of the orbit to reach the trochlea, where it bends laterally to insert into the capsule. The shorter inferior oblique muscle originates in the anterior and medial orbit and runs laterally just inferior to the inferior rectus. The levator palpebrae superioris parallels the superior rectus along much of its course. Lying just above the rectus, it has several fascial attachments to it, but inserts into the skin of the upper lid.[5]

The recti are easily defined by CT. However, the extent to which each muscle is evaluated depends on the plane of sectioning. For example, in the usual axial scanning angle ($-10°$), the medial and lateral recti are best visualized, because the scan slice runs longitudinally down the course of each muscle (see Fig 17–1,C). The inferior and superior recti, on the other hand, run obliquely through this scanning plane. As a result, only serial portions of these muscles are seen on scans (see Fig 17–1,E and F). Off-axis sagittal images made by reconstruction are better to visualize these in a longitudinal fashion (Fig 17–3,A). Coronal scans, because they cut across all of the muscles except the inferior oblique, are very useful in precisely determining muscle topography (see Fig 17–2,A and B). Some caution must be used interpreting direct coronal scans. Because the muscles diverge from the direct coronal plane, different parts of each muscle are imaged, e.g., the midportion of the medial rectus is imaged at the same time as the anterior portion of the lateral rectus. Therefore, it is often difficult to compare muscle size and contour within one orbit unless off-axis coronal images can be obtained by reconstruction (see Fig 17–3,B and C).

Generally, the recti have either rectangular or fusiform shapes. They are homogeneous both before and after contrast. The superior rectus and levator palpebrae superioris usually cannot be distinguished as sep-

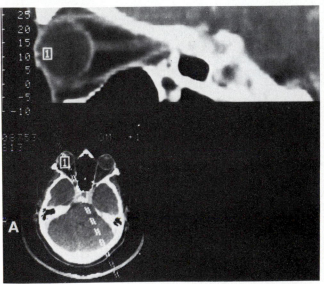

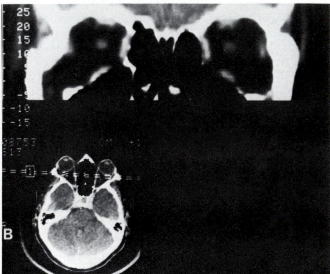

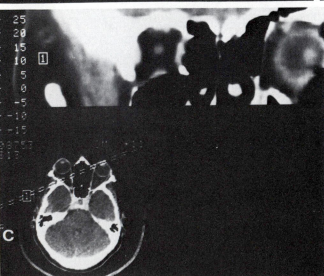

Fig 17–3.—A, normal orbit, off-axis sagittal reconstruction. The fusiform inferior rectus and superior rectus/superior levator palpebrae complex are seen optimally along their longitudinal axes. The optic nerve is also visualized longitudinally. B, normal orbit, coronal reconstruction. The midportions of the medial recti are imaged; however, simultaneously the more anterior portions of the lateral recti are imaged. This projection is useful when comparing the appearance of one orbit against the other. C, normal orbit, off-axis coronal reconstruction. The midportion of each muscle is projected. This technique is useful when it is necessary to compare structures within the same orbit.

arate muscles. The inferior oblique is commonly unrecognizable as a distinct entity, even on coronal scans. At the orbital apex, the muscles, optic nerve, and vascular structures are so compact that no one entity can reliably be resolved from the others.

The Orbital Fat

The orbital "fat" is really a collection of fibroareolar tissue that invests well-defined areas of the orbit. By convention, the orbit is separated into intraconal and extraconal compartments. The intraconal compartment is the larger and is formed by the recti and posterior globe. The extraconal fat lies between the recti and periorbita and abuts the orbital septum anteriorly. In old age, the orbital septum weakens, and fat may protrude through it. On CT scan, the fat is homogeneous except where vessels and nerves pass through it. There is clear delineation of the muscle-fat interface. The orbital septum is variably outlined, depending on the amount and turgor of the extraconal fat pressing against its posterior aspect.

The Optic Nerve

Because of its sinuous course within the orbit, the optic nerve may have a nonuniform, distorted appearance on thin axial and sagittal scan sections. The midportion of the nerve is the most common part to show CT caliber or density variation, because it is here that the nerve makes simultaneous vertical and horizontal bends. These bends can become accentuated or effaced by changes in eye position away from primary gaze.[8] Age, too, affects the tortuosity of the optic nerve, which is greater in elderly patients with less retro-orbital fat.

Exiting from the supermedial aspect of the globe, the optic nerve courses slightly laterally and inferiorly. Further posteriorly, the nerve makes a rather marked bend, forming a knee directed outward and downward.[9] It then courses upward and medially to enter the optic canal. The intracanalicular nerve continues in a superomedial direction, approximately 40° from the orbitomeatal line.[10]

The appearance of the nerve will vary, depending on the angle of scanning and the thickness of the scan slice.[9] Axial scan sections made at −10° from the orbitomeatal baseline are most apt to display the entirety of the nerve from papilla to optic canal. If a thin section cuts directly down the nerve, it will make the nerve appear uniform in density and thickness (Fig 17–1,C). However, if the section includes the portion of the nerve that bends, partial volume averaging of fat occurs and that portion of the nerve is imaged as less dense and less wide (Fig 17–1,D). Similar distortions are present in sagittally reconstructed views, even when made obliquely along the course of the nerve.

Clearly, evaluation of the exact size, density, and contour of the optic nerve should take into account scan angle, slice thickness, patient eye position, and patient age. Comparison with the contralateral nerve and scrutiny of suspect areas with other reformatted or direct planes are necessary to overcome the inherent problems of thin-section techniques.

The Optic Nerve Sheath Complex

While the preceding section has described the features of the normal "optic nerve," this term is actually a misnomer. What the CT scan images is the optic nerve sheath *complex;* that is, the nerve and its surrounding pial, arachnoidal, and dural coverings, not simply the optic nerve itself. All three of these membranes are continuous with comparable intracranial membranes and extend along the entire course of the intraorbital nerve. Thus, intracranial and intraorbital subarachnoid spaces are contiguous.[11]

Vascular and Nervous Structures

High-resolution scanners are able to resolve a number of different veins, arteries, and nerves within the orbit.[12] Obviously, the structures most easily recognized are those that are surrounded by appreciable amounts of fat, those that enhance to the greatest degree, or those that are largest. The superior and inferior ophthalmic veins, ophthalmic artery, and isolated branches of cranial nerves III and V meet these criteria.

The superior ophthalmic vein can be identified on most axial scans. The vein originates anteriorly in the medial orbit, then courses posteriorly and laterally below the superior rectus-levator palpebrae muscle complex to cross over the optic nerve. At the orbital apex, it swings medially and dives through the annulus of Zinn to enter the superior orbital fissure.[13] It is the midportion of the vein that is most commonly seen on axial scans (see Fig 17–1,E). The diameter of the vein is 2.0 to 3.5 mm.[14]

The inferior ophthalmic vein is identified much less frequently than the superior ophthalmic vein.[12] Its course, which is between the inferior rectus and optic nerve, roughly parallels that of the superior ophthalmic vein; it also enters the superior orbital fissure. The anterior and midportions are the easiest to recognize on CT scan.

The ophthalmic artery passes through the optic canal below the optic nerve to enter the orbital apex. It then swings laterally over the optic nerve. Finally, it follows a sinuous course toward the superomedial orbit, terminating in nasal, frontal, and palpebral branches.[13] On CT scan, the most apparent portions of the ophthalmic artery are where it courses through medial orbital fat and where it passes over the optic nerve (see Fig 17–

1,D). The major branches of the artery are variably seen on axial sections.[12]

In general, nerves can be differentiated from vascular structures by virtue of their straighter course. The nervous structures most commonly identified by high-resolution scanning are the frontal branch of the ophthalmic division of the fifth cranial nerve and the inferior division of the third cranial nerve.[12] The former is seen on superior scans running above the levator palpebrae; the latter on inferior scans running lateral and inferior to the optic nerve.

THE USE OF CONTRAST ENHANCEMENT

Because of inherently large density differences in the orbit, normal structures and pathologic masses are relatively well outlined without the use of contrast enhancement. This is especially true with the use of high-resolution scanners. Intravenous contrast does cause a change in attenuation values of structures within the orbit. Most notable are the rectus muscles, which show the largest amount of enhancement, followed by the sclera and optic nerve. However, the change in density is small when compared with the density differences that already exist within the orbit.[15] It would seem, then, that the routine use of contrast in all patients is unwarranted.

When should contrast be used? Clear guidelines have not evolved and still await large clinical series. There are certain contexts in which the use of contrast would seem to be appropriate. A few of these are as follows:

1. Vascular lesions: Although vascular structures, particularly if enlarged, are delineated without contrast, their nature and extent is better evaluated after contrast. For example, an arteriovenous malformation will be highlighted after contrast. A varix can be more easily delineated before or after provocative (Valsalva) maneuvers that follow contrast enhancement.

2. Neoplastic or inflammatory lesions with suspected intracranial involvement: Contrast enhancement is crucial in defining intracranial extension.

3. Optic nerve thickening: Enhancement of the optic nerve sheath would indicate a meningioma or an inflammatory condition separate from the optic nerve itself.

4. Certain retrobulbar masses: Contrast enhancement may help in distinguishing one type of well-circumscribed mass from another (e.g., hemangioma from neurilemmoma).

In summary, although most pathology of the orbit can be recognized on CT without contrast, some lesions require the use of contrast for further characterization.

ROUTINE SCANNING TECHNIQUE

With the presently available technology, patients are most effectively evaluated by direct 5.0-mm scans or 1.5-mm scans with reconstruction.[16] Direct scans comprise five to six sections each in the axial and coronal planes. Although faster to perform, direct coronal scans are limited by the patient's ability to extend his neck and by metallic artifacts from dental fillings. Also, they do not give true perpendicular views of each orbit. Sections of 1.5 mm, on the other hand, take longer to perform and require significant patient cooperation so that images are adequately reformatted from the 20 to 25 sections needed. The reformatting capability gives flexibility, in that off-axis coronal and sagittal images can be obtained that more closely match the true anatomy of the orbit.

Axial scans are routinely performed at $-10°$ to the orbitomeatal baseline. This is the best angle for imaging the intraorbital optic nerve[9, 17] and displays the intraorbital contents well. Little alteration of the angle is necessary, except when the optic canal or the intracanalicular optic nerve needs to be closely examined. In such an instance, scans at $-40°$ to the orbitomeatal baseline provide better anatomical information.[2] Coronal scans are performed in either prone or head-hanging positions so that the head is extended to about 70°. The gantry may then be tilted appropriately to avoid tooth artifacts.

Which projections are obtained depend on the nature of the suspected orbital pathology. Complex orbital trauma often requires reformatted sagittal and coronal images to learn extent and relationship of fracture fragments. Orbital infection usually requires axial and coronal sections to determine location of involvement and to evaluate any associated sinus disease. Retro-ocular masses need at least axial and coronal views. Off-axis sagittal and coronal reconstructions usually help to determine the relationship of a mass to contiguous optic nerve, extraocular muscle, and orbital wall. Optic nerve lesions are best evaluated with thin sections, because these may be able to differentiate sheath from nerve. Muscle disease is optimally evaluated with axial and (direct or off-axis) coronal views. The possibility of intracranial disease associated with orbital pathology may necessitate supplemental axial or coronal scans.

REFERENCES

1. McCotter R.E., Fralick F.B.: *A Comprehensive Description of the Orbit, Orbital Content and Associated Structures With Clinical Applications.* Omaha, Douglas Printing Co., 1943, pp. 3–13.

2. Hammerschlag S.B., O'Reilly G.V.A., Naheedy M.: Computed tomography of the optic canals. *A.J.N.R.* 2:593–594, 1981.

3. Jacobs L., Weisberg L.A., Kinkel W.R.: *Computed Tomography of the Orbit and Sella Turcica*. New York, Raven Press, 1980, pp. 38–44.

4. Hilal S.K., Trokel S.L.: Computerized tomography of the orbit using thin sections. *Semin. Roentgenol.* 12:137–147, 1977.

5. Wolff E., Last R.J.: *Anatomy of the Eye and Orbit*, ed. 6. Philadelphia, W.B. Saunders Co., 1968, pp. 256–271.

6. Poirier P., Charpy A.: Les Organes du sens, in *Traite d' Anatomie Humanie*. Paris, Masson, 1911, vol. 5, fasc. 2, pp. 558–559.

7. Koorneef L.: Details of the orbital connective system in the adult. *Acta Morphol. Neerl. Scand.* 15:1–34, 1977.

8. Salvolini U., Cabanis E.A., Rodallec A., et al.: Computed tomography of the optic nerve: I. Normal results. *J. Comput. Assist. Tomogr.* 2:141–149, 1978.

9. Unsold R., DeGroot J., Newton T.H.: Images of the optic nerve: Anatomical-CT correlation. *A.J.N.R.* 1:317–325, 1980.

10. Potter G.D., Trokel S.L.: Optic canal, in Newton T.H., Potts D.G. (eds.): *Radiology of the Skull and Brain: The Skull*. St. Louis, C.V. Mosby Co., 1971, vol. 1, book 2, pp. 487–489.

11. Whitnall S.E.: *Anatomy of the Human Orbit and Accessory Organs of Vision* (facsimile of 1921 edition). New York, Robert E. Krieger Pub. Co., Inc., 1979, pp. 376–377.

12. Weinstein M.A., Modic M.T., Risius B., et al.: Visualization of the arteries, veins, and nerves of the orbit by sector computed tomography. *Radiology* 138:83–87, 1981.

13. McCotter R.E., Fralick F.B.: *A Comprehensive Description of the Orbit, Orbital Content and Associated Structures With Clinical Applications*. Omaha, Douglas Printing Co., 1943, pp. 53–56.

14. Bacon K.T., Duchesneau P.M., Weinstein M.A.: Demonstration of the superior ophthalmic vein by high resolution computed tomography. *Radiology* 124:129–131, 1977.

15. Watanabe T.J., LeMasters D., Turski P.A., et al.: Contrast enhancement of the normal orbit, in Felix R., Kazner E., Wegener O.H. (eds.): *Contrast Media in Computed Tomography*. Amsterdam, Excerpta Medica, 1981, pp. 130–136.

16. Forbes G.S., Franklin E., Waller R.R.: Computed tomography of orbital tumors, including late-generation scanning techniques. *Radiology* 142:387–394, 1982.

17. Van Damme W., Kasmann P., Wackenheim C.I.: A standardized method for computed tomography of the orbits. *Neuroradiology* 13:139–140, 1977.

18

Orbital Trauma and Infection

WILLIAM E. ROTHFUS, M.D.

ORBITAL TRAUMA

Computed tomography is now a well-established method of evaluating the orbit in direct and indirect trauma.[1-3] In fact, with high resolution and image reformation capabilities, it is becoming the evaluative standard, surpassing conventional radiography and complex motion tomography.[4] This is especially true in the context of complex maxillofacial fractures, which require multiplanar imaging to evaluate extent and localization of all fractures. By making it possible to determine damage to the soft tissue (globe, optic nerve, extraocular muscles, and retrobulbar fat), CT has a marked advantage over other radiographic techniques. Detection and location of intraorbital foreign bodies have been greatly facilitated by the CT scan.

Mechanical injuries to the eye and orbit can be categorized under two main headings: (1) perforating missile and nonmissile injuries and (2) concussions by blunt objects. The role of the CT radiologist in evaluating either of these is to determine the anatomical extent of soft-tissue and bony injury, characterize the type of injury (e.g., hematoma, avulsion), and identify possible sources of post-traumatic complication (e.g., retained foreign body as source of infection).

Penetrating Missile and Nonmissile Injury

Up to half of traumatic eye injuries are caused by penetrating objects.[5] Some of the objects remain within the globe or orbits as retained foreign bodies. These usually are metal, but organic materials such as wood may also be retained. Identification and localization of the object are crucial for therapeutic planning. Prior to CT, localization was imprecise and cumbersome, often requiring multiple radiographs and contact lens techniques.[6] Because of its ease, accuracy, and definition of anatomical detail,[7] CT has become the mainstay of localization. The ability of CT to detect a foreign body depends upon the object size and composition. Exper-

imental work performed by Tate and Cupples[8] proves that steel and copper bodies as small as 0.06 cu mm can be detected by high-resolution scan. Aluminum and glass bodies need to be larger, 1.5 to 1.8 cu mm, to be detected. Wooden bodies are often difficult to localize.

Foreign bodies may be extraocular, intraocular, or retro-ocular (Figs 18–1 to 18–3). Extraocular bodies are easily detected on physical examination, but CT scan may be done to rule out deeper penetration. Intraocular bodies are usually from flying particles entering the eye through the cornea, iris, pupil, or sclera. Because most of the flying particles are metal and carry significant momentum, they usually penetrate to the posterior globe, lodging in the retina, choroid, or sclera.[6] Particles with less momentum (i.e., less velocity or less mass, like plastic or wood) travel a shorter distance into the globe and remain in the anterior chamber or lens.[9] Particles may course through or around the globe to come to rest behind it or in or near the optic nerve, extraocular muscle, or bony wall.

Missile or nonmissile penetrating trauma is frequently associated with local hemorrhage. As expected, hematoma appears as a high-density mass.[10] Generally, the larger the hematoma, the more heterogeneous it looks.[11] The hematomas may be local, confined to the globe wall, vitreous cavity, or optic nerve sheath, or more diffuse, spreading over the retrobulbar space. Orbital emphysema may be present, usually as small collections of air along the tract of penetration (see Fig 18–3). Structures in the path of the offending object are seen to be disrupted on CT scan. For example, the lens may be displaced, a chamber decompressed, or the optic nerve severed.

Concussion Injury

Concussions of the orbit result from the impact of a blunt force, as from a large object or fall.[12] The force may be directed at the globe itself or at its bony sur-

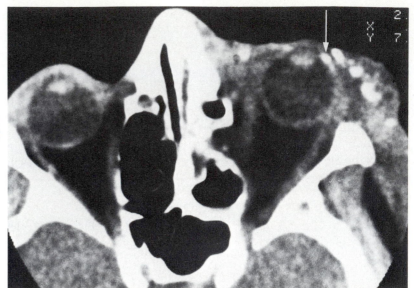

Fig 18–1.—Missile trauma. Multiple small radiodensities are seen in the swollen eyelid and preseptal soft tissues. A single small fragment *(arrow)* is embedded in the cornea.

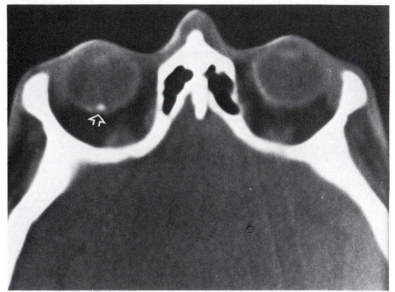

Fig 18–2.—Missile trauma. A small metallic foreign body *(arrow)* is lodged in the posterior globe wall. No significant hematoma is present.

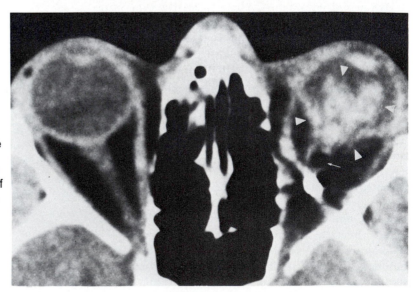

Fig 18–3.—Missile trauma. A large metallic foreign body has passed through the globe into the retrobulbar space. Exuberant hematoma is identified within the vitreous cavity and the posterior globe wall *(arrowheads)*. The optic nerve head is also involved by hematoma. A small collection of air is seen along the fragment tract *(arrow)*.

roundings; thus, orbital soft-tissue injury may be from direct or indirect forces.

When the striking force lands directly on the globe, the globe is pushed backward, and intraorbital pressure increases. If this pressure is high enough, it will fracture the thinnest portions of the bony wall[13] and "blow them out" away from the orbit. Usually, the orbital floor is the site of such a fracture because of its delicate bony structure. Bone fragments and orbital soft tissues are pushed inferiorly into the maxillary sinus, often with resultant hemorrhage. Varying amounts of orbital contents may protrude through the defect in the wall, with varying degrees of enophthalmos resulting. Orbital fat and the inferior rectus and/or inferior oblique muscles are displaced through the floor defect. They may be kinked or entrapped in the herniation, causing impairment of globe motility and diplopia.

The use of CT is ideal for evaluation of these inferior wall blow-out fractures. Coronal and oblique sagittal images are particularly well suited to delineating the bone fragments and prolapsed muscle or fat (Fig 18–4).[2, 14] Determining the location and amount of muscle herniation and kinking is of great importance. Assessment of the relationship of muscle to bony wall will help indicate if a muscle is truly entrapped and thus requires surgical intervention. The nature of the fracture itself is also important to assess, because it may have prognostic significance to the clinician. It has been stated that focal or markedly displaced fractures would have a high likelihood of entrapping and incarcerating

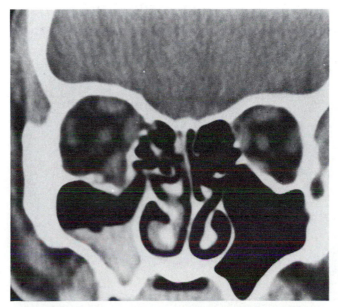

Fig 18–4.—Blunt trauma, orbital floor blow-out fracture. Coronal view shows fracture and depression of the orbital floor. The inferior rectus is displaced slightly into the fracture, but is not entrapped. There is an air-blood level in the maxillary sinus.

orbital contents because of their sharp margins and acute angles.[15] Fractures with bowed margins and obtuse angles would not be so prone to entrapment but rather would be associated with enophthalmos, which also requires surgery but may not be manifest in the acute phase.

Medial orbital wall blow-out fractures are less common than floor fractures, but frequently accompany them.[15, 16] These fractures occur through the thin lamina papyracea, displacing bony fragments, fat, or muscle into the ethmoid sinuses. To evaluate these fractures, axial and coronal CT sections are most useful (Fig 18–5). As in the floor fractures, muscle entrapment can occur, and scans in these projections can best evaluate the true position of the medial rectus and superior oblique muscles in relation to bone. The other major clinical problem with medial wall fracture is enophthalmos. In fact, the degree of medial wall blow-out seems to be a major determinant of clinically significant enophthalmos.[17] Again, CT scans provide the essential information in establishing the need and planning for cosmetic surgery.

Orbital walls can be fractured in combination with extensive maxillofacial injury. Le Fort types II and III fractures most notably involve the orbits, because they traverse lines of weakness in the midfacial skeleton.[13, 18] The Le Fort type II fracture extends bilaterally from the nasal bones, across the frontal processes of the maxillae, along the medial wall and the floor of the orbits, through the infraorbital rims, through the anterior and lateral maxillary sinus walls, and finally to the posterior maxillary sinus walls and pterygoids. Le Fort type III fractures also involve the nasal bones and frontal process of the maxillae, but extend more posteriorly through the medial wall of the orbit to involve the infraorbital fissures and lateral orbital walls, then zygomaticofrontal sutures and zygomatic arches. These Le Fort fractures need not be pure, and combinations of the fractures may exist in the same patient.

Another major facial fracture affecting the orbit is the zygomatic complex, or malar tripod, fracture. The zygoma is separated downward, inward, and posteriorly, with resultant fractures through the inferior orbital rim, zygomaticofrontal suture, and zygomatic arch. Severe fractures of this type cause comminuted fracture of the orbital floor and herniation of orbital structures into the maxillary sinus (Fig 18–6).[13]

Other fractures may involve the orbit in crucial areas. Orbital roof, basal skull, and sphenoid wing fractures are especially important in that they may involve the optic canal. Confined by its bony surroundings and held rigidly by its dural attachment, the optic nerve is most susceptible to injury at this location. Fractures may damage the optic nerve either directly with bony frag-

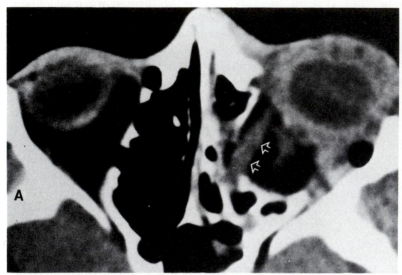
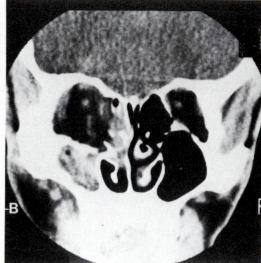

Fig 18–5.—Blunt trauma, medial wall blow-out fracture. **A,** axial scan demonstrates marked fracture of the left medial orbital wall. The medial rectus *(arrows)* is displaced into the fracture. Hematoma and emphysema are present in the lateral orbit. **B,** coronal scan illustrates fractures of the medial and inferior orbital walls. The medial rectus is displaced into the fracture, and the inferior rectus is significantly distorted.

ments or indirectly by nerve concussion or perineural hemorrhage, resulting in blindness.

Clearly, the complexity of all of these fractures makes evaluation and surgical planning difficult. A critical role is played by CT in defining both bony and soft-tissue abnormalities. Images in conventional axial and coronal projections should be supplemented by direct or reformatted images in other planes to adequately assess the extent of injury.[4] Under most circumstances, high-resolution CT scans eliminate the need for conventional tomography because of their comparable ability to detect fractures.

As in penetrating trauma, concussion injury results in a variety of soft-tissue abnormalities. These are easily detected by CT scan. Orbital emphysema is a frequent concomitant of blow-out fractures, but may be seen in malar and Le Fort fractures because of sinus involvement (see Figs 18–5 and 18–6).[13] The air is readily distinguished from air trapped behind the eyelid, a distinction sometimes difficult with radiographs alone.

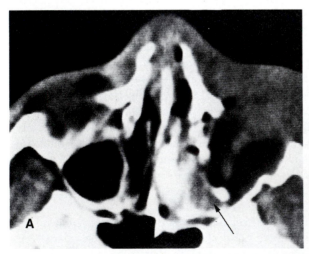
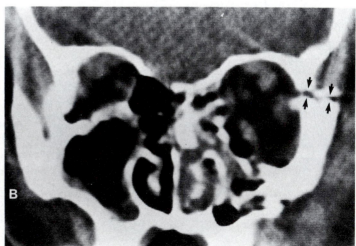

Fig 18–6.—Blunt trauma, zygomatic complex fracture. **A,** axial scan shows significant depression of orbital contents into the maxillary sinus. Some orbital floor fragments are seen posteriorly just anterior to a small portion of the fluid-filled maxillary sinus *(arrow).* **B,** coronal scan shows depression of the entire malar complex with separation of the zygomaticofrontal suture *(arrows)* and fractures of the orbital floor and lateral maxillary sinus wall. Depression of the inferior rectus and orbital air are also seen.

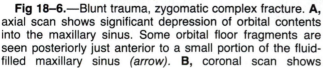

Orbital emphysema should be expected to resolve fairly rapidly and have no mass effect. These features distinguish it from the more serious complication of intraocular aerocele, an encapsulated collection of air under pressure.[19]

Severe blunt trauma is accompanied by shearing forces that lead to tears of the globe walls, rupture of the globe, subluxation of the lens, or avulsion of the optic nerve. Hemorrhages are common and occur focally in the aqueous or vitreous chambers, globe wall, optic nerve sheath, or extraocular muscles (Fig 18–7). Diffuse hemorrhage may also occur. As in penetrating trauma, CT is excellent in defining these abnormalities and their degree of severity.

ORBITAL AND PERIORBITAL INFECTION

Acute orbital or periorbital infection is rarely subtle clinically. Eyelid swelling is manifest early in infection, whether it be from reactive edema, cellulitis, or abscess. However, swelling may become so tense that physical evaluation of the globe and vision is hindered. Thus, it may be impossible to clinically determine the extent of disease and to take appropriate therapeutic measures.[20, 21] The use of CT scanning is integral in evaluating the orbit in this circumstance. Not only can the presence or absence of deeper involvement be assessed, but associated bony and intracranial disease can be evaluated.[21–23] A large percentage of cases of periorbital and orbital cellulitis are secondary to sinusitis[24] or trauma. The use of CT again becomes essential in determining the location and presence of sinus disease or an intraorbital foreign body serving as the nidus of infection.[21]

Clinically and radiologically, infectious disease can be separated into two basic anatomical groups—*preseptal* or *postseptal*—based on the location of the infection in relation to the orbital septum, the tough fascial projection extending from the periosteum of the orbital margin toward the tarsal plates.[25] The septum is a well-recognized barrier to the spread of various orbital pathologic processes, including infection.[24]

Preseptal Inflammation

By definition, preseptal or "periorbital" inflammation does not affect the orbital contents.[23] It may arise from local infection, such as cellulitis or abscess. Alternatively, it may stem from sinusitis, usually ethmoid sinusitis.[24–27] The mechanism of the latter is believed to be reactive edema, caused by elevated pressure in valveless veins that connect the sinuses with the soft tissues of the face and lids.[28]

The CT manifestation of preseptal inflammation is swelling of the soft tissue of the lid and face. The orbital septum forms a clear line of demarcation between the expanded soft tissue of the lid and the normal extraconal fat (Fig 18–8). The appearance of the swelling is identical in cellulitis, abscess, or reactive edema.[21] Location of swelling and presence of sinus opacity are therefore important features in assessing the CT scan. Soft-tissue edema is usually most prominent near the affected sinus. In ethmoid sinusitis, maximum swelling is commonly over the frontal process of the maxilla; in frontal sinusitis, it is in the upper lid. Progressively severe sinus infection causes extensive swelling, which spreads over the nose, cheek, and brow.

In general, preseptal inflammatory disease runs a much more benign course than postseptal disease.[24]

Postseptal Inflammation

Postseptal inflammation, commonly referred to as "orbital cellulitis," actually constitutes a spectrum of in-

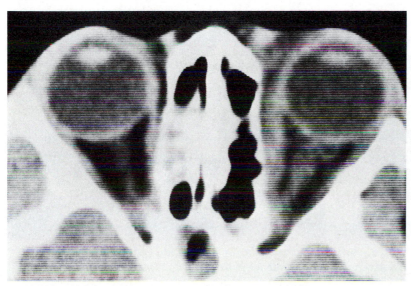

Fig 18–7.—Blunt trauma, axial scan. The left medial rectus and optic nerve sheath are thickened by hemorrhage.

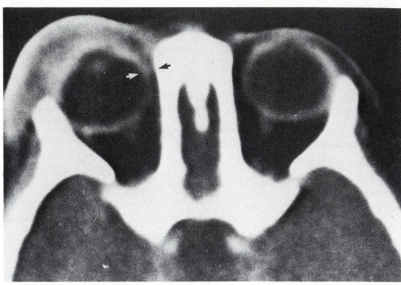

Fig 18–8.—Preseptal inflammation. The soft tissues anterior to the globe are markedly swollen. The orbital septum *(arrrows)* is displaced posteriorly, but forms a line of separation between the extraconal fat and swollen tissues.

fection located in various anatomical compartments. Diagnostically and therapeutically, it is helpful to separate this group into anatomically distinct categories based on the major location of disease. Thus, the major subgrouping is (1) subperiorbital, (2) retrobulbar, and (3) bulbar.

Subperiorbital (subperiosteal) cellulitis or abscess usually propagates from contiguous sinus inflammation, either by direct spread through the sinus wall or by progressive thrombophlebitis.[28] Edema fluid and pus accumulate within the subperiosteal space. They form an expanding mass that bows the periorbita away from the orbital wall. Because the periorbita is relatively tethered at the sutures and foramina,[29, 30] the subperiorbital collection usually attains a convex shape. Adjacent structures, e.g., extraconal fat and rectus muscle, are pushed away from the orbital walls as well.

The CT scan shows the subperiorbital collection as a convex homogeneous or heterogeneous density along the orbital wall (Figs 18–9 to 18–11). The collection has a sharp inner border, which is defined by the periorbita. The periorbita may be visualized because it enhances or because it is thickened by inflammation. When the collection is totally confined by the periorbita and has not spread into the orbit proper, a thin lucent cleavage plane of normal extraconal fat is present between the collection and the displaced rectus muscle (Fig 18–9).[25] The collection may range in size (see Figs 18–9 and 18–10) and may have an air-fluid level (see Fig 18–10).

The periosteum and orbital septa are major deterrents to the spread of inflammatory disease, but can be breached in severe infection (e.g., sinusitis, osteomyelitis, masseteric abscess). Additionally, the primary fo-

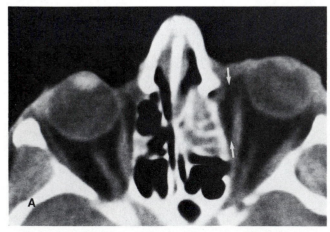
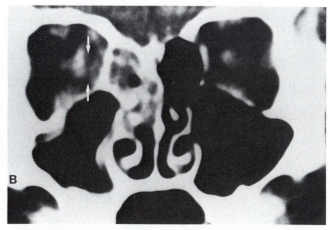

Fig 18–9.—Subperiorbital abscess. Axial **(A)** and coronal **(B)** scans show a small subperiorbital collection adjacent to ethmoid sinus infection. The medial rectus is displaced lat- erally. It is separated from the collection by a thin plane of extraconal fat *(arrows)*.

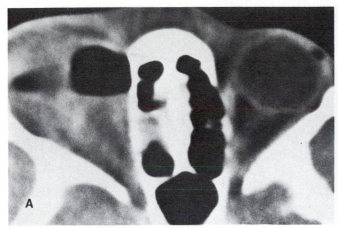
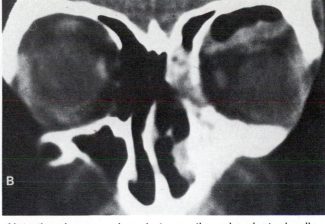

Fig 18–10.—Subperiorbital abscess. **A,** axial scan shows a large air-fluid level in the superior orbit. Posterior ethmoid opacification is from sinusitis. **B,** coronal scan shows the air-fluid level to be confined within the elevated periosteum. Note the cleavage plane between the subperiosteal collection and the superior rectus/superior levator palpebrae muscle complex.

cus of infection may begin within the periosteum. In either case, *retrobulbar* inflammation occurs. This is potentially more dangerous and less surgically accessible than subperiorbital infection, but fortunately less frequent.[31] The CT findings of infection in this compartment include obscuration of normal soft-tissue planes,[21] increased density of retro-ocular fat,[13] and swelling and enhancement of involved extraocular muscles (Figs 18–11 and 18–12). When inflammation matures from cellulitis to actual abscess, a definable mass, ring enhancement, or air collection occurs.[23, 32] Proptosis may be marked.

Deep *bulbar* infection (endophthalmitis) can be present with or without other forms of postseptal disease. The most common CT appearance is ocular wall thickening of either a nodular or uniform character with homogeneous enhancement (Fig 18–13).[21] When retrobulbar disease is present, bulbar swelling is marked in the region of the most active cellulitis. The soft-tissue density of the globe wall most likely represents a combination of actual scleral swelling and effusion distending Tenon's capsule.[32]

REFERENCES

1. Grove A.S.: Orbital trauma evaluation by computed tomography. *Comput. Tomogr.* 3:267–278, 1979.
2. Grove A.S., Tadmor R., New F.F.J., et al.: Orbital fracture evaluation by coronal computed tomography. *Am. J. Ophthalmol.* 85:679–685, 1978.
3. Rowe L.D., Miller E., Brant-Zawadzki M.: Computerized tomography in maxillofacial trauma. *Laryngoscope* 91:745–757, 1981.

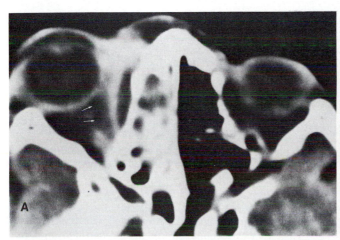
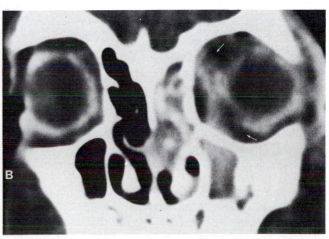

Fig 18–11.—Subperiorbital and retrobulbar cellulitis. Axial **(A)** and coronal **(B)** scans show a homogeneous collection beneath the enhancing periorbita. Lateral to this the orbital fat is increased in density *(arrows)*, consistent with cellulitis.

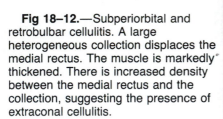

Fig 18–12.—Subperiorbital and retrobulbar cellulitis. A large heterogeneous collection displaces the medial rectus. The muscle is markedly thickened. There is increased density between the medial rectus and the collection, suggesting the presence of extraconal cellulitis.

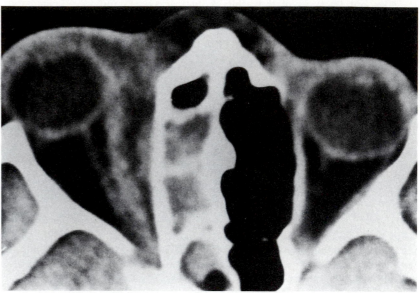

Fig 18–13.—Bacterial endophthalmitis. The posterior globe wall is thickened and enhances homogeneously *(arrows)*. There appears to be involvement of the insertion of the lateral rectus by adjacent inflammation.

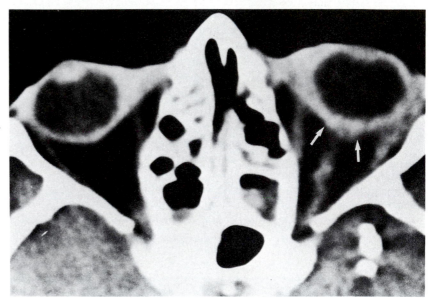

4. Brant-Zawadzki M.N., Minagi H., Federle M.P., et al.: High resolution CT with image reformation in maxillofacial pathology. *A.J.N.R.* 3:31–37, 1982.

5. Nirnanen M.: Perforating eye injuries—a comparative epidemiological prognostic and socioeconomic study of patients treated 1930–1939 and 1950–1959. *Acta Ophthalmol. Suppl.* 135:1–87, 1978.

6. Lloyd G.A.S.: *Radiology of the Orbit.* Philadelphia, W.B. Saunders Co., 1975, pp. 197–210.

7. Kadir S., Aronow S., Davis K.R.: The use of computerized tomography in the detection of intraorbital foreign bodies. *Comput. Tomogr.* 1:151–156, 1977.

8. Tate E., Cupples H.: Detection of orbital foreign bodies with computed tomography: Current limits. *A.J.N.R.* 2:363–365, 1981.

9. Coleman D.J., Lizzi F.L., Jack R.: *Ultrasonography of the Eye and Orbit.* Philadelphia, Lea & Febiger, 1977, p. 264.

10. Salvolini U., Menichelli F., Pasquini U.: Computer assisted tomography in 90 cases of exophthalmos. *J. Comput. Assist. Tomogr.* 1:81–100, 1977.

11. Jacobs L., Weisberg L.A., Kinkel W.R.: *Computerized Tomography of the Orbit and Sella Turcica.* New York, Raven Press, 1980, pp. 195–222.

12. Duke-Elder Sir, S., MacFaul P.A.: *System of Ophthalmology, vol. XIV: Injuries,* pt. 1. London, Henry Kimpton, 1972, pp. 63–291.

13. Lloyd G.A.S.: *Radiology of the Orbit.* Philadelphia, W.B. Saunders Co., 1975, pp. 180–188.

14. Hammerschlag S.B., Hughes S., O'Reilly G.V., et al.:

Blow-out fractures of the orbit: A comparison of computed tomography and conventional radiography with anatomical correlation. *Radiology* 143:487–492, 1982.

15. Zilkha A.: Computed tomography of blow-out fracture of the medial orbital wall. *A.J.N.R.* 2:427–429, 1981.

16. Dodick J.M., Galin M.A., Littleton J.T., et al.: Concomitant medial wall fracture and blow-out fracture of the orbit. *Arch. Ophthalmol.* 85:273–276, 1971.

17. Hammerschlag S.B., Hughes S., O'Reilly G.V., et al.: Another look at blow-out fractures of the orbit. *A.J.N.R.* 3:331–335, 1982.

18. Gerlock A.J., Sinn D.P., McBride K.L.: *Clinical and Radiographic Interpretation of Facial Fractures.* Boston, Little, Brown & Co., 1981, pp. 137–144.

19. Holler M.L., Brockup A.H., Shiffman F.: Intraorbital aerocele. *Arch. Ophthalmol.* 98:1612–1613, 1980.

20. Goldberg F., Berne A.S., Oski F.A.: Differentiation of orbital cellulitis from preseptal cellulitis by computed tomography. *Pediatrics* 62:1000–1005, 1978.

21. Zimmerman R.A., Bilaniuk L.T.: CT of orbital infection—its cerebral complications. *A.J.R.* 134:45–50, 1980.

22. Leo J.S., Halpern J., Sackler J.R.L.: Computed tomography in the evaluation of orbital infections. *Comput. Tomogr.* 4:133–138, 1980.

23. Fernback S.K., Naidich T.P.: CT diagnosis of orbital inflammation in children. *Neuroradiology* 22:7–13, 1981.

24. Gellady A.M., Shulman S.T., Ayoub E.M.: Periorbital and orbital cellulitis in children. *Pediatrics* 61:272–276, 1978.

25. Putterman A.M., Urist M.J.: Surgical anatomy of the orbital septum. *Ann. Ophthalmol.* 6:290–294, 1974.

26. Smith T.F., O'Day D., Wright P.F.: Clinical implications of preseptal (periorbital) cellulitis in childhood. *Pediatrics* 62:1006–1009, 1978.

27. Gamble R.C.: Acute inflammations of the orbit in children. *Arch. Ophthalmol.* 10:483–497, 1922.

28. Chandler J.R., Langenbrunner D.J., Stevens E.R.: The pathogenesis of orbital complications in acute sinusitis. *Laryngoscope* 80:1414–1428, 1970.

29. Whitnall W.E.: *Anatomy of the Human Orbit and Accessory Organs of Vision* (facsimile of 1921 edition). New York, Robert E. Krieger Pub. Co., Inc., 1979, pp. 85–86.

30. Rothfus W.E.: Unpublished data, 1983.

31. Morgan P.R., Morrison W.V.: Complications of frontal and ethmoid sinusitis. *Laryngoscope* 90:661–666, 1980.

32. Harr D.L., Quencer R.M., Abrams G.W.: Computed tomography and ultrasound in the evaluation of orbital infection and pseudotumor. *Radiology* 142:395–401, 1982.

19

Orbital Masses

WILLIAM E. ROTHFUS, M.D.

MOST CLINICAL SERIES of orbital masses are enumerative. That is, they either list a wide variety of masses, simply describing their features entity by entity, or they present a single clinical entity, then list its multiple CT scan appearances. Few series are oriented toward differential diagnosis of the CT scan findings themselves.

Several authors point out difficulties in making histologic diagnoses of orbital masses based solely on CT scan appearance.[1-5] Indeed, it is not surprising that CT falls short in differentiating processes in which histology, method of spread, and anatomical preference are similar, as is the case in many orbital tumors and pseudotumors. However, some groups of orbital masses do have similarities on CT scan that seem to separate them from other groups of masses.

Thus, we have endeavored to combine pathologic entities with similar CT appearances into differential categories: (1) The *well-circumscribed* mass has distinct margins separate from the surrounding orbital structures. This type is usually round or oval in shape; histologically, it usually has a capsule. (2) The *infiltrative*, or less well-marginated mass, has less definite margins than the well-circumscribed mass. It characteristically involves multiple orbital structures and is not encapsulated. Although a portion of the mass may be fairly distinct, other portions blend into the surrounding structures. (3) The *serpiginous mass* has a knobby exterior, but has well-defined margins. (4) The *thickened optic nerve sheath complex* has tubular, fusiform, or excrescent enlargement of the optic nerve or its sheath.

WELL-CIRCUMSCRIBED MASSES

Cavernous Hemangiomas

Cavernous hemangiomas are common tumors, being among the five most common orbital neoplasms.[6] They are encapsulated and have smooth or mildly lobulated exteriors. Slow growing, they usually remain isolated from other orbital structures; invasion of the optic nerve or extraocular muscles is uncommon.[6] These tumors are made up of multiple vascular channels, thus containing a large blood pool.

As predicated by its histology, the hemangioma is a well-delineated round or oval mass on CT scan.[7-10] Because of its highly vascular composition, its inherent density is high, and it enhances following contrast administration. This enhancement is homogeneous or heterogeneous,[7] depending on the size of vascular channels within the tumor (Fig 19–1). Calcified phleboliths may be present. Although the characteristic location is intraconal and superolateral, hemangiomas may occur anywhere, intraconally or extraconally. The optic nerve may be displaced, but rarely invaded. The tumor may cause adjacent orbital wall remodelling.

Hemangiopericytoma

Pathologically, hemangiopericytomas have vascular channels, are well circumscribed, and may have a fibrous coat.[11] It is easy to see, then, why these tumors have a CT appearance that is similar to hemangiomas.[3] Enhancement may be heterogeneous or homogeneous, but is usually prominent (Fig 19–2). These tumors grow slowly, so they too may cause expansion of bony walls. The natural history of these tumors is different than hemangiomas, in that local invasion of muscles and bone is more common, and recurrences (local and metastatic) more frequent.[11]

Neurofibroma, Neurilemmoma

Neurilemmoma and the isolated form of neurofibroma are benign, encapsulated tumors that are well defined when presenting in the orbit. They are often, but not invariably, associated with other features of neurofibromatosis. In general, they become apparent in the adult years. They tend not to be vascular and are made up of a fairly uniform population of cells.[12] On CT, they are oval-shaped, easily delineated

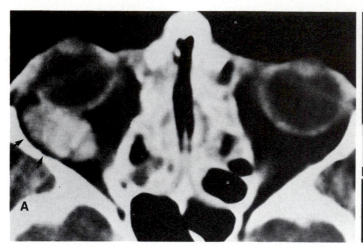

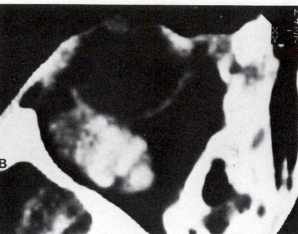

Fig 19–1.—Cavernous hemangioma. **A,** a well-defined oval mass sits in the superolateral retrobulbar space. Diffuse, though inhomogeneous enhancement is noted. Notice slight remodelling of the lateral orbital wall *(arrows).* **B,** magnified view at different window setting brings out tumor heterogeneity.

masses[9] with uniform texture and enhancement, unless central necrosis has occurred. Enhancement is less pronounced than in hemangioma or hemangiopericytoma (Fig 19–3).

This CT appearance is decidedly different than in the plexiform type of neurofibroma, the other major form of neurofibroma. Grossly cord-like, the plexiform type is nodular on CT scan. It is more vascular and diffuse than the isolated form[12] and can be seen to entangle itself around normal orbital structures. Plexiform neurofibroma is discussed with serpiginous masses.

Dermoid

Of the well-defined masses, dermoid cysts have the most unique CT scan characteristics.[1, 13, 14] The interior of the cyst is very low in absorption number, usually near fat density. The smooth thin cyst wall is clearly visible; the contiguous bony wall is commonly remodelled into a smooth sclerotic rim. Occasionally, debris is seen within the cyst (Fig 19–4).

Other Tumors

Fibromas, extradural meningiomas, and fibrous histiocytomas are also types of well-defined orbital masses.[1, 15] They are homogeneous high-density lesions that enhance with contrast. Occasionally, an orbital varix will have a round contour that simulates a neoplasm.[16] Contrast enhancement is pronounced and homogeneous. As discussed later (under serpiginous masses), provocative maneuvers may significantly alter the shape of a varix, thus helping to distinguish it from other vascular masses.

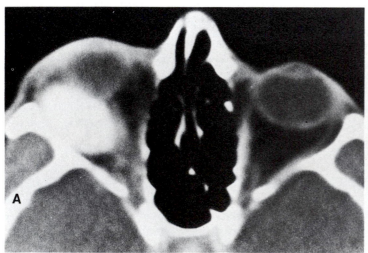

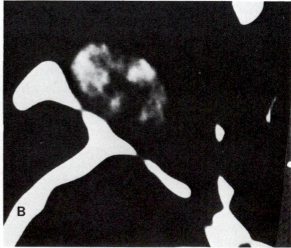

Fig 19–2.—Hemangiopericytoma. **A,** this enhancing mass is quite similar to Figure 19–17, being well marginated and oval. **B,** magnified view with different window setting establishes the inhomogeneous nature of enhancement.

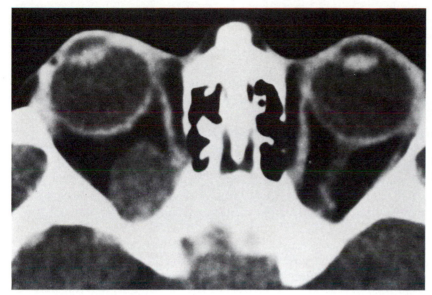

Fig 19–3.—Neurofibroma. This well-defined mass is like Figures 19–1 and 19–2, but enhancement pattern is much more homogeneous and is less pronounced.

In summary, the well-circumscribed masses may be separated into three major groups based on their CT appearance. Dermoids constitute one group and are distinguished by their thin wall and low-absorption interior. Hemangiomas and hemangiopericytomas are distinguished by their high density before contrast administration and intense enhancement after contrast. The enhancement is frequently heterogeneous, with small "pools" of contrast within the mass. For practical purposes, the tumors are indistinguishable by CT scan alone, unless there is evidence of aggressive behavior (erosion of bone, invasion of contiguous muscle or nerve), which is more characteristic of hemangiopericytoma. Varices also enhance prominently, but are homogeneous.

The final group comprises those masses that usually enhance moderately and are more homogeneous in tex-

ture. Neurofibroma may be recognized as part of a generalized neurofibromatosis, but separating these tumors from fibromas, fibrous histiocytomas, and extradural meningiomas is probably impossible.

INFILTRATIVE MASSES

Pseudotumor

Orbital pseudotumor is a reactive inflammatory lesion that in many ways simulates a neoplasm. The etiology of the reactive process is unknown, and its clinical course is unpredictable. Pseudotumors are common, being the fourth most-frequent orbital mass in a large Mayo Clinic series.[17] Clinical presentation, especially in the acute phase, suggests the inflammatory nature of the disease, with proptosis, chemosis, limitation of eye motion, pain, and lid swelling. Proptosis, however, may

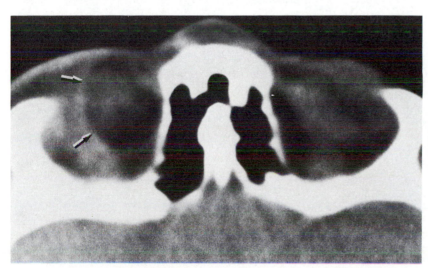

Fig 19–4.—Dermoid. This thin-walled mass *(arrows)* has a low-absorption interior measuring in the fat range. Some high-density material (debris) is seen within the mass.

dominate the more inflammatory-type symptoms, and thus the clinical presentation is more like tumor.[18] Pseudotumor usually is unilateral. Corticosteroid therapy and low-dose radiotherapy have been effective in most cases in alleviating or curing symptoms.[17, 19, 20]

Pathologically, pseudotumor may be diffuse, affecting many orbital structures, or local by mainly affecting muscle (myositis), lacrimal gland (dacryoadenitis), posterior globe (episcleritis), or orbital fat. Histologically, lymphocytic infiltration predominates, often being so extensive that the underlying tissue is replaced. The maturity of the lymphocytes and presence of other cell types, e.g., polymorphonuclear leukocytes and plasma cells, emphasizes the inflammatory nature of the disease.[17, 18]

Various authors have described CT findings in orbital pseudotumor.[1, 2, 20–24] Being a disease with multiple expressions, pseudotumor can manifest a host of different scan appearances. However, some classification is possible when based on the regional nature of disease involvement.[24] That is, pseudotumor largely limited to the muscle can be separated from pseudotumor of the lacrimal gland, which can be separated from pseudotumor of the retrobulbar and extraconal fat.

The dominant CT characteristic of a pseudotumor mass, wherever it is located, is its tendency toward homogeneous texture. This correlates well with the pathologic process, which is a relatively uniform inflammation that obliterates normal structures. The periphery of the mass spreads irregularly through orbital fat when it originates behind or around the globe.[17] Thus, on CT the mass usually has irregular, sometimes quite indistinct margins. Because the retrobulbar inflammatory process invariably involves contiguous muscle, fat, and connective tissue,[18] the CT scan shows obscuration of

soft-tissue planes by the mass. Thus, the mass seems to combine the affected structures into one homogeneously enhancing conglomerate (Fig 19–5). Occasionally, the pseudotumor mass is relatively confined to the extraconal or intraconal space. As such, the muscles and their associated fascial structures limit the mass, giving it a more defined appearance (Fig 19–6). In these cases, some part of the mass may be marginated while another part may show a more typical ill-defined margin.

Nugent and colleagues[24] have noted the tendency for acute retrobulbar pseudotumors to be located either anteriorly, posteriorly, or diffusely in the orbital cone. The anterior masses relate closely to the back of the globe and are associated with swelling and enhancement of the scleral margin. Such scleral involvement is believed to be highly characteristic of pseudotumor.[23] The posterior type originates at the apex, obliterating the tissue planes near the annulus of Zinn. Diffuse-type involvement obscures all structures from the back of the globe to the apex. Because localized disease has been observed to progress to the diffuse type, it is likely that the latter represents the severest stage of disease progression. Bilateral retrobulbar pseudotumor can exist, but may be a concomitant of a systemic disorder, such as Wegener's granulomatosis, polyarteritis nodosa, sarcoidosis, multifocal fibrosclerosis, or thyroiditis.[17] Bony wall erosion or expansion is rarely seen.

Lymphoma and Lymphoid Hyperplasia

Orbital lymphoma is a common cause of proptosis, in one series following only inflammatory conditions and hemangiomas in frequency.[25] It occurs principally in and after middle age and usually presents clinically as a mass with swelling and proptosis. Occasionally, symptoms and signs may be more inflammatory, making dis-

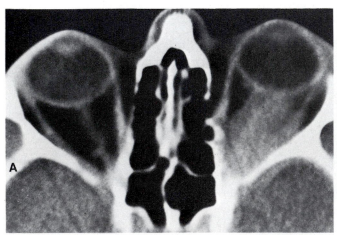 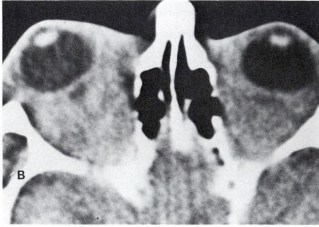

Fig 19–5.—Pseudotumor with progression. **A,** a fairly homogeneous mass spreads predominantly through the posterior intraconal space, obscuring the fat planes around the left optic nerve and lateral rectus. Although the medial border is fairly distinct, the lateral and anterior borders fade gradually without defined borders. **B,** two years later, the disease progressed to involve both orbits. The masses involve the retrobulbar structures diffusely.

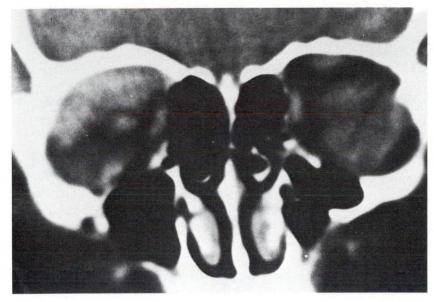

Fig 19–6.—Pseudotumor. The large homogeneous mass in the superolateral orbit appears to have fairly distinct margins. These margins seem to be following known orbital fascial planes, which divide the intraconal from the extraconal space.

tinction from pseudotumor difficult. As well, it may be difficult histologically and radiologically to distinguish lymphomas from pseudotumor. Microscopically, the conditions look alike, having a predominance of lymphocytes. Special immunopathologic techniques may be necessary to help separate the two. Similarly, the microscopic appearance of lymphoid hyperplasia mimics a well-differentiated lymphoma. Often, the only way to distinguish these is by searching for other evidence of systemic lymphoma.[26]

Because of this pathologic similarity, lymphoma and lymphoid hyperplasia have many of the same CT features as pseudotumors.[1–3] In particular, the lymphomatous mass has an homogeneous texture both before and after contrast administration. It may be intraconal or extraconal. The mass also obscures nearby muscle because of the contiguity of similar CT densities and, in some cases, frank invasion of muscle. Lymphomas may be primarily irregular, with poorly delineated margins on CT corresponding with gross appearance of lumpy, ill-defined tumor (Fig 19–7). On the other hand, the gross and CT characteristics may be more defined, especially in the superior orbit.[27] In such a case, the tumor mass conforms more to the orbital space, forming a cast within the orbital fat (Fig 19–8). Lymphomas may show a tendency to "coat" the globe. The homogeneous mass of tumor is seen to extend in a blanket-like manner around the periphery of the globe (Fig 19–9). Diffuse spread of tumor throughout the orbit, contiguous extraorbital spread, and bony destruction, although un-

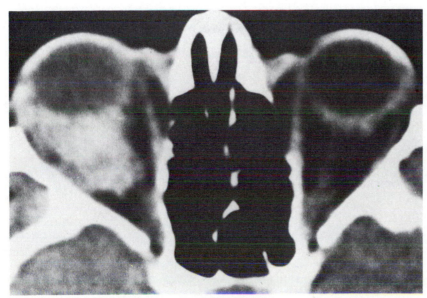

Fig 19–7.—Lymphoma. The periphery of the tumor mass is lumpy and irregular, without a clear sulcus between it and surrounding structures.

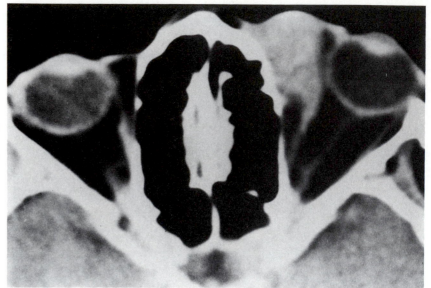

Fig 19–8.—Lymphoma. The mass appears fairly well defined because of its being confined within the extraconal space. The posterior aspect of the mass, however, shows a typical irregular border.

common, are indicative of highly malignant forms of lymphoma.[3]

Metastatic Tumor

Most metastatic involvement of the orbit is by carcinoma, particularly adenocarcinomas, with breast and lung being the most frequent primary sites. Incidence is chiefly in the adult age group, with a peak in the seventh decade. Interestingly, in a significant number of cases, the orbit is the first site of presentation, with the primary tumor being found later. Proptosis, diplopia, pain, eyelid swelling, and ophthalmoplegia are all common symptoms.[28, 29]

Metastases occur in the bony wall, globe, retrobulbar soft tissues, or optic nerve sheath. When involving the soft tissues alone, tumor may be located intraconally or extraconally, focally or diffusely (Fig 19–10). On CT, the margins of the metastatic tumor mass are usually irregular, reflecting their infiltrative nature.[1, 14] Enhancement is variable; texture is commonly inhomogeneous.

Most retrobulbar metastases have mass effect, causing proptosis of the globe. Uniquely, scirrhous adenocarcinoma, regardless of the primary site of origin, causes a retraction of orbital contents (enophthalmos) as it infiltrates them.[28] Thus, an infiltrative mass associated with enophthalmos is likely to be a scirrhous type of metastatic adenocarcinoma.

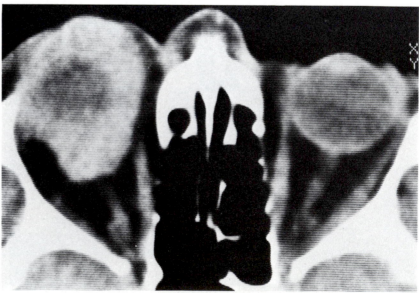

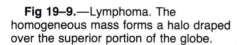

Fig 19–9.—Lymphoma. The homogeneous mass forms a halo draped over the superior portion of the globe.

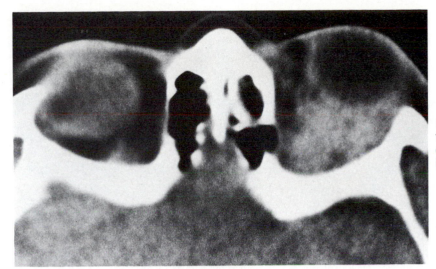

Fig 19–10.—Metastatic carcinoma. Relatively homogeneous, ill-defined tumor spreads over the posterior orbit, obscuring fat planes. The appearance is identical to pseudotumor.

Capillary Hemangioma

Capillary hemangiomas occur at an earlier age than cavernous hemangiomas and do not have true capsules. They tend to be more aggressive, infiltrating local structures, which makes surgical removal difficult.[6] Some of these tumors involve the face, eyelids, or scalp and extend back into the orbit for a variable distance. The cutaneous lesions are easily seen and may change in size with alteration in intravascular pressure.

The CT scan delineates the extent of these tumors well. Because capillary hemangiomas possess more stromal tissue and fewer vascular channels than cavernous hemangiomas, they have a more homogeneous pattern before and after contrast. The tumors insinuate through and around orbital structures. They may pass through the orbital septum and present as an enhancing mass over the involved portions of the face and scalp (Fig 19–11). This type of tumor has a tendency to involute.[30] As it does, it may develop a capsule and thus become more circumscribed on CT.

Lymphangioma

Lymphangioma is a benign tumor of childhood that clinically may simulate features of hemangioma—proptosis, fluctuation in size, strabismus, orbital enlargement, and cutaneous lesions. Histologically, it is made up of numerous lymph-filled channels surrounded by a stromal framework.[31] The proportion of lymph channels to stroma may vary. Bleeding into the cysts is common and may be enough to compromise vision. Difficult to remove surgically, these infiltrative tumors may extend through large portions of the orbit, intraconally or extraconally, and have a tendency to recur locally.

Because of the variable histologic makeup of the tumor, the CT appearance of lymphangiomas is likewise variable. The spectrum ranges from relatively homogeneous density to highly irregular density, probably depending on the uniformity of vascular spaces and the presence or absence of bleeding within the tumor cysts. Although one end of the CT spectrum is toward tumor homogeneity, lymphangiomas are not usually as uniform in texture as lymphomas or pseudotumor (Fig 19–12). Only half of lymphangiomas show enhancement;[7] when they do, it is usually not prominent.

Most lymphangiomas have indistinct margins because

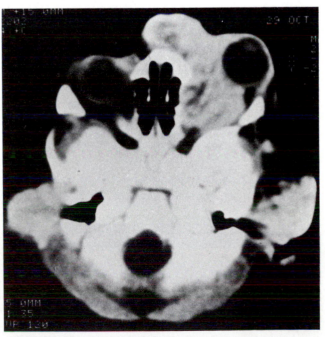

Fig 19–11.—Capillary hemangioma. A large enhancing tumor extends from the nose and face through the orbital septum into the retrobulbar space. It extends irregularly through the retro-ocular fat.

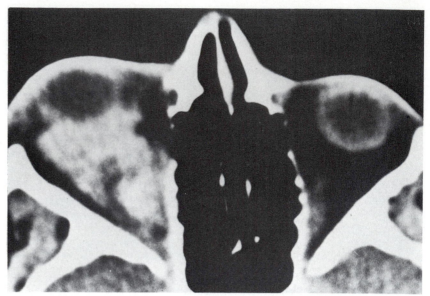

Fig 19–12.—Lymphangioma. The irregularly enhancing mass is confined to the intraconal space, giving it a somewhat defined periphery.

of their invasive character and lack of a capsule. When the tumor is limited by the muscle cone or there is frank hematoma formation, the periphery becomes more delineated.

There is no particular location in which orbital lymphangiomas occur. They may be entirely intraconal or extraconal or bridge between the spaces. They may even extend through large portions of the orbit and may be diffuse.[7] Calcification may occur and is usually focal and dense. Expansion of the orbital walls can sometimes be demonstrated by CT and documents the slow growth of this tumor.

Other Neoplastic or Neoplastic-Like Conditions

Multiple myeloma is an unusual tumor of the orbit and may be either primary or secondary.[32] As would be expected by the monotonous cellular composition of the myeloma infiltrate, CT scan of the mass shows homogeneity. It may be localized to the retro-ocular spaces or involve contiguous globe, bone, and facial soft tissues.[33]

Wegener's granulomatosis fairly commonly involves the orbital structures.[34] When presenting as a retrobulbar mass, the CT scan shows a local or diffuse infiltrative mass with homogeneous density and variable enhancement,[5, 35] which is indistinguishable from pseudotumor. Involvement may be unilateral or bilateral. One distinguishing characteristic of Wegener's granulomatosis is the presence of a sinus mass or sinus bone destruction, neither of which need to be contiguous with the orbital mass. A similar CT appearance, except for sinus disease, can be seen in other granulomatous diseases, such as sarcoidosis and histiocytosis.[36] As in Wegener's granulomatosis, the processes may be unilateral or bilateral.

To summarize, infiltrative masses have irregular margins, except where they may be confined by normal anatomical boundaries (e.g., orbital septum). They often obscure the soft-tissue planes within the orbit, making normal structures "melt" into the density of the mass itself. Simply, they can be thought of as comprising two major groups: childhood and adulthood. Hemangiomas and lymphangiomas predominate in the childhood group. Of these two, hemangiomas tend to be more vascular and enhance vigorously. Lymphangiomas enhance less than hemangiomas and may be quite variable in texture. The adult infiltrative masses—pseudotumor, lymphoma, lymphoid hyperplasia, and metastasis—can appear similar on CT scan. Metastasis may be less homogeneous than the others and may cause enophthalmos. Otherwise distinguishing metastasis from the other types of mass may be impossible.

SERPIGINOUS MASSES

Arteriovenous Malformation

Arteriovenous malformations (AVM) may occur anywhere in the orbit. When in the retrobulbar space, they can present with exophthalmos, chemosis, bruit, ophthalmoplegia, or visual loss. Supplied by branches of the ophthalmic and/or external carotid arteries, they have the typical appearance of enlarged, serpiginous vessels.[37] Usually, an AVM wraps around the normal structures, but may penetrate them as well.

The CT scan appearance of intraorbital AVM is fairly characteristic.[1, 38] Tortuous densities are seen, which represent dilated arteries and veins (Fig 19–13). These enhance very prominently, especially when rapid dynamic scanning is done. Portions of the AVM may be composed of tightly entwined vascular channels that

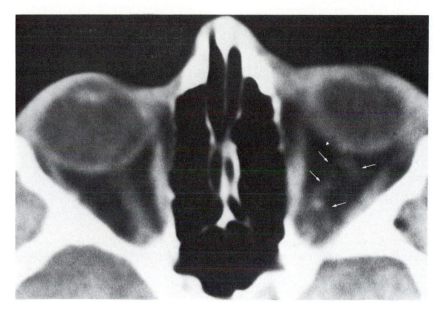

Fig 19–13.—AVM. A small AVM is seen in the posterior retrobulbar space. It is identified by a multiplicity of small serpiginous densities *(arrows)*.

cannot be individually distinguished. Rather, they appear as a densely enhancing mass with a multinodular periphery. Calcifications occasionally occur within AVM. Muscle enlargement may be an accompanying finding (Fig 19–14), especially if the AVM intimately involves the muscle. Rarely, AVM may cause bony wall remodelling.

Some of the above findings (enlarged, prominently enhancing vascular structures and muscle enlargement) can be seen with another arteriovenous communication, carotid-cavernous fistula. Usually, a distinction between the two can be made. Carotid-cavernous fistulas enlarge only venous structures, especially the superior ophthalmic vein.[39] They have no definable vascular "mass"; muscle enlargement affects multiple muscles rather than one.

Venous Varix

Venous malformations, specifically varices, characteristically cause intermittent exophthalmos. Exophthalmos can be provoked by such maneuvers as jugular compression, the Valsalva maneuver, straining, or dropping the head. The malformations may be developmental or associated with an AVM.[40]

On CT in the resting patient, the varix may be inapparent or only a small lobulated linear or round density. Even contrast administration will fail to make it stand out sufficiently. Provocative maneuvers done at the

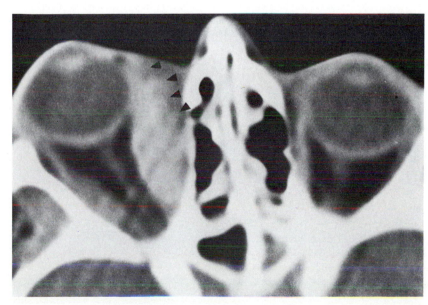

Fig 19–14.—AVM. The medial rectus is intimately involved by an AVM, which forms a dense conglomerate with a nodular periphery *(arrowheads)*. There is remodelling of the medial orbital wall.

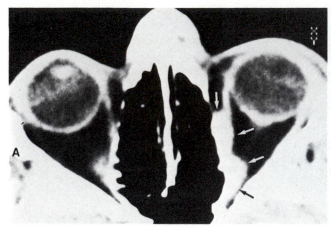

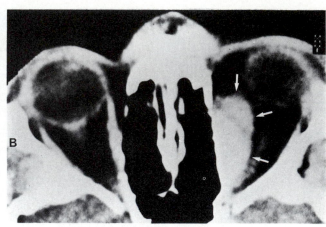

Fig 19–15.—Varix. **A,** in normal head position, the varix is seen as a thin, slightly tortuous enhancing density along the medial orbit *(arrows).* **B,** scan in head-hanging position illustrates marked dilatation of the varix *(arrows).* Note associated flattening of the orbital wall, probably a result of chronic pulsatile pressure.

time of scanning with contrast enhancement can accentuate the volume of the varix, sometimes strikingly (Fig 19–15).[41] Obviously, clinical suspicion must be high to anticipate the need for such maneuvers. Varices, like AVM, may have phlebolithic calcification and can cause deformity of the orbit wall.

Plexiform Neurofibroma

Plexiform neurofibromas are invariably associated with neurofibromatosis. As previously stated, they are knobby, rope-like tumors that can be quite diffuse. They envelope normal structures like the optic nerve, extraocular muscles, and lacrimal gland.[12, 42] On the CT scan, nodular thickening occurs longitudinally along the object affected by the tumor. Because the tumor is relatively vascular, enhancement occurs, but not nearly to the same degree as in AVM (Fig 19–16). Associated bony dysplasia of the sphenoid bone, another common finding in neurofibromatosis, may be seen with these tumors.

THE THICKENED OPTIC NERVE SHEATH COMPLEX

Enlargement of the optic nerve sheath complex presents a differential diagnosis encompassing a wide variety of disease processes. The most dramatic are primary optic nerve gliomas and meningiomas, but nonneoplastic conditions, like papilledema or Grave's disease, can similarly expand the sheath. As yet, the resolution of thin-section CT is not sufficient to consistently distinguish the optic nerve from its surrounding sheath. Thus, differentiating primary optic nerve pathology from pathology of the nerve sheath or the enclosed ce-

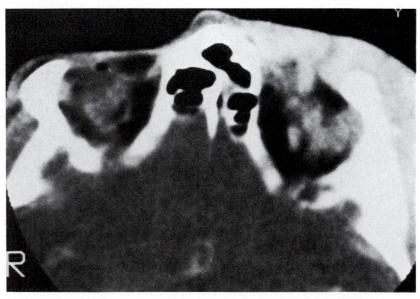

Fig 19–16.—Plexiform neurofibroma. A knobby enhancing mass spreads over the superior left orbit, obscuring normal muscular and vascular structures. There is a large component of tumor over the face and temporal regions. (*R* = right.)

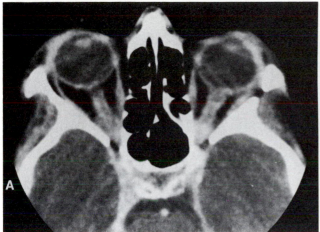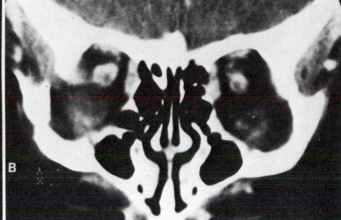

Fig 19–17.—Bilateral optic nerve meningioma. Nearly the entire length of each optic nerve is surrounded by enhancing tumor. Each optic nerve is seen as a longitudinal lucency in axial scan **(A)** and as a round lucency in coronal scan **(B)**.

rebrospinal fluid (CSF) spaces becomes difficult. Most often, differential diagnosis is accomplished by evaluating size, shape, enhancement characteristics, growth patterns, and patient age.

Optic Nerve Sheath Meningioma

Although most series of orbital tumors contain large numbers of meningiomas, they do not differentiate primary sheath meningiomas from those originating from the orbital walls. Indeed, compared with sphenoid wing meningiomas, sheath meningiomas are relatively rare. Clinically, they present with early visual loss with atrophy and late proptosis in a middle-aged patient. Understanding of their CT appearance comes from consideration of their site of origin and nature of growth.[43]

Intraorbital meningiomas arise from the arachnoid attached to the dura of the sheath. Early growth is usually confined to the area between the optic nerve and sheath, so that the tumor spreads in a sheet-like manner along the CSF space surrounding the nerve. With progressive growth, there is compression of the optic nerve. Finally, the enlarging tumor breaks through the dura, producing an exophytic intraconal tumor mass.

The CT appearance of intraorbital meningiomas tends to fall into two patterns, one corresponding to the "subdural" mode of growth and the other to the "exophytic" mode. Subdural growth, which is limited by the dura, produces tubular enlargement of the nerve sheath complex. This enlargement may affect the entire intraorbital length of the nerve (Fig 19–17) or be more segmental, depending on the extent of tumor extension through the perineural space (Fig 19–18). Extension into the optic canal is often associated with canal widening and hyperostosis. Occasionally, these menin-

giomas calcify, giving a smooth, sleeve-like focal calcification surrounding the nerve (Fig 19–19).[44]

Exophytic meningiomas show wide-based tumor extending from the optic nerve sheath complex and projecting into the surrounding orbit. Though sometimes lobulated, the mass is always well defined. Enhancement is homogeneous and generally of a greater degree than other tumor types.[9] These tumors, too, may extend into and through the optic canal, causing widening and sclerosis of adjacent sphenoid. With thin sections (e.g., 1.5 mm), the enhancing tumorous optic nerve sheath can usually be distinguished from the lucent optic nerve (Figs 19–17, 19–18, and 19–20).[45] Occasion-

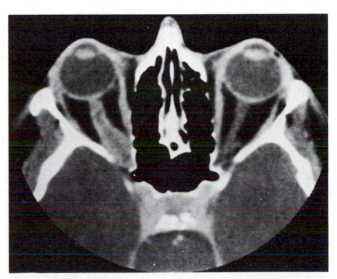

Fig 19–18.—Optic nerve meningioma. The posterior aspect of the intraorbital optic nerve is surrounded by enhancing tumor, forming a fusiform enlargement of the nerve sheath complex.

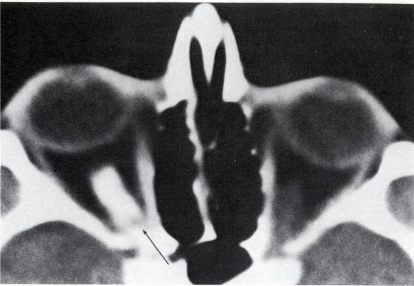

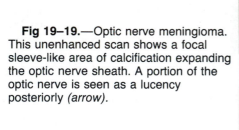

Fig 19–19.—Optic nerve meningioma. This unenhanced scan shows a focal sleeve-like area of calcification expanding the optic nerve sheath. A portion of the optic nerve is seen as a lucency posteriorly *(arrow)*.

ally, the meningioma may become so large as to encompass the nerve completely, giving the image of the optic nerve "ghost" (see Fig 17–36). The tumor may become eccentric enough to displace the nerve, but keeps a broad attachment to it.

Intraorbital Optic Nerve Glioma

Primary optic nerve gliomas usually present in a younger age group than meningiomas, being one of the most prevalent orbital tumors in children. Diminished visual acuity and some proptosis are common clinical findings. Often seen in the context of von Recklinghausen's disease, gliomas may be bilateral.

One typical CT appearance is of smooth, fusiform widening of the optic nerve[46] relating to a pattern of circumferential growth of tumor and/or circumferential proliferation of adjacent arachnoid.[47] The widening may be focal in early stages, but slowly progresses to diffuse bulging in later stages (Fig 19–21). Occasionally, the tumor may lose its characteristic spindle shape and develop bulbous, rounded excrescences where it has stretched or penetrated the dura.[48] Even so, the tumor remains well defined and uniform in density. If tumor growth is primarily longitudinal, that is, along the nerve axis, the CT image becomes one of a uniformly thickened nerve.[46] When this happens, the nerve often becomes tortuous or kinked (Fig 19–22).

Optic nerve gliomas are sometimes difficult to differentiate from meningiomas. In general, they have lower precontrast density than meningiomas and enhance to a lesser degree.[49] They do not exhibit a central lucency within the tumor mass, as do meningiomas, and thus are homogeneous in enhancement.[45] Calcification, al-

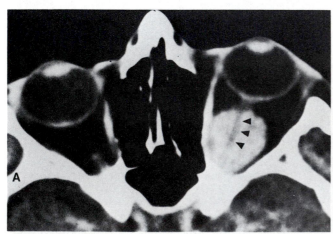

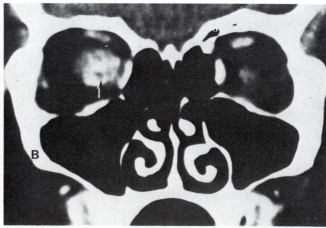

Fig 19–20.—Large optic nerve meningioma. Axial **(A)** and coronal **(B)** scans show the extensive exophytic tumor. The optic nerve (**A,** *arrowheads;* **B,** *arrow*) is clearly seen as a lucency running longitudinally through the tumor.

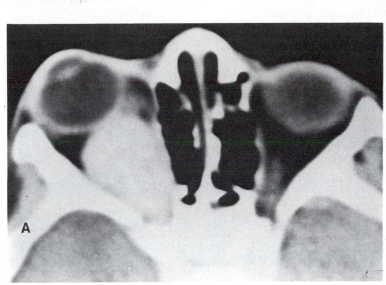
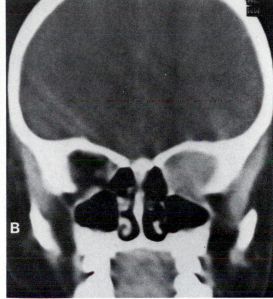

Fig 19–21.—Optic nerve glioma. Large fusiform homogeneously enhancing tumor in axial **(A)** and coronal **(B)** scans fails to disclose any optic nerve lucency. The tumor extends all the way to the posterior globe.

though more frequent in meningiomas, can occur in optic gliomas.

When optic glioma is being considered in the diagnosis, it is essential to evaluate the intracanalicular and intracranial portions of the optic nerve, because contiguous tumor spread into the chiasm and even optic tracts is common.[50] Metrizamide cisternography is particularly useful in delineating subtle thickening of the intracranial nerve, chiasm, or tracts.

Other Neoplasms

Metastatic involvement of the optic nerve or nerve sheath is uncommon. It represents about 1% of all orbital and ocular metastases.[51] Breast, stomach, and lung account for most cases. Deposits occur more frequently in the nerve sheath than the nerve parenchyma.[52] For this reason, it would be more common to see a metastasis encircling the lucent nerve than expanding the nerve on CT scan (Fig 19–23).

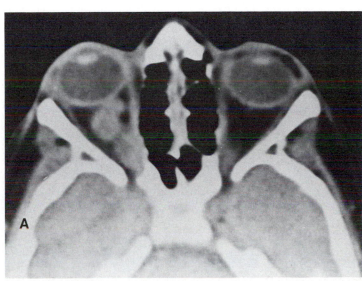
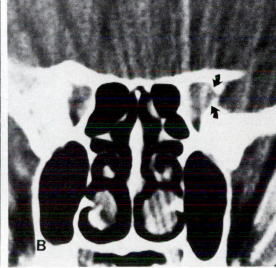

Fig 19–22.—Optic nerve glioma. **A,** there is tubular expansion of the right optic nerve along with tortuosity and kinking. Note the absence of the optic nerve lucency. **B,** coronal scan shows tumor expanding the optic canal *(curved arrows).*

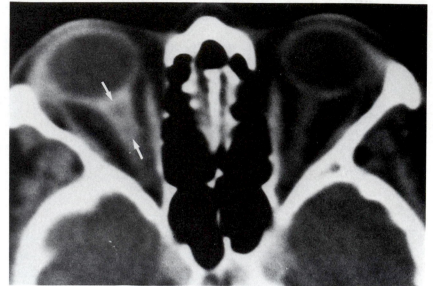

Fig 19–23.—Optic nerve sheath metastasis. An enhancing mass surrounds the optic nerve, which produces a thin longitudinal lucency *(arrows).*

Leukemias and lymphomas are pathologically different than metastases, in that they infiltrate the leptomeninges and the nerve together.[52] The CT scan appearance then has tubular expansion of the nerve sheath complex, with homogeneous involvement of both nerve and sheath and no demonstration of an optic nerve lucency.

Papilledema and Optic Neuritis

First described in 1974,[38] the CT appearance of the optic nerve in papilledema is one of uniformly increased nerve sheath caliber. Raised intracranial pressure produces optic nerve fiber swelling and vascular engorgement, which thicken the nerve itself; heightened subarachnoid space pressure distends the dural sheath.[53, 54] On CT, the resultant enlargement of the nerve sheath complex usually occurs bilaterally, but may be asymmetric. The normal tortuous curve of the optic nerve becomes accentuated as well (Fig 19–24).[54]

Similar tubular widening of the complex may occur with optic neuritis,[2, 5, 54–57] presumably from inflammatory nerve edema and cellular infiltrate, perineural fluid collection, or infiltrate of the nerve coverings. The latter may contribute to a shaggy outline of the expanded complex. Such shagginess is especially evident in granulomatous (e.g., sarcoid) neuritis.

The Patulous Subarachnoid Space

The perioptic subarachnoid space, which communicates with the intracranial subarachnoid space, can vary

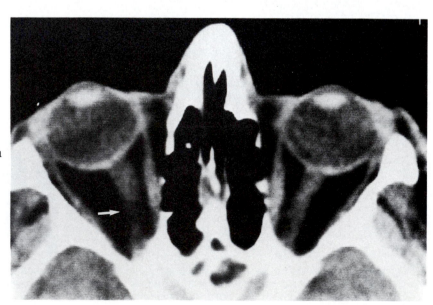

Fig 19–24.—Papilledema. There is bilateral thickening of the optic nerve sheath complexes. The right nerve has a more tortuous course than normal, bending out of the scan section posteriorly *(arrow).*

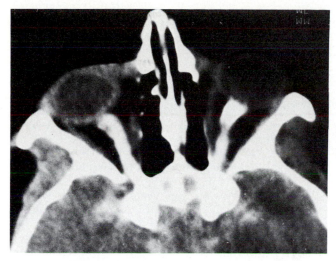

Fig 19–25.—Patulous subarachnoid space; cisternogram. Subarachnoid metrizamide extends along the entire length of both optic nerve sheaths. Portions of the optic nerves are visualized as lucencies within the metrizamide.

in size, depending on age, CSF pressure, and the extent of communication between the two spaces.[53, 58] Several authors have documented the passage of intrathecal metrizamide around the optic nerve during cisternography,[58–60] thus confirming the presence of the patulous, freely communicating perioptic subarachnoid space in some patients. Such a communication may occur normally or as the result of optic nerve atrophy (Fig 19–25).

Apical Compression

Optic nerve sheath enlargement has been reported in association with thyroid orbitopathy.[61–63] Uniform and moderate in degree, the widening is believed to be a result of edema, cellular infiltrate, and vascular engorgement, which occur as a result of apical compression from contiguous muscle enlargement (see Chapter 20, Fig 20–2). Similar apical compression can result from tumors and myositic pseudotumor.

Trauma

Direct or indirect mechanical trauma of the optic nerve can produce nerve swelling or hematoma within the nerve sheath. Both of these then produce widening of the nerve sheath complex on CT scan. Occasionally, acute blood within the sheath can be identified as hyperdensity outlining the lucent optic nerve.

REFERENCES

1. Wende S., Aulich A., Nover A., et al.: Computed tomography of orbital lesions. *Neuroradiology* 13:123–134, 1977.
2. Gyldensted C., Lester J., Fledelius H.: Computed tomography of orbital lesions—a radiological study of 144 cases. *Neuroradiology* 13:141–150, 1977.
3. Forbes G.S., Sheedy P.F., Waller R.R.: Orbital tumors evaluated by computed tomography. *Radiology* 136:101–111, 1980.
4. Knochel J., Osborne A.G., Wing D.S.: Differential diagnosis of lateral orbital masses. *J. Comput. Tomogr.* 5:11–15, 1981.
5. Gawler J., Sanders M.D., Bull J.W.D., et al.: Computer assisted tomography in orbital disease. *Br. J. Ophthalmol.* 58:571–587, 1974.
6. Henderson J.W.: *Orbital Tumors*. New York, Brian C. Decker, 1980, pp. 128–133.
7. Davis K.R., Hesselink J.R., Dallow R.L., et al.: CT and ultrasound in the diagnosis of cavernous hemangioma and lymphangioma of the orbit. *J. Comput. Tomogr.* 4:98–104, 1980.
8. Nikoskelainen E., Enzmann D.R., Sogg R.L., et al.: Computerized tomography of the orbits. *Acta Ophthalmol.* 55:885–900, 1977.
9. Forbes G.S., Earnest F., Waller R.R.: Computed tomography of orbital tumors, including late-generation scanning techniques. *Radiology* 142:387–394, 1982.
10. Lloyd G.A.S.: CT scanning in the diagnosis of orbital disease. *Comput. Tomogr.* 3:227–239, 1979.
11. Henderson J.W.: *Orbital Tumors*. New York, Brian C. Decker, 1980, pp. 136–143.
12. Henderson J.W.: *Orbital Tumors*. New York, Brian C. Decker, 1980, pp. 261–279.
13. Blei L., Chambers J., Liotta L., et al.: Orbital dermoid diagnosed by computed tomographic scanning. *Am. J. Ophthalmol.* 85:58–61, 1978.
14. Hesselink J.R., Davis K.R., Dallow R.L., et al.: Computed tomography of masses in the lacrimal gland region. *Radiology* 131:143–147, 1979.
15. Jacobs L., Weisberg L., Kinkel W.: *Computerized Tomography of the Orbit and Sella Turcica*. New York, Raven Press, 1980, p. 105.
16. Lloyd G.A.S.: Vascular anomalies in the orbit: CT and angiographic diagnosis. *Orbit* 1:45–54, 1982.
17. Henderson J.W.: *Orbital Tumors*. New York, Brian C. Decker, 1980, pp. 512–526.
18. Blodi F.C., Gass J.D.M.: Inflammatory pseudotumor of the orbit. *Br. J. Ophthalmol.* 52:79–93, 1968.
19. Kim R.Y., Roth R.E.: Radiotherapy of orbital pseudotumor. *Radiology* 127:507–509, 1978.

20. Harr D.L., Quencer R.M., Abrams C.W.: Computed tomography and ultrasound in the evaluation of orbital infection and pseudotumor. *Radiology* 142:395–401, 1982.

21. Wilner H.I., Gupta K.L., Kelly J.K.: Orbital pseudotumor: Association of orbital vein deformities and myositis. *A.J.N.R.* 1:305–309, 1980.

22. Enzmann D.R., Donaldson S.S., Marshall W.H., et al.: Computed tomography in orbital pseudotumor (idiopathic orbital inflammation). *Radiology* 120:597–601, 1976.

23. Bernardino M.E., Zimmerman R.D., Citrin C.M., et al.: Scleral thickening: A CT sign of orbital pseudotumor. *A.J.R.* 129:703–706, 1977.

24. Nugent R.A., Rootman J., Robertson W.D., et al.: Acute orbital pseudotumors: Classification and CT features. *A.J.N.R.* 2:431–436, 1981.

25. Jakobiec F.A., Jones I.S.: Lymphomatous, plasmacytic, histiocytic, and hematopoietic tumors, in Jones I.S., Jakobiec F.A. (eds.): *Diseases of the Orbit.* Hagerstown, Md., Harper & Row, 1979, pp. 309–315.

26. Knowles D.M., Jakobiec F.A.: Orbital lymphoid neoplasms: Clinical, pathologic, and immunologic characteristics, in Jakobiec F.A. (ed.): *Ocular and Adnexal Tumors.* Birmingham, Ala., Aesculapius Publishing Co., 1978, pp. 257–280.

27. Henderson J.W.: *Orbital Tumors.* New York, Brian C. Decker, 1980, pp. 344–376.

28. Henderson J.W.: *Orbital Tumors.* New York, Brian C. Decker, 1980, pp. 451–470.

29. Font R.L., Ferry A.P.: Carcinoma metastatic to the eye and orbit: III. A clinicopathologic study of 28 cases metastatic to the orbit. *Cancer* 38:1326–1335, 1976.

30. Jakobiec F.A., Jones I.S.: Vascular tumors, malformations, and degenerations, in Duane T.D. (ed.): *Clinical Ophthalmology.* Philadelphia, Harper & Row, 1981, vol. 2, pp. 1–6.

31. Henderson J.W.: *Orbital Tumors.* New York, Brian C. Decker, 1980, pp. 147–152.

32. Clarke E.: Plasma cell myeloma of the orbit. *Br. J. Ophthalmol.* 37:543–554, 1953.

33. Price H.I., Danzinger A., Wainwright H.C., et al.: CT of orbital multiple myeloma. *A.J.N.R.* 1:573–575, 1980.

34. Haynes B.F., Fishman M.L., Fauci A.S., et al.: The ocular manifestations of Wegener's granulomatosis: Fifteen years' experience and review of the literature. *Am. J. Med.* 63:131–141, 1977.

35. Vermess M., Haynes B.F., Fauci A.S., et al.: Computer assisted tomography of orbital lesions in Wegener's granulomatosis. *J. Comput. Assist. Tomogr.* 2:45–48, 1978.

36. Hilal S.K., Trokel S.L.: Computerized tomography of the orbit using thin sections. *Semin. Roentgenol.* 12:137–147, 1977.

37. Newton T.H., Troost B.T.: *Arteriovenous Malformations and Fistulae,* in Newton T.H., Potts D.G. (eds.): *Radiology of the Skull and Brain,* vol. 2, book 4. St. Louis, C.V. Mosby Co., 1974, pp. 2534–2535.

38. Ambrose J.A.E., Lloyd G.A.S., Wright J.E.: A preliminary evaluation of fine matrix computerized axial tomography (EMI scan) in the diagnosis of orbital space-occupying lesions. *Br. J. Radiol.* 47:747–751, 1974.

39. Merrick R., Latchaw R.E., Gold L.H.A.: Computerized tomography of the orbit in carotid-cavernous sinus fistula. *Comput. Tomogr.* 4:127–132, 1979.

40. Jakobiec F.A., Jones I.S.: Vascular tumor, malformations, and degenerations, in Duane T.D. (ed.): *Clinical Ophthalmology.* Philadelphia, Harper & Row, 1981, vol. 2, pp. 15–18.

41. Winter J., Centeno R.S., Bentson J.R.: Maneuver to aid diagnosis of orbital varix by computed tomography. *A.J.N.R.* 3:39–40, 1982.

42. Jakobiec F.A., Jones I.S.: Neurogenic tumors, in Duane T.D. (ed.): *Clinical Ophthalmology.* Philadelphia, Harper & Row, 1981, vol. 2, pp. 12–14.

43. Wright J.E.: Primary optic nerve meningioma: Clinical presentation and management. *Trans. Am. Acad. Ophthalmol. Otolaryngol.* 83:617–625, 1977.

44. Jacobs L., Weisberg L., Kinkel W.: *Computerized Tomography of the Orbit and Sella Turcica.* New York, Raven Press, 1980, pp. 87–100.

45. Daniels D.L., Williams A.L., Syvertsen A., et al.: CT recognition of optic nerve sheath meningioma: Abnormal sheath visualization. *A.J.N.R.* 3:181–183, 1982.

46. Byrd S.E., Harwood-Nash D.C., Fitz C.R., et al.: Computed tomography of intraorbital optic nerve gliomas in children. *Radiology* 129:73–78, 1978.

47. Hogan M.J., Zimmerman L.E.: *Ophthalmic Pathology: An Atlas and Textbook,* ed. 2. Philadelphia, W.B. Saunders Co., 1962, pp. 617–619.

48. Henderson J.W.: *Orbital Tumors.* New York, Brian C. Decker, 1980, pp. 290–306.

49. Jacobs L., Weisberg L., Kinkel W.: *Computerized Tomography of the Orbit and Sella Turcica.* New York, Raven Press, 1980, pp. 127–137.

50. Savoiardo M., Harwood-Nash D.C., Tadmor R., et al.: Gliomas of the anterior optic pathways in children. *Radiology* 138:601–610, 1981.

51. Ferry A.P., Font R.L.: Carcinoma metastatic to the eye and orbit: I. A clinicopathologic study of 227 cases. *Arch. Ophthalmol.* 92:276–286, 1974.

52. Eggers H., Jakobiec F.A., Jones I.S.: Optic nerve gliomas, in Duane T.D. (ed.): *Clinical Ophthalmology.* Philadelphia, Harper & Row, 1981, vol. 2, pp. 1–14.

53. Hayreh S.S.: Pathogenesis of edema of the optic disc. *Doc. Ophthalmol.* 24:298–411, 1968.

54. Cabanis E.A., Salvolini U., Rodallec A., et al.: Computed tomography of the optic nerve: II. Size and shape modifications in papilledema. *J. Comput. Assist. Tomogr.* 2:150–155, 1978.

55. Krohel G.B., Charles H., Smith R.S.: Granulomatous optic neuropathy. *Arch. Ophthalmol.* 99:1053–1055, 1981.

56. Howard C.W., Osher R.H., Tomsok R.L.: Computed tomographic features in optic neuritis. *Am. J. Ophthalmol.* 89:699–702, 1980.

57. Som P.N., Sacher M., Weitzner I., et al.: Sarcoidosis of the optic nerve. *J. Comput. Assist. Tomogr.* 6:614–616, 1982.

58. Chambers E.F., Manelfe C., Cellerier P.: Metrizamide CT cisternography and perioptic subarachnoid space imaging. *J. Comput. Assist. Tomogr.* 5:875–880, 1981.

59. Fox A.J.: Intrathecal metrizamide enhancement of the optic nerve sheath. *J. Comput. Assist. Tomogr.* 3:653–656, 1979.

60. Manelfe C., Pasquini U., Bank W.O.: Metrizamide demonstration of the subarachnoid space surrounding the optic nerves. *J. Comput. Assist. Tomogr.* 2:545–547, 1978.

61. Healy J.R., Rosenkrantz H.: Enlargement of the optic nerve sheath complex in thyroid ophthalmopathy. *J. Comput. Tomogr.* 5:8–10, 1981.

62. Trokel S.L., Hilal S.K.: Recognition and differential diagnosis of enlarged extraocular muscles in computed tomography. *Am. J. Ophthalmol.* 87:503–512, 1979.

63. Kennerdell J.S., Rosenbaum A.E., El-Hoshy M.H.: Apical optic nerve compression of dysthyroid optic neuropathy on computed tomography. *Arch. Ophthalmol.* 99:807–809, 1981.

20

Differential Problems in Orbital Diagnosis

WILLIAM E. ROTHFUS, M.D.

EXTRAOCULAR MUSCLE ENLARGEMENT

No specific measurements have been made on a wide population of patients to determine normal ranges of extraocular muscle size or density. Therefore, labeling a muscle as "enlarged" requires comparison with the opposite side and close scrutiny of the muscle in more than one projection.

Muscle thickening in one disease process is often similar radiographically to that in other pathologically different processes, but the associated findings, e.g., changes in orbital fat, bony wall, or globe, can narrow the differential diagnostic possibilities.[1]

Graves' Disease

Muscular involvement in Graves' disease can be unilateral or bilateral, symmetric or asymmetric, singular or multiple, subtle or marked. However, bilateral, symmetric thickening of multiple muscles is most frequent;[2] single muscle involvement is unusual.[1] Pathologically, the muscles are infiltrated with mucopolysaccharides, edema fluid, and round cells from a diffuse inflammatory reaction.[3] As expected, enhancement of the affected muscle is commonly seen on CT scan.[4] Characteristically, the enhancement is uniform (Fig 20–1). The muscle becomes more fusiform in shape as degree of enlargement increases. Enzmann and coworkers[5] have shown that correlation exists between clinical severity of disease and extent of muscle involvement.

Graves' disease is a diffuse disease of the orbital contents. As such, muscle swelling is usually accompanied by CT alterations in other structures in the orbit. Orbital fat, for instance, may increase in volume, causing proptosis of the globe and prolapse of the orbital fat anteriorly (Fig 20–1).[1–3, 6] In addition, the character of the fat may change, showing a finely reticulated, "dirty-fat" appearance, presumably reflecting edema and cellular infiltrate. Interestingly, these findings can occur in the absence of muscle thickening. The globe, besides being displaced forward, may rarely show episcleral enhancement at the point of attachment of an inflamed muscle tendon. When multiple muscles are enlarged, especially at the orbital apex, the optic nerve can become swollen, either from associated inflammatory change or compression (Fig 20–2).[7, 8]

The lacrimal glands and eyelids can also become swollen and displaced in severe disease (Fig 20–3). Rarely, orbital wall erosion results from chronic direct pressure and hyperemia.[9] Superior ophthalmic vein engorgement from vascular compression at the orbital apex may be apparent on CT (Fig 20–4). The combination of muscle thickening and superior ophthalmic vein enlargement may therefore rarely mimic carotid-cavernous fistula.

Myositic Pseudotumor

In many ways, the CT appearance of pseudotumor myositis mimics that in Graves' ophthalmopathy. In fact, clinically and radiographically it may be impossible to distinguish them. Because it too originates from reactive inflammation, muscle swelling in myositis is fusiform[10] and accompanied by uniform enhancement. The inflammatory response may also involve the contiguous muscle tendon and sclera (Fig 20–5).[6, 11] Usually, muscle thickening is moderate in degree. Although myositis has been reported to have an irregular muscle contour,[1] this has not been a reliable indicator of myositis vs. Graves' disease.

The pattern of muscle swelling varies in the two diseases. While solitary muscle swelling is uncommon in thyroid ophthalmopathy, it is said to be the rule in pseudotumor myositis.[1] Pseudotumor is not usually associated with fat bulging the orbital septum[1] or changes of fat density so characteristic of Graves' disease. Unfortunately, exceptions do exist, and pseudotumor may present with multiple muscle involvement, proptosis, and even "dirty fat" (Fig 20–6). In these cases, clinical

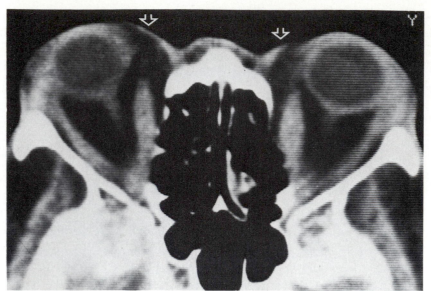

Fig 20–1.—Graves' disease, axial scan. There is marked proptosis. Orbital fat bulges the septa forward *(arrows).* The medial and lateral recti are symmetrically enlarged and homogeneously enhanced.

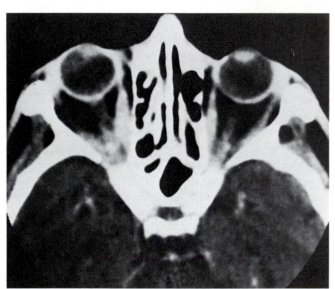

Fig 20–2.—Graves' disease. There is asymmetric muscle enlargement, more severe on the right. Because of more severe apical compression, the right optic nerve sheath is distended.

Fig 20–3.—Graves' disease. Marked exophthalmos is accompanied by eyelid swelling and pronounced enhancement of the lacrimal glands.

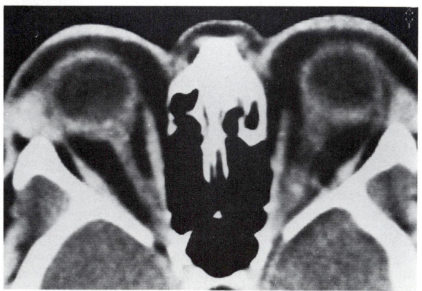

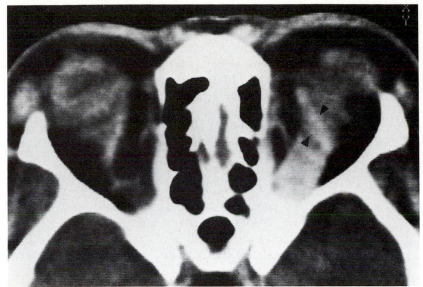

Fig 20–4.—Graves' disease. A high slice through asymmetrically involved orbits shows distention of the left superior ophthalmic vein *(arrowheads)*.

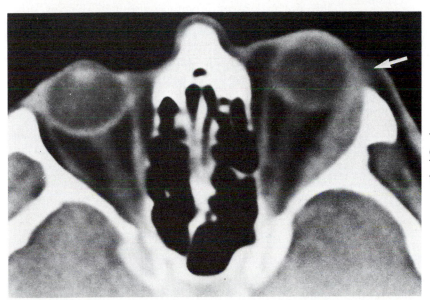

Fig 20–5.—Myositic pseudotumor. The left lateral rectus is markedly enlarged and enhances homogeneously. There is involvement of the muscle tendon and adjacent globe wall *(arrow)*.

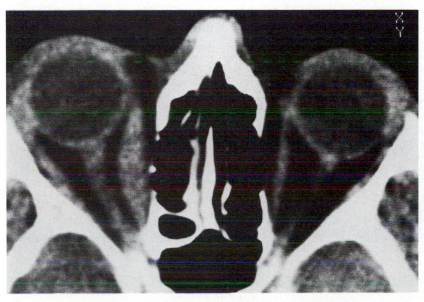

Fig 20–6.—Myositic pseudotumor. The medial and lateral recti are moderately enlarged on the right. Note involvement of the lateral rectus tendon. The optic nerve is thickened. The right orbital septum bulges, but not to a pronounced degree.

information provides the key to differential diagnosis.[12, 13]

Acromegaly

Diffuse extraocular muscle enlargement can occur in acromegaly.[14, 15] The findings mimic those of Graves' disease, but proptosis is not a prominent feature. The degree of muscle enlargement is usually moderate and shows no direct correlation with growth hormone levels.[16]

Primary and Secondary Neoplasm

The enlargement of a rectus muscle that results from tumor can be from direct extension of neoplasm within or around the muscle or from venous outflow compression.[1] Primary tumors, i.e., rhabdomyosarcoma, which occur most commonly in children,[17] directly infiltrate the muscle, forming a local or diffuse, usually enhancing mass (Fig 20–7).[18, 19] With further growth, the aggressive nature of the tumor is demonstrated by contiguous bone destruction.[20]

Secondary neoplasms may occasionally be deposited and grow within an extraocular muscle,[6, 21] appearing quite similar on CT to a primary muscle tumor or myositis. More commonly, a metastatic neoplasm infiltrates or compresses the muscle from contiguous bony, sinus, or foraminal spread. The use of CT clearly illustrates the extraorbital portion of the tumor and proves the "passive" nature of muscle involvement. Thus, CT is usually accurate in distinguishing neoplastic muscle enlargement from that of Graves' disease or pseudotumor.[1]

Arteriovenous Malformations and Fistulas

Arteriovenous malformations (AVM) and fistulae, as emphasized by Trokel and Hilal,[1] produce uniform enlargement of rectus muscle or muscles. The muscle swelling seems to be a result of increased venous pressure, supported by the commonly associated findings of a dilated superior ophthalmic vein (Fig 20–8).[1, 22] In fact, this latter finding is important in distinguishing the AVM-fistula category of muscle swelling from thyroid and pseudotumor swelling, which also cause uniform, diffuse muscle thickening and proptosis. Contrast-enhanced scanning is crucial in making this distinction, because an AVM or arteriovenous fistula will commonly produce serpiginous vascular channels, and carotid-cavernous fistula might show dilatation of the ipsilateral cavernous sinus. Shunt-based muscle enlargement does not characteristically have fat prolapse, so frequent in Graves' ophthalmopathy.[1] Superior ophthalmic vein dilatation is not pathognomonic of arteriovenous shunting, but may occur in any disease (e.g., Graves' orbitopathy, apical tumor) in which apical compression is significant.

Other Orbital Inflammations

Although not emphasized in the literature, swelling of an extraocular muscle may result from contiguous orbital or sinus infection. Ordinarily, muscle thickening is just one of a constellation of CT findings related to the orbital abscess or cellulitis (see Chapter 18, Orbital and Periorbital Infection). In this context, moderate uniform swelling and enhancement arise from cellular infiltrate, edema, and hyperemia (see Fig 18–12).

THE ENLARGED SUPERIOR OPHTHALMIC VEIN

As previously discussed, the normal superior ophthalmic vein is frequently seen on CT scans of the

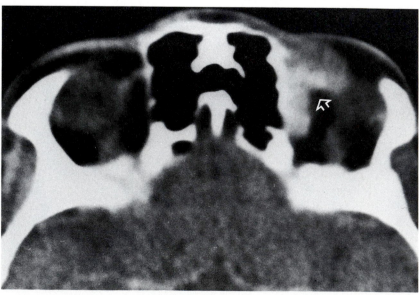

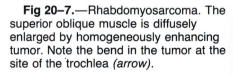

Fig 20–7.—Rhabdomyosarcoma. The superior oblique muscle is diffusely enlarged by homogeneously enhancing tumor. Note the bend in the tumor at the site of the trochlea (arrow).

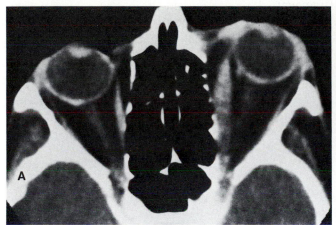 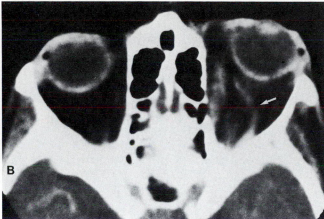

Fig 20–8.—Carotid-cavernous fistula. **A,** unilateral muscle enlargement and proptosis are present with no appreciable fat prolapse. **B,** distension of the superior ophthalmic vein *(arrow)* results from the high-flow state.

orbit. With high-resolution scanners, the rate of visualization is around 100%.[23] The vein has a tortuous course and increases in width from anterior to posterior. Measurements of the normal vein have been made with CT scan, giving a diameter of 2.0 mm anteriorly and 3.5 mm posteriorly.[24] The superior ophthalmic vein can be enlarged in a number of pathologic processes. Basically, however, there are two main etiologic categories for the dilatation—increased flow through the vein or congestion of venous outflow.

Those lesions with increased flow include carotid-cavernous fistulae, AVM, and highly vascular tumors.[24, 25] Carotid-cavernous fistula is suggested on CT scan by associated findings of proptosis, extraocular muscle enlargement, and dilatation of the cavernous sinus. Clinically, chemosis and engorged conjunctival vessels are seen, and bruit may be heard (see Fig 20–8).[22, 26, 27] While AVM might clinically simulate carotid-cavernous fistula, the CT scan appearance of irregular, serpiginous enhancing densities would distinguish them. A vascular tumor large enough to cause significant shunting through the superior ophthalmic vein would be readily apparent on CT scan, making differential diagnosis simple.

The lesions causing venous congestion may be compressive or destructive. The most common area of venous compression is at the orbital apex, where orbital structures are most confined and in closest proximity. Apical tumors and enlarged muscles at the annulus of Zinn, such as are present in Graves' disease, may extrinsically compress the superior ophthalmic vein enough to cause venous congestion (see Fig 20–4); so too, an obstructed or compressed cavernous sinus may rarely result in venous congestion that dilates the vein.[24] High-resolution scans can, in most cases, separate apical tumor from apical muscle thickening. This is especially easy when there is supportive evidence of Graves' ophthalmopathy or myositic pseudotumor on the scan (see preceding, Extraocular Muscle Enlargement).

LACRIMAL GLAND ENLARGEMENT

Masses of the lacrimal gland are largely confined to the superolateral aspect of the anterior orbit. The lacrimal gland fossa, bounded by the orbital septum anteriorly, the globe and levator palpebrae medially, the periorbital surface of the frontal bone laterally, and extraconal fat posteriorly,[28] provides a significant restrictive barrier to other than the most aggressive disease processes. Easily palpated, these masses displace the globe medially and inferiorly. Lacrimal globe tumors are the commonest primary extraconal tumors.[29]

Unilateral Enlargement

Tumors comprise about half of lacrimal gland masses. Benign (pleomorphic or mixed) types tend to remain localized to the fossa, although they may enlarge the bony walls of the fossa.[30] Well defined, these tumors variably enhance.[19, 27, 31] Malignant tumors (primary and metastatic) show no consistent enhancement pattern. When small, they are usually confined, but with growth they may invade the orbital wall or extend posteriorly, encasing the lateral rectus muscle and displacing the optic nerve.[31]

Inflammatory conditions, like acute or chronic dacryoadenitis and pseudotumor, may radiographically mimic the appearance of benign tumor.[31, 32] Inflammatory masses are well defined and generally show some enhancement. A rim-like enhancement pattern can be seen in chronic dacryoadenitis (Fig 20–9), although the usual appearance is more homogeneous.

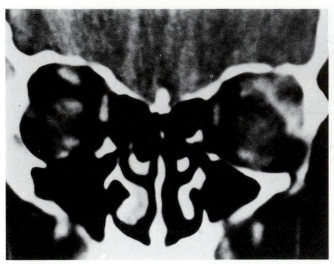

Fig 20–9.—Lacrimal gland, chronic dacryoadenitis. The right lacrimal gland is enlarged. A thin enhancing rim surrounds a well-defined lucent area in the lateral portion of the gland.

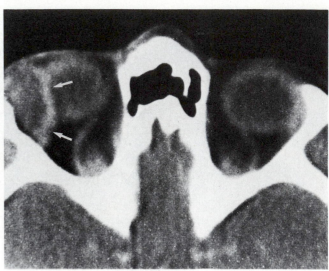

Fig 20–10.—Lacrimal gland, dermoid cyst. There is a thin, well-defined wall (arrows) surrounding a lucent, fat-density interior.

Dermoid cyst is the only lacrimal gland mass that has an unequivocal CT scan appearance—well defined, oval wall, cystic interior of low absorption (often fat density), and smooth erosion of the contiguous bony wall (Fig 20–10).[27, 31, 33, 34] A fluid level is sometimes seen in the cyst.[35]

Bilateral Enlargement

Bilateral lacrimal gland enlargement may be a manifestation of sarcoidosis, Mikulicz's syndrome, Sjögren's syndrome, Graves' disease, myxedema, amyloidosis, blood dyscrasias, and occasionally pseudotumor and lymphoid hyperplasia.[36] Because most of these are composed of a round-cell infiltrate with accompanying inflammatory changes, CT scan appearance of these numerous entities is similar, that is, well-defined, homogeneous enlargement of both glands (Fig 20–11). Mikulicz's syndrome and Sjögren's syndrome may show prominent enhancement.[31]

MASSES OF THE POSTERIOR GLOBE

Although CT scanning is useful in demonstrating a variety of ocular disease processes,[26, 27, 37–40] funduscopic examination and ultrasound are presently the standard methods of examination. Even with high resolution, CT scans can neither reach the level of sensitivity of ultrasound regarding detail of the chambers, lens, and globe wall, nor give the same level of tissue characterization of masses in the globe.

One of the primary uses for CT in ocular disease is for delineating masses of the posterior globe walls, specifically in determining the presence and extent of ex-

traocular spread. Such an evaluation is especially crucial for neoplasms, because it largely determines their subsequent course of management. Ultrasound alone may be unsatisfactory, especially if the mass contains calcium or if there is extensive retro-orbital spread.

Retinoblastoma

Retinoblastoma is by far the most common intraocular malignancy of childhood. Usually presenting in the first 2 years of life, it is multicentric, occurring bilaterally in about one third of patients. It is highly malignant and spreads by local invasion and hematogenous metastasis. Locally, the tumor extends from the retina through the other layers of the globe wall, along the perivascular and perineural tissue planes, and into the subarachnoid space. Determination of the extent of extraocular tumor is critical in these patients, because its presence forebodes a poor prognosis.[41, 42]

Characteristics of retinoblastoma on CT scan include a well-defined, high-density global wall mass, conglomerate areas of calcification, and slight contrast enhancement.[41–44] The mass may protrude a variable distance into the vitreous and be flat or papillated. Generally, calcification is more common in the intraocular portions of the tumor (Fig 20–12).[42] Extrascleral spread presents as a soft-tissue mass of slight-to-moderate enhancement, commonly relating to the optic nerve.

The differential diagnosis of retinoblastoma is limited. Pigmented hyperplastic primary vitreous, a congenital vascular malformation, can mimic retinoblastoma clinically and by CT, but does not usually calcify.[45] Phthisic inflammatory changes associated

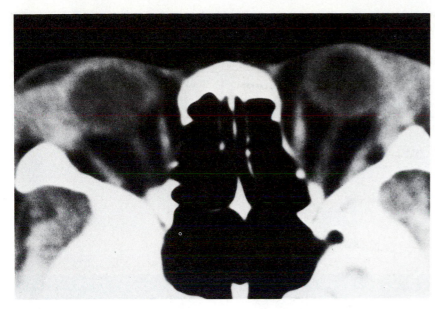

Fig 20–11.—Lacrimal gland sarcoidosis. Both lacrimal glands are enlarged and show homogeneous enhancement.

with chronic retinal detachment and hemorrhage can also produce a posterior wall soft-tissue mass (Fig 20–13).

Malignant Melanoma

Malignant melanoma is the most common primary intraocular tumor of adulthood. Originating in the choroid layer of the wall, it spreads quickly and metastasizes early. The tumor can extend through the wall, forming a retrobulbar mass in 15% of cases.[46] By CT, melanoma presents a nodular or convex eccentric thickening of the global rim.[26, 39, 47] It is high density on the unenhanced scan and enhances moderately following contrast administration. Calcification is not present (Fig 20–14).

Metastatic and Other Tumors

Metastatic disease of the eye is probably more common than primary malignant melanoma. In adults, the richly vascularized choroid layer is the most common site of implantation. Spread of tumor into the orbit from the globe is seen in a significant number of patients. Breast, lung, and kidney carcinomas have the highest incidence of ocular involvement.[21] The CT scan may show a globular thickening of the wall or a more diffuse, smooth expansion. There may be a combination of the two appearances in the same globe. Enhancement is usually prominent and can simulate an inflammatory condition of the wall such as retinitis (Fig 20–15).

Lymphoma, lymphoid hyperplasia, and leukemia may involve bulbar and peribulbar structures[46] similar to metastases. Fairly smooth, homogeneous, moder-

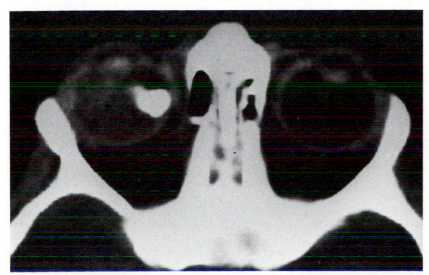

Fig 20–12.—Retinoblastoma. Dense calcification is seen in the wall of the globe. High-density tumor fills the posterior chamber. There is no retrobulbar mass. (Courtesy of Victor Haughton, M.D., Milwaukee.)

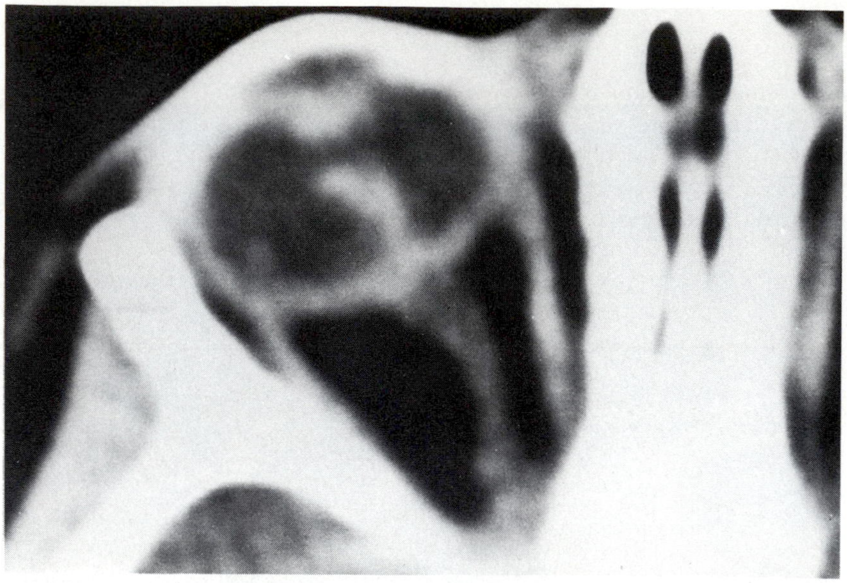

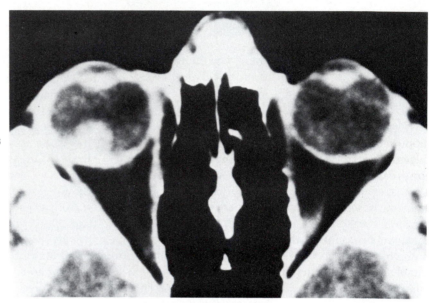

Fig 20–13.—Phthisic inflammation. A noncalcified soft-tissue mass in the posterior right globe protrudes into the vitreous cavity.

Fig 20–14.—Malignant melanoma. A contrasted scan shows a dome-like mass of the posterior wall protruding into the vitreous cavity. There is no retrobulbar mass.

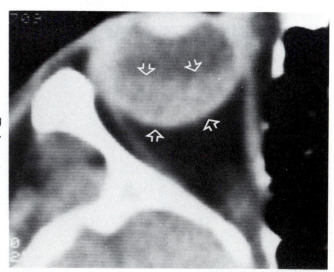

Fig 20–15.—Globe metastasis. An irregular enhancing mass *(arrows)* extends across most of the posterior orbit. This breast carcinoma metastasis has no retrobulbar component. (Courtesy of Reza Raji, M.D., Pittsburgh.)

ately enhancing expansion of the globe wall is seen on CT in these disorders.

A benign tumor, choroid angioma, can simulate an ocular melanoma. It appears as a well-defined enhancing mass, restricted to and thickening the wall of the eyeball. Sturge-Weber-Krabbe syndrome is present in some of these patients.[48] Retinal angioma in von Hippel-Lindau syndrome may also present a focal enhancing mass of the wall.

NONTRAUMATIC DISEASE AFFECTING THE ORBITAL WALLS

The orbital walls may be abnormal as a result of a wide variety of congenital, developmental, or acquired diseases. Because of this variety, some categorization of disease manifestation is useful and helps to limit differential diagnosis. One approach to orbital wall disease is as follows: (1) the small orbit; (2) the large orbit; (3) lucent abnormalities of the wall; and (4) sclerotic abnormalities of the wall (after S.A. Kieffer, 1971).[49]

The Small Orbit

The vast majority of small orbits result from congenital and developmental disease. Microphthalmos and anophthalmos, both congenital diseases, have well-formed orbits that are disproportionately small in relation to the rest of the head. On CT, anophthalmos is seen as bilaterally small bony orbits, containing soft-tissue structures that represent rudimentary orbital parts. Microphthalmos, which is unilateral or bilateral, has more defined internal structures, often with a perceptible globe and muscles. The optic nerve may be missing or the globe partially calcified (Fig 20–16).[50]

Craniosynostosis and diseases associated with craniosynostosis (e.g., Crouzon's disease) are distinguished by foreshortening of the bony orbits.[51] The CT scan shows shallow orbits with proptosis of the globe, as well as the oddly shaped calvarium. Of the craniosynostoses, oxycephaly and plegiocephaly most often produce orbital abnormalities.[52]

Because growth of the orbital contents stimulates development of the bony orbit, enucleation takes away the stimulus for orbital expansion. Therefore, if an adequate prosthesis is not provided, the orbit becomes proportionally smaller.[53]

Mucocele, by slowly expanding and reforming the walls of a paranasal sinus, can contract the size of the orbit without causing an obvious lytic defect. Easy identification of the mucocele is possible by CT, which shows outward bowing of the thin sinus walls by a water-density mass. The orbit is otherwise normal.[54]

Fibrous dysplasia, by virtue of the thickening caused

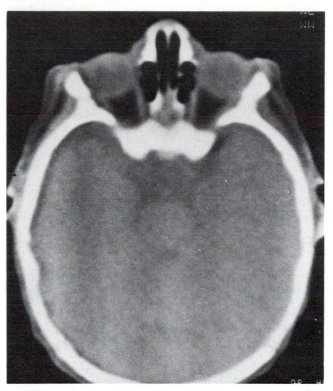

Fig 20–16.—Microphthalmos. Both globes and orbits are small in relation to head size. A hypoplastic optic nerve is barely seen in the right orbit; none is present in the left orbit.

by bony involvement, may compromise the size of the orbit. Especially when involvement is diffuse, the orbital space becomes shrunken and exophthalmos pronounced (Fig 20–17). The CT features of fibrous dysplasia are discussed later with sclerotic lesions.

The Large Orbit

Enlargement of the orbit usually results from an intraorbital mass.[49] It may be diffuse or local, depending on the underlying etiologic process. Diffuse orbital expansion occurs in congenital glaucoma, serous cysts, and neurofibromatosis. In congenital glaucoma, or buphthalmos, heightened intraocular pressure causes enlargement of the globe, which then serves to enlarge the entire orbit. This condition is easily identified by CT (Fig 20–18). Serous cysts occur in the context of anophthalmos or microphthalmos. Orbital wall dysplasia from neurofibromatosis may lead to generalized expansion of the entire orbit.[55] There is a defect of the greater wing of the sphenoid bone of varying size, illustrated well by CT. Herniation of a portion of the temporal lobe into the orbit may also contribute to orbital enlargement.

Tumors may cause diffuse or focal wall expansion. Generally, younger patients and patients with intra-

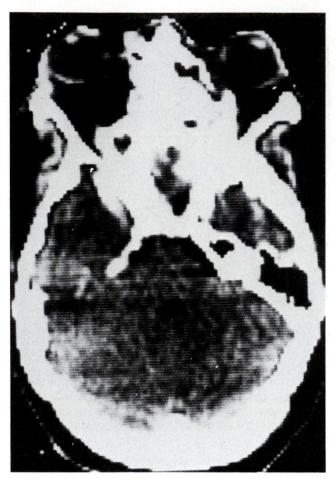

Fig 20–17.—Fibrous dysplasia. A homogeneously dense bony mass obscures the ethmoid sinus and expands the ethmoid and sphenoid bones, causing marked bilateral proptosis. (Courtesy of Manfred Boehnke, M.D., Pittsburgh.)

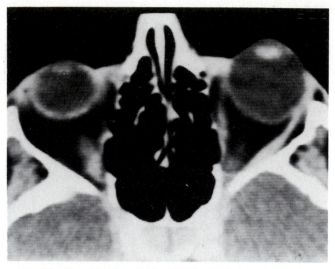

Fig 20–18.—Buphthalmos. The left globe is markedly enlarged, and there is atrophy of the globe wall. The orbital walls are slightly expanded by the enlarged globe. (Courtesy of Reza Raji, M.D., Pittsburgh.)

Lucent Abnormalities of the Wall

Congenital lucencies of an orbital wall are noted in neurofibromatosis and encephalocele. As previously described, neurofibromatosis may be manifest by absence of a portion of the greater sphenoid wing. A dysplastic change, this bony defect has a smoothly tapered margin, no associated mass, and affects the medial aspect of the bone (Fig 20–19). Long-standing temporal fossa masses, e.g., subarachnoid cyst, can produce a similar plain radiographic picture, but CT scanning easily identifies these. Encephaloceles have well-defined, circumscribed bony defects, usually near the midline. A mass may protrude into the medial orbit.[49] Computed tomographic scanning illustrates the defect containing CSF or brain density and any associated anomaly of the globe or brain. Other well-defined defects of bone may result from slow-growing orbital tumors like dermoids, lacrimal gland adenomas, hemangiomas, or neurofibromas.[49] The accompanying tumor is readily apparent on scan.

Secondary tumors from local or distant neoplasia are the most common source of lucent defects. Sinus, nasal cavity, and nasopharyngeal tumors frequently invade the orbit, usually by direct extension through the orbital walls. Thus, destruction of the bony walls occurs at the medial wall and floor in ethmoid and maxillary sinus, nasal cavity, and nasopharyngeal tumors and at the orbital roof in frontal sinus tumors. Tumors may also extend through orbital foramina to enter the orbit.[58] Orbital involvement by malignant tumor is characterized by irregular, permeative destruction of bone and an invasive soft-tissue mass, while benign tumor has less irregular destruction and a well-defined mass.[59]

conal rather than extraconal masses have a greater tendency to have diffusely enlarged orbits. So, too, long-standing, slow-growing tumors are more prone to remodel their bony surroundings. Thus, hemangiomas, optic gliomas, and pseudotumors have a propensity to cause enlargement of the entire orbit.[49] Focal remodelling is more likely in adult tumors and in those with an extraconal location. Hemangiomas, hemangiopericytomas, neurofibromas, and lacrimal gland tumors can all focally affect the wall (see Fig 18–14). Venous varix, a tumor-like condition in many ways, can by its chronic pulsations erode the orbital wall.

Maxillary sinus hypoplasia or aplasia results in orbital enlargement because of depression of the orbital floor. This diagnosis can be confirmed by CT findings that include thickening of the antral wall, lateral expansion of the ipsilateral nasal cavity, hypoplasia of the zygomatic recess of the antrum, and ipsilateral inferior turbinate hypertrophy.[56, 57]

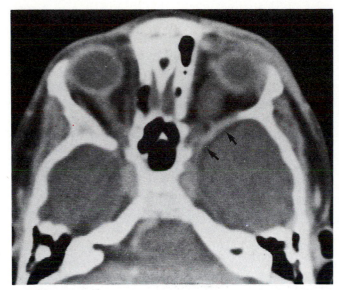

Fig 20–19.—Neurofibromatosis. There is a well-defined defect of the greater wing of the left sphenoid bone *(arrows).* In this particular case, the temporal lobe does not herniate through the defect; the enhancing dura covers the defect. The posterior optic nerve is involved by glioma. (Courtesy of Reza Raji, M.D., Pittsburgh.)

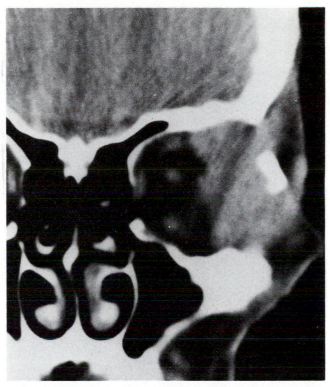

Fig 20–20.—Metastasis to the orbital wall. The lateral wall of the orbit is mostly destroyed, and there is a large soft-tissue mass protruding into the orbit and displacing the lateral rectus.

Metastatic spread from distant primary sites to the orbital wall comprises about 12% of all metastatic orbital and ocular disease.[21] Most of these deposits are from breast, lung, and kidney carcinomas in the adult and from neuroblastoma and Ewing's sarcoma in children. These metastases are primarily lytic rather than sclerotic. Destruction of the wall is usually irregular on the CT scan and has an associated enhancing soft-tissue component (Fig 20–20). Varying amounts of orbital invasion are seen; the tumor mass may be confined by the periorbita or break through it, involving fat and muscle by a fairly defined or irregular mass.

Eosinophilic granuloma and histiocytosis X may be difficult to distinguish from metastatic disease by CT. The bony defect is fairly well delineated; usually only a small soft-tissue mass is present. Although the frontal bone is most often affected, other bones of the orbit can be involved.

Osteomyelitis may result from sinusitis, trauma, or hematogenous spread. Lytic defects are usually irregular with acute disease, but can be sclerotic with chronic disease. A soft-tissue mass from adjacent cellulitis or abscess is likely to accompany the bony changes. When orbital bone destruction accompanies mucosal thickening of several sinuses in the absence of air-fluid levels, fungus disease (i.e., mucormycosis or aspergillosis) should be suspected.[60]

Extensive lysis of bone may accompany very aggressive meningiomas that extend directly into the orbit.[58]

Generally, the soft-tissue component is large. Such tumors may become so extensive that they obliterate all definable bony and soft-tissue structures (Fig 20–21).

Rarely, intraorbital malignancies such as rhabdomyosarcoma will invade the adjacent bony wall. The resultant bony destruction and mass are easily identified by CT scan.

Sclerotic Abnormalities of the Wall

Sphenoid wing meningiomas generally cause hyperostosis and thickening. They often have a high-density soft-tissue component that protrudes into the posterior orbit and/or middle cranial fossa. On CT, homogeneous enhancement is characteristic. The extraconal tumor, displacement of extraocular muscles, and proptosis are apparent (Fig 20–22). These meningiomas may be extensive, compromising the superior orbital fissure and optic foramen and associated neurovascular structures. Meningiomas of the orbital roof, also sclerotic, are less likely than sphenoid wing meningiomas to invade the orbit.[49] Those meningiomas that arise in the parasellar region and from the medial sphenoid wing may gain access to the orbit by invading the superior orbital fissure.[58]

Fibrous dysplasia may involve any of the bones of the

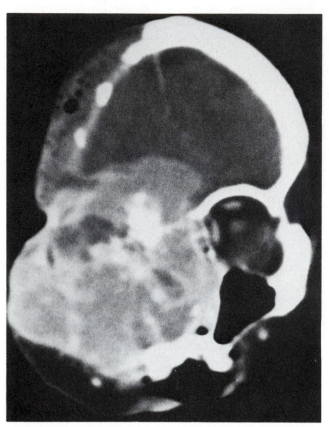

Fig 20–21.—Extensive wall meningioma. This large tumor has grown to such an extent that it has obliterated the normal structures of the orbit.

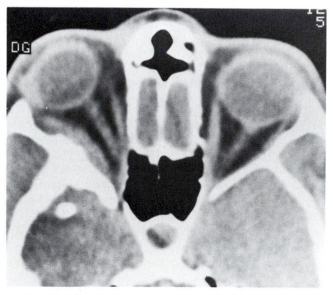

Fig 20–22.—Sphenoid wing meningioma. The right sphenoid wing is thickened and sclerotic. Homogeneous extraconal tumor displaces the lateral rectus into the orbit. (Courtesy of Lawrence Gold, M.D., Minneapolis.)

orbit. With its thickened, sclerotic appearance, it may in some instances simulate meningioma. Bone involved with fibrous dysplasia tends to have extremely high density and homogeneous texture on CT (see Fig 20–17). There is no significant soft-tissue component as in meningioma.[61, 62] Fibrous dysplasia also occurs at a younger age group than meningioma.

Paget's disease unusually affects the orbit and only rarely in a solitary fashion. The involved bone is expanded and shows both lytic and sclerotic areas. On CT, sclerosis is irregular, with areas of low density interspersed within the thickened bone.[63] Foraminal openings may be severely compromised.

Metastases to the orbital wall can be sclerotic as well as lytic. Carcinomatous implants from the prostate or breast are the most common blastic metastasis to the orbit. As in Paget's disease, sclerosis is irregular. Bony thickening, however, is not as prominent as in Paget's disease, and enhancing soft-tissue mass is almost always present. By CT, the most difficult differential possibility to exclude is an aggressive meningioma, which may have sclerotic and lytic areas and a prominent soft-tissue mass.

CT-GUIDED FINE-NEEDLE BIOPSY

Fine-needle aspiration biopsy techniques have proved to be useful and safe in orbital diagnosis.[64–66] Whether done blindly or guided by ultrasound or CT, they have applicability in several clinical contexts, most notably inoperable orbital masses or masses presenting diagnostic (and thus therapeutic) dilemmas.

When done with CT guidance, the biopsy is performed with a 22- or 23-gauge needle usually placed through the lower lid just below the outer canthus. Once the needle is inserted, its position is checked by contiguous 5-mm (or less) scans (Fig 20–23). If needed, repositioning and rescanning are performed. The biopsy is made by a combination of suction to and agitation of the needle.[64, 66] Cytologic analysis is then made on the specimen. It is emphasized that this is a cytologic test. As such, it is limited by specimen sampling.

As various techniques have been attempted and modified, indications for CT-guided biopsy have developed. Thus, CT guidance has been found to be unnecessary for relatively superficial lesions and extraconal lesions, which can be biopsied without CT localization. Large intraconal masses, especially if anteriorly placed, are more easily biopsied with ultrasound guidance.[67] Additionally, aspiration biopsy is not indicated in well-circumscribed intraconal or extraconal masses. Some of these masses, e.g., hemangiopericytoma and mixed lacrimal gland tumor, can become locally aggressive if their capsule is violated.[64]

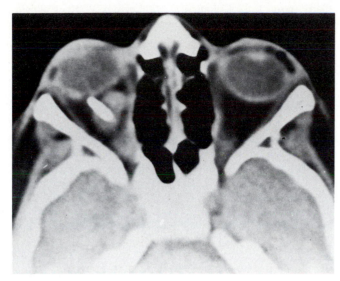

Fig 20–23.—Fine-needle aspiration biopsy. A biopsy needle has been placed into the enlarged optic nerve. The scan confirms needle position. Biopsy established the diagnosis of optic nerve glioma (same patient as in Figure 19–22).

Optic nerve lesions are most amenable to CT localization and biopsy techniques. Indeed, fine-needle aspiration has led to histologic diagnoses of a host of optic nerve lesions, including meningioma, astrocytoma, leukemia, and perineural inflammation.[65]

In summary, although fine-needle aspiration biopsy is limited by the amount of specimen obtained and inability to determine extent of disease, in the appropriate clinical setting diagnostic information may be gained easily and safely, saving the patient major surgery.

REFERENCES

1. Trokel S.L., Hilal S.K.: Recognition and differential diagnosis of enlarged extraocular muscles in computed tomography. *Am. J. Ophthalmol.* 87:503–512, 1979.
2. Enzmann D.R., Donaldson S.S., Kriss J.P.: Appearance of Graves' disease on orbital computed tomography. *J. Comput. Assist. Tomogr.* 3:815–918, 1979.
3. Robbins S.: *Pathologic Basis of Disease.* Philadelphia, W.B. Saunders Co., 1974, p. 1336.
4. Brismar J., Davis K.R., Dallow R.L., et al.: Unilateral endocrine exophthalmos: Diagnostic problems in association with computed tomography. *Neuroradiology* 12:21–24, 1976.
5. Enzmann D.R., Marshall W.H., Rosenthal A.R., et al.: Computed tomography in Graves' ophthalmopathy. *Radiology* 118:615–620, 1976.
6. Trokel S.L., Jakobiec F.A.: Correlation of CT scanning and pathologic features of ophthalmic Graves' disease. *Ophthalmology* 88:553–564, 1981.
7. Healy J.F., Rosenkrantz H.: Enlargement of the optic nerve sheath complex in thyroid ophthalmopathy. *J. Comput. Tomogr.* 5:8–10, 1981.
8. Kennerdell J.S., Rosenbaum A.E., El-Hoshy M.H.: Apical optic nerve compression of dysthyroid optic neuropathy on computed tomography. *Arch. Ophthalmol.* 99:807–809, 1981.
9. Healy J., Metcalf J.H., Brahme F.J.: Thyroid ophthalmopathy: Bony erosion on CT and increased vascularity on angiography. *A.J.N.R.* 2:472–474, 1981.
10. Nugent R.A., Rootman J., Robertson W.D., et al.: Acute orbital pseudotumors: Classification and CT features. *A.J.N.R.* 2:431–436, 1981.
11. Bernardino M.E., Zimmerman R.D., Citrin C.M., et al.: Scleral thickening: A CT sign of orbital pseudotumor. *A.J.R.* 129:703–706, 1977.
12. Jellinek E.H.: The orbital pseudotumor syndrome and its differentiation from endocrine exophthalmos. *Brain* 92:35–58, 1969.
13. Blodi F.C., Gass J.D.M.: Inflammatory pseudotumor of the orbit. *Br. J. Ophthalmol.* 52:79–93, 1968.
14. Mastaglia F.L., Barwick D.D., Hall R.: Myopathy in acromegaly. *Lancet* 2:907–909, 1970.
15. Nagulesparen M., Trickey R., Davies M.J., et al.: Muscle changes in acromegaly. *Br. Med. J.* 2:914–915, 1976.
16. Dal Pozzo G., Boschi M.C.: Extraocular muscle enlargement in acromegaly. *J. Comput. Assist. Tomogr.* 6:706–707, 1982.
17. Jones I.S., Reese A.B., Kraut J.: Orbital rhabdomyosarcoma: An analysis of 62 cases. *Am. J. Ophthalmol.* 61:721–736, 1966.
18. Knochel J.Q., Osborn A.G., Wing D.S.: Differential diagnosis of lateral orbital masses. *J. Comput. Tomogr.* 5:11–15, 1980.
19. Forbes G.S., Sheedy P.F., Waller R.R.: Orbital tumors evaluated by computed tomography. *Radiology* 136:101–111, 1980.
20. Jacobs L., Weisberg L.A., Kinkel W.R.: *Computerized Tomography of the Orbit and Sella Turcica.* New York, Raven Press, 1980, pp. 137–140.
21. Ferry A.P., Font R.L.: Carcinoma metastatic to the eye and orbit: I. A clinicopathologic study of 227 cases. *Arch. Ophthalmol.* 92:276–286, 1974.
22. Merrick R., Latchaw R.E., Gold L.H.A.: Computerized tomography of the orbit in carotid-cavernous sinus fistulae. *Comput. Tomogr.* 4:127–132, 1980.
23. Weinstein M.A., Modic M.T., Risius D., et al.: Visualization of the arteries, veins, and nerves of the orbit by sector computed tomography. *Radiology* 138:83–87, 1981.
24. Bacon K.T., Duchesneau P.M., Weinstein M.A.: Demonstration of the superior ophthalmic vein by high resolution computed tomography. *Radiology* 124:129–131, 1977.
25. Dubois P.J., Kennerdell J.S., Rosenbaum A.E.: Advantages of a fourth generation CT scanner in the management of patients with orbital mass lesions. *Comput. Tomogr.* 3:279–290, 1979.
26. Hilal S.K., Trokel S.L.: Computerized tomography of the

orbit using thin sections. *Semin. Roentgenol.* 12:137–147, 1977.

27. Wende S., Aulich A., Nover A., et al.: Computed tomography of orbital lesions. *Neuroradiology* 13:123–134, 1977.

28. Whitnall E.S.: *The Human Orbit and Accessory Organs of Vision* (facsimile of 1921 edition). New York, Robert E. Krieger Pub. Co., Inc., 1979, pp. 208–214.

29. Lloyd G.A.S.: CT scanning in the diagnosis of orbital disease. *Comput. Tomogr.* 3:227–239, 1979.

30. Lloyd G.A.S.: *Radiology of the Orbit.* Philadelphia, W.B. Saunders Co., 1975, pp. 132–134.

31. Hesselink J.R., Davis K.R., Dallow R.L., et al.: Computed tomography of masses in the lacrimal gland region. *Radiology* 131:143–147, 1979.

32. Nugent R.A., Rootman J., Robertson W.D., et al.: Acute orbital pseudotumors: Classification and CT features. *A.J.N.R.* 2:431–436, 1981.

33. Salvolini U., Menichelli F., Pasquini U.: Computer assisted tomography in 90 cases of exophthalmos. *J. Comput. Tomogr.* 1:81–100, 1977.

34. Blei L., Chambers J., Liotta L., et al.: Orbital dermoid diagnosed by computed tomographic scanning. *Am. J. Ophthalmol.* 85:58–61, 1978.

35. Wright J.E., Stewart W.B., Krohel G.B.: Clinical presentation and management of lacrimal gland tumors. *Br. J. Ophthalmol.* 63:600–606, 1979.

36. Duke-Elder Sir, S., McFaul P.A.: Diseases of the lacrimal gland in the ocular adenexa: Part II, in *System of Ophthalmology.* St. Louis, C.V. Mosby Co., 1974, pp. 595–674.

37. Momose J.K., New P.F.J., Grove A.S. Jr., et al.: The use of computed tomography in ophthalmology. *Radiology* 115:361–368, 1975.

38. Dallow R.L.: Reliability of orbital diagnostic tests: Ultrasonography, computerized tomography and radiography. *Ophthalmology* 85:1218–1228, 1978.

39. Bernardino M.E., Danzinger J., Young S.E., et al.: Computed tomography in ocular neoplastic disease. *A.J.R.* 131:111–113, 1978.

40. Brandt-Zawadski M., Enzmann D.R.: Orbital computed tomography: Calcific densities of the posterior globe. *J. Comput. Assist. Tomogr.* 3:503–505, 1979.

41. Hilal S.K., Trokel S.L., Coleman D.J.: High resolution computerized tomography and β-scan ultrasonography orbits. *Trans. Am. Acad. Ophthalmol. Otolaryngol.* 81:601–617, 1976.

42. Danzinger A., Price H.I.: CT findings in retinoblastoma. *A.J.R.* 133:783–785, 1979.

43. Price H.I., Batnitzky S., Danzinger A., et al.: The neuroradiology of retinoblastoma. *RadioGraphics* 2:7–24, 1982.

44. Goldberg L., Danzinger A.: Computed tomographic scanning in the management of retinoblastoma. *Am. J. Ophthalmol.* 84:380–382, 1977.

45. Mafee M.F., Goldberg M.F., Valvassori G.E., et al.: Computed tomography in the evaluation of patients with persistent hyperplastic primary vitreous (PHPV). *Radiology* 145:713–715, 1982.

46. Grimson B.S., Cohen K.L., McCartney W.H.: Concomitant ocular and orbital neoplasms. *J. Comput. Assist. Tomogr.* 6:617–619, 1982.

47. Jacobs L., Weisberg L.A., Kinkel W.R.: *Computerized Tomography of the Orbit and Sella Turcica.* New York, Raven Press, 1980, pp. 281–291.

48. Guibert-Tranier F., Pitron J., Calabet A., et al.: Orbital syndromes—CT analysis of 100 cases. *Comput. Tomogr.* 3:241–265, 1979.

49. Kieffer S.A.: Orbit, in Newton T.H., Potts D.G. (eds.): *Radiology of the Skull and Brain.* St. Louis, C.V. Mosby Co., 1971, vol. 1, book 2, pp. 463–485.

50. Jacobs L., Weisberg L.A., Kinkel W.R.: *Computerized Tomography of the Orbit and Sella Turcica.* New York, Raven Press, 1980, pp. 275–278.

51. Blodi F.C.: Pathologic changes of the orbit bones. *Trans. Am. Acad. Ophthalmol. Otolaryngol.* 81:26–57, 1976.

52. Jacobs L., Weisberg L.A., Kinkel W.R.: *Computerized Tomography of the Orbit and Sella Turcica.* New York, Raven Press, 1980, pp. 255–257.

53. Kennedy R.E.: The effect of early enucleation on the orbit in animals and humans. *Am. J. Ophthalmol.* 60:277–306, 1965.

54. Hesselink J.R., Weber A.L., New P.F.J., et al.: Evaluation of mucoceles of the paranasal sinuses with computed tomography. *Radiology* 131:397–400, 1979.

55. Binet E.F., Kieffer S.A., Martin S.H., et al.: Orbital dysplasia in neurofibromatosis. *Radiology* 93:820–833, 1969.

56. Mancuso A.A., Hanafee W.N.: *Computed Tomography of the Head and Neck.* Baltimore, Williams & Wilkins Co., 1982, pp. 210–211.

57. Modic M.T., Weinstein M.A., Berlin A.J., et al.: Maxillary sinus hypoplasia visualized with computed tomography. *Radiology* 135:383–385, 1980.

58. Hesselink J.R., Weber A.L.: Pathways of orbital extension of extraorbital neoplasms. *J. Comput. Assist. Tomogr.* 6:593–597, 1982.

59. Parsons C., Hodson N.: Computed tomography of paranasal sinus tumors. *Radiology* 132:641–645, 1979.

60. Centeno R.S., Bentson J.R., Mancusok A.A.: CT scanning in rhinocerebral mucormycosis and aspergillosis. *Radiology* 140:383–389, 1981.

61. Jacobs L., Weisberg L.A., Kinkel W.R.: *Computerized Tomography of the Orbit and Sella Turcica.* New York, Raven Press, 1980, pp. 251–254.

62. Glydensted C., Lester J., Fledelius H.: Computed tomography of orbital lesions: A radiological study of 144 cases. *Neuroradiology* 13:141–150, 1977.

63. Jacobs L., Weisberg L.A., Kinkel W.R.: *Computerized Tomography of the Orbit and Sella Turcica.* New York, Raven Press, 1980, pp. 258–259.

64. Kennerdell J.S., Dekker A., Johnson B.J., et al.: Fine needle aspiration biopsy: Its use in orbital tumors. *Arch. Ophthalmol.* 97:1315–1317, 1979.

65. Kennerdell J.S., Dekker A., Johnson B.J.: Orbital fine needle aspiration biopsy: The results of its use in 50 patients. *Neuro-ophthalmology* 1:117–121, 1980.

66. Dubois P.J., Kennerdell J.S., Rosenbaum A.E., et al.: Computed tomographic localization for fine needle aspiration biopsy of orbital tumors. *Radiology* 131:149–152, 1977.

67. Spoor T.C., Kennerdell J.S., Dekker A., et al.: Fine needle aspiration biopsy with β-scan guidance. *Am. J. Ophthalmol.* 89:274–277, 1980.

Dementia

21

Computed Tomography and Positron Emission Tomography in Aging and Dementia

AJAX E. GEORGE, M.D.
MONY J. DE LEON, ED.D.

HISTORICAL BACKGROUND

It is an ancient belief that specific areas of the brain have specific functions.[1] As early as 1870, Fritsch and Hitzig[2] produced movement of body parts by electrically stimulating the motor cortex of the brain. Today, the motor homunculus is accepted as an accurate representation of specific motor functions of the cerebral cortex. Cognitive functions, however, such as memory, awareness, personality, and intelligence continue to pose baffling questions that challenge us to identify their site and mechanism of function. Such knowledge would permit us to evaluate the significance of structural and functional changes demonstrated by CT and positron emission tomography (PET).

Popular and scientific belief assumes that the cortex is the essential organ of thinking and consciousness. After all, there is extraordinary enlargement of the human cortex especially in the temporal, parietal, and frontal regions when compared with that of lower animals.[3] If the cerebral cortex is the site of cognition, then the cognitive impairment and memory loss phenomena seen in aging and dementia must have a counterpart in the cerebral cortex.

Today, Alzheimer's disease, originally described in 1907[4] as a presenile dementia, is recognized as the most common cause of dementia in the elderly (senile dementia of the Alzheimer type or SDAT), accounting for more than 50% of cases. Alzheimer's disease, both in the presenile and elderly populations, manifests *initially as loss of recent memory and progresses eventually to disorientation, loss of affect and personality, urinary and fecal incontinence, and ultimately to death.*[5] It has been assumed that the key to the diagnosis of Alzheimer's disease must lie in cortical changes. Indeed, neuropathologic studies[6,7] have shown increased incidence of cortical atrophy as well as ventricular enlargement in the brains of patients who died suffering from Alzheimer's disease[7] when compared with the brains of normal control groups.[6]

The histologic features of SDAT (senile plaques, neurofibrillary tangles, and granulovacuolar degeneration) are also seen in normal aging, but are much more common in the brains of Alzheimer patients who demonstrate extensive involvement of the cortex, especially of the frontal and temporal lobes.[7] *Plaque counts have been found to correlate with cortical atrophy, but not ventricular dilatation.* In the group with the highest plaque count, marked temporal lobe atrophy was observed. Furthermore, Blessed and colleagues[8] demonstrated a correlation between plaque counts and the severity of dementia.

In the first in vivo studies, correlations between cerebral atrophy, as seen by pneumoencephalography (PEG), and normal and pathologic aging produced inconsistent results. This was in part due to the difficulty in acquiring normative data, which is underscored by the following policy statement made in 1929 by the American Roentgen Ray Society Committee on standardization of encephalography: "It was realized that we cannot expect encephalographic procedures to be carried out on normal individuals and the best that we can do is to declare our judgment as to what is approximately normal from a large number of negative encephalographic studies."[9]

In an early PEG study using planimetry, Heinrich[10] found that ventricular area increased with age. Enlargement was most marked after age 65. The subarachnoid spaces were also noted to enlarge. Andersen and coworkers[11] (cited by Jacobsen and coworkers[12]), reviewing the results of PEG performed on healthy male criminals aged 17 to 64, found that 43 studies were "normal," only one demonstrating moderate "internal" atrophy. Iivanainen,[13] on the other hand, noted *cortical atrophy* increasing with age, but found no correlation between ventricular size and age.

In summary, a consistent relationship between ventricular or sulcal enlargement and aging had not been established in the PEG literature.

Studies by PEG of dementia also led to differing conclusions.

Engeset and Lonnum,[14] as well as Nielsen and colleagues,[15] demonstrated a correlation between the degree of ventricular dilatation at PEG and intellectual impairment, but the scatter was marked.[16] The width of the third ventricle and height of the left lateral ventricle appeared to be the individual measurements that corresponded best with intellectual impairment. The same authors found that cognitive impairment showed a closer correlation with sulcal than ventricular dilatation. On the other hand, Huber[17–19] found that PEG brain atrophy associated with organic personality changes was usually central and involved the white matter and the nuclei.

Gosling[20] reported that generalized cerebral atrophy was occasionally found in patients without impairment of intellectual functions. Mann[21] also showed that radiologic cortical atrophy at PEG could not be equated with dementia and that a third of the patients with demonstrable radiologic cortical atrophy were free of any evidence of dementia at 5- and 10-year follow-up.

In summary, the PEG studies raised several questions, but seemed to confirm that a relationship exists between dementia and sulcal as well as ventricular enlargement. Some studies supported a closer correlation with cortical atrophy.

The advent of CT promised the realization of a heretofore impossible task—the noninvasive visualization of the *in vivo* functioning brain. In the study of memory impairment and dementia, it was assumed on the basis of the pathology and PEG literature that cortical atrophy and ventricular enlargement would represent the in vivo anatomical correlates of dementia. Confidence in this preconceived notion was so strong that early CT interpretations, despite the lack of established norms, frequently included the diagnosis of "cerebral atrophy." It soon became apparent that there were problems with this basic concept: (1) Many patients with cerebral atrophy were not demented; (2) many patients with dementia did not demonstrate obvious atrophy; and (3) early CT studies of dementia produced inconsistent results

(see following). Some studies correlating CT changes with cognitive impairment showed a relationship between atrophy and cognitive impairment, but only for ventricular enlargement,[22] whereas other studies[23–25] showed no significant correlation between cerebral atrophy and quantitative cognitive decline. As a consequence of the above inconsistencies and in view of the controversies in the pathology and the PEG literature, a consensus began to emerge that perhaps neither ventricular nor sulcal changes were relevant to clinical dementia.

Neuropsychological Literature

In order to interpret the above apparent discrepancies between the anticipated structural brain changes and the early CT findings in dementia, it may be worthwhile to review the literature on experimental brain lesions in search of the brain-behavior relationships that may help us localize the site(s) of memory and cognition. First of all, unilateral removal of a large part of the frontal lobe produces no loss of memory and no obvious disability.[1] The patient, however, does to a variable degree lose the ability to take initiative and plan activities. According to Bricken,[26] *bilateral* removal of the frontal lobes *does* result in personality change and memory impairment for recent events.[26] Pennfield and Rasmussen[3] also noted that removal of practically the whole frontal lobe anterior to the precentral gyrus resulted in an "amazing" lack of obvious defect. In a series of bilateral frontal gyrectomies, however, Pennfield and Rasmussen found increasing impairment of mental performance as bilateral removals were carried further back into the intermediate frontal cortex.

Stimulation of the temporal cortex in an epileptic discharge may produce complex psychological phenomena and hallucinations. The patient may feel that a present experience becomes suddenly a familiar one. Stimulation by electrode of the temporal cortex may bring to consciousness life experiences from dreaming or from previous readings.[3] Ablation of the temporal cortex limited to the anterior 5 cm is apparently associated with no memory impairment. Bilateral temporal lobectomy was described by Klüver and Bucy[27] in an animal model. A lobectomized monkey was no longer afraid of a snake that he had previously been terrified of, apparently having lost memory of previous experiences. Babkin (quoted by Pavlov[28]) also showed that a dog that has lost both temporal lobes no longer responds to his or her name. Bilateral temporal lobectomies in humans have been associated with severe antegrade amnesia.[29]

Ojemann and coworkers[30, 31] have shown that electrical stimulation of the ventrolateral thalamus *improved* short-term memory performance, but only with stimulation of the *left* thalamus. These experiments were performed during thalamotomy for dyskinesia. Left thalamic insult by stroke or hemorrhage may result in *thalamic aphasia* and short-term verbal memory disturbance. It is clear that bilateral thalamic infarcts are associated with profound memory loss and dementia.[32] This phenomenon, termed "thalamic dementia," is exemplified by the following case history: A 44-year-old mildly hypertensive man (Fig 21–1) suddenly became mute, staring without expression into the distance. The patient slowly regained speech over the next few weeks, but was left with a profound and incapacitating loss of memory for recent events, though he did retain certain memories of events in the distant past. Scans by CT revealed bilateral thalamic infarcts (see Fig 22–1). Thorough subsequent evaluation of metabolic, cardiac, and vascular status, including cerebrovascular angiography, produced negative results. The infarcts at this point are presumed to be of hypertensive origin, and the case has been classified as an example of thalamic dementia.

The concept of thalamic dementia has also received attention in the lay literature. The *Los Angeles Times*

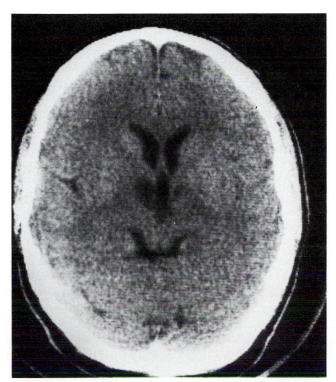

Fig 21–1.—Thalamic dementia in 44-year-old man. Bilateral thalamic infarcts of sudden onset. A 2-cm diameter radiolucency involves the dorsomedial and anterior aspects of the right thalamus consistent with infarction. There is no associated mass effect. The third ventricle is somewhat dilated for age. Smaller left thalamic infarct is also present in the same region. The study is otherwise unremarkable. (Courtesy of C. Anayiotos, M.D., Long Branch, N.J.)

in 1979[33] reported the story of a 20-year-old man who sustained a freak accident when a fencing foil entered his nostril with the tip lodging in the thalamus. The patient had severe loss of recent memory. Since then, he has been able to function at the level required to take care of himself. A CT scan confirmed the presence of thalamic injury as a consequence of the previous trauma.[34]

Further evidence of the importance of the thalami and subcortical nuclei is suggested by the well-known selective involvement of the mamillary bodies, the thalami, and hypothalami in Korsakoff's disease.[35] Selective loss of recent memory characterizes this condition common in alcoholics. In a study of 82 brains of patients with Wernicke-Korsakoff syndrome, Victor and colleagues[35] found a high degree of correlation between the memory defect and involvement, primarily neuronal loss, of the mamillary bodies, the medial dorsal nucleus of the thalamus, and the medial part of the pulvinar. In five patients with attacks of Wernicke's disease consisting of ophthalmoparesis, ataxia, and confusional apathetic state and in whom the memory defects completely cleared, the medial dorsal nucleus was normal. These were the only five cases in the series in which the nucleus was spared. Involvement to a lesser degree (minimal to moderate) was also noted of the midbrain, pons, and medulla.

In view of the experimental literature, Pennfield and Rasmussen[3] proposed the intriguing hypothesis that memories are stored in either or both temporal cortices, that the frontal cortex is utilized in the elaboration of thought, but that the important coordinator of these functions actually exists in subcortical centers, notably the mesencephalon and diencephalon, that the diencephalon is in fact "the seat of consciousness" and the center that summons and coordinates memory.[3] In this hypothesis, the mesencephalon and diencephalon in effect represent the central processing unit, and the frontal and temporal cortices represent memory banks, with right or left being used interchangeably. Removal of both leaves the central processing unit with no memory storage capacity.

Neurotransmitter Deficits in Senile Dementia

In keeping with the intriguing hypothesis of a subcortical center of cognition and memory, recent findings have provided evidence that senile dementia, though disruptive of higher cortical functions, indeed may not be a disease of the neocortex. Several studies have demonstrated neurotransmitter deficits in senile dementia. Loss of cortical acetylcholine transferase has been shown in the brains of senile dementia patients,[36–39] apparently secondary to loss of subcortical neurons of the basal nucleus of Meynert, located below the ventral globus pallidus; the axons of this nucleus provide cholinergic innervation to the frontal and hippocampal cortex.[40] This connection has been confirmed in animal models.[41] Whitehouse and associates[42] showed a profound (> 75%) loss of neurons of the basal nucleus of Meynert in the brains of patients with Alzheimer's disease.

Significant reduction of norepinephrine concentration has also been shown in the gyrus frontalis and putamen of senile dementia patients.[43] Mann and coworkers[44] found norepinephrine reduced in several regions of the cerebral cortex, which they attributed to failure of the nucleus locus ceruleus in the brain stem. Bondareff and colleagues,[45] studying the brains of 20 elderly dementia patients and 10 controls, found a loss of more than 80% of the locus ceruleus neurons in a subgroup with high dementia scores, indicating a deficit of adrenergic innervation to the cortex.

The above studies suggest that the disintegration of cortical functions may result from the degeneration of brain stem and basal ganglia nuclei that project to the cortex.

In summary, clinical, anatomical, and neuroendocrine work to date suggests that not only the cerebral cortex (primarily frontal and temporal cortices), but also several important subcortical sites of the diencephalon and midbrain, are involved in the function of memory and cognition. The advent of CT has offered us the unique opportunity to explore the structure of the in vivo functioning brain both in normal aging and in dementia; scanning by PET has provided us with the capability to study function itself of living brain with emphasis on glucose metabolism.

CT AND PET IN SENILE DEMENTIA AND AGING

It is now accepted that both cognitive and structural changes occur with normal aging. The structural and cognitive changes of senile dementia must, therefore, be thought of as additive phenomena superimposed on the aging process.

Neuropathologic studies as noted above have demonstrated a relationship between ventricular size as well as cortical atrophy and intellectual impairment in Alzheimer's disease.[6, 7]

Early CT reports failed to establish consistent brain-behavior (structural-cognitive) relationships in Alzheimer's disease, i.e., between brain structure as demonstrated by CT and brain function as quantitated by tests of cognition and memory. Diagnostic and prognostic criteria for senile dementia could not be established. In our own center, we undertook a series of CT studies including PET in order to determine what relationships, if any, exist between brain structure as demonstrated by CT, and brain function as demonstrated clinically by psychometric testing and radiologically by PET scanning.

It may be useful to break down the structural and functional changes expected in aging and senile dementia into specific questions.

1. Does *brain structure* change with normal aging? Does the brain structure of senile dementia patients differ from elderly normal controls? Are CT measures of brain pathology related to the extent of cognitive deficit? To answer these questions, measures of gross anatomy have been used, which include linear measures of the ventricular system and sulci as well as volumetric ventricular and sulcal estimates.

2. Are there *parenchymal changes* associated with the aging process? Are there parenchymal changes in the brains of senile dementia patients? These CT evaluations of white and gray matter have included subjective assessment of *gray-white discriminability* and derivation of CT attenuation values.

3. Are there *functional derangements* of brain metabolism as determined by PET scanning using the glucose analogue 2-fluorodeoxyglucose (FDG) in senile dementia? Are these functional deficits part of the aging process?

In order to answer the above questions, groups of normal volunteers were studied in addition to the dementia patients. In our studies, volunteer medical students (mean age 26.1 ± 5.1 years) made up the groups of young normals. Volunteer spouses of the dementia patients served as the elderly normal controls.

All patients studied received a CT scan of the head as well as an extensive psychometric battery and a medical and neurologic evaluation. Several patients also received a PET scan. All data from cognitive testing, PET, and CT studies were intercorrelated in search of structure-function relationships.

Normal Aging

Studies of normal aging by PET and CT have shown that the normal brain undergoes significant atrophic changes (Figs 21–2 and 21–3) without significant metabolic changes (Fig 21–4).[46]

Using the glucose analogue FDG and PET, we have found no significant difference between the glucose utilization of young volunteers (average age 26.1 ± 5.1 years) and 22 elderly normals (see Fig 21–4). Breaking down the 22 elderly patients to 11 young-old (average age 60.3 ± 4.2 years) and 11 old-old (average age 72 ± 3.1 years), none of the glucose metabolic rates showed any significant differences.

Studies of normal groups using several methods of CT scan evaluation have consistently concluded that the

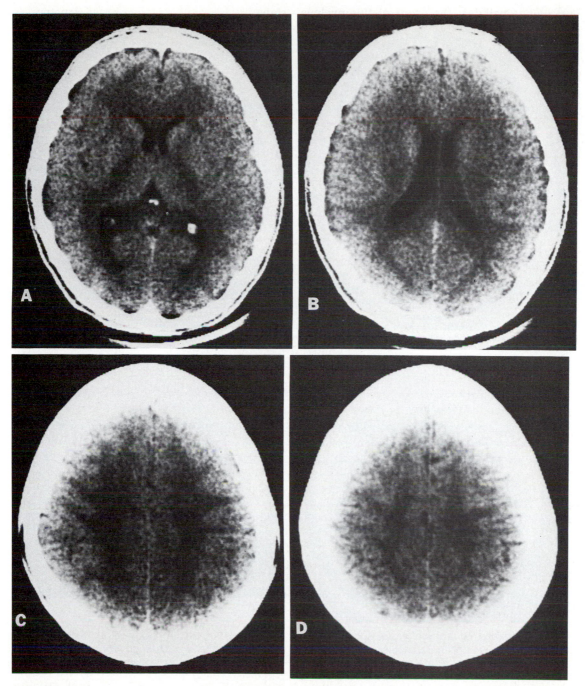

Fig 21–2.—Young normal CT in a 25-year-old man. Composite ventricular volume is 2.8% of brain. **A,** basal ganglia level: exquisite demonstration of gray and white structures with clear differentiation of the cortex from central white matter. The internal capsule is clearly defined, as is the external capsule. Sulci are only faintly visualized. **B,** ventricular body level: excellent visualization of gray and white structures. The bodies of the caudate nuclei are silhouetted as dense rims between the lateral ventricles and the adjacent white matter. **C,** centrum semiovale level. **D,** high convexity level. Note faint visualization of sulci. Gray-white matter discriminability is excellent.

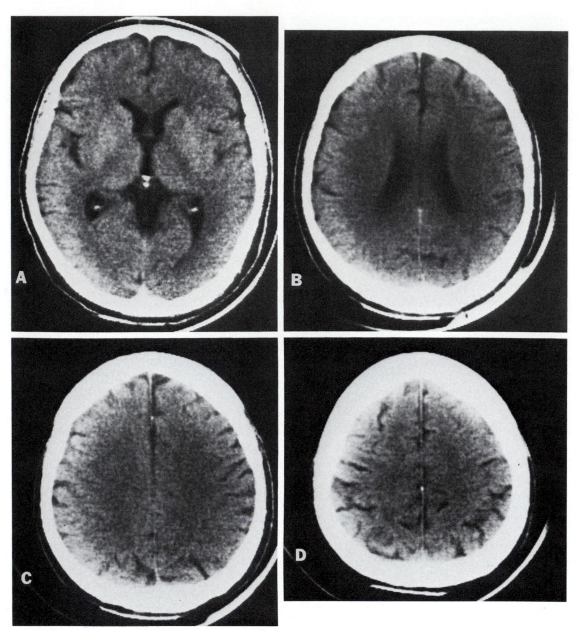

Fig 21–3.—Old normal control (volunteer spouse). This 65-year-old man has a composite ventricular volume of 5% of brain. **A,** basal ganglia level. There is enlargement of the third ventricle when compared with young normals (see Fig 21–2) as well as enlargement of sulci and fissures of mild degree. **B,** ventricular body level: sulcal prominence. **C,** centrum semiovale. **D,** high convexity. Discrimination of gray and white matter structures is diminished when compared with young normals.

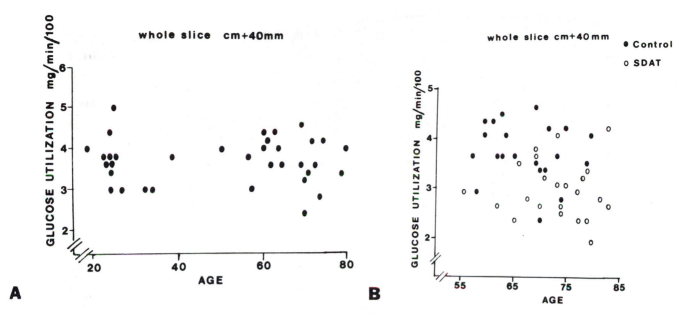

Fig 21–4.—Scattergrams. **A,** PET metabolic values, young vs. old normals. Difference is noted in the glucose utilization values for young vs. old. **B,** PET metabolic val-

ues, Alzheimer patients vs. normal control spouses. A significant difference is present in the two groups: *P* < .01 of 7% to 25%.

size of both the ventricles and cortical sulci increase with age (see Figs 21–2 and 21–3).[46–55] In our own data,[46] we have found of particular interest the very strong relationship between age and the prominence of cortical sulci (*r* = .85; Pearson Product Correlation Coefficient; *P* < −.01) determined by a ranking method, suggesting that cortical atrophy best reflects the effects of age. In previous studies of senile dementia (see following), cortical atrophy was a weak associate of cognitive impairment, and several reports in the literature found no relationship between cortical atrophy and Alzheimer's disease.[22, 24] Thus, evaluation of generalized cortical atrophy (separate from ventricular assessment) is the best means of identifying age. Of the linear ventricular measures, the width of the third ventricle is the strongest associate of normal aging.[46]

Zatz and coworkers[56] studied CT attenuation values in normal volunteers. Attenuation values for white matter in the centrum semiovale decreased with age in subjects over the age of 54. This result agrees with the findings of Cala and coworkers,[52] who found no age-related changes in the attenuation values of either white or gray matter in normal volunteers aged 15 to 40 years. In our own studies of normal volunteers, the centrum white matter attenuation values of 19 young normals and 23 normal subjects over the age of 65 were not significantly different.

Results for gray matter have not been conclusive because of the technical difficulties inherent in a determination of reliable gray matter attenuation values, in part because of the artifical increase of attenuation val-

ues adjacent to the calvarium secondary to beam hardening.

Thus, studies currently indicate that CT structural changes clearly occur with aging (see Figs 21–2 and 21–3), whereas glucose metabolism does not change significantly with the aging process (see Fig 21–4).

Alzheimer's Disease (Senile Dementia)

Ventricular and Sulcal Assessments
(Figs 21–5 and 21–6)

In studies to date, measures of CT structural change represent attempts to quantitate cerebral atrophy by estimating the amount of cerebrospinal fluid within the cranial cavity. Several investigators[23–25] have found no significant correlation between psychometric scores and CT assessments of cerebral atrophy. Nathan and Frumkin[25] studied community-residing persons over 65 years of age with CT and subtests of the Wechsler Adult Intelligence Scale (WAIS). For CT groups rated as showing minimal, moderate, or advanced atrophy, no differences were found for any of the cognitive measures except one, the Mental Health Rating Scale. The authors do not specify whether sulci were evaluated in the atrophy rating. Similarly, Claveria and associates[24] tested 81 patients diagnosed on the basis of CT as having cerebral atrophy and found no correlations between ventricular and sulcal atrophic changes seen on CT and psychometric test performance. More recently, Hughes and Gado[23] found no significant correlation between psychometric scores (the Clinical Dementia Rating) and

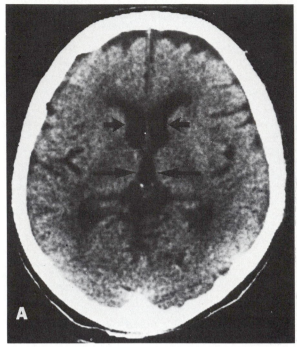
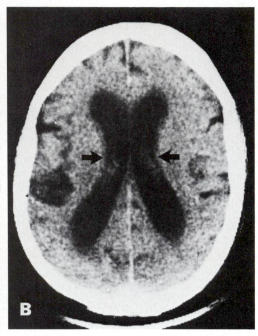

Fig 21–5.—Linear ventricular measurements utilized for CT analyses. **A,** basal ganglia level. The width of the third ventricle *(long arrows),* bicaudate diameters *(short arrows),* bifrontal span, and diagonal widths of the frontal horns were derived from this level. The maximal width of the cranium as measured from inner table to inner table was used for brain correction. **B,** ventricular body level. The cut showing the largest representations of the lateral ventricles was utilized. The waist of the two ventricles was measured at their narrowest point *(arrows).* The width of the cranium from inner table to inner table was utilized for brain correction.

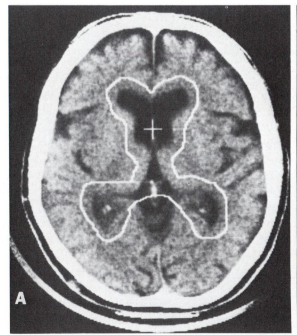
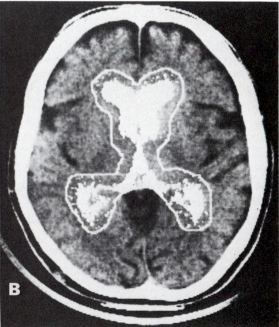

Fig 21–6.—Software derivation of ventricular volume. This procedure was utilized at every level showing ventricular structures, and summations of the ventricular volumes were obtained corrected for brain by dividing by the sum of the five greatest brain volumes. **A,** the region of interest is operator-defined to include the ventricular structures of interest. A cerebrospinal fluid range is then indicated by the operator. For these analyses, the range −11 to +25 Hounsfield units was utilized. **B,** computer-generated highlighting of the pixels falling within the range designated in **A.**

CT measurements of ventricular and sulcal enlargement in a group of 100 hospital patients over the age of 65.

Other CT studies, including our own[22, 57–65] (see Figs 21–5 and 21–6), *have* found significant relationships between ventricular size and cognitive deficit. The correlations, however, have been relatively weak. Measuring ventricular area by a planimeter, Roberts and Caird[22] demonstrated a "broad" relationship between increasing ventricular dilatation and intellectual impairment as measured by the Crichton Behavioral Rating Scale and the 30-point memory test. No relationship was demonstrable between measures of cortical atrophy and the psychometrics.

Earnest and coworkers[57] studied a group of 59 subjects over the age of 60 with CT and subtests of the WAIS. After allowing for the effects of age, the authors concluded that CT evidence of atrophy only weakly predicted impaired mental function.[57] Jacoby and Levy[58] studied 40 senile dementia patients and 50 normal controls over the age of 60 with CT and psychometrics. Demented subjects showed significantly more CT evidence of atrophy than the normal controls, but there was considerable overlap.

In our initial studies, we derived a large number of linear and subjective measures in search of the best descriptors of structural change in Alzheimer's disease (see Fig 21–6).[59–63] All linear measures were corrected for brain size by dividing the width of the brain at that level. In order to test the influence of methodology on the results, we rank-ordered scans according to increasing ventricular size and separately for increasing sulcal size and also used subjective rating procedures.[65] Correlations with psychometrics revealed consistent relationships between ventricular as well as sulcal enlargement and cognitive impairment; however, these correlations were again relatively weak ($P < .03$). Contrary to expectations, but in keeping with the subcortical cognition hypothesis, ventricular dilatation was a significantly better correlate of dementia than cortical atrophy. Of the linear measures, the width of the third ventricle was the strongest correlate, lending further support to the hypothesis that significant alterations occur at the level of the basal ganglia and the base of the brain in dementia.

These findings, therefore, reaffirmed that relationships do exist between structural (ventricular and sulcal) changes as demonstrated by CT and cognitive impairment and that the structural changes of Alzheimer's disease are superimposed on and overlap with the structural changes of normal aging (Figs 21–3 and 21–7).

Encouraged in part by the above results, but unclear as to the significance of the weak correlations obtained, we decided to determine whether three-dimensional estimates of ventricular size would produce stronger correlations with dementia scores than linear and subjective measures. We therefore undertook a subsequent study using a new generation scanner (General Electric 8800) of 35 senile dementia patients and 29 normal controls (volunteer spouses).[63, 66] We found ventricular volume determined by algorithm summation of pixels falling within a specified range (see Fig 21–6) and corrected for brain size (ventricular-brain ratio) to be significantly larger (44%) in the senile dementia patients than in the normal controls (two-tailed *t* test; $P < .01$), but with considerable overlap (Fig 21–8). The mean for the normal elderly group was 5.2% (± 3) and for the Alzheimer group, 7.5% (± 3). Furthermore, ventricular volume increased with increasing cognitive deficit ($P < .05$). The Pearson Product Correlation Coefficient between ventricular volume and the Mental Status Questionnaire, a test for global function,[67] was .42 ($P < .01$) and for the Global Deterioration Scale,[68] .37 ($P < .05$). Thus, the strength of the correlations with psychometrics remained weak despite the use of more precise estimates of ventricular size.

Gado and coworkers,[69] using a similar method, determined the ventricular volume of 20 senile dementia patients and 27 normal controls. All patients in the study were community-residing volunteers. Sulcal size was also quantitated using the same technique. Highly significant ($P < .0001$) differences were found between the normal and impaired groups. Ventricular volume corrected for brain size was 5.3% (± 1.9) in controls and 10.5% (± 4.8) in the impaired group. Sulcal size was 6.1% (± 2.5) and 10.6% (± 3.3), respectively. The authors also analyzed a subgroup of 29 scans using linear as well as volumetric measures. The linear measures showed less pronounced differences between the normal and impaired groups. The authors concluded that the conflicting results in the literature concerning variations in ventricular and sulcal size in dementia and normal aging were in part a reflection of the insensitivity of linear measures. Our own results, however, show far less pronounced differences between the normal and impaired groups, with considerable overlap. It is of some interest that in our normal elderly group we found essentially the same mean ventricular volume ratio as Gado and coworkers, 5.2% vs. 5.3%. However, our mean for the Alzheimer group was 7.5% vs. 10.5%, implying that the two pathologic groups are somehow different.

Regional Cortical Changes

In severely demented Alzheimer patients, CT findings are characterized by *focal* atrophic changes (Fig 21–9) with severe enlargement of the Sylvian fissures and marked shrinkage of the temporal and frontal lobes

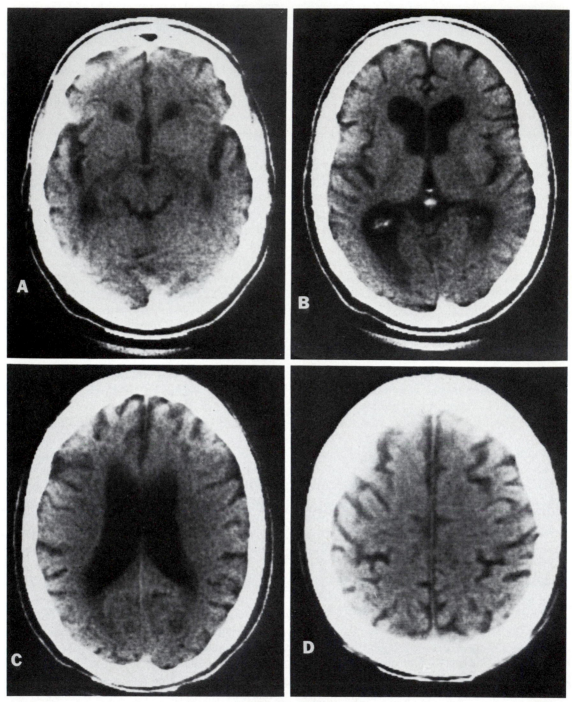

Fig 21–7.—Alzheimer's disease, moderately advanced. This 70-year-old man had a composite ventricular volume of 7.5% of brain. **A,** base of brain level: shrinkage of the temporal lobes with enlargement of the Sylvian fissures and third ventricle. **B,** basal ganglia level. Discrimination of gray and white structures is diminished markedly when compared with old controls and young controls. Poor-to-fair discrimination of gray and white structures. **C,** ventricular body level. **D,** high convexity level.

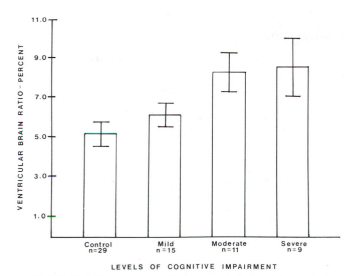

Fig 21–8.—Bar graphs of mean ventricular volume (ventricular brain ratio %) and standard error of the mean for different levels of cognitive impairment. Global Deterioration Scale (GDS) scores of 1 and 2 = control group; GDS of 3 = mild impairment group; GDS of 4 = moderate impairment; GDS of 5, 6, and 7 = severe group. The largest increment in ventricular volume is noted between the mild group (n = 15) and the moderate group (n = 11).

(Figs 21–10 and 21–11); in these cases, generalized atrophic changes may be less pronounced than the temporal and frontal changes. Two characteristic examples are shown in Figures 21–10 and 21–11. The 83-year-old patient in Figure 21–10 was severely demented at the time of CT scanning and was able to utter only unintelligible sounds. Marked enlargement of the Sylvian fissures was demonstrated by CT, indicating *very severe* temporal lobe shrinkage bilaterally (see Fig 21–10,A and C). There was moderately severe generalized cortical atrophy and moderately severe ventricular enlargement. The patient expired 1 month following the CT scan. At pathology (see Fig 21–10,B), marked shrinkage of the temporal lobes was noted with large numbers of senile plaques and tangles present in the shrunken cortex. A method for quantitation of focal temporal atrophy is shown in Figure 21–9. Advanced focal changes of Alzheimer's disease closely resemble the known focal changes of Pick's disease (see following), which represents the major CT differential diagnosis.

CT Parenchymal Measures

GRAY-WHITE MATTER DISCRIMINABILITY.—Impressed by the variability that exists in the density differences between gray and white matter structure in different patients (see Figs 21–3 and 21–7), we decided to test a variable that we called "gray-white matter

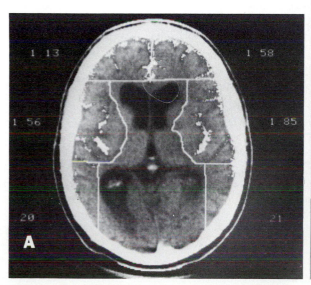
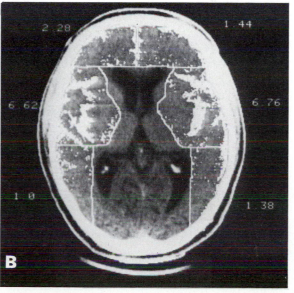

Fig 21–9.—Quantitation of regional cortical atrophic changes, temporal atrophy. **A,** example of mild Sylvian fissure dilatation and sulcal prominence. **B,** severe Sylvian fissure enlargement with temporal tip atrophy. The same method is utilized to quantitate cortical atrophy as used in Figure 21–6 to determine ventricular volume. Within the regions of interest, a cerebrospinal fluid range is designated that best highlights the sulci and fissures. The numbers indicate the volume of highlighted pixels for each region of interest. In **A,** the Sylvian fissures demonstrate a volume of 1.56 and 1.85 cm; in **B,** the corresponding volumes are 6.62 and 6.76. Temporal cortical atrophies are significantly correlated with cognitive measures (P < .01).

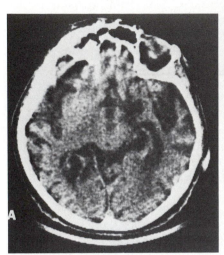 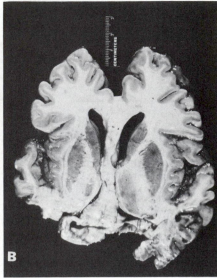 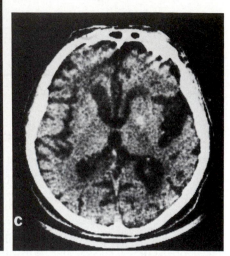

Fig 21–10.—Alzheimer brain CT neuropathologic correlation in an 83-year-old woman with severe Alzheimer's disease. The patient was only able to utter unintelligible sounds. **A,** basal CT cut; marked shrinkage of the temporal lobes and dilatation of the Sylvian fissures. The temporal horns are also enlarged, and the anterior third ventricle is dilated. **B,** pathologic section through the basal ganglia; marked shrinkage of the temporal gyri bilaterally. The cortical ribbon of gray matter is markedly shrunken. A large number of plaques and tangles were shown histologically to involve the entire temporal and frontal cortex. **C,** basal ganglia CT cut; moderate enlargement of the ventricular system and moderately severe dilatation of sulci. The gaping Sylvian fissures, especially on the left side, are again demonstrated.

discriminability"[62] and to assess its relationship to cognitive impairment. Gray-white matter discriminability, defined as the subjective contrast between central white matter and cortical gray matter, was rated on a five-point scale as poor, poor-to-fair, fair, fair-to-good, and good at three brain levels (basal ganglia, centrum semiovale, and high convexity) in a group of 26 Alzheimer patients studied with a Philips 200 translation-rotation scanner.[62] Loss of gray-white matter discriminability was significantly ($P < .05$) related to the severity of cognitive impairment, but also to ventricular size. At the high convexity level, nine of 11 cognitive measures (91%, $P < .05$) were correlated with discriminability loss. No correlation between loss of discriminability and age was found. This study, the first to our knowledge, suggested the presence of parenchymal CT changes in senile dementia that were more pronounced at the cortical level.[62]

CT ATTENUATION VALUES IN DEMENTIA.—Studies by CT of attenuation values in normal aging (see preceding)[52, 56] have shown a decrease in white matter attenuation values after the age of 56. As an extension of the gray-white discriminability results (see preceding), we attempted to quantitate gray as well as white matter attenuation values. The CT values derived from the basal ganglia and the cuts above the ventricular system in the same group of patients described in Gray-White Matter Discriminability[62] produced a few significant correlations with psychometrics, more so for the left hemisphere; interestingly, increasing attenuation values were associated with increasing deficit. This finding was in conflict with an earlier report of 7 senile dementia patients, 10 presenile patients, and 7 controls by Naeser and colleagues,[70] who found decreasing attenuation values with increasing dementia. The authors used a 169-pixel tissue sample that included apparently both white and gray structures, as well as dilated sulci, in the dementia patients. Because all of the dementia patients also demonstrated atrophy, it is very likely that the decrease in attenuation values simply reflected a sampling of increasing sulcal cerebrospinal fluid. In a subsequent study by Gado and associates[71] using a Siemens Somatom II, no difference was found between the attenuation values of 25 dementia patients when compared with those of 33 controls. However, some correlations were obtained between psychometrics and attenuation values for the *right* hemisphere. Furthermore, attenuation values were found to increase with increasing deficit. In order to quantitate gray-white matter discriminability, white matter attenuation values were subtracted from gray matter values. The gray-white matter difference scores thus obtained did not correlate with cognitive scores, but *were* significantly related to ventricular size. Thus, increasing ventricular

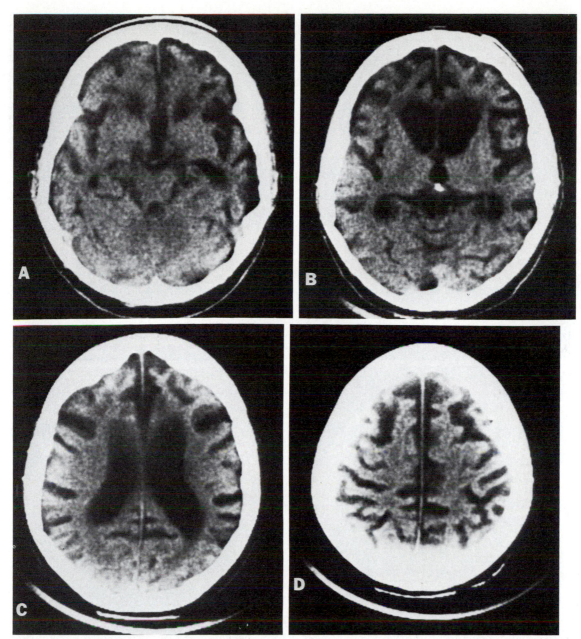

Fig 21–11.—Alzheimer's disease: advanced CT changes. **A,** basal cut. Note marked dilatation of the third ventricle, shrinkage of the temporal lobes, and enlargement of the Sylvian fissures and temporal horns. **B,** basal ganglia cut. Marked dilatation of sulci and fissures, especially frontally with marked enlargement of the frontal horns. This pattern is essentially indistinguishable from Huntington's disease and Pick's disease. Visualization of gray and white structures is very poor. **C,** ventricular body level. Note asymmetric enlargement of the ventricular system with the left lateral ventricle somewhat larger than the right, accentuating the frequently seen normal variation. **D,** high convexity level. The frontal as well as parietal and central sulci are markedly dilated. The frontal fissures and sulci, however, are involved to a somewhat greater degree than the remaining sulci.

size was associated with a diminution of the gray-white difference score. This result was in agreement with our previous finding that (subjective) gray-white matter discriminability was significantly ($P < .05$) related to ventricular enlargement and especially the width of the third ventricle. These two studies therefore lend support to the concept that gray-white changes are related to ventricular enlargement. The magnitude of this correlation, however, is low, which speaks against a cause-and-effect relationship.

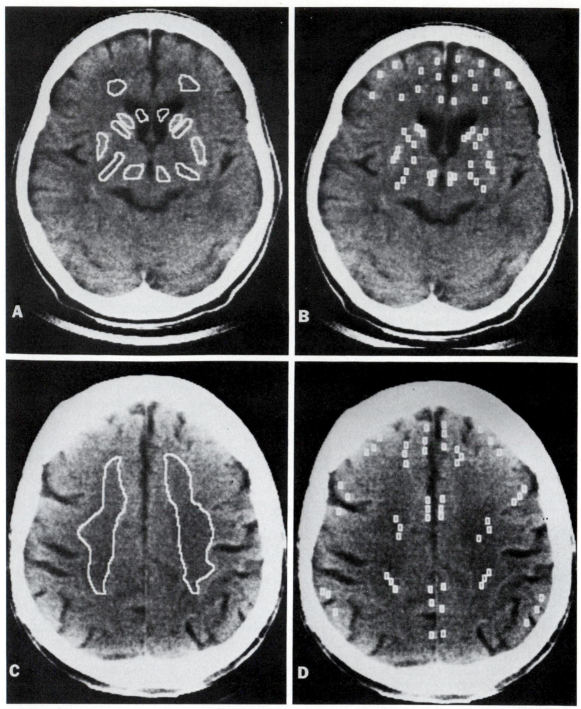

Fig 21–12.—Derivation of CT attenuation values. **A,** basal ganglia level regions of interest included frontal white matter, the heads of the caudate nuclei, the anterior and posterior limbs of the internal capsules, the thalami, and the striate body. **B,** three pixel regions of interest were utilized in order to obtain cortical gray measures. **C,** at the centrum semiovale level, large regions of interest were utilized to obtain a measure of central white matter. **D,** three pixel regions of interest were used to derive medial and lateral cortical measures.

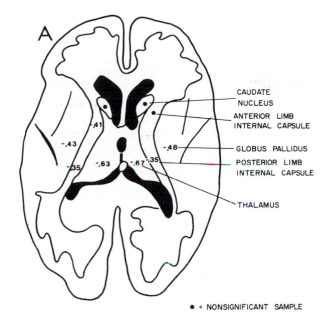

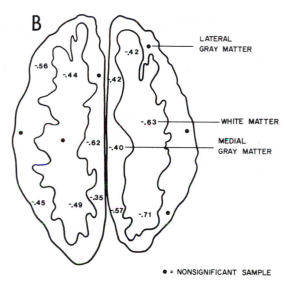

● = NONSIGNIFICANT SAMPLE

Fig 21–13.—Significant correlation coefficients (mean values) between CT attenuation values as derived in Figure 21–12 and psychometric scores. **A,** basal ganglia level. Significant correlations (*P* < .05) were obtained for both thalami, the internal capsule, and striate body attenuation values. **B,** centrum semiovale level. Significant correlations were obtained both from medial and lateral cortical gray matter as well as for central white matter bilaterally.

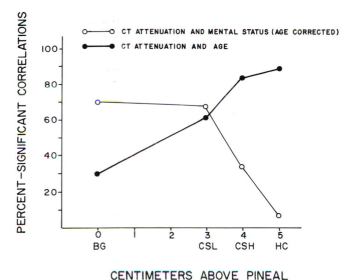

Fig 21–14.—Percent significant correlations between CT attenuation values and psychometrics and between CT attenuation values and age for brain levels. (*BG* = basal ganglia; *CSL* = centrum semiovale; *CSH* = level 1 cm above *CSL*; *HC* = high convexity [level 1 cm above *CSH*].) The data points are derived by summating the number of significant correlations at each level. Thus, at the basal ganglia level, 70% of the correlations between CT attenuation values and mental status were significant. Only 24% of the attenuation value correlations with age were significant at the same level. The number of significant correlations increases for age between the basal ganglia and the high convexity. The number of CT attenuation-psychometric correlations decreased at the higher cuts. These findings suggest that age-related changes may be more significant at the cortical level for CT, whereas dementia changes may be more relevant at the subcortical level.

In our subsequent studies using a rotation-rotation scanner (General Electric 8800), attenuation values were derived from the basal ganglia structures as well as gray and white structures at the level of the ventricular system and above (Figs 21–12 to 21–14).[66] Significant correlations were found between CT attenuation values in both gray and white structures and cognitive measures (see Fig 21–13) (*P* < .05). In this study, however, contrary to the original gray-white discriminability study, increasing cognitive deficit was associated with *decreasing* CT values. We noted with interest a progressive increase in the number of significant psychometric CT correlations between the high convexity and the basal ganglia, whereas the number of age correlations with attenuation values decreased from the high convexity to the basal ganglia (see Fig 21–14). This finding, in contrast to the discriminability results,[62] again suggests that the aging process is more closely reflected by cortical changes, whereas dementia is better represented by ventricular change.

Other studies have addressed the question of attenuation changes in dementia[72, 73] with variable results. Bondareff and associates,[72] using an EMI 1010 scanner and 388-pixel regions of interest, found lower attenuation values in various regions of the brain in the dementia group when compared with those of controls. Wilson and coworkers[73] found no correlation between attenuation values of the thalamus, cortex, and cerebellum and the presence or degree of dementia.

Thus, the question of whether attenuation value changes exist or not in senile dementia and in which direction remains to be settled. Several studies to date have been performed with a wide variety of technologically older as well as newer scanners using widely differing reconstruction algorithms and differing attenuation value corrections. Some of these studies[62, 71] point to a ventricular-parenchymal relationship. Ventricular enlargement may thus be a secondary phenomenon reflecting changes in adjacent white matter. Whether the white matter changes are primary or secondary to cortical gray neuronal loss remains to be demonstrated. In such a chain of events, the original lesion may be subcortical, e.g., at the basal nucleus of Meynert, with secondary cortical degeneration of projection areas, leading to white matter changes and hence to ventricular enlargement. This sequence of cortical gray-central white changes may also explain the phenomenon of gray-white discriminability loss as cortical gray shrinks and becomes less differentiated from central white.

Finally, differences in published results may reflect inhomogeneity of subject samples and specifically the admixture of Alzheimer's and vascular disease cases (multiinfarct dementia/Binswanger's disease).

Planned nuclear magnetic resonance studies will address these questions in an effort to differentiate between diagnostic categories and to elucidate the significance of the parenchymal manifestations of cognitive deficit.

PET: Studies of Brain Metabolism

Over 90 studies have been performed to date using the Brookhaven National Laboratory PET III and more recently the PET VI scanner, which have included 44 senile dementia patients and 22 spouse controls. In addition, 30 young normals have been studied. The glucose analogue FDG tagged with the positron-emitting fluorine 18 was administered in all cases by intravenous route. The shorter half-life carbon 11 being used in current studies permits multiple studies, e.g., before and after medication or other perturbation.[74–81] Brain cells take up FDG in the same way as glucose. The FDG is phosphorylated, but undergoes no further metabolism; therefore, unlike glucose, the tracer remains trapped. The half-life for ^{18}F is 112 minutes. Glucose utilization is derived with the use of an operational equation described by Sokoloff and is expressed in milligrams per 100 cc of tissue per minute.[82]

The results of these studies (Figs 21–14 and 21–15) have shown a consistent diminution in the glucose metabolic rate both at the basal ganglia as well as centrum semiovale levels in the senile dementia patients when compared with normal controls. The degree of diminution ranged between 17% and 25% in the pathologic group. Though individual anatomical structures such as basal ganglia and thalami demonstrated diminished activity, the phenomenon is apparently diffuse; whole

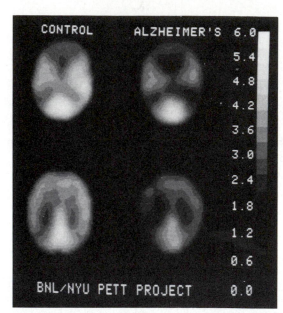

Fig 21–15.—PET scanning: senile dementia vs. elderly spouse control. In the 2-FDG method, glucose utilization is expressed in milligrams per 100 cc of tissue per minute (gray scale). *Top row,* PET III scans, basal ganglia level. The dementia patient shows lower metabolic activity for the temporal and frontal lobes and basal ganglia when compared with control. *Bottom row,* centrum semiovale 7 cm above canthomeatal line. Metabolic values for the dementia patient show a marked difference for the entire hemisphere when compared with control.

hemisphere metabolic values were also reduced by the same amount when compared with those of normal controls. Comparison of the young normals with the old normals demonstrated no difference in glucose uptake (see Fig 21–4 and Normal Aging). This is particularly interesting in view of reported diminution in local cerebral blood flow with normal aging demonstrated by stable xenon CT studies.[83] Amano and coworkers[83] also found further local cerebral blood flow reduction (11% to 22%) in the cortex and thalamic regions of dementia patients when compared with that in elderly controls.

Thus, certain questions arise from these findings that are not as yet clarified: (1) Is the diminished metabolic activity seen in the dementia group a quantitative or qualitative finding (i.e., does the diminished activity reflect reduced uptake because of a diminished number of cells, or is the activity per cell diminished)? and (2) Is the reduction in metabolic function a reflection of diminished blood flow, or is the diminished blood flow a reflection of reduced metabolic activity?

Though many questions remain to be answered on this subject, we continue to search for additional relationships. In this context, CT attenuation values and PET metabolic values were intercorrelated at the level of the basal ganglia in order to search for further structure-function relationships.[78] This intercorrelation produced significant correlations ($P < .05$) at the level of the basal ganglia. Diminution in attenuation values was related to diminution in metabolic activity.[78] The meaning of this finding is entirely speculative, but does apparently underscore the structure-function relationships in dementia.

Multiinfarct Dementia/Binswanger's Disease (Figs 21–16 and 21–17)

The most common cause of senile dementia after Alzheimer's disease is cerebrovascular disease. Multiple infarcts, especially if bilateral, are often associated with dementia (multiinfarct dementia or MID). Clinically, MID is characterized by the association of dementia and stroke symptoms. The infarctions, however, may be subclinical but apparent on CT. Certain infarcts, especially the lacunar type, may be difficult to identify by CT and may be equally obscure to clinical scrutiny (see Fig 21–17).

An interesting variety of cerebrovascular disease is subcortical atherosclerosis or Binswanger's disease. Binswanger[84] described a slowly progressing disease beginning in the fifth and sixth decades, presenting with intellectual impairment and loss of memory associated with recurrent or transient neurologic deficits. Because the atherosclerotic changes primarily affect the deep penetrating white matter arteries, Jellinger and Neumayer[85] assumed this to be a special form of atherosclerosis affecting the basal ganglia and white matter. Clinically, it is difficult to differentiate between Binswanger's disease and the usual hypertensive atherosclerotic cerebrovascular disease. We find it useful to consider cortical as well as subcortical changes as part of a spectrum of (often hypertensive) *atherosclerotic cerebrovascular disease often associated with MID.* Scans by CT demonstrate multiple periventricular lucencies corresponding to demyelinated patches of white matter (see Figs 21–16 and 21–17). Lacunar infarcts are common both on CT and at pathology. In the typical case, the presence of diffuse white matter patches and cortical or lacunar infarcts differentiates MID from Alzheimer's disease.

Other Causes of Dementia

Several nonatherosclerotic causes of vascular disease may also be associated with dementia, including the various arteritides and postirradiation vasculitis. Nonvascular causes of dementia are numerous and varied; especially common is post-traumatic dementia, including the variety associated with boxing. A partial list of the many other diseases associated with dementia includes Huntington's chorea, Parkinson's disease, metabolic disorders, infectious diseases including progressive multifocal leukoencephalopathy, Jakob-Creutzfeldt disease, kuru and lues, multiple sclerosis, and muscular dystrophy.[5]

Pick's Disease

Pick's disease is a rare cause of progressive, usually presenile dementia of unknown etiology[86] first described in 1892.[87] Familial occurrence is known.[88] In advanced cases, the atrophy characteristically affects the anterior portions of the frontal and temporal lobes.

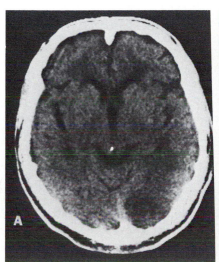 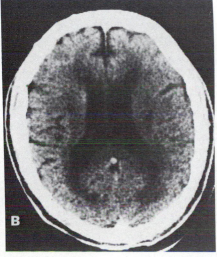 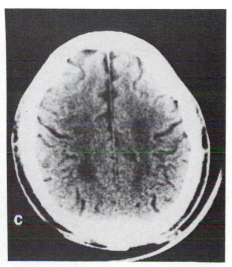

Fig 21–16.—Multiinfarct dementia: enlarged ventricles in an elderly man. **A,** basal ganglia level. A left occipital infarct is present. There are also lucencies in the frontal white matter bilaterally. **B,** ventricular body level. Patchy radiolucencies throughout the white matter are consistent with the demyelinated patches of subcortical atherosclerosis. Note more discrete lucencies indicating presence of lacunar infarcts. **C,** high centrum semiovale cut. Scattered white matter lucencies are again seen, as well as lacunar infarcts.

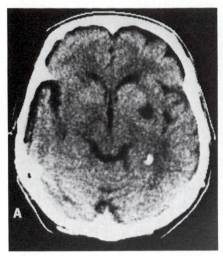 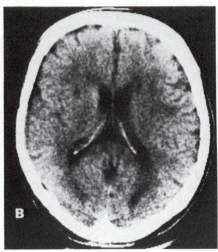 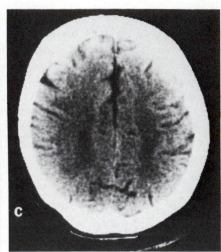

Fig 21–17.—Multiinfarct dementia (normal ventricular system) in an elderly man. **A,** basal ganglia level. A large lacunar infarct is situated in the left striate region. **B,** ventricular body level. Findings are similar to Figure 21–16,B. Patchy radiolucencies are scattered throughout the white matter, but the ventricular system is not enlarged. **C,** centrum semiovale level. Multiple lucencies indicate presence of demyelinated patches.

Therefore, CT may show marked shrinkage of the frontal and temporal poles with widening of the Sylvian fissures and the interhemispheric fissure. The CT changes may be indistinguishable from advanced Alzheimer's disease and also bear similarity to Huntington's chorea; in the typical case, the frontal horns are dilated out of proportion to the enlargement of the rest of the ventricular system both at CT[86] and pathology.[89] Histologic sections of the involved cortex show severe nerve cell loss and intracytoplasmic argentophilic bodies (Pick's bodies). Eosinophilic inclusions (Hirano bodies) and granulovacuolar changes are also seen.[86]

SUMMARY

The CT and PET assessments to date in normal aging and in the dementias of aging may be summarized as follows:

1. There is primarily sulcal and secondarily ventricular enlargement as part of the normal aging process. Ventricular size (ventricular volume corrected for brain size) is approximately 5% of brain in normal elderly controls. This measure is approximately 100% larger than that of normal young volunteers. Sulcal volume, on the other hand, increases by approximately 200% between young and old.

2. Ventricular and, to a lesser degree, sulcal enlargement occurs in Alzheimer dementia. Because Alzheimer's disease is a disease of the elderly, both processes are at work in the senile dementia patient. An additional 44% ventricular enlargement occurs in senile dementia patients when compared with controls. A ventricular/brain measurement greater than 10% is associated with an 83% chance of senile dementia.

3. Ventricular enlargement on CT, especially in early dementia, may more closely reflect the cognitive deficit of senile dementia than cortical atrophy, which may more accurately reflect the normal aging process. *Focal, often marked enlargement of the Sylvian fissures and temporal and hippocampal atrophy, however, are commonly seen in severe Alzheimer cases* in association with marked ventricular enlargement, especially of the third ventricle.

4. The importance of the third ventricle in multiple studies underscores the involvement of subcortical structures, notably the basal ganglia, hypothalamus, and thalamus in Alzheimer's disease.

5. Glucose utilization as demonstrated by *positron emission tomography* does not diminish significantly with age. Senile dementia patients, however, show a 17% to 25% diminution in glucose metabolism when compared with their normal spouses. This diminution is in proportion to deficits. This phenomenon is both focally demonstrated, e.g., in the basal ganglia, as well as diffuse, reflecting diminished activity of the entire hemisphere.

6. Parenchymal changes exist in senile dementia concurrently with ventricular enlargement. There is subjective loss of CT gray-white discriminability in relationship to cognitive deficit. Changes in CT attenuation value have also been shown, but the results are conflicting. The ventricular changes may reflect a secondary phenomenon related to parenchymal (gray and white matter) changes. Further structure-function relationships are suggested by the discovery of significant correlations between PET metabolic and CT attenuation values.

7. Use of CT can reliably differentiate the Alzheimer

group from dementias secondary to a wide variety of causes including cerebrovascular disease (MID/Binswanger's disease) and post-traumatic dementia.

The evidence from the experimental and clinical literature and from the above CT and PET studies indicates that cognition and memory are highly complex and diffuse phenomena with multiple subcortical key sites that may represent either centers or relay stations. A center of memory per se remains undefined. In Alzheimer's disease, subcortical (diencephalic) cell loss may lead to cortical degeneration and secondary white matter changes manifesting as a spectrum of gross structural and parenchymal CT changes, along with diffuse and focal PET metabolic deficits.

The use of CT is an invaluable clinical tool, and PET with CT is an invaluable research tool that has permitted us a first glimpse in the study of cognition, the aging process, and the cognitive afflictions of aging. The introduction of new research technologies such as nuclear magnetic resonance promises to shed new light on many mysteries and unanswered questions in the very complex and fascinating subject of cognition and age-related brain change.

Acknowledgment

This work was supported in part by the National Institute of Mental Health grant 36969.

The authors would like to express their special appreciation to Joan Askew for her invaluable assistance and secretarial work in the preparation of this manuscript.

REFERENCES

1. Ranson S.W., Clark S.L.: The anatomy of the nervous system: Its development and function, in *The Cerebral Cortex*, ed. 8. Philadelphia, W.B. Saunders Co., 1947, p. 291.
2. Fritsch G.: Uber die elektrische erregbarkeit des grosshirns. *Arch. F. Anat. Physiol.* 1870, p. 3000.
3. Pennfield W., Rasmussen T.: The cerebral cortex of man, in *Cortex and Diencephalon*. New York, Macmillan Publishing Co., 1950, pp. 204–206.
4. Alzheimer A.: Uber eine eigenartige Erkrankung der Hirninde. *Allg. Z. Psychiat.* 64:146, 1907.
5. Haase G.R.: Disease presenting as dementia, in Wells C.E. (ed.): *Dementia*, ed. 2. Philadelphia, F.A. Davis Co., 1977, p. 27.
6. Tomlinson B.E., Blessed G., Roth M.: Observations on the brains of non-demented old people. *J. Neurol. Sci.* 7:331–356, 1968.
7. Tomlinson B.E., Blessed G., Roth M.: Observations on the brains of demented old people. *J. Neurol. Sci.* 11:205–242, 1970.
8. Blessed G., Roth M., Tomlinson B.E.: The association between quantitative measures of dementia and of senile change in the cerebral grey matter of elderly subjects. *Br. J. Psychiatry* 114:797, 1968.
9. American Roentgen Ray Society: Report of committee on standardization of encephalography. *A.J.R.* 22:474–480, 1929.
10. Heinrich A.: Das normale enzephalogramm in seiner abhangigkeit vom lebersalter. *Z. Alternsforsch.* 1:345–354, 1939.
11. Andersen E., Vive Larsen J., Jacobsen H.H.: Atrophia cerebri. *Ugeskr. Laeg.* 125:86–91, 1963.
12. Jacobsen H.H., Melchior J.C.: On pneumoencephalographic measuring methods in children. *A.J.R.* 101:188–194, 1967.
13. Iivanainen M.: Pneumoencephalographic and clinical characteristics of diffuse cerebral atrophy. *Acta Neurol. Scand.* 51:310–327, 1975.
14. Engeset A., Lonnum A.: Third ventricles of 12 mm width or more: A preliminary report. *Acta Radiol. Diagn.* 50:5–11, 1958.
15. Nielsen R., Peterson O., Thygesen P., et al.: Encephalographic cortical atrophy: Relationships to ventricular atrophy and intellectual impairment. *Acta Radiol. Diagn.* 4:437–448, 1966.
16. Nielsen R., Peterson O., Thygesen P., et al.: Encephalographic ventricular atrophy. *Acta Radiol. Diagn.* 4:240–256, 1966.
17. Huber G.: Die bedentung der neuroradiologic fur die psychiatrie. *Fortsch. Med.* 81:705, 1963.
18. Huber G.: Zur diagnose, prognose und typologic hirnatrophischer syndrome. *Radiologe* 5:456, 1965.
19. Huber G.: Hirnatrophische prozesse im mittleren Lebensalter. *Munch. Med. Wschr.* 114:429, 1972.
20. Gosling R.H.: The association of dementia with radiologically demonstrated cerebral atrophy. *J. Neurol. Neurosurg. Psychiatry* 18:129–133, 1955.
21. Mann A.H.: Cortical atrophy and air encephalography: Clinical and radiological study. *Psychol. Med.* 3:374–378, 1973.
22. Roberts M.A., Caird F.I.: Computerized tomography and intellectual impairment in the elderly. *J. Neurol. Neurosurg. Psychiatry* 39:986–989, 1976.
23. Hughes C.P., Gado M.: Computed tomography and aging of the brain. *Radiology* 139:391–396, 1981.
24. Claveria L.E., Moseley I.F., Stevenson J.F.: The clinical significance of cerebral atrophy as shown by CAT, in Du Boulay F.G., Moseley I.F. (eds.): *The First European Seminar on Computerized Tomography in Clinical Practice*. Berlin, Springer-Verlag, 1977, pp. 213–217.
25. Nathan R.J., Frumkin K.: Cerebral atrophy and independence in the elderly. Read before the Annual Meeting of the *American Psychiatric Association*, Atlanta, May 8–12, 1978.
26. Bricken R.M.: *The Intellectual Functions of the Frontal Lobe*. New York, Macmillan Publishing Co., 1936.
27. Klüver H., Bucy P.C.: Preliminary analysis of functions of the temporal lobes of monkeys. *Arch. Neurol. Psychiatry* 42:979–1000, 1939.
28. Pavlov I.P.: *Conditioned Reflexes*, Anrep G. (trans.-ed.). Oxford, England, Oxford University Press, 1927, p. 430.
29. Scoville W.B., Milner B.: Loss of recent memory after

bilateral hippocampal lesions. *J. Neurol. Neurosurg. Psychiatry* 20:11–21, 1957.

30. Ojemann G.A., Blick K., Ward A. Jr.: Improvement and disturbances of short term verbal memory with human ventrolateral thalamic stimulation. *Brain* 94:255–240, 1971.

31. Ojemann G.A.: Mental arithmetic during human thalamic stimulation. *Neuropsychologia* 12:1–10, 1974.

32. Tomlinson B.E.: The pathology of dementia, in Wells, C.E. (ed.): *Dementia*, ed. 2. Philadelphia, F.A. Davis Co., 1977, p. 117.

33. Chen E.: Amnesia: A daily battle in isolation. *Los Angeles Times*, 1979.

34. Kuhl D.: Personal communication, 1981.

35. Victor M., Adams R.D., Collins G.H.: *The Wernicke-Korsakoff Syndrome*. Philadelphia, F.A. Davis Co., 1971, pp. 88–132.

36. Bowen D.M., Smith C.B., White P., et al.: Neurotransmitter-related enzymes and indices of hypoxia in senile dementia and other abiotrophies. *Brain* 99:459–496, 1976.

37. Davis P., Maloney A.J.R.: Selective loss of central cholinergic neurons in Alzheimer's disease. *Lancet* 2:1403, 1976.

38. Perry R.D., Pena C.: Experimental production of neurofibrillary regeneration: II. Electron microscopy, phosphatase histochemistry and electron probe analysis. *J. Neuropathol. Exp. Neurol.* 24:200–210, 1965.

39. White P., Goodhart M.J., Keet S.P., et al.: Neocortical cholingeric neurons in elderly people. *Lancet* 1:668–670, 1977.

40. Emson P.C., Lindvall O.: Distribution of purative neurotransmitters in the neocortex. *Neuroscience* 1:1–30, 1979.

41. Johnston M.V., McKinney M., Coyle J.: Evidence for a cholinergic projection to neocortex from neurons in basal forebrain. *Neurobiology* 76:5392–5396, 1979.

42. Whitehouse P.J., Price D.L., Struble R.G., et al.: Alzheimer's disease and senile dementia: Loss of neurons in the basal forebrain. *Science* 215:1237–1239, 1982.

43. Adolfsson R., Gottfries C.G., Roos B.E., et al.: Changes in the brain catecholamines in patients with dementia of Alzheimer's type. *Br. J. Psychiatry* 135:216–223, 1979.

44. Mann D.M.A., Lincoln J., Yates P.O., et al.: Changes in the monoamine containing neurones of the human CNS in senile dementia. *Br. J. Psychiatry* 136:533–541, 1980.

45. Bondareff W., Mountjoy C.Q., Roth M.: Loss of neurons or origin of the adrenergic projection to the cerebral cortex (nucleus locus ceruleus) in senile dementia. *Neurology* 32:164–168, 1982.

46. de Leon M.J., George A.E., Ferris S.H., et al.: Positron emission tomography and computed tomography assessment of the aging human brain. *J. Comput. Assist. Tomogr.* 8:88–94, 1984.

47. Glydensted C., Kosteljanetz M.: Measurements of the normal ventricular system with computed tomography: A preliminary study on 44 adults. *Neurology* 10:205–215, 1976.

48. Hahn F.J.Y., Rim K.: Frontal ventricular dimensions on normal computed tomography. *A.J.R.* 126:593–596, 1976.

49. Haug G.: Age and sex dependence of the size of normal ventricles on computed tomography. *Neuroradiology* 14:201–204, 1977.

50. Jacoby R.J., Levy R., Dawson J.M.: Computed tomography in the elderly: I. The normal population. *Br. J. Psychiatry* 136:249, 1980.

51. Yamamura H., Ito M., Kubota K., et al.: Brain atrophy during aging: A quantitative study with computed tomography. *J. Gerontol.* 4:492–498, 1980.

52. Cala L.A., Thickbroom G.W., Black J.I., et al.: Brain density and cerebrospinal fluid space size: CT of normal volunteers. *A.J.N.R.* 2:41–47, 1981.

53. Barron S.A., Jacobs L., Kindel W.: Changes in size of normal lateral ventricles during aging determined by computerized tomography. *Neurology* 26:1011–1013, 1976.

54. Hatazawa J., Ito M., Yamamura H., et al.: Sex differences in brain atrophy during aging: A quantitative study with computed tomography. *J. Am. Geriatr. Soc.* 3:1–11, 1982.

55. Zatz L.M., Jernigan T.L., Ahumada A.J. Jr.: Changes on computed cranial tomography with aging: Intracranial fluid volume. *A.J.N.R.* 3:1–11, 1982.

56. Zatz L.M., Jernigan T.L., Ahumada A.J. Jr.: White matter changes in cerebral computed tomography related to aging. *J. Comput. Assist. Tomogr.* 6:19–23, 1982.

57. Earnest M.P., Heaton R.K., Wilkenson W.E., et al.: Cortical atrophy, ventricular enlargement and intellectual impairment in the aged. *Neurology* 29:1138–1143, 1979.

58. Jacoby R.J., Levy R.: Computed tomography in the elderly: II. Diagnosis and functional impairment. *Br. J. Psychiatry* 136:256–269, 1980.

59. de Leon M.J., Ferris S.H., George A.E., et al.: A new method for the CT evaluation of brain atrophy in senile dementia. *I.R.C.S. Medical Science* 7:404, 1979.

60. de Leon M.J., Ferris S.H., Blau I., et al.: Correlations between computerized tomographic changes and behavioural deficits. *Lancet* 2:538, 1979.

61. de Leon M.J., Ferris S.H., George A.E., et al.: Computed tomography evaluations of brain-behavior relationships in senile dementia of the Alzheimer's type. *Neurobiol. Aging* 1:69–79, 1980.

62. George A.E., de Leon M.J., Ferris S.H., et al.: Parenchymal CT correlates of senile dementia: Loss of gray-white discriminability. *A.J.N.R.* 2:205–213, 1981.

63. George A.E., de Leon M.J., Rosenbloom S., et al.: Ventricular volume and cognitive deficit: A computed tomographic study. *Radiology* 149:493–498, 1983.

64. Mersky H., Ball M.J., Blume L.S.T., et al.: Relationships between psychological measurements and cerebral organic changes in Alzheimer's disease. *Le Journal Canadien des Sciences Neurologicquel* 7:45–49, 1980.

65. George A.E.: Structural CT correlates of senile dementia. Presented at the 18th Annual Meeting of the American Society of Neuroradiology, Los Angeles, March 1980.

66. George A.E., de Leon M.J., Rosenbloom S., et al.: Parenchymal and structural CT changes in senile dementia:

A. Grey and white matter attenuation values; B. Ventricular volume. Presented at the 19th Annual Meeting of the American Society of Neuroradiology, Chicago, April 1981.

67. Kahn R.L., Goldfarb A., Pollack M., et al.: Brief objective measures for the determination of mental status in the aged. *Am. J. Psychiatry* 117:326–328, 1960.

68. Reisberg B., Ferris S.H., de Leon M.J., et al.: The global deterioration scale for the assessment of primary degenerative dementia. *Am. J. Psychiatry* 139:1135–1139, 1982.

69. Gado M.H., Hughes C.P., Danziger W., et al.: Volumetric measurements of the cerebrospinal fluid spaces in subjects with dementia and in controls. *Radiology* 144:535–538, 1982.

70. Naeser M.A., Gebhardt C., Levine H.L.: Decreased computerized tomography numbers in patients with senile dementia. *Arch. Neurol.* 37:401–407, 1980.

71. Gado M., Danziger W.L., Chi D., et al.: Brain parenchymal density measurements by CT in demented subjects and normal controls. *Radiology* 147:703–710, 1983.

72. Bondareff W., Baldy R., Levy R.: Quantitative computed tomography in senile dementia. *Arch. Gen. Psychiatry* 38:1365–1368, 1981.

73. Wilson R.S., Fox J.H., Huckman M.S., et al.: Computed tomography in dementia. *Neurology* 32:1054–1057, 1982.

74. Ferris S.H., de Leon M.J., Wolf A.P., et al.: Positron emission tomography in the study of aging and senile dementia. *Neurobiol. Aging* 1:127–131, 1980.

75. Ferris S.H., de Leon M.J., Christman D., et al.: Positron emission tomography (PET) studies of regional brain metabolism in elderly patients, in Perris C., Struw G., Jansson B. (eds.): *Biological Psychiatry 1981.* New York, Elsevier North-Holland Biomedical Press, 1981.

76. Farkas T., Ferris S.H., Wolf A.P., et al.: ^{18}F-2-deoxy-2-fluoro-D-glucose as a tracer in the positron emission tomographic study of senile dementia. *Am. J. Psychiatry* 139:352–353, 1982.

77. de Leon M.J., George A.E., Ferris S.H.: Computed tomography and positron emission tomography in the study of senile dementia of the Alzheimer's type, in Alter I.

(ed.): *The Limits of Functional Localization.* New York, Raven Press, 1982.

78. de Leon M.J., George A.E., Ferris S.H., et al.: Positron emission tomography (PET) and computed tomography (CT) evaluations combined in the study of senile dementia. *A.J.N.R.* 4:553–556, 1983.

79. de Leon M.J., Ferris S.H., George A.E., et al.: Positron emission tomography (PET) studies of aging and Alzheimer's disease. *A.J.N.R.* 4:568–571, 1983.

80. de Leon M.J., Ferris S.H., George A.E., et al.: Computed tomography and positron emission transaxial tomography evaluations of normal aging and Alzheimer's disease. *J. Cereb. Blood Flow Metab.* 3:391–394, 1983.

81. Ferris S.H., de Leon M.J., Wolf A.P., et al.: *Neurobiology II: PET Scan in AD.* New York, Raven Press, (in press).

82. Reivich M., Kuhl D., Wolf A., et al.: The[18]fluorodeoxyglucose method for the measurement of local cerebral glucose utilization in man. *Circ. Res.* 44:127–137, 1979.

83. Amano T., Meyer J.S., Okabe T., et al.: Stable xenon CT cerebral blood flow measurements computed by a single compartment-double integration model in normal aging and dementia. *J. Comput. Assist. Tomogr.* 6:923, 1982.

84. Binswanger O.: Die Abrenzung der allgemeinen progressiven paralyse. *Berl. Klin. Wachenschr.* 31:1103–1105, 1137–1139, 1180–1186, 1894.

85. Jellinger K., Neumayer E.: Progressive subcorticale vasculare Encephalopathie Binswanger. *Arch. Psychiatr. Cesamte. Neurol.* 205:523–554, 1964.

86. McGeachie R.F., Fleming J.O., Sharer L.R., et al.: Diagnosis of Pick's disease by computed tomography. *J. Comput. Assist. Tomogr.* 3:113, 1979.

87. Pick A.: Ueber die Benziehungen der senile n Hirnatophiel zur Aphasie. *Prager Med. Wochenschr.* 17:165, 1892.

88. Groen J.J., Hekster R.F.M.: Computed tomography in Pick's disease. *J. Comput. Assist. Tomogr.* 6:907, 1982.

89. Corsellis J.A.N.: Aging and the dementias, in Blackwood W., Corsellis J.A.N. (eds.): *Greenfield's Neuropathology,* ed. 3. Chicago, Edward Arnold Publishing Co., 1976, pp. 817–821.

Congenital Anomalies

22

Congenital Anomalies of the Brain

Richard E. Latchaw, M.D.

A NUMBER of classifications of congenital abnormalities of the CNS have been suggested.[1,2] Unfortunately, most such classifications are based upon a greater presumption of embryogenesis and/or etiology than is currently known for the majority of the malformations. A radiologist is a specialist in visual images and bases his differential diagnosis on specific visual findings or image patterns. Therefore, we have produced the classification of congenital cerebral abnormalities presented in Table 22–1, which organizes the abnormalities upon the presence of specific visually determined pathologic features. Such a classification will allow the radiologist or neuroscience clinician to establish the most appropriate differential diagnosis, given the pattern of findings on the CT scan.

The most striking visual finding is used as the basis of organization. For example, dilatation of the third and lateral ventricles is the most dramatic aspect of aqueductal stenosis, and therefore the entity is listed with those conditions in which the most prominent finding is that of third and lateral ventricular dilatation. While schizencephaly may be associated with enlarged ventricles, the most dramatic radiographic finding is the presence of the hemispheric clefts. This entity is therefore listed under abnormalities presenting with hemispheric defects within the category of craniocerebral malformations. It is obvious that a particular anomaly could be placed into a number of categories. For example, the Chiari malformations, particularly Chiari II and Chiari III, obviously have gross distortion of multiple portions of the brain and therefore could be categorized with the craniocerebral malformations. However, the most dramatic finding of the Chiari II and III malformations at the time of *initial presentation* is the pronounced ventricular dilatation of the third and lateral ventricles. The Chiari II and III malformations are therefore listed under abnormalities presenting with increased ventricular size as a basis for differential diagnosis. The Chiari I

malformation, however, may present with little or no ventricular dilatation and is therefore listed under the cerebellar craniocerebral malformations, again for purposes of differential diagnosis.

Categories I through IV will be discussed at length in this chapter, as will arachnoid cysts from Category VI. The congenital tumors listed in Category V are discussed in Chapters 9 and 11 of this volume. The Sturge-Weber syndrome is likewise discussed in Chapter 11, while the rest of the vascular lesions are dealt with in Chapter 5. Craniopharyngioma and Rathke's pouch cyst are discussed in Chapter 16.

NORMAL VARIANTS

Three normal variants that are well known from pneumoencephalographic studies and that are now seen with CT scanning are the cavum septum pellucidum, cavum vergae, and cavum velum interpositum. The cavum septum pellucidum is a cerebrospinal fluid (CSF) collection located between the leaves of the septum pellucidum. The cavum generally communicates with one or both of the lateral ventricles, so that it fills with air at the time of pneumoencephalography. It is commonly seen on the CT scan of an infant (Fig 22–1). Autopsy studies have demonstrated a cavum septum pellucidum in 82% of newborns, with a progressive decrease in the incidence with increasing age. Ten percent of infants have a cavum septum pellucidum on CT scan, with that number decreasing to 5% by age 2 years, paralleling the decreased visualization at autopsy.[3]

The cavum vergae is much less frequent than the cavum septum pellucidum, being found in only 30% of newborns.[3] It may be seen as a posterior extension of the cavum septum pellucidum, and the two are frequently found together (see Fig 22–1). The constriction between the two cava results from compression by the

TABLE 22–1.—A RADIOLOGIST'S APPROACH
TO CONGENITAL CEREBRAL ABNORMALITIES

I. Normal midline variants
   A. Cavum septum pellucidum
   B. Cavum vergae
   C. Cavum velum interpositum
II. Increased ventricular size
   A. Lateral and third ventricles
      1. Aqueductal stenosis
      2. Chiari II and III malformations
      3. Inflammatory obstruction
      4. Atrophy
   B. All ventricles
      1. Dandy-Walker syndrome
      2. Inflammatory obstruction
      3. Atrophy
III. Craniocerebral malformations
   A. Midline cerebrum
      1. Holoprosencephaly
      2. Septo-optic dysplasia
      3. Agenesis of the corpus callosum
   B. Lateral cerebral hemispheric defects
      1. Porencephaly
      2. Schizencephaly
   C. Combined midline and lateral cerebrum: Hydranencephaly
   D. Cerebellum
      1. Chiari I malformation
      2. Hypoplasia/Aplasia
         a. Vermis
         b. Hemisphere
         c. Entire cerebellum
   E. Cerebral cortex
      1. Lissencephaly
      2. Pachygyria
      3. Polymicrogyria
   F. Brain size
      1. Microcephaly
      2. Megalencephaly
   G. Dura and cranium
      1. Encephalocele
      2. Craniosynostosis
IV. Ectopias: Heterotopic gray matter
V. Congenital tumors
   A. Teratomatous tumors: Teratoma, germinoma, dermoid, epidermoid
   B. Hamartomas
      1. Hamartoma of the tuber cinereum
      2. Tuberous sclerosis
   C. Lipoma
   D. Neuroectodermal tumors
      1. Astrocytoma
      2. Primitive neuroepithelial tumor (PNET)
         a. Primary intracranial neuroblastoma
         b. Pineoblastoma/pineocytoma
         c. Medulloblastoma
      3. Ependymoma
VI. Cysts
   A. Arachnoid cyst
   B. Craniopharyngioma
   C. Rathke's pouch cyst
VII. Abnormal vasculature
   A. Arteriovenous malformation (including vein of Galen aneurysm)
   B. Encephalotrigeminal angiomatosis (Sturge-Weber syndrome)
   C. Aneurysm

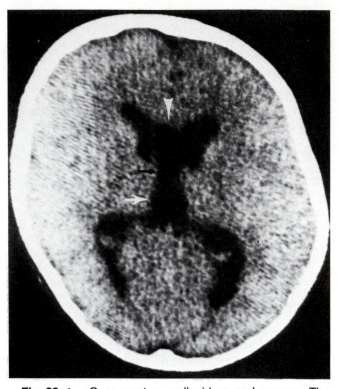

Fig 22–1.—Cava septum pellucidum and vergae. The cavum septum pellucidum *(white arrowhead)* is seen between the frontal horns, while the cavum vergae *(white arrow)* is located more posteriorly. The constriction between the two *(black arrow)* is from the fornices.

fornices. The posterior margin of the cavum vergae is the splenium of the corpus callosum.

The cavum velum interpositum is a collection of CSF within the velum interpositum, that cistern lying above the third ventricle and below the corpus callosum. Air typically fills this latter cavum from the ambient and quadrigeminal cisterns rather than from the ventricles, which occurs with the cava septum pellucidum and vergae.

INCREASED VENTRICULAR SIZE

Lateral and/or Third Ventricles

Aqueductal Stenosis

Congenital stenosis of the aqueduct of Sylvius may be divided into three categories. The first is that of a true stenosis without evidence of gliosis to suggest a postinflammatory etiology of the narrowed diameter. The second condition is referred to as forking of the aqueduct. In this condition, there are two small channels separated by normal tissue, with one channel making a fork in its course. The third type is that of a neuroglial septum at the caudal end of the aqueduct.[4, 5]

Whatever the form of aqueductal stenosis, the resulting CT scan appearance is the same. There is dilatation of the third and lateral ventricles, with a small fourth ventricle (Fig 22–2). Such a disparity in ventricular size strongly suggests the presence of an aqueductal block. An enhanced scan fails to show evidence of neoplasm or other enhancing lesions in the region of the aqueduct.

Chiari Malformations

Three types of Chiari malformations are recognized, with classification dependent upon the degree of downward displacement of the cerebellum and fourth ventricle. The Chiari I malformation consists of caudal displacement of the medulla into the upper spinal canal and herniation of the cerebellar tonsils or inferior processes arising from the tonsils to cover the dorsolateral surfaces of the displaced medulla. The fourth ventricle is in normal location; there is either no hydrocephalus or mild ventricular enlargement secondary to slight elongation of the aqueduct; and there may be no associated spinal dysraphism. Generally, symptoms do not present until adulthood, at which time there may be vague posterior fossa signs and symptoms suggesting intrinsic cerebellar or brain stem disease.

The Chiari II malformation is nearly always associated with spinal or cranial dysraphism such as meningocele, meningomyelocele, or encephalocele. There is caudal displacement of the medulla, cerebellar tonsils, and vermis, while the fourth ventricle is inferiorly displaced and elongated, producing hydrocephalus. In the Chiari III malformation, the medulla, fourth ventricle, and most, if not all, of the cerebellum are displaced caudally into an upper cervical and occipital encephalocele. Both Chiari II and Chiari III malformations are seen in childhood, as opposed to the Chiari I malformation. There are also numerous associated congenital abnormalities involving the cerebellar hemispheres, upper brain stem, dural coverings of the brain, and spinal cord. The multiplicity of these associated findings, as discussed below, reveal the Chiari II and III malformations to be more than just abnormalities of the hindbrain.

Various theories as to the origin of the Chiari malformations have been proposed. These theories include abnormal traction of the spinal cord to pull the hindbrain through the foramen magnum; hydrocephalus in utero producing transtentorial herniation of the hindbrain; overgrowth of the hindbrain; and a primary dys-

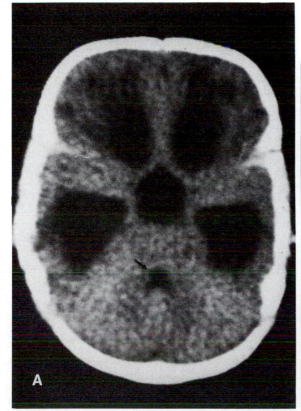
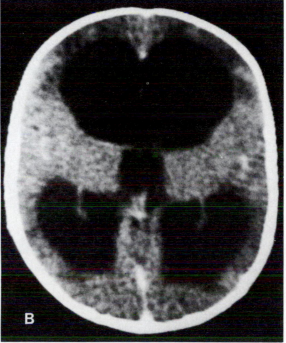

Fig 22–2.—Aqueductal stenosis. There is marked dilatation of the third and lateral ventricles **(B)**, but a normal-sized fourth ventricle **(A,** *arrow*). Periventricular edema anterior to the frontal horns indicates transependymal flow of CSF secondary to increased intraventricular pressure. The discrepancy between the size of the third and fourth ventricles signals an obstruction between them.

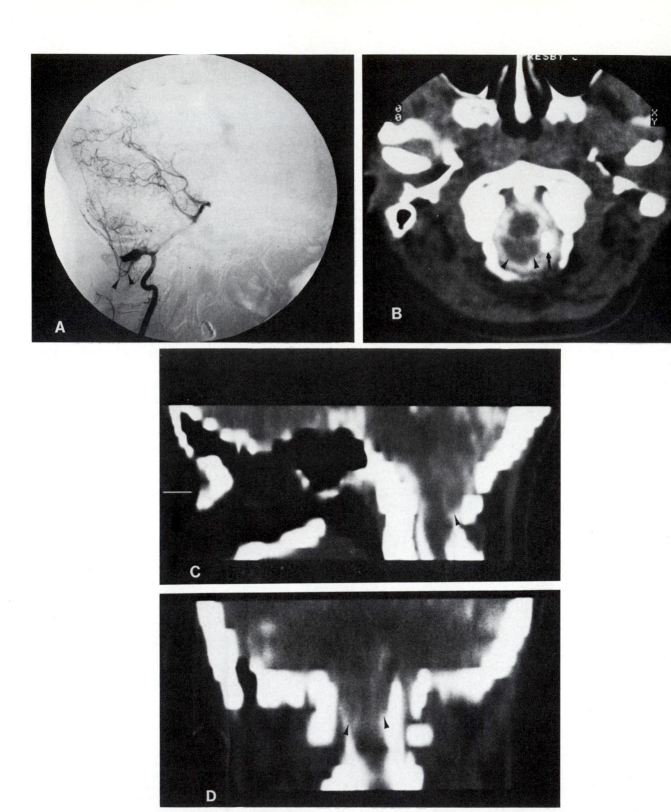

Fig 22–3.—Chiari I malformation. This 36-year-old woman presented with progressive gait disturbance and a presumptive diagnosis of multiple sclerosis. The lateral view of the vertebral angiogram **(A)** demonstrates inferior displacement of the tonsillohemispheric branches *(arrowheads)* of the posterior inferior cerebellar arteries. There is no evidence of a posterior fossa mass lesion. The tips of the tonsillar pegs are as low as the inferior margin of C-1. Axial CT scanning at the level of the odontoid following the intrathecal placement of metrizamide **(B)** demonstrates the two tonsillar pegs *(arrowheads)* located behind the spinal cord. A small droplet of Pantopaque *(arrow)* is noted. Sagittal **(C)** and coronal **(D)** reformations demonstrate to good advantage the position of the tonsils *(arrowheads)* relative to the spinal cord and bony structures. The bulge of the spinal cord just below the tonsillar tips represents some kinking of the cord in this malformation.

442

genesis of the hindbrain.[1, 6–11] Objections raised against these theories include the presence of the malformation in the absence of a spinal cord lesion, the lack of hydrocephalus in the presence of a Chiari malformation so that intrauterine hydrocephalus cannot be invoked, the lack of experimental evidence for the ability of increased intracranial pressure in utero to produce such hindbrain abnormalities, and the lack of experimental evidence of hindbrain overgrowth. An abnormality of the closure of the neural tube is most likely responsible.[6] This is particularly true in view of the diffuse anomalies found throughout the cerebrum, hindbrain, and spinal cord in the more severe Chiari malformations.

The significant radiographic finding in the Chiari I malformation is that of inferior displacement of the cerebellar tonsils, or abnormal tissue attached to those tonsils, without evidence of a localized intracranial lesion that could produce tonsillar herniation. Previous neuroradiologic techniques for this diagnosis included pneumoencephalography and vertebral angiography, with the latter technique demonstrating the inferior displacement of the tonsillohemispheric branches of the posterior-inferior cerebellar arteries (Fig 22–3). A far easier method of evaluation today is the instillation of a low dose of metrizamide into the spinal canal, with CT imaging in the axial and, more importantly, in the coronal and sagittal projections (Figs 22–3 and 22–4).[12] This technique, utilizing 5 ml of 190 mg/ml metrizamide in an adult, is extremely easy to perform and is definitive after the CT scan exclusion of a focal intracranial mass. Occasionally, slight ventricular enlargement may accompany the tonsillar herniation, and basilar

impression is a related anomaly in 20% to 50% of cases.[13] There must be sensitivity to a diagnosis of possible Chiari I malformation on the part of both the clinician and the radiologist when a patient presents with cerebellar findings such as ataxia or vestibular and/or oculomotor signs and symptoms suggesting a disturbance in the brain stem. Such patients have frequently been given a clinical diagnosis of multiple sclerosis or degenerative disease of the cerebellum or brain stem when a focal mass lesion is not discovered. Following the CT scan diagnosis of the Chiari I malformation, occipital and high cervical decompression may relieve the symptomatology, so that a high degree of suspicion of this condition may yield significant rewards.

In the Chiari II and III malformations, the pronounced caudal herniation of the posteroinferior portion of the cerebellum and fourth ventricle leads to a variable appearance of the fourth ventricle on the CT scan. In 70% of the cases, no fourth ventricle will be seen (Figs 22–5 and 22–6), while in 15% of cases a fourth ventricle that is flattened from side to side will be seen in normal position or slightly caudal in position; an additional 10% of cases will demonstrate a small but normally positioned fourth ventricle, while in 5% the fourth ventricle appears to be enlarged.[14] These findings contrast with the typical appearance in aqueductal stenosis, where a small fourth ventricle is almost always seen. The cerebellar tonsils and nodulus of the inferior vermis are herniated into the spinal canal with effacement of the cisterna magna. There is an elongated or, less commonly, frankly occluded aqueduct leading to dilatation of the lateral ventricles. In particular, the posterior portions of the lateral ventricles may be di-

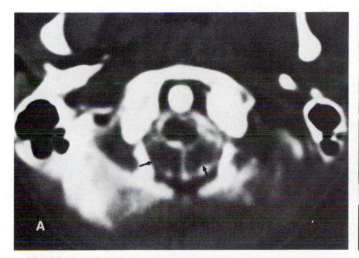
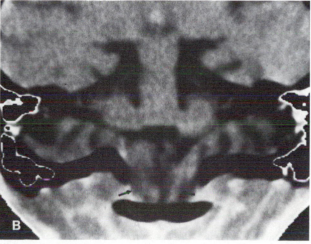

Fig 22–4.—Chiari I malformation. This 16-year-old male presented with a 3-year history of blurred vision, nystagmus, broad-based gait, and hyperreflexia. The initial concern was for a posterior fossa tumor. CT scanning did not reveal any evidence of an intracranial mass. Rather, CT scanning in the axial projection **(A)** demonstrated the cerebellar tonsils *(arrows)* to be inferiorly displaced to the level of the odontoid. Direct coronal scanning **(B)** with reversed window demonstrates the position of the tonsils *(arrows)* relative to the foramen magnum.

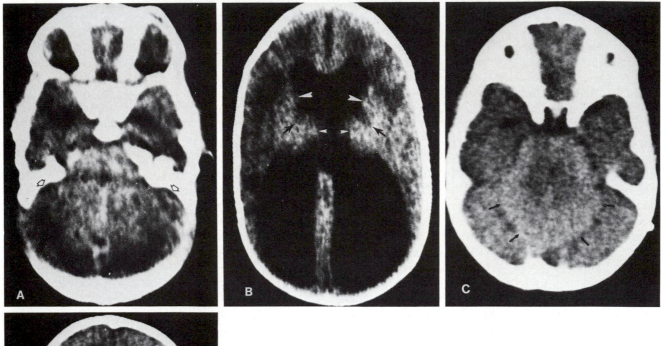

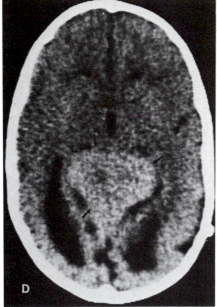

Fig 22–5.—Chiari II malformation. Cuts throughout the posterior fossa **(A)** did not demonstrate a definite fourth ventricle. There is scalloping of the petrous bones *(open arrows)* by the compressed cerebellum within the small posterior fossa. A cut through the third and lateral ventricles **(B)** demonstrates moderately severe enlargement of the ventricular system, particularly the posterior portions of both lateral ventricles. The "points" of the frontal horns *(black arrows)* are produced by prominent impressions of enlarged caudate nuclei *(large white arrowheads)* and thalami *(small white arrowheads);* the third ventricle appears disproportionately small because of the thalamic impressions. The frontal horn pointing and thalamic-caudate impressions produce a "figure-3" configuration. **C, D,** the compressed cerebellum grows anterolaterally into the cerebellopontine angles, and the vermis *(black arrows)* is displaced superiorly through a widened tentorial incisura to produce a "bullet-shaped" density.

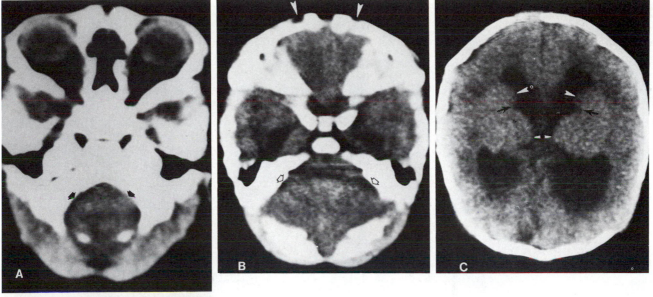

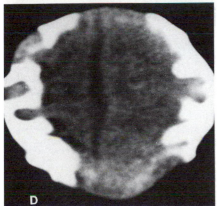

Fig 22–6.—Chiari II malformation. Bony changes include enlargement of the foramen magnum (**A,** *black arrows*), scalloping of the petrous bones (**B,** *open arrows*), and craniolacunia (lückenschädel) (**B,** *white arrowheads;* **D**). Ventricular changes include lack of visualization of the fourth ventricle **(B),** and the "figure-3" configuration of the frontal horns and third ventricle **(C).** This "figure-3" configuration is produced by enlargement of the caudate nuclei *(large white arrowheads),* enlargement of the thalami *(small white arrowheads),* a relatively small third ventricle secondary to the thalamic enlargement, and "pointing" of the frontal horns *(black arrows).*

lated out of proportion to the frontal horns, which may be relatively normal in size (see Fig 22–5). The third ventricle, however, appears to be dilated to only a mild degree, if at all. This is because of large massa intermedia, which produce a biconcave appearance of the third ventricle (Figs 22–5 and 22–7).[14] The third ventricle may also have a large suprapineal recess (see Fig 22–7) that may herniate through the tentorial notch into the posterior fossa.[6] An accessory commissure (Meynert's commissure) lies between the anterior commissure and the optic chiasm, but is typically not visualized with CT scanning unless sagittal projections are obtained.

The frontal horns have an unusual configuration that results from impressions by enlarged caudate nuclei. In the axial projection, the impression along the lateral aspect of the frontal horn produces a lateral "point," and when combined with the prominent concavity of the third ventricle, a "figure-3" configuration is obtained (see Figs 22–5 and 22–7). The caudate impression also

produces "pointing" of the floor of the lateral ventricle in the coronal projection.[14] The septum pellucidum may be totally or partially absent.

In virtually all patients with the Chiari II malformation, there is some degree of fusion of the colliculi of the quadrigeminal plate, with chronic pressure in the deformed and compacted posterior fossa and tentorial incisura producing a "beaked" appearance of the mesencephalon, which may be more apparent following a shunting procedure (Figs 22–7 and 22–8).[15] There is a notch in the superior cerebellar vermis to accommodate this mesencephalic beak (see Figs 22–7 and 22–8). There is confluence of the cisterns of the velum interpositum, superior vermis, and ambient wings, frequently forming a diamond appearance (Figs 22–7 and 22–9).[14] Following a shunting procedure, not only may large posterior portions of the lateral ventricles remain, but there may be a relative lack of cerebral substance in the medial parietal regions bilaterally (Fig 22–10). This latter finding may be due to the intrauterine dis-

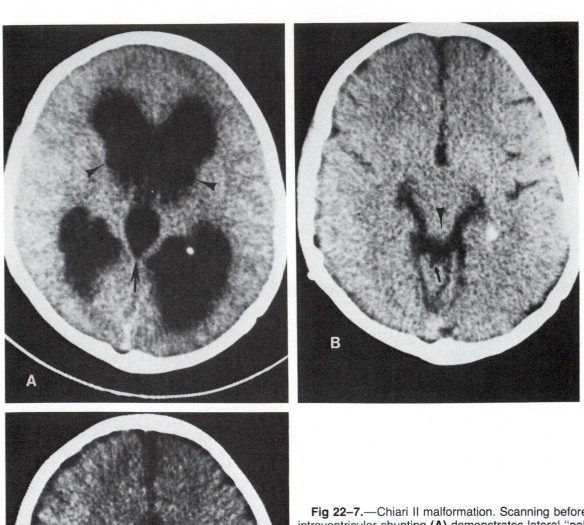

Fig 22–7.—Chiari II malformation. Scanning before intraventricular shunting **(A)** demonstrates lateral "points" of the frontal horns *(arrowheads),* enlarged thalami, and a prominent suprapineal recess of the third ventricle *(arrow).* **B, C,** following intraventricular shunting, it is easier to visualize the fusion of the colliculi of the quadrigeminal plate and the "beaked" appearance of the mesencephalon and colliculi **(B,** *arrowhead).* There is a notch in the superior cerebellar vermis *(arrow),* which accommodated the mesencephalic beak in the preshunted state. There is confluence of the superior cerebellar cistern, ambient cisternal wings, and velum interpositum to form a diamond appearance **(C,** *curved arrow).* Note the shunt in the right frontal horn **(C).**

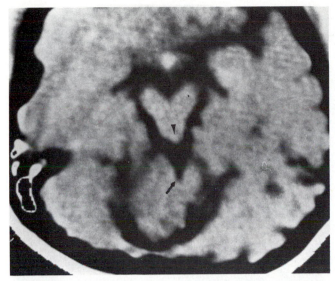

Fig 22–8.—Chiari II malformation. An axial slice through the quadrigeminal plate and superior cerebellar vermis, depicted with a reversed window, nicely demonstrates the combined collicular fusion and mesencephalic beaking *(arrowhead)* and the notch in the superior cerebellar vermis *(arrow).*

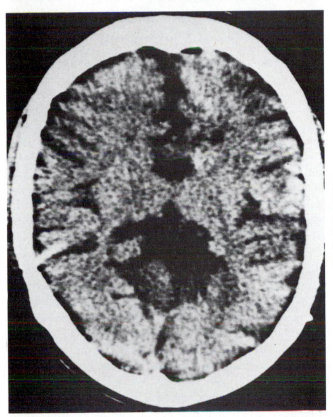

Fig 22–9.—Chiari II malformation. This axial slice was performed above the ventricular system in this 15-year-old patient who had been previously shunted for the Chiari II malformation associated with meningomyelocele. There is a loss of the medial portions of the parietal lobes that may have been secondary to the disproportionate enlargement of the posterior portions of the lateral ventricles in the preshunted state.

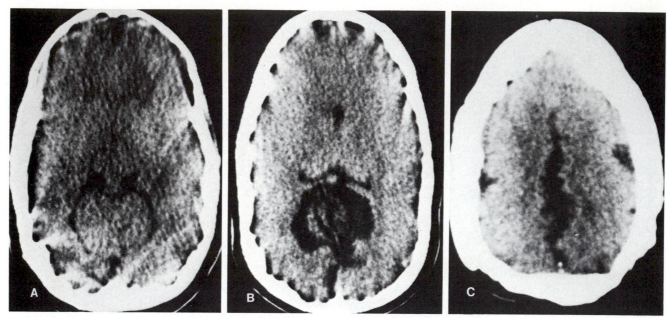

Fig 22–10.—Chiari II malformation. A cut through the level of the tentorial incisura **(A)** shows upward displacement of the cerebellum through the widened tentorial incisura. A slightly higher level **(B)** in this shunted patient shows confluence of the subarachnoid cisterns and decreased volume of the parietal lobes. A cut high over the convexities **(C)** demonstrates interdigitation of the gyri along the medial aspects of both cerebral hemispheres and hypoplasia of the falx.

proportionate enlargement of the posterior horns, so that the medial parietal lobes do not develop. Other parenchymal changes include interdigitation of cerebral gyri high over the convexity, with either hypoplasia or fenestration of the falx (Figs 22–10 and 22–11).[16]

Bony and dural abnormalities include craniolacunia (lückenschädel) (see Fig 22–6), which are areas of relative thinning of the neonatal calvarium having sharper margins on skull films than the impressions because of increased intracranial pressure. The craniolacunia are part of the dysplasia and are not due to increased intracranial pressure, as denoted by their spontaneous disappearance during the first 6 months of life. Not only is there hypoplasia or fenestration of the falx, but the tentorium has a low insertion on the petrous bones, producing a small posterior fossa. Over time, the compressed cerebellum produces scalloping of the posterior aspects of the petrous bones (see Figs 22–5, 22–6, and 22–11), and herniation of the inferior cerebellum and brain stem caudally produces enlargement of the foramen magnum (see Fig 22–6).[16] The tentorial notch is widened, with upward displacement of the cerebellum to produce a "bullet-shaped" tissue density projecting through the widened tentorial incisura (see Figs 22–5, 22–8, and 22–10).[15]

The cerebellum also grows around the brain stem, overlapping both the cerebral peduncle and the lateral aspect of the pons, filling the cerebellopontine angle, and wedging between the lateral aspect of the brain stem and tentorial margin (see Fig 22–5).[15]

The medulla is displaced caudally through the foramen magnum into the spinal canal, and in 50% of patients there is an S-shaped bend or kink in the cervicomedullary junction.[1] Spinal dysraphism is present in essentially all patients with a Chiari II malformation, with the most common type being meningomyelocele in the lumbar region, but cervical meningocele or meningomyelocele, encephalocele, diastematomyelia, and hydromyelia may also be found.[1]

The radiographic evaluation of this wide spectrum of anomalies includes CT scanning of the head, preferably in both the axial and coronal projections, and sagittal imaging if obtainable. Metrizamide cisternography is of value in demonstrating the caudal extent of the cerebellar herniation (see Figs 22–3 and 22–4), while metrizamide myelography with CT scanning is useful for evaluation of the various abnormalities of the spinal cord and canal (see Chapter 33). Scanning of the spinal column without an intrathecal contrast agent may demonstrate various abnormalities that include tethering of the cord, lipomatous tissue, and meningomyelocele. At this institution, we prefer to perform CT scanning of the head before proceeding with evaluation of the spinal cord abnormalities, which is usually done with complete metrizamide myelography following lumbar puncture above the meningomyelocele.

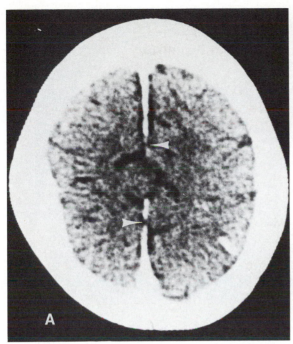

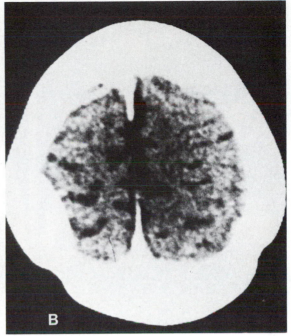

Fig 22–11.—Chiari II malformation. There is fenestration (**A**, *arrowheads*) of portions of the falx and hypoplasia of its midportion (**B**). There is interdigitation of cerebral gyri in the midline.

Inflammatory Obstruction

Increase in the size of only the lateral ventricles or both the lateral and third ventricles may be due to obstruction of the foramen of Monro or the aqueduct, respectively, secondary to intrauterine inflammatory disease. Intrauterine infectious diseases affecting the brain are denoted by the mnemonic STORCH (*S*, syphilis; *T*, toxoplasmosis; *O*, other; *R*, rubella; *C*, cytomegalic inclusion virus; *H*, herpes). Any of these disease entities may produce calcifications that are punctate, nodular, or confluent, and that may be located in cortical, subcortical, or periventricular regions or a combination of these locations (Figs 22–12 to 22–15). Ventricular enlargement may be secondary to obstruction (see Fig 22–12), but atrophy can also be present (see Fig 22–13) with extensive encephalomalacia that may be cystic (see Fig 22–15).[17]

It is extremely difficult in any one case to specify which inflammatory disease is responsible for the constellation of CT findings. The presence of the multiple calcifications will require the start of the STORCH protocol, including serologic tests for syphilis, rubella, and herpes; evaluation of the retinae for the classic findings of toxoplasmosis; evaluation of the urine for cytomegalic virus, etc. Calcification occurs in syndromes with a congenital metabolic basis such as Fahr's, Cockayne's, and Kearn-Sayre syndromes.[18] However, the calcifications do not generally appear until later in childhood.

Intraventricular membranes may be congenital in origin as a result of intrauterine inflammatory disease (Fig 22–16).[19] Such membranes may be extremely difficult to see on the CT scan, because they are so thin relative to the large volume of CSF. It is important to detect the membranes, because multiple loculations within the ventricular system will require several shunts for ventricular decompression. When membranes are visualized, ventriculography with a water-soluble contrast agent is of great value in determining the degree of communication of the various compartments.

Atrophy

Atrophic processes involving primarily the cerebrum will lead to dilatation of the lateral ventricles only or both the third and lateral ventricles. The most common etiology is that of perinatal hypoxia, with the CT scan demonstrating ventricular enlargement with multiple areas of encephalomalacia (Fig 22–17). There may or may not be enlargement of cortical sulci in the neonatal period. Other congenital etiologies of diffuse atrophy include intrauterine infection and the intrauterine exposure to toxic chemicals.

All Ventricles

Dandy-Walker Syndrome

The Dandy-Walker syndrome consists of aplasia or hypoplasia of the cerebellar vermis, cystic dilatation of the fourth ventricle, and generalized hydrocephalus. Originally, it was thought that this anomaly resulted from atre-

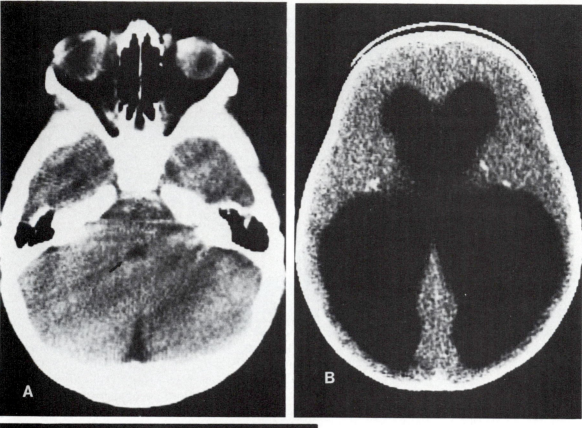

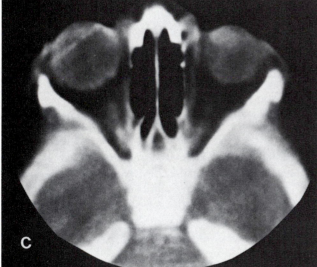

Fig 22–12.—Congenital rubella. This 15-month-old child had an enlarging head and positive titers for rubella. There is a small fourth ventricle (**A,** *arrow*), while there is marked enlargement of the third and lateral ventricles (**B**), indicative of an aqueductal obstruction by inflammatory tissue. Periventricular calcifications are present (**B**), indicating foci of inflammation. The left globe is small (**C**), and there is a prominent lens.

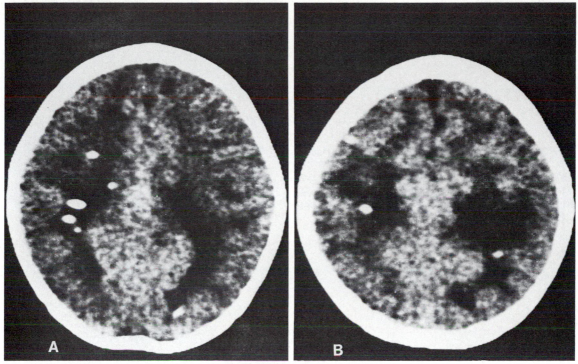

Fig 22–13.—STORCH syndrome. This 11-month-old child had microcephaly, developmental delay, and a left hemiparesis. Scans at the level of the bodies of the lateral ventricles (**A**) and centrum semiovale (**B**) demonstrate multiple periventricular and parenchymal calcifications along with multiple areas of encephalomalacia. The infectious agent is unknown.

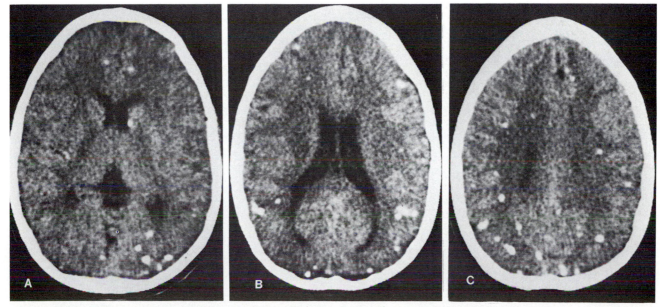

Fig 22–14.—Congenital toxoplasmosis. The CT scan demonstrates multiple parenchymal calcifications throughout both cerebral hemispheres (**A, B, C**). A few periventricular calcifications (**A, B**) are also present. The patient had high toxoplasmosis titers and the findings of chorioretinitis typical of toxoplasmosis, which is one of the congenital infections within the STORCH syndrome.

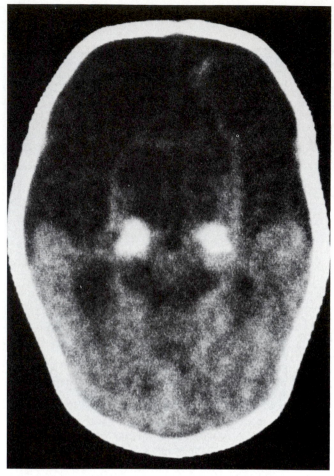

Fig 22–15.—Congenital herpes encephalitis. This 4-month-old child had cutaneous herpes and was born of a mother with genital herpes. The scan demonstrates extensive cystic encephalomalacia involving both frontal lobes, dilatations of the frontal horns, and thalamic calcifications bilaterally.

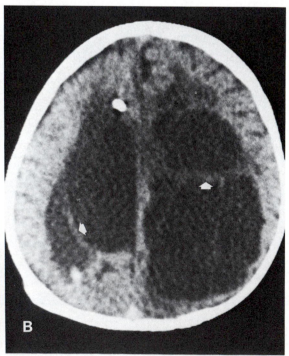

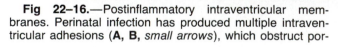

Fig 22–16.—Postinflammatory intraventricular membranes. Perinatal infection has produced multiple intraventricular adhesions (**A, B,** *small arrows*), which obstruct portions of the lateral ventricles. A single shunt tube (**A,** *large arrow*) is ineffectual at decompressing the entire ventricular system.

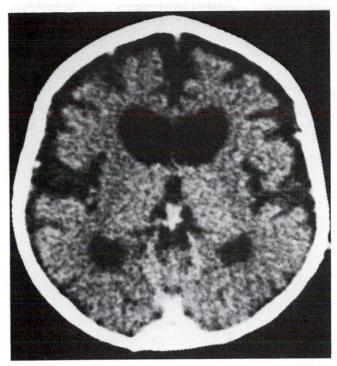

Fig 22–17.—Diffuse cerebral atrophy. This young child had microcephaly and developmental delay. The scan demonstrates ventricular enlargement and increased size of sulci diffusely, indicative of diffuse cortical and deep periventricular atrophy.

sia of the foramina of Luschka and Magendie, producing dilatation of the fourth ventricle and secondary hypoplasia or aplasia of the cerebellum caused by compression during intrauterine development.[20, 21] Because the foramina are patent in a number of cases, this theory is now considered untenable.[1] Multiple alternative theories have been suggested, including cleavage of the embryonic neural tube, with the defective development of the roof of the fourth ventricle leading to progressive cystic dilatation of this ventricular structure.[1, 22] The Dandy-Walker malformation may be part of a more generalized embryologic disturbance as evidenced by its presence in other family members[23] and the presence of other congenital anomalies including agenesis of the corpus callosum, holoprosencephaly, cortical heterotopia, and occipital encephalocele.[1, 6, 22, 24]

The radiographic features of the classic form of Dandy-Walker syndrome include an enlarged posterior fossa containing a large cystic mass (Figs 22–18 and 22–19). The fourth ventricle opens directly into the cyst. Small nodules of cerebellar tissue are frequently seen anteriorly and inferiorly (see Fig 22–18). These may be the only portions of cerebellum that develop, although larger portions of the anteroinferior aspects of the cerebellum may also be present (see Fig 22–19). Angiography demonstrates blood supply to this remaining cer-

ebellum from the anterior-inferior cerebellar arteries, with hypoplasia or absence of the posterior-inferior cerebellar arteries.[24] The posterior fossa expansion produces a high position of the torcula, transverse sinuses, tentorium, and lambdoid sutures (see Fig 22–19). Dilatation of the third and lateral ventricles varies considerably from mild to severe (see Figs 22–18 and 22–19).

An important presurgical consideration is the communication between the lateral ventricles and the posterior fossa cyst. A large cyst may produce sufficient compression of the aqueduct that shunting of only the lateral ventricles will not decompress the posterior fossa; placement of a shunt into the posterior fossa cyst may be required in addition to ventricular shunting. Two approaches to solve this question of communication may be used. First, shunting of the lateral ventricles may be performed, with postoperative scanning to detect any change in the cyst size besides decompression of the lateral ventricles. Metrizamide ventriculography may then be performed through the shunt tubing to assess communication and the need for subsequent shunting of the posterior fossa cyst (see Figs 22–18 and 22–19). Alternatively, metrizamide ventriculography may be performed following temporary ventriculostomy; if inadequate communication is demonstrated, a Y-shunt may be placed for simultaneous shunting of both the lateral ventricles and posterior fossa cyst.

Part of the spectrum of the Dandy-Walker syndrome is the Dandy-Walker variant. The variant consists of dilatation of the posterior portion of the fourth ventricle with a diverticulum extending from this structure; the anterior portion of the fourth ventricle is normal (Fig 22–20). The inferior cerebellar vermis is hypoplastic in such instances. The diverticulum varies in size and shape, but is not as large as the classic Dandy-Walker cyst. The appearance of the variant as a lack of development of the posterior portion of the roof of the fourth ventricle gives added support to the theory of maldevelopment of the entire fourth ventricular roof in the classic Dandy-Walker syndrome.

The Dandy-Walker cyst is to be distinguished from other cystic abnormalities within the posterior fossa. In particular, a large arachnoid cyst may simulate a Dandy-Walker cyst, but generally a fourth ventricle is visualized, although it is flattened and displaced. While the Dandy-Walker cyst may fill with air or contrast material following placement of the contrast agent into a lateral ventricle, an arachnoid cyst may not fill from either the intraventricular or intrathecal route. Vertebral angiography in the presence of an arachnoid cyst will demonstrate displaced posterior-inferior cerebellar arteries of a normal caliber, while these arteries are generally hypoplastic or absent in the Dandy-Walker syndrome because of its development early in gesta-

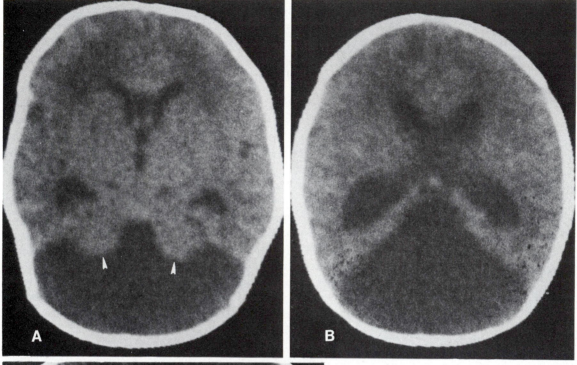

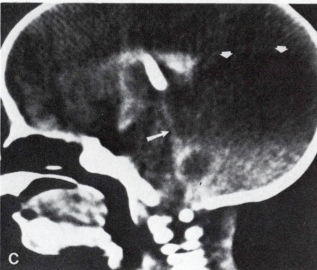

Fig 22–18.—Classic Dandy-Walker syndrome. A cut through the posterior fossa **(A)** demonstrates a large cystic structure of CSF density occupying almost all of the posterior fossa. There are small vestigial cerebellar hemispheres *(arrows)* with a wide space between them. A separate fourth ventricle is not present; rather, the aqueduct communicates directly with the cyst representing the "blown-out" fourth ventricle. A higher cut **(B)** demonstrates the large cystic expansion extending superiorly above the usual level of the tentorium. The lateral and third ventricles are only mildly to moderately dilated, considering the size of the cyst. A direct sagittal view **(C)** following intraventricular shunting, through which metrizamide was placed, demonstrates the aqueduct *(large arrow),* which is anteriorly displaced by the cystic expansion, the top of which is denoted by the *small arrows.* The metrizamide layers in the inferior portion of the cyst, demonstrating rapid communication between the third ventricle and the cyst.

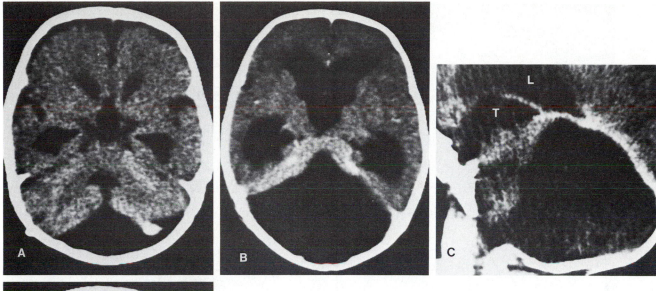

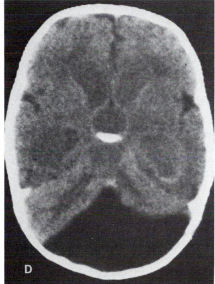

Fig 22–19.—Dandy-Walker cyst with poor communication between ventricular system and cyst. Scans through the posterior fossa **(A, B)** demonstrate a large cyst that communicates directly with a fourth ventricle. There is more cerebellar tissue than in Figure 22–18. There is moderately severe dilatation of the third and lateral ventricles. An enhanced direct sagittal scan **(C)** demonstrates elevation of the tentorium, as defined by the straight sinus, because of the large cyst. The dilated third *(T)* and lateral *(L)* ventricles are seen. Following intraventricular shunting and deposition of metrizamide through the shunt **(D)**, a metrizamide-CSF level is seen in the third ventricle. The third and lateral ventricles are opacified almost to the density of surrounding parenchyma by the intraventricular metrizamide. There was no detectable contrast material within the posterior fossa cyst on scanning over a 12-hour period. This indicated poor communication between the third ventricle and the cyst, most likely the result of aqueductal compression by the cyst and requiring shunting of both the cyst and the ventricular system.

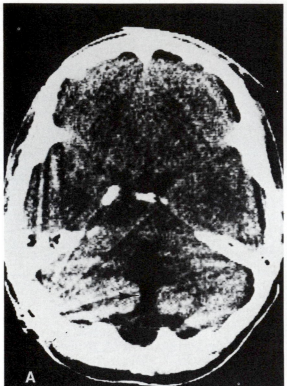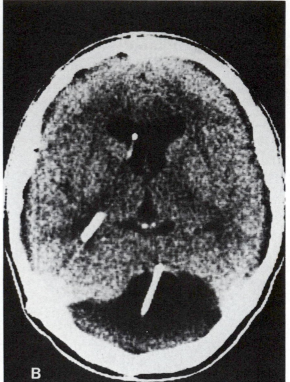

Fig 22–20.—Dandy-Walker variant. The lowest cut **(A)** demonstrates an enlarged vallecula *(arrowhead)*, with communication between an enlarged fourth ventricle and a retrocerebellar cyst. A higher cut **(B)** demonstrates the cyst to be of a smaller size than in Figures 22–18 and 22–19. The

Dandy-Walker variant has a more normal fourth ventricle, with communication between the roof of the fourth ventricle and a cystic expansion that is smaller in size than the classic Dandy-Walker cyst. There are shunts within both the ventricular system and the cyst.

tion.[25, 26] Another differential consideration is the enlarged cisterna magna, although it is never the size of the classic Dandy-Walker cyst. The enlarged cisterna magna is generally confused with an arachnoid cyst and not, with the Dandy-Walker syndrome, because the fourth ventricle is visualized, is in a normal location, and there is no hydrocephalus.[26, 27] The entire subject of arachnoid cyst and the enlarged cisterna magna will be discussed later in this chapter.

A final differential possibility is the enlarged fourth ventricle that results from outlet obstruction. The foramina of Luschka and Magendie may be obstructed from inflammation, surgical adhesions, local hemorrhage, etc. In such cases, there may be diffuse enlargement of the entire ventricular system, simulating the appearance of a communicating hydrocephalus caused by convexity block. When there is also an aqueductal obstruction secondary to previous inflammation, there may be an isolated fourth ventricle (Fig 22–21).[28] In such cases of acquired disease, the cerebellum is not hypoplastic, the fourth ventricle is not enlarged to the degree of the Dandy-Walker cyst, nor is there enlargement of the posterior fossa.[6]

Inflammatory Obstruction

Obstruction to the flow of CSF over the cerebral convexities will produce dilatation of the entire ventricular system. In such cases, there is communication between the ventricular system and the subarachnoid space of the spinal canal, thereby acquiring the term "communicating hydrocephalus." Such convexity obstruction may be from one of the intrauterine inflammatory diseases (Fig 22–22), including those of the STORCH group. Other etiologies include intrauterine subarachnoid hemorrhage producing arachnoid scarring, and congenital hypoplasia or absence of the arachnoid granulations leading to decreased CSF resorption.[29] It should be emphasized that many cases of communicating hydrocephalus (approximately 60%) do not have dilatation of the fourth ventricle associated with dilatation of the third and lateral ventricles; a diagnosis of communicating hydrocephalus cannot be based solely on the presence of dilatation of the entire ventricular system.

Atrophy

The various causes of atrophy have been previously discussed. To produce dilatation of the entire ventricu-

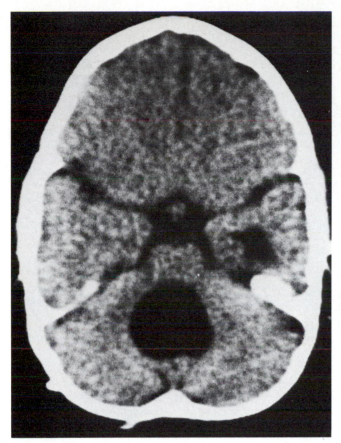

Fig 22–21.—Isolated fourth ventricle. This child had neonatal intraventricular hemorrhage producing adhesions throughout the ventricular system and a need for ventricular shunting. The left temporal horn is dilated. In addition, there is pronounced dilatation of the fourth ventricle as a result of adhesion within the aqueduct and involving the foramina of the fourth ventricle. Such adhesions isolate the fourth ventricle and prevent its decompression from ventricular shunting.

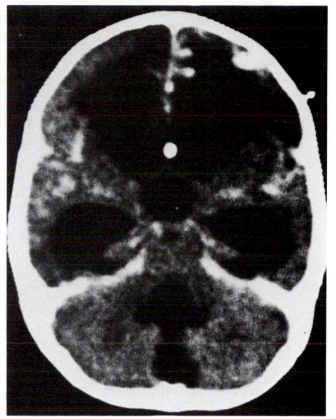

Fig 22–22.—Neonatal meningitis producing communicating hydrocephalus. *Hemophilus influenzae* meningitis has produced a communicating form of hydrocephalus, as denoted by enlargement of the lateral, third, and fourth ventricles. There is enhancement of inflammatory tissue within the subarachnoid spaces of multiple supratentorial cisterns and sulci.

lar system, atrophy would involve both the cerebrum and cerebellum.

CRANIOCEREBRAL MALFORMATIONS

Midline Cerebrum

Holoprosencephaly, septo-optic dysplasia, and agenesis of the corpus callosum present a spectrum of overlapping pathologic findings. All three involve structures derived from the diencephalon and telencephalon. Relatively mild changes of "squaring" of the frontal horns and absence of the septum pellucidum may be present in the lobar form of holoprosencephaly, findings identical to those in septo-optic dysplasia. Some cases of lobar and semi-lobar holoprosencephaly have associated diencephalic cysts, mimicking the appearance of agenesis of the corpus callosum with associated interhemi-

spheric cyst. Differentiation of these overlapping syndromes can be difficult; the pathologic and CT appearances described below should help in this differentiation.

Holoprosencephaly

The holoprosencephalies are a spectrum of congenital abnormalities in which there is incomplete cleavage of the prosencephalon into the normal diencephalon and telencephalon. There is also absent or incomplete separation of the telencephalon into cerebral hemispheres and lobes. The malformation may be divided as follows into three varieties with a descending degree of severity: alobar, semilobar, and lobar holoprosencephaly.[30]

In alobar holoprosencephaly, there is a small cerebrum without division into lobes or hemispheres. There is a monoventricular cavity, and the thin cerebral parenchyma is located primarily anteriorly and laterally (Fig 22–23). The basal ganglia and thalami are fused in the midline (Fig 22–24). The interhemispheric fissure,

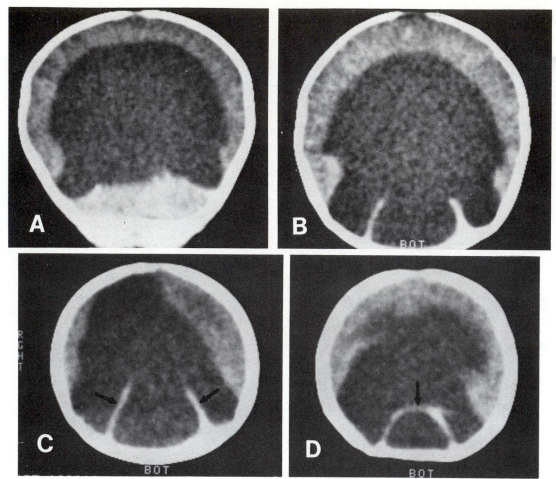

Fig 22–23.—Alobar holoprosencephaly. The lowest cut **(A)** demonstrates brain covering a monoventricle anteriorly and laterally. Cerebellar tissue is seen posteriorly. A slightly higher cut **(B)** demonstrates communication of the supratentorial monoventricle with a cyst located within the posterior fossa. Cerebellar hypoplasia and posterior fossa cysts have been reported with holoprosencephaly. The higher cuts **(C, D)** demonstrate the high position of the tentorium *(arrows)* resulting from the expansion of the posterior fossa cyst. There is no evidence of an interhemispheric fissure or falx. (Courtesy of Charles Fitz, M.D., Toronto.)

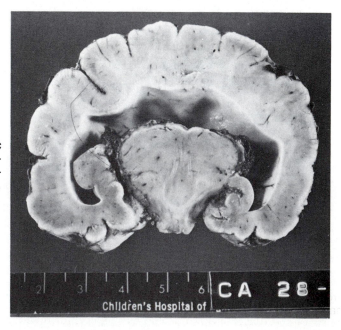

Fig 22–24.—Alobar holoprosencephaly. This pathologic specimen demonstrates the classic findings of alobar holoprosencephaly, including fusion of the thalami, a monoventricle, and the lack of interhemispheric and Sylvian fissures.

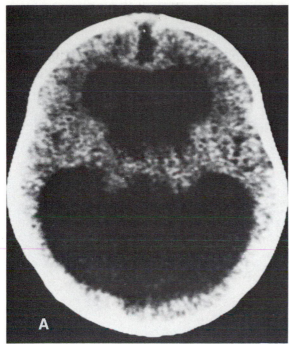
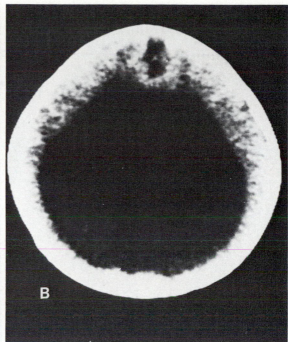

falx cerebri, and corpus callosum are not formed (see Fig 22–24), nor are the olfactory bulbs and nerves.[31–34] The only significant differential diagnostic consideration with alobar holoprosencephaly is hydranencephaly. In that condition, the cortex and white matter of the majority of the cerebral hemispheres is absent and replaced by a large fluid-filled cavity (see Figs 22–42 and 22–43), but the falx is present and the basal ganglia are separated.[31]

In semilobar holoprosencephaly, there is an attempt at separation into two cerebral hemispheres, with some portion of the interhemispheric fissure usually seen anteriorly. There is also some attempt at formation of individual frontal horns, although the ventricular system

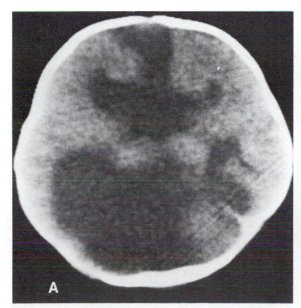
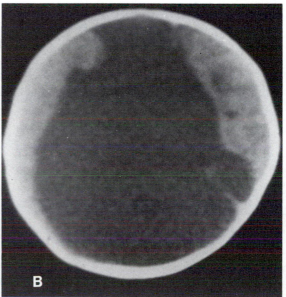

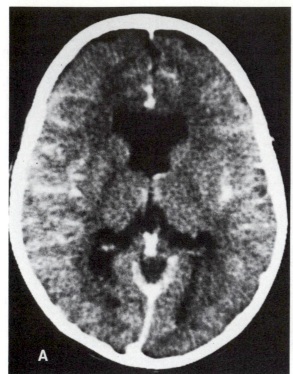
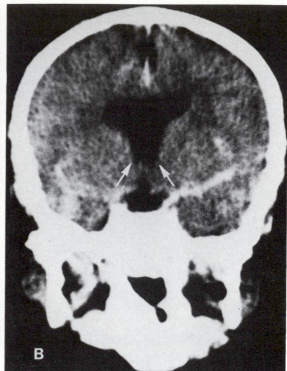

Fig 22–27.—Septo-optic dysplasia. Axial **(A)** and coronal **(B)** scans demonstrate lack of formation of the septum pellucidum, "squaring" of the frontal horns with flattening of the roofs of the lateral ventricles, and "points" of the inferior margins of the lateral ventricles **(B, arrows)**.

remains, by and large, a monoventricle. The corpus callosum is unformed, and the thalami and basal ganglia are fused (Fig 22–25).[31]

In lobar holoprosencephaly, separation into two cerebral hemispheres is nearly complete. There may be a "squaring" of the frontal horns and a flattening of the ventricular roof, as is seen with septo-optic dysplasia (see Figs 22–27 and 22–28), as a result of hypoplasia of the corpus callosum. Likewise, the septum pellucidum may be absent. The thalami and basal ganglia may be

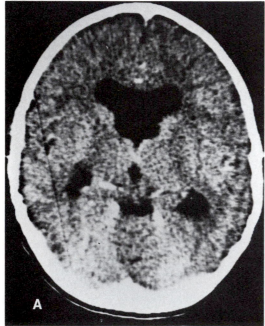
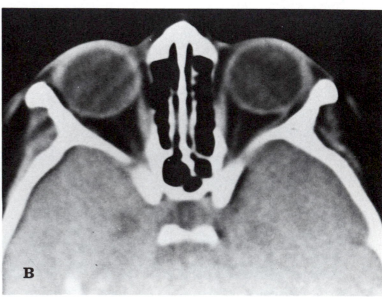

Fig 22–28.—Septo-optic dysplasia with hypoplastic optic nerves. The axial scan of the brain **(A)** demonstrates a missing septum pellucidum and "squaring" of the frontal horns. The axial scan of the orbits **(B)** demonstrates small optic nerves bilaterally.

either fused or separated. The interhemispheric fissure and falx may be incomplete; these subtle changes may be the only findings that differentiate mild degrees of lobar holoprosencephaly from agenesis of the septum pellucidum and septo-optic dysplasia.[6, 31]

A number of cases of holoprosencephaly are associated with superior extension of the monoventricular cavity to form a midline cyst (Fig 22–26). There is little difficulty in diagnosis when the typical findings of holoprosencephaly are found, including continuity of the ventricular system, fused thalami, and missing interhemispheric fissure and falx (see Fig 22–26). However, in the more subtle forms of holoprosencephaly, the presence of an interhemispheric cyst may suggest the diagnosis of agenesis of the corpus callosum with associated interhemispheric cyst. In the former case, there is no impression on the cystic cavity by a falx nor visualization of the falx on the CT scan. In the latter condition, the normally formed falx is seen on the CT scan and produces an impression on the midline cyst.[31, 35]

Anomalies of the face parallel the degree of cerebral dysplasia.[36] In alobar holoprosencephaly, facial deformities include cyclopia, ethmocephaly, cebocephaly, median cleft lip and palate, and bilateral cleft lip and palate. The semilobar holoprosencephaly is accompanied by median cleft lip and palate and bilateral cleft lip, while lobar holoprosencephaly may have only mild facial deformities including hyper- or hypotelorism. Facial deformities, however, do not always accompany holoprosencephaly. Seventeen percent of patients with alobar holoprosencephaly have been found to have no obvious facial deformities, and certainly a large percentage of patients with less severe forms of holoprosencephaly may have normal facies.[37]

The prognosis is extremely poor for alobar holoprosencephaly, and most patients do not survive infancy. The semilobar malformation is associated with marked mental retardation, while the lobar variety is accompanied by lesser degrees of psychomotor retardation. Hydrocephalus is generally present in 80% of lobar forms.[31]

The etiology of the holoprosencephalies is unknown, but the condition appears to occur between the fourth and eighth weeks of intrauterine life.[1, 31] There is association with several chromosomal syndromes, including trisomy 13–15 and trisomy 18. There is also an association with the Dandy-Walker malformation.[38]

Septo-Optic Dysplasia (deMorsier Syndrome)

Septo-optic dysplasia consists of agenesis of the septum pellucidum and hypoplasia of the optic discs, optic chiasm, optic nerves, and pituitary infundibulum. The diagnosis is generally made on a clinical basis after finding hypoplastic discs, impaired vision, and nystagmus in a patient with short stature.[6]

The pathologic findings in this syndrome are best evaluated with both the axial and coronal CT projections.[39–41] The septum pellucidum is missing, the frontal horns have a "square" appearance, and the roof of the ventricles is flat (Figs 22–27 and 22–28). The frontal horns are usually dilated to a mild degree and are "pointed" along their inferior margins (see Fig 22–27) as in the Chiari II malformation. There is a bulbous optic recess of the third ventricle, the "optic ventricle," with a hypoplastic infundibular recess. These latter findings usually require pneumoencephalography for visualization. The optic nerves may appear hypoplastic (see Fig 22–28), although care must be exercised in avoiding partial volume errors.

Agenesis of the Corpus Callosum

Agenesis of the corpus callosum may be partial or complete and may result from either an abnormality in embryogenesis or possibly destruction of a normally formed corpus callosum by an intrauterine insult.[6] An early injury to the prosencephalon leads to holoprosencephaly, while a more localized insult will lead to abnormal development of specific structures such as the corpus callosum. In addition, a mass such as a tumor or cyst may cause or be associated with agenesis of the corpus callosum.[1, 42]

The pathologic and CT findings consist of separation of the lateral ventricles and thalami and dorsal extension of the third ventricle (Fig 22–29).[1, 6, 43] Superior extension of the third ventricle may be subtle on axial scans, however, with suspicion of this abnormality prompted by separation of the internal cerebral veins (Fig 22–30), separation of the bodies of the lateral ventricles (Figs 22–29 to 22–32), and a typical "bat-wing" configuration to the frontal horns (see Figs 22–29, 22–31, and 22–32). This latter appearance is due to impression upon the medial aspects of the frontal horns by longitudinal bundles of myelinated fibers, the bundles of Probst.

Coronal views are particularly important in substantiating the presence of dorsal extension of the third ventricle (Figs 22–31 to 22–33), particularly in subtle cases (see Fig 22–31). The characteristic bat-wing configuration is well visualized on such coronal projections (see Figs 22–31 and 22–32). The leaves of the septum pellucidum may be widely separated, or they may be absent. Absence of the septum pellucidum is also associated with septo-optic dysplasia and holoprosencephaly or may occur as an isolated finding.[1]

Agenesis of the corpus callosum may be associated with an interhemispheric cyst. The cyst may communicate with the ventricular system and therefore represent a midline extension of that ventricular system. In such a case, the appearance may mimic holoprosencephaly with a dorsal cyst (see Fig 22–26). The pres-

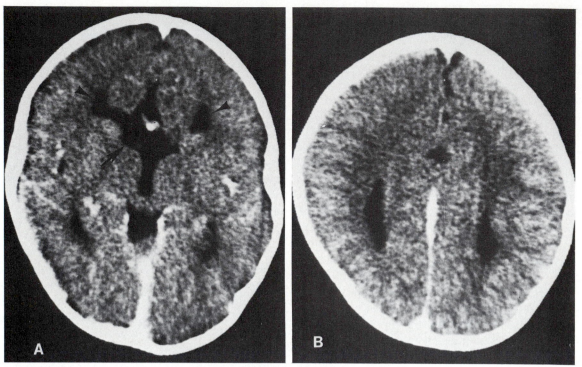

Fig 22–29.—Agenesis of the corpus callosum. A scan at the level of the frontal horns **(A)** demonstrates an enlarged third ventricle *(arrow)* extending superiorly, separating the frontal horns *(arrowheads)*. These frontal horns assume a "bat-wing" configuration. A high cut **(B)** demonstrates separation of bodies of the lateral ventricles.

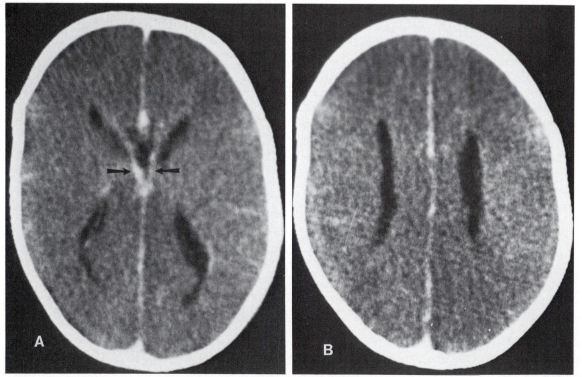

Fig 22–30.—Agenesis of the corpus callosum. The degree of superior extension of the third ventricle is more subtle in this case than in Figure 22–29. In this case, the elevated third ventricle produces separation of the internal cerebral veins **(A,** *arrows)*. The frontal horns are flared rather than assuming a classic "bat-wing" configuration. A high cut **(B)** demonstrates the classic separation of the bodies of the lateral ventricles.

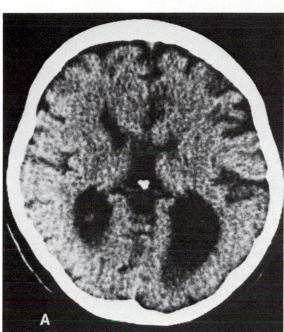

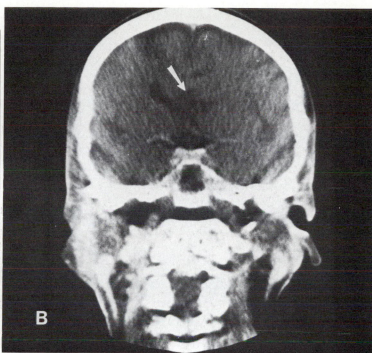

Fig 22–31.—Agenesis of the corpus callosum. The axial scan **(A)** demonstrates the "bat-wing" configuration of the frontal horns, with that on the right particularly well seen. The coronal scan **(B)** shows the same configuration of the right frontal horn and is particularly effective at showing the relationship of the superiorly displaced third ventricle *(arrow)* relative to the frontal horns.

ence of the falx and an impression on the cystic structure by that falx differentiates agenesis of the corpus callosum from holoprosencephaly.[35] However, the cyst may not communicate with the ventricular system, in which case it is most likely an arachnoid cyst.[44] In such a case, the placement of metrizamide into the cystic cavity will help in the evaluation of ventricular communication (Fig 22–34) and aid in the presurgical planning of a shunting procedure or resection.

Agenesis of the corpus callosum is associated with a lipoma that may be located either anteriorly near the rostral corpus callosum (see Fig 11–6) or more posteriorly near the splenium (see Fig 11–7). Other congenital anomalies that accompany agenesis of the corpus callosum include holoprosencephaly, encephalocele, heterotopic gray matter, and the Dandy-Walker cyst (see Fig 22–33).[6, 45] The function of the corpus callosum is poorly understood, but agenesis of the corpus callosum is probably asymptomatic. Symptoms are probably caused by other congenital cerebral malformations present in association with this malformation.[1, 46, 47]

Lateral Cerebral Hemispheric Defects

The term "porencephaly" originally meant a defect extending from the subarachnoid space through the cerebral parenchyma into the underlying ventricle. That meaning has been modified over the years, so that the term now denotes a cystic space that communicates with the ventricular system, with the subarachnoid space, with both, or with neither.[6] The most common use of the term today denotes a cystic space that communicates with the ventricular system.

It may be difficult to differentiate between developmental malformations and lesions caused by destruction of normal tissue resulting from intrauterine insult. Both types of lesions may have a similar pathologic appearance, particularly because necrosis from a destructive lesion that occurred early in intrauterine life may not be evident after birth and further development.[1] Even with these problems in determining pathogenesis, the hemispheric defects are divided into the encephaloclastic type, with the term denoting an intrauterine destructive process, and the schizencephalic type, representing a malformation of embryogenesis.[48, 49] Porencephaly generally denotes the former category and will be so used in this discussion.

Porencephaly

Intrauterine porencephaly may be secondary to any insult that produces destruction of tissue. A common denominator, however, may be decreased blood flow to a localized area, with subsequent infarction.[50] A porencephalic cyst usually communicates with the ventricular system, with the cystic fluid having absorption coeffi-

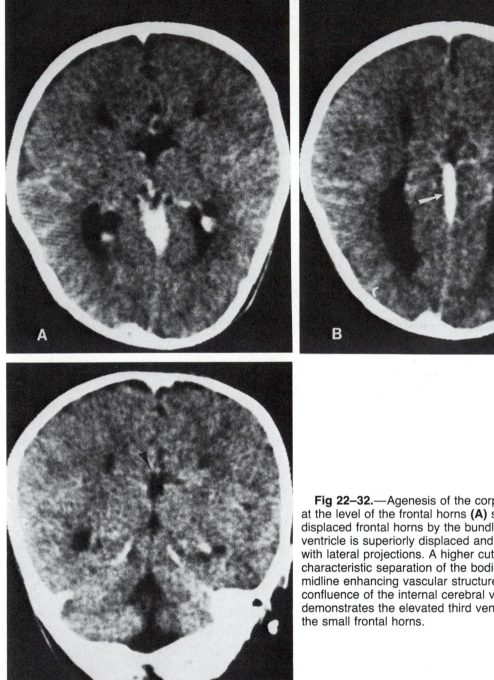

Fig 22–32.—Agenesis of the corpus callosum. The axial scan at the level of the frontal horns **(A)** shows small and laterally displaced frontal horns by the bundles of Propst. The third ventricle is superiorly displaced and has an unusual configuration with lateral projections. A higher cut **(B)** demonstrates the characteristic separation of the bodies of the lateral ventricles. A midline enhancing vascular structure *(arrow)* probably represents confluence of the internal cerebral veins. A coronal cut **(C)** demonstrates the elevated third ventricle *(arrowhead)* relative to the small frontal horns.

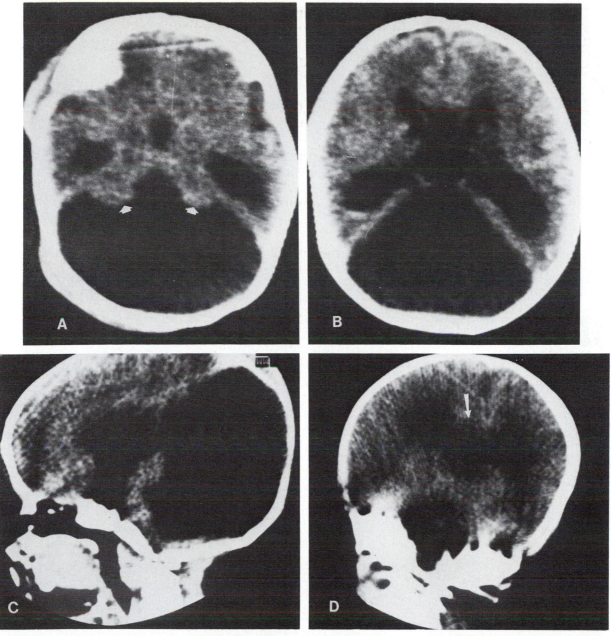

Fig 22–33.—Agenesis of the corpus callosum with associated Dandy-Walker malformation. There is a huge cyst of the posterior fossa with small vestigial cerebellar hemispheres (**A,** *arrowheads*), the classic appearance of the Dandy-Walker cyst. The third ventricle is elevated in position, with lateral flaring of the frontal horns (**B**). A direct sagittal scan (**C**) demonstrates the enormous cyst that elevates the tentorium and straight sinus. A direct coronal scan (**D**) demonstrates the relationship of the elevated third ventricle *(arrow)* relative to the dilated frontal horns.

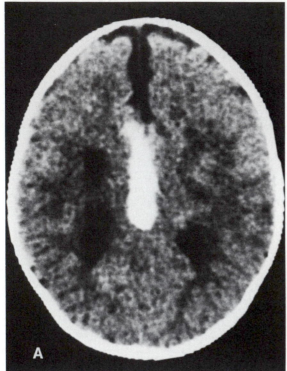

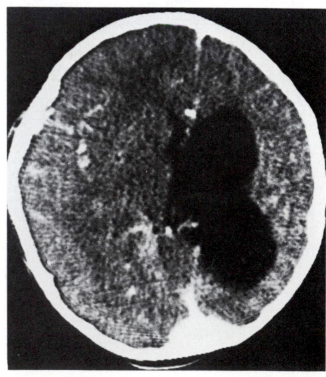

Fig 22–34.—Agenesis of the corpus callosum with interhemispheric arachnoid cyst following the direct placement of metrizamide into a large midline cystic cavity. An axial scan through the most inferior portion of the metrizamide-filled cyst **(A)** demonstrates lateral displacement of the bodies of the lateral ventricles. The coronal scan **(B)** demonstrates the enormity of the cyst and its lack of communication with the third and lateral ventricles. Such a lack of communication indicates the need for resection or direct shunting of the cyst, because shunting of the ventricular system will not decompress the cyst.

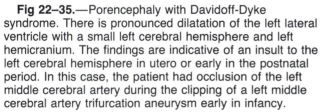

Fig 22–35.—Porencephaly with Davidoff-Dyke syndrome. There is pronounced dilatation of the left lateral ventricle with a small left cerebral hemisphere and left hemicranium. The findings are indicative of an insult to the left cerebral hemisphere in utero or early in the postnatal period. In this case, the patient had occlusion of the left middle cerebral artery during the clipping of a left middle cerebral artery trifurcation aneurysm early in infancy.

cients equal to CSF (Figs 22–35 to 22–38). Occasionally, the defect will also extend to the cortical surface (see Fig 22–36). There is frequently associated cerebral atrophy because of the parenchymal insult, resulting in a shift of the ventricular system towards the side of involvement (see Fig 22–35). When associated with an extensive degree of atrophy of a hemisphere, there may be secondary changes of the skull during development, including elevation of the petrous ridge, thickening of the calvarium, and increased pneumatization of the paranasal sinuses (Davidoff-Dyke syndrome).

The porencephalic cavity may act as a mass and produce thinning of the overlying calvarium (see Fig 22–37), most likely from the "water-hammer" pulsation of CSF within the cyst. There may also be a ball-valve action of the communication between the body of the lateral ventricle and the cyst cavity. Such a ball-valve action would allow the cavity to enlarge to a size greater than the rest of the ventricular system, again creating mass effect rather than an appearance of atrophy, enlargement of a hemisphere, and displacement of midline structures to the opposite side (see Fig 22–38).

It may be difficult to differentiate a porencephalic cavity from any other type of intracranial cystic mass such as an arachnoid cyst. Tissue interposed between the body of a lateral ventricle and the porencephalic cavity may suggest that the cystic mass is separate from the ventricular system, such as would occur with arachnoid cyst (see Fig 22–38); conversely, attenuated parenchyma interposed between an extra-axial arachnoid cyst and the ventricular system may be difficult to define on the CT scan, making differentiation of porencephaly from extra-axial cyst impossible. In such cases, it is extremely important to evaluate the size of the cystic space following ventricular shunting to determine the degree of communication. In addition, the placement of metrizamide into either the cystic space or the ventricular system with CT scanning over time is an excellent method of determining communication. The porencephalic cavity, which is separated from the rest of the ventricular system by either membranes or normal tissue, thereby acting as a mass, may require direct therapy such as shunting, similar to an extraventricular arachnoid cyst.[51]

Schizencephaly

Schizencephaly is considered to be a true malformation, because the hemispheric defects are usually bilateral and symmetric and there is agenesis of the septum pellucidum.[52] In addition, other malformations are frequently present, such as polymicrogyria at the margins of the defects.[1] The condition probably originates at or prior to the sixth week of gestation.[48, 49]

Scans by CT demonstrate defects extending from the

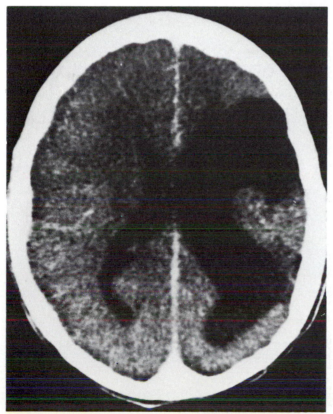

Fig 22–36.—Porencephaly. This patient presented with the clinical findings of cerebral palsy. A scan demonstrates porencephalic dilatation of the left lateral ventricle, with the porencephaly extending to the surface of the brain both anteriorly and posteriorly. The left cerebral hemisphere is small, indicative of an insult early in development.

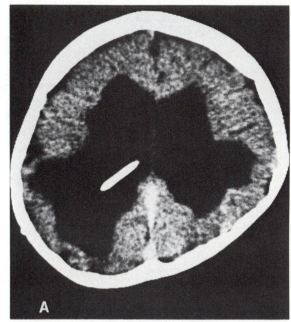

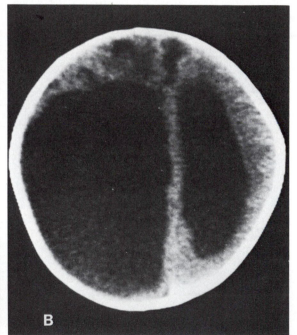

Fig 22–37.—Porencephalic cyst acting as a mass. There is pronounced dilatation of both lateral ventricles **(A),** with the dilatation of the posterior portion of the right lateral ven- tricle being most dramatic. This area of porencephaly acts as a mass with pronounced deformity of the overlying skull **(B).**

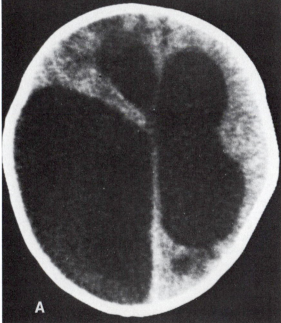

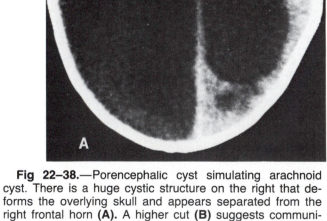

Fig 22–38.—Porencephalic cyst simulating arachnoid cyst. There is a huge cystic structure on the right that de- forms the overlying skull and appears separated from the right frontal horn **(A).** A higher cut **(B)** suggests communi- cation between the ventricular system and the cyst. It is dif- ficult to distinguish between a porencephalic cyst of the right lateral ventricle, which is separated from the right frontal horn, and an arachnoid cyst, which is contiguous to the ven- tricular system. Following ventricular shunting, metrizamide placed through the shunt was quickly visualized within the right-sided cystic structure, indicating that this was a poren- cephalic dilatation of the right ventricle.

ventricular system to the cortical surface. The defects may be localized to only a small portion of each hemisphere, such as the frontal lobes bilaterally (Fig 22–39). The defects may be larger, however, involving a large portion of the cortical surfaces bilaterally (Fig 22–40), or there may be multiple but more localized defects involving each of the hemispheres (Fig 22–41). "Pointing" of the floors of the lateral ventricles, as seen in Figure 22–41, is also seen with other conditions associated with agenesis of the septum pellucidum, including septo-optic dysplasia, and in the Chiari II malformation. This latter finding is further evidence for schizencephaly being a true malformation and not a product of an intrauterine insult.

Combined Midline and Lateral Cerebrum: Hydranencephaly

Hydranencephaly consists of the absence of the majority of the cerebral hemispheres except for the occipital lobes, basal portions of the temporal lobes, and thalami. A large membranous sac containing CSF occupies the rest of the intracranial space. The wall of this

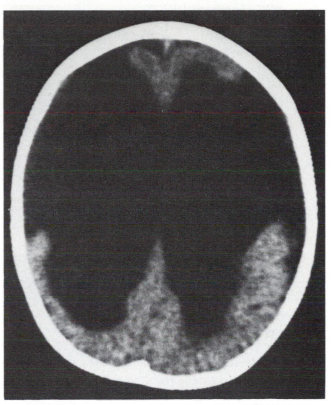

Fig 22–40.—Schizencephaly. Whereas the hemispheric defects were relatively localized to small portions of the frontal lobes in Figure 22–39, the defects in this case are extensive, with the ventricular system opening directly to the subarachnoid spaces over the convexities.

sac is pia-arachnoid overlying glial fibers devoid of neurons. This is an important finding, in that with even the most severe forms of hydrocephalus, some neural parenchyma persists. In addition, the falx is present, while in holoprosencephaly the falx is absent.

Various theories as to the origin of hydranencephaly have been proposed, including intrauterine infection, a defect in embryogenesis, and bilateral occlusion of the internal carotid arteries.[6]

Scans by CT demonstrate CSF density throughout the supratentorial space (Fig 22–42). Two soft-tissue densities at the base of the skull represent the persisting thalami. Occipital and temporal lobe tissue may also be visualized, along with normal tissue density in the posterior fossa (Fig 22–43).

It must be emphasized that reliable differentiation of hydranencephaly from severe hydrocephalus cannot be made on a CT scan alone. While the classic findings of hydranencephaly may strongly suggest this diagnosis,[53] severe hydrocephalus may have a similar picture. In addition, hydrocephalus is treated with an intraventricular shunt, which may allow recovery of a great deal of function even in the most severe forms of hydrocepha-

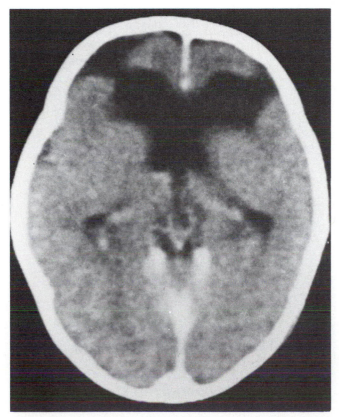

Fig 22–39.—Schizencephaly. There are bilateral and symmetric defects of the frontal lobes, extending from the frontal horns to the surfaces of the brain. The septum pellucidum is missing. The bilaterality of the condition and the associated agenesis of the septum pellucidum are classic findings for schizencephaly.

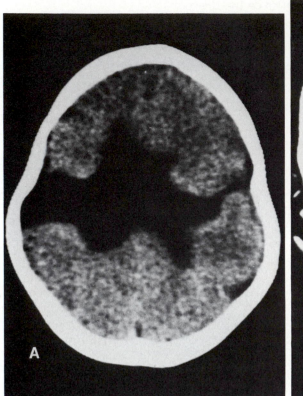

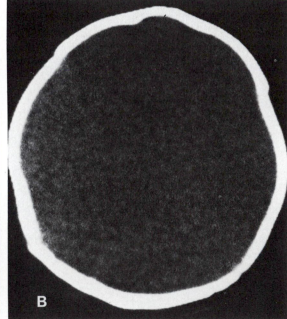

Fig 22–41.—Schizencephaly. The axial **(A)** and coronal **(B)** scans demonstrate bilateral hemispheric defects and a missing septum pellucidum, characteristic of schizence-phaly. The margins of the frontal horns appear "pointed," and there is probably agenesis of the corpus callosum in addition to agenesis of the septum pellucidum.

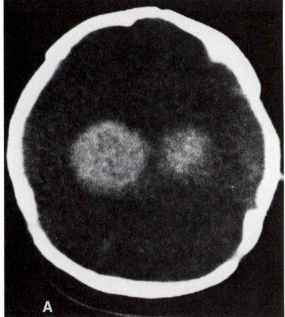

Fig 22–42.—Hydranencephaly. This scan was performed at 5 days of age because of pronounced transillumination of the head. The lower scan **(A)** demonstrates CSF occupying the majority of the head. The only cerebral tissue consists of two round structures representing thalamic tissue. A higher cut **(B)** shows fluid of CSF density occupying the en-tire intracranial space. The child lived for 17 months before dying of infection; autopsy confirmed hydranencephaly.

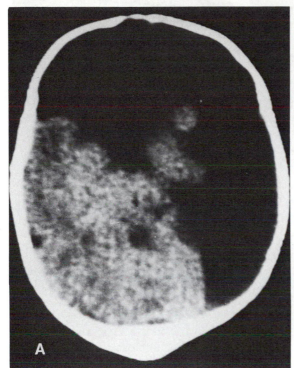 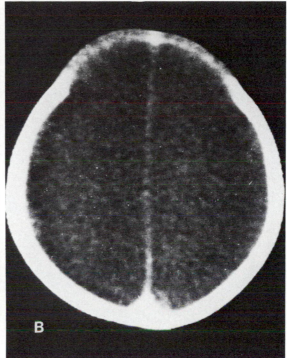

Fig 22–43.—Hydranencephaly. The scan was performed at 4 weeks of age for pronounced transillumination of the head. A lower cut **(A)** demonstrates that on the left the only visible tissue is the left thalamus and basal ganglia and tissue in the left occipital region in the distribution of the left posterior cerebral artery. There is more tissue on the right, particularly middle and posterior right temporal lobe, right occipital lobe, and thalamus. Again, the tissue that persists appears to be in the right posterior cerebral artery distribution. A higher cut **(B)** demonstrates the lack of cerebral tissue and fluid with attenuation coefficients of CSF. This higher cut demonstrates the presence of a falx, which is not seen in alobar holoprosencephaly. Tissue in the distribution of the posterior cerebral arteries may persist in hydranencephaly, while tissues in the middle and anterior cerebral distributions are not visualized.

lus. The need to distinguish between these two entities is therefore obvious. Angiography is definitive in this differentiation. In severe hydrocephalus, vascular structures are intact, albeit stretched and thinned. In hydranencephaly, vessels in the anterior and middle cerebral artery distributions are absent. Posterior cerebral arteries from the basilar artery may persist, supplying basal cerebral structures. Occasionally, alobar holoprosencephaly becomes a differential diagnostic consideration on the CT scan. The condition is characterized by an azygous anterior cerebral artery coursing far anteriorly because of the lack of separation of the brain into hemispheres.

Cerebellum

The most common malformations involving the cerebellum are the Chiari malformations. The Chiari II and III malformations also involve multiple portions of the cerebral hemispheres, whereas the Chiari I malformation is characterized on neuroradiologic examinations primarily by caudal displacement of the cerebellar tonsils. These conditions have been discussed earlier in the chapter.

Hypoplasia of the cerebellar vermis, particularly the inferior vermis, is usually associated with the Dandy-Walker malformation. However, the malformation may occasionally occur without an associated cystic dilatation of any portion of the fourth ventricle, as in the Joubert syndrome.[54–56] In this condition, there is agenesis of the inferior vermis, mental retardation, ataxia, and abnormal eye movements. Inferior vermian agenesis has also been associated with communicating hydrocephalus and port-wine nevi among family members.[57] The CT scan findings in cases of inferior vermian agenesis consist of pronounced widening of the vallecula, nonvisualization of the inferior vermis, and a large cisterna magna, but without hydrocephalus or other findings of the Dandy-Walker variant (Fig 22–44).

Agenesis of one of the cerebellar hemispheres is rare and may be associated with other cerebral anomalies.[1] Complete agenesis of the cerebellum is extremely rare, but has been reported in association with arthrogryposis

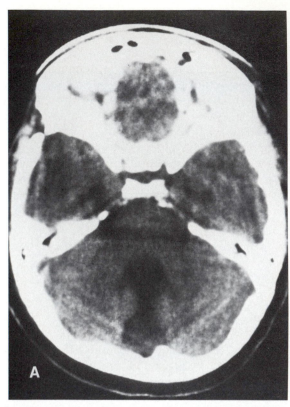

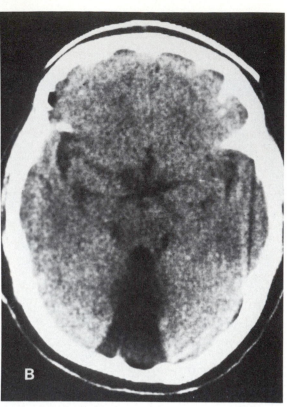

Fig 22–44.—Vermian agenesis in the Joubert syndrome. This 44-year-old patient presented with ophthalmoplegia and midline ataxia. The scan shows a lack of development of vermian tissue **(A, B)** with dilatation of the fourth ventricle **(A).** There was no dilatation of the third or lateral ventricles to suggest the Dandy-Walker variant.

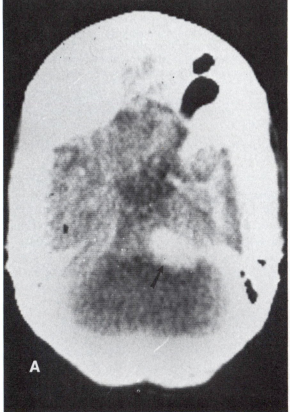

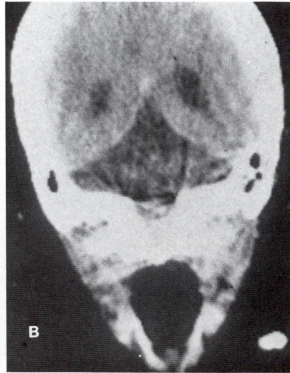

Fig 22–45.—Agenesis of the cerebellum. This 67-year-old woman presented with left-sided hearing loss. The CT scan demonstrates a well-circumscribed enhancing mass (**A**, *arrow*) in the left cerebellopontine angle. There is extensive low density throughout the rest of the posterior fossa behind the brain stem. The coronal scan **(B)** demonstrates CSF density throughout the entire posterior fossa below the tentorial leaves. At the time of craniectomy for tumor removal, no cerebellum was seen; the surgeon looked from the edge of the calvarium directly into brain stem and tumor.

multiplex congenita.[58] Figure 22–45 is that of a 67-year-old woman who complained of hearing loss. Scanning not only demonstrated the presence of an acoustic schwannoma, but there was aplasia of the entire cerebellum. Symptoms referable to that aplasia consisted of only a mild degree of midline ataxia.

Cerebral Cortex

The surface of the fetal brain is smooth during early gestation, but gyri and sulci form secondary to cellular migration that begins in the seventh gestational week. The failure of neuroepithelial cells to migrate from the periventricular germinal matrix to the cortical surface of the brain results in abnormalities in the formation of gyri, fissures, and sulci of both the cerebrum and cerebellum. The subsequent anomalies consist of polymicrogyria, agyria-pachygyria (lissencephaly), and heterotopic gray matter.

Polymicrogyria is a condition consisting of an increased number of gyri that are smaller than normal, producing a cobblestone texture to the surface of the brain. Pachygyria is characterized by a few broad gyri separated by a decreased number of sulci (Fig 22–46). An extreme degree of pachygyria is agyria or lissencephaly (smooth brain). The lack of neuronal migration produces nests of periventricular cells that project into the ventricle and are known as heterotopic gray matter.

The CT findings in the lissencephaly syndrome have been rarely described.[59, 60] There is a lack of development of the temporal and frontal opercula, leaving the insula exposed. This produces the appearance of a deep cleft in the region of the Sylvian fissure, communicating with the cerebral surface (Fig 22–47). Both axial and coronal scanning is of value in defining this cleft and the shape of the frontal and temporal lobes. The surface of the brain appears to be smoother than the usual neonatal brain, although it should be stressed that the normal infant brain appears smoother than the adult brain, particularly on the older CT scanners.

Patients with lissencephaly are characterized by severe mental retardation, seizures, and microcephaly. Associated congenital cerebral anomalies are frequent, and death usually occurs early.

Brain Size

Microcephaly

A small brain may be secondary to many different etiologies, such as destructive lesions (e.g., infectious lesions of the STORCH group), degenerative and metabolic disorders (e.g., phenylketonuria), chromosomal anomalies, and various congenital cerebral malformations. Those malformations include the lissencephaly syndrome, holoprosencephaly, and absence of the corpus callosum,[1] all of which have been discussed previously in this chapter.

Megalencephaly

Enlargement of the head may occur for many reasons, including hydrocephalus, cerebral edema from a variety of causes, extracerebral fluid collections, diffuse thickening of the skull, and megalencephaly. The term "megalencephaly" refers to an enlarged brain caused by an increase in the volume of nonedematous cerebral parenchyma.

DeMyer has produced a classification of megalen-

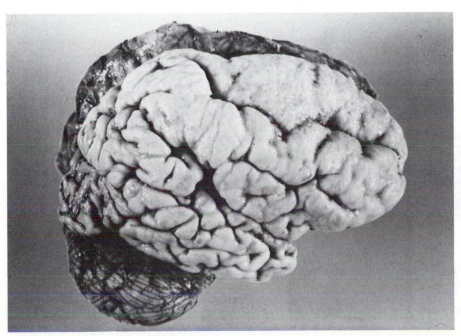

Fig 22–46.—Pachygyria. This photograph of a brain removed at autopsy shows broad gyri over the right convexity. These gyri are smooth, and there is a lack of division by sulci.

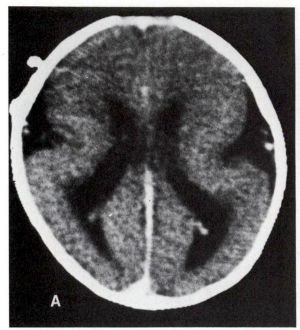
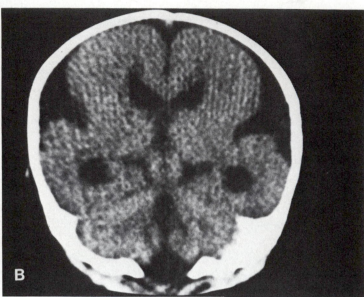

Fig 22–47.—Lissencephaly. This 4-month-old child was scanned because of a failure to thrive. The axial **(A)** and coronal **(B)** scans demonstrate small frontal lobes and deep clefts in the regions of the Sylvian fissures bilaterally. The clefts are due to lack of development of the temporal and frontal opercula, leaving the insula exposed bilaterally. The surface of the brain is smooth, which gives the name lissencephaly ("smooth brain") to the malformation.

cephaly, dividing cases into those with unilateral or those with bilateral parenchymal enlargement and also basing the classification upon anatomical or metabolic causation.[61] Unilateral megalencephaly may be secondary to abnormal cell migration in the third intrauterine month[62] and may be associated with somatic hemihypertrophy.[61] The metabolic megalencephalies include cerebral enlargement associated with aminoaciduria; leukodystrophies such as Canavan's and Alexander's diseases, Tay-Sachs disease, and metachromatic leukodystrophy; and mucopolysaccharidoses such as Hunter-Hurler's disease.

The majority of megalencephalies are bilateral with a brain that is anatomically large, but without a metabolic or infiltrative abnormality. For example, megalencephaly occurs in the gigantism syndromes, such as cerebral and pituitary gigantism. Parenchymal enlargement may also be seen with the neurocutaneous syndromes such as tuberous sclerosis and neurofibromatosis (Fig 22–48).[61, 63] Megalencephaly may be seen with syndromes producing dwarfism, most notably achondroplasia. Probably the most common conditions, however, are brains that are simply at the upper limits of normal in size or occur in multiple family members without any other associated syndromes.

Generally, CT scanning demonstrates a normal-appearing brain that is unremarkable except for the physical finding of increased size relative to age. In some cases, the ventricular system may appear to be mildly enlarged for age (see Fig 22–48). However, the ventricles appear to be proportional in size to the amount of cerebral parenchyma present. It is important to emphasize in such cases that the overall cranial enlargement is not due to hydrocephalus. Long-standing controversy has been present regarding the role of ventricular dilatation vs. nonhydrocephalic parenchymal enlargement with achondroplasia.[64] It has been suggested that while megalencephaly may be present at birth in achondroplasia, progressive CSF obstruction at the base of the skull and foramen magnum leads to progressive hydrocephalus in later life.[65]

Dura and Cranium

Encephalocele

A defect in the closure of the embryologic neural tube may cause an abnormality in the cranium and underlying meninges. There is a spectrum of the abnormalities of closure, with the most mild being cranium bifidum occultum, analogous to spina bifida occulta. A cutaneous component is frequently present, such as a dermal sinus leading through the congenital cranial defect, which may be associated with an intracranial dermoid cyst. Herniation of the meninges through the cranial defect is termed a meningocele, while herniation of both brain and meninges is termed an encephalocele.

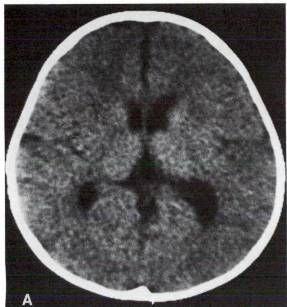

Fig 22–48.—Megalencephaly associated with neurofibromatosis. This 21-month-old child had a head circumference greater than 3 SD of the mean for his age. He had peripheral stigmata of neurofibromatosis. In an absolute sense, the lateral ventricles **(A, B)** are slightly larger than normal for this age, but are proportional to the size of the rest of the brain, characteristic of megalencephaly.

Encephaloceles are midline anomalies with an occipital location occurring in 70% of cases.[66] Encephaloceles are frequently accompanied by congenital anomalies of the brain such as the Chiari malformation. Occipital encephalocele may be associated with holoprosencephaly and/or aqueductal stenosis,[67] while agenesis of the corpus callosum is known to accompany an encephalocele at the posterior fontanel.[1] A nasofrontal encephalocele may project into the medial aspect of the orbit, producing a mass in this region, a broad base of the nose, and hypertelorism. An encephalocele passing through the cribriform plate or through a defect in the sphenoid and/or ethmoid bone may produce a mass in the nose or nasopharynx. Because both nasal polyps and adenoid tissue are rare in infants, the clinician should be wary of the diagnosis of encephalocele with a mass in such a location in the infant. Transsphenoidal encephaloceles are associated with facial anomalies such as cleft lip and cleft palate[6] and with midline malformations of the brain such as agenesis of the corpus callosum.[68]

The density of an encephalocele is variable, depending on the relative amounts of brain and CSF within the protruding sac. Multiple projections are necessary for complete evaluation of these lesions, including direct coronal and sagittal projections (Fig 22–49) or sagittal and coronal computer reformations (Fig 22–50). Close attention to the appropriate bone window will allow definition of the bony defect (see Fig 22–49), which is necessary for appropriate surgical intervention. Metrizamide cisternography may be helpful, particularly for the basal encephaloceles, to better define the communication of the encephalocele with the subarachnoid space.[68] The use of CT scanning should also be directed toward identification of accompanying cerebral malformations such as agenesis of the corpus callosum (Fig

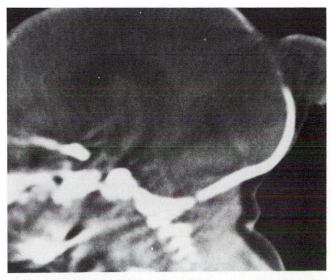

Fig 22–49.—Occipital encephalocele. A direct sagittal scan demonstrates a midline bony defect in the occipital region, with a soft-tissue mass extending posteriorly. There was an associated Chiari II malformation.

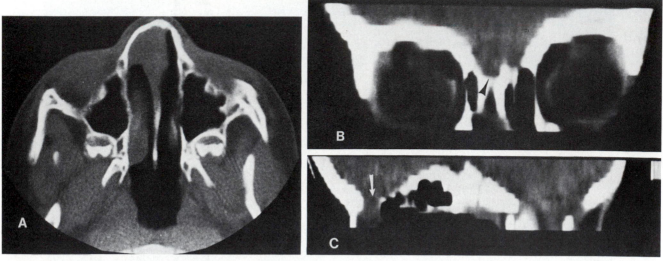

Fig 22–50.—Nasal encephalocele. This 4-year-old boy presented with hypertelorism and a mass in the nose. The axial scan **(A)** demonstrates a soft-tissue mass in the anterior aspect of the right side of the nose. A coronal reconstruction **(B)** shows asymmetry in the region of the cribri-form plate, with deepening and widening of the bony structures to the right of the midline *(arrowhead)*. A sagittal reconstruction **(C)** just to the right of the midline shows the bony defect of the cribriform plate *(arrow)* and a soft-tissue mass extending inferiorly into the nose.

22–51), holoprosencephaly, the Chiari malformation, etc.[67, 68] Angiography may be of value to demonstrate the presence of cerebral tissue within an encephalocele[69] when this is difficult to determine on CT scanning with or without metrizamide.

Craniosynostosis

Craniosynostosis is a general term for premature closure of one or multiple cranial sutures. The particular suture or sutures that close prematurely determine the subsequent shape of the head. For example, premature closure of the sagittal suture prevents lateral growth of the cranium, requiring the increasing cerebral volume to be accommodated by an increased growth in the anteroposterior diameter of the head (scaphocephaly). Premature closure of the coronal sutures prevents growth in the anteroposterior direction, resulting in growth in the lateral and cephalic directions (oxycephaly). Closure of multiple sutures may produce very unusual configurations of the head such as the kleeblattschädel skull deformity ("cloverleaf" skull) (Fig 22–52). Such complex deformities are frequently accompanied by anomalies of the face such as in Figure 22–52. When oxycephaly is accompanied by a flattening in the anteroposterior diameter of the facial structures, particularly in the orbits, bulging of the eyes results. This entire complex of cranial and facial distortions is called Crouzon's disease. The Crouzon malformation may be accompanied by anomalies of the small bones of the hands (Apert's syndrome).

Scanning by CT has been utilized in the evaluation of the various forms of craniosynostosis.[70] Such scanning requires an extensive use of bone windows to evaluate the appearance of the cranial sutures. One may see a "beaking" when there is sutural fusion and pronounced bony overgrowth (Fig 22–53). Evaluation of the cranium may be difficult, however, requiring multiple cuts to determine sutural patency. Because of the sloping of the skull, a false impression of sutural fusion may occur unless the plane of the cut is at right angles to the portion of a suture in question. Skull films undoubtedly will remain an important radiographic technique for this abnormality, although detection of infantile sutures is difficult on plain films alone. Scanning by CT is also useful for the detection of underlying cerebral anomalies.

ECTOPIA

Heterotopic gray matter represents the major ectopia to be discussed. As pointed out in the section dealing with abnormalities of the cerebral cortex (polymicrogyria, pachygyria, lissencephaly), the failure of migration of neuroepithelial cells to the cerebral surface leaves nests of ectopic neurons below the ventricular surface. There is no gliosis associated with these projections, nor is there calcification as is seen with the subependymal nodules (hamartomas) of tuberous sclerosis. While cases of cerebral malformations with pathologically proved heterotopia of gray matter have been de-

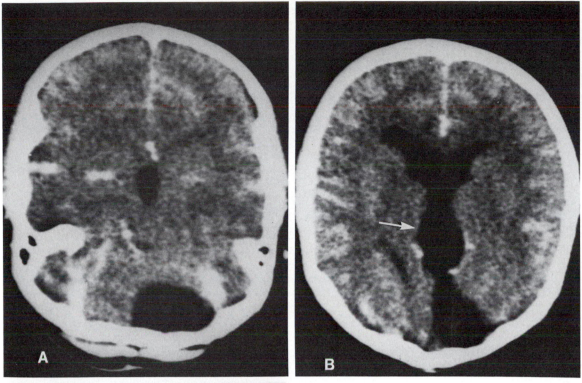

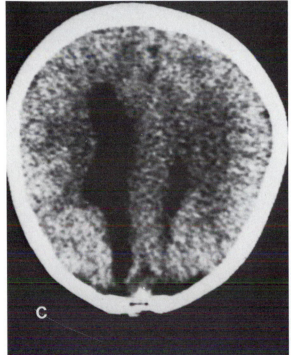

Fig 22–51.—Occipital encephalocele with associated agenesis of the corpus callosum. Photos **A** and **B** demonstrate a large CSF-containing space located in both posterior fossa and supratentorial compartments, just to the left of the midline. The patient had had an occipital encephalocele repaired early in infancy. A tentorial defect must exist to allow the cystic structure to be in both the supratentorial and infratentorial compartments. There is dilatation of the posterior portion of the third ventricle (**B,** *arrow*), which communicates directly with the cystic structure located more posteriorly. Vascular structures are contiguous to this dilated third ventricle, but are laterally displaced. The posterior portion of the corpus callosum is absent. A higher cut (**C**) shows separation of the lateral ventricles, characteristic of agenesis of the corpus callosum. The posterior portions of both lateral ventricles extend posteriorly secondary to the developmental displacement of the brain through the cranial defect.

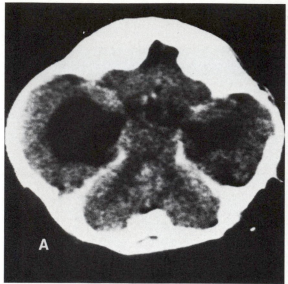
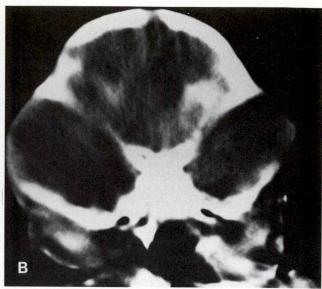

Fig 22–52.—Craniosynostosis: Kleeblattschädel skull ("cloverleaf skull"). Premature fusion of multiple cranial sutures, including the coronal and lambdoid sutures, have produced this gross deformity of the skull as seen on axial **(A)** and coronal **(B)** views. The anteroposterior diameter of the head is markedly shortened, with shallow orbits and midface hypoplasia. The lateral bowing of the temporal regions and high vertex give the name "cloverleaf skull." Ventricular dilatation is also present secondary to the Chiari malformation. The patient had multiple other systemic congenital anomalies of the gastrointestinal and genitourinary systems.

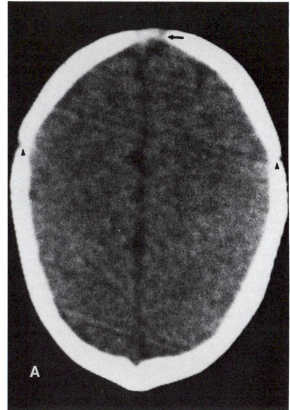
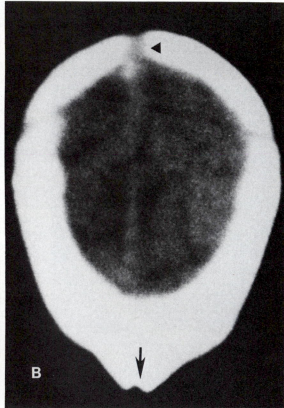
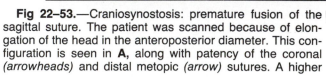

Fig 22–53.—Craniosynostosis: premature fusion of the sagittal suture. The patient was scanned because of elongation of the head in the anteroposterior diameter. This configuration is seen in **A,** along with patency of the coronal *(arrowheads)* and distal metopic *(arrow)* sutures. A higher cut **(B)** demonstrates patency of the anterior portion of the sagittal suture *(arrowhead)*, but a "beaked" configuration *(arrow)* to the cranium posteriorly. This beaking represents sutural fusion and bony overgrowth.

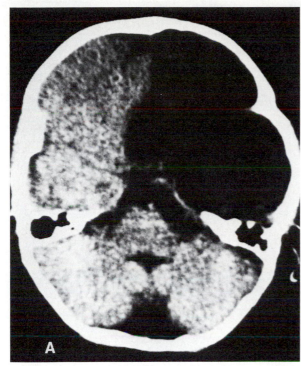

Fig 22–54.—Left frontotemporal arachnoid cyst. This is a large cystic expansion in the left frontotemporal region **(A)** with a density of CSF. The extra-axial expansion has produced thinning and deformity of the overlying calvarium. There is hypoplasia of much of the left frontal and temporal lobes, but not enough to prevent a pronounced midline shift **(B)**. The sharp margins, including the relatively "square" margin along the left basal ganglia, represents the interfaces between the cyst and the deformed frontal and temporal lobes.

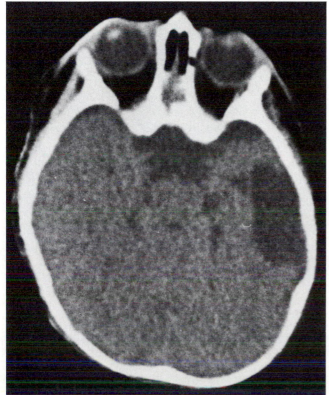

Fig 22–55.—Left temporal arachnoid cyst. The low density, well-marginated cyst in the left temporal region has a classic appearance for an arachnoid cyst. The "square" or slightly inwardly convexed posterior margin of the cyst is the interface between the cyst and the deformed residual temporal lobe.

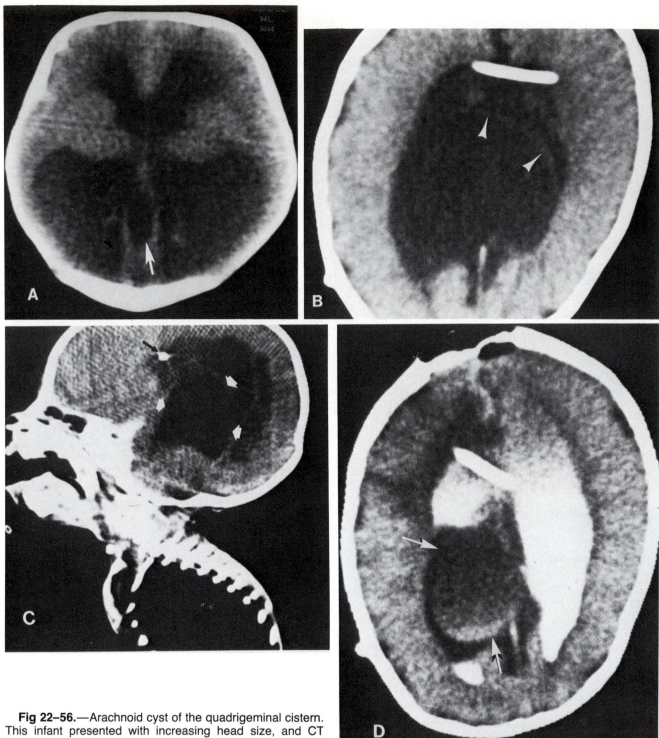

Fig 22–56.—Arachnoid cyst of the quadrigeminal cistern. This infant presented with increasing head size, and CT scanning showed pronounced dilatation of the third and lateral ventricles **(A)**. At first glance, the CSF-containing midline structure **(A,** *arrow)* may appear to be simply a dilated suprapineal recess of the third ventricle, although it is located a bit too far posteriorly. Following ventricular decompression, there has been marked enlargement of the cystic structure in the midline, which is separated from the surrounding ventricular system by a membrane **(B,** *arrowheads)*. A direct sagittal scan **(C)** nicely demonstrates the relationship of the cyst *(white arrows)* separated from the surrounding ventricular system by a membrane. The shunt within the lateral ventricles is noted *(black arrow)*. To further evaluate the anatomy of the cyst and the degree of com- munication with the ventricular system, metrizamide was instilled through the intraventricular shunt **(D).** There is slow accumulation of contrast material in the dependent posterior portion of the cyst *(arrows)* over a number of hours. This poor communication indicated the need for resection or decompressive shunting of the cyst itself. The cyst most likely originated within the quadrigeminal cistern and produced compression of the aqueduct. Surrounding ventricular enlargement kept its apparent size small, but ventricular decompression allowed it to expand rapidly. Its deep periventricular position and its density equal to CSF made it difficult to separate from the surrounding ventricular system.

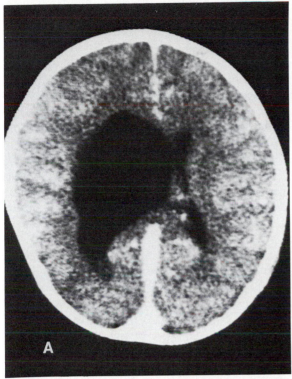

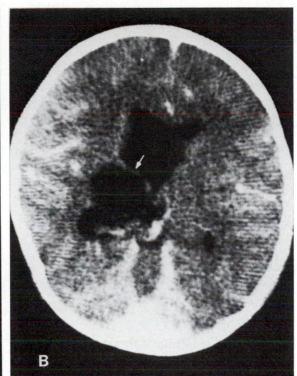

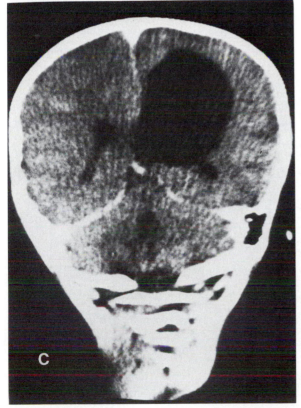

Fig 22–57.—Periventricular arachnoid cyst. A cut through the bodies of the lateral ventricles **(A)** demonstrates a large cystic structure contiguous to and inseparable from the right lateral ventricle. Membranous interfaces between the cyst and the ventricle cannot be seen, suggesting that this may be porencephalic dilatation of the ventricle. A lower cut **(B)** does show separation of the cystic structure in the right thalamic region from the rest of the ventricle by a thin portion of tissue *(arrow)*, but there is a cystic dilatation contiguous to or part of the right frontal horn. It is impossible to separate the cyst from the body of the ventricle on the coronal scan **(C)**. This was considered to most likely be an arachnoid cyst in a periventricular location because of the separation of the cyst from the ventricle in the right thalamic region. However, the occasional appearance of separation of a porencephalic cyst from the rest of the ventricle inferiorly, analogous to that seen in Figure 22–38, prompted direct puncture of the cyst with the instillation of metrizamide. No communication between the cyst and the ventricular system could be visualized (not shown). A craniotomy was performed, with marsupialization of the cyst into the right lateral ventricle and subsequent ventriculocystoperitoneal shunting.

scribed in the CT literature,[71] the heterotopic nodules themselves have not actually been identified on CT. While the newer high-resolution scanners may show these subtle nodular excrescences from the ventricular surface, particularly with the use of intraventricular water-soluble contrast agents, CT scanning is most useful for the detection and evaluation of cerebral malformations associated with gray matter heterotopia.

CONGENITAL TUMORS

The teratomatous tumors and intracranial hamartomas and lipomas are extensively discussed in Chapter 11. Various neuroectodermal tumors occur during early infancy and are considered to be on a congenital basis. These tumors, including astrocytomas, ependymomas, and the various forms of the primitive neuroepithelial tumor, are discussed extensively in Chapter 9 of this volume.

CYSTS

Craniopharyngioma and Rathke's Pouch Cyst

These congenital cystic lesions found in the sellar and suprasellar regions are discussed in Chapter 16.

Arachnoid Cyst

An arachnoid cyst is an extraparenchymal nonneoplastic fluid accumulation having a density similar to CSF. The most frequent location is the temporal fossa, with other common sites being the cerebellopontine angle, the retrocerebellar space, the ambient and quadrigeminal plate cisterns, the suprasellar cisterns, and the interhemispheric fissure. While some arachnoid cysts are most likely secondary to trauma[72] or infection, the majority appear to be congenital in nature. Controversy exists as to the pathogenesis of the congenital lesions. One theory is that the accumulation of fluid between leaves of arachnoid during cerebral development causes secondary hypoplasia of the contiguous brain tissue.[73] A contrasting theory is that of primary hypoplasia of the cerebral lobe with secondary cystic accumulation of fluid.[74] In either case, the slowly growing lesion present during skull maturation produces bony deformity (Fig 22–54).

Scanning by CT demonstrates that arachnoid cysts are sharply marginated, nonenhancing lesions of a density equal to CSF (Figs 22–54 to 22–59). There is no calcific rim as seen with some epidermoid and dermoid cysts (see Figs 11–4 and 11–5). An arachnoid cyst located in the temporal region frequently has a straight posterior margin, representing the interface between the cyst and the deformed temporal lobe (see Fig 22–55).[75] The margins of an arachnoid cyst may be difficult to separate from adjoining ventricular structures (see Figs 22–56 and 22–57).

For example, an arachnoid cyst in the quadrigeminal

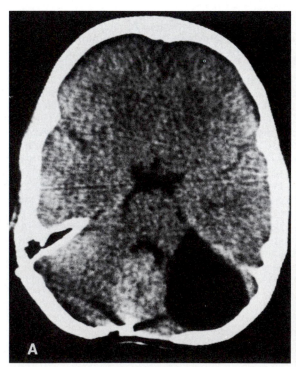
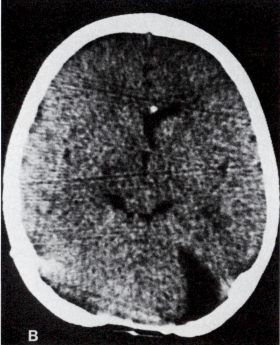

Fig 22–58.—Posterior fossa subarachnoid cyst. There is a large laterally positioned extracerebellar arachnoid cyst that displaces the fourth ventricle slightly to the right (A). A higher cut (B) demonstrates the cyst curving over the upper portion of the cerebellum, and a shunt within the decompressed lateral ventricles. A metrizamide cisternogram with scanning over 24 hours did not show any communication between the subarachnoid spaces and the cyst (not shown).

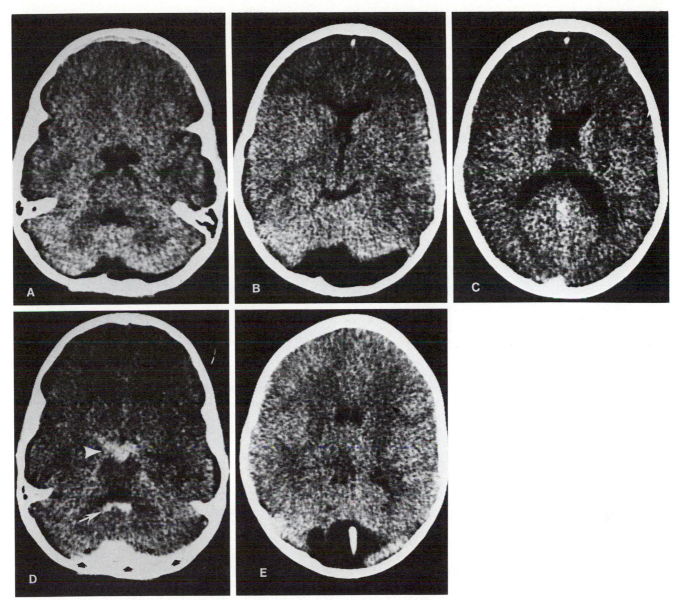

Fig 22–59.—Retrocerebellar arachnoid cyst simulating enlarged cisterna magna. This 7-year-old male presented with a history of intermittent headaches, drooping of the eyes, bilateral leg weakness, and falling to the ground. The initial scans (**A, B, C**) show a lucency behind the cerebellum without displacement of the fourth ventricle, having a configuration like an enlarged cisterna magna. The lateral ventricles (**C**) are borderline in size for a patient of this age. Metrizamide cisternography was subsequently performed via lumbar puncture and demonstrated immediate filling of the cystic structure (**D,** *small black arrows*) by the metrizamide, along with opacification of the fourth ventricle (**D,** *white arrow*) and the interpeduncular and perimesencephalic cisterns (**D,** *white arrowhead*). The degree of free communication between the subarachnoid spaces and cystic structure again suggests an enlarged cisterna magna. Because of the patient's symptoms, surgical exploration of the posterior fossa was elected. At operation, the distended dura was bluish in color, and the fluid within the cyst was under extremely high pressure. A shunt was placed between the cyst and the peritoneal cavity, and postoperatively the patient had no more symptoms. A postoperative scan (**E**) demonstrated decrease in the size of the lateral ventricles. The CT appearance of the retrocerebellar cystic structure had an appearance of an enlarged cisterna magna on both the plain scan and the cisternography, but symptoms suggested the presence of an arachnoid cyst. The presence of symptoms, the high pressure within the cyst at surgery, and the decrease in the size of the lateral ventricles confirmed the diagnosis of arachnoid cyst.

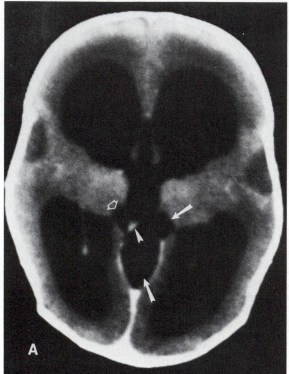
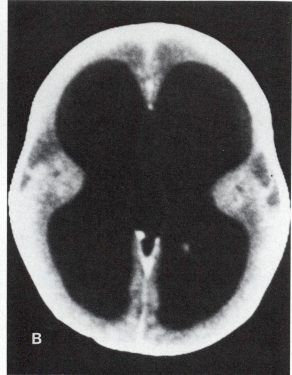

Fig 22–60.—Obstructive hydrocephalus with ventricular diverticula. There is marked dilatation of the third and lateral ventricles **(A, B)**, most likely from aqueductal obstruction. A diverticulum from the medial aspect of the left ventricular atrium **(A,** *closed arrows*) extends medially and posteriorly through the tentorial incisura to lie in the superior cerebellar cistern. A smaller diverticulum is seen on the right **(A,** *open arrow*). An enhancing vascular structure *(arrowhead)* separates both the smaller right ventricular diverticulum and the posterior portion of the third ventricle from the larger left

ventricular diverticulum. No separation is seen between the left ventricular diverticulum and the lucency in the superior cerebellar cistern, suggesting that the lucencies are in contiguity and are all a large diverticulum. An arachnoid cyst in the quadrigeminal cistern, analogous to that seen in Figure 22–56, cannot be absolutely excluded. The easiest method of confirmation is to repeat the scan following ventricular shunting to see if the posterior and medial cystic lucencies are decompressed. Metrizamide could also be placed through the shunt to look for communication.

and superior cerebellar cisterns may produce compression of the aqueduct, leading to obstructive hydrocephalus (see Fig 22–56); this appearance may be indistinguishable, however, from obstructive hydrocephalus from any other cause, such as congenital aqueductal stenosis leading to ventricular enlargement and a dilated suprapineal recess of the third ventricle or a ventricular diverticulum (Fig 22–60). Likewise, an arachnoid cyst in the intrasellar-suprasellar cisterns may be difficult to separate from a dilated third ventricle.[76] Sagittal and coronal projections are an invaluable addition to the axial view when evaluating the complex anatomy of these cysts and their relationships to contiguous parenchymal and ventricular structures (see Figs 22–56 and 22–57). Intraventricular and/or intracisternal metrizamide studies are extremely valuable in separating the cyst from contiguous portions of a ventricle (see Fig 22–56) and in the presurgical evaluation of the CSF dynamics for the appropriate intraventricular or intracystic placement of a shunt.

Arachnoid cysts may be divided into two types, those that freely communicate with the subarachnoid space and those that are relatively noncommunicating with this space. Theories for fluid accumulation in the latter type include secretions by the cyst wall, osmotic differences between cyst fluid and CSF, and ball-valve actions by slits in the cyst wall, allowing the slow entry of CSF, but no egress of fluid from the cyst.[77] Air or metrizamide may freely enter a communicating cyst (see Fig 22–59), while in the poorly communicating ones there will be only slow accumulation of metrizamide over a matter of hours as detected by CT scanning (see Fig 22–56), giving support to the ball-valve theory.[77, 78] It is difficult to understand how a freely communicating cyst might produce mass effect if it were able to decompress itself directly into adjoining subarachnoid cisterns. This author wonders if such a loculation might not represent an aspect of communicating hydrocephalus secondary to arachnoidal adhesions, with the generalized ventricular dilatation secondary to those adhe-

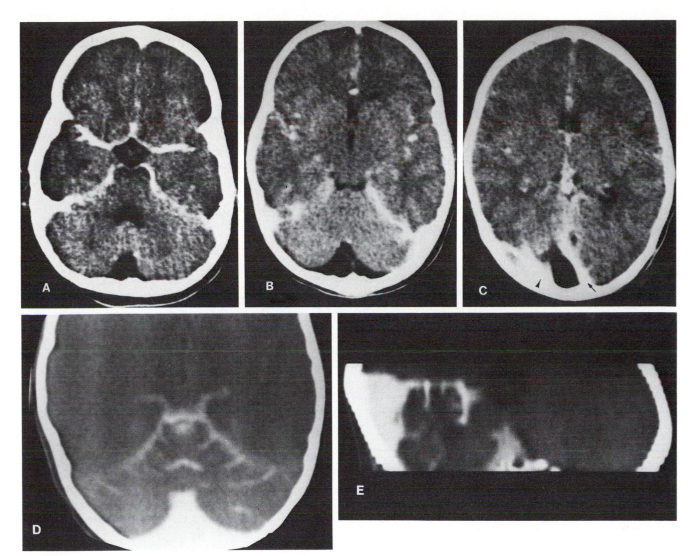

Fig 22–61.—Enlarged cisterna magna. This 9-year-old child was scanned because of head trauma, and a retrocerebellar cystic structure was seen, having the typical "figure-3" configuration of an enlarged cisterna magna (**A, B**) and not displacing the fourth ventricle. The cisterna magna invaginated between the right transverse sinus (**C,** *arrowhead*) and the displaced distal straight sinus and torcula (**C,** *arrow*). Such a finding is common with an enlarged cisterna magna. The lateral ventricles were not enlarged (**B, C**). While all of the findings supported the diagnosis of an enlarged cisterna magna, and not an arachnoid cyst, worry on the part of the referring physician for the presence of an arachnoid cyst prompted the performance of a metrizamide cisternogram via lumbar puncture. The axial scan (**D**) and sagittal reformation (**E**) demonstrate metrizamide filling the cisterna magna above and behind the cerebellum, with filling of prepontine and ambient cisterns and sulci over the cerebellum. Again, the configuration is classic for an enlarged cisterna magna. The lack of further symptoms did not suggest the need for further evaluation as in the case shown in Figure 22–59.

sions rather than from the effects of the "cyst" itself (see Fig 22–59).[51]

The type of communication is of therapeutic importance in that both the dilated ventricular system and a cyst that freely communicates with that ventricular system should be adequately decompressed with shunting of either the ventricular system or cyst (see Fig 22–59). A dilated ventricular system and a cyst with poor communication will require both shunting of the ventricular system and either shunting or resection of the cyst itself (see Fig 22–56).[51, 78]

A note of caution must be raised in the diagnosis of a retrocerebellar arachnoid cyst. The enlarged cisterna magna that is a normal variant has a "figure-3" configuration and freely communicates with the subarachnoid spaces (Fig 22–61). Such normal variants have been misdiagnosed as arachnoid cysts in patients who have no evidence of fourth ventricular displacement or hydrocephalus. On the other hand, a retrocerebellar arachnoid cyst may also have, in part, a similar configuration as it molds itself around the cerebellum (see Fig 22–59). When confusion exists, metrizamide cisternography would demonstrate the degree of communication with the subarachnoid cisterns (see Fig 22–59); the necessity of subsequent surgery would depend upon the clinical symptoms and presence of ventricular dilatation.

Low-density nonenhancing neoplasms have frequently been diagnosed as arachnoid, epidermoid, or porencephalic cysts. The distinction between a low-density glial tumor and a cyst such as an arachnoid cyst does not depend on absorption coefficients, which may be similar in either case.[79] Rather, the distinction is made on the basis of the margins of the lesion. While low-density glial tumors frequently have relatively sharp contours in many areas, some degree of irregularity is usually present (see Figs 9–14, 9–15, and 9–21). An arachnoid cyst, on the other hand, is sharply marginated in all projections; this determination requires multiple CT scanning projections.

REFERENCES

1. Ludwin S.K., Malamud N.: Pathology of congenital anomalies of the brain, in Newton T.H., Potts D.G. (eds.): *Radiology of the Skull and Brain*. St. Louis, C.V. Mosby Co., 1977, vol. 3, pp. 2979–3015.
2. DeMyer W.: Classification of cerebral malformations. *Birth Defects* 7:78–93, 1971.
3. Nakano S., Hojo H., Kataoka K., et al.: Age related incidence of cavum septi pellucidi and cavum vergae on CT scans of pediatric patients. *J. Comput. Assist. Tomogr.* 5:348–349, 1981.
4. Russell D.S.: *Observations on the Pathology of Hydrocephalus*. London, Her Majesty's Stationery Office, 1949.
5. Luduiczuk R., Dietemann J.L., Wachenheim A.: CT and pneumographic studies of membraneous occlusion of the aqueduct of sylvius. *Neuroradiology* 18:53–55, 1979.
6. Strother C.M., Harwood-Nash D.C.: Congenital malformations, in Newton T.H., Potts D.G. (eds.): *Radiology of the Skull and Brain*. St. Louis, C.V. Mosby Co., 1978, pp. 3712–3748.
7. Lichtenstein B.W.: Distant neuroanatomic complications of spina bifida (spinal dysraphism): Hydrocephalus, Arnold-Chiari deformity, stenosis of the aqueduct of sylvius, etc.; pathogenesis and pathology. *Arch. Neurol. Neurosurg. Psychiatry* 47:195–214, 1942.
8. Gardner W.J.: Myelomeningocele: The result of rupture of the embryonic neural tube. *Cleveland Clin. O.* 27:88–100, 1960.
9. Gardner W.J.: Hydrodynamic mechanism of syringomyelia: Its relationship to myelocele. *J. Neurol. Neurosurg. Psychiatry* 28:247–259, 1965.
10. Gardner W.J.: Myelocele: Rupture of the neural tube? *Clin. Neurol. Neurosurg.* 15:57–79, 1967.
11. Daniel P.M., Strich S.J.: Some observations on the congenital deformity of the central nervous system known as the Arnold-Chiari malformation. *J. Neuropathol. Exp. Neurol.* 17:255–266, 1958.
12. Woosley R.E., Wholey R.A.: Use of metrizamide in computerized tomography to diagnose the Chiari I malformation. *J. Neurosurg.* 56:373–376, 1982.
13. DeBarros M.C., Farias W., Ataide L., et al.: Basilar impression and Arnold-Chiari malformation: A study of 66 cases. *J. Neurol. Neurosurg. Psychiatry* 31:596–605, 1968.
14. Naidich T.P., Pudlowski R.M., Naidich J.B.: Computed tomographic signs of the Chiari II malformation: III. Ventricles and cisterns. *Radiology* 134:657–663, 1980.
15. Naidich T.P., Pudlowski R.M., Naidich J.B.: Computed tomographic signs of Chiari II malformations: II. Midbrain and cerebellum. *Radiology* 134:391–398, 1980.
16. Naidich T.P., Pudlowski R.M., Naidich J.B., et al.: Computed tomographic signs of the Chiari II malformation: I. Skull and dural partitions. *Radiology* 134:65–71, 1980.
17. Dubois P.J., Heinz E.R., Wessel N.B., et al.: Multiple cystic encephalomalacia of infancy: Computed tomographic findings in two cases with associated intracerebral calcifications. *J. Comput. Assist. Tomogr.* 3:97–102, 1979.
18. Seigel R.S., Seeger J.F., Gabrielsen T.O., et al.: Computed tomography in oculocraniosomatic disease (Kearn-Sayre syndrome). *Radiology* 130:159–164, 1979.
19. Savolaine E.R., Gerber A.M.: Computerized tomography studies of congenital and acquired intraventricular membranes: Report of two cases. *J. Neurosurg.* 54:388–391, 1981.
20. Dandy W.E., Blackfan K.D.: Internal hydrocephalus: An experimental, clinical and pathological study. *Am. J. Dis. Child.* 8:406–482, 1914.
21. Taggart J.K. Jr., Walker A.E.: Congenital atresia of the foramens of Luschka and Magendie. *Arch. Neurol. Psychiatry* 48:583–612, 1942.

22. Padget D.H.: Development of so-called dysraphism, with embryologic evidence of clinical Arnold-Chiari and Dandy-Walker malformations. *Johns Hopkins Med. J.* 130:127–165, 1972.

23. Lehman R.M.: Dandy-Walker syndrome in consecutive siblings: Familial hindbrain malformation. *Neurosurgery* 8:717–719, 1981.

24. Carmel P.W., Antemes J.L., Hilal S.K., et al.: Dandy-Walker syndrome: Clincopathological features and re-evaluation of modes of treatment. *Surg. Neurol.* 8:132–138, 1977.

25. Vaquero J., Carillo R., Cabezudo J.M. et al.: Arachnoid cysts of the posterior fossa. *Surg. Neurol.* 16:117–121, 1981.

26. Archer C.R., Darwish H., Smith K.: Enlarged cisternae magnae and posterior fossa cysts simulating Dandy-Walker syndrome. *Radiology* 127:681–686, 1978.

27. Adam R., Greenberg J.O.: The mega cisterna magna. *J. Neurosurg.* 48:190–192, 1978.

28. Scotti G., Musgrave M.A., Fitz C.R., et al.: The isolated fourth ventricle in children: CT and clinical review in 16 cases. *A.J.N.R.* 1:419–424, 1980.

29. Gutierrez Y., Friede R.L., Kaliney W.J.: Agenesis of arachnoid granulations and its relationship to communicating hydrocephalus. *J. Neurosurg.* 43:553–558, 1975.

30. DeMyer W., Zeman W.: Alobar holoprosencephaly (arhinencephaly) with median cleft lip and palate: Clinical, electroencephalographic and nosologic considerations. *Confinia Neurologica* 23:1–36, 1963.

31. Manelfe C., Sevely A.: Neuroradiological study of holoprosencephalies. *J. Neuroradiol.* 9:15–45, 1982.

32. Byrd S.E., Harwood-Nash D.C., Fitz C.R., et al.: Computed tomography evaluation of holoprosencephaly in infants and children. *J. Comput. Assist. Tomogr.* 1:456–463, 1977.

33. Hayashi T., Yoshida M., Kuramoto S., et al.: Radiological features of holoprosencephaly. *Surg. Neurol.* 12:261–265, 1979.

34. Derakhshan I., Sabouri-Deylami M., Lofti J.: Holoprosencephaly: Computerized tomographic and pneumographic findings with anatomic correlation. *Arch. Neurol.* 37:55–57, 1980.

35. Osaka K., Matsumoto S.: Holoprosencephaly in neurosurgical practice. *J. Neurosurg.* 48:787–803, 1978.

36. DeMyer W., Zeman W., Palmer C.: The face predicts the brain: Diagnostic significance of median facial anomalies for holoprosencephaly (arhinencephaly). *Pediatrics* 34:256–263, 1964.

37. DeMyer W.: Holoprosencephaly (cyclopia-arhinencephaly), in Vinken P.J., Bruyn G.W. (eds.): *Handbook of Neurology*. Amsterdam, North Holland Pub. Co., 1977, vol. 30, pp. 431–478.

38. Hayashi T., Takagi S., Kuramoto S.: A case of holoprosencephaly with possible association of Dandy-Walker cyst. *Brain Dev.* 3:97–101, 1981.

39. Manelfe C., Rochiccioli P.: CT of septo-optic dysplasia. *A.J.R.* 133:1157–1160, 1979.

40. O'Dwyer J.A., Newton T.H., Hoyt W.F.: Radiologic features of septo-optic dysplasia: deMorsier syndrome. *A.J.N.R.* 1:443–447, 1980.

41. Krause-Brucker W., Gardner D.W.: Optic nerve hypoplasia associated with absent septum pellucidum and hypopituitarism. *Am. J. Ophthalmol.* 89:113–120, 1980.

42. Loeser J.D., Alvord E.C. Jr.: Agenesis of the corpus callosum. *Brain* 91:553–570, 1968.

43. Marina R., Pero G., Nicoletti F.: Computed tomography findings in agenesis of corpus callosum. *Acta Neurol.* 36:435–438, 1981.

44. Solt L.C., Deck J.H., Baim R.S., et al.: Interhemispheric cyst of neuroepithelial origin in association with partial agenesis of the corpus callosum: Case report and review of the literature. *J. Neurosurg.* 52:399–403, 1980.

45. Phillips H.E., Carter A.P., Kennedy J.L. Jr., et al.: Aicardi's syndrome: Radiologic manifestations. *Radiology* 127:453–455, 1978.

46. Besigye E.: Diagnosis of agenesis of the corpus callosum by computer assisted tomography: Report of two cases presenting with epileptic seizures. *Comput. Tomogr.* 3:155–158, 1979.

47. Lynn R.B., Buchanan D.C., Fenechel G.M., et al.: Agenesis of the corpus callosum. *Arch. Neurol.* 37:444–445, 1980.

48. Yakovlev P.I., Wadsworth R.C.: Schizencephalies: A study of the congenital clefts in the cerebral mantle: I. Clefts with fused lips. *J. Neuropathol. Exp. Neurol.* 5:116–130, 1946a.

49. Yakovlev P.I., Wadsworth R.C.: Schizencephalies: A study of the congenital clefts in the cerebral mantle: II. Clefts with hydrocephalus and lips separated. *J. Neuropathol. Exp. Neurol.* 5:169–206, 1946b.

50. Lyon G., Robain O.: Etude comparative des encephalopathies circulatoires prenatales et para-natales (hydranencephalies, porencephalies et encephalomalacies kystiques de la substance blanche). *Acta Neuropathol.* 9:79–98, 1967.

51. Latchaw R.E., Albright A.L., Rothfus W.E., et al.: Physiological evaluation of arachnoid and other intracranial cysts using metrizamide and CT scanning (in preparation).

52. Aicardi J., Goutieres F.: The syndrome of absence of the septum pellucidum with porencephalies and other developmental defects. *Neuropediatrics* 12:319–329, 1981.

53. Dublin A.B., French B.N.: Diagnostic image evaluation of hydranencephaly and pictorially similar entities, with emphasis on computed tomography. *Radiology* 137:81–91, 1980.

54. Joubert M., Eisenring J.J., Robb J.P., et al.: Familial agenesis of the cerebellar vermis: A syndrome of episodic hyperpnea, abnormal eye movements, ataxia, and retardation. *Neurology* 19:813–825, 1969.

55. Curatolo P., Mercuri S., Cotroneo E.: Joubert syndrome: A case confirmed by computerized tomography. *Dev. Med. Child Neurol.* 22:362–366, 1980.

56. Lindhout D., Barth P.G., Valk J., et al.: The Joubert syndrome associated with bilateral chorioretinal coloboma. *Eur. J. Pediatr.* 134:173–176, 1980.

57. Nova H.R.: Familial communicating hydrocephalus, posterior cerebellar agenesis, mega cisterna magna, and port-wine nevi: Report on five members in one family. *J. Neurosurg.* 51:862–865, 1979.

58. Yoshida M., Nakamura M.: Complete absence of the cerebellum with arihrogyposis multiplex congenita diagnosed by CT scan. *Surg. Neurol.* 17:62–65, 1982.

59. Garcia C.A., Dunn D., Trevor R.: The lissencephaly (agyria) syndrome in siblings: Computerized tomographic and neuropathologic findings. *Arch. Neurol.* 35:608–611, 1978.

60. Ohno K., Enomoto T., Imamoto J., et al.: Lissencephaly (agyria) on computed tomography. *J. Comput. Assist. Tomogr.* 3:92–95, 1979.

61. DeMyer W.: Megalencephaly in children: Clinical syndromes, genetic patterns, and differential diagnosis from other causes of megalencephaly. *Neurology* 22:634–643, 1972.

62. Fitz C.R., Harwood-Nash D.C., Boldt D.W.: The radiographic features of unilateral megalencephaly. *Neuroradiology* 15:145–148, 1978.

63. Patronas N.K., Zelkowitz M., Levin K.: Ventricular dilatation in neurofibromatosis. *J. Comput. Assist. Tomogr.* 6:598–600, 1982.

64. Mueller S.M., Bell W., Cornell S., et al.: Achondroplasia and hydrocephalus: A computerized tomographic, roentgenographic, and psychometric study. *Neurology* 27:430–434, 1977.

65. Mueller S.M.: Enlarged central ventricular system in infant achondroplastic dwarf. *Neurology* 30:767–769, 1980.

66. Matson D.D.: *Neurosurgery of Infancy and Childhood,* ed. 2. Springfield, Ill., Charles C Thomas, Publisher, 1969.

67. Hutchinson J.W., Stoving J., Turner P.T.: Occipital encephalocele with holoprosencephaly and aqueduct stenosis. *Surg. Neurol.* 12:331–335, 1979.

68. Manelfe C., Starling-Jardim D., Touibi S., et al.: Transsphenoidal encephalocele associated with agenesis of corpus callosum: Value of metrizamide computed cisternography. *J. Comput. Assist. Tomogr.* 2:356–361, 1978.

69. Pinto R.S., George A.E., Koslow M., et al.: Neuroradiology of basal anterior fossa (transethmoidal) encephaloceles. *Radiology* 117:79–85, 1975.

70. Brambilla G.L., Pizzotta S., Rognone F.: CT scan and craniostenosis. *J. Neurosurg. Sci.* 25:13–16, 1981.

71. Mikhael M.A., Mettar A.G.: Malformation of the cerebral cortex with heterotopia of the grey matter. *J. Comput. Assist. Tomogr.* 2:291–296, 1978.

72. Latchaw R.E., Nadell J.: Intra- and extracerebral arachnoid cyst. *A.J.R.* 126:629–633, 1976.

73. Starkman S.P., Brown T.C., Linell E.A.: Cerebral arachnoid cysts. *J. Neuropath. Exp. Neurol.* 17:486–500, 1958.

74. Robinson R.G.: Congenital cysts of the brain: Arachnoid malformations. *Prog. Neurol. Surg.* 4:133–174, 1971.

75. Banna M.: Arachnoid cysts on computed tomography. *A.J.R.* 127:979–982, 1976.

76. Leo J.S., Pinto R.S., Hulvat G.F., et al.: Computed tomography of arachnoid cysts. *Radiology* 130:675–680, 1979.

77. Hayashi T., Kuratomi A., Kuramoto S.: Arachnoid cyst of the quadrigeminal cistern. *Surg. Neurol.* 14:267–273, 1980.

78. Wolpert S.M., Scott R.M.: The value of metrizamide CT cisternography in the management of cerebral arachnoid cysts. *A.J.N.R.* 2:29–35, 1981.

79. Latchaw R.E., Gold L.H.A., Moore J.S., et al.: The nonspecificity of absorption coefficients in the differentiation of solid tumors and cystic lesions. *Radiology* 125:141–144, 1977.

CT in Otolaryngology

23

The Temporal Bone

KATHERINE A. SHAFFER, M.D.

METHODS OF EVALUATING the temporal bone and cerebellopontine angle have undergone dramatic change in recent years as CT scanner technology has advanced to provide thin-section scans with submillimeter spatial resolution. Images produced by CT now rival pluridirectional tomograms for available information, because the improved contrast resolution in CT scans compensates for the better spatial resolution of pluridirectional tomograms. The radiologist must be familiar with temporal bone anatomy to determine which projections will give the most information about a particular structure. As with conventional tomography, multiple scanning planes are necessary to see all portions of the temporal bone. Occasionally, CT in one plane can be combined with pluridirectional tomography in another plane in which it is difficult to perform CT scans. For instance, the descending portion of the facial nerve canal may not be evaluated reliably on axial CT scans, and the canal may also be hard to define on coronal scans. In these instances, a few sagittal tomographic sections will usually demonstrate the canal in its entirety.

TECHNIQUE

The axial plane is the most convenient for CT scans of the temporal bone. We usually do scans parallel to the infraorbitomeatal line, but a plane parallel to the supraorbitomeatal line has some advantages to see specific structures such as the horizontal semicircular canal.[1] Whichever scanning plane is chosen, care should be taken not to have the scanning beam pass directly through the eyes, so radiation dose to the lens is kept to a minimum.

The second plane usually chosen for CT scanning of the temporal bone is the coronal plane. Ideally, this is a true coronal plane similar to that used in pluridirectional tomography, but sometimes this cannot be achieved. We usually use a "hanging head"position, although the patient may be positioned prone with his neck hyperextended. A modified coronal plane, in which the patient lies supine and flexes his neck, can be used for those patients with limited neck extension.[1] Other planes used in pluridirectional tomography can be duplicated with CT if special equipment is available, such as an auxiliary table, tilting head holder, and angling table top.[2] The complex anatomy in the temporal bone often requires different imaging angles to demonstrate specific structures, and scanning planes can be chosen accordingly.[1, 2]

A CT scanner must have several features to make it useful for studying the temporal bone. These include the capability to do thin and/or overlapping slices (2 mm or less thick), a reconstruction algorithm that emphasizes bone detail, and a wide CT number range or edge enhancement computer processing of scan data.

A number of scanners currently on the market are satisfactory for scanning the temporal bone. We use the General Electric (GE) CT/T 8800 body scanner (General Electric Medical Systems, Milwaukee), which has a 1.5-mm collimator. This produces an actual slice thickness of 1.8 mm.[3] Scanning is always done at 120 kVp, so dense bone is easily penetrated by the x-ray beam. In conventional tomography, such a high kilovoltage setting would result in considerable scatter and an unsatisfactory image. When a narrow collimator is chosen, the number of photons reaching the detectors decreases, and the image noise increases. This is noticeable in the brain, but it is not a problem in areas of high subject contrast such as the temporal bone where air, soft tissues, and bone are in contact. If the temporal bone is the only area of interest in the scan, relatively low mAs can be used.[1] If small intracranial soft-tissue structures are being evaluated with the 1.5-mm collimator, we use the highest mA setting that produces 1,152 mAs.

Even when high mAs is used, the x-ray beam is tightly collimated so that there is little scatter. Therefore, the eyes receive insignificant radiation during coronal scanning of the temporal bone. This is also true during axial scanning if the patient is positioned so that the scanning beam does not pass directly through the eyes.[1, 4]

The spatial resolution of a CT system is determined by a number of factors. Spatial resolution, or the ability to distinguish two small dense objects that are close together, cannot be better than the pixel size of the display matrix. Two objects must usually be separated by more than one pixel width to be resolved. Smaller objects can be detected, however, if they raise the CT number of the pixel sufficiently. Therefore, spatial resolution and the size of a detectable object are not the same.[5] Factors other than pixel size influence spatial resolution. These include the following: detector aperture size; focal spot size; distance between the x-ray tube, object, and detectors; size of the reconstruction matrix; type of reconstruction algorithm; and slice thickness.

Contrast resolution is the ability to discriminate two objects that have nearly the same attenuation. In addition to the previous factors, high photon flux is important for good contrast resolution; therefore, the highest mA setting and long scanning time are used with the 1.5-mm collimator when scanning the brain.

High spatial resolution of approximately 0.6 mm can be achieved on our scanner by reconstructing raw data from scans with an algorithm designed to improve spatial resolution at the expense of contrast resolution. This process is called "target reconstruction" or "zoom reconstruction" in general terms, and ReView™ reconstruction by the manufacturer (GE). A portion of the image data is chosen for reconstruction, and this in turn causes magnification of the image and reduction of pixel size in the display. This process will improve spatial resolution only if more information is present in the raw data than was displayed in the original reconstruction. The new pixel size is directly related to the magnification factor or target factor chosen and the old pixel size of the standard reconstruction. Magnification of 3.2 times produces 0.25-mm pixels instead of the standard 0.8-mm pixels (3.2 = 0.8 ÷ 0.25). There is also an edge enhancement effect of the high contrast or "bone detail" reconstruction algorithm.[6]

A wide CT number range is also crucial for studying the temporal bone. Maximum densities in the otic capsule may exceed 2,000 Hounsfield units (HU), but CT numbers above 1,000 HU cannot be differentiated by the standard window width of −1,000 to +1,000 HU. Extension of the CT number range also makes small lucent structures like the semicircular canals visible within the dense temporal bone.[6] A wide CT number range is routinely available on some scanners. We usually view CT scans of the temporal bone at a window width of 4,000 HU, which represents a CT number range of −1000 to +3000 HU.

NORMAL ANATOMY

Two anatomical studies have compared specimen radiographs of temporal bone sections to CT images from the GE CT/T 8800 scanner. One study compared decalcified slices of the temporal bone to CT scans,[7] and the other study compared nondecalcified whole head sections to pluridirectional tomograms and CT scans.[8] Both studies concluded that there was excellent correlation between the 1.5-mm thick CT scans reconstructed with the ReView™ program and the anatomical slices. Littleton and colleagues[8] also found that standard reconstructions of the same slices did not provide adequate information about intratemporal structures and did not compare well with conventional tomograms. Although pluridirectional tomography demonstrated most structures within the temporal bone as well as CT did, false shadows occurred on the tomograms. Some thin areas or curved surfaces of bone such as the tegmen tympani and anterior boundary of the middle cranial fossa were not accurately demonstrated, because the x-ray beam did not strike a tangent to the surface during the exposure (law of tangents). Figure 23–1 illustrates normal anatomy of the right temporal bone in the axial projection, progressing from inferiorly to superiorly. Figure 23–2 shows normal coronal anatomy of the right temporal bone from posteriorly to anteriorly, with tomograms for comparison (Fig 23–3). Five recent publications also illustrate normal CT anatomy of the temporal bone.[2, 9–12]

CONGENITAL ANOMALIES

Congenital abnormalities usually involve the external and middle ear or the inner ear because of differing embryologic origins of these parts of the ear. The embryology of the ear is quite complex; in general, the pinna, tympanic bone, and middle ear develop from the first and second branchial arches and the first branchial groove, whereas the inner ear originates from the otocyst.[13] Anomalies of the middle and inner ear usually coexist only in specific situations: chromosomal abnormalities, craniofacial dysplasias, and malformations caused by maternal ingestion of thalidomide.[14] However, one series reported middle ear or external ear abnormalities in 25% of ears with inner ear malformations.[15] Some of the chromosomal abnormalities known to be associated with inner and middle ear anomalies are trisomy 13, trisomy 18, and trisomy 21. Craniofacial dysplasias include Treacher-Collins syndrome, Crouzon's disease, and Goldenhar's syndrome.

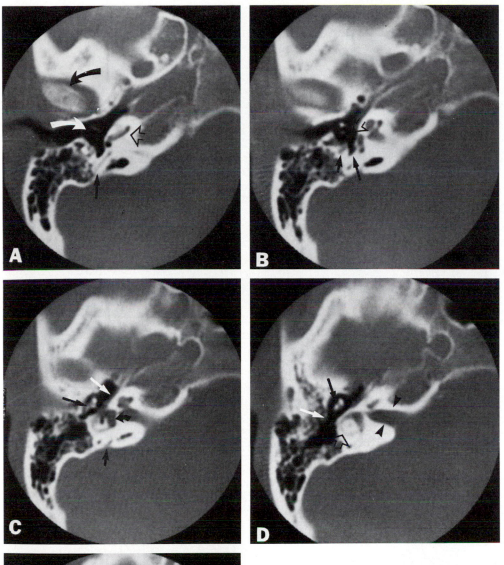

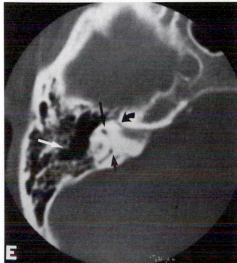

Fig 23–1.—Contiguous 1.5-mm axial scans of right temporal bone reconstructed with ReView™ program and viewed at 4,000-HU window width. Section **A** is most inferior; **E** is the highest section. **A,** handle of the malleus and long process of the incus *(curved white arrow),* cochlea *(open arrow),* posterior semicircular canal *(straight arrow)* and mandibular condyle *(curved black arrow).* **B,** descending portion of the facial nerve canal *(short arrow),* stapes *(open arrow),* and sinus tympani *(long arrow).* **C,** body and short process of the incus *(long arrow),* horizontal portion of facial nerve *(white arrow),* vestibular aqueduct *(short arrow),* vestibule *(curved arrow).* **D,** internal auditory canal *(arrowheads),* horizontal semicircular canal *(open arrow),* aditus ad antrum *(white arrow),* head of malleus and body of incus *(black arrow).* **E,** facial nerve canal *(curved arrow),* common crus *(short arrow),* superior semicircular canal *(long arrow),* mastoid antrum *(white arrow).*

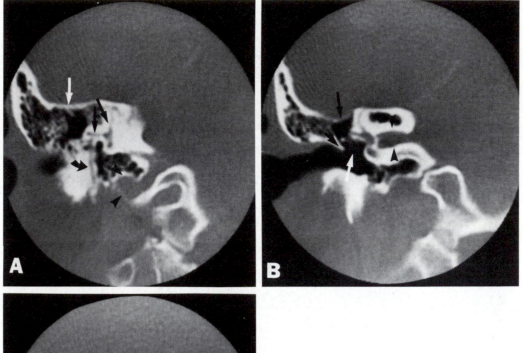

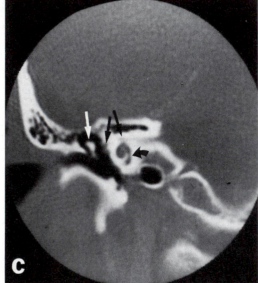

Fig 23–2.—Direct coronal 1.5-mm scans of right temporal bone, reconstructed as described in Figure 23–1. **A,** most posterior section: descending facial nerve canal *(curved arrow),* mastoid antrum with Körner's septum *(white arrow),* horizontal and superior semicircular canals *(long arrows),* jugular fossa *(arrowheads).* **B,** anterior 4.5 mm to **A:** internal auditory canal *(arrowheads),* tegmen *(long arrow),* long process of incus and incudostapedial joint *(white arrow),* drum spur *(short arrow).* **C,** anterior 3 mm to **B.** Malleus *(white arrow),* cochlea *(curved arrow),* limbs of facial nerve canal *(straight arrows).*

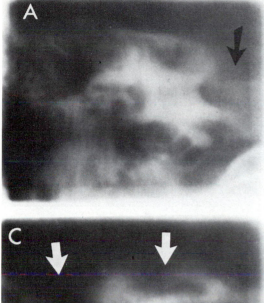
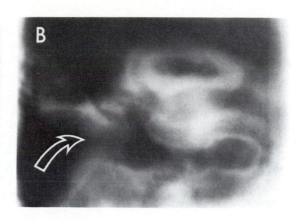
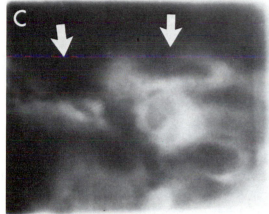

Fig 23–3.—Pluridirectional tomograms at similar levels to scans in Figure 23–2. **A,** most posterior section. There is a false shadow at the medial end of the petrous bone *(arrow).* **B,** anterior 4 mm to **A.** A false shadow is in the external auditory canal *(arrow).* **C,** anterior 3 mm to **B.** Detail of the superior surface of the temporal bone is not sharp *(arrows).*

Pluridirectional tomography has long been used to evaluate congenital abnormalities of the temporal bone, usually in deaf children.[15–19] No studies comparing high-resolution CT with pluridirectional tomography in patients with congenital abnormalities have been published, although some investigators have studied moderate numbers of patients with congenital abnormalities of the middle and external ear.[20]

Detailed radiographic evaluation of the temporal bone is essential in congenital anomalies of the external auditory canal and middle ear if surgery is contemplated. The surgeon must know the state of the middle ear space and ossicles, course of the facial nerve, and mastoid development before attempting reconstructive surgery. The tympanic bone may be atretic with no external auditory canal, or there may be a small canal filled with soft tissue. There is often a bony atresia plate of variable thickness where the tympanic membrane normally exists. The middle ear cavity is often contracted, and it may or may not be pneumatized. Ossicular malformations are common and of varying degrees of severity (Fig 23–4). Part of the malleus or incus may be fused to the bony atresia plate. The course of the facial nerve is frequently abnormal, with the vertical

portion often anteriorly positioned. Greater aberrations in its course exist with more significant atresia of the external auditory canal.[14, 19]

Most external, middle, and inner ear anomalies can be evaluated by CT as well as by pluridirectional tomography. Soft-tissue structures are more reliably identified with CT. Although minor variations in the course of the vertical portion of the facial nerve canal are not identified as well as with lateral pluridirectional tomography, this obstacle could be overcome by high-quality sagittal computer reformatted images or direct sagittal scans.

INFLAMMATORY DISEASE

Simple inflammation of the middle ear seldom requires radiologic investigation. However, chronic otitis media with granulation tissue or complications of infection such as malignant external otitis, labyrinthitis ossificans, or cholesteatoma should have tomography performed, particularly if surgery is anticipated. The role of tomography is not usually to identify the disease process, but to determine the extent of pathology, because the amount of bone destruction and soft-tissue disease

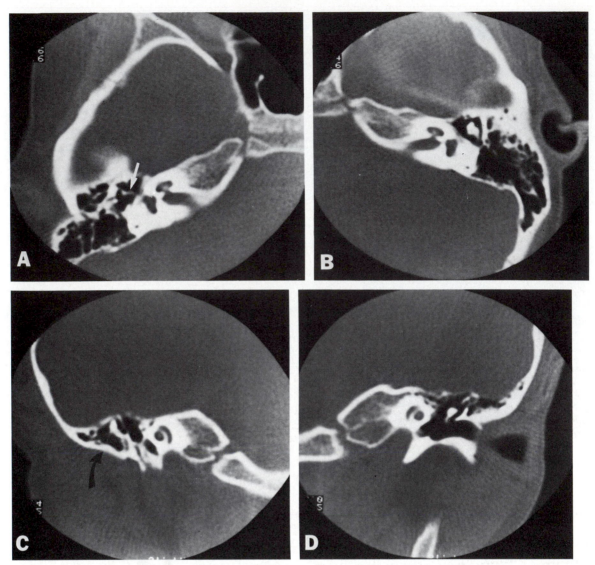

Fig 23–4.—Patient with congenital absence of the right external auditory canal and abnormal middle ear demonstrated on both axial and coronal scans. **A,** right ear, axial section. No malleus is visible, and the incus is abnormally shaped *(arrow)*. Mastoid is well pneumatized. **B,** normal left ear for comparison. **C,** right ear, coronal section. No malleus or external auditory canal is visible. Hypoplastic tympanic bone is indicated by *(arrow)*. **D,** normal left ear. (Courtesy of Saul Taylor, M.D., St. Paul.)

may influence the surgical procedure chosen by the otologist.[21]

Malignant external otitis is an infection that begins in the external auditory canal in diabetics and is usually caused by *Pseudomonas aeruginosa*. The infection is severe, causing chondritis and osteomyelitis of the temporal bone. It may spread into the jugular foramen, temporomandibular joint, and skull base and even cause an inflammatory mass in the nasopharynx. Malignant external otitis is just one of many causes of destructive lesions in the temporal bone, and the diagnosis requires clinical and radiologic correlation.

Malignant external otitis can be divided into early

and late stages radiographically by the absence or presence of bone destruction.[22] Facial nerve paralysis is usually caused by involvement of the horizontal rather than the vertical portion of the nerve,[22] but it may be caused by involvement of the nerve at or below the stylomastoid foramen.[23] Facial nerve paralysis is a grave prognostic sign; in a large series, half of those patients who had facial nerve paralysis died.[24] Bony involvement of the jugular foramen does not necessarily cause paralysis of the nerves passing through the foramen, however. Medical management with intravenous antibiotics is preferred, with surgery being reserved for treatment failures.[24]

High-resolution CT is better than conventional tomography to study malignant external otitis, because the entire head can be studied, rather than restricting the tomograms to the temporal bone and possibly missing important information such as skull base osteomyelitis (Fig 23–5). Extension of the inflammatory process into the subtemporal region can be detected easily on CT scans.[23] Sigmoid sinus thrombosis may also be inferred by doing a contrast-enhanced scan.

Labyrinthitis ossificans is an unusual complication of suppurative labyrinthitis. It can be seen with tumors, trauma, inner ear hemorrhage, and advanced otosclerosis.[25] We have recently seen a case of Paget's disease that was indistinguishable from labyrinthitis ossificans. Suppurative labyrinthitis may occur from hematogenous, meningitic, or tympanogenic routes. Although the obliteration of the normal inner ear spaces (cochlea, vestibule, semicircular canals) may occur over many years, it has been shown to occur as rapidly as in 1 year.[25]

High-resolution CT images of the temporal bone viewed with a 3,000- to 4,000-HU window width can demonstrate labyrinthitis ossificans adequately; in fact, CT is superior to pluridirectional tomography in this situation, because CT can distinguish density changes better. Scans by CT are normally performed with high kVp, so penetration of a dense temporal bone is not the problem it would be with conventional tomography.

CHOLESTEATOMA

The use of CT has several advantages over pluridirectional tomography in the study of patients with cholesteatoma. The contrast resolution of CT is superior to

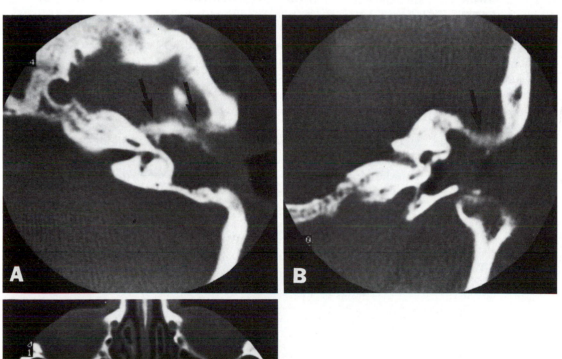

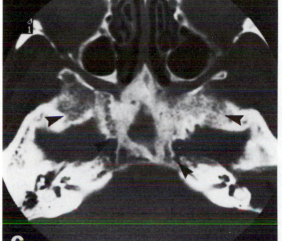

Fig 23–5.—Elderly diabetic woman with malignant external otitis caused by *Pseudomonas aeruginosa*. She had a left mastoidectomy prior to the CT scan. **A,** axial scan, left ear. Soft tissue fills the surgical defect, and there is erosion of bone anteriorly *(arrows)*. **B,** coronal scan demonstrating erosion of bone over the mastoidectomy cavity *(arrow)*. **C,** infection also spread to the skull base and sphenoid sinuses. Abnormally textured bone is involved with osteomyelitis *(arrowheads)*.

that of pluridirectional tomography, so soft tissues can be accurately distinguished from air or demineralized bony structures in the middle ear. The axial projection is much better than the standard coronal and sagittal tomographic projections to identify fistulas of the horizontal semicircular canal. The sinus tympani region, which is difficult to evaluate with standard tomographic projections or direct examination, is demonstrated well by axial CT (Fig 23–6).[26] The use of CT can also disclose unexpected extension of cholesteatoma medially into the petrous portion of the temporal bone or posteriorly into the mastoid (Fig 23–7).

Most cholesteatomas are of the acquired type, arise in the attic, and are the result of a previous tympanic membrane perforation. On both CT and pluridirectional tomography, a cholesteatoma will commonly appear as a soft-tissue density in the attic, middle ear, and/or mastoid, which has usually caused some bone erosion. Radiographic findings with cholesteatoma include erosion of the drum spur (scutum), lateral attic wall, and ossicles, particularly the incus.[27] Tegmen erosion may also occur, but this can be appreciated best in coronal or sagittal projections. Acquired cholesteatoma has even been reported to spread intracranially outside the temporal bone.[28] In these rare cases, CT is essential to plan adequate therapy.

Congenital cholesteatomas are much less common than acquired cholesteatomas. They may occur in the cerebellopontine angle, petrous pyramid, middle ear and mastoid, and jugular fossa.[27] A congenital choles-teatoma arising in the middle ear and mastoid is difficult to differentiate from an acquired cholesteatoma in which the tympanic perforation has healed.

Congenital cholesteatoma is one of a number of lesions that can produce a defect in the petrous apex.[29] Mucocele[30, 31] has recently been added to this list, which also includes giant air cell, petrositis, arachnoid cyst, aneurysm, metastasis, glomus tumor, neurinoma, lymphoma, histiocytosis, and chondroma.[29, 31–33]

It continues to be difficult to distinguish cholesteatoma in the middle ear from chronic inflammatory disease by either CT or pluridirectional tomography. If a rounded mass surrounded by air is visible, this mass is usually cholesteatoma (assuming that the clinical appearance of the mass resembles cholesteatoma).[34] Air-fluid levels may coexist with cholesteatoma.[35] The CT numbers of proved cholesteatomas have been variable and are probably unreliable.[36] If intravenous contrast is administered, chronic inflammatory disease may enhance, whereas cholesteatoma unassociated with chronic inflammation will not enhance.[37] Whether this finding is reliable and of clinical importance has not been determined yet.

The use of CT is also helpful in identifying areas of recurrent cholesteatoma in the postoperative ear (Fig 23–8).[38] Soft-tissue densities can be detected in the mastoid cavity or in parts of the middle ear not visible to the otologist. Therefore, CT scans of the temporal bone are important in the examination of patients with cholesteatoma. Axial CT scans are optimal for deter-

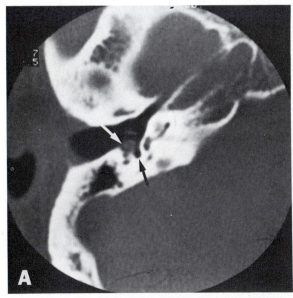 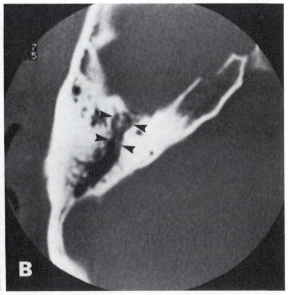

Fig 23–6.—Man with a small cholesteatoma in his right middle ear. He had had a previous left radical mastoidectomy. **A,** axial scan, right ear. Cholesteatoma is seen as a soft-tissue mass posteriorly, sparing the sinus tympani *(black arrow),* but in the facial recess *(white arrow).* Long process of the incus is absent. **B,** section 6 mm higher. Soft tissue surrounds head of the malleus and body of the incus and extends posteriorly into the aditus, but not the mastoid antrum *(arrowheads).*

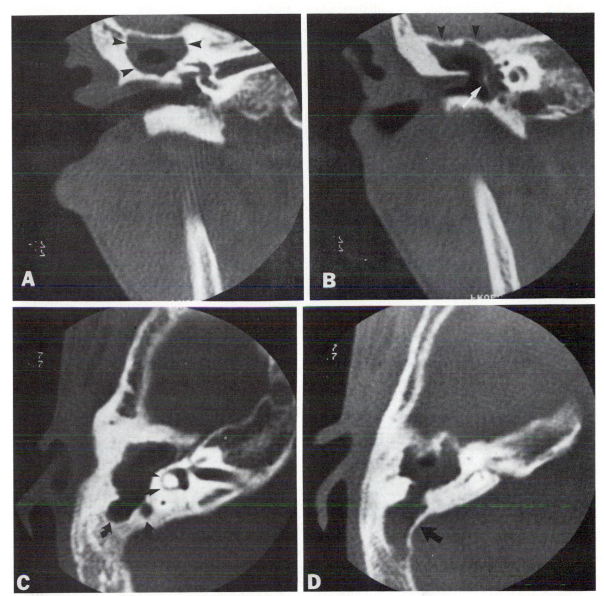

Fig 23–7.—Thirteen-year-old boy with chronic right otitis media and clinical evidence of cholesteatoma. He had not had a mastoidectomy. **A,** coronal scan, right ear, at the level of the internal auditory canal. There is a large cavity in the mastoid produced by the cholesteatoma *(arrowheads).* The middle ear and cavity contain small pneumatized areas. It is difficult to determine whether this is all cholesteatoma or there is associated chronic inflammatory disease and granulation tissue. **B,** anterior 4.5 mm to **A.** The lateral attic wall is completely eroded. A tiny remnant of malleus is visible adjacent to the tympanic membrane *(white arrow).* The tegmen is intact *(arrowheads).* **C,** axial scan, right ear. The horizontal semicircular canal retains a bony covering *(straight arrows),* while the cholesteatoma has extended posteriorly into the mastoid air pockets *(curved arrows).* **D,** higher 6 mm than **C.** Large posterior superior extension of cholesteatoma was not detected by tomography and was unsuspected. Thin bone separates cholesteatoma from the sigmoid sinus *(arrow).*

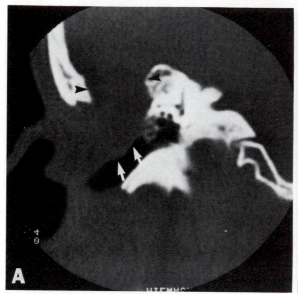

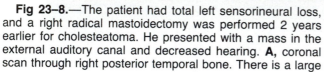

Fig 23–8.—The patient had total left sensorineural loss, and a right radical mastoidectomy was performed 2 years earlier for cholesteatoma. He presented with a mass in the external auditory canal and decreased hearing. **A,** coronal scan through right posterior temporal bone. There is a large defect in the tegmen *(arrowheads)* with temporal lobe herniating into the external auditory canal *(white arrows).* **B,** anterior 6 mm to **A.** A large defect is still present. There is a small soft-tissue mass in the middle ear that may represent recurrent cholesteatoma *(arrow).*

mining posterior extension of cholesteatoma into the mastoid and for evaluating the posterior middle ear, particularly the sinus tympani.[39] Bone destruction is detected as reliably and soft-tissue structures are demonstrated more effectively with CT than with pluridirectional tomography. At this time, increased cost of CT scans is the only drawback to replacing conventional tomography with CT in patients with cholesteatoma.

OTODYSTROPHIES

Otosclerosis

Otosclerosis is a condition of unknown etiology that initially causes spongiotic foci in the temporal bone. These are followed by sclerotic foci of thickened bone. The oval window is usually affected, with fixation of the stapes footplate leading to conductive hearing loss. There may even be bony proliferation that obliterates the entire oval window niche. Other parts of the bony labyrinth may also be involved with otosclerosis, particularly the cochlear capsule, leading to sensorineural or mixed hearing loss. The disease frequently occurs in young adults, commonly affects females, and is often hereditary.

The standard tomographic projection for evaluating the oval window and stapes footplate is the 20° semiaxial view. In this projection, the head is rotated toward the side being studied, bringing the oval window and stapes footplate perpendicular to the tomographic plane. This projection can be duplicated with CT, but both ears must be scanned separately.[2] The oval window and cochlea are also adequately seen on coronal and axial CT scans. Our experience with otosclerosis is limited, although others have demonstrated oval window obliteration and demineralized areas in the cochlear capsule with high-resolution CT.

Paget's Disease

Paget's disease, which affects the skeleton in older adults, is of unknown etiology. The disease has both lytic and proliferative phases, and the skull is involved in 28% to 70% of patients.[40] Temporal bone involvement usually coincides with calvarial Paget's disease, and it often produces hearing loss. The lytic phase of Paget's disease predominates in the temporal bone, affecting the petrous bone first and progressing laterally.[41] The dense bone of the otic capsule is most resistant to lytic foci. The reparative phase of Paget's disease produces thickened bone that narrows normal lumina. The temporal bone findings may be indistinguishable from labyrinthitis ossificans, but changes of Paget's disease elsewhere in the skull generally clarify the diagnosis.

The use of CT can demonstrate the variable bony densities in the temporal bone of patients with Paget's disease quite accurately (Fig 23–9). In some cases, CT is superior to pluridirectional tomography, because the bone is so demineralized that it is difficult to evaluate on conventional tomograms.

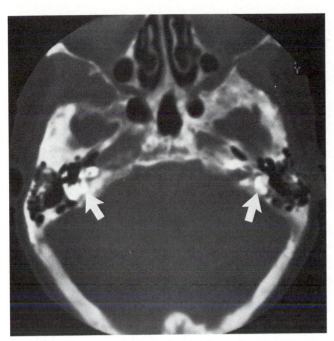

Fig 23–9.—Elderly woman with bilateral severe hearing loss. Axial scan viewed at a 4,000-HU window width detects areas of demineralized bone in both petrous pyramids with relative sparing of the otic capsules *(arrows),* findings characteristic of Paget's disease.

Other Otodystrophies

Osteogenesis imperfecta, osteopetrosis, craniometaphyseal dysostosis, and fibrous dysplasia are sufficiently rare that CT experience has not been accumulated in these diseases. The use of CT should be equal or superior to that of pluridirectional tomography in demonstrating structural abnormalities, because CT can penetrate thick dense bone that occurs in osteopetrosis or craniometaphyseal dysostosis as well as detect density differences.

TEMPORAL BONE TUMORS

Intratemporal tumors are less commonly seen by otolaryngologists than are cases of inflammatory disease and cholesteatoma or tumors of the cerebellopontine angle. Tumors affecting the temporal bone may be either benign or malignant, primary in the ear, or metastatic from a local or distant site.[42]

Benign Tumors

Glomus tumors or chemodectomas are the most common benign mesenchymal tumors of the temporal bone.[43] Glomus tumors arise from chemoreceptor cells that are found in the jugular bulb and middle ear. These benign lesions are respectively called glomus jugulare and glomus tympanicum tumors. Chemodectomas also occur in association with the vagus nerve

(glomus vagale) and carotid bifurcation (carotid body tumor). Glomus tumors rarely metastasize, but they may be locally aggressive and difficult to control. Treatment is usually surgical removal, which may be followed by irradiation.[43]

Multiple radiographic techniques have been used for evaluating patients suspected of having glomus jugulare or glomus tympanicum tumors. These procedures include plain films, hypocycloidal tomography, selective carotid arteriography with subtraction films, and retrograde jugular venography. High-resolution CT is the most important radiographic study in patients with glomus tumors, and CT can replace most of the other studies. Thick CT slices from older scanners will not detect small glomus tympanicum lesions, however (Fig 23–10).[44] Scans before and after contrast infusion will demonstrate tumor enhancement, and bone destruction can be detected readily on scans.[45] Scans by CT will also demonstrate intracranial portions of the tumor as well as caudal extension of the mass into the upper neck (Figs 23–11 and 23–12).

A technique for dynamic scanning of glomus tumors has been described recently.[46] The tumor is first identified on a 5-mm axial section without contrast; then a rapid bolus injection of 30 to 40 ml of 60% iodinated

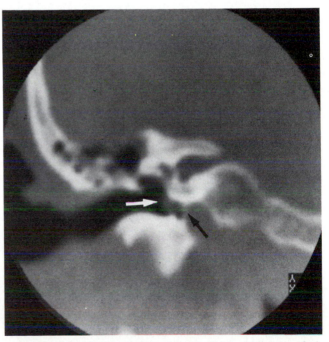

Fig 23–10.—Coronal scan through right middle ear of elderly woman with a red mass in the hypotympanum. Scan is viewed at 4,000-HU window width, but was not reconstructed with the ReView™ program. A soft-tissue mass representing a glomus tympanicum tumor is visible in the hypotympanum *(white arrow).* Bone over the carotid canal is intact *(black arrow),* so this mass does not represent an ectopic carotid artery.

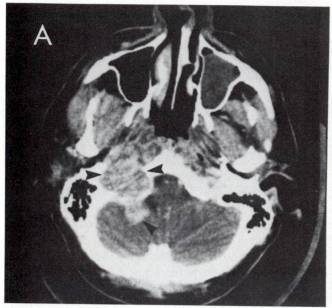

Fig 23–11.—Thirty-year-old man whose right 12th nerve paralysis and vocal cord paralysis were incidentally discovered. **A,** large enhancing mass in right jugular foramen projecting posteriorly into cerebellum *(arrowheads).* **B,** mass extending inferiorly behind and medial to the mandible *(arrows).* Large glomus jugulare tumor was resected.

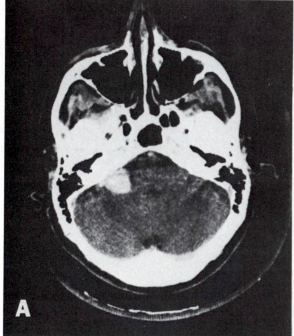
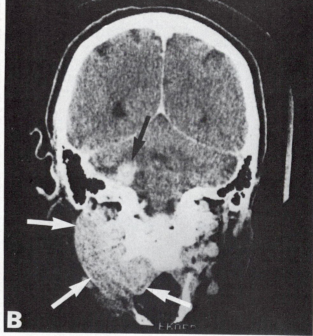

Fig 23–12.—Middle-aged man with several-year history of paralysis of right cranial nerves 8 to 12. **A,** axial scan at level of internal auditory canals. A round 2-cm enhancing mass simulates an acoustic neuroma. **B,** coronal scan posterior to the internal canals. Scan shows intracranial tumor *(black arrow)* and large tumor in the upper neck *(white arrows).* This glomus tumor arose around the vagus nerve (glomus vagale) and extended intracranially through the jugular foramen.

contrast is given over 4 seconds. Single-level dynamic scans document the arrival times of contrast in the carotid artery, jugular vein, and tumor. Graphs of attenuation values can then be constructed by positioning the cursor over the artery, vein, and tumor in turn. Using this technique, glomus tumors have peak enhancement similar to the carotid artery, but slightly delayed (Fig 23–13). A high jugular bulb in the middle ear can be differentiated by this technique. Digital angiography may also replace standard arteriography and venography to evaluate patients with glomus tumors, because arterial supply, tumor blush, and jugular vein patency can all be determined from a digital subtraction arteriogram.

Osteomas are uncommon lesions that may arise anywhere in the temporal bone; however, the mastoid is the most common site.[47] There have been no reports of the CT appearance of an osteoma of the temporal bone. Thin-section scans viewed with a wide CT number range (4,000 HU) should depict a temporal bone osteoma optimally. Its relationship to adjacent structures will be defined, and the density and homogeneity of the osteoma can be evaluated. Osteomas should be distinguished clinically from bony exostoses, which are often seen in the external auditory canals of people who swim in cold water.[42]

Hemangiomas are rare temporal bone neoplasms, comprising only 0.7% of a series of 1,430 intratemporal

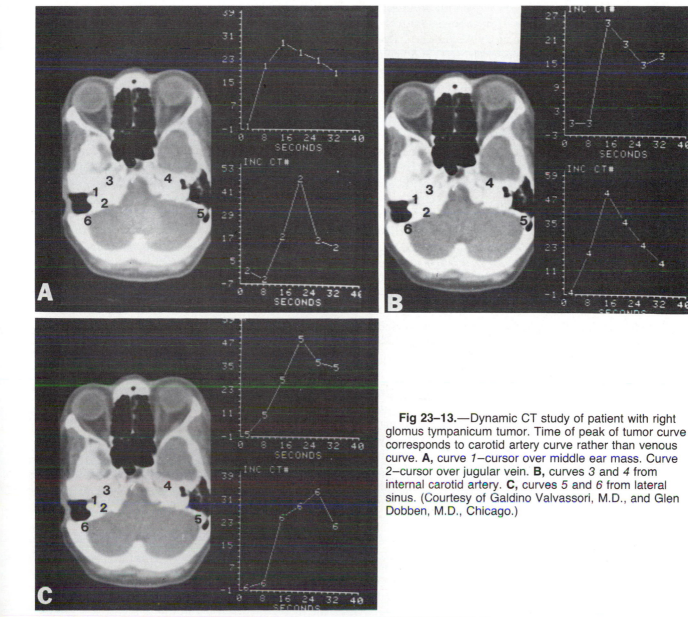

Fig 23–13.—Dynamic CT study of patient with right glomus tympanicum tumor. Time of peak of tumor curve corresponds to carotid artery curve rather than venous curve. **A,** curve 1–cursor over middle ear mass. Curve 2–cursor over jugular vein. **B,** curves 3 and 4 from internal carotid artery. **C,** curves 5 and 6 from lateral sinus. (Courtesy of Galdino Valvassori, M.D., and Glen Dobben, M.D., Chicago.)

tumors.[48] These tumors may produce bone erosion and may be indistinguishable radiographically from a facial nerve neuroma or an acoustic neuroma. A 7-mm tumor at the medial end of the internal auditory canal has been detected by CT.[48] Dynamic thin-section CT as discussed with glomus tumors may also be useful for determining the vascularity of hemangiomas.

Meningiomas rarely may arise primarily within the temporal bone, although most meningiomas affecting the temporal bone invade from intracranial sites. Meningiomas arise in arachnoid granulations, and ectopic arachnoid granulations may be found in the temporal bone.[49] Thirteen intratympanic meningiomas reported in the literature have been reviewed, and the authors added three cases believed to be primary intratympanic meningiomas. However, when these patients were subsequently studied with CT 2 to 4 years postoperatively, all were found to have intracranial meningiomas.[50] One meningioma involving the semicircular canal and internal auditory canal was not detected by pluridirectional tomography or by CT.[51] This lesion was identified by positive contrast cisternography, and it would also have been seen with air CT cisternography (see discussion under Cerebellopontine Angle Masses).

The high spatial and contrast resolution available with current CT scanners should identify any intracranial component of a middle ear meningioma or any temporal bone invasion from a meningioma in the cerebellopontine angle. The use of CT probably could not distinguish a middle ear meningioma from other small enhancing lesions in a similar location.

Tumors are estimated to produce only 5% of all cases of facial nerve paralysis.[52] Usually arising from Schwann's cells, facial nerve neuromas are uncommon tumors that may involve the nerve anywhere in its course from the cerebellopontine angle to the peripheral portions of the nerve outside the temporal bone. Most neuromas occur within the temporal bone, most commonly in the tympanic and mastoid segments.[52] A facial nerve tumor most often produces slowly developing paralysis, although some patients may have no muscular weakness. A tumor in the middle ear may cause conductive hearing loss by interfering with ossicular motion. It is important to radiographically evaluate all portions of the facial canal when trying to identify a cause for facial nerve paralysis. Other lesions that can also cause facial nerve paralysis include trauma, infarcts, cholesteatoma, primary or metastatic malignant tumors, glomus tumors, parotid tumors, meningiomas, and acoustic neuromas.

The coronal CT projection demonstrates the two limbs of the facial nerve canal above the cochlea as well as the horizontal portion of the nerve passing beneath the horizontal semicircular canal. The horizontal portion of the nerve can also be seen in the axial projection, but it is more difficult in this plane to determine whether its bony covering is dehiscent or eroded. The vertical portion of the canal is more difficult to evaluate by CT, because it is seen best in the sagittal plane. Direct sagittal CT scans of the temporal bone are very difficult to perform, however. Reformatted images will show the vertical descending portion of the facial nerve canal, but not with the same detail present on direct scans.[53] The vertical portion of the facial nerve canal is not seen in all coronal scans, probably because the scans can seldom be taken in a true coronal plane. In axial scans, the facial nerve canal can be identified posterior to the pyramidal eminence and the facial recess.[35]

Intralabyrinthine schwannomas are extremely rare and differ from the usual vestibular schwannoma or acoustic neuroma in that they do not arise in the internal auditory canal. Radiographs were normal in five of six reported cases. One patient had a loss of radiolucency at the basal turn of the cochlea.[54] Findings from CT would likely also be normal in these rare lesions.

Malignant Tumors

Malignant tumors involving the temporal bone are of four general types: primary epithelial tumors, primary mesenchymal tumors, direct extension from adjacent malignant lesions, and metastatic foci from distant primary tumors.[42]

Excluding lesions of the pinna, the most common primary epithelial malignancy of the temporal bone is squamous carcinoma of the external auditory canal. Tumors arising laterally in the membranous canal tend to spread laterally into the parotid. Many carcinomas arise deep in the external auditory canal and extend medially into the middle ear.[55] When a deep tumor is discovered, it may be difficult to determine the actual site of origin.[56] Adenocarcinoma and adenoid cystic carcinoma are much less common primary epithelial tumors of the temporal bone.[57] Melanoma may also occur primarily in the middle ear, because melanocytes have been demonstrated in the middle and inner ear.[57, 58]

Most patients with carcinoma of the external auditory canal or middle ear have symptoms including discharge, pain, hearing loss, and facial nerve paralysis.[59] Thirty to seventy percent of patients have a history of chronic otitis media.[56] Treatment of primary temporal bone malignancies usually involves temporal bone resection, if the tumor is localized, and irradiation.

Sarcomas can also occur primarily in the temporal bone. Embryonal rhabdomyosarcoma is the most common malignant tumor of the ear in children. The middle ear is the third-most-common site in the head and neck for rhabdomyosarcoma in the pediatric age group, after the orbit and nasopharynx.[60] Children with rhabdomyosarcoma of the middle ear may present with a variety of symptoms, including otorrhea. Early differential diagnosis from inflammatory disease or other lesions such as histiocytosis X is important. Treatment usually combines partial resection, irradiation, and chemotherapy.

Histiocytosis X is a complex that includes three clinical entities: eosinophilic granuloma, Hand-Schüller-Christian syndrome, and Letterer-Siwe disease. Histiocytosis X is characterized by proliferation of histiocytes, usually in children and young adults. Eosinophilic granulomas are usually well-circumscribed lesions of bone, whereas the other two syndromes have visceral disease also and an associated higher mortality. Otitis media and otitis externa are frequent clinical manifestations of histiocytosis X lesions. Destructive lesions in the mastoid may be mistaken for mastoiditis, cholesteatoma, or a malignant lesion. Although the bone lesions usually respond to irradiation, the prognosis is determined by the extent of nonosseous disease.[33]

Metastatic disease of the temporal bone may occur by direct extension of malignant neoplasms such as those arising in parotid, nasopharynx, and skin. Distant metastases occur most often from tumors that metastasize to bone, including carcinoma of the lung, breast, kidney, and prostate.[42, 61, 62] Patients with metastatic tumors to the temporal bone may have variable signs and symptoms. Often, a suspected metastasis to the temporal bone is not investigated because it is part of extensive metastatic disease, although the temporal bone can be the first recognized site of metastatic disease. The marrow spaces of the temporal bone are usually affected first by hematogenous metastases, but metastatic foci may occur in the mastoid air cells and middle ear. The otic capsule is usually spared.[61]

Obtaining axial and coronal planes by CT is useful in studying patients with carcinoma of the temporal bone to determine the extent of local disease and the feasibility of temporal bone resection. Axial CT is particularly useful for evaluating bone destruction anteriorly around the carotid artery and the eustachian tube.[56] Coronal scans will demonstrate tegmen erosion and intracranial extension of tumor better than pluridirectional tomography. More posterior tumor spread into the mastoid may be missed on conventional tomograms, but will be detected by CT.

TEMPORAL BONE FRACTURES

Temporal bone fractures have been classically divided into two main types, longitudinal and transverse. Longitudinal fractures are more common, representing about 80% of temporal bone fractures.[63] Fracture lines cross the mastoid, external auditory canal, and tegmen tympani and extend anteriorly parallel to the anterior margin of the petrous pyramid. Longitudinal fractures usually produce tympanic membrane tears, hemorrhage from the external auditory canal, and conductive hearing loss. Facial nerve injury occurs less often than with transverse fractures, and the paralysis may be immediate or delayed.[64] The region of the geniculate ganglion anteriorly and the descending portion of the facial nerve canal are frequent sites of injury to the nerve. The horizontal portion of the nerve running along the medial wall of the middle ear may also be injured, particularly if there is a congenital absence of the bony covering.

Ossicular fractures or dislocations may commonly accompany longitudinal fractures (Fig 23–14). The incus is the most vulnerable to injury, because it is rather loosely supported between the malleus (which is attached to the tympanic membrane) and the stapes (in the oval window). Malleus fracture and dislocation and crush injuries of the stapes crura also occur.[65] Cerebrospinal fluid otorrhea or rhinorrhea can result from temporal bone fractures if the dura is torn adjacent to a tegmen fracture. Brain may herniate into the mastoid through a sufficiently large bony defect (see Fig 23–14,B).

Transverse fractures are much less common than longitudinal fractures, and they usually produce damage to the inner rather than middle ear. The fracture line is perpendicular to the long axis of the petrous pyramid, and a displaced fracture may actually disrupt the seventh and eighth nerves in the internal auditory canal.

In actual practice, fracture lines may be multiple or obliquely oriented, but they still can be generally classified as longitudinal or transverse. Transverse fractures are studied ideally by CT, because the line is perpendicular to the plane of both axial and coronal CT sections. Longitudinal fractures may have fracture lines that are not detected readily, because they are parallel to the scanning planes. The lateral tomographic projection, which is the most useful for evaluating patients with longitudinal fractures, is not practical in CT. In our experience and that of others, however, CT is adequate and even preferred to conventional tomography to study both types of temporal bone fractures.[11, 35]

As with conventional tomography, more than one projection is needed to adequately demonstrate temporal bone fractures because of the direction of the fracture lines relative to the scanning planes. For example, evaluating tegmen fractures is nearly impossible without coronal scans. Ossicular dislocation can be detected in both axial and coronal projections. The incudomalleal articulation has been described as appearing like an ice cream cone in the axial projection, and disruption of

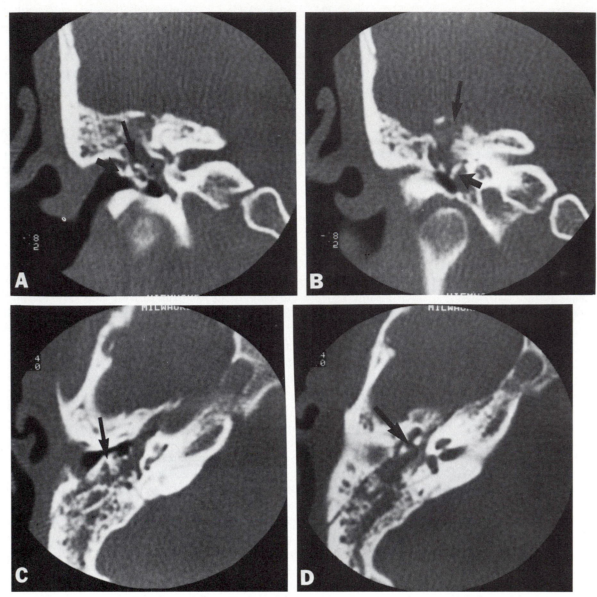

Fig 23–14.—Young man who had severe head injury and resulting facial nerve paralysis from an automobile accident. **A,** coronal scan, right ear. There are multiple tegmen fractures, and the incus is dislocated inferiorly *(long arrow).* There is a large bone fragment in the medial external auditory canal *(short arrow).* **B,** anterior 3 mm to **A.** A large tegmen fracture is present *(long arrow).* Malleus is dislocated and rotated medially *(short arrow).* Brain was found herniating into the attic at surgery. **C,** axial scan, right ear, showing multiple fracture lines and pieces of posterior wall of the external auditory canal in the lumen of the canal *(arrow).* **D,** higher 3 mm than **C.** Fracture lines and opacified air spaces are again seen. There is marked separation of the malleus and incus *(arrow).*

this relationship indicates ossicular injury (see Fig 23–14, D).[35] Fluid collections in the middle ear and mastoid are demonstrated better by CT because of its greater contrast resolution, and air-fluid levels may even be seen. Intracranial sequelae of head trauma such as extracerebral hematoma, parenchymal hematoma, and pneumocephalus can also be identified on CT scans at the same time that the temporal bone fracture is being evaluated. Undoubtedly, some tiny fractures will escape detection by CT just as they do with pluridirectional tomography.[63]

CEREBELLOPONTINE ANGLE MASSES

Cerebellopontine angle masses are usually evaluated by doing 5-mm thick contiguous axial CT sections through the posterior fossa and 1.5-mm thick sections through the internal auditory canals if acoustic neuroma is suspected. Scans are usually done after infusion of contrast containing 40 gm of iodine. To study abnormalities primarily in the posterior fossa rather than the temporal bone, the gantry is angled −15° to the infraorbitomeatal line for the axial scans, which provides scans more perpendicular to the brain stem and decreases the interpetrous streaking artifact. If a lesion is present, scans are also done in the coronal position to demonstrate the cephalocaudad extent of tumor and its relationship to structures such as the tentorium, brain stem, and skull base. The highest scan technique (1,152 mAs) is used for the 1.5-mm thick sections to provide the best contrast resolution available. This high technique is not necessary when only the temporal bone is being evaluated.

Many tumors can occur in the cerebellopontine angle, but acoustic neuroma is by far the most common neoplasm in this location. In most series, acoustic neuromas account for 80% to 90% of cerebellopontine angle tumors. Meningioma is the second-most-common cerebellopontine angle mass, and epidermoid tumor is the third.[66] Many other rare lesions may arise in the cistern or extend to involve it.[67] Some lesions, such as aneurysms, are not neoplasms.

Many articles have been written about the differential diagnosis of cerebellopontine angle masses, particularly related to their contrast enhancement. The timing of contrast enhancement of various tumors should influence the technique of scanning, e.g., whether contrast should be administered first and the patient scanned after a delay of 30 to 60 minutes. Early studies of contrast enhancement of acoustic neuromas showed that these tumors characteristically had a rapid rise of contrast enhancement followed by a significant decrease in enhancement 30 to 60 minutes after injection.[68–70] These reports are in disagreement with a more recent article, which demonstrated delayed enhancement in nine of ten acoustic neuromas scanned 35 to 45 minutes after injection of contrast.[66] We have not systematically studied this problem, but it has been our impression that enhancement of acoustic neuromas tends to decrease when the study is prolonged. Acoustic neuromas and meningiomas enhance in part because of vascularity, but an abnormal blood-brain barrier should not be related to delayed enhancement, as it is in gliomas, because acoustic neuromas and meningiomas arise outside the brain substance.

Acoustic Neuroma

It has been well documented in the literature that modern CT scanners can detect a high percentage of acoustic neuromas if careful attention is paid to scanning technique. In 1978, Valavanis and colleagues[71] reported 41 acoustic neuromas diagnosed on CT scans, 15 of which were 1 cm or less in diameter. Narrow sections (5 mm or less) and an adequate amount of intravenous iodinated contrast are necessary to detect small tumors. Narrow sections also decrease partial volume averaging and diminish the interpetrous streak artifact. A negative gantry angle also helps to decrease the interpetrous streaks.[71] Because unenhanced acoustic neuromas are usually isodense with respect to surrounding brain, we no longer do scans both before and after contrast infusion.

Most acoustic neuromas have a characteristic CT appearance. The tumor usually arises at the porus acusticus, and it nearly always enhances. The center may have decreased attenuation, which is usually due to necrosis or cyst formation (Fig 23–15). Acoustic neuromas may be spherical or somewhat lobulated with distinct margins. The normal cerebellar flocculus should not be mistaken for an acoustic neuroma. The flocculus is posterior and inferior to the porus acusticus, and no secondary signs of acoustic neuroma are present (Fig 23–16).[72]

The only direct sign of an acoustic neuroma is visualization of the tumor. The presence of indirect signs of tumor may lead to further radiographic studies, however. Indirect signs of acoustic neuroma include the following: asymmetry of the internal auditory canals, widening of the ipsilateral ambient cistern, obliteration of the ipsilateral cerebellopontine angle cistern, distortion of the fourth ventricle, rotation of the brain stem, and hydrocephalus. Indirect signs are seen more frequently with larger tumors, with the exception of widening of the internal auditory canal.[66, 71]

Acoustic neuromas have sometimes been called vestibular schwannomas, because most arise from the vestibular nerve, which is in the posterior portion of the internal auditory canal. A wide window on the CT dis-

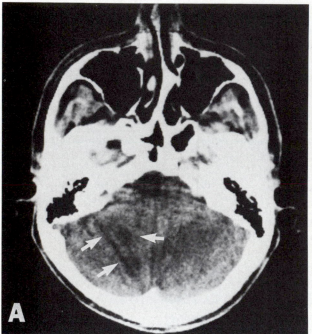
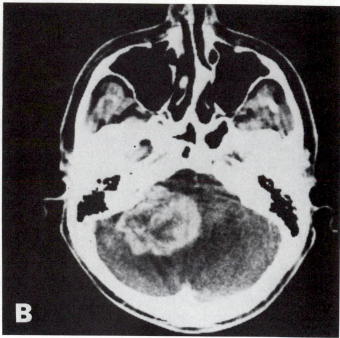

Fig 23–15.—A 28-year-old man with right sensorineural hearing loss and absent corneal reflex. **A,** axial scan through posterior fossa before contrast administration. Fourth ventricle is not seen, and there are abnormal areas of decreased attenuation in the right side of the posterior fossa *(arrows).* **B,** large mass with low-density areas centrally detected following contrast infusion, a 4-cm acoustic neuroma.

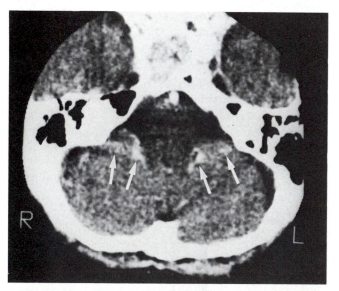

Fig 23–16.—Elderly woman with pituitary adenoma. Note enhancement of vessels and choroid of fourth ventricle and flocculus *(arrows).* (R = patient's right; L = patient's left.)

play will demonstrate flaring of the internal auditory canal or shortening of the posterior wall of the canal (Fig 23–17). Asymmetry of the internal canals alone does not necessarily mean that the patient has an acoustic neuroma, because at least 10% of the population have variations in the size and shape of the internal au-

ditory canals.[73] Clinical correlation with the patient's audiometric tests is obviously necessary before deciding to pursue more invasive tests to rule out acoustic neuroma. Bony canals can also be measured directly on the scans or by evaluating attenuation profiles across the canals to provide an objective graph.[74]

Radiologic evaluation of patients with suspected acoustic neuroma depends on the type of CT equipment available. When a newer high-resolution scanner capable of thin sections is used, CT scanning with contrast enhancement is the first study performed.[75] We do not believe, as some authors do,[76] that plain films or tomography are necessary in addition to CT. If target reconstruction is done on 1.5-mm thick scans from the GE 8800 scanner (see earlier discussion), diagnostic temporal bone images are produced without additional cost or irradiation (Fig 23–18).

If a high-quality contrast-enhanced CT scan through the cerebellopontine angle cisterns does not definitely demonstrate a tumor, then another study is indicated in those patients who have a strong clinical suspicion of tumor based on audiologic testing. In the past, the definitive contrast study for small acoustic neuromas was posterior fossa myelography using iophendylate (Pantopaque). This contrast was known to have limitations and complications, however,[77] and a technique to detect small acoustic tumors was described combining sub-

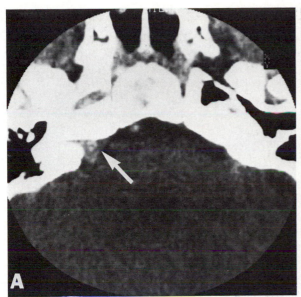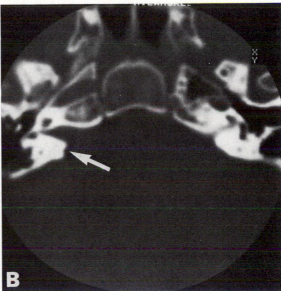

Fig 23–17.—A, enhanced 1.5-mm axial scan showing small right acoustic neuroma *(arrow)*. **B,** same section viewed at wide window demonstrating erosion of the poste- rior wall of the internal auditory canal *(arrow)* and widening of the canal.

arachnoid gas injection and complex motion tomography.[78] A variation of subarachnoid gas injection combined with CT was described more recently,[79, 80] and gas CT cisternography has now become a popular technique for excluding small acoustic neuromas. Gas cisternography will not directly demonstrate the size of large acoustic neuromas, so we require a normal contrast-enhanced CT scan before proceeding to gas cisternography.

The technique for gas CT cisternography varies slightly with description by individual authors.[81–83] The study involves lumbar puncture with a small needle (22 gauge or smaller), injection of gas (3 to 6 cc), and positioning the patient so the gas reaches the affected cerebellopontine angle cistern. Thin-section scans are then done through the internal auditory canal. Target reconstruction and an extended CT number range enable the viewer to routinely see the nerves within the internal

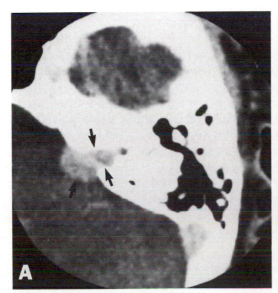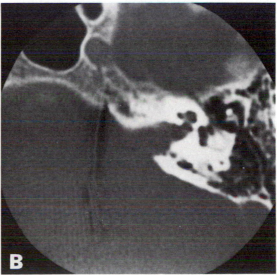

Fig 23–18.—A, magnified 1.5-mm axial scan through left internal auditory canal. Small acoustic neuroma is in the enlarged canal and projecting into the cerebellopontine angle cistern *(arrows)*. **B,** same section reconstructed with ReView™ program, viewed at 4,000-HU window width. Bone detail is improved considerably, but the tumor is barely visible.

auditory canal in the normal patient (Fig 23–19), and small intracanalicular tumors will also be outlined by gas (Fig 23–20). An edge enhancement program can also be used to identify the nerves.[81] Examination of both internal canals can be performed by turning the patient from one decubitus position to supine to the other decubitus position while the head is flexed.[84] Recently, filtered CO_2 has been recommended as the contrast agent, instead of room air or oxygen.[85] The authors found that there was a significant decrease in the major complication of the procedure, headache. This is presumably due to the rapid absorption of CO_2 from the cisternal spaces.

False-negative gas CT cisternograms are usually the result of inadequate gas in the cistern. Some authors advocate leaving the spinal needle in place during the procedure in case additional gas needs to be injected.[82, 84, 85] The patient can also be repositioned in an attempt to move more gas into the cistern.

Some false-positve studies may be encountered, just as they were with iophendylate examinations. Gas may not fill the space around the nerves in a small internal auditory canal, or a vascular loop may obstruct the flow of gas. Arachnoiditis may also simulate an acoustic neuroma and prevent filling of the internal auditory canal with gas.[86]

Water-soluble contrast has also been recommended for studying the cisternal spaces to identify small tumors when high-resolution CT is not available. The

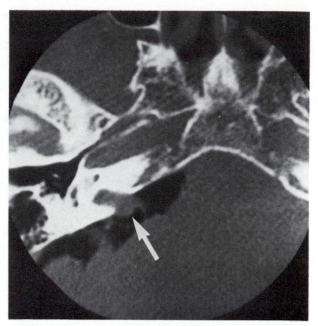

Fig 23–20.—Intracanalicular right acoustic neuroma *(arrow)* seen on 1.5-mm thick ReView™ reconstruction after injection of subarachnoid air. Patient was in the left lateral decubitus position, but the print is oriented in the conventional manner.

nerves and vascular structures in the internal auditory canal and at the porus acusticus can be identified when a small amount of metrizamide (Amipaque) is injected via C1-2 puncture, positioned in the cerebellopontine angle cistern, and pluridirectional tomograms are done through the canal (Fig 23–21).[87]

Metrizamide CT cisternography is also occasionally useful to evaluate cerebrospinal fluid spaces in the posterior fossa.[88, 89] Disadvantages of this technique are the risk of adverse reaction to the contrast and the usual practice of performing metrizamide studies only on hospitalized patients. This low-dose metrizamide technique for cisternography does not demonstrate cerebrospinal fluid spaces in the internal auditory canal unless the canal is very large. Because gas CT cisternography is more innocuous, can be performed on outpatients, is less expensive, and will demonstrate intracanalicular abnormalities, we and others[85, 88] use gas CT cisternography as the next test to detect a small acoustic neuroma after the patient has had a normal contrast-enhanced CT scan.

Meningioma

Meningioma is the second-most-common primary neoplasm in the cerebellopontine angle, accounting for fewer than 10% of tumors in this location. Meningiomas may arise along the posterior surface of the petrous bone or extend into the cerebellopontine angle from

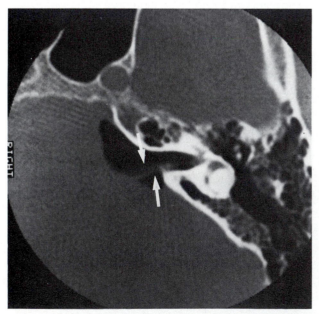

Fig 23–19.—Normal left air CT cisternogram. Patient was in the decubitus position, but the scan is oriented in the conventional manner. Nerves *(arrows)* are clearly seen crossing the cerebellopontine angle cistern and within the canal with ReView™ reconstruction.

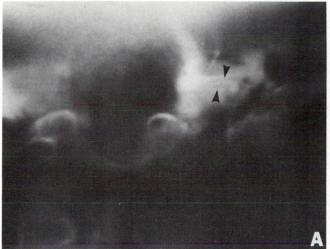 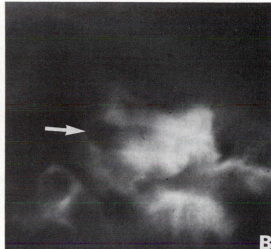

Fig 23–21.—**A,** normal metrizamide study with contrast surrounding nerves in the internal auditory canal *(arrowheads).* **B,** intracanalicular acoustic neuroma with metriza-mide capping tumor at the porus acusticus *(arrow).* (Courtesy of Hugh D. Curtin, M.D., Pittsburgh.)

other primary locations, including the tentorium, clivus, and parasellar region.[90]

Meningiomas tend to be more dense than surrouding brain before contrast infusion, and they may or may not be calcified.[90, 91] Meningiomas are usually oval in shape and have a long attachment to the temporal bone (Fig 23–22). As opposed to acoustic neuromas, meningiomas usually are centered anterior or posterior to the porus acousticus rather than at it. Contrast enhancement of meningiomas is characteristically homogeneous,[90] and the degree of enhancement often varies inversely with the extent to which the tumor is calcified. Densely calcified meningiomas may not enhance perceptibly (Fig 23–23). Hyperostosis of the temporal bone caused by meningioma is less common than hyperostosis associated with meningiomas elsewhere in the head.[90] The tumors can occasionally erode bone as well.

Cerebellopontine angle meningiomas also have characteristic features in common with acoustic neuromas indicating extra-axial location. These include widening of the ipsilateral cistern, sharp margins, and confluent margin with the temporal bone or tentorium.

Epidermoid Tumors

Epidermoid tumors are uncommon lesions that can occur at many intracranial sites, the most common of which is the cerebellopontine angle.[92] They produce variable symptoms, which were often of long duration prior to the development of CT.

Epidermoid tumors have been described as having low attenuation (near the attenuation of cerebrospinal fluid or below) on CT scans.[92–94] These tumors rarely enhance, and they may have some calcification of the rim (Fig 23–24). The low CT density is thought to be

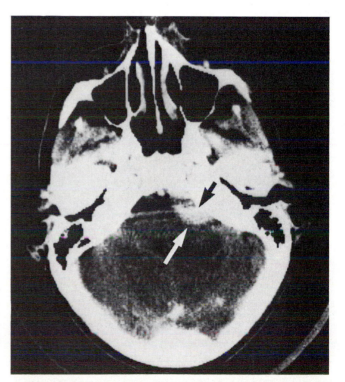

Fig 23–22.—Young woman with headaches (clinical impression of headache etiology was cervical spondylosis). Axial scan following contrast injection shows enhancing left cerebellopontine angle mass anterior to the internal auditory canal *(white arrow).* There is some hyperostosis of the petrous apex, which was seen better at a wider window *(black arrow).* The appearance is characteristic of meningioma.

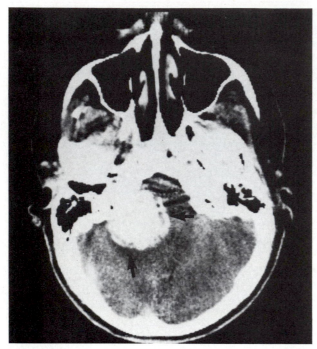

Fig 23–23.—A 50-year-old white woman with a long history of right deafness and unsteadiness. A large densely calcified right cerebellopontine angle meningioma enhances only slightly at its periphery following contrast infusion *(arrows)*.

due to a mixture of cholesterol and keratin in the mass.[95] However, three posterior fossa epidermoid tumors with high attenuation (80 to 120 HU) have been reported.[95] These masses were difficult to distinguish from meningiomas, although their densities were not as high as would be expected for a densely calcified meningioma, and the epidermoid tumors had no contrast enhancement, an unusual finding in meningiomas. Therefore, it appears that epidermoid tumors may have two distinctly different CT appearances.

It may occasionally be difficult to distinguish an arachnoid cyst from an epidermoid tumor that widens the cerebellopontine angle cistern. High-resolution CT should accurately identify epidermoid tumors. If only an older scanner is available or if there is unexplained asymmetry of the cerebellopontine angle cisterns, further radiographic procedures are necessary.[93]

Other Cerebellopontine Angle Masses

Multiple other masses can occur in the cerebellopontine angle, including arachnoid cysts, exophytic intra-axial tumors, metastases, aneurysms, tortuous basilar artery, glomus tumors, and other less common neoplasms (Fig 23–25).[66, 96] Differential diagnosis from the more common cerebellopontine angle neoplasms may sometimes be difficult. Diagnosis of rare lesions must be made by evaluating the entire lesion, as well as sur-

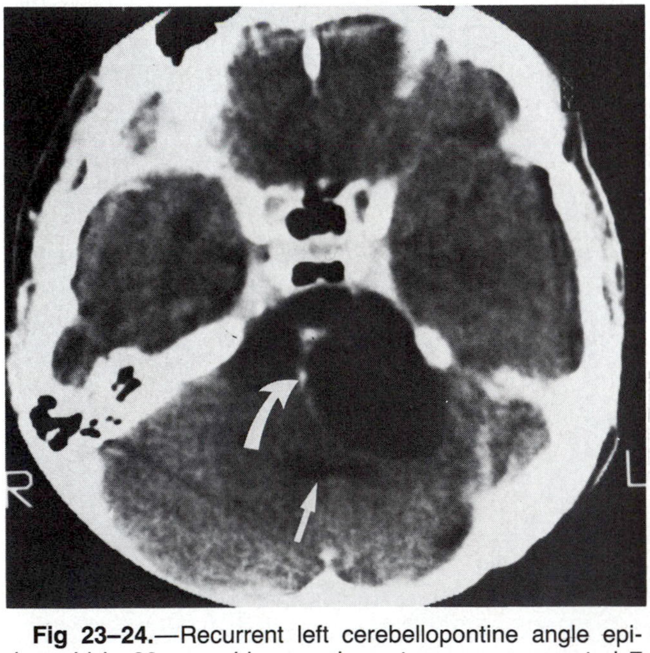

Fig 23–24.—Recurrent left cerebellopontine angle epidermoid in 30-year-old man whose tumor was resected 7 years earlier. Fourth ventricle is compressed *(straight arrow)*, and there is a small area of calcification at the edge of the tumor *(curved arrow)*. (R = patient's right; L = patient's left.)

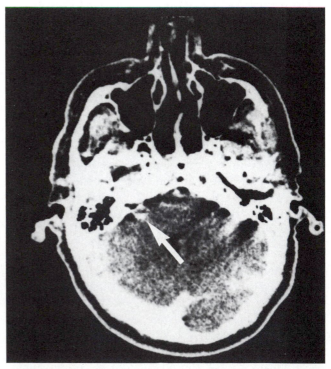

Fig 23–25.—Middle-aged man with right hearing loss and facial weakness. A poorly enhancing small mass in the cerebellopontine angle *(arrow)* was a primary extra-axial glioma.

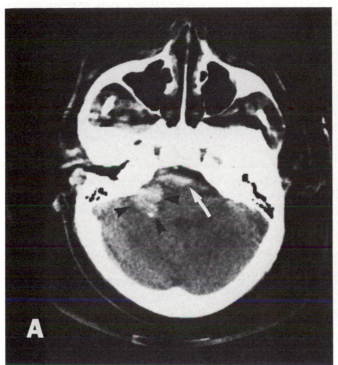

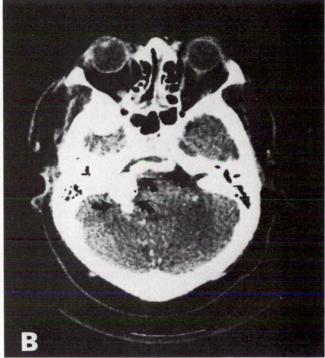

Fig 23–26.—Elderly man with multiple cranial nerve palsies. **A,** enhanced scan showing large right cerebellopontine angle mass with lobulation and a small fleck of calcium *(arrowheads).* Linear density anteriorly is a dilated basilar artery *(white arrow).* **B,** dynamic scan following bolus injection of contrast medium (different angle than **A**) showing marked enhancement of basilar artery and aneurysm *(arrows).*

rounding bony structures and brain, both before and after contrast. Vascular lesions such as aneurysm and arteriovenous malformation will be studied best by dynamic CT scanning (Fig 23–26).

Acknowledgment

Thanks to Hugh Curtin, M.D., Saul Taylor, M.D., Galdino Valvassori, M.D., and Glen Dobben, M.D., for providing CT scans to strengthen the chapter. Thanks also to Victor Haughton, M.D., and June Unger, M.D., for reviewing the manuscript and to Sandra Mundt for typing the manuscript.

REFERENCES

1. Chakeres D.W., Spiegel P.K.: A systematic technique for comprehensive evaluation of the temporal bone by computed tomography. *Radiology* 146:97–106, 1983.
2. Zonneveld F.W., Van Waes P.F.G.M., Damsma H., et al.: Direct multiplanar computed tomography of the petrous bone. *RadioGraphics* 3:400–449, 1983.
3. Barnes J.E.: Personal communication, 1982 (General Electric Medical Systems, Milwaukee).
4. Shaffer K.A., Haughton V.M., Wilson C.R.: High resolution computed tomography of the temporal bone. *Radiology* 134:409–414, 1980.
5. Zatz L.M.: Basic principles of computed tomography scanning, in Newton T.H., Potts D.G. (eds.): *Radiology of the Skull and Brain: Technical Aspects of Computed Tomography.* St. Louis, C.V. Mosby Co., 1981, vol. 5, pp. 3853–3876.
6. Shaffer K.A., Volz D.J., Haughton V.M.: Manipulation of CT data for temporal-bone imaging. *Radiology* 137:825–829, 1980.
7. Beatty C.W., Harris L.D., Suh K.W., et al.: Comparative study using computed tomographic thin-section zoom reconstructions and anatomic macrosections of the temporal bone. *Ann. Otol. Rhinol. Laryngol.* 90:643–649, 1981.
8. Littleton J.T., Shaffer K.A., Callahan W.P., et al.: Temporal bone: Comparison of pluridirectional tomography and high resolution computed tomography. *A.J.R.* 137:835–845, 1981.
9. De Smedt E., Potvliege R., Pimontel-Appel B., et al.: High resolution CT-scan of the temporal bone—a preliminary report. *J. Belge. Radiol.* 63:205–212, 1980.
10. Shaffer K.A.: CT of the temporal bone. *RadioGraphics* 1:62–72, 1981.
11. Taylor S.: The petrous temporal bone (including the cerebellopontine angle). *Radiol. Clin. North Am.* 20:67–86, 1982.
12. Virapongse C., Rothman S.L.G., Kier E.L., et al.: Computed tomographic anatomy of the temporal bone. *A.J.R.* 139:739–749, 1982.
13. Sando I., Wood R.P. II: Congenital middle ear anomalies. *Otolaryngol. Clin. North Am.* 4:291–318, 1971.

14. Hanafee W.N., Bergstrom L.: Radiology of congenital deformities of the ear. *Head Neck Surg.* 2:213–221, 1980.

15. Valvassori G.E., Naunton R.F., Lindsay J.R.: Inner ear anomalies: Clinical and histopathological considerations. *Ann. Otol. Rhinol. Laryngol.* 78:929–938, 1969.

16. Phelps P.D., Lloyd G.A.S., Poswillo D.: Congenital ear malformations and the facial nerve. Presented at the Ninth Congress of Radiology of Otolaryngology, Fontevraud, France, June 6–9, 1982.

17. Reisner K.: Tomography in inner and middle ear malformations. *Radiology* 92:11–20, 1969.

18. Unger J.M., Shaffer K.A.: The abnormal temporal bone in the "normal" deaf. *Head Neck Surg.* 3:185–192, 1981.

19. Wright J.W. Jr.: Polytomography and congenital external and middle ear anomalies. *Laryngoscope* 91:1806–1811, 1981.

20. Taylor S.: Personal communication, 1982.

21. Hanafee W.N. Mancuso A., Winter J., et al.: Edge enhancement computed tomography scanning in inflammatory lesions of the middle ear. *Radiology* 136:771–775, 1980.

22. Mendez G. Jr., Quencer R.M., Post M.J.D., et al.: Malignant external otitis: A radiographic-clinical correlation. *A.J.R.* 132:957–961, 1979.

23. Curtin H.D., Wolfe P., May M.: Malignant external otitis: CT evaluation. *Radiology* 145:383–388, 1982.

24. Chandler J.R.: Malignant external otitis: Further considerations. *Ann. Otol. Rhinol. Laryngol.* 86:417–428, 1977.

25. Hoffman R.A., Brookler K.H., Bergeron R.T.: Radiologic diagnosis of labyrinthitis ossificans. *Ann. Otol. Rhinol. Laryngol.* 88:253–257, 1979.

26. Hanafee W.N., Jenkins H.A., Mancuso A.A., et al.: Computerized tomography scanning of the temporal bone. *Ann. Otol. Rhinol. Laryngol.* 88:721–728, 1979.

27. Phelps P.D., Lloyd G.A.S.: The radiology of cholesteatoma. *Clin. Radiol.* 31:501–512, 1980.

28. Kreutzer E.W., DeBlanc G.B.: Extra-aural spread of acquired cholesteatoma: A report of two unique cases. *Arch. Otolaryngol.* 108:320–323, 1982.

29. Gacek R.R.: Evaluation and management of primary petrous apex cholesteatoma. *Otolaryngol. Head Neck Surg.* 88:519–523, 1980.

30. DeLozier H.L., Parkins C.W., Gacek R.R.: Clinical records: Mucocele of the petrous apex. *J. Laryngol. Otol.* 93:177–180, 1979.

31. Osborn A.G., Parkin J.L.: Mucocele of the petrous temporal bone. *A.J.R.* 132:680–681, 1979.

32. Komisar A., Som P.M., Shugar J.M.A., et al.: Benign chondroma of the petrous apex. *J. Comput. Assist. Tomogr.* 5:116–118, 1981.

33. McCaffrey T.V., McDonald T.J.: Histiocytosis X of the ear and temporal bone: Review of 22 cases. *Laryngoscope* 89:1735–1742, 1979.

34. Lloyd G.A.S., Phelps P.D., Du Boulay G.H.: High-resolution computerized tomography of the petrous bone. *Br. J. Radiol.* 53:631–641, 1980.

35. Mancuso A.A., Hanafee W.N.: *Computed Tomography of the Head and Neck.* Baltimore, Williams & Wilkins Co., 1982, pp. 244–287.

36. Lloyd G.A.S.: Tumors of the petro-mastoid demonstrated by high resolution CT. Presented at the Ninth International Congress of Radiology of Otolaryngology, Fontevraud, France, June 6–9, 1982.

37. Valvassori G.: Personal communication, 1982.

38. Johnson D., Vorhees R., Lufkin R., et al.: CT in the management of cholesteatomas of the temporal bone. *Radiology* 148:733–737, 1983.

39. Shaffer K.A.: Comparison of computed tomography and complex motion tomography in the diagnosis of cholesteatoma. *A.J.N.R.*, in press.

40. Petasnick J.P.: Tomography of the temporal bone in Paget's disease. *A.J.R.* 105:838–843, 1969.

41. Valvassori G., Potter G., Hanafee W., et al.: *Radiology of the Ear, Nose, and Throat.* Philadelphia, W.B. Saunders Co., 1982, pp. 12–126.

42. Zizmor J., Noyek A.: Tumors and other osseous disorders of the temporal bone. *Semin. Roentgenol.* 4:151–170, 1969.

43. Spector G.J., Maisel R.H., Ogura J.H.: Glomus tumors in the middle ear: I. An analysis of 46 patients. *Laryngoscope* 83:1652–1670, 1973.

44. Caughran M., White T.J. III., Gerald B., et al.: Computed tomography of jugulotympanic paragangliomas. *J. Comput. Assist. Tomogr.* 4:194–198, 1980.

45. Marsman J.W.P.: Tumors of the glomus jugulare complex (chemodectomas) demonstrated by cranial computed tomography. *J. Comput. Assist. Tomogr.* 3:795–799, 1979.

46. Valvassori G.E.: Vascular masses of the middle ear. Presented at the Postgraduate Course, the Ninth International Congress of Radiology of Otolaryngology, Fontevraud, France, June 5–6, 1982.

47. Denia A., Perez F., Canalis R.R., et al.: Extracanalicular osteomas of the temporal bone. *Arch. Otolaryngol.* 105:706–709, 1979.

48. Mangham C.A., Carberry J.N., Brackmann D.E.: Management of intratemporal vascular tumors. *Laryngoscope* 91:867–875, 1981.

49. Guzowski J., Paparella M.M., Rao K.N., et al.: Meningiomas of the temporal bone. *Laryngoscope* 84:1141–1146, 1976.

50. Parisier S.C., Som P.M., Shugar J.M.A., et al.: The evaluation of middle ear meningiomas using computerized axial tomography. *Laryngoscope* 88:1170–1177, 1978.

51. Brookler K.H., Hoffman R.A., Camins M., et al.: Trilobed meningioma: Ampulla of posterior semicircular canal, internal auditory canal, and cerebellopontine angle. *Am. J. Otol.* 1:171–173, 1980.

52. Neely J.G.: Neoplastic involvement of the facial nerve. *Otolaryngol. Clin. North Am.* 7:385–396, 1974.

53. Turski P., Norman D., DeGroot J., et al.: High-resolution CT of the petrous bone: Direct vs. reformatted images. *A.J.N.R.* 3:391–394, 1982.

54. DeLozier H.L., Gacek R.R., Dana S.T.: Intralabyrinthine schwannoma. *Ann. Otol. Rhinol. Laryngol.* 88:187–191, 1979.

55. Crabtree J.A., Britton B.H., Pierce M.K.: Carcinoma of the external auditory canal. *Laryngoscope* 86:405–415, 1976.

56. Phelps P.D., Lloyd G.A.S.: The radiology of carcinoma of the ear. *Br. J. Radiol.* 54:103–109, 1981.

57. Conley J., Schuller D.E.: Malignancies of the ear. *Laryngoscope* 86:1147–1163, 1976.

58. Lin C.-S., Zak F.G.: Studies on melanocytes: VI. Melanocytes in the middle ear. *Arch. Otolaryngol.* 108:489–490, 1982.

59. Chen K.T.K., Dehner L.P.: Primary tumors of the external and middle ear: I. Introduction and clinicopathologic study of squamous cell carcinoma. *Arch. Otolaryngol.* 104:247–252, 1978.

60. Dehner P., Chen K.T.K.: Primary tumors of the external and middle ear: III. A clinicopathologic study of embryonal rhabdomyosarcoma. *Arch. Otolaryngol.* 104:399–403, 1978.

61. Berlinger N.T., Koutroupas S., Adams G., et al.: Patterns of involvement of the temporal bone in metastatic and systemic malignancy. *Laryngoscope* 90:619–627, 1980.

62. Coppola R.J., Salanga V.D.: Metastatic prostatic adenocarcinoma to the temporal bone. *Neurology* 30:311–315, 1980.

63. Hobeika C.P.: Trauma involving the temporal bone. *Otolaryngol. Clin. North Am.* 2:433–447, 1969.

64. Harker L.A., McCabe B.F.: Temporal bone fractures and facial nerve injury. *Otolaryngol. Clin. North Am.* 7:425–431, 1974.

65. Wright J.W. Jr.: Trauma of the ear. *Radiol. Clin. North Am.* 12:527–532, 1974.

66. Vignaud J., Aubin M.L., Baleriaux-Waha D., et al.: CT-scan diagnosis of lesions causing an angle or internal auditory canal syndrome. *J. Belge. Radiol.* 63:295–311, 1980.

67. Olson J.E., Glasscock M.E., Britton B.H.: Lipomas of the internal auditory canal. *Arch. Otolaryngol.* 104:431–436, 1978.

68. Hatam A., Bergvall U., Lewander R., et al.: Contrast medium enhancement with time in computer tomography. *Acta Radiol. Suppl.* 348:63–81, 1975.

69. Hatam A., Bergstrom M., Moller A., et al.: Early contrast enhancement of acoustic neuroma. *Neuroradiology* 17:31–33, 1978.

70. Lewander R., Bergstrom M., Bergvall U.: Contrast enhancement of cranial lesions in computed tomography. *Acta Radiol.* 19:529–552, 1978.

71. Valavanis A., Schubiger O., Wellauer J.: Computed tomography of acoustic neuromas with emphasis on small tumor detectability. *Neuroradiology* 16:598–600, 1978.

72. Daniels D.L., Haughton V.M., Williams A.L., et al.: The flocculus in computed tomography. *A.J.N.R.* 2:227–229, 1981.

73. Weinberg P.E., Kim K.S., Gore R.M.: Unilateral enlargement of the internal auditory canal: A developmental variant. *Surg. Neurol.* 15:39–42, 1981.

74. Hatam A., Bergstrom M., Berggren B.M., et al.: Attenuation profiles of the petrous bone with acoustic neuroma. *Neuroradiology* 19:123–129, 1980.

75. O'Connor S.M., Sackett J.F.: Radiologic evaluation of the cerebellopontine cistern and the internal auditory canal. *Head Neck Surg.* 3:193–197, 1981.

76. Kaseff L.G., Perkins R., Hambley W.H.: Radiological techniques for small acoustic tumors: A re-evaluation. *Laryngoscope* 91:63–70, 1981.

77. Anderson R., Diehl J., Maravilla K., et al.: Computerized axial tomography with air contrast of the cerebellopontine angle and internal auditory canal. *Laryngoscope* 91:1083–1097, 1981.

78. Siew F.P., Kricheff I.I., Chase N.E.: Demonstration of small acoustic neuromas, using negative contrast medium with tomography. *Radiology* 91:764–769, 1968.

79. Kricheff I.I., Pinto R.S., Bergeron R.T., et al.: Air-CT cisternography and canalography for small acoustic neuromas. *A.J.N.R.* 1:57–63, 1980.

80. Sortland O.: Computed tomography combined with gas cisternography for the diagnosis of expanding lesions in the cerebellopontine angle. *Neuroradiology* 18:19–22, 1979.

81. Bentson J.R., Mancuso A.A., Winter J., et al.: Combined gas cisternography and edge-enhanced computed tomography of the internal auditory canal. *Radiology* 136:777–779, 1980.

82. Naidich T.P.: Air CT canalography for the evaluation of the internal auditory canals. *Laryngoscope* 90:526–530, 1980.

83. Penley M.W., Pribram H.F.W.: Diagnosis of cerebellopontine angle tumors with small quantities of air. *Otolaryngol. Head Neck Surg.* 89:457–462, 1981.

84. Lee S.H., Lewis E., Montoya J.H., et al: Bilateral cerebellopontine angle air-CT cisternography. *A.J.N.R.* 2:105–106, 1981.

85. Pinto R.S., Kricheff I.I., Bergeron R.T., et al.: Small acoustic neuromas: Detection by high resolution gas CT cisternography. *A.J.R.* 139:129–132, 1982.

86. Downey E.F. Jr., Buck D.R., Ray J.W.: Arachnoiditis simulating acoustic neuroma on air-CT cisternography. *A.J.N.R.* 2:470–471, 1981.

87. Curtin H.D.: Evaluation of the internal auditory canal using pluridirectional tomography with metrizamide. *Radiology* 144:115–120, 1982.

88. Huete I., Corrales M.: Computed cisternography in the diagnosis of small acoustic neurinomas. *J. Neuroradiol.* 6:335–340, 1979.

89. Rosenbaum A.E., Drayer B.P., Dubois P.J., et al.: Visualization of small extracanalicular neurilemmomas by metrizamide cisternographic enhancement. *Arch. Otolaryngol.* 104:239–243, 1978.

90. Valavanis A., Schubiger O., Hayek J., et al.: CT of meningiomas on the posterior surface of the petrous bone. *Neuroradiology* 22:111–121, 1981.

91. Moller A., Hatam A., Olivecrona H.: Diagnosis of acoustic neuroma with computed tomography. *Neuroradiology* 17:25–30, 1978.

92. Hamel E., Frowein R.A., Karimi-Nejad A.: Intracranial intradural epidermoids and dermoids. *Neurosurg. Rev.* 3:215–219, 1980.

93. Dee R.H., Kishore P.R.S., Young H.F.: Radiological evaluation of cerebellopontine angle epidermoid tumor. *Surg. Neurol.* 13:293–296, 1980.

94. Gagliardi F.M., Vagnozzi R., Caruso R., et al.: Epidermoids of the cerebellopontine angle (cpa): Usefulness of CT scan. *Acta Neurochir.* 54:271–281, 1980.

95. Braun I.F., Naidich T.P., Leeds N.E., et al.: Dense intracranial epidermoid tumors. *Radiology* 122:717–719, 1977.

96. Rao K.G., Woodlief R.M.: CT simulation of cerebellopontine tumor by tortous vertebrobasilar artery. *A.J.R.* 132:672–673. 1979.

24

Nose, Paranasal Sinuses, and Facial Bones

HUGH D. CURTIN, M.D.

THE ABILITY of CT to demonstrate the components of the soft tissue rather than just bone detail as seen on plain films and tomography has produced a dramatic change in the radiologist's role in evaluating the nose, paranasal sinuses, and face. Instead of predicting the extent of pathology by evaluating subtle bone changes, we can now demonstrate quite accurately the margins of the disease process itself.[1-4] Defining the precise extent of a lesion is the primary role of the radiologist, but in some instances a fairly specific diagnosis can be confidently suggested. The radiologist must understand the disease processes as well as the anatomy in order to determine extension of the pathology.

Before proceeding with a description of the various pathologic entities that affect the area of the paranasal sinuses, two important CT concepts will be discussed. First, while one of the major advantages of CT over the other radiographic studies is the capability of showing various components of nonbony soft tissue, CT exquisitely defines bony contours and anatomy. Because bony structures represent natural barriers to the spread of disease, the various bony changes visible on CT will be discussed. Second, because CT lends itself to efforts to define more precisely what is actually present in an opaque sinus, this problem will be briefly discussed.

Finally, the section on use of CT in various disease states will begin with neoplasm, and it is in this section that routes of spread will be emphasized. Detection of spread necessitates knowledge of the anatomy as well as potential pathologic pathways. It is here also that the anatomical landmarks important in CT evaluation of the sinuses will be presented.

This chapter is not a complete description of individual pathologic entities, but stresses general principles of CT evaluation. Congenital anomalies are not routinely evaluated with CT and are not included here, but should be kept in mind when an abnormality is detected on CT. Other areas where CT is useful in the sinus area, such as encephaloceles, are discussed elsewhere in this book.

GENERAL CT OBSERVATIONS

Bone Changes

As in plain radiography and tomography, bone changes are very important in CT. Currently, the findings in CT are often an extrapolation of the findings on plain films or tomography, which have been well described in the literature.[4-6]

Bone Destruction

Destruction of a bony wall is very significant in an aggressive process such as malignancy, mycotic infection, or granulomatous disease. In definition of bone destruction, CT is competitive with tomography. However, care must be taken not to produce apparent destruction of bone on CT by overwindowing; that is, thin bone can be made to disappear by changing window settings on the CT console (see Figs 24–5 and 24–16). Very thin bone may have density lower than typical bone because of partial volume effect if the slice orientation is slightly oblique to the bone. The correct interpretation of bone destruction is aided by the ability of CT to define the soft tissues on the outer (nonsinus) side of the bone. A fat plane is often conveniently present on the outer side of the bony wall, and obliteration of this fat plane is a very sensitive indication of progression of pathology through the bone (Fig 24–1). When a fat plane is not present, it is more difficult to detect minimal extension through the bone. In these cases, however, there is often enough density difference between the pathologic process and the soft tissues on the outer side of the bone that some assessment can be made. This will be further discussed in the section on direct extension of tumors.

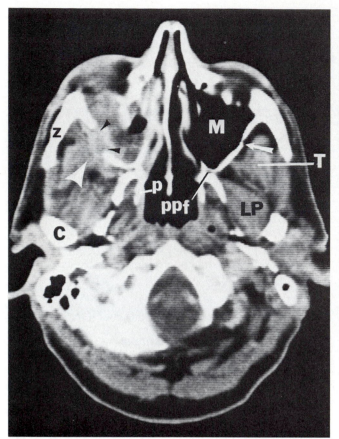

Fig 24–1.—Squamous cell carcinoma involving the maxillary sinus and infraorbital nerve. Note destruction of posterolateral wall of the sinus *(small arrowheads)* and tumor obliterating the fat plane just outside the sinus *(large arrowhead)*. Compare with normal structures on opposite side. (*M* = maxillary sinus, *arrow* denotes fat plane outside wall of maxillary sinus, *z* = zygomatic arch, *p* = pterygoid plate, *LP* = lateral pterygoid muscle, *C* = mandibular condyle, *ppf* = pterygopalatine fossa, *T* = temporalis muscle.)

Bowing or Remodelling of the Bony Wall

Bowing of the bony structures implies slow growth, with remodelling occurring as the bone reacts to the presence and the slow growth of the lesion. This is classic in mucocele formation, but is also seen in slow-growing benign neoplastic lesions. We have seen it occasionally in a slow-growing malignancy, perhaps because of softening of the bone (Figs 24–2 and 24–3). Therefore, the finding does not exclude malignancy.[7]

Enlargement of a Foramen or Neural Canal

Enlargement of a neural foramen demonstrated during the work-up of a malignancy very strongly suggests extension of tumor along the nerve. In such a case, the radiologist must carefully evaluate the more central segments of the involved nerve to properly stage a tumor. Again, the advantage of CT lies in its ability to

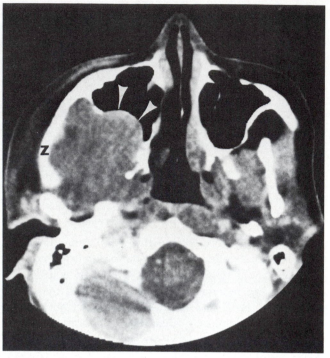

Fig 24–2.—Undifferentiated small cell carcinoma in infratemporal fossa (deep to the zygoma) bowing, but not completely destroying, the posterolateral wall of the maxillary sinus *(arrowheads)*. The tumor obliterates fat planes in the infratemporal fossa. (*z* = zygoma.)

demonstrate the soft tissues both at the entrance and the exit of the various neural foramina. Benign lesions such as neuromas can also enlarge neural foramina.

Sclerotic Walls

Thickening of the bony wall is the bone's natural reaction to any stress or insult. This sclerotic change indicates a chronic lesion and is most commonly seen in inflammatory disease (Fig 24–4) such as chronic sinusitis, but has also been described in association with tumors. Bony sclerosis and bone thickening can also be seen as a reaction to surgery or after radiation therapy (Fig 24–5).

Hyperostosis and sclerosis can be associated with meningioma and rarely will affect walls of the sinuses. This usually occurs in the region of the sphenoid, but can affect the maxillary sinus when the meningioma reaches the infratemporal fossa. Hyperostosis from meningioma is discussed in Chapter 10 of this book.

Bone Enlargement

Fibrous dysplasia represents abnormal formation and mineralization of bone. The bone is increased in size and can be very dense, resembling cortical bone, or can have a somewhat lower CT density depending on the degree of mineralized matrix. Descriptions of the CT

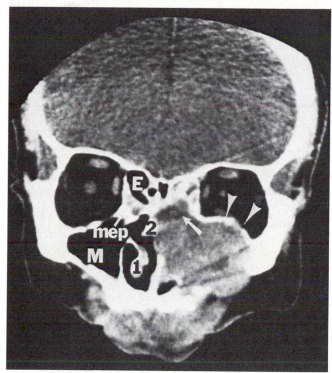

Fig 24–3.—Coronal scan. Fibrous histiocytoma of maxillary sinus bowing the orbital floor superiorly *(arrowheads),* pushing up the inferior rectus muscle. There is also destruction of the maxilloethmoidal plate *(arrow)* and lateral wall of the maxillary sinus as tumor extends into ethmoid sinus and cheek respectively. The upper ethmoid may be opacified by obstruction rather than actual tumor involvement as evidenced by residual septation. Compare with normal side. (M = maxillary sinus, E = ethmoid sinus, mep = maxillary ethmoid plate, 1 = inferior turbinate, 2 = middle turbinate.)

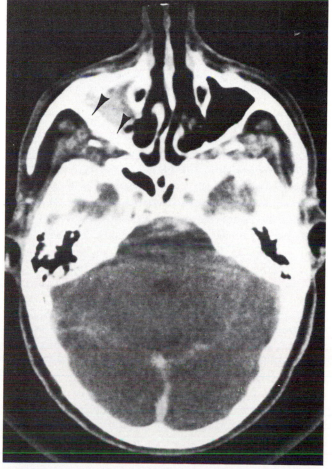

Fig 24–4.—Chronic sinusitis in maxillary antrum. The bony wall is thickened and sclerotic *(arrowheads).*

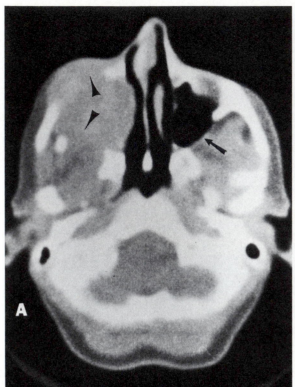

Fig 24–5.—A, squamous cell carcinoma preradiation. Tumor of maxillary sinus is "destroying" anterior and posterior walls *(arrowheads).* Note, however, how posterolateral wall of maxillary sinus on opposite side is indistinct because of "overwindowing" *(arrow).* **B,** postradiation therapy. Note thickened sclerotic bone of malar eminence *(arrowhead). (PPF* = pterygopalatine fossa, *3* = nasolacrimal duct.)

appearances of fibrous dysplasia are somewhat limited (Fig 24–6).[8]

Other bony dysplasias can result in thickening and increased density in the bones of the skeleton. These include osteopetrosis, craniometaphyseal dysplasia, sclerostosis, and cortical hyperostosis (Fig 24–7). Although the abnormalities can be detected by CT, they are easily evaluated by other methods. The radiologist may, however, see these changes incidently on CT when evaluating the patient for another problem.[9–11]

A patient with an increased blood cell turnover, such as in thalassemia, can have grossly enlarged marrow spaces that may result in an increase in bony thickness without necessarily an increase in bone density (Fig 24–8). This represents an increase in the patient's marrow as it extends into the bony walls of, for instance, the maxillary sinus. This results in a decrease in the size of the sinus, but an increase in the size of the maxilla. Paget's disease can thicken the facial bones and encroach upon the sinuses.

The "Opaque Sinus"

Opacity of a sinus can be due to inflamed mucosa, cyst, tumor, retained secretions, blood, or occasionally the result of a bony obliteration or maldevelopment. When malignancy is present, the opaque sinus becomes an even more significant diagnostic problem. The opacity can be due to extension of tumor into the sinus itself or can be related to obstruction of the outflow of the sinus. When outflow from the sinus is compromised, there is retention of secretions that eventually may lead to mucocele formation. The earliest radiographic finding, however, is opacification without any bony change. A low uniform density in the sinus on an enhanced scan suggests retained secretions. The mucosa may enhance with intravenous contrast, and this combined with a uniform low density is, in a sense, quite reassuring (Fig 24–9). The mucosal enhancement is, however, not always visualized. Often, with rapid infusion of contrast, a tumor will enhance, and the ability to see the tumor margin bordered by the low density of retained secretions allows the radiologist to define how much of an opaque sinus is tumor (Fig 24–10).

If, however, the sinus does not have a uniformly low CT density, the problem is more difficult. Tumor and inflamed mucosa can have very similar appearances on intravenously enhanced CT scans. When an obstructed sinus develops infection and the mucosa is enlarged and

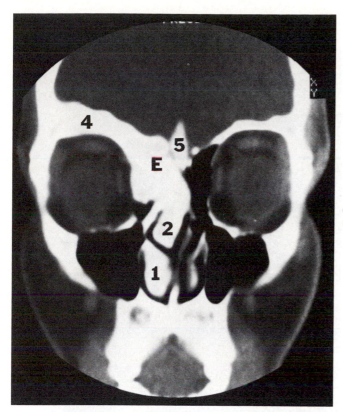

Fig 24–6.—Fibrous dysplasia involving the roof of the orbit *(4)*. (*E* = ethmoid air cells, *1* = inferior turbinate, *2* = middle turbinate, *5* = crista galli.)

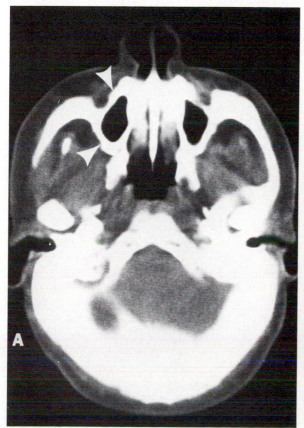

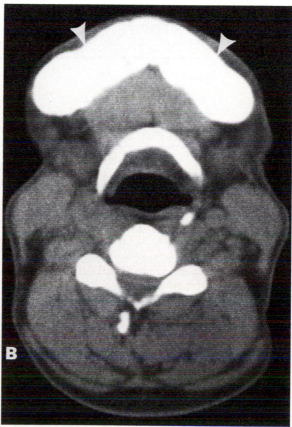

Fig 24–7.—**A,** Van Buchem's disease (hyperostosis corticalis generalisata). The skull base is thickened, as are the walls of the maxillary sinus *(arrowheads).* **B,** the mandible shows considerable hyperostosis also *(arrowheads).*

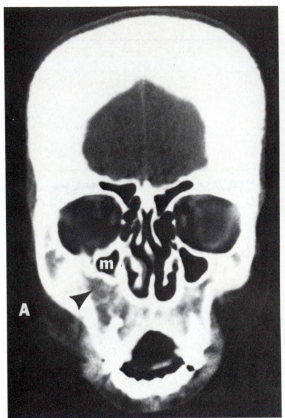

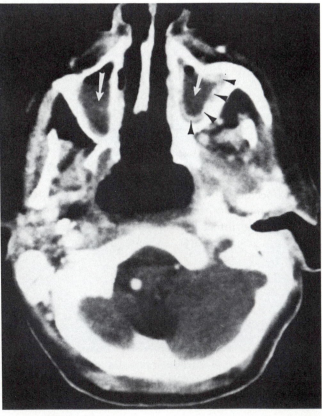

Fig 24–8.—A, thalassemia major, coronal cut. The marrow spaces in the maxilla and zygoma are enlarged *(arrowhead)* with resultant thickening of bone and decrease in size of maxillary sinuses *(m).* Note also the thickening of the skull. **B,** axial slice showing widened marrow spaces *(arrowheads).* Patient has juvenile angiofibroma extending into the infratemporal fossa and into the maxillary sinus *(arrow).*

Fig 24–9.—Opaque sinuses. Note retention of secretions that have low attenuation *(arrows).* The mucosa presumed to be inflamed enhances *(arrowheads),* outlining the sinus. Patient had had previous therapy for nasopharyngeal lesion.

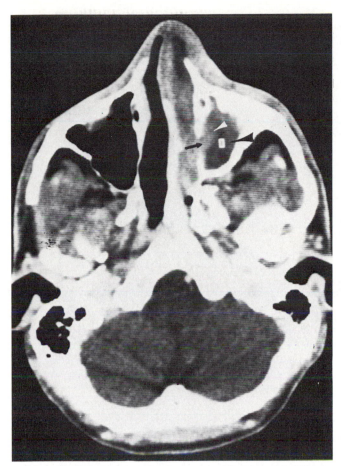

Fig 24–10.—Tumor (histiocytic lymphoma) in nasal cavity extending through maxillary ostium *(arrow)* causing obstruction. The lesion enhances, differentiating tumor *(small arrowhead)* from the retained secretions *(large arrowhead).*

inflamed, it is very difficult to differentiate where the neoplasm stops and the inflammatory mucosa begins. In the large maxillary sinus, this is not as difficult a problem, because the mucosa may be separated from the tumor by low-density secretions. It is, however, a major problem in smaller air cells such as in the ethmoid sinus, where minimal swelling of the mucosa may virtually occlude the space so that the entire sinus enhances, mimicking tumor. In such a case, one hopes to demonstrate intact bony septations, which suggest obstruction of the outflow of the sinus and perhaps subsequent infection rather than actual extension of tumor throughout the air cells (Fig 24–11). More investigation with correlation of pathologic specimens and CT findings is necessary before firm conclusions can be made with respect to the opacified sinus.

TUMOR AND TUMOR-LIKE CONDITIONS

To evaluate neoplasm in the region of the nose and sinuses, one must have a knowledge of the anatomy and

routes of spread of neoplastic processes.[5] The important methods of tumor spread are direct extension, extension along nerves, lymphatic spread to the nodes, and hematogenous spread. Hematogenous spread is very rare.

Routes of Spread

Direct Extension

While tumor extension through a bony margin of a sinus can be detected by destructive changes in the bone itself, visualizing the pathology in the soft tissue on the other (outer) side of the bone is the true advantage of CT. The density of the tissue on the outer side of the bony wall of the sinus determines the ease of detection of this transosseous spread of tumor.

MAXILLARY SINUS.—The maxillary sinus is perhaps the easiest to evaluate, because its bony margins are oriented perpendicular to either axial or coronal planes, and the tissues or spaces on the outer side of the bone lend themselves to CT investigation. Tumor can progress in any direction.

Posterior and Posterolateral Extension.—Tumor extending through the posterolateral wall spreads into the infratemporal fossa. A well-defined fat plane borders

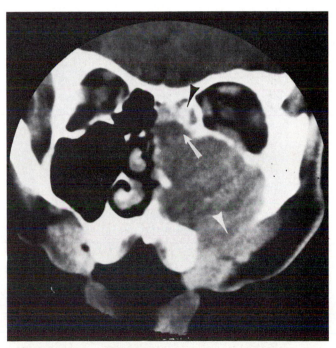

Fig 24–11.—Inverting papilloma and squamous cell carcinoma. Tumor of nasal cavity and maxillary sinus extending into lower ethmoid sinus *(arrow).* The upper ethmoids were not aerated. The septae *(black arrowhead)* are intact, suggesting obstruction rather than tumor extension, but tumor cannot be definitely excluded. Tumor also extends through anterior wall of maxillary antrum *(white arrowhead).*

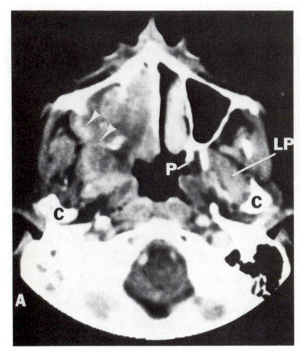
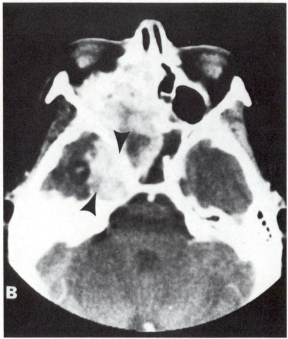

Fig 24–12.—A, adenocystic carcinoma nasal cavity and maxillary sinus extending through posterolateral wall into infratemporal fossa *(arrowheads).* The pterygoid plates are destroyed and pterygoid muscle involved. (Normal side: *P* = pterygoid plates, *LP* = lateral pterygoid muscle, *C* = mandibular condyles.) **B,** tumor eroded through skull base into middle cranial fossa *(arrowheads).*

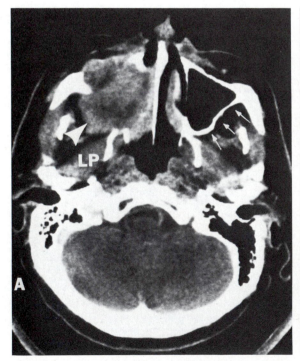
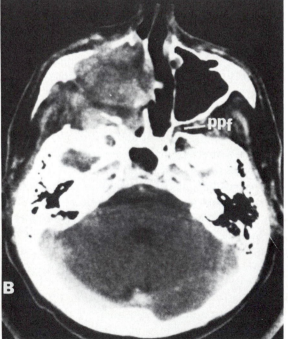

Fig 24–13.—A, tumor eroding posterolateral wall of maxillary sinus and extruding into fat of the infratemporal fossa. Tumor margin *(arrowhead).* The pterygoid muscle *(LP)* is not involved. Note the intact fat plane *(small arrows)* behind the maxillary sinus on the normal side. **B,** higher slice showing involvement of the pterygopalatine fossa. Note fat density in pterygopalatine fossa *(ppf)* on the normal side.

the bony wall of the sinus, separating it from the temporalis muscle (Figs 24–12 and 24–13). The pterygoid muscles are well seen on CT, and involvement of the muscles themselves is of great importance in determination of treatment.

Direct posterior extension gives tumor access to the pterygopalatine fossa and its cluster of nerves and vessels (see Figs 24–12 and 24–13). There is almost always enough fatty tissue in the pterygopalatine fossa itself to allow visualization on CT, both in axial and coronal projections. Obliteration of this fat indicates extension into the area, but bone destruction is almost always present in cases of direct extension of malignancy. The pterygopalatine fossa can also be involved as tumor spreads along a nerve, especially the infraorbital nerve, as discussed in a later section.

Superior Extension.—Superiorly, tumor spreads from the maxillary sinus into the orbit, where oblitera-

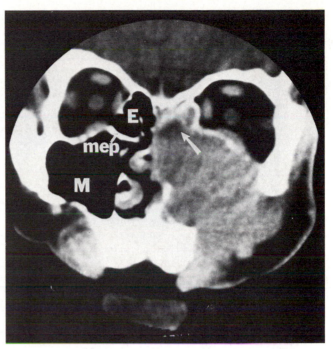

Fig 24–15.—Coronal section through tumor of maxillary sinus extending through maxilloethmoid plate into lower ethmoid *(arrow)*. (Normal side: *mep* = maxillary ethmoid plate, *M* = maxillary sinus, *E* = ethmoid sinus).

tion of the extraconal fat near the inferior rectus is a good indicator of tumor extension (Fig 24–14). Superomedial extension is through the bony maxilloethmoidal plate into the ethmoid sinus (Fig 24–15). Again, the difficulty in attempting to differentiate tumor involving the ethmoid sinus from an obstructive process must be emphasized. The maxilloethmoidal plate is usually thick enough to allow evaluation of destruction.

Coronal scans are used to evaluate subtle changes in the orbital floor and extension into the ethmoid sinuses. On axial scans, the superior recess of the maxillary sinus is often seen at the same level as the orbital contents, and tumor involvement of this recess should not be confused with extension into the orbit. The bony floor of the orbit is angled at this level and so is often not visible on axial CT (Fig 24–16). Coronal views can be used to make the differentiation.

Medial, Anterior, and Inferior Extension.—Medial extension from the maxillary sinus is into the nasal cavity, destroying the common wall between the nasal cavity and the sinus (Fig 24–17). This wall can be thin, making assessment of its integrity difficult. Anterior extension can be readily seen as tumor encroaches on the fat planes of the cheek (Fig 24–18).

Inferiorly, the tumor can destroy the alveolar ridge and form a mass in the oral cavity. Performing a scan with the mouth slightly open can be helpful, because

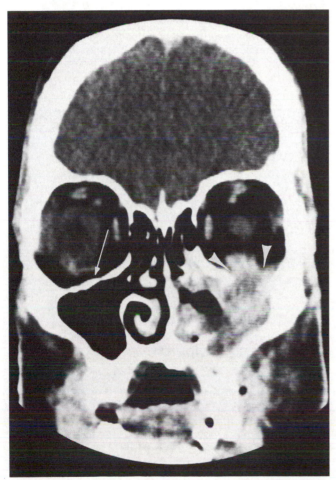

Fig 24–14.—Tumor involving upper maxillary sinus with destruction of orbital floor and involvement of the orbit. The lesion obliterates the fat just above the floor *(arrowheads)*. Note normal fat plane *(long arrow)* just above the orbital floor on the normal side.

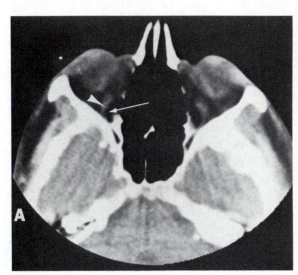

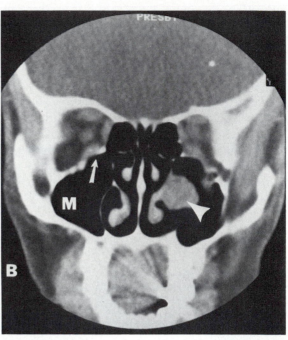

Fig 24–16.—A, axial scan through superior recess of the maxillary sinus *(arrow)* at the level of the lower orbit. Tumor extending into this region can be confused with involvement of the orbit, especially as in this case, when the bony wall is indistinct *(arrowhead)*. **B,** coronal scan showing relationship of the superior recess *(arrow)* of the maxillary sinus *(M)* to the orbit. Tumor of maxillary sinus is indicated by *arrowhead*.

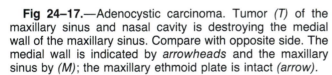

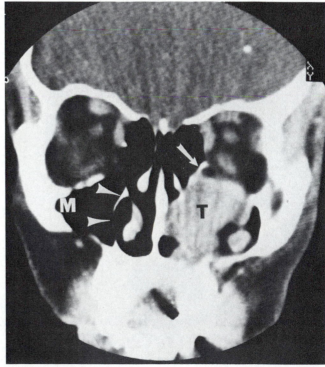

Fig 24–17.—Adenocystic carcinoma. Tumor *(T)* of the maxillary sinus and nasal cavity is destroying the medial wall of the maxillary sinus. Compare with opposite side. The medial wall is indicated by *arrowheads* and the maxillary sinus by *(M)*; the maxillary ethmoid plate is intact *(arrow)*.

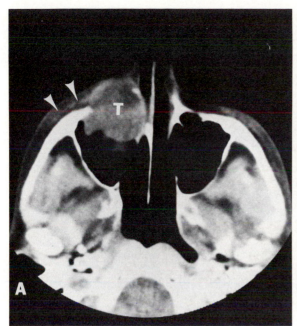

Fig 24–18.—A, tumor *(T)* involving anterior maxillary sinus wall and anterior cheek with destruction of the anterior wall of the maxillary sinus. The superficial muscle of the face is indicated by *arrowheads.* **B,** coronal scan with tumor extending into the fat planes of the cheek *(small arrow).* Also note erosion of orbital rim.

air bordering the palate will act as a natural contrast agent. Extension by this route is, however, easily evaluated clinically (Fig 24–19).

ETHMOID SINUSES.—Extension from the ethmoid can be inferiorly into the maxillary sinus through the maxilloethmoidal plate or into the nasal cavity. All are well evaluated by CT. Tumor destroys the bone, and the mass is seen encroaching on the airspaces.

Evaluation of the extension into the orbits from the ethmoid is also quite accurate as tumor extends into the orbital fat, this time medial to the medial rectus (Fig 24–20).

Superior extension is indicated by destruction of the cribriform plate and roof of the ethmoid. Tumor extending through the dura involves the frontal lobe, and the tumor margin can usually be identified on a coronal scan with contrast enhancement (Figs 24–21 and 24–22).

Posterior extension leads the tumor into the sphenoethmoidal recess and sphenoid sinus (Fig 24–23). The sphenoethmoidal recess is a narrow extension of the nasal cavity between the ethmoid and sphenoid sinuses. More laterally, only a bony wall separates the two sinuses. Bone destruction indicates tumor extension. Because of the position of the draining ostium of the sphenoid, tumor extending posteriorly from ethmoid into sphenoethmoid recess may obstruct the sphenoid sinus. Again, differentiation of tumor extension from obstructive changes is difficult without frank bone de-

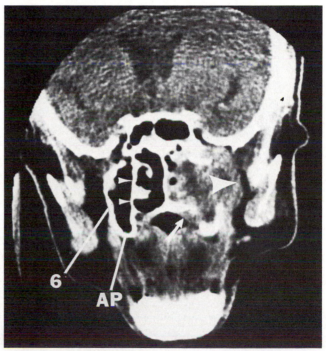

Fig 24–19.—Coronal slice of tumor of the maxillary sinus destroying medial wall and lateral wall. Tumor extends into fat planes of the infratemporal fossa *(large arrowhead).* The tumor breaks through into the mouth *(arrow).* Normal side: Medial wall of maxillary sinus is indicated by *small arrowheads,* lateral wall by *6,* and alveolar process by *AP.*

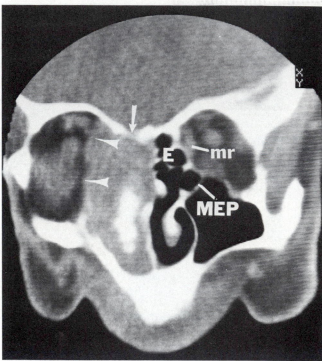

Fig 24–20.—Adenocystic carcinoma of the ethmoid extending laterally into the orbit, obliterating fat planes near medial rectus. Tumor margin is indicated by *arrowheads*. There is erosion of, but not extension through, the roof of the ethmoid *(arrow)*. Normal side: *E* = ethmoid, *MEP* = maxillary ethmoid plate, *mr* = medial rectus.

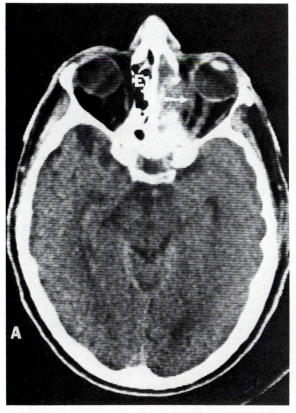

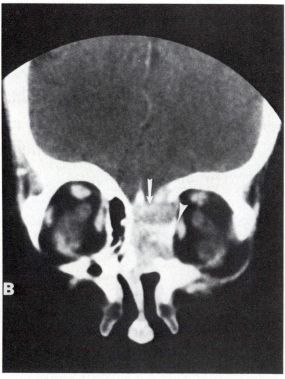

Fig 24–21.—**A,** tumor of ethmoid. Axial scan shows tumor extending laterally, deviating the medial rectus *(arrow)*. (*E* = ethmoid) **B,** coronal shows early lateral extension, but fat plane is intact *(arrowhead)*, suggesting lesion is limited by periosteum at this level. The cribriform is eroded *(arrow)*.

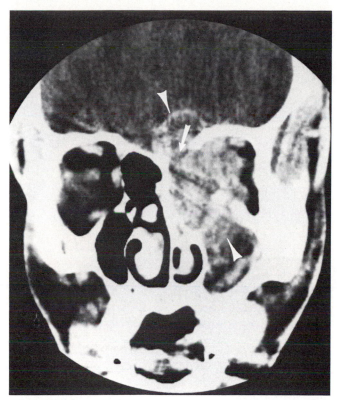

Fig 24–22.—Rhabdomyosarcoma of ethmoid and orbit extending through roof of ethmoid. Also note extension into the maxillary sinus. Tumor margin is indicated by *arrowheads*. *Arrow* denotes defect in roof of ethmoid.

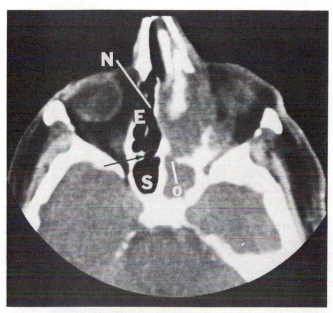

Fig 24–23.—Tumor of ethmoid extending posteriorly into sphenoethmoid recess and sphenoid sinus as well as into the orbit. (Normal side: *E* = ethmoid, *S* = sphenoid, *arrow* indicates sphenoethmoid recess, *o* = ostium of sphenoid sinus, *N* = upper nasal cavity.)

struction. This will be also discussed in the mucocele section.

SPHENOID SINUS.—Tumors arising in the sphenoid are quite rare in our experience, and the problem is more commonly one of nasopharyngeal or ethmoid tumor extending into and at times through the sphenoid. Bone destruction is the key to demonstrating extension, but again, CT is able to effectively visualize the structures outside the sinus. It may be very difficult to determine if a tumor is extending into the brain or limited by dura.

Superiorly, tumor extends into the pituitary fossa and suprasellar cisterns; posteriorly, into the prepontine and crural cisterns. These areas normally are filled with cerebrospinal fluid and can be evaluated well using coronal and axial scans respectively.

Tumor extends laterally into the cavernous sinus and eventually into the region of the temporal lobe. Examination performed with intravenous enhancement will show lateral bowing of the lateral margin of the cavernous sinus and can differentiate tumor from normal brain quite well (Fig 24–24). Without displacement of the cavernous sinus or extension into the temporal lobe, however, emphasis is made again on the difficulty in differentiating bone loss resulting from tumor extension from that caused by early mucocele formation secondary to sinus obstruction. Low density can suggest mucocele formation, but central necrosis in the tumor will also produce an area of low density.

FRONTAL SINUS.—The frontal sinus is rarely a site of primary malignancy, but may be along the route of spread of another malignancy (Fig 24–25). Detection of tumor spread posteriorly into the dura and brain can be detected both by the bone destruction and by the differential density between tumor and brain on an intravenously enhanced scan.

NASAL CAVITY.—Tumors of the nasal cavity tend to extend into the sinuses, where they can be seen in contrast to the air in the sinuses. Obstruction of the sinus ostium by the tumor is also quite common, returning us to the problem of the opaque sinus (Fig 24–26). Rapid infusion of contrast material may be helpful in demonstrating the margin of the tumor, thus differentiating neoplasm from the obstructed areas within the sinus.

Lymphatic Spread

Lymphatic spread from sinus and nasal cavity lesions is relatively infrequent. The nodal groups most commonly involved should be included in the radiologic examination. They include the lateral pharyngeal nodes, the jugulodigastric nodes, and deep cervical nodes. The

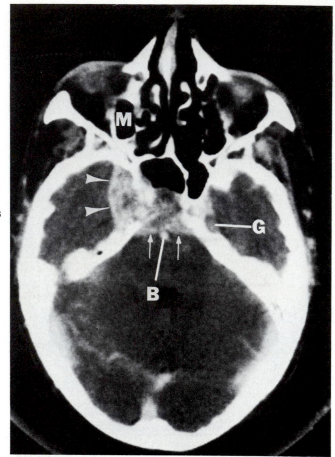

Fig 24–24.—Nasopharyngeal tumor involving posterior and lateral wall of sphenoid. Laterally, tumor extends through gasserian ganglion and cavernous sinus and abuts on temporal lobe *(arrowheads).* Posteriorly, tumor extends into prepontine cistern *(arrows)* and pushes the basilar artery *(B).* (*G* = gasserian ganglion [normal], *M* = superior recess of maxillary sinus.)

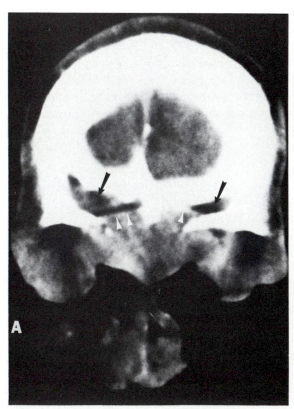

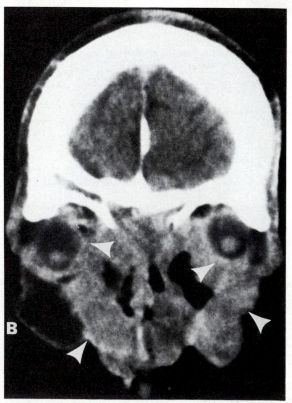

Fig 24–25.—**A,** basal squamous cell carcinoma, tumor of face extending through anterior wall of the frontal sinus. Tumor margin is indicated by *arrowheads.* The position of the tumor would prevent drainage of the sinuses through the nasofrontal ducts, causing mucous retention *(arrows).* **B,** more posterior slice shows involvement of the orbits with deviation of eyes. Tumor margin is indicated by *arrowheads.*

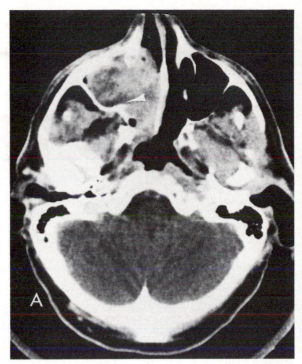
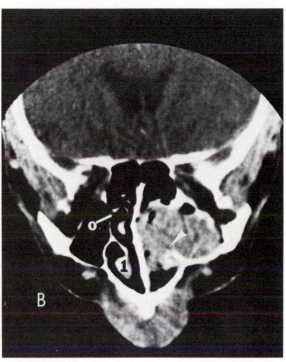

Fig 24–26.—A, inverting papilloma, tumor of nasal cavity extending into the maxillary sinus. The tumor passes through the natural ostium, but also destroys a portion of the medial wall of maxillary sinus and turbinate *(arrow-head)*. **B,** coronal scan. Tumor erodes bone minimally *(ar-rowhead)*. (Normal side: *o* = maxillary ostium, *1* = inferior turbinate.)

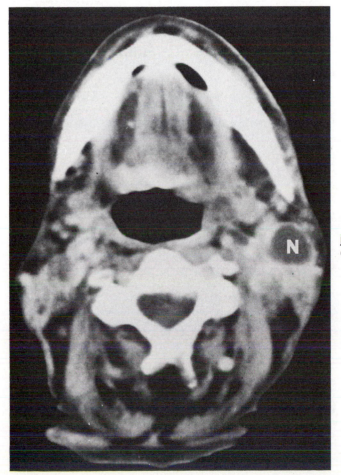

Fig 24–27.—Typical appearance of an involved jugulodigastric lymph node with enhancing margin and low-density center (squamous cell carcinoma). (*N* = node.)

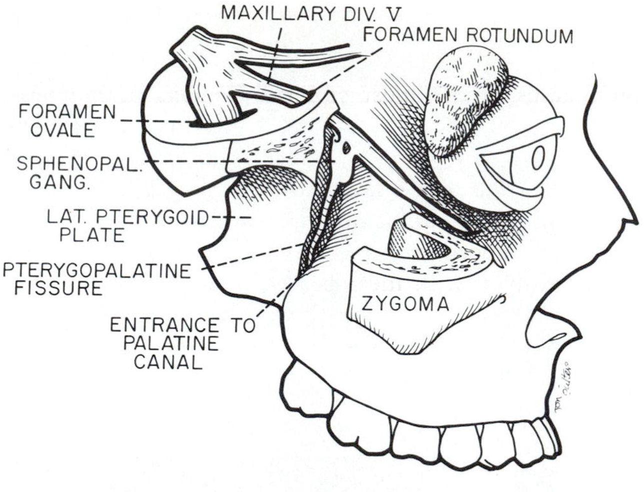

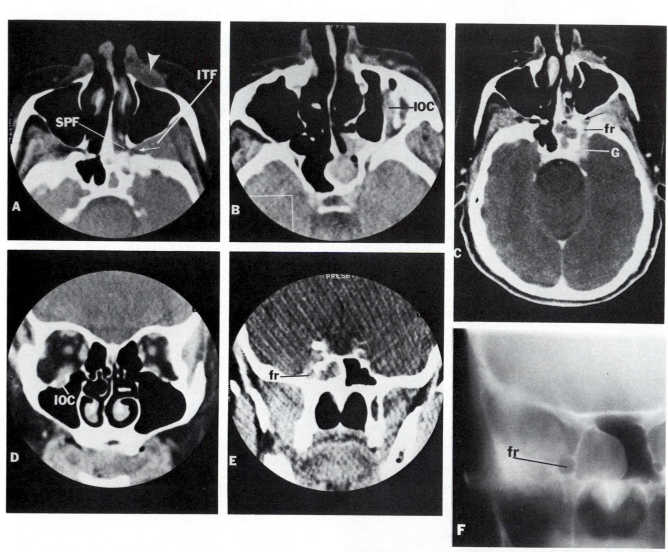

Fig 24–28.—Diagram of maxillary division of trigeminal intraorbital nerve, which is seen along floor of orbit.

Fig 24–29.—**A,** mixed histiocytic lymphocytic lymphoma, tumor of cheek *(white arrowhead)* and infratemporal fossa *(ITF)* obliterating fat plane in pterygopalatine fossa *(short arrow).* Tumor extends through sphenopalatine foramen *(SPF)* into posterior nasal cavity. **B,** axial view. The infraorbital canal is enlarged as it passes along orbital floor. *(IOC = infraorbital canal.)* **C,** tumor in pterygopalatine fossa *(short arrow).* Tumor extends through and enlarges foramen rotundum *(fr).* Enhancement is seen in the gasserian ganglion region *(G).* **D,** coronal slice through enlarged infraorbital canal *(IOC).* **E,** coronal slice showing enlarged foramen rotundum *(fr).* **F,** confirmatory tomogram of enlarged foramen rotundum *(fr).*

532

lymphatics of the most superior regions of the nasal cavity can travel on both sides of the cribriform plate and can also drain to the retropharyngeal nodes. A superficial lesion of the face or the vestibule of the nose can drain to the submandibular and parotid nodes.

In our experience, a common CT appearance of a node involved with metastatic disease is a low-density center with peripheral enhancement (Fig 24–27).

Transforaminal Spread

Tumor spread along a nerve trunk is an ominous sign (Fig 24–28). Adenocystic carcinoma is well known for extending along nerves, but other malignancies can also metastasize in this manner.[12–15] Tumor following the infraorbital nerve spreads to the pterygopalatine fossa (Fig 24–29). The alveolar and palatine nerves can also carry a malignancy to the pterygopalatine fossa (Fig 24–30). Involvement of this fossa is demonstrated by obliteration of the normal fat density within the fossa. The foramen rotundum connects the pterygopalatine fossa with the middle cranial fossa and, therefore, tumor can follow the maxillary division of the trigeminal nerve through the foramen rotundum to the region of the gasserian ganglion, cavernous sinus, and middle cranial fossa (Fig 24–31). The basal foramina, including their entrances and exits, can be well evaluated with CT using both axial and coronal projections.

Although enlargement of a foramen is a good indication of transforaminal spread, a word of caution must be added that demonstration of a normal foramen may not exclude extension through a foramen. So-called perineural extension may not enlarge a nerve and, therefore, may not enlarge the foramen. Distant recurrences, however, may be present, so the most common destination of this type of spread should still be radiographically evaluated. More data is required before firm statements can be made about the role of CT in detection of perineural metastasis.

Pterygopalatine Fossa Involvement

Before leaving our discussion of the types of spread of tumor, special emphasis should be made of the importance of the pterygopalatine fossa. This small area is situated between the posterior wall of the maxillary sinus and the anterior cortex of the pterygoid plate (Fig 24–32).

Axial sections show definite fat density within the fossa in normal situations. Visualization is optimal when slices are perpendicular to the posterior wall of the maxillary sinus (Fig 24–33). Coronal scans show the fat density, which extends slightly toward midline in its superior portion. Small densities within the fat are neural and vascular structures. The importance of tumor spread into the pterygopalatine fossa relates not so much to any vital structures contained within the fossa as to the ease with which tumor can spread from the fossa to involve local or distant structures. Tumor extends into the fossa either directly or by transneural spread, usually along the infraorbital or palatine nerves.

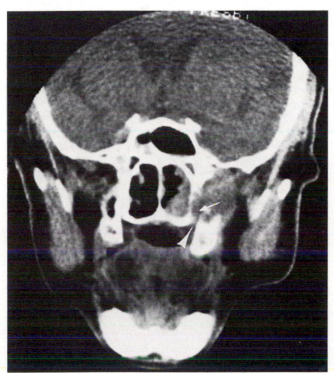

Fig 24–30.—Adenocystic carcinoma of the maxillary sinus eroded into the lower portion of the pterygopalatine canal *(arrow)* just above the greater palatine foramen *(arrowhead)*. The pterygopalatine canal (palatine nerve) carried the tumor to the pterygopalatine fossa and eventually to the gasserian ganglion.

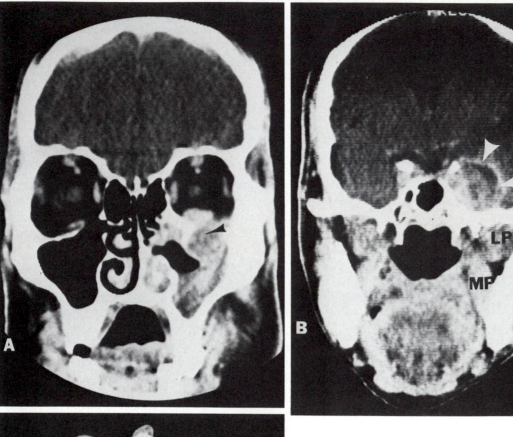

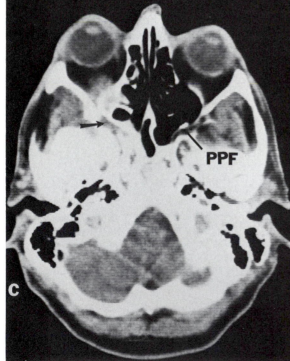

Fig 24–31.—A, squamous cell carcinoma. Tumor involves cheek, sinus, and infraorbital nerve. There was also involvement of the infraorbital nerve *(arrowhead).* **B,** coronal slice through the middle cranial fossa shows large tumor involving gasserian ganglion and temporal lobe *(arrowheads).* (*LP* = lateral pterygoid muscle, *MP* = medial pterygoid muscle.) **C,** axial slice through upper pterygopalatine fossa shows obliteration of fat planes *(arrow);* compare with opposite side. (*PPF* = upper pterygopalatine fossa.) No destruction of the base of the skull around the foramen rotundum was seen.

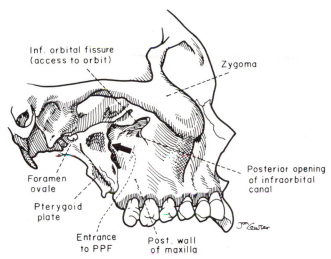

Fig 24–32.—Pterygopalatine fossa *(PPF)* between posterior wall of maxillary sinus and the anterior surface of pterygoid plates.

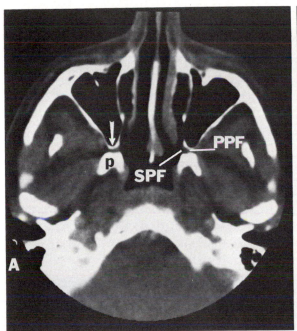

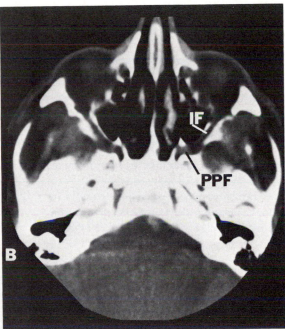

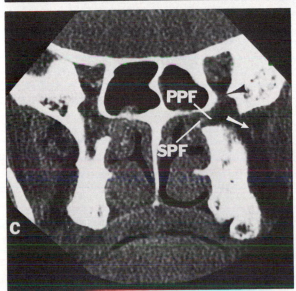

Fig 24–33.—**A,** normal axial slice low in pterygopalatine fossa *(PPF).* (*p* = pterygoid plate, *arrow* indicates posterior wall of maxillary sinus, *SPF* = sphenopalatine foramen.) **B,** higher axial slice. Pterygopalatine fossa *(PPF)* meets the inferior orbital fissure *(IF).* **C,** coronal slice through the pterygopalatine fossa *(PPF),* which communicates medially with the nasal cavity through the sphenopalatine foramen *(SPF)* and laterally with the infratemporal fossa *(arrow).* Superiorly, the fossa connects with the orbital apex *(arrowhead).*

From the pterygopalatine fossa, tumor has easy access to contiguous structures by way of the numerous foramina and fissures with which it connects. Superiorly, tumor extends through the inferior orbital fissure into the orbit.[16] Laterally, the fossa opens into the infratemporal fossa beneath the zygoma (Fig 24–34). Medially, the sphenopalatine foramen leads to the nasal cavity. These routes are important, but not quite as ominous as spread posteriorly through the foramen rotundum, which gives access to the cavernous sinus and middle cranial fossa as mentioned in the previous section.

Evaluation of the pterygopalatine fossa and its connections should be considered as an important part of a CT study of the sinuses.

Types of Tumors

Neoplasms[17, 19]

Squamous cell carcinoma represents about 80% of malignant tumors of the sinuses and nasal cavity. Glandular tumors are less common, accounting for 10% to 14% of malignancies, and are broken down into adenocystic carcinoma, adenocarcinoma, pleomorphic adenoma, mucoepidermoid, and undifferentiated carcinoma. Rarer still are melanomas, lymphomas, plasmocytomas, oncocytomas, hemangiopericytomas, fibrohistiocytomas, and sarcomas. Neurogenic tumors include the olfactory neuroblastoma (esthesioneuroepithelioma), which usually arises high in the nasal cavity. At the time of this writing, a tissue-specific diagnosis of sinus and nasal cavity tumors cannot be made by CT, but the radiologist can estimate the aggressiveness of the tumor by the extent of the lesion and by how much bone is destroyed or remodelled. In some cases, bone or cartilage formation in the tumor can indicate an osteomatous or chondromatous lesion, but these represent a minority of cases (Fig 24–35). Osteomas (compact bone) may be single or may be multiple in Gardner's syndrome associated with colon polyps and skin lesions. Calcifications can be seen in some odontogenic tumors also.

Other tumors arising in the bony skeleton of the sinuses are very rare. Giant cell tumors have been described, though most authors conclude that almost all of these are giant cell reparative granulomas. Giant cell tumor may be seen in older patients associated with Paget's disease.[20–22]

Polyps and Papillomas

Benign lesions such as polyps and papillomas can be confused with malignancies, because they are seen as masses causing obstruction and with some bone changes.

Polyps are usually seen incidentally on CT and may or may not obstruct a sinus (Figs 24–36 and 24–37). They tend to cause bony remodelling rather than destruction if any bone change is present at all (Fig 24–38). Polyps can often be bilateral, especially when related to allergy, and can obstruct multiple sinuses without destroying large segments of bone. If a malignant tumor obstructs multiple sinuses, especially on both

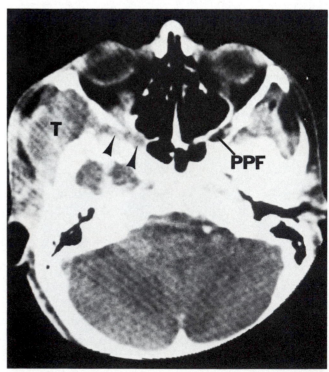

Fig 24–34.—Tumor (T) of the infratemporal fossa extending directly into the pterygopalatine fossa, obliterating the fat (arrowheads). Compare with opposite normal side. (PPF = pterygopalatine fossa.)

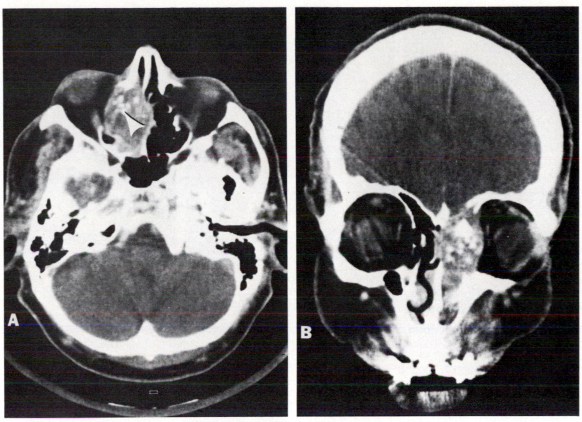

Fig 24–35.—A, chondrosarcoma. Axial slice through ethmoid tumor showing calcification of organic matrix *(arrowhead).* **B,** coronal slice.

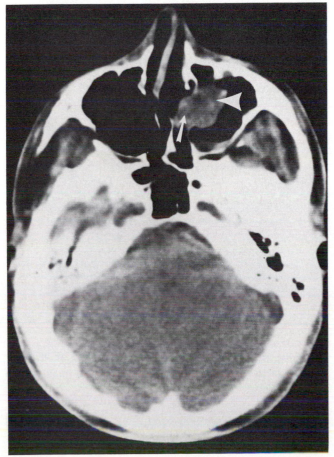

Fig 24–36.—Polyp, axial slice through maxillary sinus. Polyp in sinus *(arrowhead)* protrudes through the ostium with nasal cavity *(arrow).*

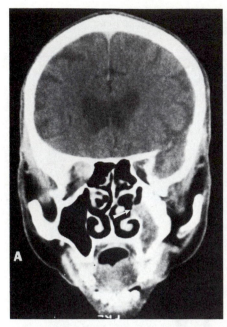
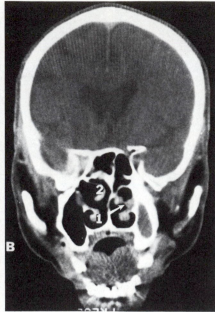
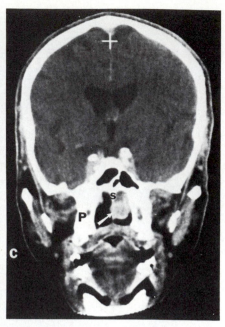

Fig 24–37.—A, antral choanal polyp, coronal slice. Soft-tissue density is demonstrated in ostium *(arrow)* with opacity of sinus. **B,** slightly posterior cut shows mass *(arrow)* just beneath the middle turbinate. (*1* = inferior turbinate, *2* = middle turbinate.) **C,** polyp seen in cross section *(arrow)* as it protrudes through the choana as marked by the pterygoid plate *(P).* (*S* = nasal septum.)

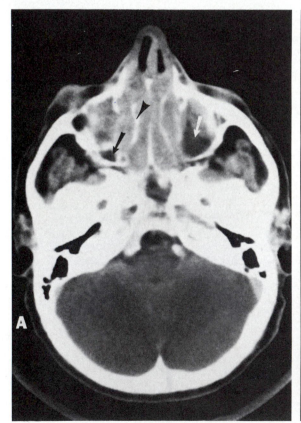
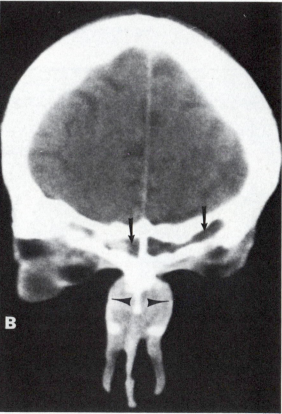

Fig 24–38.—A, multiple polyps, axial slice. Diffuse enhancement fills the air spaces of nasal cavity, but the bony turbinates are not destroyed *(arrowhead).* Note obstructed areas of maxillary sinus, which shows characteristic low density *(arrows).* **B,** coronal slice shows obstructed frontal sinuses *(arrows).* There is remodelling of the nasal bones *(arrowheads).*

sides of the midline, the large destructive mass should be obvious on CT.

Inverting papilloma is locally invasive and can cause bone destruction (Fig 24–39). Although the diagnosis may be suggested from the extent of the lesion and the position (almost all arise from the lateral wall of the nasal cavity), the diagnosis must be established by biopsy. Again, CT is used to define the extent of the tumor and postoperatively to exclude recurrence.

Juvenile Angiofibroma of the Nasopharynx[23, 24]

Although not actually of the nasal cavity or sinus, this tumor can present with nasal obstruction and often affects the sinuses and nasal airway secondarily. Producing epistaxis in adolescent males, the tumor has CT findings that are usually characteristic. There is enlargement of the pterygopalatine fossa, usually with anterior displacement of the posterior maxillary wall (Figs 24–40 and 24–41). The tumor enhances intensely when the scan is performed with intravenous enhancement. The pterygopalatine fossa normally can be unusually large when there is a hypoplastic maxillary sinus. In this case, the pterygopalatine fossa should contain usual fat density.

Dental-Related Neoplasms and Cysts

Lesions arising in dental structures are seen during CT evaluation of the paranasal sinuses either as the pri-

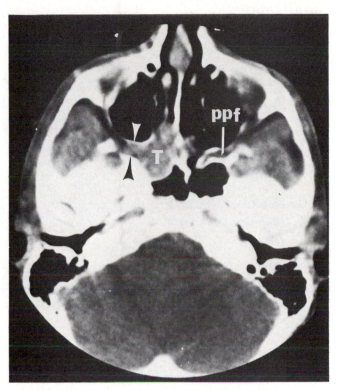

Fig 24–40.—Juvenile angiofibroma. Tumor *(T)* is seen in posterior nasal cavity with enlargement of the pterygopalatine fossa *(arrowheads)*. Compare with normal side. *(ppf = pterygopalatine fossa.)* Tumor enhances.

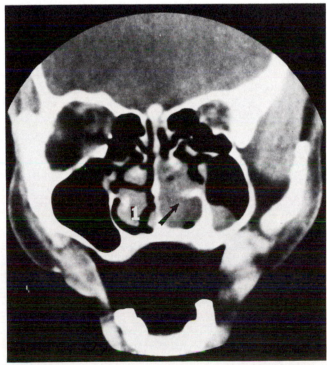

Fig 24–39.—Inverting papilloma with minimal destruction of the inferior turbinate *(arrow)*. Compare with inferior turbinate *(1)* on opposite side.

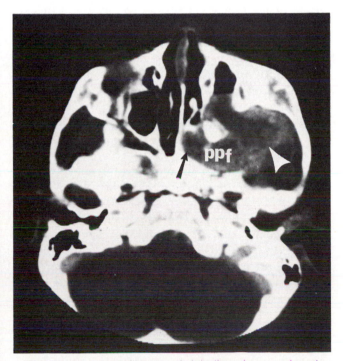

Fig 24–41.—Angiofibroma. Axial slice shows enhancing tumor in posterior nasal cavity *(arrow)*, enlarging the pterygopalatine fossa *(ppf)* and extending into the infratemporal fossa *(arrowhead)*.

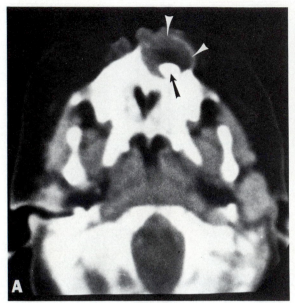

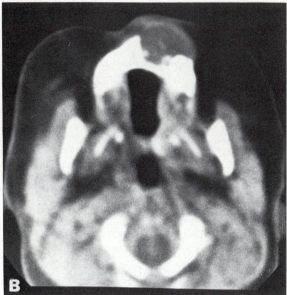

Fig 24–42.—A, ameloblastic fibro-odontoma. Hypodense odontogenic tumor of anterior maxilla *(arrowheads). Arrow* indicates tooth remnant. **B,** lower section showing small amount of calcification in lower part of lesion.

mary pathology or as an incidental finding. Odontogenic tumors, benign or malignant, develop from cells that are related to the formation of the tooth. These must be considered in evaluation of lesions of the alveolar process and floor of the maxillary sinus as well as of the mandible. Scans by CT can define very well the extent of the lesion and suggest the nature of the central matrix of the abnormality.

The appearance of an odontogenic neoplasm is variable, depending on its cell origin and degree of differentiation. It can have a purely cystic appearance on plain films or may have varying amounts of calcification resembling a chondromatous lesion (Figs 24–42 and 24–43). Teeth in or bordering a lesion are also indicative of a dental origin, but the finding is not present in all cases.

The appearance of odontogenic tumors is well described in literature dealing with plain films. When a lesion is seen on CT, correlation with plain films, including dental films, is very important. Little has been written about the CT findings in odontogenic neoplasms, but as further experience is accumulated, the ability of CT to give useful diagnostic information about the internal characteristics of these odontogenic neoplasms may allow for more precise preoperative diagnosis.

Odontogenic and nonodontogenic cysts are also seen during CT of the sinuses. Odontogenic cysts can be recognized by the retained crown of the tooth (Fig 24–44). Some odontogenic tumors that do not calcify, such as ameloblastoma, odontogenic myxoma, and ameloblastic fibroma, can give a similar low-density appearance.

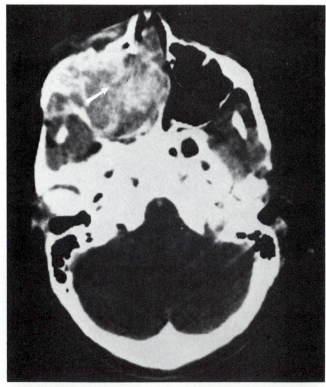

Fig 24–43.—Cemento-ossifying fibroma enlarging maxillary sinus with central calcifications *(arrow).* The pterygopalatine fossa is "pushed" posteriorly, but the foot planes are maintained.

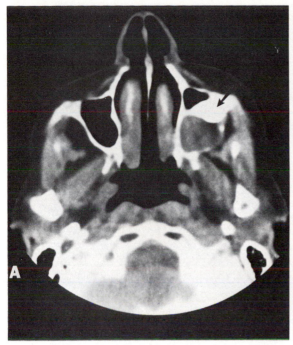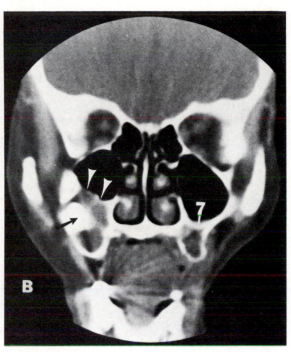

Fig 24–44.—A, odontogenic cyst, hypodense lesion expanding into the maxillary sinus. The cyst actually arises in the alveolar ridge. *Arrow* denotes tooth remnant. **B,** coronal slice showing cyst and tooth remnant *(arrow).* The superior margin represents the superior cortex of the bony alveolar process *(arrowheads).* Compare with normal side. (7 = upper cortex of alveolar process.)

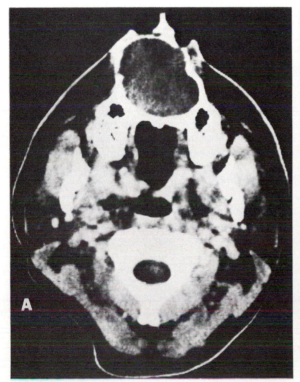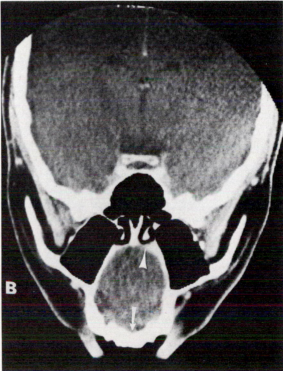

Fig 24–45.—A, nasopalatine cyst (exceptionally large). Hypodense expansile lesion involves anterior alveolar ridge and hard palate. **B,** coronal slice (angled because of metal fillings). Lesion is in midline and extends into septum. Upper bone margin *(arrowhead)* represents the superior cortex of the palate. The cyst arose in nasopalatine canal between central incisors *(arrow).*

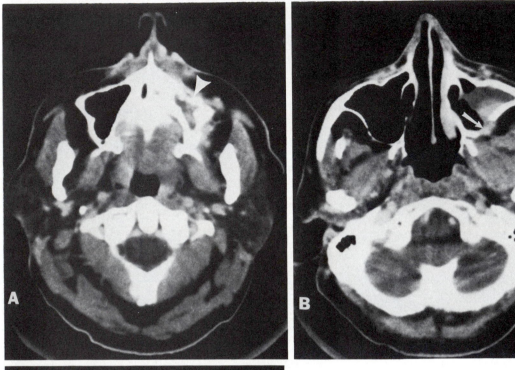

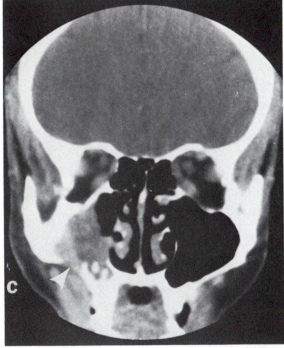

Fig 24–46.—A, inverting papilloma with carcinoma in situ. Axial slice shows irregular bone destruction of antrum alveolar ridge *(arrowhead)*. This is usual position of a Caldwell-Luc defect. B, higher slice showing defect in the posterolateral wall *(arrow)* with slight impingement on the fat plane just outside the wall. This is not the usual defect and so was biopsied showing inverting papilloma with carcinoma in situ. C, coronal slice through defect from surgery just above alveolar ridge. Defect is indicated by *arrowhead*.

Nonodontogenic epithelial-lined cysts do not arise from the tooth elements, but from an epithelial remnant near the teeth (Fig 24–45). The incisive canal cyst (nasopalatine cyst) arises in the midline and widens or shortens the incisive canal between the central incisors. Most are small incidental findings, but very rarely one can grow large enough to present as a mass in the floor of the nose. The globulomaxillary cyst arises between the lateral incisor and the canine tooth.

This brief description of some of the more common odontogenic entities that can occasionally be seen on CT is far from complete. Perhaps the most important thing to remember is how helpful correlation with dental films, as well as with routine sinus views, can be in these cases. An excellent description of the plain film findings correlated with Pindborg's classification may be found in *Oral Roentgenographic Diagnosis* by Stafne and Gibilisco.[25]

Post-therapy Scanning

A brief note should be made about the role of CT in the post-therapy patient. Familiarity with the various types of partial and total maxillectomy and ethmoidectomy, as well as Caldwell-Luc defects, can be helpful when trying to detect destruction from recurrent tumor (Fig 24–46).[26, 27] The best method, however, is to obtain a CT scan in the postoperative period, allowing future comparison and detection of subtle recurrences.[28] This postoperative scan should be done after several weeks to allow swelling to decrease.

When a neoplasm is irradiated, tumor response or recurrence can be accurately assessed by CT. Bone reaction is quite variable, from osteonecrosis to bony sclerosis. There may be reappearance of bone that had been "destroyed" by tumor (Fig 24–47).

INFECTION AND INFLAMMATORY PROCESS

Sinusitis

Routine sinusitis is not usually evaluated with a CT scan. When a secondary problem occurs, such as orbital cellulitis or intracranial extension from frontal sinusitis, the secondary problem may be well evaluated with CT scan using the same principles for detection of spread as are used in staging tumors. In the same way that CT shows the extension of tumor into the fat bordering the outer side of a bony wall, so too will CT show extension of infection into the orbit. The infection may re-

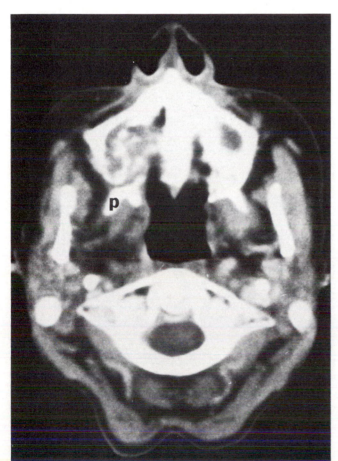

Fig 24–47.—Axial CT after radiation of adenocystic carcinoma (preradiation scan, Fig 24–12). Note return of pterygoid plates *(P)*.

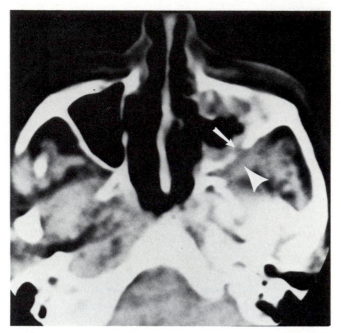

Fig 24–48.—Mucormycosis, axial slice with defect in posterolateral wall and obliteration of normal fat plane outside maxillary sinus. Defect is indicated by *arrow*. Soft-tissue involvement in infratemporal fossa is indicated *(arrowhead)*. Compare with normal side.

main confined by the periosteum or can break through into the orbital fat. Precise localization can be made using CT.

Mucormycosis and Aspergillosis

Sinusitis can break through the lamina papyracea or follow the vessels to extend to tissues outside the sinuses. Mucor and other fungal infections, however, can destroy significant amounts of bone, enough so that they may be mistaken for malignancy (Fig 24–48). Again, the radiologist must define as precisely as possible the extent of the lesion, using the same principles as in malignancies. Especially dangerous is extension through the orbital apex into the cavernous sinus. Here the invasive nature of the microorganism can cause occlusion of the ophthalmic and even the internal carotid arteries. Evaluation of the brain for evidence of infarction should also be performed during CT evaluation.[29]

Granulomatous Disease

Wegener's granulomatosis can cause bony changes, as can midline lethal granuloma. The bone destruction may suggest malignancy on CT scan. Bony replacement of the sinuses has been recently described in Wegener's granulomatosis.[30] At this time, however, more experi-

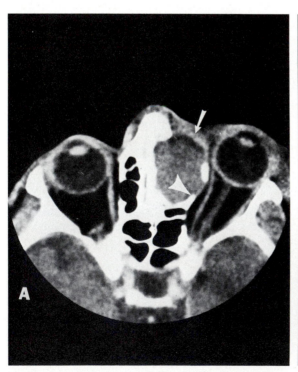

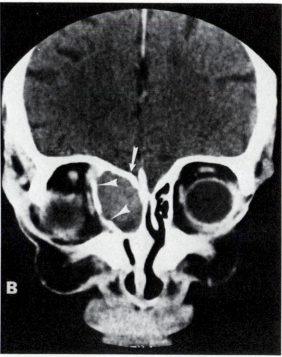

Fig 24–49.—**A,** ethmoid mucocele. Axial slice through expanded mucocele with displacement and actual defects in the bony wall. Note the low density within the mucocele and the displaced globe. Outward bowing of bone is indicated by *arrowhead* and the defect in bone by *arrow*.

B, coronal section with expansion of ethmoid and outward bowing of the lateral wall of ethmoid *(arrowheads)*. Note remodelling of the roof of ethmoid and olfactory groove *(arrow)*.

ence is needed to determine the CT changes in this disease.

Mucocele[31-33]

A mucocele forms when an entire sinus is obstructed. The obstruction is usually related to sinusitis and inflammatory change, but can also be associated with tumor. The bony walls of the sinus are remodelled as pressure builds behind the obstruction. In the usual case, this results in ballooning of the bony wall with some associated thinning (Fig 24–49). We have also seen thinning of the bony wall without definite enlargement of the sphenoid sinus, which was obstructed by malignant neoplasm (Fig 24–50). Presumably, the more rapid course of the malignancy led to evaluation of the sinus before considerable expansion could occur.

Usually, the mucocele has a uniformly low density, but this is not universal. With concurrent infection, a mucopyocele is formed that often shows enhancement on the postinfusion scan.

Any sinus can be affected. Involvement of the frontal and ethmoid sinuses is most common, followed by the sphenoid, which is less common, and maxillary antrum, which is quite rare. In the ethmoid, one air cell may be grossly enlarged with isolated expansion, or the entire

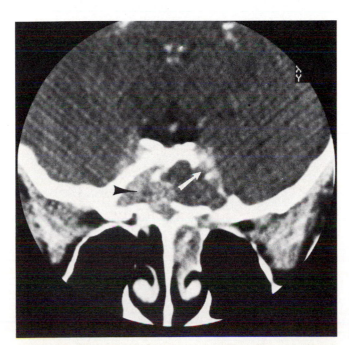

Fig 24–50.—Coronal CT in patient with obstructed sphenoid, tumor in region of ostium. Note loss of lateral bony wall of sphenoid *(arrow)* and hypodense opacification of the sinus on that side. There is some enhancement on the opposite side *(arrowhead)*. At surgery, there was no tumor in the sphenoid, and the erosion of the lateral wall was from early mucocele formation. It was not clear whether the opposite side represented inflamed mucosa or slight extension of tumor into anterior sphenoid on that side.

ethmoid can be enlarged with intact cell walls.[32] This latter situation is usually seen in association with multiple polyps (Fig 24–51).

The mode of CT is ideally suited for defining the margin of the mucocele and also in detecting any complications related to "breakout" of the mucocele, be it into the orbit or into the anterior cranial fossa. Perhaps the most often-asked question about a mucocele is in regard to its separation from the cranial contents. An intact bony cortex is reassuring to the surgeon, whereas detection of defects in the cortex, especially with enhancement of the dura, can forewarn the surgeon of a more difficult surgical problem (Fig 24–52).

Brief mention is made here of the retention cyst, which like a mucocele can have a uniform internal density, but unlike a mucocele does not involve the entire sinus. Rather, it has a smooth-domed margin and usually presents in the maxillary antrum (Fig 24–53).

BONE DYSPLASIAS

These are briefly covered in the section on bone changes presented earlier in this chapter.

TRAUMA[34, 35]

Facial fractures are routinely evaluated at our institution, using plain films and pluridirectional tomography. Aside from being more readily available than CT, tomography demonstrates anatomy in two key orientations: coronal and sagittal. These orientations are important in assessing inferior displacement. The shortcomings of axial CT include difficulty in assessment of the pterygoid plates, because the usual fracture of the pterygoid is in the horizontal axis and, as such, falls in the plane of axial scanning. Superior and inferior displacement of either tripod or Le Fort's fracture is also difficult to evaluate in the axial orientation. Fractures of the orbital floor may also be missed. Coronal CT images can be obtained, but good coronal positioning can be very difficult in patients with severe fractures of the face.

In a severely traumatized patient, however, axial cuts through the facial bones can be readily obtained at the same time the patient undergoes CT examination of the head. In such a case, performing pluridirectional tomography would require further patient transport and manipulation. Indeed, lateral projection tomography may well be impossible in these patients. Axial CT can give a very accurate survey of the fracture.

Useful information can be gained by doing coronal and sagittal reconstructions of original axial image data. However, at present, it may be difficult to obtain good reformatted views in severely traumatized patients, be-

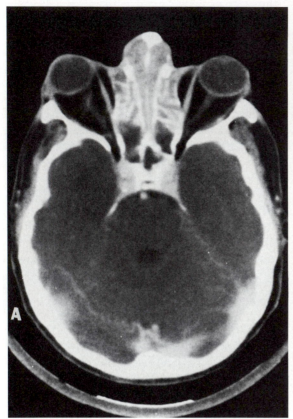

Fig 24–51.—A, patient with multiple polyps and diffuse opacification of the ethmoids and sphenoid. There is apparent expansion of the ethmoids, though the shape of the lateral wall of the ethmoids may be quite variable. **B,** coronal slide showing opacification of nasal cavity and ethmoids. Note also mucocele of the orbital roof *(arrow),* which was a continuation of a mucocele involving the frontal sinus.

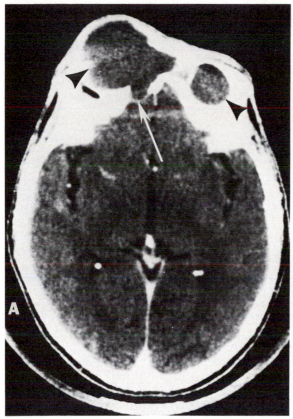

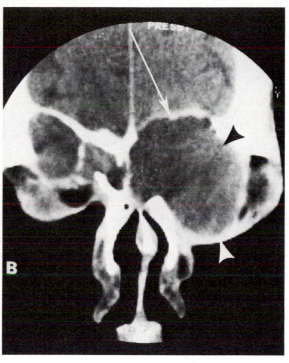

Fig 24–52.—**A,** axial CT of huge bilateral mucocele *(arrowheads).* There is "breakthrough" of the posterior wall, with enhancement of the dura or wall of mucocele *(arrow).* At surgery, the dura and wall of mucocele were adherent.

B, coronal CT showing mucocele *(arrowheads)* and loss of bony margin and enhancement of wall of mucocele or dura *(arrow).*

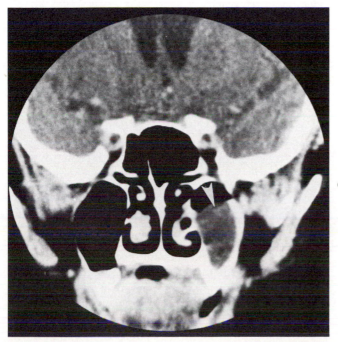

Fig 24–53.—Retention cyst in maxillary sinus. Note low density and upper "domed" margin *(arrowhead).*

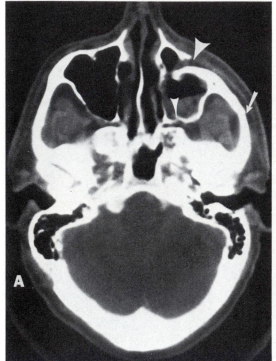

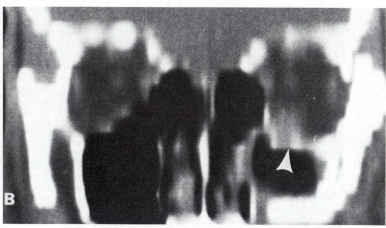

Fig 24–54.—A, axial CT through a tripod fracture with fracture of the anterior wall *(large arrowhead)* and posterior wall *(small arrowhead)*. There is a buckle fracture of the zygoma *(arrow)*. **B,** coronal reformatted image shows inferior displacement of the floor, but the image quality is not as good as tomography or direct coronal CT. *Arrowhead* indicates displaced floor.

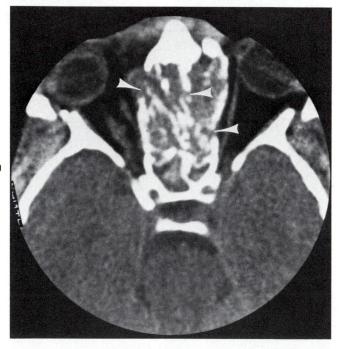

Fig 24–55.—Comminuted fracture through ethmoid with multiple fracture lines *(arrowheads)* and opacification.

cause there is often slight movement between CT slices, producing step artifacts on the reconstructed images that mimic fractures (Fig 24–54). Faster dynamic scanning could well address this problem.

Scans by CT are useful in following fractures through the ethmoid, where opacification of the air cells can aid in detection of the fracture site (Fig 24–55). Small frac-

tures through the ethmoid and lamina papyracea are often very difficult to visualize on conventional tomography. Also, posterior displacement of the malar eminence and anterior maxillary wall are easily detected on CT, as are fractures of the zygomatic arch and lateral wall of the orbit. Fractures of the posterior wall of the frontal sinus are quite well evaluated using CT.

An added value of CT in facial trauma is the demonstration of the soft tissues. This is especially useful in a blow-out fracture of the orbit, because herniation of the orbital musculature can be easily evaluated. In such a case, direct coronal scanning can be performed because the patient is not as severely traumatized, so positioning is easier. Evaluation of hematomas and foreign bodies also benefit from the ability of CT to demonstrate soft tissues, thereby demonstrating the relationship of the abnormality to vital structures not seen on plain films.

SUMMARY

Scanning by CT has become a very important mode of investigation in the region of the sinuses. In our institution, almost all lesions are biopsied, and the ability of CT to define the precise extent of the lesion has been more helpful than our ability to make a specific diagnosis. As experience increases, more definitive diagnoses may be made as CT characteristics become more specific.

REFERENCES

1. Forbes W., Fawcitt R., Isherwood I., et al.: Computed tomography in the diagnosis of the paranasal sinuses. *Clin. Radiol.* 29:501–511, 1978.
2. Mancuso A.A., Hanafee W.N.: *Computed Tomography of the Head and Neck*. Baltimore, Williams & Wilkins Co., 1982.
3. Parsons C., Hodson N.: Computed tomography of paranasal sinus tumors. *Radiology* 132:641–645, 1979.
4. Valvassori G.E., Potter G.D., Hanafee W.N., et al: *Radiology of the Ear, Nose and Throat*. Philadelphia, W.B. Saunders Co., 1982.
5. Dodd G.D., Jing B.S.: *Radiology of the Nose, Paranasal Sinuses and Nasopharynx*. Baltimore, Williams & Wilkins Co., 1977.
6. Samuel E., Lloyd G.A.S.: *Clinical Radiology of the Ear, Nose and Throat*. Philadelphia, W.B. Saunders Co., 1978.
7. Som P.M., Shugar J.M.A., Cohen B.A., et al.: The nonspecificity of the antral bowing sign in maxillary sinus pathology. *J. Comput. Assist. Tomogr.* 5:350–352, 1981.
8. Higashi T., Iguchi M., Shimura A., et al.: Computed tomography and bone scintigraphy in polyostotic fibrous dysplasia. *Oral Surg.* 50:580–583, 1980.
9. Beighton P., Durr L., Hamersma H.: Clinical features of sclerosteosis—a review of the manifestations in twenty-five affected individuals. *Ann. Intern. Med.* 84:393–397, 1976.
10. Beighton P., Hamersma H., Horan F.: Craniometaphyseal dysplasia variability of expression within a large family. *Clin. Genet.* 15:252–258, 1979.
11. Hamersma H.: Facial nerve paralysis in the osteope-

troses, in Fisch V. (ed.): *Proceedings of the 3rd Symposium on Facial Nerve Surgery*. Zurich, Switzerland, 1976, p. 555.
12. Ballantyne A.J., McCarten A.B., Ibanez M.L.: The extension of cancer of the head and neck through peripheral nerves. *Am. J. Surg.* 106:651–667, 1963.
13. Conley J., Dingman D.L.: Adenoid cystic carcinoma in the head and neck (cylindroma). *Arch. Otolaryngol.* 100:81–90, 1974.
14. Dodd G.D., Dolan P.A., Ballantyne A.J., et al.: The dissemination of tumors of the head and neck via the cranial nerves. *Radiol. Clin. North Am.* 8:445–461, 1970.
15. Spiro R.H., Huvos A.G., Strong E.W.: Adenoid cystic carcinoma of salivary origin: A clinicopathologic study of 242 cases. *Am. J. Surg.* 128:512–520, 1974.
16. Hesselink J.R., Weber A.L.: Pathways of orbital extension of extraorbital neoplasms. *J. Comput. Assist. Tomogr.* 6:593–597, 1982.
17. Batsakis J.G.: *Tumors of the Head and Neck: Clinical and Pathological Considerations*, ed. 2. Baltimore, Williams & Wilkins Co., 1979.
18. Paparella M.A., Shumrick D.A.: *Otolaryngology*. Philadelphia, W.B. Saunders Co., 1973, vol. 3.
19. Sisson G.A., Becker S.P.: Cancer of the nasal cavity and paranasal sinuses, in Suen J.Y., Myers E.N. (eds.): *Cancer of the Head and Neck*. New York, Churchill Livingstone, Inc., 1981, pp. 242–279.
20. Handler S.D., Savino P.J., Peyster R.G., et al.: Giant cell tumor of the ethmoid sinus: An unusual cause of proptosis in a child. *Otolaryngol. Head Neck Surg.* 90:513–515, 1982.
21. Jaffe H.L.: Giant cell reparative granuloma, traumatic bone cyst and fibrous (fibro-osseous) dysplasia of the jaw bones. *Oral Surg.* 6:159–175, 1953.
22. Spjut H.J., Dorfman H.D., Fechner R.E., et al.: *Tumors of Bone and Cartilage*. Armed Forces Institute of Pathology, 1970.
23. Bryan R.N., Sessions R.B., Horowitz B.L.: Radiographic management of juvenile angiofibroma. *A.J.N.R.* 2:157–166, 1981.
24. Weinstein M.A., Levine H., Duchesneau P.M., et al.: Diagnosis of juvenile angiofibroma by computed tomography. *Radiology* 126:703–705, 1978.
25. Stafne E.C., Gibilisco J.A.: *Oral Roentgenographic Diagnosis*, ed. 4. Philadelphia, W.B. Saunders Co., 1975.
26. Goodman W.S.: The Caldwell-Luc procedure. *Otolaryngol. Clin. North Am.* 9:187–195, 1976.
27. Lore J.M.: Partial and radical maxillectomy. *Otolaryngol. Clin. North Am.* 9:255–267, 1976.
28. Som P.M., Shugar J.M.A., Biller H.F.: The early detection of antral malignancy in the post maxillectomy patient. *Radiology* 143:509–512, 1982.
29. Centeno R.S., Bentson J.R., Mancuso A.: CT scanning in rhinocerebral mucormycosis and aspergillosis. *Radiology* 140:383–389, 1981.
30. Paling M.R., Roberts R.L., Fauci A.S.: Paranasal sinus obliterations in Wegener's granulomatosis. *Radiology* 144:539–543, 1982.

31. Hesselink J.R., Weber A.L., New P.F.J., et al.: Evaluation of mucoceles of the paranasal sinuses with computed tomography. *Radiology* 133:397–400, 1979.

32. Jacobs M., Som P.: The ethmoidal "polypoid mucocele." *J. Comput. Assist. Tomogr.* 6:721–724, 1982.

33. Som P.M., Shugar J.A.: CT classification of ethmoid mucoceles. *J. Comput. Assist. Tomogr.* 4:199–203, 1980.

34. Grove A.: Orbital trauma evaluation by computed tomography. *Comput. Tomogr.* 3:267–278, 1979.

35. Zilkha A.: Computed tomography in facial trauma. *Radiology* 144:545–548, 1982.

25

Nasopharynx and Paranasopharyngeal Space

HUGH D. CURTIN, M.D.

THE USE of CT represents a new dimension in diagnosis of lesions involving the nasopharynx and related structures. Although the mucosal surfaces are best evaluated by direct visualization, the deeper parapharyngeal and retropharyngeal areas are inaccessible to the clinician and are ideal subjects for CT imaging.[1-8]

ANATOMY

The nasopharynx extends from the choana to the level of the soft palate. The most prominent landmark of the lateral wall is the torus tubarius, which with the salpingopharyngeal fold surrounds the opening of the eustachian tube on three sides (Fig 25–1). The fossa of Rosenmüller is a recess that parallels the outer circumference of the torus. In the midline, the mucosa and submucosa of the roof of the nasopharynx are closely applied to the base of the skull (sphenoid). More posteriorly (posterior wall of the nasopharynx), the mucosa and submucosa are separated from the basiocciput by the prevertebral muscles. The posterior wall and the roof may form a smooth curve or may form a right angle.

The structures deep to the mucosa can be grouped according to muscle and fat planes, which are well seen on CT (Figs 25–2 and 25–3).

The *deglutitional muscles* make up the soft-tissue densities immediately lateral to the nasopharynx airway. Low in the nasopharynx, according to some authors, the superior constrictor muscles merge with fibers from the palatal muscles to form a complete ring around the nasopharynx called Passavant's ring (see Fig 25–3,A). Above the ring, the superior constrictors are absent along the lateral wall of the nasopharynx, though they do continue up to the base of the skull posteriorly. The "gaps" in the lateral wall are closed by the pharyngobasilar fascia, a thin but very tough fibrous sheath attached to the base of the skull. This fascia holds the nasopharynx open. At this level, the soft-tissue densities lateral to the airway on CT are made up by the levator and tensor veli palatini muscles and by the wall of the eustachian tube (see Fig 25–3,B).

The *masticator muscles* include the pterygoids, masseter, and temporalis muscles and form a second muscle group separated from the deglutitional muscles by the parapharyngeal spaces. These muscles are enclosed in a fascia that may "direct" the spread of disease and thus make up the *masticator space*. This area is often referred to as the infratemporal fossa, defined as an area deep to the zygomatic arch and immediately inferior to the skull base. Some authors include the parapharyngeal space in the infratemporal fossa, and some separate the two areas.

The *parapharyngeal space* separates the muscles of mastication from the muscles of deglutition. The parapharyngeal space approximates an inverted pyramid extending from the skull base to the hyoid. It is wider posteriorly than anteriorly, so obliquity of a patient must be considered in judging symmetry on coronal views. The fascia around the styloid muscles extends anteromedially toward the tensor veli palatini, separating the parapharyngeal space into pre- and poststyloid compartments, which are actually anterolateral and posteromedial respectively (see Fig 25–2). The poststyloid space contains the carotid artery, the jugular vein, and the associated cranial nerves. The anterior space contains nothing vital, but tumors from the parotid can grow into this space by passing between the styloid process and the posterior margin of the mandible through the stylomandibular tunnel. As will be discussed later, the effect of the tumor on the parapharyngeal spaces is the key to localization of tumor origin and also determines what further radiologic work-up is necessary.

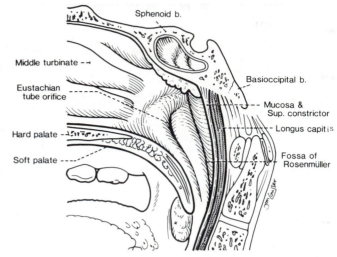

Fig 25–1.—Lateral wall of the nasopharynx viewed from midline. Fossa of Rosenmüller is the crease paralleling the outer margin of the torus tubarius, which partially surrounds the eustachian tube orifice. The prevertebral musculature inserts on the base of the skull, roughly separating the roof from the posterior wall of the nasopharynx. (From Curtin H.D.: Infratemporal fossa, nasopharynx, and parapharyngeal spaces, in Carter B. [ed.]: *Computed Tomography of the Head and Neck.* New York, Churchill-Livingstone, 1984.)

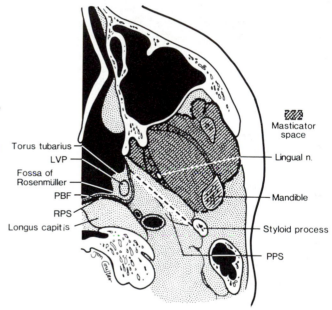

Fig 25–2.—Horizontal section depicting the nasopharynx and related deeper structures. Only one side is shown. The parapharyngeal space *(PPS)* is between the pharyngobasilar fascia and the masticator space. The *dotted line* approximates the separation between pre- and poststyloid compartments. The structures in the poststyloid compartment represent carotid artery and jugular vein. (*LVP* = levator veli palatini, *PBF* = pharyngobasilar fascia, *RPS* = retropharyngeal space.) (From Curtin H.D.: Infratemporal fossa, nasopharynx, and parapharyngeal spaces, in Carter B. [ed.]: *Computed Tomography of the Head and Neck.* New York, Churchill-Livingstone, 1984.)

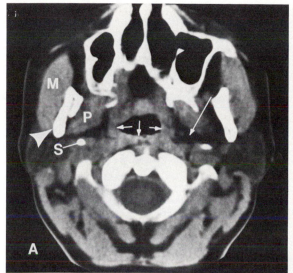

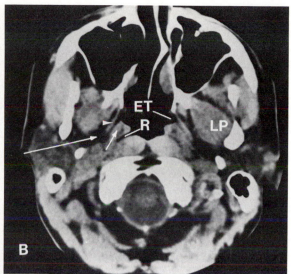

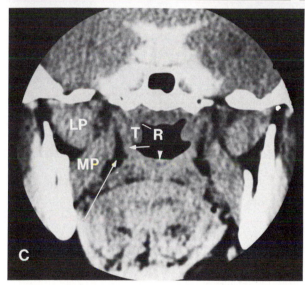

Fig 25–3.—A, axial slice through the nasopharynx at the level of Passavant's ring. *Small white arrows* depict Passavant's ring. (*P* = medial pterygoid, *M* = masseter, *S* = styloid.) Mandibular ramus is indicated by *large white arrowhead* and the parapharyngeal space by the *long white arrow.* **B,** higher slice through the nasopharynx. (*LP* = lateral pterygoid, *R* = fossa of Rosenmüller, *ET* = eustachian tube orifice.) Tensor veli palatini is indicated by *arrowhead,* the levator veli palatini by the *short white arrow* and the parapharyngeal space by the *long white arrow.* **C,** coronal view through the nasopharynx. (*T* = torus tubarius, *R* = fossa of Rosenmüller.) Deglutitional muscles are represented by the levator veli palatini *(short white arrow).* This extends into the soft palate *(white arrowhead).* The masticator muscles are represented by the lateral pterygoid *(LP)* and medial pterygoid *(MP).* The parapharyngeal space *(long white arrow)* separates the deglutitional muscles from masticator muscles. Image was taken during a metrizamide cisternogram done for unrelated problem. (From Curtin H.D.: Infratemporal fossa, nasopharynx, and parapharyngeal spaces, in Carter B. [ed.]: *Computed Tomography of the Head and Neck.* New York, Churchill-Livingstone, 1984.)

The *retropharyngeal space* is a potential space between the pharyngobasilar fascia and the prevertebral musculature posterior to the nasopharynx. According to some authors, this space can be separated into two compartments by an extrafascial layer called the alar fascia.[9]

CT TECHNIQUE

Axial scans are taken from the sphenoid to a level below the hard palate. In cases of malignancy, the nodal areas most likely to be involved are included. Slices are taken approximately 5 mm apart. A contrast agent is administered intravenously during the actual performance of the scan, which defines the vessels and gives an idea of the nature of a lesion. Axial scans are taken at Reid's base line or approximately parallel to the hard palate. Coronal sections are often helpful. As the posterior wall and roof of the nasopharynx are somewhat variable in their configuration, the use of a scan angle perpendicular to the bony wall in a questionable area can also be helpful.

Opening the mouth or blowing against pinched nostrils (Valsalva maneuver) may help by distending the fossa of Rosenmüller and the eustachian tube orifice.

PATHOLOGY

Tumors

The effect of a tumor on the parapharyngeal fat is key to determination of the origin of a tumor.

Nasopharynx

Nasopharyngeal tumors can obliterate the airway. Lateral extension first widens the deglutitional ring and then impinges on the parapharyngeal fat from the medial side (Fig 25–4). Involvement of the eustachian tube orifice causes a middle ear effusion, which when appearing for the first time in an older individual should direct the physician's attention to the nasopharynx. On CT, obstruction of the eustachian tube can be suspected when there is fluid in an otherwise normal mastoid and middle ear. Deeper involvement results in cranial nerve palsies and in skull base erosion.

Masses in the lumen of the nasopharynx, including choanal polyps and adenoidal tissue, may obliterate the airway, but do not compromise the parapharyngeal fat or erode bone (Fig 25–5). With rapid infusion of intravenous contrast during the scan, the mucosa may blush, and thus an intraluminal location of a lesion can be confirmed. Adenoid tissue, though usually in midline, can be quite asymmetric.

NASOPHARYNGEAL CARCINOMA.—Approximately 90% of nasopharyngeal malignancies are squamous cell carcinoma.[10, 11] Early lesions may efface the fossa of Rosenmüller and eustachian tube or widen the deglutitional muscle ring. Small asymmetries can be normal and should be evaluated by direct visualization and biopsy.

As stated, deeper involvement deforms the parapharyngeal space from the medial aspect, and if the direction of extension is posterior or superior the skull base can be eroded (Fig 25–6,A).

Extension to the dura first causes an enhancing "bulge" in the dura, impinging on the cerebrospinal fluid spaces anterior to the brain stem (Fig 25–6,B). Tumors may extend through the foramen lacerum or petro-occipital suture to gain access to the intracranial compartment. Anterior extension involves the ethmoid sinuses and nasal cavity.

Nasopharyngeal carcinoma can spread to several nodal groups. The upper spinal accessory nodes high in the posterior triangle of the neck are particularly important, because enlargement of these nodes is highly suggestive of squamous cell carcinoma of the nasopharynx (Fig 25–7). Jugulodigastric nodes (angle of the mandible), jugular nodes, and retropharyngeal nodes may also be involved. Nodes involved with squamous cell carcinoma often show low-density centers (necrotic areas) and peripheral enhancement.

OTHER MALIGNANCIES.—Rhabdomyosarcoma occurs in children, and by the time of presentation it may in-

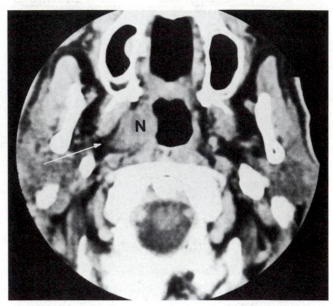

Fig 25–4.—Neurilemmoma *(N)* involving the nasopharyngeal wall and pushing laterally into the parapharyngeal space on the normal side. Parapharyngeal space is indicated by *long white arrow.* (From Curtin H.D.: Infratemporal fossa, nasopharynx, and parapharyngeal spaces, in Carter B. [ed.]: *Computed Tomography of the Head and Neck.* New York, Churchill-Livingstone, 1984.)

volve the ear and skull base as well as the nasopharynx. The point of origin may therefore be unclear. Adenoid cystic carcinoma, melanoma, lymphoma, plasmocytoma, and other rarer lesions can also arise in this area.

Tumor may extend into the nasopharynx from the skull base or nasal area. Tumors of the oral cavity and soft palate can extend superiorly to involve the submucosal area of the nasopharynx. The fossa of Rosenmüller may be affected without actual involvement of the mucosa.

BENIGN LESIONS.—*Juvenile angiofibromas* are discussed in Chapter 24.

Tornwaldt's cyst can form in the pharyngeal bursa and present in the second or third decade. The cyst would be in the midline high in the nasopharynx.

Choanal polyps protrude into the nasopharynx. They do not disturb the parapharyngeal spaces. The nasal cavity is involved on one side, and the maxillary sinus is usually opacified (see Fig 25–5).

Chordomas arise from notochordal remnants. They usually arise in the clivus, but occasionaly remnants of the notochord can be found in the posterior wall of the nasopharynx.[12] Chordomas can therefore arise rarely in the nasopharyngeal wall.

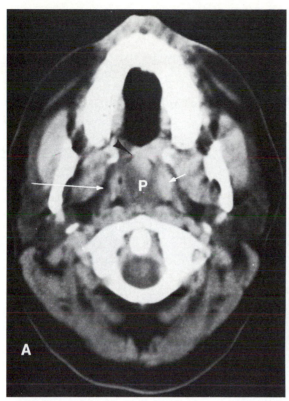

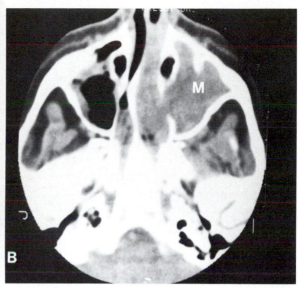

Fig 25–5.—A, intraluminal mass (choanal polyp). The polyp (P) appears to blend in with the deglutitional muscles (small white arrow). The parapharyngeal spaces are, however, not deformed (long white arrow). Small amount of air is seen between the polyp and the soft palate (arrowhead).

B, higher cuts show obliteration of the nasal cavity and involvement of the maxillary sinus (M). (From Curtin H.D.: Infratemporal fossa, nasopharynx, and parapharyngeal spaces, in Carter B. [ed.]: Computed Tomography of the Head and Neck. New York, Churchill-Livingstone, 1984.)

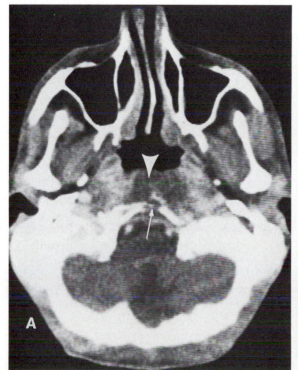

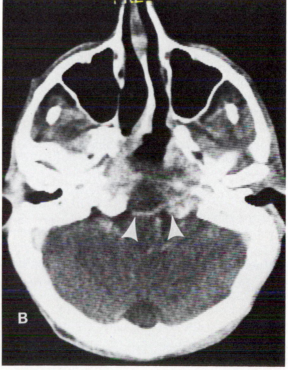

Fig 25–6.—A, tumor of the nasopharynx (arrowhead) eroding the base of the skull (white arrow). B, the tumor bulges the dura (arrowheads), compromising the subarachnoid cistern anterior to the brain stem. (From Curtin H.D.:

Infratemporal fossa, nasopharynx, and parapharyngeal spaces, in Carter B. [ed.]: Computed Tomography of the Head and Neck. New York, Churchill-Livingstone, 1984.)

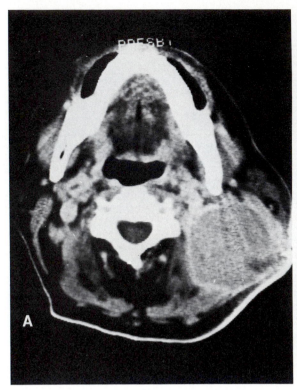

Fig 25–7.—A, large mass with peripheral enhancement and central hypodense area, which represents spinal accessory node involved with squamous cell carcinoma. **B,** coronal scan showed asymmetry of the soft tissues in the nasopharynx. Biopsy of the abnormal side *(small white arrow)* revealed nasopharyngeal carcinoma. No bone erosion was identified. (From Curtin H.D.: Infratemporal fossa, nasopharynx, and parapharyngeal spaces, in Carter B. [ed.]: *Computed Tomography of the Head and Neck.* New York, Churchill-Livingstone, 1984.)

Rathke's pouch tumors (craniopharyngiomas) can occur high in the nasopharyngeal vault, but are much more commonly intracranial than extracranial. Calcification is very common.

Encephaloceles can extend into the nasopharynx. They are covered elsewhere in this volume.

Neuromas and other benign lesions are uncommon.

Parapharyngeal Space[13, 14]

Tumors of the *prestyloid (anterolateral) compartment* are usually extensions from the deep lobe of the parotid. These tumors often extend through the narrow gap between the mandible and styloid called the stylomandibular tunnel (Fig 25–8). This gives a characteristic "dumbbell" appearance. The fat in the parapharyngeal space is pushed medially. Occasionally, CT sialography may be helpful, because the finger of the parotid tissue extending through the tunnel can be opacified, showing the relationship of the tumor to the gland.

Primary tumors of the prestyloid parapharyngeal space would be very rare. Most tumors involve this space secondarily.

Poststyloid (posteromedial) tumors are related to the neurovascular elements associated with the jugular vein and carotid artery. Lesions arising here push the parapharyngeal fat anteriorly and slightly laterally (Fig 25–9). A fat plane may separate the tumor from the nasopharyngeal mucosa (Fig 25–10). As the tumor expands and is limited posteriorly by the bony elements, the bulk of the tumor may actually be located further anteriorly than is the styloid process.

PARAGANGLIOMAS.—*Paragangliomas* (*glomus tumors*) (see Fig 25–9) arise in the poststyloid compartment and enhance prominently with rapid-flow contrast administration. Glomus vagale tumors arise in the vagal ganglion inferior to the temporal bone. Glomus jugulare tumors can extend from the jugular fossa inferiorly into the poststyloid space. Differentiation is made by looking for destruction of the jugular foramen. Glomus vagale pushes the carotid artery anteriorly on arteriog-

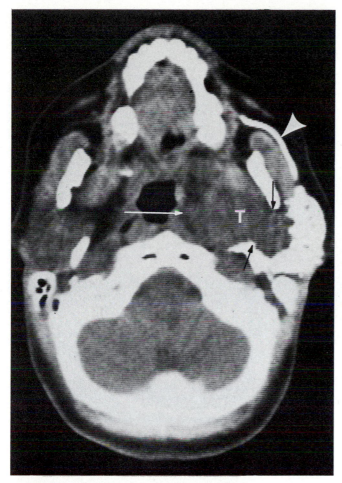

Fig 25–8.—Pleomorphic adenoma arising in the deep lobe of the parotid gland. The tumor impinges upon the parapharyngeal space, pushing the fat *(white arrow)* medially. The tumor has a typical dumbbell shape, being constricted (between *small black arrows*) as it passes through the stylomandibular tunnel between the mandibular ramus and styloid. (*T* = tumor.) The image is taken during CT sialogram. Parotid duct is indicated by *white arrowhead.* Contrast is seen in the parotid. (From Curtin H.D.: Infratemporal fossa, nasopharynx, and parapharyngeal spaces, in Carter B. [ed.]: *Computed Tomography of the Head and Neck.* New York, Churchill-Livingstone, 1984.)

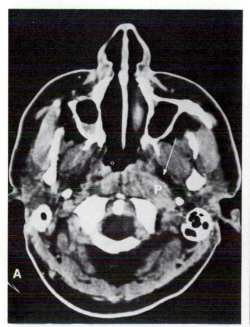
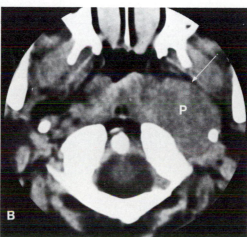
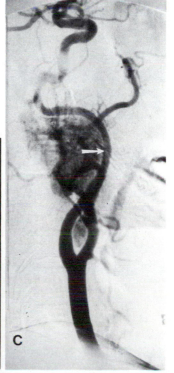

Fig 25–9.—**A,** axial slice through the paraganglioma *(P).* The parapharyngeal space *(white arrow)* is pushed anteriorly and laterally. **B,** slightly lower cut shows bulk of the paraganglioma *(P),* further displacing the parapharyngeal fat *(small white arrow).* **C,** arteriogram shows tumor blood pushing the carotid anteriorly *(arrow).*

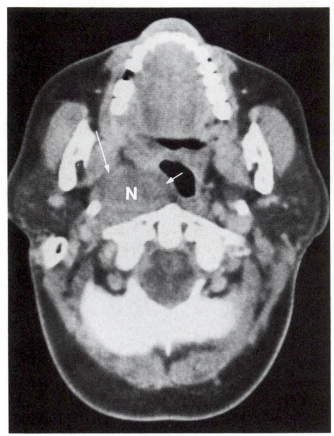

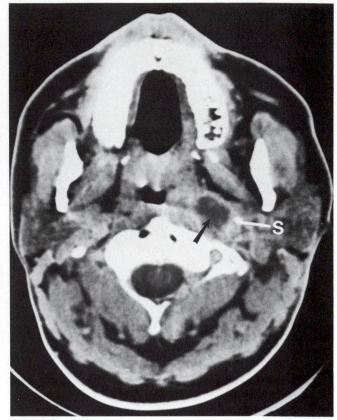

Fig 25–10.—Neurilemmoma *(N)* arising in the poststyloid parapharyngeal space. The parapharyngeal fat *(long white arrow)* is pushed anteriorly and laterally. Small fat plane *(short white arrow)* is seen between the tumor and the pharyngeal mucosa. (From Curtin H.D.: Infratemporal fossa, nasopharynx, and parapharyngeal spaces, in Carter B. [ed.]: *Computed Tomography of the Head and Neck.* New York, Churchill-Livingstone, 1984.)

Fig 25–11.—Squamous cell carcinoma involving the retropharyngeal node *(arrow).* The parapharyngeal fat is pushed anteriorly. The bulk of the lesion is medial to the styloid process. Note the necrotic center. (*S* = styloid.) (From Curtin H.D.: Infratemporal fossa, nasopharynx, and parapharyngeal spaces, in Carter B. [ed.]: *Computed Tomography of the Head and Neck.* New York, Churchill-Livingstone, 1984.)

raphy. Paragangliomas may be multiple, but are rarely malignant.

NEUROMAS.—*Neuromas* also often enhance and can be confused with paragangliomas. They have a different appearance on angiography (see Fig 25–10).

LATERAL RETROPHARYNGEAL NODES.—*Lateral retropharyngeal nodes* arise just medial to the carotid and behave as poststyloid masses.[15] They usually have a necrotic center, which is hypodense on CT scan (Fig 25–11).

MENINGIOMAS.—*Meningiomas* may involve the pre- or poststyloid spaces as well as the masticator area. They cause hyperostosis of the bone and may calcify (Fig 25–12).

When a lesion involves the poststyloid parapharyngeal space, arteriography is performed to help differentiate the various tumors and to define the relationship of the tumor to the great vessels. This is not usually necessary in prestyloid masses, and angiography is not usually done.

Infratemporal Fossa (Masticator Space)

Tumors of the infratemporal fossa are usually extensions from primaries in the surrounding areas. The most common is probably the maxillary sinus (see Chapter 24). Primary tumors may arise in the mandible or in the associated musculature. Tumors may leave the infratemporal fossa by extending into the middle cranial fossa via the foramen ovale or into the pterygopalatine fossa. Extension into these areas can be detected because of the difference in density between the tumor and the normal soft tissue (fat in the pterygopalatine fossa and brain in the middle cranial fossa).

Mandibular and lingual nerves pass through the infratemporal fossa and can be enlarged by perineural ex-

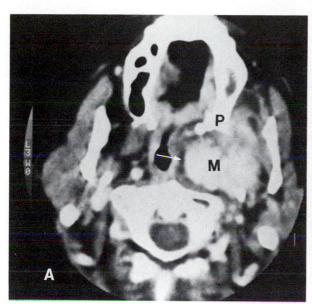

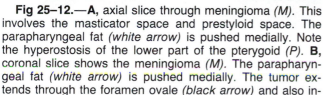

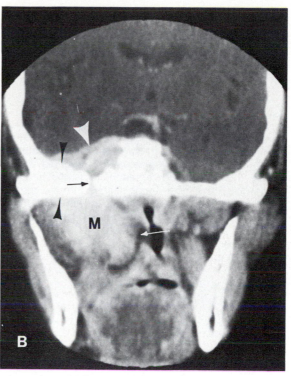

Fig 25–12.—A, axial slice through meningioma *(M)*. This involves the masticator space and prestyloid space. The parapharyngeal fat *(white arrow)* is pushed medially. Note the hyperostosis of the lower part of the pterygoid *(P)*. **B,** coronal slice shows the meningioma *(M)*. The parapharyngeal fat *(white arrow)* is pushed medially. The tumor extends through the foramen ovale *(black arrow)* and also involves the middle cranial fossa *(large white arrowhead)*. Note the hyperostosis of the skull base *(black arrowheads)*. (From Curtin H.D.: Infratemporal fossa, nasopharynx, and parapharyngeal spaces, in Carter B. [ed.]: *Computed Tomography of the Head and Neck.* New York, Churchill-Livingstone, 1984.)

tension (see Chapter 24). This would be very rare as an initial finding, and other manifestations of the tumor would certainly be present.

Hematogenous metastasis can reach the mandible usually from the breast, kidney, lung, colon, or prostate (Fig 25–13).

Infection

The fascial planes of the area may direct the spread of an infectious process. The infection may be of dental or tonsillar origin. Infection may also drain in the retropharyngeal nodes, where an abscess can form in the retropharyngeal or the poststyloid parapharyngeal space.

Infection of the masticator space can spread easily into the temporal space, which is actually the superior extension of the masticator space (Fig 25–14). The buccal space, lateral to the buccinator muscle, can be involved, but is usually separated from the masticator space. Retropharyngeal infection can spread down into the mediastinum. The spaces are not impervious, but may limit the spread of infection to some extent.

Malignant external otitis is a persistent *Pseudomonas* infection, usually in an elderly diabetic. There is bone destruction with a granulation-like growth. Disease may extend down into the soft tissues beneath the temporal bone. This usually involves the area just beneath the external auditory canal, but occasionally the disease can extend medially into the region of the nasopharynx, obliterating the fat planes.[16]

MISCELLANEOUS

Atrophy of the muscles bordering the nasopharynx can accentuate the normal recesses in the elderly. If cranial nerve V is destroyed, the muscles of mastication atrophy (Fig 25–15). When this is seen on CT, the more central connections of the trigeminal nerve should be evaluated.

In a patient undergoing hemimandibulectomy, the condyle and part of the ramus may be left on the resected side. Because there are no teeth to limit the motion of the fragment, the pterygoid muscles pull the bone anteriorly. This may result in a pseudoenlargement of the muscle when compared with the opposite side. This apparent enlargement is due to shortening of the muscle and may minimize tumor recurrence.

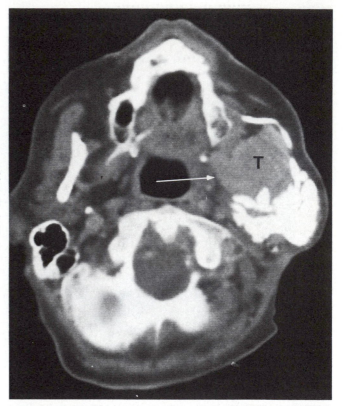

Fig 25–13.—Metastatic tumor from lung to mandible. (*T* = tumor.) The tumor replaces the coronoid process. The tumor was thought to represent a parotid tumor, but is actually deep to it. The tumor pushes into the parapharyngeal fat *(white arrow),* pushing it medially (parotid sialogram). (From Curtin H.D.: Infratemporal fossa, nasopharynx, and parapharyngeal spaces, in Carter B. [ed.]: *Computed Tomography of the Head and Neck.* New York, Churchill-Livingstone, 1984.)

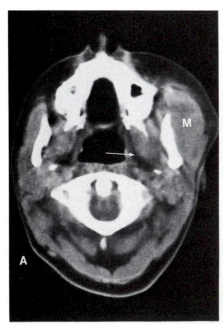

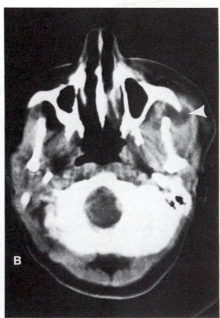

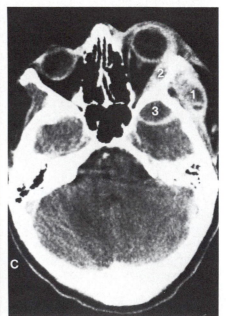

Fig 25–14.—A, infection from a molar extraction. The masseter muscle appears to be enlarged because of the abscess in the masticator space. (*M* = enlarged masseter.) The parapharyngeal space *(arrow)* is normal. **B,** higher slice shows abscess just beneath the zygomatic arch *(arrow-* *head).* This represents the junction of the masticator and temporalis spaces. **C,** higher slice shows abscess in the temporal space *(1),* orbit *(2).* There is also an epidural abscess *(3).*

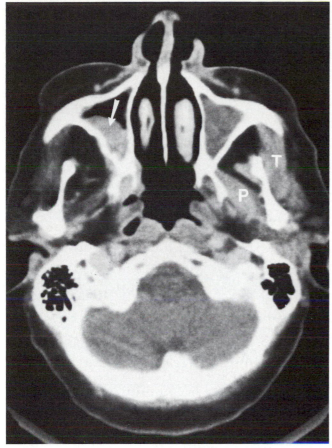

Fig 25–15.—Adenoid cystic carcinoma of the maxillary sinus *(arrow)*. Tumor involves the maxillary division of the trigeminal nerve, causing atrophy of the masticator muscles. Compare with the opposite normal side. (*P* = normal pterygoid, *T* = normal temporalis muscle.) The maxillary sinus on the uninvolved side showed an obstructive phenomena with mucous retention.

SUMMARY

The symmetric muscles and fat planes make the nasopharynx and surrounding structures ideal for CT imaging. The effect of a tumor on the parapharyngeal space is especially important in definition of tumor origin. The radiologist's primary role is to determine the extent of the disease.

REFERENCES

1. Bohman L., Mancuso A., Thompson J., et al.: CT approach to benign nasopharyngeal masses. *A.J.R.* 136:173–180, 1981.
2. Carter B.: Computed tomography, in Valvassori G.E., Potter G.D., Hanafee W.N., et al. (eds.): *Radiology of the Ear, Nose and Throat.* Philadelphia, W.B. Saunders Co., 1982.
3. Doubleday L.C., Jing B., Wallace S.: Computed tomography of the infratemporal fossa. *Radiology* 138:619–624, 1981.
4. Mancuso A., Bohman L., Hanafee W., et al.: Computed tomography of the nasopharynx: Normal and variants of normal. *Radiology* 137:113–121, 1980.
5. Mancuso A., Hanafee W.: *Computed Tomography of the Head and Neck.* Baltimore, Williams & Wilkins Co., 1982.
6. Silver A.J., Mawad M.E., Hilal S.K., et al.: Computed tomography of the nasopharynx and related spaces: I. Anatomy. *Radiology* 147:725–731, 1983.
7. Silver A.J., Mawad M.E., Hilal S.K., et al.: Computed tomography of the nasopharynx and related spaces: II. Pathology. *Radiology* 147:733–738, 1983.
8. Som P.M., Biller H.F., Lawson W.: Tumors of the parapharyngeal space (preoperative evaluation, diagnosis, and surgical approaches). *Ann. Otol. Rhinol. Laryngol.* 90:3–15, 1981.
9. Grodinsky M., Holyoke E.A.: The fascia and fascial spaces of the head, neck and adjacent regions. *Am. J. Anat.* 63:367–408, 1938.
10. Choa G.: Cancer of the nasopharynx, in Suen J.Y., Myers E.N. (eds): *Cancer of the Head and Neck.* New York, Churchill Livingstone, Inc., 1981.
11. Goldstein J.C., Sisson G.A.: Tumors of the nose, paranasal sinuses, and nasopharynx, in Paparella M.M., Shumrick D.A. (eds.): *Otolaryngology.* Philadelphia, W.B. Saunders Co., 1980, vol. 8, pp. 2078–2114.
12. Bonneville J., Belloir A., Mawazini H., et al.: Calcified remnants of the notochord in the roof of the nasopharynx. *Radiology* 137:373–377, 1980.
13. Bass R.: Approaches to the diagnosis and treatment of tumors of the parapharyngeal space. *Head Neck Surg.* 4:281–289, 1982.
14. Som P.M., Biller H.F.: The combined CT-sialogram. *Radiology* 135:387–390, 1980.
15. Mancuso A.A., Harnsberger H.R., Muraki A.S., et al.: Computed tomography of cervical and retropharyngeal lymph nodes: Normal anatomy, variants of normal, and applications in staging head and neck cancer: I. Normal anatomy. *Radiology* 148:709–714, 1983.
16. Curtin H.D., Wolfe P., May M.: Malignant external otitis: CT evaluation. *Radiology* 145:383–388, 1982.

26

The Normal and Abnormal Neck

R. Nick Bryan, M.D.
Charles W. McCluggage, M.D.
Barry L. Horowitz, M.D.

CT EVALUATION OF THE CERVICAL REGION

The technique of CT is significantly changing and increasing the value of radiographic evaluation of the neck. This is primarily a consequence of two factors: (1) the relative ease of the examination and (2) the vastly superior information available as compared with that from earlier imaging techniques. The neck, which extends from the inferior border of the mandible and foramen magnum to the thoracic inlet, is a relatively small, thin area that is amenable to direct clinical observation and palpation externally and direct endoscopic observation internally. Most masses within this area are clinically detectable, while relatively small in size. However, this is not to say that additional morphological information is not needed by the clinician.

While the neck is a small anatomical area, it is very complex, with many small critical structures and tissues closely approximated. While lesions might be easily detectable, their precise anatomical location and relationships are not always obvious by clinical means alone. Unfortunately, prior radiographic techniques usually did not provide the necessary anatomical and pathologic resolution that the clinician wanted. In fact, traditional radiographic techniques often mimicked or duplicated clinical observations. Plain x-rays of the neck demonstrated little beyond the air-contrasted respiratory tract, bone of the cervical spine, and, to a lesser degree, the cartilaginous anatomy of the larynx. For most lesions, the plain x-rays offered only gross, indirect anatomical information. Even the more invasive techniques such as laryngography, air-contrast pluridirectional tomography, and barium studies of the digestive tract yielded only information concerning gross displacements or the appearance of the mucosal surfaces, which in most cases could be obtained by direct and indirect endoscopy. In only a limited number of cases did contrast opacification of visceral structures by lymphangiography, angiography, or sialography provide direct information about internal soft tissues. In selected cases, high-resolution ultrasound provided some intrinsic information, particularly about the thyroid gland. On the other hand, CT now allows very high-resolution anatomical images that display the major muscles, viscera, vessels, and associated intervening spaces. Indeed, CT provides far more information concerning the anatomy, and even occasionally the pathology, of lesions than can be obtained by clinical examination. Furthermore, the examination is essentially noninvasive and easy to perform. It should now be considered the primary imaging technique for most neck pathology.

Unfortunately, clinical application of the technique has been excessively slow. One of the main reasons has been the lack of knowledge and hence interest in this area by many radiologists. Because of the previous limited demand by clinicians for radiographic studies of the neck, appropriate anatomical knowledge of the area by the radiologist has been forgotten, if ever learned. Likewise, the more important pathophysiology of this region has not been extensively taught or studied by radiologists. However, now that the usefulness of the technique is becoming obvious, it is imperative that the imaging physician refamiliarize himself with the fine anatomy of this area and reacquaint himself with the important pathology.

With this background, this chapter will concentrate on the anatomy of the neck and attempt to relate the traditional topographic and surgical anatomy of the neck with the cross-sectional anatomy as displayed by CT. This correlation is extremely important because the traditional clinician remains anatomically oriented and does not usually transfer cross-sectional anatomy to the clinical, gross anatomical situation. Subsequently, a few of the major pathologic processes in the neck will be discussed and correlated with appropriate CT images. Because one cannot attempt to cover all of the widely diverse pathologic conditions in this area in a single chapter, we will concentrate on lesions involving the salivary glands, larynx, and lymphatic system, as well as a few other miscellaneous topics.

While the cervical spine is obviously a large and important component of the neck, its anatomy and pathology are basically a different topic that will be covered elsewhere. In addition, the dorsal neck (to be later defined) will be minimally discussed in this section because it contains the relatively simple anatomy of the paraspinal muscles and is involved with little pathology independent of the cervical spine. Therefore, we will concentrate on the soft tissues of the anterior two thirds of the neck.

ANATOMY

Cervical Triangles

The anterior neck has traditionally been divided into triangular regions that are defined and separated by major muscles (Fig 26–1). This descriptive subdivision of the neck has been of great clinical usefulness because (1) various regions can usually be defined by observation and palpation, (2) the regions are related to relatively consistent underlying anatomy that allows postulation of location and origin of contained lesions, and (3) important surgical approaches are suggested.[1]

The posterior extent of the "triangular" neck is the anterior border of the trapezius muscle. Anything posterior to this plane is in the dorsal neck and will not be discussed in this section. Each right and left half of the neck has symmetric and essentially identical triangular regions.

The major division is into an anterior and a posterior triangle, which are separated by the sternocleidomastoid (SCM) muscles. These large, easily palpable muscles that extend from the mastoid process to the medial end of the clavicle and adjacent manubrium define the posterior border of the anterior triangle, which extends to the ventral midline, and the anterior border of the posterior triangle, which extends back to the trapezius muscle. The posterior triangle is subdivided into a subclavian and occipital triangle by the intervening posterior belly of the omohyoid muscle. The omohyoid muscle has two bellies, the posterior of which originates from the area of the suprascapular notch of the scapula and extends to an intermediate tendon, which is attached to the medial clavicle and first rib. The anterior belly then proceeds superiorly to insert on the body of the hyoid bone. The occipital triangle lies between the trapezius muscle posteriorly, the SCM muscle anteriorly, and the posterior belly of the omohyoid inferiorly. The subclavian triangle lies inferior to the posterior belly of the omohyoid muscle, posterior to the SCM muscle, and rostral to the clavicle.

The large anterior cervical triangle can be subdivided into an upper and lower portion separated by the hyoid bone. The upper portion contains two triangular regions. The digastric triangle lies below the inferior border of the mandible and between the anterior and pos-

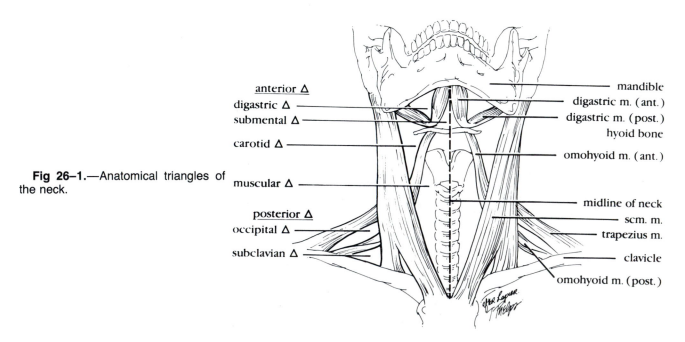

Fig 26–1.—Anatomical triangles of the neck.

anterior △
digastric △
submental △
carotid △
muscular △
posterior △
occipital △
subclavian △

mandible
digastric m. (ant.)
digastric m. (post.)
hyoid bone
omohyoid m. (ant.)
midline of neck
scm. m.
trapezius m.
clavicle
omohyoid m. (post.)

terior bellies of the digastric muscle. Anteriorly, the digastric muscle is attached to the inner surface of the mandibular symphysis. The anterior belly then passes posterolaterally to a tendinous sling attached by an aponeurosis to the lateral aspect of the body of the hyoid bone. The posterior belly extends posteriorly to the base of the skull at the digastric notch just medial to the mastoid tip. The smaller submental triangle lies between the anterior belly of the digastric muscle and the midline, below the symphysis of the mandible and above the hyoid bone.

The lower portion of the anterior cervical triangle is subdivided into an upper carotid triangle and a lower muscular triangle, which are separated from each other by the anterior belly of the omohyoid muscle. The carotid triangle is bounded by the posterior belly of the digastric muscle superiorly, the SCM muscle posteriorly, and the anterior belly of the omohyoid muscle anteroinferiorly. The muscular triangle lies between the anterior belly of the omohyoid muscle superiorly, the SCM muscle posteriorly, and the midline anteriorly.

Each of the cervical triangles contain certain critical structures (Figs 26–2 to 26–4). The posterior triangle has a deep floor of muscles, which are basically the anterior and lateral paravertebral muscles and are contained within the tough prevertebral fascia. From anterior to posterior, these muscles are the anterior, middle, and posterior scalene and levator scapula muscles. This is a relatively continuous sheath of muscles, except for a gap between the anterior and middle sca-

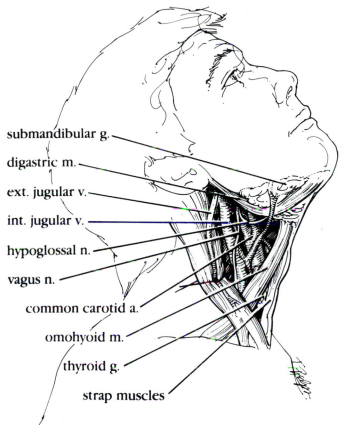

submandibular g.
digastric m.
ext. jugular v.
int. jugular v.
hypoglossal n.
vagus n.
common carotid a.
omohyoid m.
thyroid g.
strap muscles

Fig 26–3.—Contents of the anterior cervical triangle, lateral view.

lene through which pass the cervical and upper brachial nerve plexuses and the subclavian artery. The subclavian vein passes anterior to the anterior scalene muscle at the medial aspect of the clavicle. In the occipital triangle, the floor then consists of the above muscles and the cervical plexus. The branches of the cervical plexus (which supply essentially all of the muscles of the cervical region as well as the overlying skin) loop about the posterior border of the SCM before they course to their respective muscles and cutaneous territories. Only a few superficial cervical lymph nodes are located in the occipital triangle. The 11th cranial nerve crosses the midaspect of the occipital triangle as it passes from behind the SCM muscle to the undersurface of its termination in the trapezius muscle. Crossing the anterior aspect of the occipital triangle and extending down across the subclavian triangle is the external jugular vein, which lies outside of the investing layer of the deep cervical fascia.

Within the subclavian triangle, the subclavian vein lies just anterior to the anterior scalene muscle, while the subclavian artery and brachial plexus proceed laterally between the anterior and middle scalene muscles.

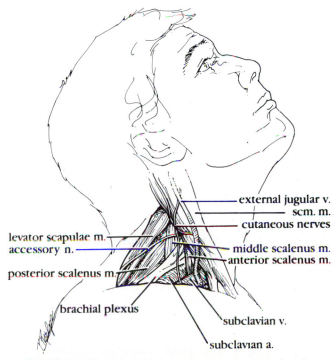

levator scapulae m.
accessory n.
posterior scalenus m.
brachial plexus
external jugular v.
scm. m.
cutaneous nerves
middle scalenus m.
anterior scalenus m.
subclavian v.
subclavian a.

Fig 26–2.—Contents of the posterior cervical triangle.

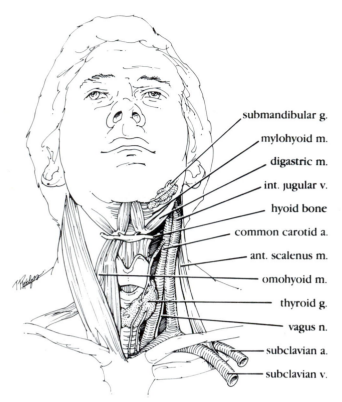

submandibular g.

mylohyoid m.

digastric m.

int. jugular v.

hyoid bone

common carotid a.

ant. scalenus m.

omohyoid m.

thyroid g.

vagus n.

subclavian a.

subclavian v.

Fig 26–4.—Contents of the anterior cervical triangle, frontal view.

The digastric triangle has as its floor the mylohyoid muscle anteriorly, while lateral pharyngeal wall structures form the floor more posteriorly. Within the triangle lie the superficial portion of the submandibular gland, submandibular lymph nodes, and the facial artery. The small submental triangle has the mylohyoid muscle as the floor and contains only a few submental lymph nodes. The carotid triangle has the middle and inferior constrictor muscles of the pharynx and the pretracheal strap muscles as its floor. It contains the carotid artery, cervical sympathetic plexus, vagus nerve, internal jugular vein, and deep cervical lymph nodes.

The muscular triangle has the inferior portion of the carotid sheath, pretracheal fascia, and pretracheal strap muscles as its floor. It contains the inferior portions of the internal jugular vein, common carotid artery, vagus nerve, cervical sympathetic plexus, inferior thyroidal vessels, inferior laryngeal nerve, and inferior deep cervical lymph nodes.

Visceral Columns

Another conceptual approach to the anatomy of the neck is that of a concentric columnar structure (Fig 26–5). The neck can be viewed as consisting of a median visceral column, lateral visceral column, and surrounding musculofascial sheath. The median visceral column primarily consists of pharyngeal derivatives, including the hypopharynx, larynx, trachea, and esophagus. It is a concentrically tight, fascially isolated compartment, but is open superiorly and inferiorly.

Anterolateral to the median visceral column is the lateral visceral column, which is an intermediate fascial space that consists primarily of the major vascular structures of the neck and components of pharyngeal arch derivatives. This column includes the carotid sheath (which contains the internal jugular vein, carotid arteries, and vagus nerve), deep cervical lymph nodes, and, in a subdivided anterior inferior compartment, the thyroid and parathyroid glands. The salivary glands, particularly the parotid and submandibular glands, might also be included in this compartment, although in a somewhat artificial manner.

Enveloping the central columns is a strong V-shaped musculofascial sheath consisting primarily of the deep cervical fascia and the SCM and trapezius muscles, which this strong fascia envelopes. Posterolaterally, the deep cervical fascia is continuous with the prevertebral fascia, which basically separates the posterior aspect of the neck. The anatomical boundaries between these three anatomical columns are relatively strong, and therefore lesions external to the deep cervical fascia or posterior to the prevertebral fascia tend to be excluded from the deeper spaces. The lateral visceral column, while effectively separated from the median visceral column and the overlying musculofascial sheath, is relatively open throughout its length, including top and bottom. This forms a potential conduit for disease to spread throughout the length of the neck and beyond.

Lymphatic System

With respect to spread of disease in the cervical region, one must also consider the lymphatic system of this area, which may be subdivided into four main groups: (1) superficial cervical nodes, (2) deep cervical nodes, (3) junctional nodes, and (4) anterior cervical nodes (Fig 26–6). The superficial cervical nodes are relatively few in number and lie external to the deep cervical fascia, primarily over the parotid region, and along the external jugular vein. The deep cervical nodes are more numerous and are far more important. They basically all lie along the carotid sheath-jugular vein region and hence are sometimes called jugular nodes. They may be subdivided into an upper group, which is above the anterior belly of the omohyoid muscle, and an inferior group caudal to that plane. The upper group includes jugulodigastric nodes near the middle tendon of the digastric muscle, which receive lymph from the tonsillar region; the jugulo-omohyoid nodes, which drain the anterior tongue and submental nodes; the

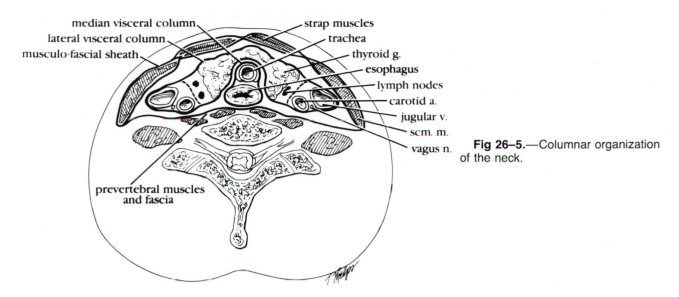

median visceral column
lateral visceral column
musculo-fascial sheath

strap muscles
trachea
thyroid g.
esophagus
lymph nodes
carotid a.
jugular v.
scm. m.
vagus n.

prevertebral muscles
and fascia

Fig 26–5.—Columnar organization of the neck.

retropharyngeal nodes near the base of the skull, which drain the nasopharynx and the eustachian region; and the deep parotid nodes, which lie within the parotid gland. The inferior group of deep cervical nodes receive efferent vessels from the superior deep cervical channels as well as apical axillary nodes.

Junctional nodes lie at the junction of the head and neck and include one or two occipital nodes, several mastoid nodes, the nodes in relationship to the parotid gland, approximately five nodes near the submandibular gland, and one to four submental nodes.

The anterior cervical nodes generally lie along the ventral midline and include infrahyoid nodes on the thyrohyoid membrane, prelaryngeal nodes near the cricothyroid membrane, and pre- and paratracheal nodes. It is important that one not only remembers the general location of these nodes, but also notes their usual drainage patterns.

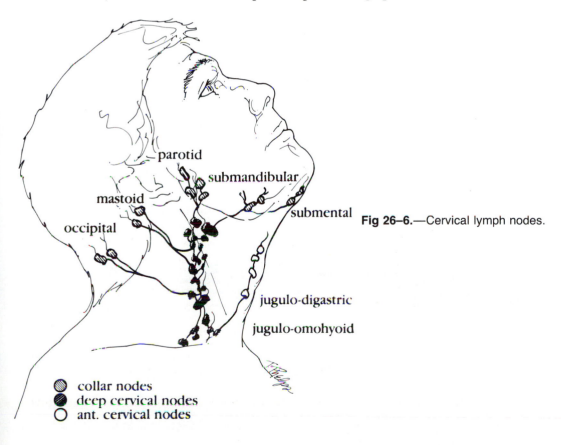

parotid
submandibular
mastoid
submental
occipital

jugulo-digastric

jugulo-omohyoid

Fig 26–6.—Cervical lymph nodes.

⊘ collar nodes
● deep cervical nodes
○ ant. cervical nodes

Salivary Glands

While only part of the salivary glands are in the cervical region, we will include a discussion of these structures as they do relate to the upper neck and are seen and evaluated on CT scans of this region. Only the parotid and submandibular glands are well demonstrated by CT, and descriptive anatomy and pathology will be limited to these salivary structures (Figs 26–7 and 26–8).

The parotid gland is the largest of the major salivary glands and is roughly triangular in shape both in the lateral and axial projections. It is a fatty glandular tissue that is encased in a dense capsule. Because of this, the parotid gland on CT is consistently more lucent than surrounding muscles and likewise is distinctly more radiodense than adjacent fat in the subcutaneous tissues, infratemporal fossa, and lateral pharyngeal space. The parotid duct is not routinely visualized on CT without intraductal contrast opacification.

The gland is arbitrarily and indistinctly divided into a medial and lateral portion by the facial nerve. The facial nerve enters the gland posteriorly as it exits from the stylomastoid foramen. The nerve then passes lateral to the styloid process and anteriorly through the gland lateral to the external carotid artery and retromandibular vein to break up into its major trunks lateral to the mandible. One can routinely define the styloid process and retromandibular vein. The facial nerve itself cannot be seen passing through the gland.

The medial portion of the parotid extends behind the mandible to occupy the retromandibular space. More medially, it abuts the pterygoid muscles anteriorly and the lateral pharyngeal space medially. The deep portion of the gland is separated posterolaterally from the major neurovascular bundle by the styloid diaphragm and stylopharyngeus ligament. Because of the tough fascial, ligamentous, and membranous capsule, lesions of the parotid tend to remain localized within the gland.

The parotid gland is intimately related to two groups of lymph nodes. The superficial group lies along the surface of the gland, while the deep nodes lie scattered within the gland itself.

The submandibular gland is approximately one-half the size of the parotid gland. It is a hockey-stick shaped structure with the larger superficial portion of the gland covered by platysma and lying below the mylohyoid muscle, which is the major muscle supporting the floor of the mouth. The gland then passes around the back of the mylohyoid muscle, where its smaller deep portion lies on top of the mylohyoid muscle. The submandibular duct passes forward from this deep portion beneath and adjacent to the sublingual gland to its opening in the papilla in the anterior floor of the mouth. The submandibular gland is adjacent to numerous lymph nodes throughout its course, but contains no nodes within its capsule.

On CT scans, the bulk of the superficial portion of the gland is seen as a globular soft-tissue structure along the superolateral aspect of the hyoid bone. The submandibular glands are more radiodense than the parotid glands and are approximately the same as adjacent muscles. The deeper portions and the ducts of the submandibular glands are best seen on coronal scans.

Larynx

The larynx is obviously one of the most important structures in the neck. Because of its relatively small

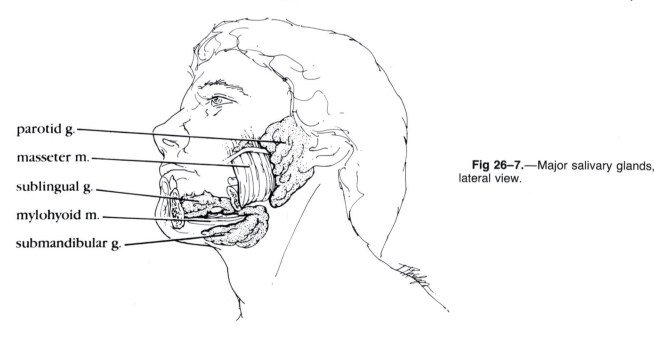

parotid g.
masseter m.
sublingual g.
mylohyoid m.
submandibular g.

Fig 26–7.—Major salivary glands, lateral view.

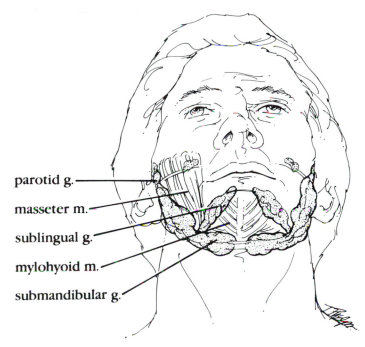

parotid g.
masseter m.
sublingual g.
mylohyoid m.
submandibular g.

Fig 26–8.—Major salivary glands, frontal view.

and complex structure, it deserves a few specific comments. Both from a gross anatomical as well as CT viewpoint, the larynx can best be understood by first appreciating its bony and cartilaginous skeleton (Fig 26–9). This consists, from superiorly to inferiorly, of the hyoid bone and the major cartilages—thyroid, arytenoid, and cricoid. The hyoid bone is the U-shaped bone suspended from the floor of the mouth mainly by the geniohyoid, mylohyoid, styloid, and digastric muscles. Suspended from it by the thyrohyoid membrane is the V-shaped thyroid cartilage, with broad lateral laminae extending from the midline anteriorly to the free posterior borders where the smaller superior and inferior cornu arise. The superior cornu ascends to articulate with the hyoid bone, while the inferior cornu extends behind the cricoid cartilage. The thyroid cartilage cal-

cifies in an extremely variable fashion, usually its internal and external cortices first, with the central medullary portion last.

The signet-ring shaped cricoid cartilage is the foundation of the larynx. It is suspended anteriorly from the thyroid cartilage by the thyrocricoid ligament, but posteriorly the posterior lamina ascends to reach the level of the midthyroid lamina, where the two small L-shaped arytenoid cartilages articulate with the upper surface of the cricoid cartilage. The vocal ligament extends from the thyroid cartilage anteriorly just below the thyroid notch to the anteriorly projecting vocal processes of the arytenoids posteriorly. The superior processes of the arytenoids extend to the posteroinferior aspects of the aryepiglottic folds. The cricoid cartilage tends to calcify earlier and more intensely than the

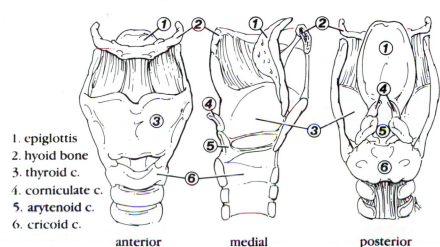

1. epiglottis
2. hyoid bone
3. thyroid c.
4. corniculate c.
5. arytenoid c.
6. cricoid c.

anterior   medial   posterior

Fig 26–9.—Osseous and cartilaginous skeleton of the larynx.

thyroid cartilage. All of these laryngeal skeletal structures may be identified on CT.

The soft tissue of the larynx may be simplified by considering it to be a suspended stocking-like sheath open superiorly at its attachment to the posterior inferior epiglottis and aryepiglottic folds and interiorly where it is continuous with the tracheal mucosa (Fig 26–10). This relatively simple column of mucosa and underlying submucosal areolar tissue then has a lateral tuck or fold near its midportion at the level of the glottis between the false and true vocal cords. This lateral fold is the laryngeal ventricle, which lies just superior to the true vocal cords and beneath the false vocal cords. The true and false vocal cords then bulge toward the midline above and below the ventricle itself. The false vocal cord lies at the plane of the superior-most portion of the arytenoid cartilage and extends anteriorly to the inferior-most aspect of the epiglottis and preepiglottic space just above the thyroid notch. It contains relatively loose areolar tissue as well as mucous glandular tissue and has a relatively distinctive fatty lucent triangular appearance on CT. The true vocal cord, on the other hand, lies at the plane of the cricoarytenoid joint and the anteriorly projecting vocal process of the arytenoid. The vocal cord itself is relatively dense by CT (as compared with the false cord), because it consists of the relatively solid vocal muscle and the vocal ligament that extends forward to attach to the posterior aspect of the thyroid cartilage just below the thyroid notch. This junctional area between the two true vocal cords and the thyroid cartilage is the anterior commissure, which is little more than a thin tendinous insertion.

The false vocal cord is approximately 6 mm in vertical height, while the true vocal cord is 5 to 6 mm. There is a fairly sharp transition from true vocal cord to subglottic space at the level of the midcricoid cartilage. It must be remembered that the true vocal cord is at the plane of and closely related to the upper cricoid cartilage posteriorly. However, the true vocal cord is well above the more inferiorly positioned anterior portion of the cricoid ring. The preepiglottic space anterior to the epiglottis and behind the thyrohyoid ligament is primarily filled with fat and is therefore relatively lucent on CT.

An abbreviated atlas of normal cross-sectional anatomy of the neck is presented in Figure 26–11.

PATHOLOGY

Developmental

Developmental anomalies of the cervical region are not common, although one, the "branchial cyst," is not rare. It, like other anomalies, is best understood by review of the embryology of the cervical region. This, of course, is basically the story of the pharyngeal pouch system (Fig 26–12).[2] The most striking developmental structures in the cervical region are the mesodermal pharyngeal arches. These solid, bilaterally symmetric, horizontal pillars of soft tissue develop in relationship to the original six pharyngeal arch arteries as the adjacent mesodermal tissues differentiate and coalesce about the vessels. Between the solid-tissue arches, entodermal pouches of the primitive pharynx extend laterally to approach, but not reach, shallow depressions of the superficial ectodermal surface of the embryo.

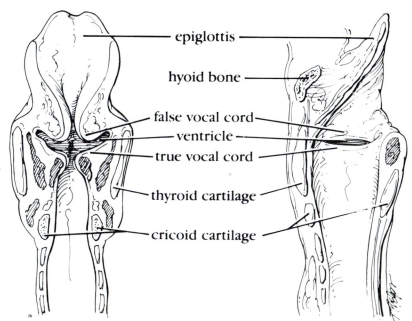

Fig 26–10.—Pharyngeal soft tissues.

epiglottis

hyoid bone

false vocal cord

ventricle

true vocal cord

thyroid cartilage

cricoid cartilage

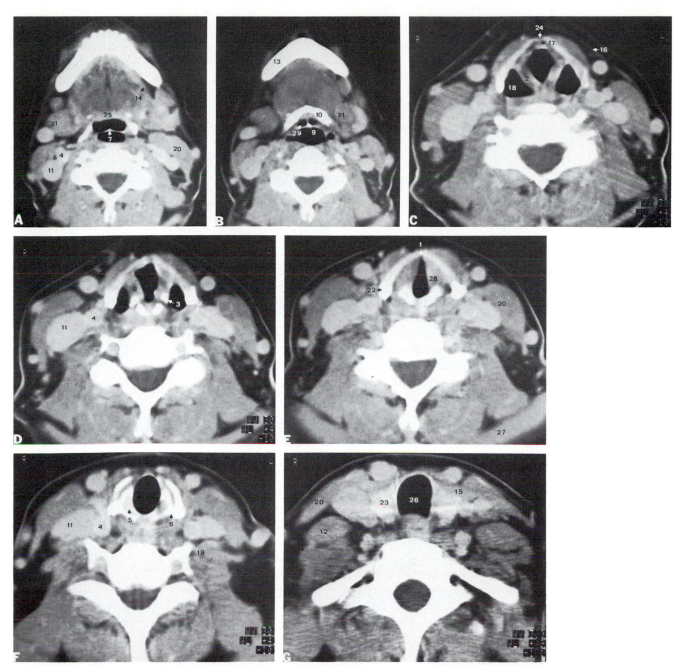

Fig 26–11.—Normal cervical CT scans. Levels of the slices are the epiglottis **(A)**, the vallecula **(B)**, thyroid notch **(C)**, arytenoid cartilage **(D)**, true vocal cord **(E)**, cricoid cartilage **(F)**, and trachea **(G)**. Anatomical legend for Figure 26–11. (1 = anterior commissure, 2 = aryepiglottic fold, 3 = arytenoid cartilage, 4 = carotid artery, 5 = cricoid cartilage, 6 = cricothyroid articulation, 7 = epiglottis, 8 = false vocal cord, 9 = glossoepiglottic ligament, 10 = hyoid bone, 11 = jugular vein, 12 = levator muscle of scapulae, 13 = mandible, 14 = mylohyoid muscle, 15 = omohyoid muscle, 16 = platysma muscle, 17 = preepiglottic space, 18 = pyriform sinus, 19 = scalene muscles, 20 = sternocleidomastoid muscle, 21 = submandibular gland, 22 = thyroid cartilage, 23 = thyroid gland, 24 = thyroid notch, 25 = tongue base, 26 = trachea, 27 = trapezius muscle, 28 = true vocal cord, 29 = vallecula)

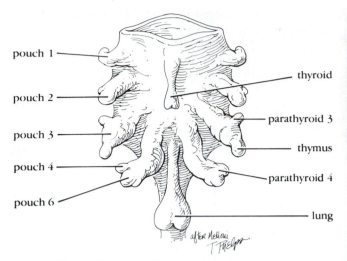

Fig 26–12.—Branchial pouch embryogenesis.

These early ectodermal depressions are termed pharyngeal clefts. Important structures develop in relationship to ectodermal pharyngeal clefts, mesodermal arches, and entodermal pouches.[3] During later development, the pharyngeal pouches become pinched off and discontinuous with the final central pharyngeal derivatives. They may evolve into tubular structures such as the middle ear and eustachian tube from the first and second pouches, solid lymphatic structures such as the palatine tonsil from the second pouch, or glandular structures such as the parathyroid glands from the third and fourth branchial pouches.

There may be a persistent epithelial-lined tract in the developmental course of a pharyngeal pouch, which will become a branchial cyst in the adult. Approximately 95% of such branchial cysts are remnants of the second branchial pouch. They may be a continuous fistula from skin to pharyngeal wall or anything in between, including a small cutaneous fistula, internally isolated cyst, or sinus tract of the pharyngeal wall. At any rate, the lesion will lie somewhere along a path from the anterior border of the SCM, inferior to the hyoid and above the sternum, through the deep cervical fascia just beneath the SCM muscle, along the carotid sheath—between the external carotid artery and the more posterior internal carotid artery—to the pharyngeal wall near the tonsillar region or into the tonsillar fossa itself.

Most of these cysts present as painless fluctuant swellings just below the angle of the mandible along the anterior border of the SCM muscle. They may become infected, with signs of inflammation. They are relatively distinct from adjacent structures, thinwalled, filled with yellowish fluid, and lined by squamous epithelium. If of sufficient size, they are well demonstrated by CT

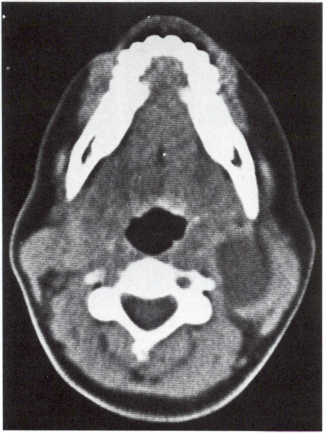

Fig 26–13.—Branchial cyst. Well-defined, thin-walled, cyst-like mass lies directly beneath the left SCM.

(Fig 26–13). They are usually sharply marginated, centrally lucent masses with some enhancement of the adjacent capsule. The primary radiographic differential diagnosis is abscess, but the history usually suggests a more chronic course.

One of the most common congenital tumors of the neck is cystic hygroma. This is a benign, but often large, locally insinuating lesion that usually occurs in the posterior triangle of the neck. Pathologically, cystic hygroma is of lymph vessel origin, which is dominated by large cysts at lesser parts of discrete lymph vessels. It usually originates in the subclavian triangle and extends superiorly, posterior to the SCM. If it occurs higher in the neck, it usually involves the region of the tail of the parotid gland. These tumors appear as irregularly marginated, lucent masses on CT, with internal mesh-like soft-tissue densities (Fig 26–14). The appearance is fairly characteristic, because most other tumors are more radiodense, and cysts and abscesses lack the internal architecture. Other congenital vascular tumors with mass are not common in the neck except in relationship to the inferior face and mouth.

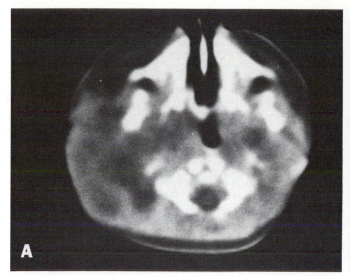

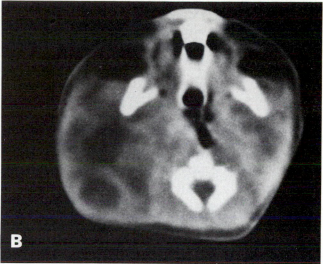

Fig 26–14.—Cystic hygroma. Three-day-old child presented with dyspnea. Multiloculated cystic mass is grossly deforming right cervical anatomy at the levels of the mid **(A)** and lower **(B)** aspects of the mandibular ramus.

Salivary Glands

While many patients with diseases of the major salivary glands can be easily evaluated clinically because of the superficial location of the glands, there remains a significant number of cases where radiologic consultation is required to establish and define the pathologic process. Until recently, imaging of the major salivary glands has primarily involved plain film demonstration of calcification, radionuclide scanning for evidence of "hot or cold" masses, angiography for delineation of rare vascular lesions, and, most importantly, sialography for definition of intraductal lesions and demonstration of masses within the parotid or submandibular gland. Sialography has been shown to be highly accurate in demonstrating intraductal lesions, relatively accurate in demonstrating masses, but poorly predictive of histology, except in certain types of chronic inflammatory lesions such as sialectasis.[4] Sialography, however, may be tedious to perform, associated with some patient discomfort, and difficult to interpret with precision.

Over the past 3 years, we have used CT to evaluate over 100 patients for possible salivary gland lesions.[5] Analyzing those patients who had previous surgical exploration, biopsy, or an obvious clinical diagnosis, the overall sensitivity of CT in detecting salivary gland lesions was over 95%. In addition, the anatomical relation of the lesion to adjacent crucial structures such as the facial nerve was excellent.

While sensitivity was quite good, specificity of the CT scan alone, without clinical information, was only 75% when categorizing lesions as to benign neoplasia,

malignant neoplasia, or diffuse or focal inflammatory disease with or without calculi. When combined with clinical information and laboratory findings, the overall specificity was 90%. The main diagnostic difficulty is differentiating focal sialadenitis, without calculi, from malignant neoplasia. The clinical history of acute swelling, fever, and tenderness aids in the differentiation. Extension of the disease beyond the capsule of the gland indicates neoplasm rather than inflammatory disease. Though not systematically evaluated, intense contrast enhancement seemed to suggest inflammatory disease.

We believe that conventional sialography is seldom, if ever, needed in neoplastic disease and probably not often necessary in inflammatory processes except to show obstructive lesions, though others disagree.[6–8] A conventional sialogram is not as anatomically precise as CT in showing the size and location of tumors, or demonstrating extension beyond the gland. This is based on the limited number of CT-sialogram comparisons in our study and literature sialogram statistics of sensitivity of 85% and specificity of approximately 60%. In nonobstructive inflammatory disease, the sialogram may give more precise anatomical information concerning ductal sialectasis; however, the CT and history can usually differentiate this disease from neoplasia and normal glandular tissue. It is probably unnecessary to demonstrate the sialectasis. In fact, it is preferable to avoid the irritating sialogram. In cases of obstructive inflammatory disease, the sialogram is clearly superior in anatomical detail, and if demonstration of ductal anatomy is clinically necessary, sialography is indicated.

With high-resolution CT scanners, we believe CT-sialography is unnecessary in all but a few cases. Using a scanner that can spatially define the salivary glands and adjacent compartments, as well as resolve their relative density, obviates the necessity of injecting the gland. In addition, the high radiodensity of most sialographic agents creates artifacts that obscure anatomical detail that is normally present.

Based on our experience, CT with a high-resolution CT scanner is the initial radiographic procedure of choice in evaluating salivary gland masses, particularly if neoplasia is the prime consideration. Only in selected tumor cases and patients with inflammatory disease is sialography necessary.

A complete detailed classification of diseases of the salivary glands may be found in Work and Batsakis;[9] however, these detailed classification systems are not particularly practical for the radiologist, because they include many clinical lesions that require no radiographic imaging and many rare lesions without distinctive radiographic findings. An abbreviated and more workable classification is from Work and Hecht[2] and is included in Table 26–1. Even this simplified outline includes numerous conditions that do not require radiographic diagnosis, such as mumps and metabolic atrophy of the salivary glands. A summary of the salivary gland lesions that we have evaluated by CT is contained in Table 26–2 and provides a reasonable statistical approximation of the most common salivary gland lesions that are amenable to CT analysis.

Scans by CT are most often requested and are most useful in patients with tumors of the major salivary glands. Approximately three fourths of salivary gland tumors will occur in the parotid gland and approximately 20% in the submandibular gland. In the parotid gland, approximately three fourths of the tumors will be benign, while this three-to-one benign/malignant ratio is reversed in the submandibular gland. By far and away the most common benign tumor of the parotid gland is the mixed tumor (Fig 26–15), which accounts for approximately 60% of neoplasms of the parotid. Approximately 90% of mixed tumors are benign, with the remainder being malignant, the latter fact being determined more by tumor behavior than histology. No more than 30% of these tumors occur in the submandibular gland. The other common benign tumor of the major salivary glands is the Warthin's tumor (papillary adenocystoma lymphomatosum). This tumor accounts for between 5% and 10% of parotid tumors and rarely occurs elsewhere. These benign tumors are readily demonstrable by CT. They appear as hyperdense (in comparison with the relatively lucent parotid tissue), sharply marginated masses within the gland (Fig 26–16). Essentially all benign neoplasms have this same

TABLE 26–1.—Salivary Gland Diseases*

I. Nonneoplastic disorders
  A. Acute inflammatory disorders
    1. Mumps (epidemic parotitis)
    2. Sialodochitis fibrinosa (Kussmaul's disease)
    3. Acute abscess (acute suppurative sialadenitis)
  B. Chronic inflammatory disorders
    1. Recurrent
      a. Nonobstructive
        (1) Chronic recurrent sialadenitis
        (2) Chronic sialectasis (sialodochitis)
      b. Obstructive
        (1) Sialolithiasis
        (2) Duct stricture
    2. Progressive
      a. Granulomatous
      b. Lymphoepithelial sialadenopathy
  C. Metabolic and endocrine disorders
    1. Benign hypertrophy
    2. Benign atrophy
    3. Gouty parotitis
  D. Congenital disorders
  E. Traumatic disorders
  F. Cystic disorders
II. Neoplastic disorders
  A. Neoplasms of supporting tissue origin
    1. Benign
      a. Lymphangioma
      b. Hemangioma
      c. Lipoma
      d. Neuroma
    2. Malignant (sarcomas)
  B. Neoplasms of epithelial tissue origin
    1. Benign
      a. Mixed tumors
      b. Mucoepidermoid "tumor"
      c. Adenomas
        (1) Papillary cystadenoma lymphomatosis (Warthin's tumor)
        (2) Acidophilic cell adenoma (oncocytoma)
        (3) Serous cell adenoma (acinic cell)
    2. Malignant
      a. Squamous cell carcinoma
      b. Gland cell carcinoma
        (1) Adenoid cystic adenocarcinoma
        (2) Acinic cell adenocarcinoma
        (3) Acidophilic cell adenocarcinoma
      c. Mucoepidermoid "tumor"
      d. Unclassified

*From Work W.P., Hecht D.W.: Congenital malformations and trauma of the salivary glands, in Paparella M.M., Shumrick D.A. (eds.): *Otolaryngology.* Philadelphia, W.B. Saunders Co., 1973, vol. 3, pp. 253–257.

appearance and cannot be differentiated from each other by CT. An exception to this statement is when multiple lesions are seen, in which case the diagnosis is usually Warthin's tumor. These tumors are frequently multiple and bilateral in older males.

In most pathologic series, the most frequent malignant tumor of the salivary glands is the mucoepidermoid carcinoma, followed by various types of adenocarcinoma including adenocystic carcinoma and squamous cell carcinoma. The typical CT image of any malignant salivary gland tumor is a poorly defined area of in-

TABLE 26–2.—SALIVARY GLAND
LESIONS DEMONSTRATED BY CT*

LESION	NO.
Neoplastic	
Benign	
Mixed tumor	8
Warthin	5
Other	2
Subtotal	15
Malignant	
Mixed tumor	2
Adenocarcinoma	4
Squamous carcinoma	2
Mucoepidermoid carcinoma	1
Lymphoma	1
Metastasis	2
Subtotal	12
Inflammatory	
Obstruction with calculus	6
Localized sialadenitis	9
Diffuse sialectasis	2
Sarcoid	1
Inflammatory nodes	2
Subtotal	20
Trauma: hematoma	1

*From Bryan R.N., Miller R.H., Ferreyro R.I., et al.: Computed tomography of the major salivary glands. *A.J.R.* 139:547, 1982.

creased density within the gland, often with obscuration of the fatty-fascial planes about the gland (Fig 26–17). The loss of the glandular margins suggests extension of the disease into adjacent structures. Very small, low-grade malignancies of the salivary glands may,

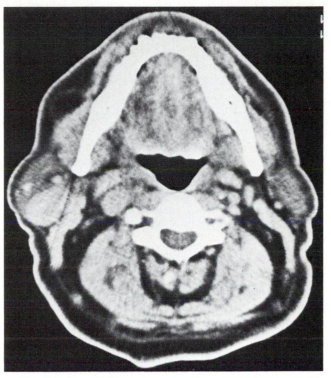

Fig 26–16.—Warthin's tumor. Note hyperdense, multicentric neoplasm of the right parotid gland.

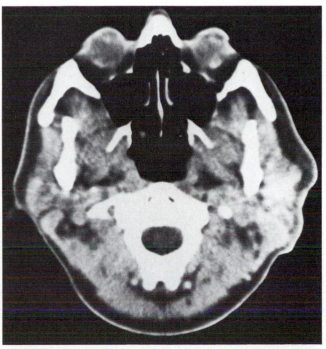

Fig 26–17.—Malignant parotid neoplasm. Note poorly defined, hyperdense parotid mass with violation of the capsule of the gland and invasion of the surrounding tissues.

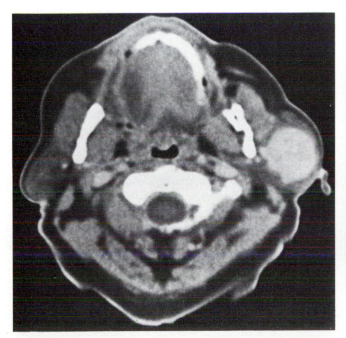

Fig 26–15.—Benign mixed tumor. Note hyperdense, sharply marginated encapsulated lesion of the left parotid gland.

however, have a very similar appearance to benign tumors (Fig 26–18).

Of clinical importance in any parotid tumor is the relationship to the facial nerve and involvement of the deep lobe of the parotid. Deep lobe involvement is better shown by CT than any other method, including clinical examination (Fig 26–19). Involvement of the facial nerve can only be inferred, because the nerve itself cannot be identified by CT.

Any disease process that results in lymph node enlargement may mimic benign salivary neoplasm by CT, because the nodes, either on the surface or within the parotid gland, are usually hyperdense and well marginated. Both inflammatory, as well as neoplastic nodal enlargement, can result in discrete CT masses (Fig 26–20).

In children, the differential diagnosis of neoplasms is different in that they have a far higher percentage of congenital vascular neoplasms such as hemangioma, lymphangioma, and cystic hygroma. These benign lesions account for approximately one third of the total childhood salivary neoplasms. Benign mixed tumor remains the most common tumor after those of developmental origin, with mucoepidermoid carcinoma being the most common malignant neoplasm.

Inflammatory disease of the salivary glands is clinically far more common than neoplasia, but less frequently requires radiographic evaluation. The more common inflammatory conditions may be subdivided into those that are noninfectious and infectious, with the latter being subdivided into acute and chronic conditions. The most common noninfectious condition that the radiologist may be asked to investigate is sialectasis from a benign lymphoepithelial sialadenopathy. This occurs in Sjögren's syndrome, in which the salivary disease occurs in conjunction with keratoconjunctivitis sicca and often a rheumatoid-type arthritis. Pathologically, there is a periductal infiltrate of lymphocytes with subsequent replacement of glandular tissue by lymphoepithelial collections, ductal dilatation, and finally replacement of the gland by lymphoid and fibrous tissue surrounding large dilated cysts. The disease commonly occurs in middle-aged females and is usually bilateral. The CT appearance is that of a diffusely increased radiodense gland with many small lucent cystic collections (Fig 26–21). Sarcoid also frequently involves the parotid gland and has the opposite appearance of chronic sialectasis in that there are many small focal hyperdense collections scattered throughout the relatively normal lucent gland.[8]

Acute infections of the salivary glands, either viral or bacterial in origin, seldom require radiographic diagnosis, which is required only when the inflammatory condition becomes more chronic or clinically confusing. Chronic sialadenitis is usually bacterial in origin and usually is associated with some ductal obstruction. By CT, the involved region is a poorly defined, hyperdense area. It may be confused with malignant neoplasia of the gland; however, it ofttimes enhances after contrast injection much more intensely than neoplasms, and it also assiduously observes the glandular boundaries (Fig 26–22).

Sialolithiasis is both the cause and consequence of chronic recurring sialadenitis and can be a cause of acute disease. The stones, composed of inorganic calcium and sodium phosphate, are far more common in the submandibular gland (90%) than in the parotid gland. Because of its increased sensitivity to calcium, CT can be very accurate in detecting these stones. It also can demonstrate the associated sialadenitis (Fig 26–23). While CT may demonstrate many inflammatory lesions, sialography may still be important, because it demonstrates the fine ductal anatomy and location of strictures and obstructions far more accurately than CT.

Larynx

For practical purposes, radiographic evaluation of the larynx—CT, laryngography, etc.—is primarily for evaluation of carcinoma of the larynx. At least 90% of "tu-

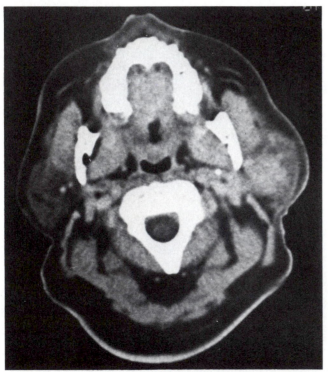

Fig 26–18.—Adenocarcinoma of left parotid gland. Moderately well-defined, slightly hyperdense mass with slightly irregular lateral borders suggests malignancy.

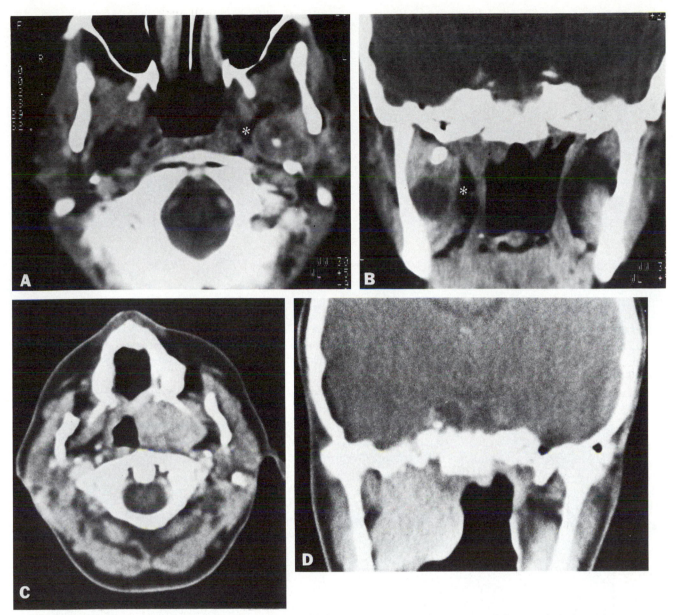

Fig 26–19.—Malignant mixed tumor in deep lobe of left parotid gland. **A, B,** cystic, inhomogeneous, and partially calcified mass lateral to the lateral pharyngeal space *(*)* in a 31-year-old woman. Patient had a 4-month history of left seventh nerve palsy. **C, D,** schwannoma occurring as a left parapharyngeal mass, medial to the fatty lateral pharyngeal space bordering the parotid gland. These lesions and the anatomically distinct lesions of the deep lobe of the parotid **(A)** may present a similar endoscopic appearance.

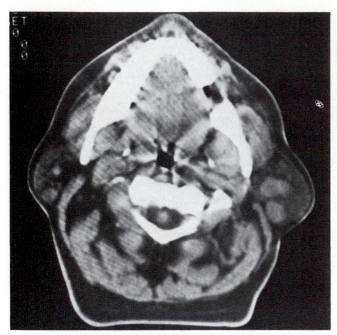

Fig 26–20.—Enlarged parotid lymph nodes. Two hyper-dense, well-demarcated masses within the left parotid gland are shown in a patient with lymphoma.

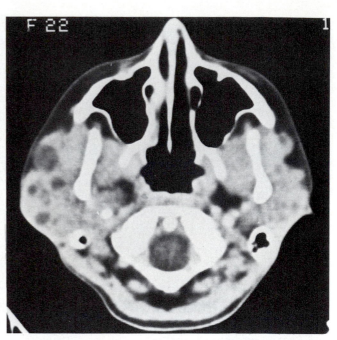

Fig 26–21.—Sjögren's syndrome. Bilateral multicystic degeneration of the parotid glands demonstrates greater involvement on the right.

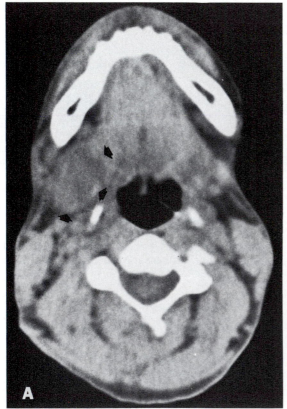

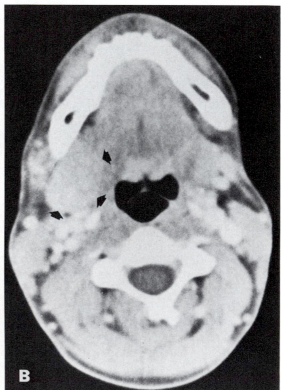

Fig 26–22.—Chronic submandibular sialadenitis. Unenhanced **(A)** and enhanced **(B)** scans show well-defined, enhancing right submandibular mass *(arrows)* in patient with chronic, recurrent sialadenitis, who had left submandibulectomy for same disease.

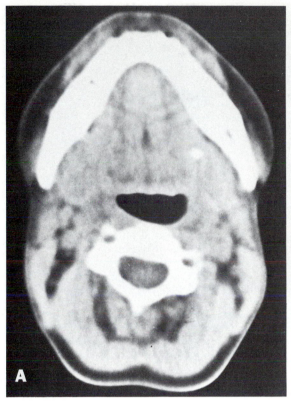
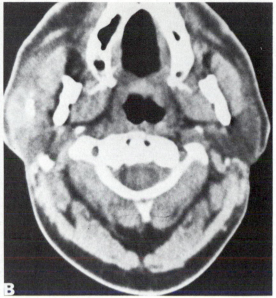

Fig 26–23.—Sialolithiasis. **A,** left submandibular stone. **B,** right parotid stone. Note associated sialadenitis in **B** characterized by swelling and increased radiodensity of the gland.

mors" of the larynx requiring radiographic aid are squamous cell carcinomas. Furthermore, diagnosis of this tumor is clinical, and the radiologist is merely helping to stage the tumor for subsequent treatment. Therefore, it is important to understand the basic concepts of squamous cell carcinoma of the larynx.

First, one must understand the staging of larynx cancer. The lesions are anatomically divided into infraglottic, glottic, supraglottic, and transglottic lesions. The lesions are then subcategorized as to their extent as shown in Table 26–3. The purpose of this classification is to statistically organize them for determination of optimum treatment modality. It should be remembered that there are really two major types of larynx cancer. The first and most common is glottic cancer with or without supra- or infraglottic extension. These tumors are clinically diagnosed relatively early, because involvement of true vocal cords results in early symptoms (such as hoarseness) that precipitate the initial clinical visit. Most of these tumors are relatively small and are stage I or II tumors. On the other hand, supraglottic tumors do not involve critical structures that lead to early presentation. As a result of this, they tend to be much larger tumors, less well restricted, and are stage III and IV. These patients do not present with hoarseness, but rather with symptoms of a mass in the hypopharynx. There is likewise a great difference in the metastatic pattern in that glottic tumors have a rela-

TABLE 26–3.—T CLASSIFICATION: LARYNX*

Supraglottis
TIS   Carcinoma in situ
T1   Tumor confined to region of origin with normal mobility
T2   Tumor involving adjacent supraglottic site(s) or glottis without fixation
T3   Tumor limited to larynx with fixation and/or extension to involve postcricoid area, medial wall of pyriform sinus, or preepiglottic space
T4   Massive tumor extending beyond the larynx to involve oropharynx, soft tissues of neck, or destruction of thyroid cartilage

Glottis
TIS   Carcinoma in situ
T1   Tumor confined to vocal cords(s) with normal mobility (including involvement of anterior or posterior commissures)
T2   Supraglottic and/or subglottic extension of tumor with normal or impaired cord mobility
T3   Tumor confined to the larynx with cord fixation
T4   Massive tumor with thyroid cartilage destruction and/or extension beyond the confines of the larynx

Subglottis
TIS   Carcinoma in situ
T1   Tumor confined to the subglottic region
T2   Tumor extension to vocal cords with normal or impaired cord mobility
T3   Tumor confined to the larynx with cord fixation
T4   Massive tumor with cartilage destruction, extension beyond the confines of the larynx, or both

*Reproduced in part from Paparella M.M., Shumrick D.A.: *Otolaryngology.* Philadelphia, W.B. Saunders Co., 1973, vol. 3, p. 2514.

tively low percentage of nodal metastasis at original diagnosis, while supraglottic tumors have a high percentage of nodal metastasis primarily to the prelaryngeal and jugular nodes.[10]

In general, stage I tumors are treated with radiation therapy, stage II tumors with local surgery with voice preservation, while stage III and IV tumors usually require extensive surgery including laryngectomy and loss of voice function.

The role of radiographic evaluation of carcinoma of the larynx is to precisely define its extent and optimally define those lesions that can be treated with conservative therapy vs. those that require more extensive resection. The mucosal surface of the lesion is of little importance to the radiologist, because the endoscopist can usually visualize this aspect of the tumor. It is the deep extension that is of primary importance. While laryngography has been helpful in the past and is occasionally useful at the present time in evaluation of these tumors, it is primarily a duplication of the endoscopic evaluation, because it primarily images the mucosa. On the other hand, CT much more adequately displays the deeper components of the tumor, including involvement of cartilaginous structures.[11–16]

Performing CT of the larynx is relatively easy, because it simply involves thin sections of the larynx from the hyoid to the bottom of the cricoid bone. We routinely use 5-mm sections with the patient in quiet respiration. It is important that the patient not move during the examination and particularly that he not swallow or otherwise move the larynx. In general, it is best not to tell the patient anything during the procedure. An instruction to the patient to "hold your breath" usually results in a Valsalva maneuver and motion on the scan. Contrast injection is very important in the evaluation of lymph nodes and may be helpful in evaluation of the boundaries of the lesion, though the tumors tend not to enhance in any clinically useful fashion.

Stage I lesions are focal mucosal lesions that diagnostically lie in the realm of the clinical endoscopist. These lesions are too small, shallow, and superficial to be reliably demonstrated by CT. The purpose of CT scans in these patients is to make sure that they are indeed stage I lesions rather than more occult, higher-grade tumors. If at all demonstrated by CT, these tumors are seen as minimal asymmetry of the true and/or false vocal cords, where they usually occur (Fig 26–24). However, one must not overcall minimal laryngeal asymmetries. The verrucous-type carcinoma of the larynx may be stage I, but demonstrable by CT, because it tends to be a more discrete mass protruding off the vocal cord (Fig 26–25).

Stage II tumors, regardless of location, are usually demonstrable by CT, and it is the differentiation be-

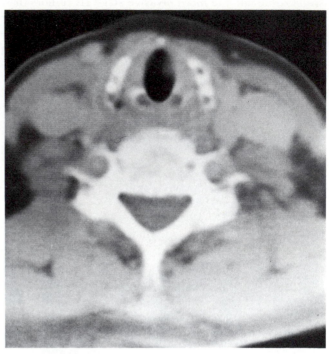

Fig 26–24.—Carcinoma of the left true vocal cord, stage I. Shallow nodular mucosal elevation confined to the true vocal cord.

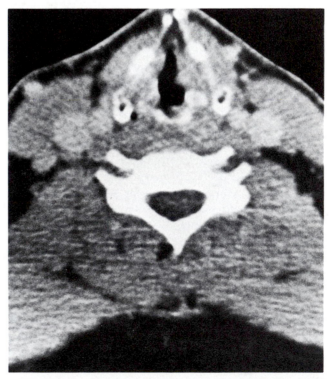

Fig 26–25.—Verrucous carcinoma of the left true vocal cord, stage I.

tween these and the more invasive stage III tumors that is the challenge to the radiologist. When confined to the vocal cord, the lesion is seen as increased bulk in the cord and occasionally has slightly increased density, though this is not consistent (Fig 26–26). One must closely evaluate its anterior extent in relationship to the anterior commissure, which is normally the thinnest soft-tissue density behind the thyroid notch. In looking for deep extension of the tumor and thyroid destruc-

tion, one should carefully note the usually present thin lucent band right along the inner surface of the carti- lage. Obliteration of this line (which is presumably per- ichondrium) raises the possibility of cartilage invasion and therefore a stage III or IV tumor. However, for definitive diagnosis of cartilage destruction to be pres- ent, there must be obvious, frank destruction of the thyroid lamina (Fig 26–27). One cannot rely on asym- metry of calcification within the thyroid cartilage for

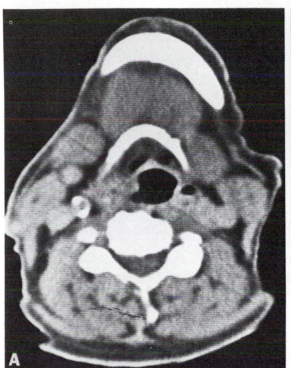

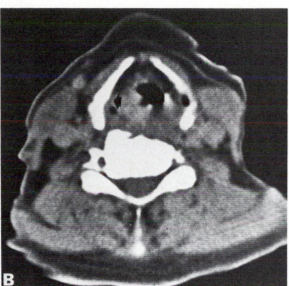

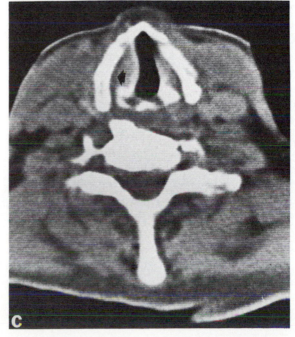

Fig 26–26.—Transglottic stage II carcinoma of the right true and false cords with pyriform sinus invasion. Scans are at the levels of the epiglottis and vallecula **(A)**, supraglottis **(B)**, and true vocal cord **(C)**. Note preservation of the lucent line adjacent to the inner margin of the thyroid cartilage **(B, C,** *arrows*).

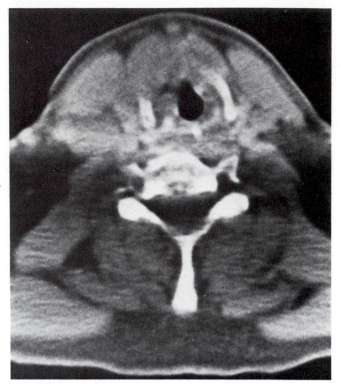

Fig 26–27.—Carcinoma of the larynx, stage IV, with bilateral invasion and destruction of the thyroid lamina.

this diagnosis, because there is significant normal asymmetry from side to side in calcification.[17]

Subglottic extension of these tumors is also critical. While radiologists have often used a "magic number" for subglottic extension, i.e., 10 mm, of far more importance is the relationship of the inferior extension to the cricoid cartilage. For voice conservation surgery, the skeletal base of the larynx—the cricoid—must be preserved. Because the cricoid cartilage lies at a much higher level posteriorly than anteriorly, subglottic extension should be evaluated in terms of cricoid involvement rather than absolute millimeters below the true cord. Scans by CT, performed as we have described them, can accurately delineate subglottic extension to 5 mm or less, and for practical purposes this is adequate. Thinner sections can increase this accuracy. In general, more than 5-mm subglottic extension posteriorly and 10-mm subglottic extension anteriorly may obviate conservation surgery (Fig 26–28).

Supraglottic spread of glottic tumor is reflected by obliteration of the ventricular cavity and invasion of the false cord with loss of its normally lucent interior densities and increased bulk (Fig 26–29). While subtle supraglottic spread of tumor into the ventricle might seem very difficult to evaluate by CT, we have found it to be feasible in most cases.

Contralateral spread of disease is also critical in evaluation of these tumors. As classified in Table 26–3, T1 and T2 true cord lesions can be conservatively treated as long as there is not significant contralateral spread. This means that no more than one fourth to one third of the opposite true cord may be involved with tumor. These anatomicosurgical conditions are a function of the basic types of conservative laryngectomy that can be performed. Either vertical or horizontal partial laryngectomies may be performed. Horizontal or supraglottic laryngectomies involve resection of tumor above the true vocal cords at the plane of the ventricle, while vertical laryngectomies are hemilaryngectomies with resection of one side of the larynx. The vertical hemilaryngectomy can only minimally cross the midline to the side opposite the tumor.

In general, then, T2 tumors are mucosal and submucosal tumors with minimal deep extension that do not cross the important anatomical boundaries that would be the margins of partial laryngectomies.

Tumors classified as T3 are larger tumors that extend deep into underlying muscle with fixation of adjacent tissue and often metastatic nodal spread. They and the larger, more invasive T4 lesions are not particularly common at the glottic level except in patients who have neglected them, whereas they are quite common in the supraglottic region. Conservative therapy, as a rule, cannot be done, but laryngectomy with or without additional radiation therapy may still be curative, though in a lower percentage. The use of CT is very helpful in defining the margins of these larger tumors so that the surgeon can better anticipate the extent of resection.

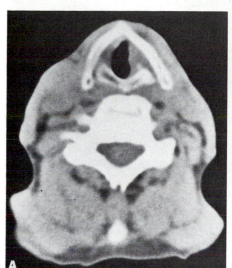
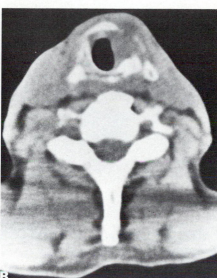
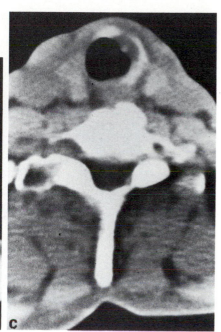

Fig 26–28.—Carcinoma of the left true cord, stage III, with subglottic extension. Scans are at the levels of the true cord **(A)**, lower margin of the cricoid cartilage **(B)**, and upper trachea **(C)**. The neoplasm extends for a distance of ap- proximately 2 cm below the glottis and invades adjacent cartilage. Voice conservation surgery is not possible with this lesion.

This is particularly important in lesions in the supra-glottic region related to the tongue base. The larger tumors also have a high percentage of occult nodes that can often be detected by CT, though radical neck dissection may be performed on clinical grounds.

Supraglottic cancers rostral to the false vocal cords are basically hypopharyngeal cancers and may be subdivided into posterior pharyngeal wall, pyriform sinus, and hypopharyngeal tumors (Fig 26–30).[18, 19] The latter primarily involve the epiglottis and are the most likely to involve the tongue base. Tumors that present on the laryngeal surface of the epiglottis without anterior extension into the radiolucent fatty preepiglottic space have much better prognosis than those with anterior extension and those that extend down to the anterior commissure near the petiole, which is the base of the epiglottis just superior to the thyroid notch.

In our experience, CT of the larynx has replaced laryngography because of its greater ease and convenience as well as its greater diagnostic usefulness. It must, however, be carefully performed with close clinical correlation for optimum results.

Lymph Nodes

An important use of CT in the cervical region is evaluation of the lymph nodes. With high-resolution CT scanning, one may see numerous small (less than 1-cm) densities scattered in the usual regions of nodal occurrence, particularly along the carotid sheath. According to Mancuso and coworkers,[20] if the nodes are less than 1 cm in diameter, they are usually normal or are at least not involved with malignancy. The nodes that are greater than 2 cm in diameter are usually malignant, although focal infectious disease can cause similar enlargement. Such inflammatory nodal enlargement is far more common in children than in adults, and the clinical history usually clarifies the situation. Lymph nodes between 1 and 2 cm in diameter are indeterminate, but in the presence of known malignancy should be considered as suspicious. Several representative cases of normal lymph nodes, as well as nodes involved with metastatic disease, are shown in Figure 26–31. Lymph node disease in the parotid region has already been discussed, and one must remember the close relationship between the submandibular gland and submandibular lymph nodes, which can usually be well differentiated.

Miscellaneous

There are many additional lesions of the cervical region that can be displayed by CT, of which only a few representative cases will be shown. Lipomas are one of the more distinctive lesions demonstrated by CT anywhere in the body because of their negative Hounsfield units. Figure 26–32 is such a case, and there is usually little difficulty in diagnosis. From a clinical viewpoint, these tumors may be more infiltrative or insinuating than is obvious, and the CT can be quite helpful in preoperative evaluation.

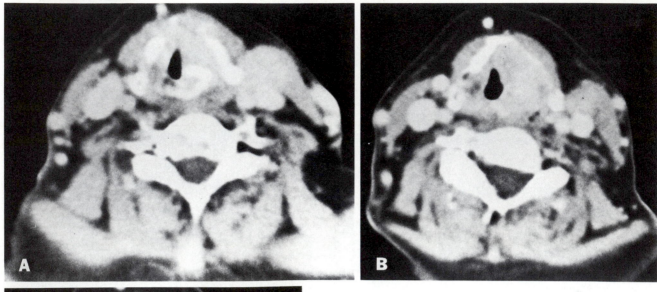

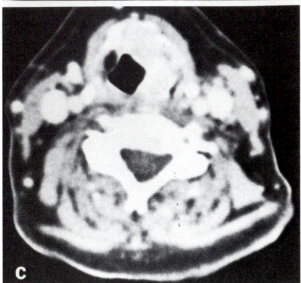

Fig 26–29.—Supraglottic invasive carcinoma of the larynx with cartilage destruction and extension above the plane of the glottis. Scans are at the levels of the arytenoid **(A)**, 1 cm above **B,** and 2 cm above the arytenoid **(C).**

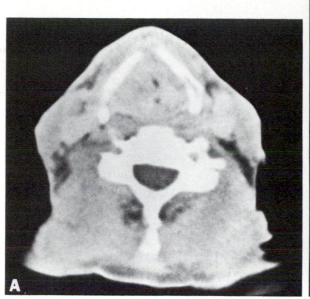

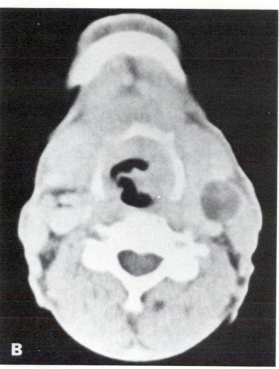

Fix 26–30.—Stage IV carcinoma of the larynx with bilateral involvement and supraglottic extension into the epiglottis. There is almost total obliteration of the glottis **(A)**. Nu-merous nodal metastases are present with a large, centrally lucent necrotic node obvious on the left **(B)**.

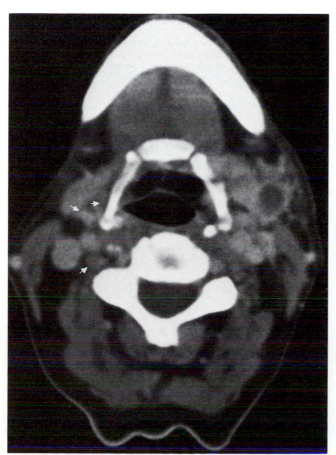

Fig 26–31.—Metastatic lymph nodes. Examples of both solid and necrotic enlarged lymph nodes are present in the left neck, while the contralateral side exhibits examples of normal nodes *(arrows)*.

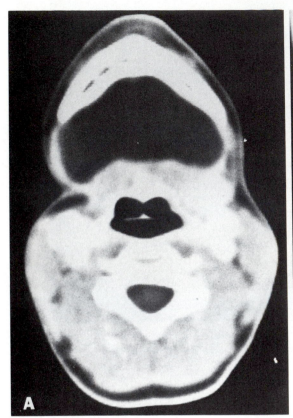

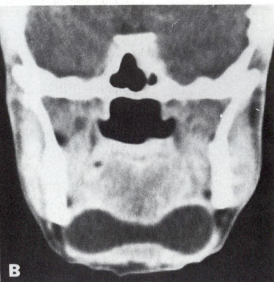

Fig 26–32.—Submental lipoma. Axial **(A)** and direct coronal **(B)** scans demonstrate the large well-circumscribed lesion with a density of fat.

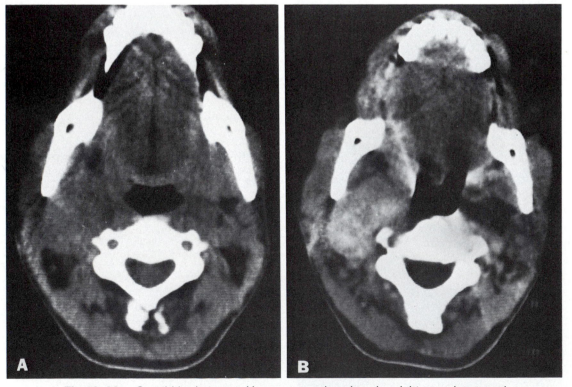

Fig 26–33.—Carotid body tumor. Homogeneously enhancing right parapharyngeal mass obliterating details in the carotid sheath on unenhanced **(A)** and enhanced **(B)** scans.

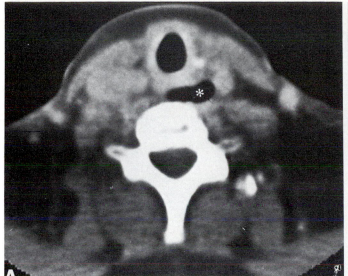
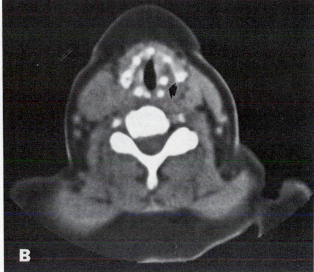

Fig 26–34.—Zenker's diverticulum (**A**,*), an incidental finding in a patient examined for paralysis of the left vocal cord. Note the asymmetry of the glottis with slight adduction of the left true cord and cricoid-arytenoid separation (**B**, *arrow*).

The classic vascular neoplasms of the cervical region include the nonchromaffin paragangliomas such as glomus tumors and carotid body tumors. They appear as relatively well-marginated, intensely enhancing lesions, particularly if drip infusion is used. They occur primarily in the expected areas along the carotid sheath, and their clinical relationships at the skull base are well demonstrable, but ofttimes requiring coronal scans (Fig 26–33).

Hemangiomas also occur in the cervical region, though as previously mentioned, usually occur near the lower face in the oral region. In contrast to the vascular paragangliomas, hemangiomas may not enhance any more than adjacent tissue, because the blood vessels within them are very slow-flow vessels that may not contain any more contrast than normal muscle. Because of this, they may be more difficult to see and their margins more indistinct.

In children, the various soft-tissue sarcomas are infrequent in the neck and usually present as large, rapidly growing, ill-defined tumors obliterating fascial planes and destroying bone in the neighborhood. The CT scan often demonstrates the greater extent of these tumors than is clinically appreciable.

While the upper esophagus lies within the cervical region, it is seldom evaluated by CT, because barium studies usually suffice, and malignancies of the upper esophagus extending into adjacent tissues are not common. Figure 26–34 is a curiosity case—a Zenker's diverticulum incidentally found in a patient with a paralyzed right true vocal cord.

The thyroid gland and parathyroid glands occur in the cervical region, but have been minimally evaluated by CT.[21–23] This may be somewhat surprising in the case of the thyroid gland because of its inherent increased iodine content and subsequent radiodensity. One suspects this is due to the adequacy of other imaging techniques as well as reluctance to use this type of ionizing radiation to evaluate the gland. One can, however, well demonstrate pathology of the thyroid gland, as shown in Figure 26–35. Doppman and coworkers[24] have discussed CT scanning for the parathyroid glands, which may be clinically useful in selected cases.

The thyroid gland develops from epithelial tissue

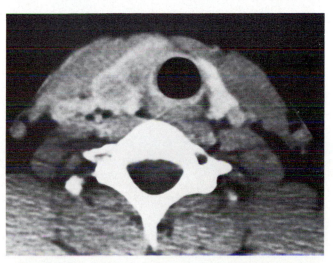

Fig 26–35.—Follicular adenoma, right thyroid lobe. Note the multicystic character of this well-defined lesion.

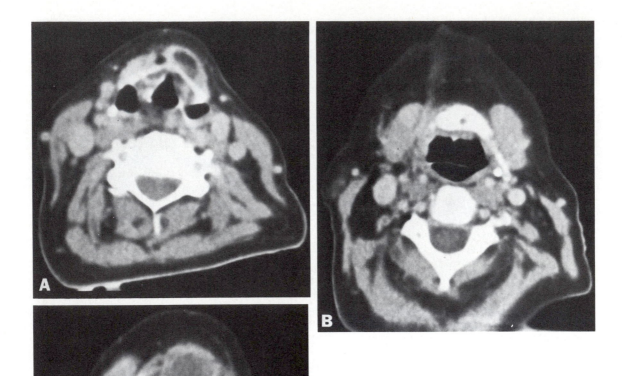

Fig 26–36.—Thyroglossal duct cyst. Note the extension of the lesion from the left lobe of the thyroid **(A)** through the hyoid bone **(B)** to the base of the tongue **(C).** The lesion is superficial to the thyroid cartilage and does not communicate with the larynx.

subsequently related to the site of the foramen cecum near the tongue base. The thyroid tissue descends in relation to the thyroglossal duct through or intimately near the hyoid bone, anterior to the larynx and to the paratracheal region in the lower neck. Ectopic tissue or remnant duct cysts may occur anywhere along this course, but two thirds occur just inferior to the hyoid bone and anterior to the thyrohyoid ligament with or without a fibrous connection to the foramen cecum (Fig 26–36).[25]

REFERENCES

1. Paff G.H.: *Anatomy of Head and Neck.* Philadelphia, W.B. Saunders Co., 1973.

2. Paparella M.M., Shumrick D.A. (eds.): *Otolaryngology.* Philadelphia, W.B. Saunders Co., vol. 3, 1973.

3. Chandler J.R., Mitchell B.: Branchial cleft cysts, sinuses, and fistulas. *Otolaryngol. Clin. North Am.* 14:175–186, 1981.

4. Gates G.A.: Sialography and scanning of the salivary glands. *Otolaryngol. Clin. North Am.* 10:379–390, 1977.

5. Bryan R.N., Miller R.H., Ferreyro R.I., et al.: Computed tomography of the major salivary glands. *A.J.R.* 139:547–554, 1982.

6. Carter B.L., Karmody C.S., Blickman J.R., et al.: Computed tomography and sialography: I. Normal anatomy. *J. Comput. Assist. Tomogr.* 5:42–45, 1981.

7. Rice D.H., Mancuso A.A., Hanafee W.N.: Computerized tomography with simultaneous sialography in evaluating parotid tumors. *Arch. Otolaryngol.* 106:472–473, 1980.

8. Som P.M., Biller H.F.: The combined CT-sialogram. *Radiology* 135:387–390, 1980.

9. Work W.P., Batsakis J.G.: Classification of salivary gland diseases. *Otolaryngol. Clin. North Am.* 10:287–296, 1977.

10. Batsakis J.G.: *Tumors of the Head and Neck,* ed. 2. Baltimore, Williams & Wilkins Co., 1979.

11. Archer C.R., Yeager V.L., Friedman W.H., et al.: Computer tomography of the larynx. *J. Comput. Assist. Tomogr.* 2:404–411, 1978.

12. Archer C.R., Friedman W.H., Yeager V.L., et al.: Evaluation of laryngeal cancer by computed tomography. *J. Comput. Assist. Tomogr.* 2:618–624, 1978.

13. Archer C.R., Sagel S.S., Yeager V.L., et al.: Staging of carcinoma of the larynx: Comparative accuracy of CT and laryngography. *A.J.R.* 136:571–575, 1981.

14. Mancuso A.A., Hanafee W.N., Julliard G.J., et al.: The role of computed tomography in the management of cancer of the larynx. *Radiology* 124:243–244, 1977.

15. Mancuso A.A., Hanafee W.N.: A comparative evaluation of computed tomography and laryngography. *Radiology* 133:131–138, 1979.

16. Scott M., Forsted D.H., Rominger C.J., et al.: Computed tomographic evaluation of laryngeal neoplasms. *Radiology* 140:141–144, 1981.

17. Lloyd G.A., Michaels L., Phelps P.D.: The demonstration of cartilaginous involvement in laryngeal carcinoma by computerized tomography. *Otolaryngol. Head Neck Surg.* 88:726–733, 1980.

18. Gamsu G., Webb W.R., Shallit J.B., et al.: CT in carcinoma of the larynx and pyriform sinus: Value of phonation scans. *A.J.R.* 136:577–584, 1981.

19. Larsson S., Mancuso A.A., Hoover L., et al.: Differentiation of pyriform sinus cancer from supraglottic laryngeal cancer by computed tomography. *Radiology* 141:427–432, 1981.

20. Mancuso A.A., Maceri D., Rice D., et al.: CT of cervical lymph node cancer. *A.J.R.* 136:381–385, 1981.

21. Machida K., Yoshikawa K.: Aberrant thyroid gland demonstrated by computed tomography. *J. Comput. Assist. Tomogr.* 3:689–690, 1979.

22. Wolf B.S., Nakagawa H., Yeh H.C.: Visualization of the thyroid gland with computed tomography. *Radiology* 123:368, 1977.

23. Sekiya T., Tada S., Kawakami K., et al.: Clinical application of computed tomography to thyroid disease. *Comput. Tomogr.* 3:185–193, 1979.

24. Doppman J.L., Brennan M.F., Koehler J.O., et al.: Computed tomography for parathyroid localization. *J. Comput. Assist. Tomogr.* 1:30–36, 1977.

25. Noyek A.M., Friedberg J.: Thyroglossal duct and ectopic thyroid disorders. *Otolaryngol. Clin. North Am.* 14:187–201, 1981.

The Spine

Introduction

RICHARD E. LATCHAW, M.D.

A few words of introduction are appropriate before beginning this section, especially regarding the use of contrast material to diagnose diseases of the spinal column and cord. There is controversy regarding the most efficacious way to diagnose herniated disc, spinal stenosis, and degenerative osteoarthritic changes (spondylosis) that impinge on the spinal cord and/or nerve roots. Some authors advocate the use of the CT scan without intrathecal contrast material, particularly in view of the high-quality scans that are derived from the new high-resolution scanners, while others believe that CT scanning following myelography with a water-soluble contrast agent gives the most complete evaluation. While the diagnosis of a herniated disc or a degenerative spur may be straightforward in the nonoperated young patient, the superimposition of degenerative changes and spinal stenosis makes evaluation more difficult. Certainly, the addition of scarring and distorted anatomy from previous surgery makes evaluation of the plain CT scan even more difficult.

Because of the controversy, we have elected to divide the analysis of herniated disc, spondylosis, and spinal stenosis into three separate chapters. The first chapter deals with an analysis of the plain CT scan, without the use of intrathecal contrast material, for the evaluation of all of these diseases. The second chapter discusses the diagnosis of herniated discs, spinal stenosis, and spondylosis in the nonoperated patient with the CT scan following water-soluble contrast myelography. The third chapter is a discussion of the difficult task of evaluating the patient who has had previous surgery and who possesses all of the superimposed changes that are the result of previous operations.

The succeeding chapters center on specific disease states. The chapter on the CT scan evaluation of trauma to the spine focuses on the use of dynamic scanning to rapidly evaluate a specific area of the spine involved in trauma. A low dose of a water-soluble contrast agent may be an important addition to evaluate abnormality of the spinal cord. Tumors and infections of the spinal column and cord are evaluated either with the plain CT scan or scan with water-soluble myelographic contrast, while cysts of the spinal cord are particularly well analyzed following the instillation of a water-soluble myelographic medium. Finally, the complex anatomy of congenital malformations of the spine is discussed, using CT scanning, plain films, and myelography.

27

CT of the Normal and Abnormal Spine

SAUL TAYLOR, M.D.

WITH THE DEVELOPMENT of high-resolution CT, its use has become routine in the investigation of most spine and spinal cord problems. Several recent texts and articles have been published demonstrating the significant amount of information that can be obtained from this noninvasive study.[1-5]

LUMBAR ANATOMY

Intervertebral Foramen

The intervertebral or neural foramen (Figs 27–1 and 27–2) extends from the pedicle above to the pedicle below. It is helpful to arbitrarily divide the intervertebral foramen into three segments to aid in its description.

1. The upper part of the intervertebral foramen is the largest and contains the exiting nerve root. Its borders are the vertebral body anteriorly, the pedicle above, and the pars interarticularis and lamina posteriorly. The articular facets are not seen at this level.

2. The midportion of the foramen corresponds to the level of the disc space and lies below the exiting nerve. The superior articular facets (SAF) arising from below appear at this level and become larger with progressively lower cuts.

3. The third and most inferior portion of the intervertebral foramen is very small and lies just above the pedicle below, bordered by the SAF behind and the vertebral body in front.

Behind the vertebral bodies at the level of the pedicles is a complete bony ring consisting of vertebral body, pedicles, and laminae.

Intervertebral Disc

The normal disc at L2–3 and L3–4 is concave (Fig 27–3) or flat (Fig 27–2,E), at L4–5 usually flat or minimally convex (Fig 27–4), and at L5-S1, flat or convex. The intervertebral disc is denser than the cerebrospinal fluid (CSF)-containing dural sac posterior to it (see Fig 27–3). It is essential to be able to resolve this small difference in attenuation in order to visualize the interface between the disc and the dural sac (see Fig 27–15). When the disc space is narrow, or when slices are nonparallel to the disc, it may not be possible to image the total disc from front to back in a single slice without including part of the vertebral end plate.

Nerve Roots

To appreciate whether a nerve root (see Figs 27–1 and 27–2) is involved in a pathologic process, it is important to know where it should lie at each level, because in many instances it cannot be visualized directly. The lumbar and sacral nerve roots are best described as either "exiting" or "traversing." The exiting root passes under the pedicle of the corresponding level and through the upper part of the neural foramen above the level of the disc. The traversing roots start within the dural sac. Preparing to exit, they move anterolaterally and may be seen as increased-density focal bulges of the sac at the level of the disc. At L5-S1, they may be well separated from the sac (Figs 27–5 and 27–6). At the level of the lower neural foramen, they lie against the pedicle in the lateral recess. Traversing nerves become exiting nerves when they pass laterally under the pedicle and out the neural foramen. The relationship of the nerves to a herniated disc and to the various types of stenoses will be discussed later. Having exited the foramen, the roots enlarge to form the dorsal root ganglia. There is considerable individual variation in the size of the dural sac. Even though surrounded by low-density CSF, individual roots within the dural sac cannot be seen without intrathecal metrizamide. Above the cauda equina, the conus may occasionally be seen delineated by CSF, but here too intrathecal metrizamide is often necessary. Superior to the conus, the thoracic cord can only occasionally be seen without metrizamide.

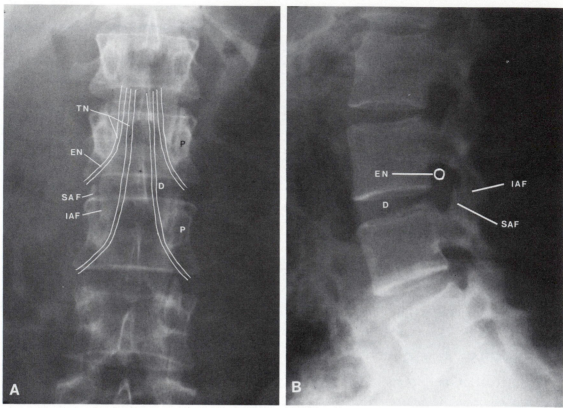

Fig 27–1.—A, normal AP and **B,** lateral plain films. The intervertebral foramen extends from pedicle to pedicle. The exiting nerve *(EN)* is high in the neural foramen, just below the pedicle. The disc *(D)* lies at the level of the midforamen and below the exiting nerve. The lower part of the foramen has a very narrow AP diameter. *(TN* = traversing nerve, *SAF* = superior articular facet, *IAF* = inferior articular facet, *P* = pedicle.)

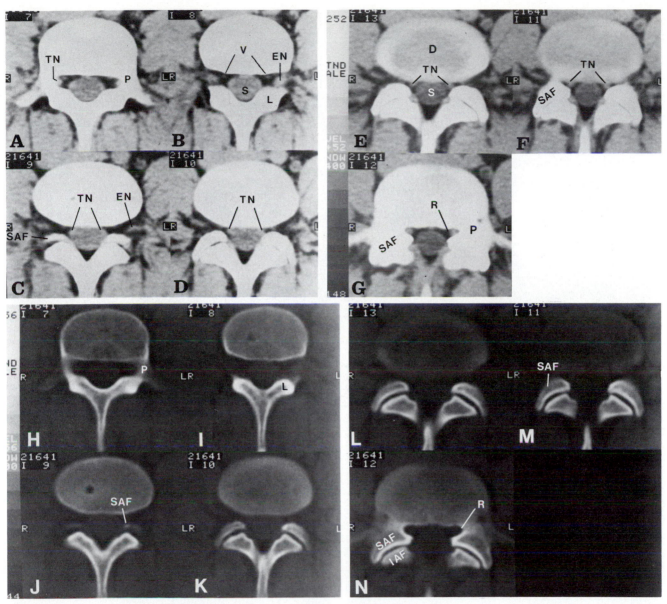

Fig 27–2.—Normal sequence of axial slices from pedicle to pedicle: **A** to **G,** soft-tissue setting; **H** to **N,** bone setting. **A** and **H,** lower aspect of pedicle (*P*) with the traversing nerve *(TN)* about to become an exiting nerve. **B** and **I,** upper neural foramen. The exiting nerve *(EN)* is seen in this large part of the foramen. Note that the articular facets are not yet seen. (*V* = anterior internal vertebral veins in epidural space, *L* = lamina, *S* = dural sac.) **C** and **J,** lower in the foramen. The exiting nerve *(EN)* is more lateral, and the top of the superior articular facet *(SAF)* has appeared. The traversing nerves *(TN)*, which will exit below, have moved to the anterolateral part of the dural sac. They are slightly increased in density, because they are not surrounded by as much CSF as when in the dural sac. **D** and **K,** Larger SAF. The slice is still above the disc. The traversing nerves *(TN)* are a little more separated from the sac. **E** and **L,** disc level. The disc *(D)* is of higher attenuation than the dural sac *(S)*. The traversing nerves *(TN)* have completely separated from the dural sac. They lie in this position when compressed by a classic posterolateral herniated nucleus pulposus. **F** and **M,** the *SAF* starting to merge into the pedicle below. *(TN =* traversing nerve.) **G** and **N,** upper pedicle. This is the level of the lateral recess *(R)* in which the traversing nerve is medial to the pedicle *(P)* and anterior to the superior articular facet *(SAF)*. *(IAF* = inferior articular facet.)

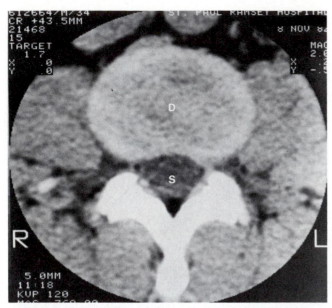

Fig 27–3.—Normal concave disc at L3-4. The disc is denser than the dural sac. (*D* = disc, *S* = dural sac.)

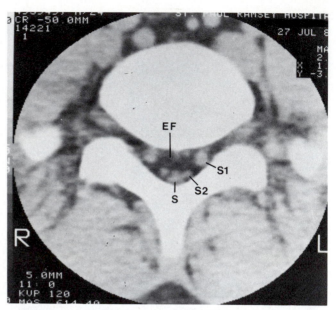

Fig 27–5.—Epidural fat. At L5-S1, the epidural fat *(EF)* is often prominent, and the traversing roots are well seen separated from the dural sac *(S)*. (*S1* = S-1 root, *S2* = S-2 root.)

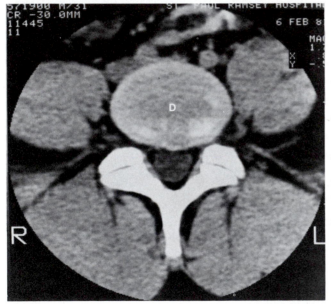

Fig 27–4.—Normal minimally convex disc at L4-5. (*D* = disc.)

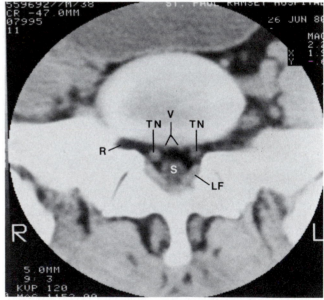

Fig 27–6.—Anterior internal vertebral veins *(V)*. The lateral recess *(R)* may normally be deep transversely. A herniated disc could extend into the extensive epidural fat, compress a traversing nerve, and still be missed with myelography. (*TN* = traversing nerves, *S* = dural sac, *LF* = ligamenta flava.)

Epidural Fat

Epidural fat surrounds and delineates the structures within the spinal canal and neural foramen, but may be obliterated by disc herniation, degenerative changes, or by previous surgery. The paired anterior internal vertebral veins are often seen and should not be confused with the traversing nerve roots (see Figs 27–2,B and 27–6). The intravertebral venous plexus or basivertebral veins communicate with the epidural veins and appear as a defect in the back of the vertebral body in the midline (Fig 27–7). Epidural fat may be prominent particularly at L5-S1 (see Fig 27–5), or it may be scant. If the anterior epidural space contains a prominent epidural venous plexus, it may appear as a homogenous increased density anterior to the dural sac and be confused with a herniated disc (Fig 27–8).[6] A rapid bolus of intravenous contrast often enhances these epidural venous structures.

Ligamenta Flava

The ligamenta flava appear as a thin strip of soft tissue between the articular facets in the posterolateral part of the spinal canal (see Fig 27–6).[7] They may become thickened or bulge into the canal and contribute to spinal stenosis. They may occasionally be calcified.

Articular Facets

The articular facets (see Figs 27–1 and 27–2) begin to appear at the midlevel of the intervertebral foramen. The SAF from the vertebra below lies anterior and lat-

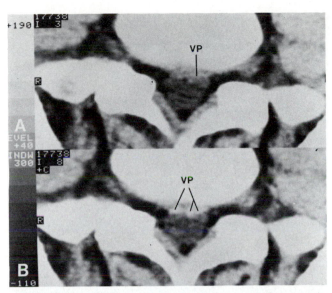

Fig 27–8.—Epidural venous plexus. **A,** without contrast, the high-density structure *(VP)* anterior to the dural sac could be confused with a L5-S1 midline HNP. **B,** after bolus intravenous contrast, marked enhancement confirms a normal venous plexus *(VP)*.

eral to the inferior articular facet (IAF) of the vertebra above. As the slices pass inferiorly through the neural foramen, the IAF becomes smaller, and the SAF enlarges. At the inferior border of the intervertebral foramen, the SAF becomes continuous with the pedicle below (see Fig 27–2,M and N). The SAF forms the posterior border of the lateral recess (see Fig 27–2,N). The joint space and articular cortex are clearly seen with axial CT images, which are excellent in evaluating lumbar facet joint disease as a cause of low back pain and sciatica (Fig 27–9).[8]

TECHNICAL CONSIDERATIONS

Gantry Angulation

There is a difference of opinion as to whether it is necessary to try to scan parallel to the disc space. Because of the lordosis at L5-S1, a nonparallel cut may falsely display what appears to be disc extending posterior to the back of the vertebral body (Fig 27–10). This is caused by "shortening" of the back of the vertebra. Angling the gantry parallel to the disc may provide a better anatomical relationship between the posterior edge of the vertebral body and the disc to determine if the disc is posteriorly displaced.[9] However, more important than the vertebral body-disc relationship is the relationship of the disc to dural sac, epidural fat, and traversing nerves (Fig 27–11), and this changes little with angulation. Thus, it is probably not necessary to angle the gantry parallel to the disc. Because many patients have a lordosis of 30° to 40°, it is

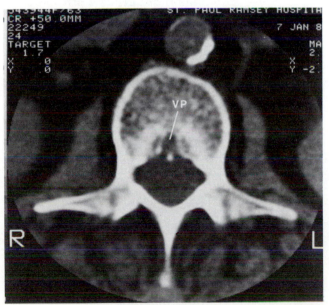

Fig 27–7.—Defect at the back of the vertebral body for the intravertebral venous plexus *(VP)*. At this level of the complete bony ring, there may be little epidural fat to aid in defining tissue planes; therefore, optimal soft-tissue resolution is very important.

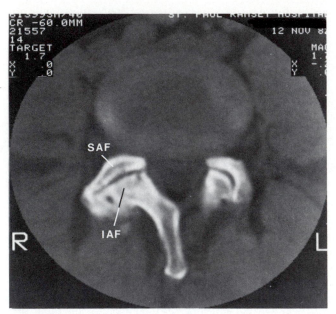

Fig 27–9.—Hypertrophic degenerative changes of the right facet joint. (*SAF* = superior articular facet, *IAF* = inferior articular facet.)

doubtful that the 15° that gantries are capable of really makes any difference, and for those patients with only mild lordosis at L5-S1, angulation is probably not important. If reformatting is anticipated, all slices should be taken at 0° (no angulation), because reformatting with gantry angulation requires additional manipulation of data and results in further degradation of the image.

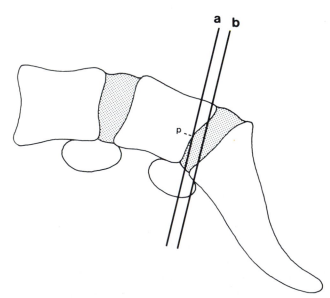

Fig 27–10.—Slice nonparallel to the disc space. When the scanning plane is nonparallel to the disc, there may be a false impression of the disc extending posterior to the vertebral body. In slice *a*, the posterior edge of the vertebral body appears to stop at point *p*. Slice *b* includes the posterior edge of S-1.

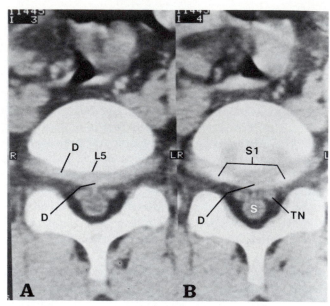

Fig 27–11.—Analysis of nonparallel slices through a normal L5-S1 disc. **A,** passing through the posterior part of the disc. **B,** a few millimeters lower to include the posterior edge of S-1: In **A,** note the "flattening" of the back of L-5 *(L5)*, and the symmetric shape of the disc *(D)* ending at the posterolateral edges of *L5* and, most importantly, the normal relationship between the disc and the spinal canal contents with no encroachment on the dural sac or roots. In **B** part of the posterior edge of *S1* shows the true relationship of the disc to the vertebral body. (*TN* = traversing nerve, *S* = dural sac, *D* = disc.)

Elimination of Lordosis

Elimination of lordosis can aid in achieving a slice roughly parallel to the disc space. However, this requires an actual rotation of the pelvis accomplished by a conscious contraction of the abdominal muscles. In fact, only the rare patient will be able to cooperate in this way. Two methods have been recommended to minimize the lordosis at L5-S1. The first, flexion of the hips, is probably effective only when the flexion approaches 90°, but at this point the knees will strike the gantry. A wedge under the pelvis tends only to elevate the pelvis rather than actually rotate it. The reader can make his own decision as to the effectiveness of these methods. Whatever techniques are used, the patient must be made comfortable so that there will be no movement. Tying the knees together and supporting the thighs allows muscle relaxation, which is particularly important in lengthy examinations.

Reformatting

Reformatting refers to the generation of sagittal, coronal, or oblique images from the data obtained in a series of transverse slices (Fig 27–12).[10] Because both spatial and soft-tissue resolution are degraded from the

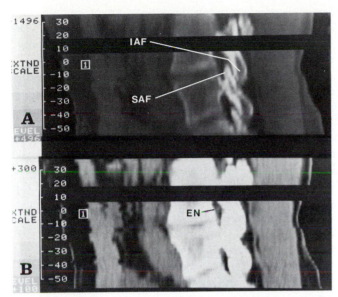

Fig 27–12.—Normal reformatted image through the neural foramen: **A,** bone. **B,** soft-tissue setting. (*EN* = exiting nerve surrounded by fat in the neural foramen, *IAF* = inferior articular facet, *SAF* = superior articular facet.)

original direct image in the reformatting process, it is necessary to collect extra data either by overlapping slices or, for better spatial resolution of bone, by using thinner collimation (e.g., 1.5 mm), both of which in turn require a greater number of slices. On the other hand, display in other planes may provide an additional spatial orientation that can be helpful in situations such as the evaluation of the neural foramina in the sagittal plane in spinal stenosis. Movement of the patient during any part of the series of axial cuts will result in misregistration artifact or the inclusion of a slice with artifact in the sequence. Both of these will further degrade the reformatted image.

Positioning Within the Gantry

Careful positioning within the gantry avoids reconstruction artifacts. The body should be positioned so that it does not extend beyond the field of view (FOV). This can be achieved by scanning with a wide FOV (large-body calibration) and using a "target" mode of reconstruction. Scanning with a small-diameter FOV gives a magnified image based on a larger number of pixels in the area of interest, but positioning is more critical, because it is easier for a body part to extend beyond the FOV. The spine is a posterior structure and should be positioned off-center or low in the FOV.

Digital Localizers and Plain Films

A digital radiograph used as a localizer is invaluable in identifying the level of the slices. However, if the patient moves or if the table is moved up or down in an angled gantry, the position of the localizer will not correspond exactly to the actual level scanned. Therefore, when viewing the slices, attention should be paid to the actual anatomy scanned within each level rather than to the initial localizer. If plain films are not available, an AP as well as the lateral localizer are helpful. Plain films are especially useful in older patients to help predict the presence of degenerative changes and stenoses. Congenital anomalies and spondylolisthesis should first be assessed on plain films. In older patients with osteoporosis or in obese patients, the localizer may not clearly demonstrate the bony anatomy, and the plain films together with the localizer are useful in determining the levels. The importance of a good clinical history cannot be overemphasized, and if previous surgery has been performed, the side and level must be known.

SCANNING PROTOCOLS

There is probably no other area in CT scanning in which there is such a wide variety of opinion as to what constitutes the best scanning protocol as in the examination of the lumbar spine. The most fundamental requirement is the ability to optimize soft-tissue contrast in order to differentiate the various soft-tissue structures within the spinal canal and intervertebral foramen. A 5-mm collimation satisfies this requirement very well. High spatial resolution may be necessary at times to visualize smaller structures such as the upper neural foramen to avoid partial volume phenomenon (PVP). In these cases, thin slices of 1.5 or 2 mm can be used, but the increased noise level from decreased photon flux may prevent adequate discrimination of soft tissues, even with very high mAs settings.

Here is a brief description of some protocols that are commonly in use (Figs 27–13 and 27–14):

1. Five-millimeter slices at 5-mm increments (no overlap) from L2-3 to S-1, without angulation: Sequential scans pass through all parts of the spinal canal from L2-3 to S-1, which provides an uninterrupted continuous display of all anatomical structures. This can aid interpretation. This approach is useful in patients with degenerative changes and stenoses at several levels and in whom a classic history of disc herniation is not present. The use of zero angulation allows for subsequent reformatting, although the reformatted detail will not be optimal, because there is no overlapping. Because all the anatomy is included, this type of scan may be performed without physician monitoring; however, this decision precludes the ability to repeat or add an intervening slice to confirm a subtle or ambiguous finding. One variation is to routinely add extra slices through the disc. Such an extensive study may not be indicated

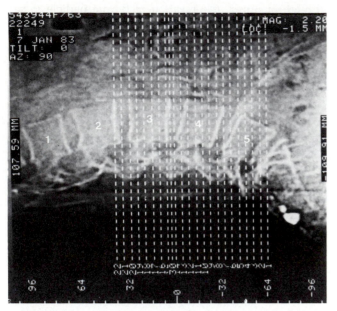

Fig 27–13.—Lateral localizer with contiguous slices from L2-3 to S-1. (*1–5* = lumbar vertebrae.)

in every case. For example, in a young patient with a history of obvious acute disc herniation, fewer slices emphasizing the most likely area for pathology (pedicle to pedicle) may be faster, more effective, and give less radiation.

2. Five-millimeter slices at 3-mm increments from L2-3 to S-1 without angulation: This is similar to the

first, but overlapping of slices provides more data both for reformatting and for evaluating soft tissues and bone in the transverse slices. Even more cuts are necessary, and this protocol should not be routine in every case.

3. Five-millimeter slices at 3- or 4-mm increments with or without gantry angulation, restricted to the interpedicular region: This study is more specific for evaluating the disc space and is useful in most cases, especially for younger patients without diffuse degenerative changes and stenoses. The study should extend above and below the actual disc to include the upper part of the intervertebral foramen and the upper border of the pedicle below so that stenoses and/or an unusual herniated disc presenting only above or below the actual disc level can be evaluated (Figs 27–15 and 27–16). It is important to note that the structures lying behind the vertebral bodies at the bony ring level are not visualized. Because of the short segmental nature of the scan, reformatting is not practical.

4. One-and-one-half millimeter slices at 1.5-mm increments confined to the disc space: This technique is used by some for very narrow disc spaces. Because of the narrow collimation, the decreased photon flux gives poor soft-tissue resolution, especially in obese patients, and the disc may not be reliably distinguished from the dural sac. Much more is lost in soft-tissue resolution than is gained in spatial resolution. Overlapping 5-mm slices provide better quality images even with narrowed discs. Compensation with higher mAs settings results in excessive radiation and tube wear. Furthermore, to

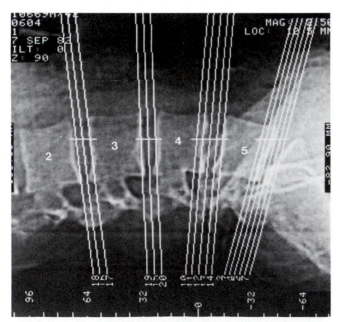

Fig 27–14.—Lateral localizer to scan the disc levels. Note that the scans include the upper neural foramen as well as the disc. L2-3 and L3-4 were scanned with fewer slices, because a large disc was found at L5-S1. (*2–5* = lumbar vertebrae.)

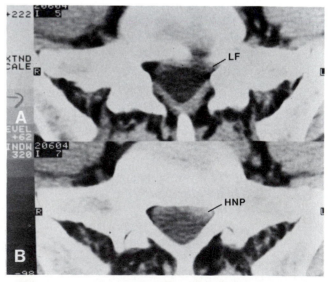

Fig 27–15.—Importance of scanning beyond the disc space. **A,** at the L5-S1 disc level, there is subtle loss of epidural fat on the left (*LF*). **B,** 5 mm lower at the S-1 pedicle, the inferiorly migrated disc is seen (*HNP*). Note the importance of maintaining soft-tissue resolution, particularly at the level of the bony ring where epidural fat is normally scant.

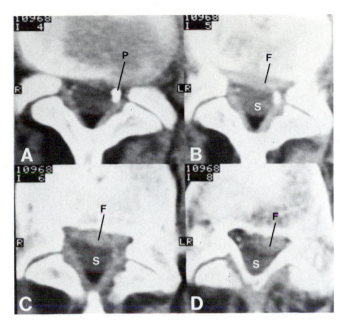

Fig 27–16.—Large migrated HNP. **A,** at the level of the disc, a drop of Pantopaque *(P)* confirms little or no posterior extension of the disc. **B,** a large fragment *(F)* is seen extending far inferiorly, gaining in size on contiguous, caudally positioned scans **(C, D).** It is unusual not to have some protrusion at the disc level when an HNP is present. This emphasizes the importance of scanning beyond the level of the disc. (*S* = dural sac.)

cover the pedicle-to-pedicle distance at several different levels, an excessive number of cuts are required.

Many variations of these protocols are possible, each with its advantages and disadvantages. It is not effective to examine every patient identically. Ideally, slice thickness and overlap, angulation, mAs, and region of emphasis should be adapted to each particular case. Checking the scan before the patient is removed from the table will greatly improve the quality of the scan. Only one or two additional or repeat slices often make a significant difference in clarifying or confirming a subtle or ambiguous finding.

I have found the following two approaches reliably accurate and sufficiently flexible. The first is for those patients who usually, but not always, are younger, with well-preserved disc spaces without degenerative changes on the plain films. They have good preservation of epidural fat and usually have more focal pathology.

The lower four intervertebral foramen levels are scanned starting with L5-S1 and then moving to the levels above. If the history or a previous myelogram strongly indicates pathology elsewhere, that level will be scanned first, hopefully to minimize the number of slices required at the other levels. Five-millimeter slices, usually with angulation, are used every 3 mm at

L5-S1, or 4 mm at L4-5, scanning from pedicle to pedicle at each level. Because pathology is very uncommon at L3-4 and L2-3 in these patients, these levels are scanned at 5-mm increments, especially if pathology has been found at a lower level. If the plain films suggest spondylolisthesis or other unusual bony abnormality, then, in anticipation of reformatting, no gantry angulation is used, and the slices are overlapped every 3 mm for better detail. The scan is checked, and any equivocal slices resulting from artifact or possible pathology are clarified by repeat or adjacent slices before the patient is taken off the table. The upper intervertebral foramen and lateral recess, as well as the disc, should be clearly visualized.

Patients with moderate or marked degenerative changes with possible multilevel stenoses are scanned from L2-3 to S-1. Five-millimeter collimation is used with 5-mm incrementation. The scan is checked, and additional cuts are performed if necessary, because at increments of 5 mm, subtle anatomy or pathology may be missed, especially in evaluating for bony stenosis. The check will also permit repeating a slice with motion artifact, which is not uncommon in older patients with degenerative changes.

CT DIAGNOSIS OF LUMBAR DISC DISEASE

High-resolution CT has rapidly become an important tool in the diagnosis of a herniated nucleus pulposus (HNP).[11-14] If carefully performed and interpreted, CT is usually superior to myelography, especially if previous surgery has not been performed. Scans by CT allow direct visualization of soft-tissue structures within the spinal canal and intervertebral foramina, whereas myelography fills only the dural sac and proximal root sleeves, leaving an important area lateral to the spinal canal nonvisualized. A prominent L5-S1 epidural space (see Fig 27–6), another blind area in myelography, is more readily evaluated with CT, particularly with the use of intravenous contrast enhancing the epidural venous plexus (see Fig 27–8).

With few exceptions, CT is the first and only study required prior to surgery. In very obese patients, the soft-tissue resolution may be inadequate to visualize a herniated disc, and myelography may be necessary (Fig 27–17). Central stenosis (see Fig 27–30) or previous surgery with loss of the epidural fat and fibrotic changes may obliterate the soft-tissue planes and preclude visualization of an HNP. At the level of the bony ring behind the vertebral body, there is less epidural fat, and the normal tissue planes may not be well seen with CT (see Figs 27–7 and 27–15). In such cases, myelography or CT with metrizamide may be necessary to image the dural sac (see Fig 27–17).

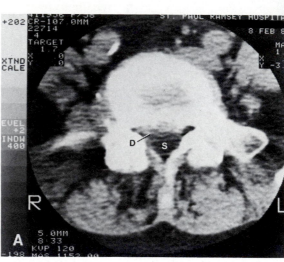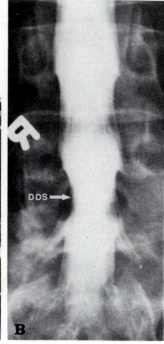

Fig 27–17.—HNP poorly seen on CT because of a noisy scan of an obese patient. **A,** CT. **B,** myelogram. **A,** the increased density disc *(D)* anterior to the dural sac *(S)* was not clearly defined. **B,** myelography was necessary to confirm an HNP. *(DDS* = deformed dural sac.)

Caution must be exercised in the use of CT. Rarely, a tumor or other lesion of the conus medullaris may clinically mimic an HNP at a lower level, and for this reason the classic myelogram is normally performed at least up to the level of the conus. Therefore, CT will fail if the study does not extend sufficiently high. A soft-tissue mass above the cauda equina may also be missed on CT without metrizamide, because the spinal canal contents tend to be homogeneous in density. This results from the lack of epidural fat around the dural sac and from the absence of the low-attenuating CSF within the sac. Thus, careful clinical correlation is mandatory to localize the area involved. In scanning for a herniated disc, an extruded disc fragment will occasionally lie above or below the disc space and may be missed if the scan does not extend beyond the actual disc level (see Figs 27–15 and 27–16).[15] It is rare, however, to have a migrated fragment without some hint of abnormality at the level of the disc. For this reason and also to evaluate for stenoses, the scan should extend from pedicle to pedicle if individual disc levels are scanned.

CT Signs of Lumbar Disc Herniation

It may be difficult to distinguish between a mild disc herniation and a bulging disc (Fig 27–18).[16, 17] The latter is an extension of the disc and annulus fibrosus beyond the edge of the vertebral body, but pathologically the annulus fibrosus is still intact. This occurs in older patients as degenerative changes develop in the disc. Usually, a bulging disc is seen as a diffuse, circumfer-ential extension of the disc beyond the vertebral body, but may occasionally be focal and indistinguishable from a small HNP. A bulging disc is probably not clinically significant *per se,* but as will be seen later, can contribute to central stenosis or lateral recess stenosis.

An HNP most commonly occurs posterolaterally (Fig 27–19). The traversing nerve is usually compressed, causing signs and symptoms at the level below. Less commonly, a large midline HNP may compress tra-

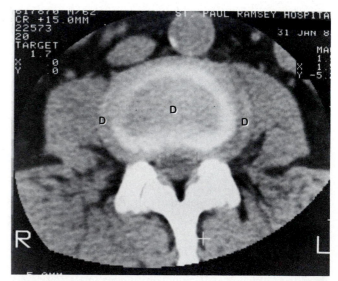

Fig 27–18.—Bulging disc. The diffuse appearance is characteristic of degenerative bulging. There is no encroachment on the dural sac and probably no compression of the traversing roots. *(D* = disc.)

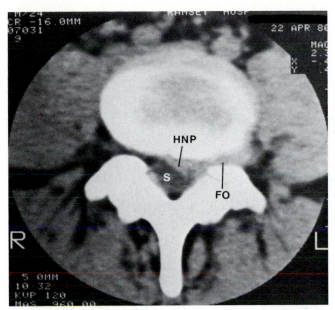

Fig 27–19.—Typical posterolateral *HNP* obliterating the epidural fat, deforming the dural sac, and extending laterally into the inferior aspect of the intervertebral foramen. This would compress the traversing root. The exiting root higher in the foramen, not shown, is free. (*S* = dural sac, *FO* = lower intervertebral foramen.)

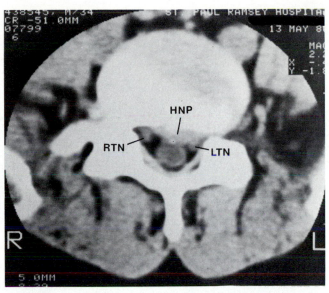

Fig 27–21.—Posterolateral *HNP* displacing the left traversing root posteriorly. Note focal loss of epidural fat. (*RTN* = right traversing nerve, *LTN* = left traversing nerve.)

versing nerves more medially to produce findings at any of several levels below (Fig 27–20). The most common CT finding is the direct visualization of the relatively increased density disc extending posterolaterally or, less commonly, directly posterior in the midline

with encroachment on the neural elements (see Figs 27–15, 27–16, 27–19 to 27–22). There may be a straight edge medially, which is the posterior longitudinal ligament (see Fig 27–19). The lower-attenuating dural sac may be indented or deformed (see Fig 27–19). The traversing nerve may be displaced posteriorly, and comparison with the position of the nerve on the opposite side is helpful (see Fig 27–21). This finding is best seen at the L5-S1 level, where the roots are farther separated from the dural sac than at the other levels.

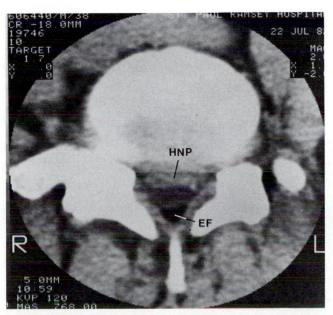

Fig 27–20.—Midline HNP at L5-S1, which resembles the venous plexus. Note that even in the presence of a large *HNP* the posterior epidural fat (*EF*) may still be present.

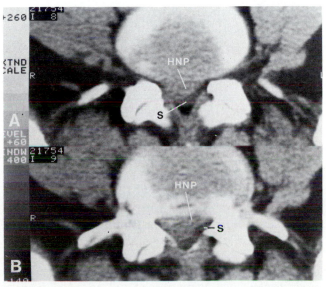

Fig 27–22.—**A,** huge *HNP* almost completely obliterating the dural sac. **B,** 5 mm lower. When a disc is this large, it may be missed, particularly if the contrast resolution between the dural sac (*S*) and the HNP is poor.

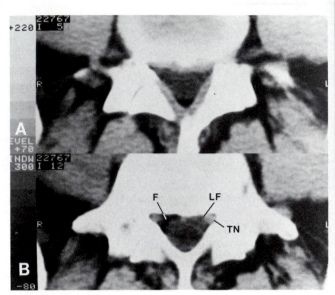

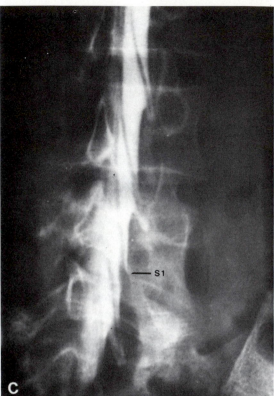

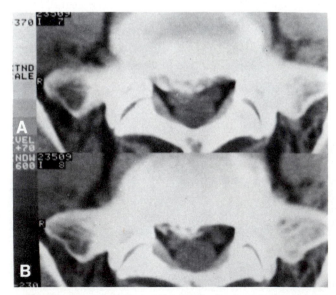

Fig 27–23.—Asymmetric epidural fat because of HNP at L5-S1. **A,** at the level of disc. **B,** 6 mm below **A. C,** myelogram. **A,** this was the best image of the disc that could be obtained because of a narrowed disc space. There is scant epidural fat bilaterally. **B,** epidural fat is normal on the right *(F)* and absent on the left *(LF)* around the traversing S-1 root *(TN).* Even though this represents a positive finding, myelography was requested for confirmation. Previous surgery, which had not been performed, causes a similar loss of fat. **C,** note very subtle flattening of the S-1 root *(S1).*

Asymmetry or obliteration of the epidural fat in the spinal canal or in the intervertebral foramen is an important sign of HNP (see Figs 27–19 and 27–21; Fig 27–23). Because the fat provides excellent contrast, a noisy scan in an obese patient may be successful even though the soft-tissue densities of the disc and dural sac cannot be differentiated. On the contrary, diagnosis may be very difficult in older patients with degenerative changes and stenosis where the epidural fat is lacking or where the fat is destroyed from previous surgery (see Figs 27–30 and 27–36). A herniated disc may be calcified in part or may be associated with an avulsed fragment of bone, producing an irregular posterior edge of the vertebral body (Figs 27–24 and 27–25).

Occasionally, a disc herniated far laterally will compress the exiting nerve of the same level either by extending superiorly in the neural foramen (Fig 27–26) or, rarely, by herniating laterally beyond the foramen to compress the exiting nerve when it has passed inferiorly to the level of the disc (Fig 27–27).[18, 19] The far lateral herniations are not seen with myelography. The HNP may be very small and seen on only one slice;

Fig 27–24.—Calcified right HNP. **A,** 5 mm below disc level. **B,** 3 mm below **A.**

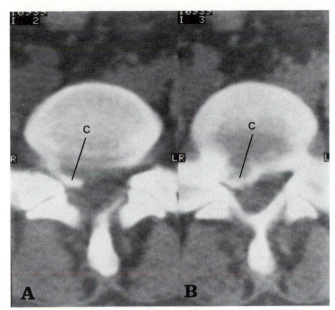

Fig 27–25.—Calcified HNP associated with avulsion of part of the back of the vertebral body. **A,** disc level. **B,** a few millimeters below **A.** (*C* = calcified HNP and fragment of vertebral body.)

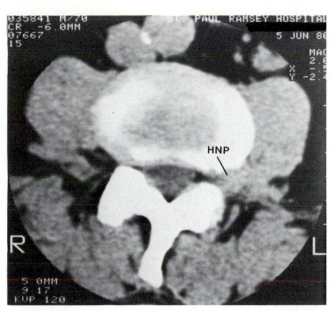

Fig 27–27.—*HNP* lateral to the intervertebral foramen. This is an uncommon presentation. The myelogram was completely normal, as would be expected with an HNP this far lateral.

there may be a subtle flattening or posterior displacement of the exiting root.

Several problems in interpretation may arise. In the image created by a nonparallel slice, a normal disc may appear to be herniated, but the epidural fat, traversing

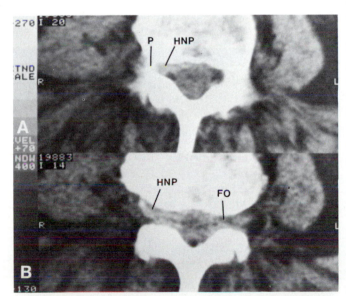

Fig 27–26.—Uncommon *HNP* migrated superiorly into the right intervertebral foramen. **A,** high-density superiorly migrated disc fragment at the level of the pedicle above. **B,** upper intervertebral foramen filled with HNP compressing the exiting nerve. Most HNP that extend laterally into the neural foramen lie below the exiting nerve. (*P* = pedicle above *HNP, FO* = normal intervertebral foramen.)

nerves, and dural sac are normal. The "disc" will have a symmetric appearance ending at the lateral edges of the vertebral body, and the back of the vertebral body may be flattened—evidence that its true posterior edge is not included in the cut. In some cases, a 1.5-mm slice a few millimeters higher or lower will show the true posterior body-disc relationship (see Fig 27–11).

The epidural venous plexus behind the vertebral body may be of the same relatively high density as the disc and be confused with a midline HNP. Absence of compression of the neural elements excludes an HNP. Intravenous contrast given as a rapid bolus and followed by immediate scanning is often helpful, because an HNP does not enhance (see Fig 27–8). Enhancement of the plexus may be homogeneous, or individual veins may be seen, either of which can be distinguished from a herniated disc. If the enhanced plexus or veins are not displaced posteriorly, it is unlikely that an HNP is present. A filling defect in the enhanced plexus produced by the herniated disc is a helpful finding (Fig 27–28).

An enlarged, swollen nerve may occur with an HNP, but as is known from myelography and CT, the root or sleeve may normally vary in size at the same level. In the presence of other findings, this may be a helpful sign.

If the HNP is very large, it may obliterate so much of the spinal canal that the interface between the disc and the dural sac may not be recognized, causing the disc in the canal to be missed (see Fig 27–22). A dis-

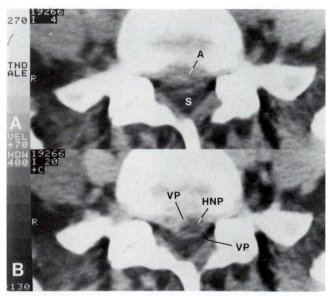

Fig 27–28.—Epidural venous plexus plus HNP. **A,** the high-density structure *(A)* anterior to the dural sac *(S)* could be a venous plexus or HNP. **B,** bolus contrast shows enhancing epidural venous plexus *(VP)* displaced posteriorly and indented by an *HNP,* which remains relatively low density. Note deformity of the anterior dural sac.

turbing streak artifact passing transversely across the spinal canal between the articular facets may simulate an HNP with a false disc-dural sac interface (Fig 27–29). Its very straight edge and sharp contrast usually favor an artifact. Repeat cuts, possibly with 1.5-mm collimation, usually will eliminate it, but in rare instances

intrathecal metrizamide may be necessary to demonstrate the true anterior margin of the dural sac.

Conjoined nerve roots represent an uncommon variation in which two roots exit from the dural sac within a single root sleeve and may mimic an HNP on CT. However, in addition to being asymptomatic, the conjoined roots tend to be less dense than an HNP.[20]

SPINAL STENOSIS

Spinal stenosis refers to encroachment on the neural elements caused by narrowing of the spinal canal or of the intervertebral foramen. This narrowing can be bony, soft tissue, or a combination of both. The use of CT is well suited for the evaluation of spinal stenosis.[21–23] Previously, lower back pain caused by spinal stenosis often went undiagnosed because of the limitations of myelography. Three main types of spinal stenosis will be discussed. Further discussion of spinal stenosis may be found in the excellent work of Macnab.[24]

Central Stenosis

Central stenosis refers to narrowing of the central canal (Fig 27–30). There may be a preexisting bony narrowing caused by thick, medially convex laminae, which may present no problem throughout life until superimposed prominent soft tissues develop associated with degenerative changes. Degenerative osteophytes at the back of the vertebral body cause further encroachment. The bony narrowing may be severe as a result of congenitally short pedicles, such as in achon-

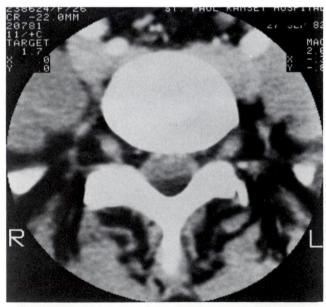

Fig 27–29.—Streak artifact causing increased attenuation in the anterior part of the canal. This could be confused with an HNP or epidural venous plexus.

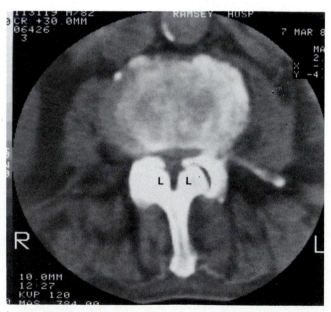

Fig 27–30.—Central spinal stenosis. The prominent medially convex laminae *(L)* are close together. The epidural fat and dural sac cannot be distinguished because of tightness in the central canal.

droplastic dwarfs, who are very sensitive to the slightest additional soft-tissue component.[25] The soft-tissue component consists of prominent ligamenta flava posterolaterally and a bulging or herniated disc anteriorly. Thus, the narrowing is usually greatest at the disc level, which accounts for the "hourglass" appearance seen on myelography. Scans by CT demonstrate both the small bony canal and the prominent soft tissues. There is usually obliteration of the epidural fat, but not always. In severe examples, the dural sac may be so compressed that CT cannot distinguish the dural sac from the surrounding tissues, and without intrathecal contrast it may be impossible to know how complete is the block. In the individual case, unless the stenosis is severe, it still may be difficult to know if it is clinically significant.

Lateral (Foraminal) Stenosis

Lateral or foraminal stenosis involves the exiting nerve as it passes under the pedicle in the upper part of the intervertebral foramen. Degenerative disc dis-

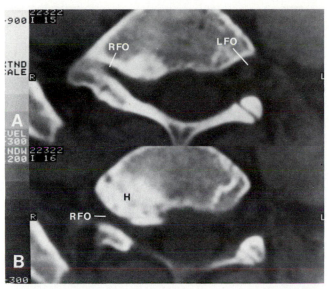

Fig 27–32.—Foraminal stenosis from scoliosis. **A,** level of the pedicle. **B,** a few millimeters below **A.** There is foraminal narrowing on the right from hypertrophy of the adjacent vertebral body caused by abnormal stresses. (*H* = hyperostosis of the vertebral body, *RFO* = narrowed right neural foramen, *LFO* = large left neural foramen.)

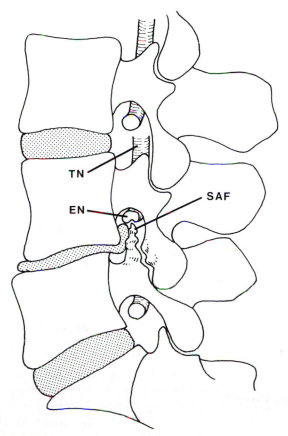

Fig 27–31.—Changes producing foraminal (lateral) stenosis. With loss of the disc space, the *SAF* moves superiorly toward the upper neural foramen to compress the exiting nerve. Posterior spondylolisthesis of the body above and osteophytes on the *SAF* cause further narrowing. (*TN* = traversing nerve, *EN* = exiting nerve in upper neural foramen.)

ease produces several anatomical changes that narrow this large upper part of the intervertebral foramen (Fig 27–31). As the disc space narrows, the upper vertebra moves inferior and posterior, causing the superior articular facet from below to move up into the upper part of the intervertebral foramen. Osteophytes on the superior and anterior aspect of the SAF result in even more encroachment on the exiting nerve. Occasionally, a laterally herniated disc, which usually lies below the exiting nerve, will extend upward from the disc level to encroach on the nerve, but usually foraminal stenosis is not associated with the disc directly. Foraminal stenosis may result from a fracture where a vertebral body fragment extends posterolaterally into the neural canal. Other causes are spondylosis and scoliosis with stress hypertrophy of the vertebral body (Fig 27–32).

Both axial and reformatted images can be used, each having advantages and disadvantages. In the axial slices, attention should be given to the upper part of the foramen where the nerve exits, and not to the lower part where the foramen is normally narrow in its AP diameter. With 5-mm slices, especially without overlapping, partial volume phenomenon may include the bottom of the pedicle above or part of the superior articular process from below, depending on where the slice lies in the foramen, and give a false narrowing of the foramen. In either case, the true upper part of the foramen may not be seen properly. A few additional 5-mm (or preferably 1.5-mm) slices through the upper foramen are extremely helpful to demonstrate the upper part of the foramen (Fig 27–33). Loss of normal epidural fat around the exiting nerve and a narrow AP diameter of the neural foramen are helpful findings, but not absolute (Fig 27–34). It may still be difficult to be certain whether there is a clinically significant compression of the nerve in the foramen. There have been numerous cases of an extremely narrow foramen with loss of fat that are completely silent clinically.

The neural canal also has a vertical component between the pedicle and superior articular facet that may not be completely appreciated on 5-mm axial slices without overlapping. Theoretically, the nerve could be compressed from below by the superior articular facet or its osteophytes, even though the AP diameter on the axial slices is adequate. This can usually be appreciated better with a few 1.5-mm axial cuts. To overcome these problems, many believe that the intervertebral foramen should be imaged with reformatting in the sagittal and possibly coronal planes.[26, 27] To preserve adequate detail of soft tissues and bone in these reformatted images, overlapping 5-mm contiguous slices every 3-mm should be made without gantry angulation. It should be remembered that this important sagittal information is well seen on conventional lateral tomography, which still has excellent spatial (bony) resolution even though soft tissues are not seen. As with axial images, the clinical significance of the narrowing may still not be definite, because wide variations exist.

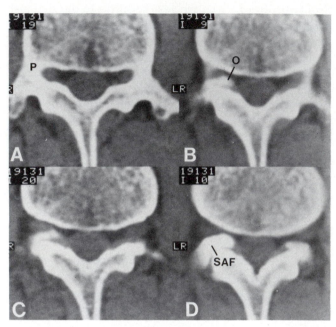

Fig 27–34.—Foraminal (lateral) stenosis. **A,** level of the pedicle *(P)*. **B** and **C,** a few millimeters below at the upper foramen where the exiting nerve passes. The osteophyte *(O)* from the SAF produces definite narrowing on the right. The left foramen is normal. **D,** lower foramen, which normally has a small sagittal diameter. Note the large *SAF* on the right. The normal left side would appear narrowed if evaluated at this level.

Subarticular (Lateral Recess) Stenosis

Subarticular stenosis refers to entrapment of the traversing nerve in the lateral recess, which is formed by the disc and vertebral body anteriorly, the upper border of the pedicle laterally, and the superior articular facet posteriorly (see Figs 27–2,E, 27–19, 27–23, and 27–35).[28, 29] A deep channel transversely with a narrow AP diameter can result from the following degenerative changes: anteriorly, a bulging or herniated disc or osteophytes at the back of the vertebral body; and posteriorly, a hypertrophied SAF (Fig 27–36). Note that in this form of stenosis the disc is directly involved, because it forms the anterior border of the lateral recess (see Fig 27–2,F). The exiting nerve has already left the foramen and is not usually involved. There may be a predisposing anatomical configuration called the "trifoil canal" (Fig 27–34,A) in which the lateral recesses are deep transversely and later become narrowed with the above changes. A superimposed central stenosis may tend to compress the traversing nerve laterally and deeper into the narrowed lateral recess. Scans by CT demonstrate this anatomy very well on the axial image. As with central and foraminal stenosis, unless it is severe, it may be difficult to be certain whether a deep lateral recess with a narrow AP diameter is really com-

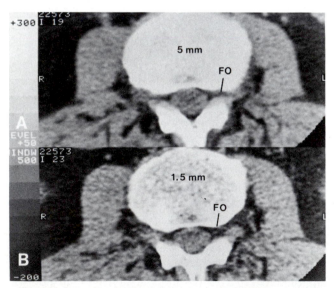

Fig 27–33.—Evaluation of the intervertebral foramen. **A,** a 5-mm slice gives the appearance of narrowing of the upper foramen *(FO)*. **B,** a 1.5-mm slice at the same level reveals fat in an adequate foramen *(FO)*. Similar findings are seen on the right side. A slice made too inferior in the foramen will give a false impression of narrowing (see Fig 27–2, **B** and **E**).

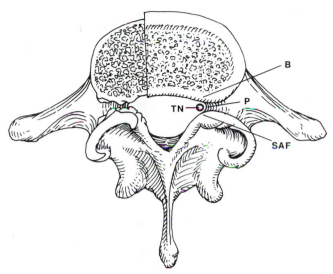

Fig 27–35.—The lateral recess. Note normal left side, lateral recess stenosis on the right. The boundaries of the lateral recess are the vertebral body (B), upper border of the pedicle (P), and base of the SAF. (TN = traversing nerve.)

pressing the nerve. Work still has to be done in quantifying the normal size of these areas. Even after surgery, it may be difficult to know the significance of a particular type of stenosis, because discectomy is often accompanied by partial foraminotomy and decompression of the lateral recess to free the nerve. Thus, even with surgical correlation, it still may be difficult to know the actual contribution of the stenosis to the patient's pain.

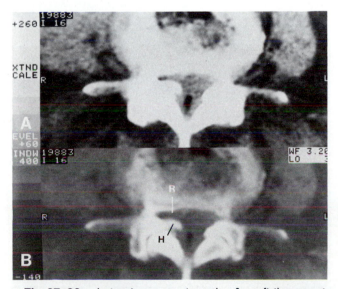

Fig 27–36.—Lateral recess stenosis. **A,** soft-tissue setting. **B,** bone setting. The lateral recess (R) is deep transversely and narrow sagittally because of a hypertrophied SAF (H). This patient also has central stenosis, which tends to push the nerve laterally into the narrowed recess.

SPONDYLOLYSIS AND SPONDYLOLISTHESIS

Spondylolysis refers to a break in the pars interarticularis, usually of L-5. It is usually bilateral and may be associated with various degrees of anterior slippage (spondylolisthesis) of the superior vertebra upon the one below. The pars interarticularis forms the posterior-superior margin of the neural foramen. At the break, there may be a pseudoarthrosis associated with hypertrophic bone or fibrocartilaginous proliferation. Either of these may narrow the neural foramen from above or behind and result in a form of foraminal stenosis. By recognizing spondylolysis beforehand from the plain films, scanning may be planned for adequate overlapping (every 3 mm) and zero gantry angulation to permit reformatting.

The axial image is often confusing because of marked lordosis. With slippage, the posterior edge of the vertebral body above will lie anterior to the posterior border of the disc and give the appearance of an HNP. The spinal canal is elongated, and the neural foramina are difficult to evaluate. Reformatting helps to determine the size and shape of the neural foramina and also to see the slippage (Fig 27–37). The use of CT allows us to see a thin nonseparated pars fracture line or lysis more easily than with plain films (Fig 27–38). The break occurs immediately adjacent to the facet joints and may be mistaken for a joint space if the scan is not carefully viewed in sequence with special attention to the location of the facet joints (Fig 27–39). The lysis and intervertebral foramina are also seen on the reformatted images.

CERVICAL SPINE

The same principles used to scan the lumbar spine apply to the cervical spine, with similar trade-offs of collimation, KVP, photon flux, and mAs. A few special considerations do apply to the cervical region. Absorbing material around the neck will improve the visualization of soft-tissue structures and spinal cord by allowing a higher mAs and preventing overranges.[30] Because of

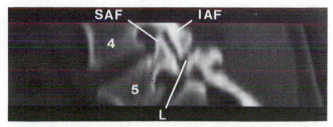

Fig 27–37.—Reformatted image showing spondylolysis of the pars of L-5. (4 and 5 = lumbar vertebrae, S = SAF of L-5, I = IAF or L-4, L = lysis of L-5 pars.)

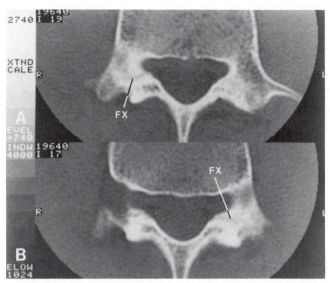

Fig 27–38.—A, B, bilateral stress fracture of the pars *(FX).* These subtle fractures would be very difficult to see on plain films.

the smaller body size, the mAs can be lower than for the lumbar spine, and rapid dynamic scanning may be more practical. Because the cervical spine is short compared with the lumbar spine, it is sometimes possible to scan the entire spine with a large, but not unreason-

able, number of cuts, although it is still preferable to identify one or more areas of importance and to scan as few levels as possible. Metallic fillings in the teeth may prevent contiguous scanning from the craniovertebral junction inferiorly without changing the angulation of the gantry (Fig 27–40). The study may have to be done in two parts, one of which will need to be angulated to work around the fillings. In such a case, the more important area, whether higher or lower, may be scanned with zero angulation to obtain optimal reformatting.

It is often not possible to see soft-tissue detail below C-5 or C-6 because of artifact generated by the shoulders lying outside the FOV (Fig 27–41). A large FOV (large-body calibration) tends to give less streak artifacts with better cord and soft-tissue detail. The patient should be encouraged to keep the shoulders low, but trying too aggressively may result in movement artifact or misregistration. Five-millimeter collimation with 4- or 5-mm increments works well for soft-tissue detail, but 1.5-mm slices are often helpful for fine bony detail (Fig 27–42).

The soft-tissue structures around the foramen magnum may be difficult to image clearly because of the streak artifact from the occipital squama, which presents as very thick bone tangential to the x-ray beam. This problem may be improved with the use of 1.5-mm slices. The upper cervical cord is often well seen sur-

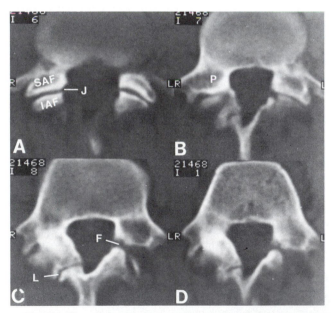

Fig 27–39.—Spondylolysis of L-5. **A,** facet joint *(J).* *(SAF = superior articular facet, IAF = inferior articular facet.)* **B,** a few millimeters below **A,** lower part of the facet joints. *(P = pedicle of L-5.)* **C,** classic lysis or fracture *(F)* of the pars interarticularis on the left and an unusual fracture or lysis of the lamina *(L)* on the right. **D,** the lower aspect of the fractures are seen. Careful attention to the sequence of anatomy is necessary in order not to confuse the lysis with the facet joints.

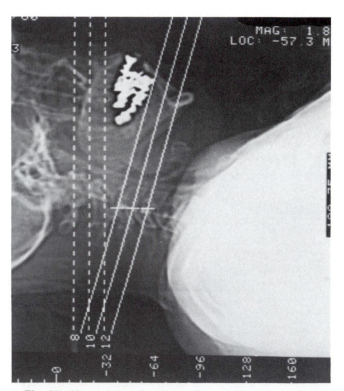

Fig 27–40.—Lateral localizer. For contiguous scanning from the foramen magnum inferiorly, it may be necessary to angle part of the study to avoid artifacts from the teeth.

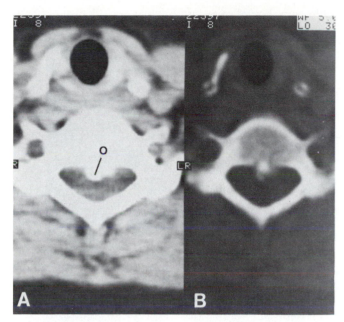

Fig 27–41.—Midline cervical osteophyte at C5-6. **A,** soft-tissue setting. **B,** bone setting. There is significant narrowing of the spinal canal because of the large osteophyte (O). The full extent of the osteophyte is usually better seen with CT than with plain lateral films, particularly if the osteophyte is not dense. Soft-tissue resolution of the cord and CSF is not often possible at C5-6 because of artifact from the shoulders.

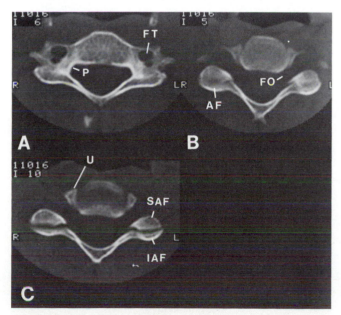

Fig 27–42.—Normal bony anatomy. **A,** level of body and complete ring. (FT = foramen transversarium, P = pedicle.) **B,** level of the intervertebral foramen (FO) at 5-mm collimation. The articular facets (AF) and joint spaces cannot be clearly distinguished. **C,** same level as **B** at 1.5-mm collimation. The uncinate processes (U) of the body below are clearly seen. (SAF = superior articular process, IAF = inferior articular process.)

rounded by CSF at C-1 and C-2, particularly when the slice passes between the bony posterior arches. With intrathecal metrizamide, the region of the cisterna magna and foramen magnum are extremely well visualized, both with axial slices and with coronal and sagittal reformatting (Fig 27–43). The brain stem and tonsils are clearly delineated. Unless the needle is removed and the patient turned supine, myelography is restricted to the anterior and lateral aspects of the foramen magnum, whereas CT, which is much simpler to perform, gives a complete 360° view.

The lateral mass of C-1 is wedgeshaped. A slice at this level will pass through both the occipital condyle and C-1, and a fracture may be simulated (Fig 27–44,A). It is also possible that the groove behind the lateral mass for the vertebral artery can be confused with a fracture (Fig 27–44,D). Because of the complex bony anatomy at the craniovertebral junction, it is often better to use 1.5-mm slices to evaluate the bony detail, but even very thin slices will not completely prevent the appearance of false fractures that are due to the anatomical configuration. A few conventional tomograms may give better bony detail faster and more simply than multiple thin CT slices with reformatting. Such is the case with a thin fracture line at the base of the odontoid, where in CT the original axial slices must be made in the same plane, that is, parallel to the fracture.

The levels C-3 through C-7 are anatomically similar and are usually scanned with 5-mm collimation. The cervical cord below C-3 is often clearly delineated by CSF (Fig 27–45), but usually not as clearly or reliably as at the C1-C2 level. As in the lumbar spine, it is often helpful to evaluate the intervertebral foramina with one or two 1.5-mm slices to avoid PVP of the pedicle above or below. This allows a more accurate evaluation of the size of the foramina, particularly if they are small. Below the pedicles lie the intervertebral foramina. The uncinate processes from the vertebra below are seen laterally, and if asymmetric, should not be confused with a fracture. The neural foramina are best seen at this level, posterolateral to the uncovertebral joints (see Fig 27–45). The facet joints lie at an angle of 45° to the x-ray beam, and because of PVP, fine detail is much better seen with 1.5-mm slices. With the gantry angled more perpendicular to the joint, the facets and joint spaces become more visible, the SAF anterior and the IAF posterior.

Even though the cord is clearly outlined with CSF or metrizamide, details of the actual internal structure cannot be resolved unless there is a lesion of very high or low attenuation, such as a cyst. If there is visualization of CSF around the cord, a significant compressive lesion can be excluded (Fig 27–46). Failure to outline the cord with CSF may be due to a compressive lesion

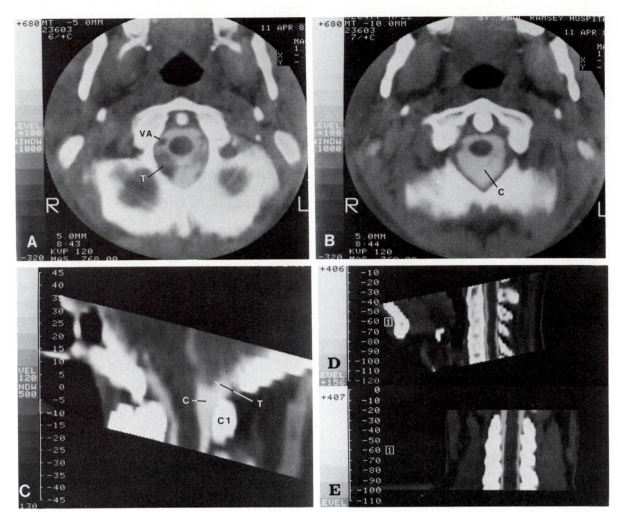

Fig 27–43.—Intrathecal metrizamide. **A,** level of the foramen magnum. **B,** 5 mm below **A. C,** sagittal reformatting at the craniovertebral junction. **D** and **E,** sagittal and coronal reformatting of the cervical spine below C-2. (*C1* = posterior arch of atlas, *T* = cerebellar tonsil, *C* = cisterna magna, *VA* = vertebral artery.)

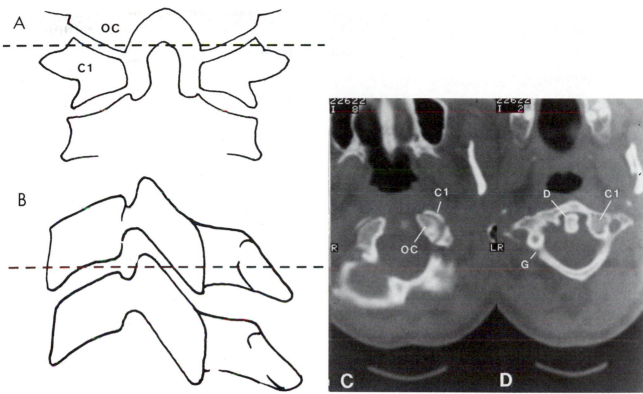

Fig 27–44.—Diagrams and scans to illustrate the relationship of scanning plane and bony anatomy. **A** and **C,** false fracture as scan passes through both occipital condyle *(OC)* and the articular mass of C-1 *(C1).* **B,** the articular facets lie at about 45° to the scanning plane. **D,** the groove *(G)* for the vertebral artery behind the lateral mass of C-1 should not be confused with a fracture. This "defect" occurs even in thin slices. *(D = dens, C1 = lateral mass of C-1.)*

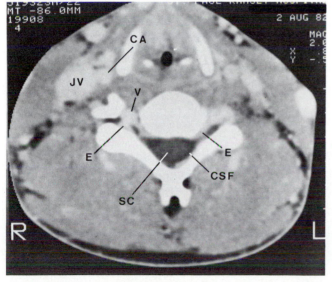

Fig 27–45.—C-3 intervertebral level with intravenous contrast. *(V = vertebral artery, E = epidural enhancement, JV = internal jugular vein, CA = carotid artery, SC = spinal cord surrounded by CSF, CSF = cerebrospinal fluid.)*

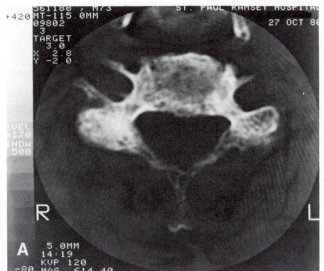

Fig 27–46.—Metastatic carcinoma of the prostate to C-6. **A,** diffuse mottling of the vertebral body and posterior arch. **B,** small mass *(M)* extending into the adjacent epidural space. Note that the CSF space is well preserved around the cord *(SC)* with no evidence of compression of the cord.

(Fig 27–47), but because the cord is not always seen in normal cases, the quality of the slice must first be evaluated to exclude artifact and poor contrast resolution. In such cases, it may be helpful to see if the cord is visualized at other levels. Similarly, a real pathologic loss of the CSF around the cord on CT still does not definitely confirm a complete block, and contrast may still be necessary, either using CT with metrizamide or myelography.

CERVICAL DISC DISEASE

The use of CT without intrathecal metrizamide for the evaluation of cervical disc disease is still not as successful as that in the lumbar spine.[31, 32] There is less epidural fat, and the cord and soft-tissue structures are less reliably seen. Individual roots cannot be followed as clearly in the central canal and out the neural foramina. However, posterior osteophytes extending into the spinal canal are well seen (see Fig 27–41). Others believe plain CT is very sensitive in demonstrating small disc herniations.[33] Compression of the cervical cord can often be appreciated if the CSF, and the cord can be resolved. Below C-5 or C-6, it is more likely that only the osteophyte will be seen because of decreasing soft-tissue resolution caused by artifact from the shoulders.

Axial slices give good detail of the neural foramina, especially at 1.5-mm collimation (see Fig 27–42). The size of the bony foramina can often be evaluated in spite of the artifact caused by the shoulders. Scans by CT are probably more sensitive than conventional

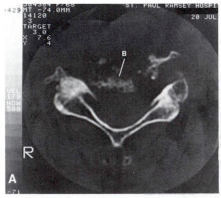
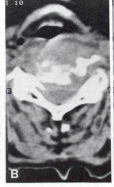
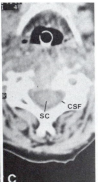
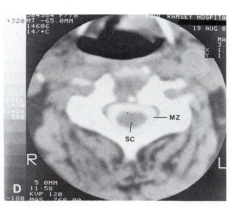

Fig 27–47.—Osteomyelitis of C-5. **A,** destruction of C-5 vertebral body **(B). B,** soft-tissue setting showing absence of CSF around cord from extension of the process into the spinal canal. **C,** after surgery at the same level, CSF now seen around the cord *(SC).* **D,** same level as **C,** metrizamide *(MZ)* surrounding the SC.

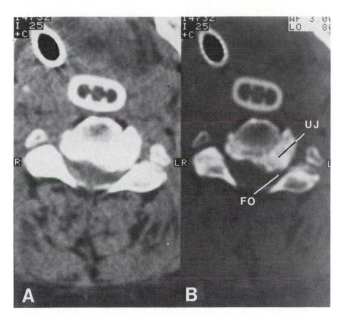

Fig 27–48.—Central and foraminal stenosis. **A,** soft-tissue. **B,** bone setting. There is marked narrowing of the left intervertebral foramen *(FO)* because of extensive bony overgrowth of the uncovertebral joint *(UJ)*. Similar but lesser changes are present on the right side. There is also narrowing of the central spinal canal.

oblique views to evaluate subtle osteophytic narrowing of the neural foramen from overgrowth of the uncovertebral joints (Fig 27–48). Epidural fat in the foramen will occasionally provide additional help in deciding whether there is foraminal stenosis. The use of intravenous contrast is helpful, because the epidural space enhances, providing delineation of the soft-tissue structures. High-circulating levels of contrast can be achieved by a very rapid bolus injection, which should be followed immediately by scanning.

In the majority of cases, intrathecal metrizamide will be necessary to define soft-tissue detail. Because a needle puncture and contrast injection are necessary for both metrizamide CT and myelography, CT loses its greatest advantage, i.e., of being noninvasive. There is no doubt, however, that with increased experience CT will gain importance in the diagnosis of cervical disc disease. Today, CT is an important noninvasive screening study, and in many instances a technically good examination will eliminate the need for myelography. Adequate clinical information is essential in deciding which levels are implicated and whether the information gained through CT is likely to prevent the necessity of myelography.

Acknowledgment

The author wishes to express his appreciation to Jim Latteier for his meticulous and dedicated technical and editorial assistance and to Ellen Werth for her secretarial help in the preparation of this manuscript.

REFERENCES

1. Genant H.K., Chafetz N., Helms C.A. (eds.): *Computed Tomography of the Lumbar Spine*. San Francisco, University of California, Department of Radiology, 1982.
2. Haughton V.M., Williams A.L.: *Computed Tomography of the Spine*. St. Louis, C.V. Mosby Co., 1982.
3. Newton T.H., Potts D.G. (eds.): *Modern Neuroradiology: Computed Tomography of the Spine and Spinal Cord.*, San Anselmo, Clavadel Press, vol. 1, 1983.
4. Gado M.H., Hodges F.J., Patel J.I.: Spine, in Lee J.K.T., Sagel S.S., Stanley R.J. (eds.): *Computed Body Tomography*. New York, Raven Press, 1983, pp. 415–462.
5. Dorwart R.H., DeGroot J., Sauerland E.K., et al.: Computed tomography of the lumbosacral spine: Normal anatomy, anatomic variants and pathologic anatomy. *RadioGraphics* 2:459–499, 1982.
6. Meijenhorst G.C.H.: Computed tomography of the lumbar epidural veins. *Radiology* 145:687–691, 1982.
7. Haughton V.M., Syvertsen A., Williams A.L.: Soft-tissue anatomy within the spinal canal as seen on computed tomography. *Radiology* 134:649–655, 1980.
8. Carrera G.F., Haughton V.M., Syvertsen A., et al.: Computed tomography of the lumbar facet joints. *Radiology* 134:145–148, 1980.
9. Hirschy J.C., Leue W.M., Berninger W.H., et al.: CT of the lumbosacral spine: Importance of tomographic planes parallel to vertebral end plate. *A.J.N.R.* 1:551–556, 1980.
10. Raskin S.P.: Demonstration of nerve roots on unenhanced computed tomographic scans. *J. Comput. Assist. Tomogr.* 5:281–284, 1981.
11. Williams A.L., Haughton V.M., Syvertsen A.: Computed tomography in the diagnosis of herniated nucleus pulposus. *Radiology* 135:95–99, 1980.
12. Haughton V.M., Eldevik O.P., Magnaes B., et al.: A prospective comparison of computed tomography and myelography in the diagnosis of herniated lumbar disks. *Radiology* 142:103–110, 1982.
13. Roberts W.D., Nugent R.A., Lapointe G.S., et al.: Comparison of CT scanning and metrizamide Amipaque myelography in lumbar disc disease. *J. Neuroradiol.* 1:368, 1980.
14. Raskin S.P., Keating J.W.: Recognition of lumbar disk disease: Comparison of myelography and computed tomography. *A.J.R.* 139:349–355, 1982.
15. Williams A.L., Haughton V.M., Daniels D.L., et al.: Differential CT diagnosis of extruded nucleus pulposus. *Radiology* 148:141–148, 1983.
16. Williams A.L., Haughton V.M., Meyer G.A., et al: Computed tomographic appearance of the bulging annulus. *Radiology* 142:403–408, 1982.
17. Kieffer S.A., Sherry R.G., Wellenstein D.E., et al.: Bulging lumbar intervertebral disk: Myelographic differentiation from herniated disk with nerve root compression. *A.J.R.* 138:709–716, 1982.

18. Williams A.L., Haughton V.M., Daniels D.L., et al.: CT recognition of lateral lumbar disk herniation. *A.J.R.* 139:345–347, 1982.

19. Novetsky G.J., Berlin L., Epstein A.J., et al.: The extraforaminal herniated disk: Detection by computed tomography. *A.J.N.R.* 3:653–655, 1982.

20. Helms C.A., Dorwart R.H., Gray M.: The CT appearance of conjoined nerve roots and differentiation from a herniated nucleus pulposus. *Radiology* 144:803–807, 1982.

21. Verbiest H.: The significance and principles of computerized axial tomography in idiopathic developmental stenosis of the bony lumbar vertebral canal. *Spine* 4:369–378, 1979.

22. Postacchini F., Pezzeri G., Montanaro A., et al.: Computerized tomography in lumbar stenosis. *J. Bone Joint Surg.* 62-B:78–82, 1980.

23. Ullrich C.G., Binet E.F., Sanecki M.G., et al.: Quantitative assessment of the lumbar spinal canal by computed tomography. *Radiology* 134:137–143, 1980.

24. Macnab I.: *Backache.* Baltimore, Williams & Wilkins Co., 1977, pp. 98–104.

25. Gelman M.I.: Cauda equina compression in acromegaly. *Radiology* 112:357–360, 1974.

26. McAfee P.C., Ullrich C.G., Levinsohn E.M., et al.: Computed tomography in degenerative lumbar spinal stenosis: The value of multiplanar reconstruction. *RadioGraphics* 2:529–554, 1982.

27. Glenn W.V., Rhodes M.L., Altschuler E.M., et al.: Multiplanar display computed body tomography applications in the lumbar spine. *Spine* 4:282, 1979.

28. Mikhael M.A., Ciric I., Tarkington J.A., et al.: Neuroradiological evaluation of lateral recess syndrome. *Radiology* 140:97–107, 1981.

29. Ciric I., Mikhael M.A., Tarkington J.A., et al.: The lateral recess syndrome. *J. Neurosurg.* 53:433–443, 1980.

30. Orrison W.W., Johansen J.G., Eldevik O.P., et al.: Optimal computed-tomographic techniques for cervical spine imaging. *Radiology* 144:180–182, 1982.

31. Badami J.P., Norman D., Barbaro N.M., et al.: Determination of objective criteria for abnormal CT examination of the cervical spine. Presented at the 21st Annual Meeting of the American Society of Neuroradiology, San Francisco, June 5–9, 1983.

32. Schonfeld S., Pinto R.S., Kricheff I.I., et al.: Metrizamide CT myelography in the evaluation of cervical myelopathy. Presented at the 21st Annual Meeting of the American Society of Neuroradiology, San Francisco, June 5–9, 1983.

33. Coin C.G., Coin J.T.: Computed tomography of cervical disk disease: Technical considerations with representative case reports. *J. Comput. Assist. Tomogr.* 5:275–280, 1981.

28

Computed Tomographic Myelography in Degenerative Disc Disease and Spinal Stenosis

JOHN D. MEYER, M.D.

COMPUTED TOMOGRAPHIC MYELOGRAPHY (CTM) following intrathecal placement of water-soluble contrast medium may be a valuable aid in diagnosis and treatment planning. A great deal of varied and detailed anatomical data is now available, most of which was not appreciated in the past. These data include subtle, normal anatomical characteristics of the subarachnoid spaces in the spinal canal, early pathologic changes, and clearer demonstration of pathologic relationships.

In general, CT scanning is performed following a standard myelogram with a water-soluble contrast medium. Currently, metrizamide is the most commonly used medium, but in the future newer and safer materials should be available. Some individuals now advocate the use of a small volume of low-concentration metrizamide for CT scanning only, eliminating the standard myelogram.[1] This procedure is performed as an adjunct to plain CT scanning and may have value in outpatient diagnostic evaluation.

The value of water-soluble contrast utilization with CT scanning was recognized early,[2–4] while recent reports confirm and enhance early impressions.[1, 5, 6] Dublin and coworkers[1] found that CTM provided more significant information than plain myelography in 40% of a series of 106 cases. When comparing plain CT scanning with CTM, these authors found that CTM "provided significant additional information as compared with plain CT in 33% of individuals examined by both techniques." These data were obtained from spinal studies in general and not confined to disc disease or spinal stenosis per se.

TECHNIQUE

While plain CT scanning will adequately reveal bony structure in all spinal areas, the subarachnoid spaces, spinal cord, and nerve root sleeves are better seen with contrast material present. Optimum concentration of contrast material is critical in order to opacify, but not obscure, the subarachnoid space. The CT examination can be performed generally up to 4 hours following a myelogram without difficulty. Scanning beyond this point usually results in suboptimal concentrations of contrast material. Scanning by CT should be performed with contrast material *homogeneously* distributed instead of *pooled*. This assures accurate and easy identification of nerve roots, small spaces, and the spinal cord. Pools of contrast material tend to produce lucent artifacts adjacent to the pool, which completely obscure subtle density differences. Intradural contents are also poorly seen (Fig 28–1). Trying to reposition pooled contrast may allow some of it to enter the intracranial subarachnoid space directly, a hazardous result. Cervical CT myelography can be performed easily in the prone or supine position after letting the bulk of the pooled contrast material flow into the lumbosacral subarachnoid space following the plain myelogram. This will leave enough of it dissolved or homogeneously distributed for adequate CT examination. For lumbar CT scanning, turning the patient once or twice will distribute much of the pooled contrast medium. In addition, waiting an hour or so following a lumbar myelogram will allow for some absorption of the contrast pool and give better scanning results.

Anatomical correlation between CTM findings and plain myelographic findings may be significantly *decreased* by the large differences in patient positioning for the examinations. During myelography of the lumbar spine, for example, more stress is placed on the spine with the patient erect or semierect, possibly enhancing "bulging" of the discs. Such bulging may not be seen during CT scanning, because the stresses are

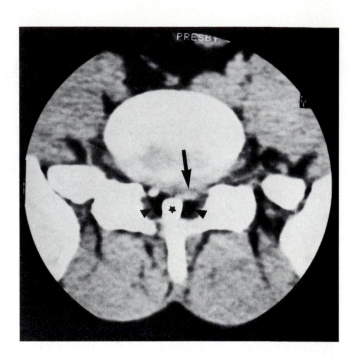

Fig 28–1.—Lucent artifact adjacent to dense metrizamide column. A herniated disc is demonstrated at L5-S1 *(arrow)*. There is nonfilling of the left S-1 nerve root sleeve. Dark triangular regions adjacent to the metrizamide column *(arrowheads)* obscure local tissue density. Concentration of retained contrast material can be reduced by waiting an hour or so following the myelogram before performing CT examination. (*star* = metrizamide within thecal sac.)

not placed along the spinal axis when the patient lies down. In addition, cervical myelography is usually performed in the prone position, which places the head in hyperextension, possibly aggravating spinal canal narrowing. Cervical CT is usually performed in the supine position and therefore may not show quite the degree of narrowing and/or relationships of soft-tissue structures as on the myelogram. These questions have not been adequately studied to date, but do warrant attention.

Quantitative measurements of the spinal canal and contents may be performed. Object size appears to vary with different window settings. Seibert and colleagues[7] found that the appropriate window center for cord size determination was the mean between the CT attenuation number of the enhanced subarachnoid space and the cord CT attenuation number. In general, wide window settings are indicated for measuring the size of the thecal sac or studying bony structures. Lack of standardization and precision while making quantitative determinations may lead to confusion in the correlation of operative and diagnostic findings.

INDICATIONS

The lumbar disc syndrome is a complex combination of disease processes including herniated disc, spondylosis, and congenital spinal stenosis. Paine and Huang[8] found that herniation of the nucleus pulposus (HNP), per se, was found in only one third of the series of 227 patients operated upon for lumbar disc syndrome. The other two thirds had spondylosis, spinal stenosis, or

some combination of spondylosis, stenosis, and HNP. The combined lesions accounted for 39% of the series. The complexity of the lumbar disc syndrome necessitates a thorough and precise approach to diagnosis, as provided with CTM. Such a diagnostic approach allows the surgeon to plan an operation with all possible information.

The older age groups present with more chronic degenerative disease, including degenerative disc problems, spondylosis, and stenosis. These patients are therefore more likely to present with complex plain CT and plain myelographic findings. Operative planning in this group may be greatly enhanced by obtaining an accurate and precise display of anatomical relationships among the disc, canal, neural arch, ligamenta flava, facets, and the subarachnoid space. These relationships may be optimally visualized with CTM.

In those patients who have an unequivocal plain CT, plain myelographic findings, or both, the additional utilization of CTM is of little diagnostic help. However, in patients with suspected herniated disc, CTM may resolve conflicts among the findings of plain CT and plain myelography. A patient with firm clinical signs and symptoms of herniated disc, but with a normal myelogram, should have a CTM regardless of plain CT findings. A possible exception is the patient with a far lateral disc herniation, which should be seen by plain CT.

The use of CTM may save a technically inadequate plain myelogram. Utilizing "dynamic" CT scanning with relatively low mAs, one may perform large numbers of adjacent thin or overlapping sections and then

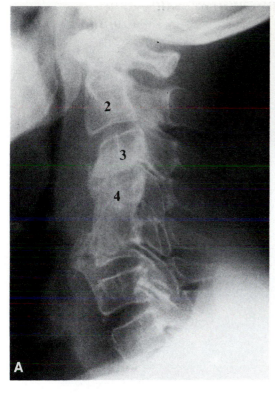

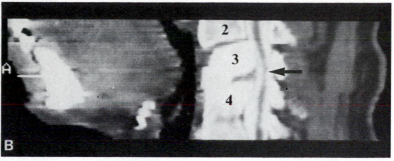

Fig 28–2.—Sagittal reconstruction of axial sections. This may save a technically inadequate plain myelogram. In photo **A**, the plain lateral cervical spine film demonstrates advanced degenerative changes accompanied by a curvature reversal at the C-3 level. Patient has had a fusion at C4-5. Contrast material will not pool easily in a spine with this configuration. A midsagittal reconstruction image is shown in **B**, obtained from multiple adjacent thin sections performed at relatively low mAs. Curvature reversal is shown centered at C-3. In addition, there is focal atrophy of the spinal cord indicated by the *arrow*. (2 = C-2, 3 = C-3, 4 = C-4.)

reformat the images to produce sagittal or coronal sections. This may be especially useful for cervical studies in which severe curvature problems exist (Fig 28–2). Although gas myelography might be helpful in this instance, reformatted CT myelography is easy to perform and provides more data. The use of CTM may also save a technically inadequate myelogram secondary to an extra-arachnoid injection. Even with injection into all three intraspinal spaces (subarachnoid, subdural, and epidural), there may be enough contrast material in the subarachnoid space to allow for diagnostic CT scanning (see Fig 28–10).

The use of CTM often reveals much more than plain myelography in patients with spinal block (Fig 28–3). Care should be taken to scan past the block by one level or so to help elucidate the cause of the block. Important data for treatment planning may result. In this regard it may be useful to maintain the patient in a position for a number of minutes that allows for the flow of a small amount of contrast medium past the block. While the amount of contrast passing the block may be insufficient for visualization on x-ray film, CT scanning may detect the contrast because of its ability to detect minute density differences.

Plain CT scanning of the entire spine or an entire subdivision of the spine is not only laborious, but gives an excessive amount of radiation to the patient. When a long segment of the spine must be evaluated or when the site of diffuse symptomatology cannot be localized, routine myelography should be performed, followed by CT scanning at a specific site or sites to resolve specific questions.

The postoperative lumbar spine presents special problems, and the next chapter is devoted to this subject. In general, CTM usually provides more significant data in the evaluation of the postoperative spine than myelography or plain CT alone.

LUMBAR SPINAL ANATOMY

The lumbar thecal sac and nerve root sleeves are very often well visualized by plain CT, but sometimes they are not. This problem tends to occur in the smaller spinal canal and in the older spine, which contains less epidural fat and more degenerative changes. In addition, there are numerous artifacts, anatomical variations, and pitfalls to make matters more difficult. Various authors have described these difficulties on plain CT.[9-13] The list includes the normal epidural venous plexus and its variations, conjoined nerve roots, root sleeve diverticulae, streak artifacts, synovial cysts from the facet joints, and intraspinal nerve root ganglia. Conjoined roots (Fig 28–4) are more commonly seen than previously appreciated. In the author's series, conjoined roots were found on 5% of all lumbar myelograms. They are commonly noted at S1-2, as well as L5-S1, may be bilateral, and are often asymptomatic in that they are found incidentally and unrelated to clinical

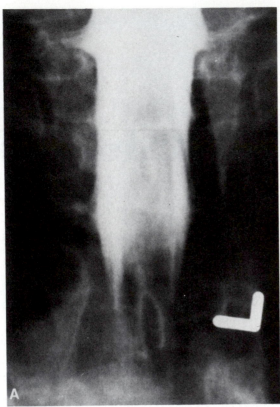

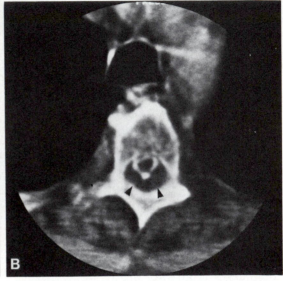

Fig 28–3.—CT scanning through a spinal block. Photo **A** demonstrates an upper thoracic spinal block that was myelographically complete. The lateral view, as well as this AP view, were not helpful in localizing the direction of the block. In addition, it was not certain that the block was extradural. CT scanning through the level of the block and just below **B** reveals a posterior and laterally located extradural mass *(arrowheads)* with no bone destruction displacing the thecal sac anteriorly. This kind of localizing data is vital to proper surgical planning.

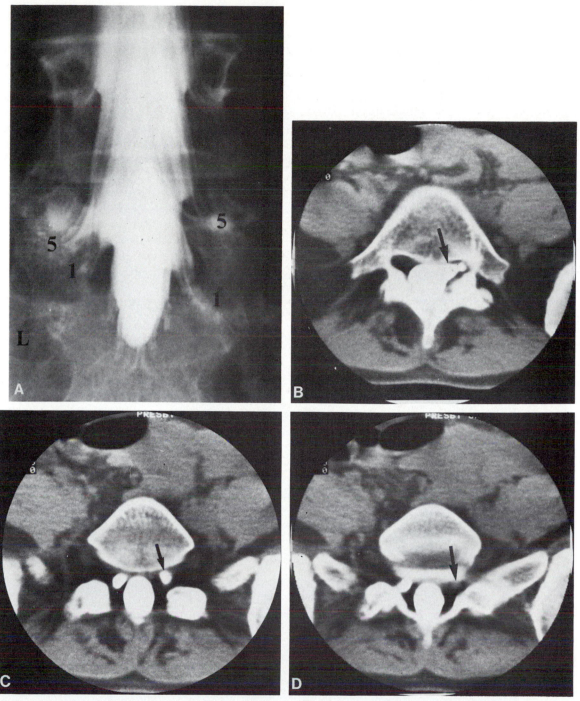

Fig 28–4.—Conjoined lumbar nerve root sleeves. Photo **A,** AP lumbar myelographic film oriented with the left (L) on the reader's left. CT scans following are oriented with the left on the reader's right side. L-5 (5) and S-1 (1) nerve root sleeves are conjoined on the left. L-5 on the left arises slightly lower, while S-1 arises slightly higher, compared with the opposite side. In photo **B,** conjoined root sleeves are indicated by a large outpouching from the thecal sac (arrow). In photo **C,** the S-1 nerve root sleeve continues caudally (arrow). In **D,** nerve root sleeve has terminated, leaving only the nerve root surrounded by fat (arrow) as it descends laterally to pass beneath the S-1 pedicle.

presentation. Lesser variations of nerve root sleeve origin (Fig 28–5) are also occasionally seen and appear to represent minor position differences of root sleeves. Nerve root diverticulae (Fig 28–6) are variations of normal and without significance.

In general, nerve roots lie in the posterior part of the thecal sac and descend anteriorly as they approach the exiting sleeves (Fig 28–7). The subarachnoid space extends to about the level of the midpoint of the pedicle or just medial to the midpoint. Beyond this point, the metrizamide does not pass, and the nerve root itself may be visualized on CT if there is sufficient fat surrounding it. The conus and cauda equina may be imaged well. Normally, horizontal roots of the cauda equina are seen at the level of the conus and have a "spider-like" appearance (Fig 28–8).

The thecal sac itself (Fig 28–9) is round or oval in shape and may be quite variable in size from patient to patient. When the oval shape is too flattened in the sagittal plane, stenosis may be present (see Fig 28–25). The thecal sac tapers caudally and ends at approximately the midportion of the sacrum; or as a variation of normal, it may end as high as the L5-S1 disc space. An intervertebral disc may be concave, flat, or somewhat convex, and its shape may be mirrored in the anterior thecal sac. While quantitative data are available for the bony spinal canal,[13] insufficient data are available for the thecal sac itself. Density measurements, per se, may be misleading, and their use must be made with caution.

The extra-arachnoid spaces (Fig 28–10) are seen by CT on occasion, even when there is no evidence of an extra-arachnoid injection on the myelogram. A small amount of contrast material may leak out of a needle tract, or the needle may puncture the dura anteriorly. At this point in time, little use of contrast in the sub-

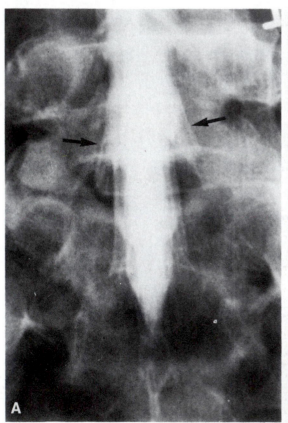

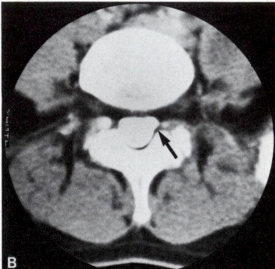

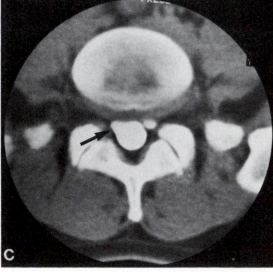

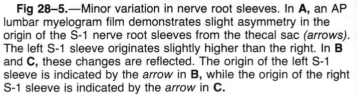

Fig 28–5.—Minor variation in nerve root sleeves. In **A,** an AP lumbar myelogram film demonstrates slight asymmetry in the origin of the S-1 nerve root sleeves from the thecal sac *(arrows)*. The left S-1 sleeve originates slightly higher than the right. In **B** and **C,** these changes are reflected. The origin of the left S-1 sleeve is indicated by the *arrow* in **B,** while the origin of the right S-1 sleeve is indicated by the *arrow* in **C.**

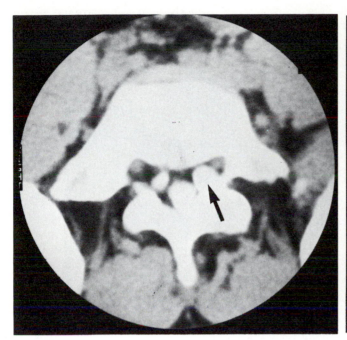

Fig 28–6.—Nerve root sleeve diverticulum. The left S-1 nerve root sleeve is larger than the right *(arrow),* a commonly noted finding considered to be a normal variation. These diverticula are usually bilateral at multiple levels in the lumbar canal.

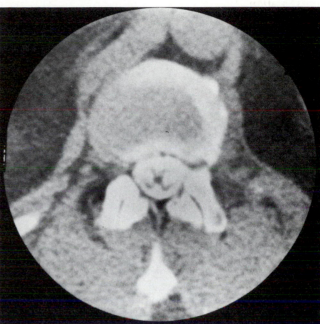

Fig 28–8.—Conus medullaris and proximal cauda equina. Sections at the caudal end of the spinal cord, the conus, often reveal a "spider-like" appearance caused by the small conus surrounded by laterally directed proximal nerve roots.

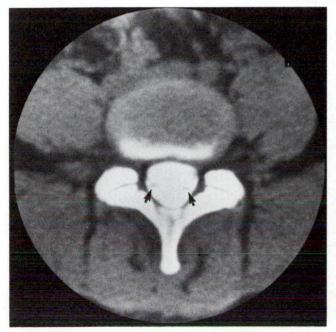

Fig 28–7.—Intrathecal nerve roots. *Arrows* indicate nerve roots within the thecal sac. They descend anteriorly proximal to the exit point (also see Fig 28–9).

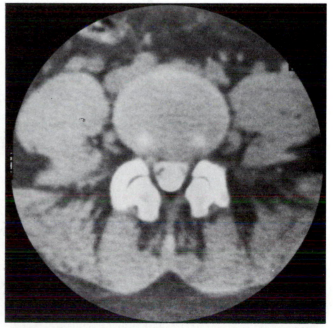

Fig 28–9.—Normal thecal sac with nerve roots. Compared with the thecal sac in Figure 28–7, this is a normal thecal sac, although smaller in size. Paired nerve roots are again noted.

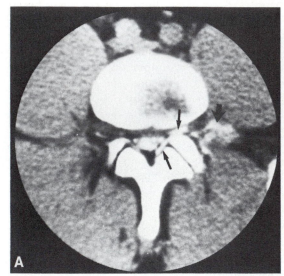
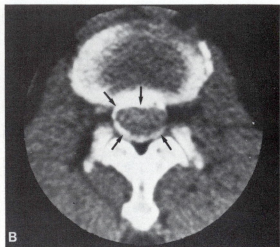

Fig 28–10.—Extra-arachnoid spaces. In photo **A,** leak-age of contrast material has occurred into the epidural space *(medial arrow)*. Contrast medium is also noted in the intervertebral foramen *(middle arrow)* and is seen in the extra-spinal space laterally *(large arrow)*. In **B,** the myelogram revealed subdural contrast medium. CT section obtained af-ter demonstrates a band of contrast medium *(arrows)* sur-rounding the thecal sac. No contrast medium was observed in the extradural location.

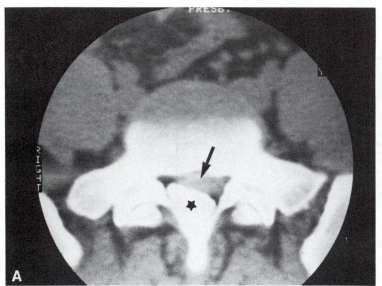
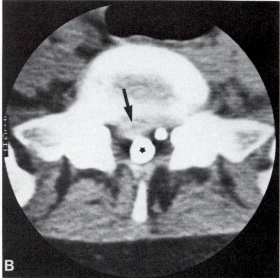

Fig 28–11.—Lumbosacral herniated disc, two different patients. In **A,** the *arrow* indicates a large L5-S1 herniated disc that distorts the thecal sac *(star)* and displaces the left S-1 root sleeve posteriorly. The thecal sac is relatively larger in this patient than in **B,** where similar findings are noted. In **B,** herniated disc material is indicated by the *ar-row,* but the thecal sac *(star)* shows little distortion. The her-niated disc material does not allow filling of the right S-I nerve root sleeve in **B,** however. The normal S-1 sleeve on the left side is filled. CTM adds little diagnostic information in instances such as these, but may be useful for therapeu-tic planning if a plain CT scan had not been performed prior to the myelogram.

CTM AND HERNIATED DISC

dural or epidural spaces has been found on CT. Care must be taken not to confuse epidural contrast with volume averaging of the junction between the lamina and transverse process.

A disc herniation of sufficient size to be well seen by plain CT, or one producing an unequivocal myelographic defect will also produce unequivocal findings on CTM (Fig 28–11). However, as noted earlier, CTM adds data concerning the bony canal and precise relations of the herniation to it. This may be useful in planning an operation, perhaps more so if microsurgical techniques are used.

A large disc herniation may make plain CT findings confusing, because the epidural fat planes, thecal sac, and root sleeves are more distorted. This may be a greater problem in a small spinal canal, or at levels higher than L5-S1, because the canal tends to be larger at the lumbosacral junction. In some cases, myelography may reveal only a block to contrast flow and not suggest a cause. If tortuous intradural nerve roots are seen, an element of spinal stenosis is present, but the disc itself must be studied by CTM (Fig 28–12).

Disc herniations (Figs 28–13 to 28–16) may present diagnostic difficulty on either plain CT, plain myelography, or both. The herniated disc may be associated with chronic degenerative changes or a small spinal canal (Fig 28–17). A small herniation may be indistinguishable from a "bulging" disc (Fig 28–18), which, although possibly symptomatic, may warrant only nonoperative therapy. In some cases, there is an equivocal plain CT, and myelography shows only a single unfilled root sleeve. Because root sleeve asymmetry may be pathologic, CTM is indicated to determine the cause (Fig 28–19). Another cause of confusion on the plain myelography or CT is central herniation (Fig 28–20), especially at L5-S1, where the anterior epidural venous plexus may simulate a herniation.

A normal myelogram preceded by an equivocal plain CT scan may be seen in a patient with a relatively lateral "bulge" or herniation and an element of lateral recess stenosis (Figs 28–21 and 28–26). This problem may not easily be solved by *any* modality or combination currently utilized. Relations of the lateral recess and lateral aspect of the disc may need to be studied by thin (1- to 2-mm) sections closely spaced. Multiplanar reconstruction may be of additional help. This group of patients represents a minority in the overall problem of herniated disc, but it is a significant minority nonetheless.

Some patients benefit from the utilization of a disc injection, with an enzyme to decrease the mass of disc

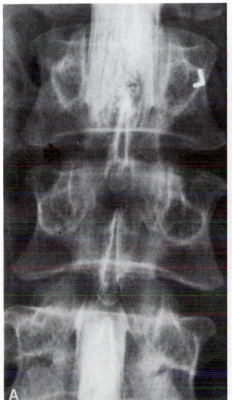
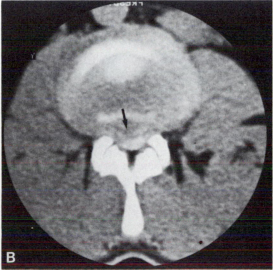

Fig 28–12.—L3-4 spinal stenosis accompanied by acute herniated disc. In **A,** the myelographic AP film reveals a high-grade stenosis to the caudal flow of contrast medium at the level of the *arrow.* In **B,** a CT section was obtained at this level. This CTM reveals an asymmetry of the thecal sac caused by herniated disc material *(arrow).* While the myelographic findings are more typical of spinal stenosis alone, this CTM finding alerts the surgeon to explore the disc space on the right anteriorly. Decompressive laminectomy alone would be an incomplete treatment.

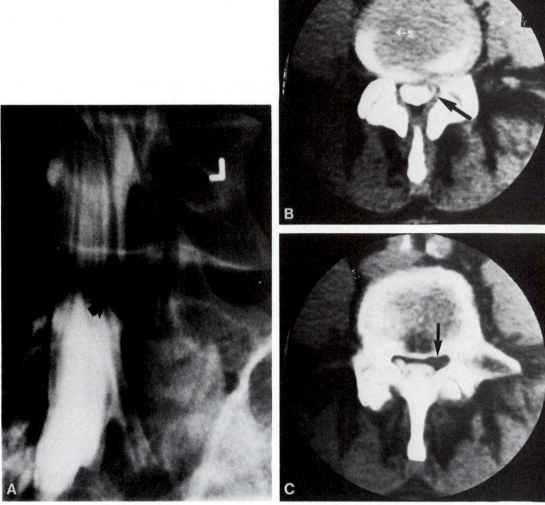

Fig 28–13.—Herniated disc with caudal migration of a free fragment. In **A,** an oblique myelographic spot film reveals nonfilling of the left L-5 nerve root sleeve with some distortion of the root *(arrow).* This finding is nonspecific and could be produced by disc bulge or disc herniation. In **B,** CTM section through the L4-5 *(4-5)* disc space reveals incomplete filling of the L-5 nerve root sleeve as it exits the thecal sac *(arrow).* In addition, there is some lateral bulging of the disc. Five millimeters below in section **C,** there is nonfilling of the L-5 nerve root sleeve and slight distortion of the thecal sac. This was secondary to a caudal and lateral migration of a free disc fragment *(arrow).* Nerve root sleeves usually fill in cases of bulging disc alone. CTM in this instance alerted the surgeon to search for a migrating free fragment.

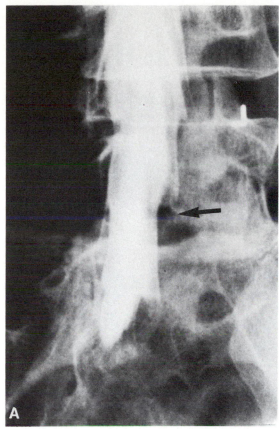

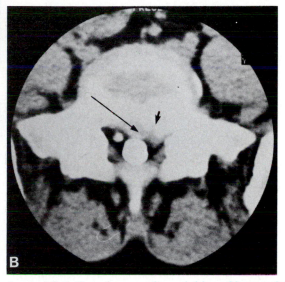

Fig 28–14.—Herniated disc accompanied by a lateral recess stenosis. In **A,** an oblique myelographic spot film reveals nonfilling of the left S-1 nerve root sleeve *(arrow)* accompanied by slight indentation of the thecal sac. Herniated disc alone might be suspected to cause the finding. In **B,** the section obtained after the myelogram through the upper level of S-1, there is a roughened ridge of bone arising from the superior and posterolateral aspect of the S-1 vertebral body *(small arrow)* accompanied by soft-tissue material, which represented herniated disc *(long arrow).* The small size of the thecal sac in relation to surrounding tissues explains in part a lack of defect upon it.

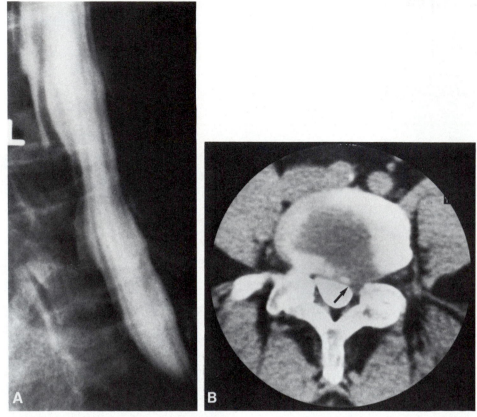

Fig 28–15.—Herniated disc with free fragment and lateral recess stenosis. In **A,** an oblique myelographic spot film is demonstrated with the left side on the reader's left. Distortion of the thecal sac is accompanied by nonfilling of the nerve root sleeve and widening of the L-5 nerve root possibly secondary to edema. CTM in **B** demonstrates similar finding with distortion of the thecal sac *(arrow).* At operation, a free fragment was found, and there was accompanying lateral recess stenosis. Both of these are not entirely clear from the CT examination and point out a possible limitation of CT scanning. While findings of herniated disc can be identified, it is not always simple to identify free fragments of disc material.

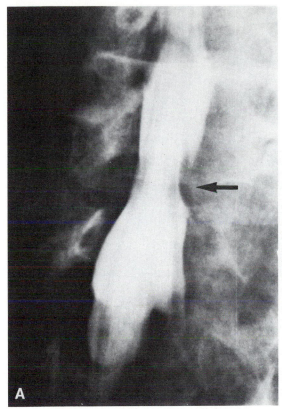

Fig 28–16.—Focal spinal stenosis without herniated disc fragment. In **A,** an oblique myelographic spot film reveals widening of the L-5 nerve root with nonfilling of the sleeve *(arrow).* In addition, there is posterior indentation of the thecal sac presumably secondary to hypertrophic facets. The findings are nonspecific, and herniated disc cannot be excluded. CTM in **B** demonstrates no evidence of herniated disc. Bilateral symmetric facet hypertrophy causes en-croachment on the canal centrally, resulting in spinal stenosis. In this instance, the myelographic finding of possible disc herniation is not supported by the CT scan. Plain CT scanning in spinal stenosis may be fraught with difficulty because of the stenotic condition itself and difficulty isolating the various components of the soft-tissue densities within the spinal canal and in relation to the discs.

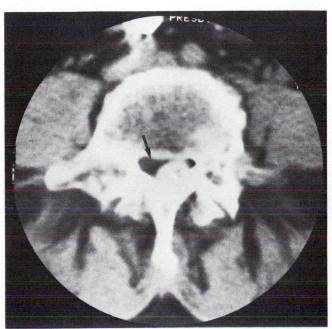

Fig 28–17.—Migrating free fragment in a patient with chronic degenerative disease. The myelographic films not reproduced here reveal multiple bilateral defects with poor filling of several nerve root sleeves and indentations on the contrast column. The findings were believed secondary to chronic degenerative disease alone. The CTM, however, revealed that one area of distorted root and thecal sac was caused by soft-tissue density confirmed at operation to represent a migrated free fragment *(arrow).*

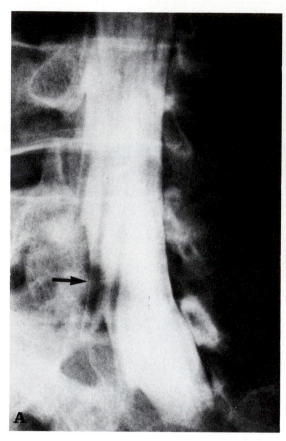

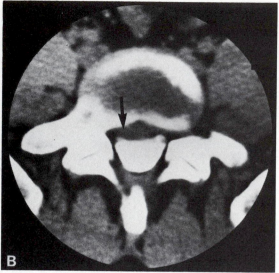

Fig 28–18.—Symptomatic "bulging" disc. In **A,** an oblique myelographic spot film reveals slight widening of the S-1 nerve root sleeve *(arrow)*. The root sleeve is well filled, however. In **B,** a CTM reveals an anterolateral epidural density *(arrow)* with slight posterior displacement of the S-1 nerve root sleeve as it exits the thecal sac. This patient responded to conservative therapy alone. Compare with Figure 28–19.

Fig 28–19.—Small free fragment of herniated disc material. The myelographic films are not reproduced, but demonstrated no distortion of the thecal sac and only slightly suboptimal filling of the right S-1 nerve root sleeve. The findings were equivocal, but CTM reveals a soft-tissue density *(arrow)* with nonfilling of the S-1 nerve root sleeve. At operation, a small free fragment was demonstrated. Operation has revealed in many instances that free fragments alone may be smaller than bulging discs. Therefore, identification of free fragments may be quite difficult.

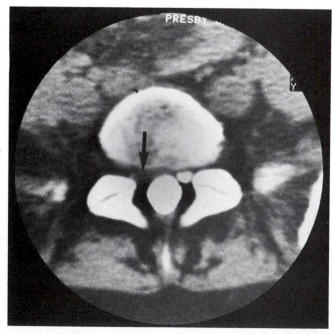

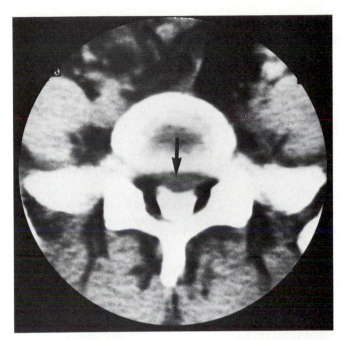

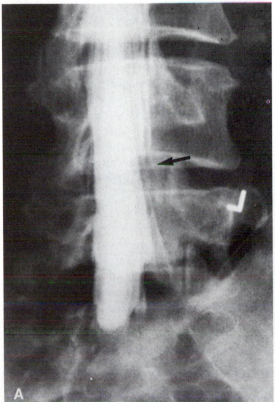

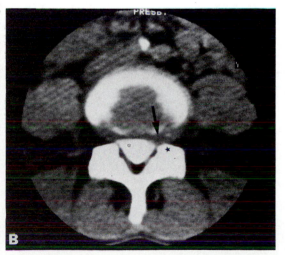

Fig 28–20.—Central herniated disc at L5-S1. The myelogram, not reproduced here, revealed a central indentation of the contrast column at L5-S1 with good filling of the S-1 nerve root sleeves. In addition, CTM revealed a central soft-tissue density *(arrow)* related to the L5-S1 disc and not characteristic of the lumbar epidural veins. Central herniation was confirmed at operation.

Fig 28–21.—Lateral bulging disc with lateral recess stenosis identified at operation. In **A,** an oblique myelographic spot film revealed slight distortion of the left L-5 nerve root sleeve *(arrow).* This finding is minimal and usually nonspecific, often having little significance. In **B,** a CTM reveals a lateral bulging disc *(arrow).* No distortion of the thecal sac is noted, but there is slight distortion of the nerve root sleeve as it exits the thecal sac. The *star* marks the superior artic-ular process of L-5. At operation, the L-5 nerve root was tethered in the lateral recess by a combination of the bulging disc and the bony projection of the superior articular process, which itself was not degenerative. Lateral bulging disc such as this is a relatively common finding, having no definite radiologic significance. In the final analysis, the significance of any given patient's symptoms may be determined clinically and not necessarily by solely radiologic means.

material. Scanning by CT, metrizamide myelography, and CTM may provide definitive methods to allow a more accurate prediction of which patients may benefit the most from disc injection. In this regard, classifying herniated disc or bulging disc by plain CT or CTM findings might enable the examiner to recognize those candidates with large fragments of herniated material that might not benefit from disc injection.

In summary, CTM provides useful and conclusive data for the diagnostic evaluation of herniated disc in a patient whose other radiologic studies are equivocal or confusing. In addition, it may be valuable for choosing a mode of therapy (conservative vs. operative) and for planning an operation.

CTM AND LUMBAR SPINAL STENOSIS

Spinal stenosis, a common problem, is complex and multifaceted. Table 28–1 lists a classification of the many causes derived by the participants of a recent symposium.[14] In this chapter, concentration is on the acquired type of spinal stenosis, specifically the "degenerative" and "combined" subgroups, while excluding the others.

The common denominator in spinal stenosis is narrowing of the spinal canal, which may be central, peripheral, or both, depending upon that portion of the canal having more stenosis. "Central" refers to the portion of the bony spinal canal bounded by the pedicles laterally, facet joints, laminae, and spinous process posteriorly, and the disc anteriorly. "Peripheral" refers to the root exit zone proximal to the intervertebral fora-

TABLE 28–1.—CLASSIFICATION OF LUMBAR
SPINAL STENOSIS*

I. Congenital-developmental stenosis
  A. Idiopathic
  B. Achondroplastic
II. Acquired stenosis
  A. Degenerative stenosis
    1. Central portion of canal
    2. Peripheral portion of canal and nerve canals
    3. Degenerative spondylolisthesis
  B. Combined stenosis: Any possible combination of developmental stenosis, degenerative stenosis, and HNP.
  C. Spondylolisthetic stenosis
  D. Postoperative stenosis
    1. Postlaminectomy
    2. Postfusion
    3. Postchemonucleolysis
  E. Post-traumatic stenosis (late changes)
  F. Miscellaneous
    1. Paget's disease
    2. Fluorosis

*From Arnoldi C.C., Brodsky A.E., Cauchoix J., et al.: *Lumbar Spinal Stenosis and Nerve Root Entrapment Syndromes: Clinical Orthopaedics and Related Research*, no. 115. Philadelphia, J.B. Lippincott, Co., 1976, pp. 4–5.

men. The root exit zone includes that portion of a spinal nerve between its point of exit from the thecal sac and the intervertebral foramen, lying in the lateral recess of the spinal canal. Central stenosis results from a decrease in the size of the sagittal and/or coronal dimensions of the spinal canal. Large facet joints, thickened laminae, short pedicles, and bulging disc material all may coexist in various combinations to cause the canal to be small. Differing patterns of symptoms may result, depending on which portions of the canal are stenotic. In addition, central and peripheral (lateral recess) stenosis commonly occur together.

It must be emphasized that these cases of spinal stenosis have a small or small-normal canal on a congenital and developmental basis. The pedicles are short and laminae thick early in life without producing symptoms. When degenerative changes are superimposed upon this small spinal canal later in life, symptoms develop. This is a common presentation and is to be differentiated from the small spinal canal associated with constitutional bone disorders such as achondroplasia, in which there is involvement of long segments of the canal or the entire canal, producing symptoms relatively early in life.

Several reports have reviewed the pathologic changes in spinal stenosis and correlated those findings with the plain CT scan.[15–21] Lancourt and colleagues,[16] and later Glenn and coworkers,[21] have emphasized the value of multiplanar reconstruction in studying the pathologic anatomy of the lumbar canal. These reports, however, have not evaluated the use of CTM in spinal stenosis, and there is little data available at this time comparing CTM with multiplanar plain CT imaging.

Metrizamide myelography without CT is a relatively good technique for studying the stenotic spinal canal. Alterations at several levels having complex pathologic anatomy can all be seen at once. However, it is nonspecific in that the causes of multiple and complex extradural defects seen on the myelogram in spinal stenosis are not always readily apparent. In addition, lumbar puncture in a stenotic canal may be difficult, with the possibility of a partial extra-arachnoid injection of contrast material. On the other hand, CTM is extremely helpful in clarifying the causes of the defects seen on the metrizamide myelogram. It may also save an otherwise poor myelogram.

Central stenosis tends to occur at multiple levels, more frequent and advanced at L4-5 (Figs 28–22 and 28–23). At the higher levels, L2-3 and L3-4, stenosis is commonly observed, but to a lesser degree and less frequently. Symptomatic stenosis may exist alone at L4-5 (Fig 28–24). At the lumbosacral junction, the bony canal tends to be larger, and while involved in the central stenosing process, the lumbosacral junction is less

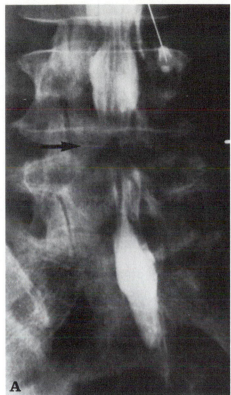

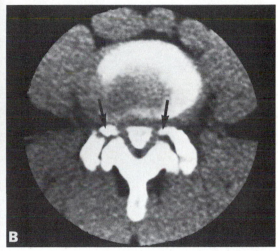

Fig 28–22.—Spinal stenosis, both central and lateral recess. In **A,** AP myelographic film reveals very poor filling of the thecal sac and the L-5 nerve root sleeves at the L4-5 level *(arrow)*. Filling is somewhat better, although still abnormal, at L5-S1 below and at L3-4 above. These are classic findings of spinal stenosis. CTM in **B** better reveals a combination of generalized disc bulge and markedly degenerative facet joints. The facet joints cause narrowing of the canal and the transverse plane. In addition, hypertrophic changes in the facets cause the superior and medial aspects to enlarge and partly project medially *(arrows)*. With decreasing height of the disc space secondary to degenerative chronic changes, the hypertrophic superior articular process from the vertebra below tends to encroach upon the lateral recess of the spinal canal. This finding is not always easily demonstrable by CT scanning, either plain or CTM. Multiplanar reconstructive methods may add a great deal of vital diagnostic data.

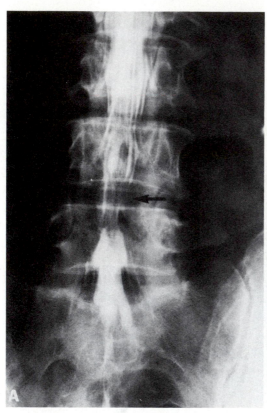

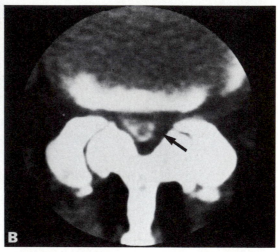

Fig 28–23.—Spinal stenosis, both central and lateral recess, with relative hypertrophy of the left ligamentum flavum. In **A,** the classic myelographic findings of spinal stenosis are demonstrated. There is poor filling of the thecal sac of L4-5 accompanied by nonfilling of the L-5 nerve root sleeves. Compare with Figure 28–22. The L5-S1 level is better demonstrated in this particular instance. In addition, there is a lateral indentation upon the thecal sac starting at the level of the *arrow* and extending inferiorly about 5 or 7 mm. CTM in **B** demonstrates that this is secondary to a relative enlargement of the left ligamentum flavum *(arrow).* Both L4-5 facet joints are markedly enlarged and hypertrophic and compress the thecal sac from the sides. The cause of the nonspecific finding is explained by CTM.

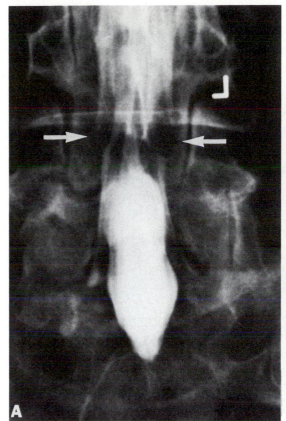

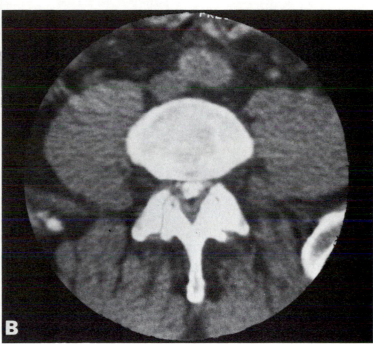

Fig 28–24.—Focal spinal stenosis at L4-5. **A,** AP myelographic film reveals poor filling of the thecal sac at L4-5 with nonfilling of the L-5 nerve root sleeves *(arrows).* The levels above and below are intact. CTM in **B** reveals large facet joints causing decreased transverse canal diameter. The AP diameter is reduced as well. Defects on the nerve root sleeves demonstrated at myelography are not secondary to herniated disc, but to enlarged facet joints.

compromised (see Figs 28–22 and 28–23). Focal disc protrusion or herniation may be observed at stenotic levels and is better appreciated by CTM than myelography (Fig 28–25). Central stenosis tends to produce complicated radicular signs and symptoms, and neurogenic claudication may result if the stenosis has progressed sufficiently.

Lateral recess stenosis,[22, 23] or peripheral stenosis, is now more appreciated as a cause of radicular signs and symptoms either alone or in combination with central stenosis or herniated disc. Reports by Epstein and coworkers[24, 25] and Ciric and associates[26] have demonstrated the role of the facets in producing radiculopathy. Ciric defined the anteroposterior height of the lateral recess as the distance between the most anterior portion of the superior articular facet and the posterior border of the vertebral body at the level of the superior margin of the corresponding pedicle. Utilizing this criterion, measurements of the height of the lateral recess were performed by CT. The data indicated that a height of 4 mm or less was associated with symptoms in all but one of 16 patients. Most occurred at L4-5, and some were associated with herniated disc.

Reynolds and coworkers[27] reported 22 patients presenting with signs and symptoms of lumbar monoradiculopathy, in whom none had a herniated disc. Nerve root compression was caused by facet hypertrophy in all cases, most commonly at L4-5. At operation, three areas of root compression were found: first, in the anteromedial canal by *either* the inferior or superior facet; second, laterally in the lateral recess by the superior facet from the level below; and third, inferior to the pedicle by the hypertrophic superior facet. This last type was least common. In addition, plain CT scanning was not particularly useful. While plain CT scanning may be diagnostic in such a process, the need for CTM indicates the difficulty of imaging the peripheral portion of the spinal canal. Glenn and colleagues[21] advocate the multiplanar method and have standardized a grading system for facet degeneration and compromise of the intervertebral foramen.

In the author's experience as well, there have been

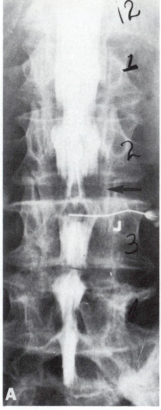
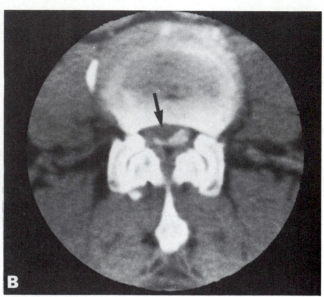

Fig 28–25.—Spinal stenosis and herniated disc. The AP myelographic film reveals poor filling of the thecal sac at L2-3, L3-4, and L4-5. Four lumbar vertebrae are present (*12* = T$_{12}$; *1–4* = lumbar vertebrae). CT section obtained at the level of the *arrow* on the myelographic film reveals a well-defined density anterior and slightly lateral *(arrow)* to the thecal sac in addition to the enlarged facet joints and central encroachment upon the canal. This was a confirmed herniated disc fragment at operation. Plain CT, while not performed in this instance, cannot clearly define herniated disc in many instances of stenotic spinal canals.

several patients who have had firm clinical findings of monoradiculopathy, but also have had myelograms and CTM of a normal or equivocal nature (Figs 28–21 and 28–26). In this group, operations were performed after a failure of conservative therapy, and a lateral recess was found to be stenotic, partly because of "bulging" of the disc without herniation. These patients have improved after operation. Examinations by CTM were performed in this group by 5-mm sections without overlap and without sagittal or coronal reconstruction. In retrospect, the diagnosis of lateral recess stenosis was not always apparent. It might be necessary to perform thinner sections or perhaps sagittal or coronal reconstruction to make the appropriate diagnosis. In addition, careful measurements of the lateral recess might need to be performed and some standards of evaluation applied. Discrepancies between radiologic findings and operative findings are not uncommon. In this regard, the recent work of Eldevik and colleagues[28] concerning discrepancies between the anatomical findings at oper-

ation and the morphology on radiologic images may be enlightening.

In conclusion, CTM is useful in spinal stenosis for evaluating confusing findings seen at myelography. Additional work appears to be necessary to resolve difficult diagnostic dilemmas arising from evaluation of the lateral recess.

CTM AND THORACIC DEGENERATIVE DISEASE

Symptomatic degenerative alterations of the thoracic spine are less frequently observed than in either the lumbar or cervical spine. Thoracic disc herniation is much less frequent than either lumbar or cervical herniation. Other symptomatic degenerative processes including spondylosis and spinal ligament calcification, while possibly causing myelopathy, are also less frequently seen. Marzluff and associates,[29] however, believe that "thoracic spondylosis" may not only be a def-

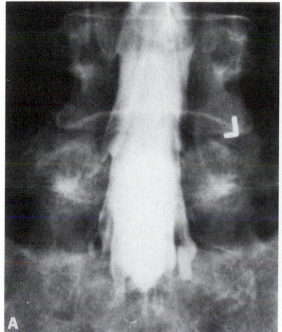

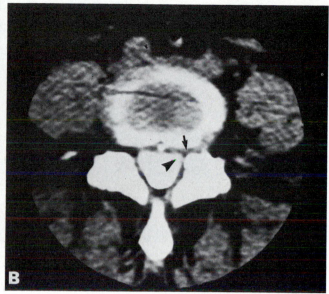

Fig 28–26.—Lateral recess stenosis. In **A,** a myelographic film reveals poor visualization of the left L4-5 nerve root sleeve (adjacent to the "left" marker). Compare with the opposite side. CTM in **B** reveals better filling of the root sleeve *(arrowhead)* with slight lateral disc bulge *(arrow).* The myelographic finding of an unfilled nerve root sleeve seems out of proportion to the CTM findings. At operation, the nerve root was tethered in the lateral recess by the bulging disc and the facet. This illustrates once again the difficulty of diagnostic evaluation in lateral recess stenosis.

inite cause of myelopathy, but may also be seen more frequently than reported.

In addition to small extradural defects on a myelogram, pathologic processes in the thoracic subarachnoid space tend to cause a high grade of block, and they are somewhat more difficult to image by plain myelography, where details are often lost. All that is often observed is an extradural block, but the cause may not be apparent (see Figs 28–3 and 28–27). The mode of CTM is especially useful in this regard and may supply critical information to the surgeon regarding the exact location of a lesion. Operative planning (transthoracic vs. posterior) may be simplified.

The method of CTM is performed by 5-mm sections, possibly overlapping by 2 mm if necessary. Radiologic studies may be confusing in these thoracic conditions, and all three examinations (plain CT, myelography, CTM) may be necessary to understand the alterations.

The spinal cord and surrounding structures are well seen in thoracic CTM (Fig 28–28). Normally, the spinal cord occupies from 50% to 80% of the available subarachnoid space and occupies the portion of the subarachnoid space nearest to the predominant curvature of the dorsal spine. Because the normal curvature is usually somewhat kyphotic, the cord is often anterior in position. In scoliosis, the cord will occupy the portion of the subarachnoid space closest to the major curvature. Blood vessels along the thoracic cord are usually not seen, but nerve roots and their sleeves may be seen. Little data is available concerning the precise anatomical appearance of the nerve root sleeves in the dorsal spine. The bony spinal canal is well defined by either plain CT or CTM. In general, the position of the facet joints in the coronal plane is within the posterior half of the spinal canal.

Thoracic discs herniate most frequently at the T10-12 levels (Fig 28–27). Herniated discs may occur at other thoracic locations, but are rare. Trauma may be a precipitating factor, but the development of symptoms may be insidious (and hence confusing). A tendency for calcification of the nucleus pulposis of a herniated disc is observed as well. Because other degenerative symptomatic thoracic conditions also tend to calcify, CTM may clarify the problem. Either an extradural defect or a block may be observed at plain myelography. On occasion, a thoracic disc ruptures through the dura and may be seen in the subarachnoid space. Although no data are published yet, CTM should help distinguish thoracic spurs from herniated disc.

Thoracic radicular and myelopathic symptoms may be produced by ossification of the ligamentum flavum,[30, 31] posterior longitudinal ligament, or both.[32–36]

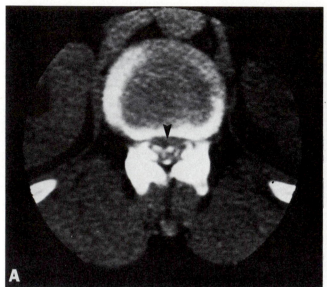

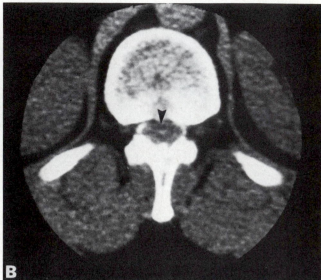

Fig 28–27.—Herniated thoracic disc at T12-L1. The myelogram, not reproduced here, revealed a complete extradural block at T12-L1. The patient was a 32-year-old man with abrupt onset of lower thoracic spinal cord symptoms. In **A**, the lower portion of the block, a curvilinear anterior epidural density is noted *(arrowhead)*. Continuing 5 mm cephalad

(B), the anterior density *(arrowhead)* is again noted. The exact borders of the subarachnoid and epidural spaces are not clear; however, it was nonetheless believed that this represented an anterior extruded disc fragment that was in the extradural space. This was operatively confirmed.

While the nature of ligamentum flavum calcification should be apparent at CT or CTM, calcification of the posterior longitudinal ligament may be confused with disc herniation or an intradural mass. The ligament calcification is usually extensive and may be visible on plain lateral films or pluridirectional tomography. Posterior longitudinal ligament calcification may also be noted in the cervical spine and cause myelopathic changes.

EVALUATION OF THE CERVICAL SPINE

Technical Notes

As previously noted, sufficient contrast material for CT scanning will remain in the cervical spinal canal when the patient is placed in the erect position and the pooled material is allowed to flow into the lumbosacral canal. Repositioning the contrast in the neck would then be ill advised, because control of the remaining bolus would be difficult.

Clinical presentation of lesions in the craniovertebral junction or in the upper cervical spine may be a diagnostic problem, and the plain metrizamide myelogram often does not image this region well enough to exclude an abnormality. When clinical signs and symptoms are confusing, difficult to localize, or indicate upper cervical cord pathologic changes, a few CT sections from the craniovertebral junction to C-2 should be performed. Such an examination may be helpful in excluding the Chiari malformation or a mass in the region of the foramen magnum or upper spinal canal.

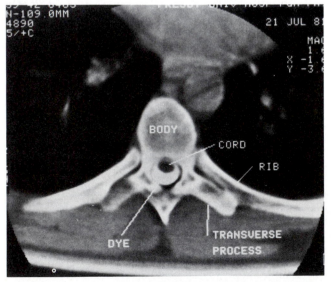

Fig 28–28.—Thoracic anatomical structures. The basic anatomical structures have been labeled. Notice that the spinal cord tends to occupy the anterior aspect of the subarachnoid space. In general, the volume of the thoracic subarachnoid space is smaller.

Selection of CT slice thickness may be a problem. Cervical pathologic entities are usually smaller than lumbar abnormalities, and the alterations occur within less tissue volume. Therefore, thinner sections (1.5 to 2 mm) or at least a 1- to 2-mm overlap of a 5-mm section may be needed to study a segment. Difficulty with this technique arises when the myelogram reveals multiple bilateral abnormalities involving more than one segment, a common problem in spondylosis, thereby requiring many sections. It is best to attempt to focus attention to as small an area as possible, i.e., one in which radicular signs and symptoms or cord compression are apparent. The myelogram should be used to indicate the levels for intensive evaluation with thin-section CT.

Currently, it is not unusual to scan four cervical interspaces, the ones in which degenerative changes are more commonly seen. This is the region covered by C3-4 through C6-7. Sections are usually obtained at 5-mm intervals, and, as noted above, an overlap of 1 to 2 mm may be necessary. The "lateral recess" of the cervical spinal canal and the intervertebral foramen may undergo significant alteration that may cause pressure defects on cervical roots. Sagittal and/or coronal reformatting of the image, as well as thin sections, may be necessary to evaluate these areas. Unfortunately, the cervical intervertebral foramina are oblique in their course, unlike the lumbar foramina. Sagittal and coronal reformations may add little to the evaluation of the cervical foramina. Development of high-resolution oblique reformatted images will probably be necessary for adequate evaluation of these structures.

Cervical CTM Anatomy

The vertebral bodies of C-1 and C-2 have characteristic shapes allowing for easy recognition. To a lesser degree, the seventh cervical vertebra is singular in shape in that its spinous process is longer than the others, and its bony ring somewhat rounder. The vertebral bodies C3-C6 are more like each other, making recognition of a level difficult without a localization image. Spinal canal size may vary from small to large in normal patients. The smaller spinal canals are associated in later life with a greater likelihood of developing symptomatic spondylosis. Pedicles may vary in size and length, and the lamina may vary as well in thickness. The mode of CTM shows the spinal cord well. The spinal cord diameter should not be less than approximately one half of the subarachnoid space diameter. When greater than approximately 80%, the cord may be abnormally large. Root sleeves and nerve roots proximal to the root sleeves are apparent on CT (Fig 28–29). In later life, degenerative changes are commonly noted in the cervical spine. These may be reflected in the CTM studies as poor filling of some of the nerve root sleeves.

Acute Cervical Disc Disease

Acute cervical disc herniation is less common than acute lumbar herniated disc. Symptoms may develop after trauma or may be unrelated to trauma. In severe neck trauma, a large herniated fragment may accompany the fracture of a vertebral body and be responsible for symptoms. This entity is not considered in this chapter, but rather the smaller disc herniations will receive our attention. The C6-7 and C5-6 levels are most commonly involved, and symptoms are usually unilateral, consisting of radiculopathy involving one root secondary to pressure from a posterolateral herniation of disc material. Central disc herniation may occur also, and either central or peripheral herniations may be associated with myelopathic findings, depending upon the size of the herniation, the size of the bony spinal canal, and the presence of superimposed degenerative changes.

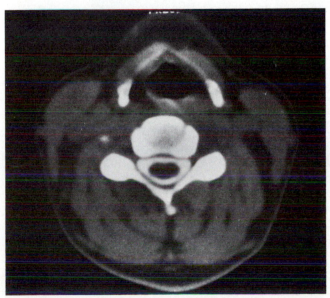

Fig 28–29.—Normal cervical canal at C4-5. Note that the spinal cord is surrounded by a pool of contrast-enhanced spinal fluid. Although not photographically reproduced, the nerve rootlets are usually well demonstrated. Note also that the intervertebral "foramen" is actually a canal along which slightly differing processes can occur.

Plain myelography is often diagnostic, because only one root may be involved (Fig 28–30). This type of herniation without any superimposed degenerative change is fairly well evaluated by plain myelography alone. The use of CTM confirms the myelographic findings and enhances the appreciation of precise anatomical relations. With concomitant degenerative changes, the significance of any single unfilled root sleeve on the myelogram becomes more difficult to evaluate, because there are other unfilled sleeves that may be secondary to formation of spurs arising from the joints of Luschka or other bony regions. The use of CTM may clearly reveal a noncalcified or nonbony extradural density representing the herniated disc (Fig 28–31). On occasion, a large cervical herniated disc may cause a block to the flow of contrast material by itself without superimposed degenerative change or may appear to be present in an *intradural* location. Precision of diagnosis in these cases is vital to surgical planning. The use of CTM can clearly define the axial relationships that are correlated with the myelographic lateral film. Cord widening may be apparent on the AP myelogram film and poorly appreciated on the lateral view because of overlapping structures (see Fig 28–38). While the myelogram may suggest an intramedullary expansion, CTM will reveal widening of the cord secondary to compression by the herniated disc.

CTM and Cervical Degenerative Disease (Cervical Spondylosis)

Degenerative disease of the cervical spine, like its counterpart in the lumbar spine, is a major health problem. Not only is it frequently seen, but its pathologic manifestations are often advanced before symptoms arise. Plain films and plain myelography should not be neglected in evaluating cervical degenerative disease. The curvature of the spine, possible subluxation, and the question of stability are factors that need attention in deciding the cause of symptoms and the course of therapy. Specifically, radiographs in flexion and extension may reveal bony relational changes not seen by myelography or CT scanning. An obstruction to the flow of oily contrast medium was commonly observed with degenerative changes in the past, and a similar relative "block" may be seen with a water-soluble contrast medium. The dynamic changes are influenced by the position of the head and neck and are best seen fluoroscopically.

However, cervical myelography in chronic degenerative disease is deficient for several reasons. First, poor filling of an irregular, small canal is common, even with water-soluble contrast media. Second, structures tend to overlap, especially on the critical cross-table lateral view (see Fig 28–35). Third, spinal cord size and shape

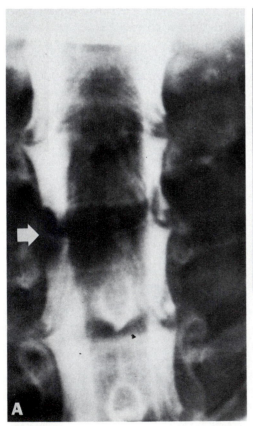
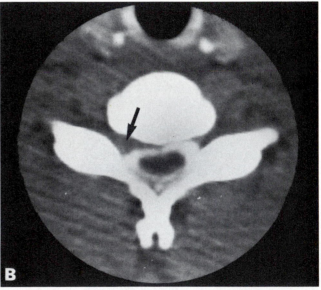

Fig 28–30.—Herniated cervical disc. **A,** an AP myelographic spot film reveals a sharply defined extradural density on the patient's right side *(arrow)*. In addition, the root sleeve is not filled at this level. The myelographic finding can conceivably represent an intradural as well as extradural process. However, CTM in **B** clearly demonstrates soft-tissue density in the right intervertebral canal *(arrow)* with posterior and slight medial displacement of the thecal sac. Compare with Figure 28–31.

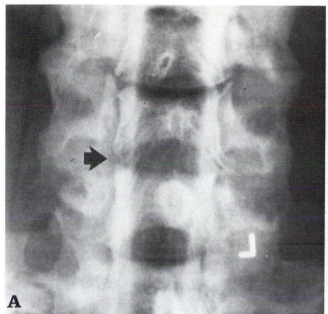

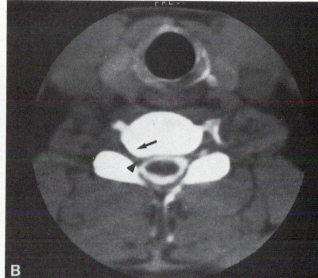

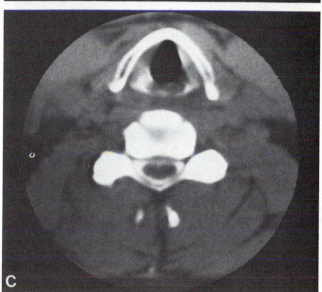

Fig 28–31.—Herniated cervical disc, smaller than the example in Figure 28–30. **A,** AP myelographic film reveals poor filling of the nerve root sleeve *(arrow)*. The opposite sleeve is well filled, but there is suboptimal filling of the two sleeves just above. This is a common myelographic problem regarding significance of unfilled cervical nerve root sleeves. In **B,** the CTM reveals not only slight spur formation arising from the inferolateral aspect of the vertebral body *(arrow)*, but also soft-tissue density within the intervertebral canal *(arrowhead)*, which represented herniated cervical disc material. In **C,** the level above the herniated disc, the root sleeves are compressed slightly by intervertebral bony canal narrowing, but no soft-tissue density is observed.

cannot be accurately assessed. Fourth, anatomical relations in the axial plane can only be inferred at best from myelography. Fifth, radiologic evaluation of symptomatic degenerative changes is a problem, because similar findings such as root sleeve irregularities are seen with normal aging. In addition, conditions that prevent pooling of contrast (reversal of the normal lordotic curve) also prevent obtaining technically adequate films. These problems are easily addressed by CTM, which may save an otherwise poor myelogram.

Plain CT offers an opportunity to evaluate complex bony alterations or those arising from calcified tissues, but even greater diagnostic advances are possible with CTM. Scotti and colleagues[37] have found that CTM better demonstrates deformity and compression of the spinal cord in cervical spondylosis than does plain CT,

while Nakagawa and coworkers[38] have observed that CT with metrizamide clearly delineates cervical disc protrusions, whereas myelography alone often shows only a block without offering data of a conclusive nature on the cause. Mawad and associates,[39] as well as Y.-L. Yu and coworkers,[40] have reported upon characteristic alterations in the shape of the spinal cord in cervical spondylosis leading to cord atrophy.

Examination of a given interspace should occur from pedicle to pedicle. Section thickness of 5 mm may not be adequate, and an overlap of 1 to 2 mm may be necessary. It may be important to obtain sections of 1.5- to 2-mm thickness in order to visualize all of the anatomical changes occurring at any given disc space without errors from partial volume averaging. For this reason, it is important that the length of a segment to be ex-

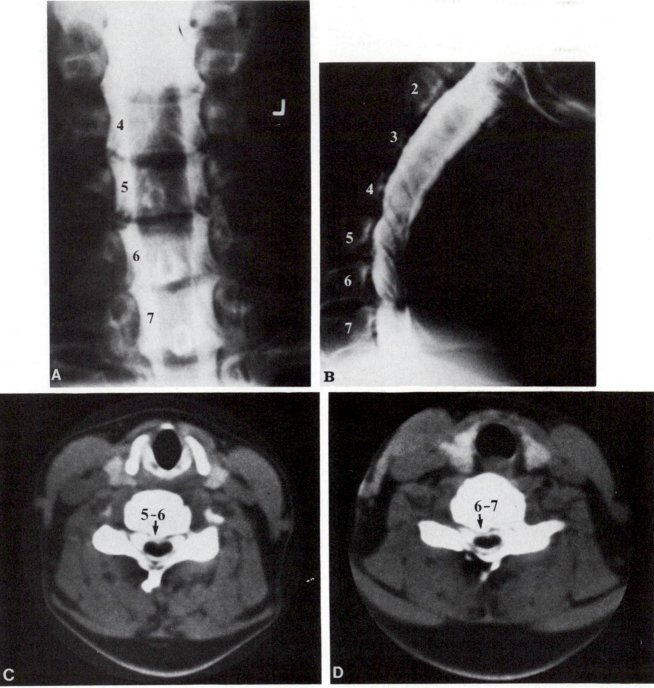

Fig 28–32.—Chronic degenerative changes with spur formation. **A** and **B** are AP and lateral myelographic films respectively (2–7 = cervical vertebrae). **C** and **D** are CTM films obtained at C5-6 *(5-6)* and C6-7 *(6-7)* respectively. In **C,** the section at C5-6, a central spur is clearly seen *(arrow)*, but is not visible on the AP or lateral myelographic films. At C6-7 **(D),** a spur is noted slightly to the right of the midline *(arrow)*, which causes slight cord compression. It is seen on the lateral myelographic film, but its exact location cannot be accurately determined from the myelogram alone. In addition, the effect from both spurs is minimal or none on the spinal cord. The precise location and size of spurs may indeed have vital significance to the future operative planning and treatment in cases of cervical spondylosis.

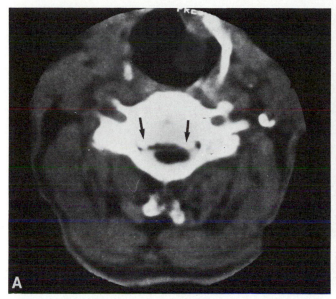

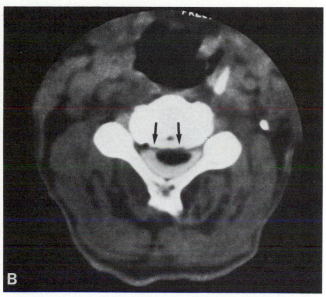

Fig 28–33.—Degenerative changes with spur formation. **A** and **B** are adjacent CTM films 5 mm apart. In **A,** uncovertebral joint spurs *(arrows)* located laterally have caused encroachment upon the lateral aspect of the spinal canal and invertebral canal. The spinal cord is slightly compressed as well. In **B,** 5 mm cephalad, degenerative changes cause bone "protrusion" encroaching upon the anterior epidural space *(arrows).*

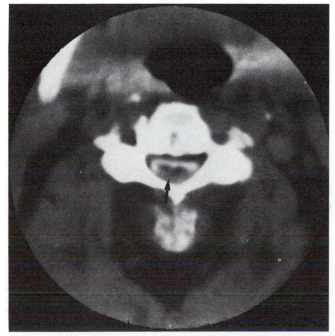

Fig 28–34.—Hypertrophic ligamentum flavum. The myelogram, not reproduced here, revealed a partial block to caudal flow of contrast medium at C3-4. A posterior defect was also noted at the C-3 level. Degenerative changes were seen anteriorly. CTM revealed nonfilling of the subarachnoid space posterior to the spinal cord *(arrow).* The spinal cord is moderately atrophic as well.

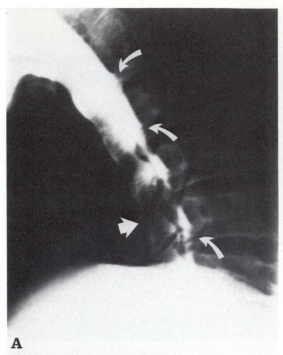

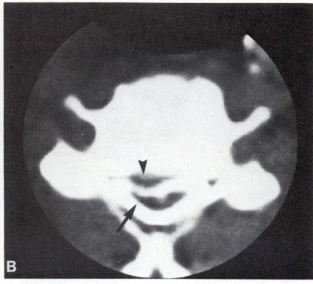

Fig 28–35.—Degenerative changes with right-sided focal atrophy. The lateral myelographic film seen in **A** demonstrates the difficulty of metrizamide myelography. Structures lying in the same axial plane are superimposed, resulting in poor visualization of any particular structure. Delineation of spurs, measurements of AP diameter, and appreciation of spinal cord configuration are difficult. Laterally located root sleeves invariably project anteriorly *(curved arrows)*. In **B,** an axial section at C4-5 *(arrow* on **A,** myelogram), focal cord atrophy is present *(arrow)* adjacent to chronically degenerative soft disc material *(arrowhead).*

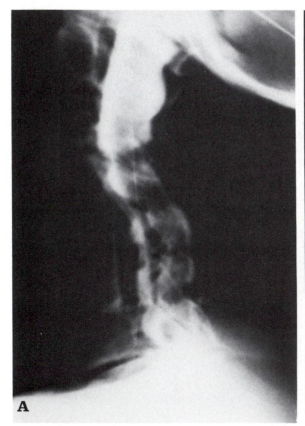

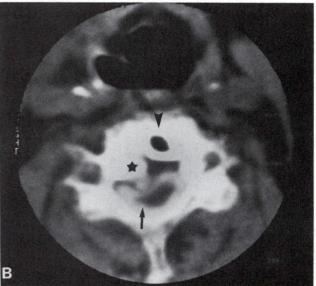

Fig 28–36.—Postoperative cervical fusion with bone plug; hemiatrophy of the spinal cord. A cross table myelographic film in **A** reveals "swan-neck" deformity of the cervical spine with confusing overlap of structures. Cord atrophy is not visible. Measurement points and the effect of the bone plug upon the spinal cord are not visualized very well. CTM in **B** clearly demonstrates hemiatrophy of the cord *(arrow)* and its relationship to the anterior spur *(star)* and the bone plug *(arrowhead).*

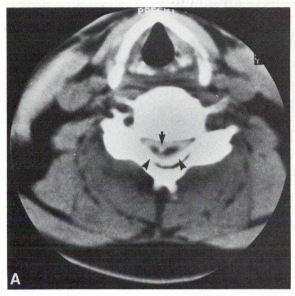

Fig 28–37.—Advanced cord atrophy; adjacent sections 5 mm apart. In **A,** atrophic cord appears nearly fragmented from thinned inner portion *(arrow)*. Subluxation of the lamina above *(arrowheads)* encroaches upon the subarachnoid space from posterior, while in **B** a large spur encroaches from anterior 5 mm caudad *(arrows)*.

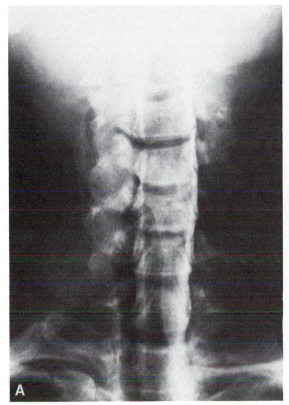

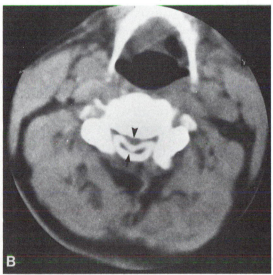

Fig 28–38.—Spurious cord widening; advanced cord atrophy. An AP myelographic film is demonstrated in **A** in this postlaminecotmy patient. Suspicious widening of the cervical spinal cord is noted with relatively little distortion of the root sleeves. The lateral view failed to settle the question. **B,** CTM, however, clearly reveals marked cord atrophy *(arrow)* and probable central disc herniation as well *(arrowhead)*.

amined be reduced to save scan time and patient exposure. The preceding cervical myelogram should act as a guide to determine the levels to be evaluated with CT scanning. Tube exposure factors can be reduced considerably during "dynamic" cervical scanning because of the inherent contrast differences between bone, metrizamide, and soft tissues.

Several examples of myelographic-CTM correlation are shown in the following figures. Bony spur formation may occur centrally or laterally (Fig 28–32). Encroachment by bony spurs arising from the joints of Luschka causes a reduction in the diameter of the intervertebral foramen (Fig 28–33). Root sleeve filling is variable, often occurring bilaterally at multiple levels. Soft-tissue changes are better seen with CTM than with myelography alone (Fig 28–34). Various atrophic changes have been observed in the cord (Figs 28–35 to 28–37). Atrophy may occur focally or generally throughout the cord, and spinal cord compression is easily assessed by CTM. Cord compression has been observed in both a relatively small spinal canal with superimposed degenerative change and in the larger spinal canal with pronounced degenerative alterations. As previously discussed, a myelographic appearance of an intramedullary expansion is occasionally observed secondary to cord compression. The use of CTM rules out an intramedullary mass and demonstrates the etiology of the cord compression (Figs 28–35 and 28–38).

In conclusion, CTM has shown great promise in augmenting the diagnostic evaluation of spinal degenerative diseases and should provide better and safer modes of therapy.

REFERENCES

1. Dublin A.B., McGahan J.P., Reid M.H.: The value of computed tomographic metrizamide myelography in the neuroradiological evaluation of the spine. *Radiology* 146:79–86, 1983.
2. DiChiro G., Schellinger D.: Computed tomography of spinal cord after lumbar intrathecal introduction of metrizamide (computer-assisted myelography). *Radiology* 120:101–104, 1976.
3. Coin C.G., Chan Y.S., Keranen V., et al.: Computed assisted myelography in disk disease. *J. Comput. Assist. Tomogr.* 1:398–404, 1977.
4. Arii H., Takahashi M., Tamakawa Y., et al.: Metrizamide spinal computed tomography following myelography. *Comput. Tomogr.* 4:117–125, 1980.
5. Anand A.K., Lee B.C.P.: Plain and metrizamide CT of lumbar disk disease: Comparison with myelography. *A.J.N.R.* 3:567–571, 1982.
6. Barrow D.L., Wood J.H., Hoffman J.C. Jr.: Clinical indications for computer-assisted myelography. *Neurosurgery* 12:47–57, 1983.
7. Seibert C.E., Barnes J.E., Dreisbach J.N., et al.: Accurate CT measurement of the spinal cord using metrizamide: Physical factors. *A.J.N.R.* 2:75–78, 1981.
8. Paine K.W.E., Huang P.W.H.: Lumbar disc syndrome. *J. Neurosurg.* 37:75–82, 1972.
9. Mall J.C., Kaiser J.A.: Computed tomography of the postoperative spine, in Genant H.K., Chafetz N., Helms C.A., (eds.): *Computed Tomography of the Lumbar Spine.* San Francisco, University of California Printing Department, 1982, pp. 245–252.
10. Thoen D.D., Halversen G.L., Satovick R.M., et al.: *Interpretation of Lumbar Spine CT Scans.* Salt Lake City, WNA Publications, vol. 1, 1982, p. 59.
11. Hirschy J.C., Leue W.M., Berninger W.H., et al.: CT of the lumbosacral spine: Importance of tomographic planes parallel to vertebral end plate. *A.J.R.* 126:47–52, 1981.
12. Teplick J.H., Teplick S.K., Goodman L., et al.: Pitfalls and unusual findings in computed tomography of the lumbar spine. *J. Comput. Assist. Tomogr.* 6:888–893, 1982.
13. Ullrich C.G., Kieffer S.A.: Computed tomographic evaluation of the lumbar spine: Quantitative aspects and sagittal-coronal reconstruction, in Post M.J.D. (ed.): *Radiographic Evaluation of the Spine: Current Advances with Emphasis on Computed Tomography.* New York, Masson Publishing USA, Inc., 1980, pp. 88–107.
14. Arnoldi C.C., Brodsky A.E., Cauchoix J., et al.: *Lumbar Spinal Stenosis and Nerve Root Entrapment Syndromes: Clinical Orthopaedics and Related Research,* no. 115. Philadelphia, J.B. Lippincott, Co., 1976, pp. 4–5.
15. Kirkaldy-Willis W.H., Wedge J.H., Yong-Hing K., et al.: Pathology and pathogenesis of lumbar spondylosis and stenosis. *Spine* 3:319–328, 1978.
16. Lancourt J.E., Glenn W.V., Wiltse L.L.: Multiplanar computerized tomography in the normal spine and in the diagnosis of spinal stenosis: A gross anatomic-computerized tomographic correlation. *Spine* 4:379–390, 1979.
17. Roberson G.H., Liewellyn H.J., Taveras J.M.: The narrow lumbar spinal canal syndrome. *Radiology* 107:89–97, 1973.
18. Verbiest H.: The significance and principles of computerized axial tomography in idiopathic developmental stenosis of the bony lumbar vertebral canal. *Spine* 4:369–378, 1979.
19. McAfee P.C., Ullrich C.G., Yuan A.H., et al.: Computed tomography in degenerative spinal stenosis. *Clin. Orthop.* 161:221–234, 1981.
20. Verbiest H.: Fallacies of the present definition, nomenclature and classification of the stenoses of the lumbar vertebral canal. *Spine* 1:217–225, 1976.
21. Glenn W.V., Rothman S.L.G., Rhodes M.L.: Computed tomography/multiplanar reformatted (CT/MPR) examinations of the lumbar spine, in Genant H.K., Chafetz N., Helms C.A., (eds.): *Computed Tomography of the Lumbar Spine.* San Francisco, University of California Printing Department, 1982, pp. 87–123.
22. Mikhael M.A., Ciric I., Tarkington J.A., et al.: Neuroradiological evaluation of lateral recess syndrome. *Radiology* 140:97–107, 1981.
23. Kirkaldy-Willis W.H., Wedge J.H., Yong-Hing K., et al.:

Lumbar spinal nerve lateral entrapment. *Clin. Orthop.* 169:171–178, 1982.

24. Epstein J.A., Epstein B.S., Rosenthal A.D., et al.: Sciatica caused by nerve root entrapment in the lateral recess: The superior facet syndrome. *J. Neurosurg.* 36:584–589, 1972.

25. Epstein J.A., Epstein B.S., Lavine L.S., et al.: Lumbar nerve root compression at the intervertebral foramina caused by arthritis of the posterior facets. *J. Neurosurg.* 39:362–369, 1973.

26. Ciric I., Mikhael M.A., Tarkington J.A., et al.: The lateral recess syndrome: A variant of spinal stenosis. *J. Neurosurg.* 53:433–443, 1980.

27. Reynolds A.F., Weinstein P.R., Wachter R.D.: Lumbar monoradiculopathy due to unilateral facet hypertrophy. *Neurosurgery* 10:480–486, 1982.

28. Eldevik O.P., Dugstad G., Orrison W.W., et al.: The effect of clinical bias on the interpretation of myelography and spinal computed tomography. *Radiology* 145:85–89, 1982.

29. Marzluff J.M., Hungerford G.D., Kempe L.G., et al.: Thoracic myelopathy caused by osteophytes of the articular processes: Thoracic spondylosis. *J. Neurosurg.* 50:779–783, 1979.

30. Omojola M.F., Cardoso E.R., Fox A.J., et al.: Thoracic myelopathy secondary to ossified ligamentum flavum: Case report. *J. Neurosurg.* 56:448–450, 1982.

31. Williams D.M., Gabrielsen T.O., Latack J.T.: Ossification in the caudal attachments of the ligamentum flavum: An anatomic and computed tomographic study. *Radiology* 145:693–697, 1982.

32. Miyasaka K., Kaneda K., Ito T., et al.: Ossification of spinal ligaments causing thoracic radiculomyelopathy. *Radiology* 143:463–468, 1982.

33. Murakami J., Russell W.J., Hayabuchi N., et al.: Computed tomography of posterior longitudinal ligament ossification: Its appearance and diagnostic value with special reference to thoracic lesions. *J. Comput. Assist. Tomogr.* 6:41–50, 1982.

34. Ono M., Russell W.J., Kudo S., et al.: Ossification of the thoracic posterior longitudinal ligament in a fixed population: Radiological and neurological manifestations. *Radiology* 143:469–474, 1982.

35. Hyman R.A., Merten C.W., Liebeskind A.L., et al.: Computed tomography in ossification of the posterior longitudinal spinal ligament. *Neuroradiology* 13:227–228, 1977.

36. Rappaport Z.H., Rovit R.: Ossification of the posterior longitudinal spinal ligament in association with anterior longitudinal ligament ankylosing hyperostosis: Case report. *Neurosurgery* 4:175–177, 1979.

37. Scotti G., Scialfa G., Pieralli S., et al.: Myeloradiculopathies in cervical spondylosis: The relative value of myelography and CT in the radiologic diagnosis. Presented at the XII Symposium Neuroradiologicum, Washington, D.C., October 1982.

38. Nakagawa H., Okumura T., Sugiyama T., et al.: The discrepancy between metrizamide CT and myelography in diagnosis of cervical soft disc protrusion. Presented at the XII Symposium Neuroradiologicum, Washington, D.C., October 1982.

39. Mawad M.E., Hilal S.K., Fetell M., et al.: Patterns of spinal cord atrophy on metrizamide CT. Presented at the XII Symposium Neuroradiologicum, Washington, D.C., October 1982.

40. Yu Y.-L., Stevens J.M., Kendall B., et al.: Cervical cord shape and measurements in cervical spondylotic myelopathy and radiculopathy (CSMR). Presented at the XII Symposium Neuroradiologicum, Washington, D.C., October 1982.

29

CT Evaluation of the Postoperative Spine

John D. Meyer, M.D.

The postoperative lumbar spine patient with symptoms may profit considerably from a thorough and comprehensive reevaluation. Myelography has been the traditional diagnostic radiographic technique for evaluating the intraspinal contents and still provides an excellent method for visualization of the lumbar spinal canal, including the region of the conus and lower dorsal spinal cord. It is often necessary to see these regions of the spine in the postoperative patient. Demonstration of regional bony anatomical relationships in the commonly used myelographic projections may be important as well in evaluating the complete picture. One cause of the "failed back" is operation at the wrong level. This commonly arises secondary to transitional vertebra formation, which is easily assessed by plain radiographic or myelographic filming. However, postmyelographic and postoperative alterations make myelographic diagnosis of recurrent herniated disc difficult. The anatomical changes of scarring and arachnoiditis on myelograms performed with either iophendylate or water-soluble contrast agents have been previously described.[1-30]

High-resolution CT scanning has extended the range of appreciation of the complexity of the spine. Developmental variations, degenerative alterations, and the changes produced by acute and chronic disc disease may now be studied routinely with CT. The anatomy of the lumbar spine may be evaluated by standard axial and reformatted techniques,[31-36] and a general awareness of the axial anatomy is growing. A great contribution to the diagnosis of disc disease has been realized,[37-46] and CT examinations may supplant, at least partially, the utilization of myelography in the diagnosis of the herniated disc in the unoperated back.

Because of the alteration of the intraspinal soft tissues by previous surgical procedures, producing scar formation and arachnoiditis, plain CT scanning of the postoperative back may be very confusing. Deformity of the thecal sac by scar tissue may simulate recurrent herniated disc; recurrent herniation may be masked by changes of the thecal sac and nerve roots from the previous surgery. Anecdotal reports referring to postoperative changes on the plain CT have appeared recently,[47-50] but a consistent and reliable set of criteria to differentiate herniated disc and scar tissue on the plain scan has been difficult to accumulate. More recently, various reports have stressed the value of CT evaluation following myelography in these confusing cases in order to better define the intraspinal anatomical structures and their alterations.[51-55] Scanning the back by CT following instillation of a water-soluble contrast material affords the most complete evaluation of the postoperative spine.

This chapter is divided into two major sections. The appearance of the plain CT scan in the postoperative patient will be thoroughly discussed. Following this, our experience in a large group of postoperative patients who have undergone both myelography and postmyelographic CT scanning will be presented. The techniques of postmyelographic CT are discussed, along with the diagnostic criteria for differentiating herniated disc from scar tissue.

THE PLAIN CT EXAMINATION

Plain CT scanning may be useful as a single diagnostic examination. Significant bony abnormalities secondary to spinal stenosis are fairly easy to image. Large herniated discs, whether recurrent or new, may be easily seen as well. Figures 29–1 and 29–2 demonstrate these points. One of the patterns observed in epidural scar formation can be fairly easily seen and identified by plain CT scan (Fig 29–3). The plain CT scan is most useful for a patient on whom only one laminectomy has been performed. In this case, the least amount of anatomical distortion is present. Usefulness, however, de-

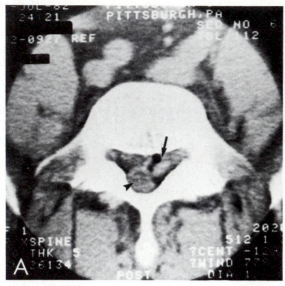

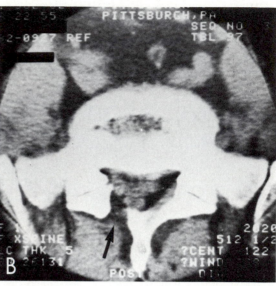

Fig 29–1.—Recurrent herniated disc—operatively proved. **A,** the section of the L-5 body level reveals extruded fragment of disc *(arrow)* containing gas found incidentally from degenerative changes in the disc. Thecal sac *(arrowhead)* shows some distortion. **B,** same patient slightly below the level of **A** reveals laminectomy site *(arrow).* At this level, configuration of intraspinal contents is confusing, a problem in noncontrasted postoperative CT scans. Note absence of ligamentum flavum on operated side.

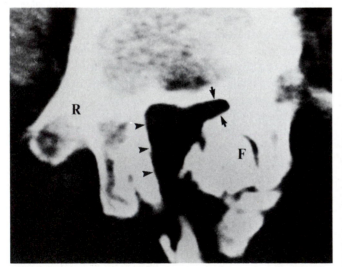

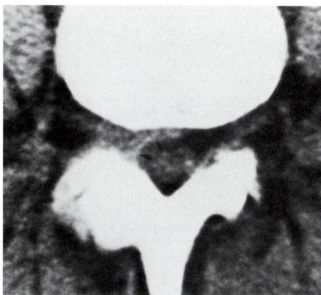

Fig 29–2.—Plain CT—partial decompression for spinal stenosis. On the patient's right side *(R),* a laminectomy and partial facetectomy have been performed. The edge of bone resection is clearly seen *(arrowheads).* On the left side, facet joint *(F)* remains enlarged secondary to degenerative changes. This facet decreases the transverse diameter of the canal from the left side. Lateral recess *(between arrows)* is somewhat narrowed.

Fig 29–3.—Extradural scar—plain CT. CT image reveals a density both anterior and lateral to the thecal sac sharply demarcated by a curved border *(arrows),* but no distortion or displacement of the thecal sac. The density extends into the intervertebral foramen.

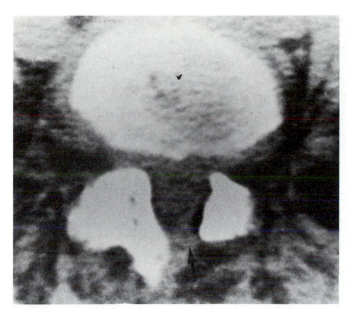

Fig 29–4.—Plain CT showing confusing pattern following multiple operations including decompressive laminectomy. *Arrow* indicates bony defect from operation. Intraspinal contents including thecal sac, extradural tissues, and disc border are indistinguishable, a common problem.

creases as the number of operations increases, because more complicated patterns of distortion are observed. These complicated distortion patterns tend to reduce visualization of the thecal sac and root sleeves. Good visualization of these structures is necessary for evaluation of the numerous and subtle alterations present in the postoperative spine. Herniated disc material may be present in the same location as scar tissue and may be difficult to differentiate from it. Herniated disc may also occur in a new location removed from an area of previous operation. In cases of multiple operation, con-

fusing patterns of scar tissue with or without herniated disc may be present (Fig 29–4).

Epidural scar tissue may be relatively radiolucent or radiodense on the plain CT scan. A tendency toward radiolucency has been observed by the author, but density difference has not seemed to be a reliable criterion (Fig 29–5). Intravenous contrast material has been advocated as a method to differentiate disc herniation from epidural scar tissue, because scar tissue tends to enhance, while disc material does not (Figs 29–6 and 29–7).[36] It is likely that the epidural veins, dura, and granulation tissue (present during healing with or without operative intervention) would likely contribute to the intraspinal enhancement pattern following intravenous infusion and make differentiation from scar tissue more difficult (Fig 29–8). To this is coupled the usual complex bony anatomy. While reliable criteria concerning the value of intravenous contrast material may be forthcoming, at present there is insufficient data to indicate its value in differentiating herniated disc from scar tissue.

Abundant literature has accumulated on spinal stenosis.[54–64] Plain CT examination may be useful in evaluating the presence and degree of stenosis in the postoperative patient. The amount and configuration of remaining abnormal bone following a limited decompression may be assessed, as seen in Figure 29–2, and careful analysis of the lateral recesses and intervertebral foramina can be performed. The technique of data reformatting may prove to be essential for these lateral portions of the canal and foramina in order to better visualize their configuration and size. It has been reported that fusion bone may occasionally produce a central spinal stenosis pattern.[64] Evaluation by plain CT is fairly straightforward in this matter. The degree of decompression of a stenotic spinal canal may be as-

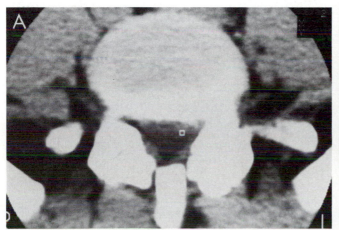
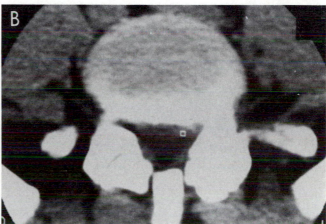

Fig 29–5.—Unreliability of CT numbers. In **A**, anterior portion of the intraspinal contents are not obviously distinguishable. Region of interest average CT number was 35. In **B**, a region of interest just a few pixels away measured 71. Separating herniated disc and scar tissue by quantitative determination is unreliable.

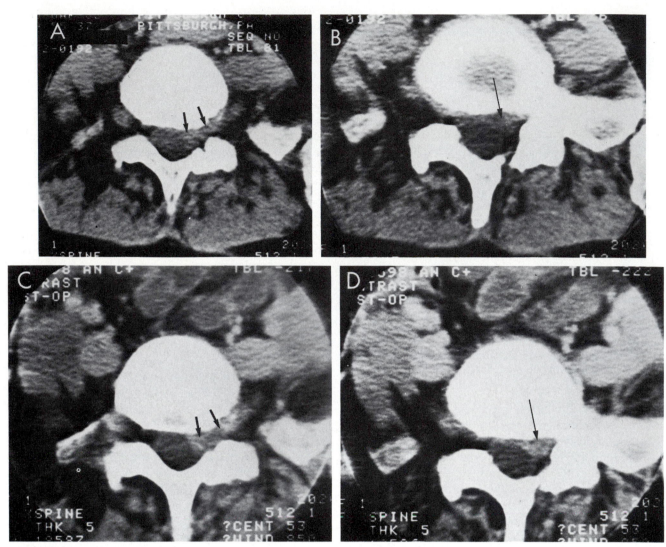

Fig 29–6.—Enhancement of presumed scar tissue. **A, B,** adjacent sections of the lumbosacral junction reveal slightly hyperdense anterolateral epidural tissue that extends into the intervertebral foramen (**A,** *short arrows;* **B,** *long arrow*). **C, D,** after intravenous contrast, the epidural tissue enhances (**C,** *short arrows;* **D,** *long arrow*). Note absence of displacement or distortion of the thecal sac.

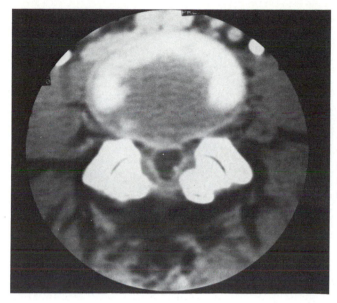

Fig 29–7.—Enhancement of scar tissue. This 45-year-old woman had had multiple laminectomies for both tumor (neurofibromatosis) and herniated disc. Attempted lumbar puncture produced exquisite pain, terminating the procedure in favor of an intravenously enhanced CT study. The scan shows diffuse enhancing epidural scar at this level, with pronounced enhancement of the margins of the thecal sac. An enhancing neurofibroma was seen at a lower level.

sessed much more accurately than in the days prior to CT examination. It may be, in fact, that many of the cases of "recurrent" stenosis secondary to new bone growth following decompression are due only to inadequate decompression in the first place.

Fusion bone may become unstable if a pseudarthrosis develops. This may not, however, be symptomatic or significant by itself.[65] Scanning by CT has limited usefulness in assessing this instability, because the plane of best evaluation lies perpendicular to the axial scanning plane. Either pluridirectional tomography or reformatted imaging with flexion and extension views might

provide a better evaluation. Axial CT scanning may detect instability from "fragmentation" or actual poor bony union of the fusion bone or other bone (Fig 29–9). In addition, evaluation of lumbar levels above the level of spinal fusion can be performed. At these levels, degenerative changes tend to occur more frequently and may be more likely to become symptomatic.

Complex anatomical variations of the facet joints can now be adequately studied. These joints themselves may be responsible for much back pain and patterns of referred pain that mimic herniated disc. Facet joint arthropathies tend to occur with aging of the spine and

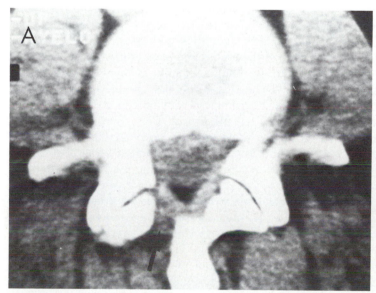
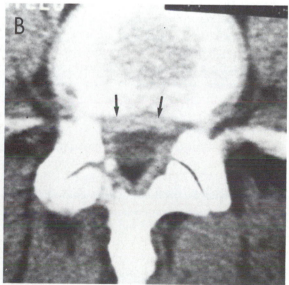

Fig 29–8.—Enhancement of the extradural space. In **A,** plain CT without contrast reveals indistinguishable anterior extradural contents. Laminectomy site marked by *arrow.* In **B,** after intravenous contrast material, anterior extradural tissue uniformly enhanced *(arrows),* but scar tissue, possible granulation tissue, veins, and position of the roots are still not distinguishable.

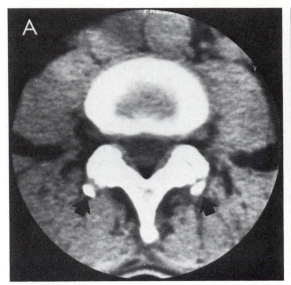 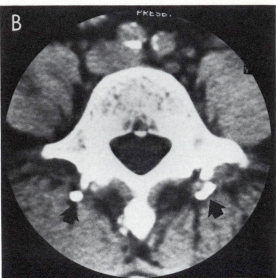

Fig 29–9.—Fusion failure. Plain CT scans through the L-5 and L5-S1 level **(A, B)** indicate no evidence of bony fu-sion. Bone placed at operation fails to show union with the spine *(arrows)*.

may certainly be associated with herniated disc. The relationship of the posterior arches to the facet joint and the spinal canal can be evaluated more precisely. This is useful in distinguishing among the various anatomical variations in the posterior arches and facets in order to elucidate the many possibilities for root entrapment. Minor congenital variations may also be studied better by CT examination than by previous methods. A recent report[66] has indicated that CT scanning was *not* useful in evaluating lumbar monoradiculopathy in cases where it would have been valuable. This may be partly due to inexperience with CT scanning of the spine, and with passage of time some of these problems may disappear.

An occasional patient will demonstrate a markedly hypertrophic ligamentum flavum. This may occur in young people and may be a cause of pain and radicular signs by itself or in combination with bony stenosis.[67] Knowledge of the normal variations in size of the ligamentum flavum is necessary at this point in time to assess its significance in the various stenosis syndromes.

An unusual cause of pain and possible neurologic deficit following operation is the formation of a pseudo-meningocele.[68–72] Plain CT examination should provide sufficient data for evaluating this pathologic entity. In doubtful or confusing cases, the addition of metriza-mide would certainly be helpful. A small outpouching of the dura following a laminectomy is very commonly noted in the postoperative spine. This needs to be distinguished from the pseudomeningocele, which is larger and possibly symptomatic.

Not only may CT aid in evaluation of the later post-operative state, but also the early period in which hemorrhage and infection are possibilities. Epidural hem-orrhage may occasionally be seen as a radiodense area that may extend along the epidural space similar to other epidural lesions and possibly produce a block to the flow of contrast medium. The use of CT may be helpful in this regard in delineating the density of the material and the extent of the compressive phenome-non. Radiographic evaluation of disc space infection, in addition to plain film and pluridirectional tomographic findings, may show intraspinal and paraspinal mass ef-fect that is better evaluated by CT scanning than other methods.

In summary, plain CT examination of the postopera-tive lumbar spine can accurately define general bony spinal canal configuration and size as well as detailed anatomy of the arches and facet joints. Large herniated discs may be noted not only at levels previously ex-plored, but also at levels not operated upon. Various scarring patterns may be demonstrated. The limitations of plain CT scanning result from complicated patterns of dural-arachnoid scarring with possible concomitant herniated disc material. In a lumbar spine of relatively small size, or one demonstrating marked degenerative changes, or both, these postoperative changes may not be interpretable without additional study utilizing me-trizamide. In such a case, the root sleeves and thecal sac may be filled with contrast material and thus allow for evaluation of subtle distortion. In the following sec-tion, the technique of metrizamide CT myelography, diagnostic criteria, and findings are discussed in a rela-tively large group of patients. As the tabular data indi-cate, this technique offers an excellent chance for a thorough reappraisal of the postoperative lumbar spine.

COMPUTED TOMOGRAPHIC MYELOGRAPHY (CTM)

Technique

Standard metrizamide lumbar myelography is performed utilizing the 190 mg/ml concentration in a volume of 10 to 12 ml. During the examination, no additional testing is performed, such as flexion or extension views, lateral bending, or weight bearing. Examination includes the conus and lower dorsal canal area. In general, delayed filming is not utilized, but in some cases it may be valuable, because metrizamide has a tendency to slowly enter spaces that are relatively "tight." It has been noted that root sleeves may fill better after waiting approximately 30 minutes, and subarachnoid spaces beyond a block may be much better visualized following a short delay.

Following the routine myelogram, the CT examination should be performed on a high-resolution scanner. This is best performed within 4 hours to avoid losing radiodensity of contrast material from the canal. An ideal time for CT scanning lies somewhere between overconcentration, seen immediately after the myelogram, and underconcentration, noted after a few hours. At this ideal time, the density of metrizamide is not so high as to obscure detail or generate excessive artifact (Fig 29–10), and spaces that might have filled slowly are filled best. Metrizamide may be uniformly distributed in the spinal canal, or it may pool in the dependent portion of the canal in some patients. This may be eliminated by turning the patient once or twice. The CT is performed supine to strictly maintain the same position during the examination. Breathing motions of the spine tend to be aggravated with the patient prone, and this position is not utilized. The legs are kept straight with the thighs unflexed.

Adjacent sections at 5-mm intervals are almost always obtained through the L5-S1 and L4-5 interspaces, with other levels scanned depending on specific needs. Scanning should be performed from pedicle to pedicle, thereby including a complete evaluation of the spine in the region examined. This is necessary, because scar tissue tends to spread along the epidural spaces adjacent to the vertebral bodies. Herniated disc material may also migrate as a free fragment. The scanner gantry is angled so that the beam is parallel to the disc, thus minimizing volume averaging. The scan may be performed by not changing the gantry angle, in which case better reformatted images are obtained. In some instances, overlapping sections or thinner sections are necessary to clarify problems arising in reference to the lateral recess or intervertebral foramen. In this instance, reformatting techniques might be applicable, depending partly on individual radiologists' needs and the needs of operating surgeons who may be more familiar with the reformatted anatomical arrangement. High-mAs images are necessary to perfectly image anatomical detail and separate tissue density differences. Density measurements, while not entirely reliable in the first place, are even less reliable lateral to the metrizamide column, where secondary beam hardening artifact occurs (see Fig 29–10). Because *mass effect* is the main parameter sought, density measurements are less important. Additional discussion concerning density measurement follows.

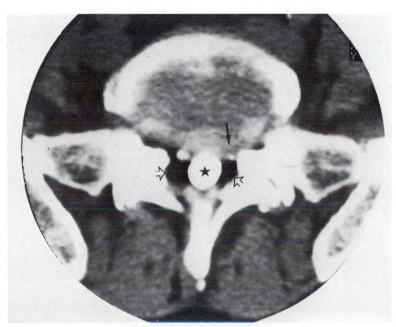

Fig 29–10.—Beam hardening lucent artifact. Dense, pooled metrizamide collection *(star)* is flanked by pronounced hypodense areas *(open arrows)* lateral to the contrast column secondary to beam hardening. This causes difficulty distinguishing tissue of lesser density, but may be eliminated by waiting longer before CT following the myelogram. A herniated disc is denoted by the *closed arrow.*

In general, canal physical measurements such as area and diameter have not been utilized, although they are easy to obtain. With respect to judging physical size in spinal stenosis, the physical appearance remains the more useful factor. Quantitative studies have been performed by others (see references in preceding chapter) on the lumbar spine and may be of some value.

Utilizing the techniques described above, over 140 postoperative patients have been studied. Of these, 56 have been operated upon. Operative results and a discussion of the data are presented below.

Diagnostic Criteria

Myelography

Myelographic findings alone are not very reliable for the differentiation of scar tissue and herniated disc in the postoperative patient. A strong tendency is observed for herniated disc material to produce a focal extradural mass on the thecal sac (Fig 29–11). Believed to be the best myelographic finding in the past for differentiation of scar and disc, this sign is fairly reliable, but conspicuous exceptions are found (see Figs 29–18 and 29–19). On the other hand, very large focal myelographic defects, those typical of extradural masses located at the disc space, are almost always secondary to herniated disc material (see Fig 29–11).

In the study group, two patients had a *second* recurrent herniated disc at the same operative site on the same side. Both of these also had some scar tissue present at operation, but large disc fragments were found as well. Both had large focal masses. Density measurements on CT were misleading in these two patients, because the focal masses were relatively radiolucent.

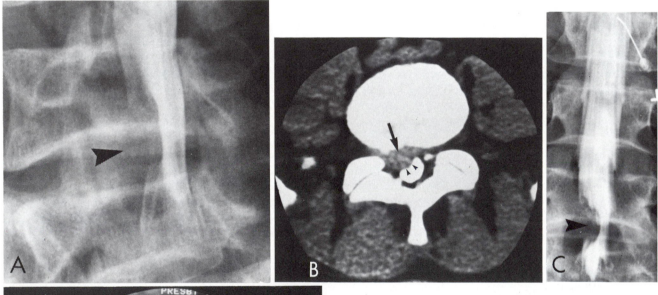

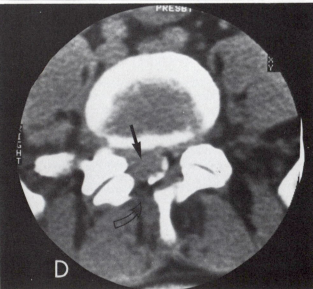

Fig 29–11.—Herniated disc in postoperative patient. **A, B,** new herniated disc at L4-5. In **A,** oblique myelographic film reveals prominent extradural defect *(arrowhead)* and no filling of the nerve root sleeve of L-5. In **B,** CT scan through the same level, the *arrow* indicates a "mass" of disc density related to the disc space with failure of filling of the root sleeve and compression of the thecal sac *(arrowheads)*. **C, D,** same patient several months later shows recurrent herniated disc at the same level—operatively proved. In **C,** very large typical extradural defect is noted *(arrowhead)*. In **D,** very large "mass" of disc density related to this disc space causes marked distortion of the thecal sac *(closed arrow)*. Laminectomy site is indicated by *open arrow*.

Preliminary studies (from unpublished data) indicate a tendency for herniated disc material and scar tissue to occur together.

Either scar tissue or disc herniation has a tendency to produce unfilled root sleeves singly or in combination. This, of course, is the main problem in diagnosis utilizing myelography alone. Metrizamide generally allows for somewhat better filling of the thecal sac and root sleeves than does the oily contrast material used in the past, but this advantage is not sufficiently reliable to allow for resolution of the problem of scar vs. disc.

All of the commonly noted myelographic deformities seen in the postoperative lumbar spine that have been described in the literature were seen in this study group. Specific myelographic findings had little predictive value in the postsurgical outcome. Complete myelographic block was observed in some patients, requiring CT scanning below the block for further evaluation. For example, the contrast in one patient was placed in the cervical subarachnoid space and allowed to pass a thoracic block secondary to arachnoiditis. It was observed below the block *24 hours* after the myelogram and allowed for elimination of recurrent herniated disc as a cause for the patient's symptoms.

CTM

HERNIATED DISC.—Disc material may be considered herniated (either because of recurrent prolapse or a new herniation) if a smooth and rounded mass of the same relative density as disc material is found in relation to the disc space (Figs 29–11 and 29–12). This description is narrowly defined, but adherence to its limits has proved to be fruitful, as the data demonstrate.

The definition, *mass of disc density related to the disc space,* differs from the definition of epidural scar in that scar tissue does not appear to be present solely as a focal mass of disc density related to the disc space itself. Epidural scar tends to spread beyond the limits of the disc space and have a rather irregular appearance. In the case of herniated disc material, the focal mass effect displaces the root sleeves and distorts or displaces the thecal sac. These findings are similar to those of the herniated disc in the nonoperated back.

When both criteria (focal mass that displaces both the thecal sac and root sleeves) are present, no difficulty is encountered in the diagnosis. If root sleeves are poorly visualized, but the thecal sac is distorted by a mass of disc-like density, no problem is generally encountered either. A problem arises, however, when root sleeves are either not seen or poorly visualized, but minimally displaced, and the thecal sac is minimally distorted. In this case, the annulus may simply "bulge" (Fig 29–13). A small number of cases of scarring also show no displacement of the thecal sac with unfilled and nondisplaced root sleeves. A diagnosis of disc herniation cannot be made in these groups. A similar problem is encountered in the unoperated spine.

A "bulging disc" by CT scan may contain herniated disc material, but not be visible as such, and it has been noted that at operation a bulging disc may certainly be related to root compression. The bulging disc may be associated with facet encroachment accompanied by a small spinal canal or a "tight" root exit zone. These findings are difficult to evaluate in the unoperated back and are even more difficult in the postoperative spine, because there is less fatty tissue present as a natural contrast agent.

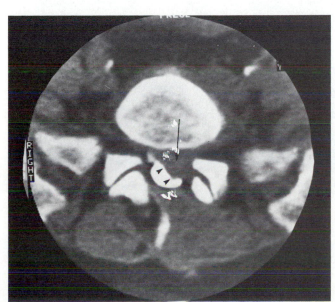

Fig 29–12.—Recurrent herniated disc—operatively proved. Myelogram is unavailable. "Mass" of disc density related to the disc space *(arrow)* causes prominent distortion of the thecal sac *(arrowheads).*

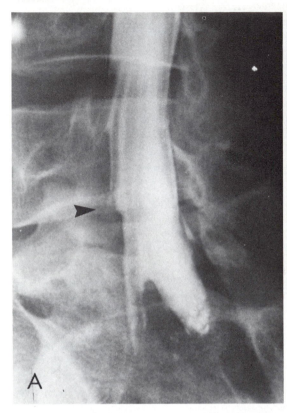

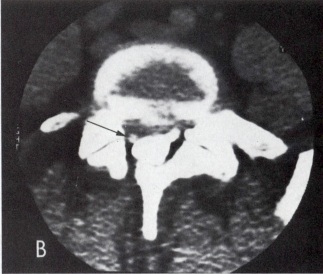

Fig 29–13.—Bulging disc without extrusion causing root pressure—operatively proved. In **A,** an oblique myelographic spot film reveals nonfilling of the L-5 root sleeve *(arrowhead).* Differential possibilities on this film alone include scar tissue or recurrent herniated disc. In **B,** the root sleeve *(arrow)* does contain contrast medium and is somewhat posteriorly displaced. At operation, a non-extruded bulging disc was found.

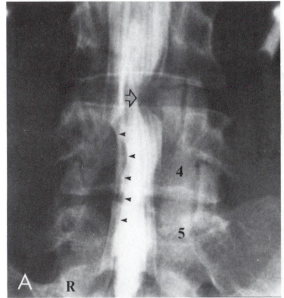

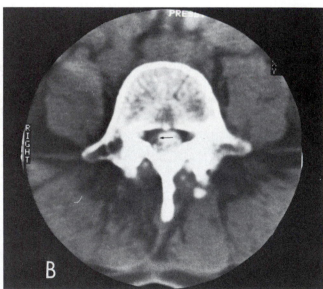

Fig 29–14.—Scar tissue only proved at operation at L-4 and L-5 on the right side. In **A,** an AP myelographic film reveals an elongated and irregular, wavy extradural density *(arrowheads)* through the L-4 *(4)* and L-5 *(5)* regions. *(R =* patient's right.) In **B** through **F,** CT images were obtained approximately at the levels of the *arrowheads* noted in **A** through the L-4 and L-5 regions. In **B,** right lateral irregular extradural density is noted and is continuous with the lateral defect through the series. This is seen in **C** and **D** and in-dicated by the *large arrow.* In **E,** *arrows* indicate the poste-rior margin of the disc space to which is related no specific focal density. Throughout the series, the *small arrows* over-lying the thecal sac reveal the intradural component of the scar pattern. On the myelogram **(A),** there is a prominent focal extradural defect on the left at L3-4 *(open arrows).* The CT scan **(G)** reveals only very minor bulging of the disc. At operation, minor disc bulging similar to the CT was found.

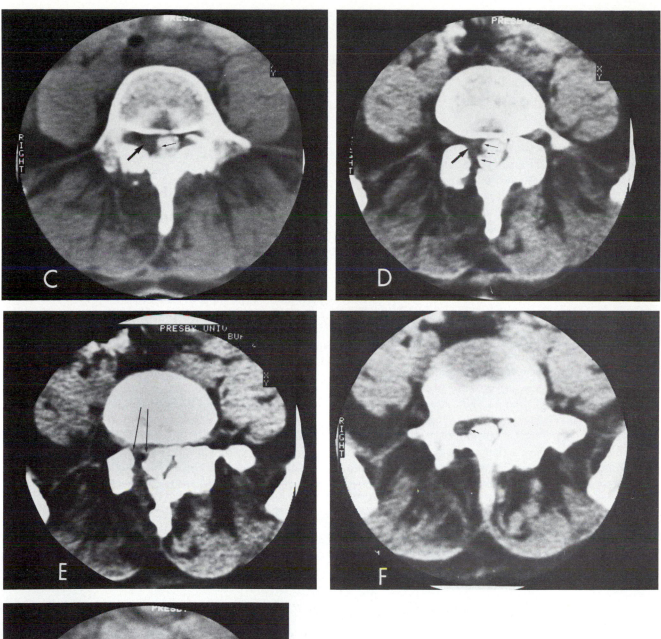

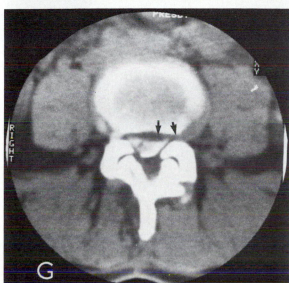

Fig 29–14 cont.

SCAR TISSUE.—Unlike herniated disc, scar tissue tends to produce elongated and irregular areas of epidural density (Fig 29–14). Although a small focal density may be present, it is continuous with epidural tissue found in relation to portions of the vertebral body and not necessarily the disc space, per se. This epidural tissue continues into the intervertebral foramen on occasion. Patterns in CT include angular and kinked distortion of the thecal sac and may involve the lateral aspects of the sac (Figs 29–15 and 29–16). The pattern seen with the herniated disc, focal density related to the disc space, is not generally seen with scar tissue.

Scar tissue occurs in both intradural and extradural locations. The intradural type (arachnoiditis) may cause matting or clumping of two or more nerve roots (Figs 29–16,B and C, and 29–17). Blunted, shortened root sleeves may occur secondary to intradural changes alone, or they may be associated with extradural scarring. A single unfilled root sleeve without displacement is difficult to evaluate, but is presumably secondary to scar tissue. This pattern is uncommon, however.

A tendency is observed for better filling of the intradural spaces on CTM than on plain myelography alone. Metrizamide flows into relatively "tight" spaces over time so that they may be better filled by the time of the CT scan. This means that root sleeves may appear to be better filled on the CT scan, allowing for a more accurate evaluation of their displacement. In addition,

intradural scar tissue may be penetrated or suffused with metrizamide. This produces an appearance of a "normal" spinal level on the CT scan following a myelogram that appears distinctly abnormal (Fig 29–18). Such a process also produces differentiation of scar tissue and disc herniation by CT.

INDETERMINATE.—The category called "indeterminate" is identified if the thecal sac is encircled by a dense and homogeneous tissue with no focal indentation on the sac and no visualization of root sleeves (Fig 29–19). Surprisingly, this pattern is unusual, allowing for classification of almost all levels scanned into a category that has treatment relevance. This indeterminate pattern may represent only epidural scar tissue possibly related to spinal stenosis; however, no firm pathologic correlation is possible at this time.

Results of the Study Group

Table 29–1 presents the findings in the 56 reoperated patients. It is apparent that the criteria describing herniated discs in the postoperative patient are reliable, because a very good operative correlation was found. In fact, all the herniated discs were identified and proved at operation. One case diagnosed as a recurrent herniated disc was found to represent a new herniation, and one suspected new herniation preoperatively was actually a recurrent herniation. Two cases of "bulging" disc were reported as epidural scarring by the surgeon.

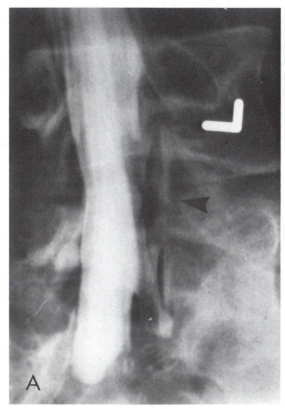
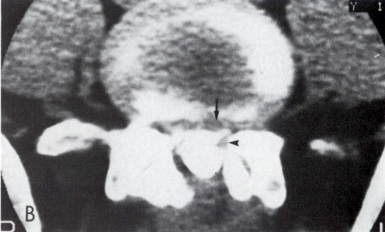

Fig 29–15.—Scar only—operatively proved. In **A,** oblique myelographic spot film, there is an unfilled L-5 nerve root sleeve *(arrowhead)*. Also noted is an irregular defect on the contour of the contrast column at the same level. These findings are nonspecific. In **B,** CT scan shows only a lateral defect *(arrowhead)* with an intact posterior disc margin *(arrow)*. At operation, no herniated disc material was found, only scar tissue along the L-5 nerve root sleeve.

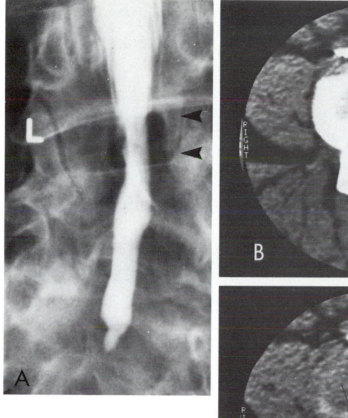

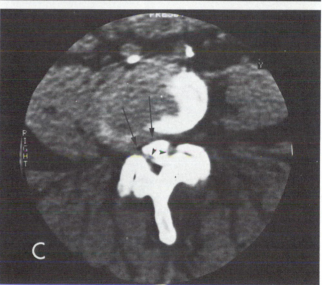

Fig 29–16.—Scar tissue pattern not operatively proved. In **A,** the AP myelographic film reveals lack of symmetry and poor filling of the thecal sac with irregular defects. *Arrowheads* indicate approximate levels of the CT scans shown in **B** and **C.** Note the patient has slight scoliosis. In both **B** and **C,** the posterior disc margin is intact *(arrows),* revealing the value of CTM. *Arrowheads* **(B, C)** indicate intradural scarring with matting of the nerve roots.

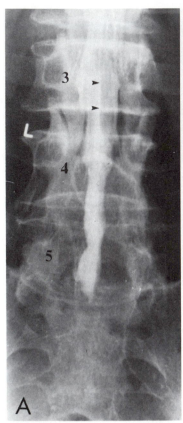

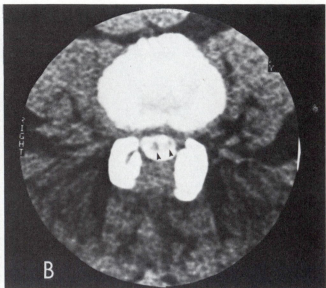

Fig 29–17.—Intradural scar. In **A,** an AP myelographic film reveals irregular poor filling of the lower portion of the thecal sac from the middle of L-4 caudally (3–5 = L₃, L₄, and L₅). At the L-3 and L3-4 level, matted nerve roots are noted also *(arrowheads).* This finding is commonly observed following operation.

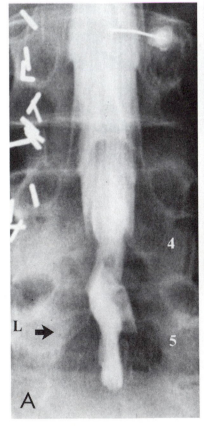

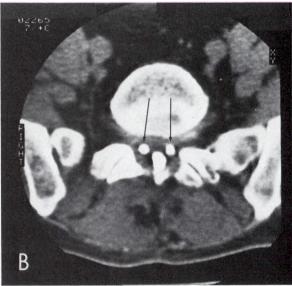

Fig 29–18.—Markedly abnormal myelogram with normal CT scan following. In **A,** an AP myelographic film reveals poor filling of the thecal sac and nerve root sleeves, nonspecific findings, however (4 and 5 = L₄ and L₅). *Arrow* indicates level of CT image in **B.** (L = patient's left.) Photo **B** reveals good filling of the root sleeves and an intact posterior disc margin *(arrows),* ruling out herniated disc. Filled nerve root sleeves are much more commonly noted at CT following metrizamide myelogram than on the myelogram itself.

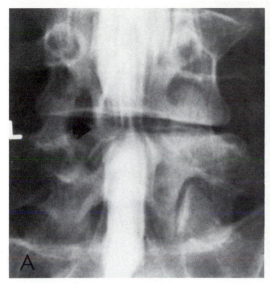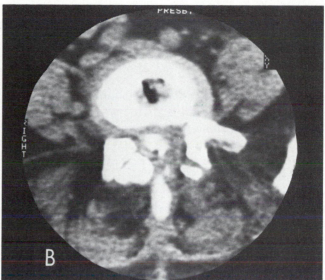

Fig 29–19.—Indeterminate pattern. In **A,** AP myelographic film reveals focal narrowing through the L4-5 level with bilateral extradural defects *(arrow).* Degenerative changes are also noted at the disc level with narrowing of the disc space more on the patient's right side. In **B,** CT scan through the level near the *arrow* in **A** reveals poor filling of the thecal sac, which is irregularly deformed by non-specific changes. These may be "fibrous," stenotic alterations accompanied by thickened extradural tissues with no distinguishing characteristics. The disc, in addition, appears to bulge. This pattern is relatively uncommon in the postoperative spine, and usually the CTM will settle questions arising at myelography.

TABLE 29–1.—Major Operative Findings at
Principal Level in 56 Patients

DIAGNOSIS	PREOPERATIVE	POSTOPERATIVE
Recurrent herniated disc	24	23
New herniated disc	6	7
"Bulging" disc	10	8
Scar	6	8
Central canal stenosis	2	2
Lateral canal stenosis	4	4
Indeterminate	4	3–Stenosis
		1–Unknown
Normal	0	0

There may be some confusion in terms when attempting correlation of operative findings and CT myelographic findings. In these two patients, it might have been difficult for the surgeon to identify a bulge in the presence of scarring. In patients who demonstrated scarring preoperatively, operations were performed because CT evaluation did not allow for a definitive diagnosis of scar *and only scar.*

In the patients not reoperated upon (84 patients), there were a few cases diagnosed radiographically as recurrent or new herniated disc. These patients were either too ill to operate upon or their herniated discs were not believed to be significant enough to warrant reexploration. There were several cases of spinal stenosis noted also. None of the patients had evidence of "postfusion" stenosis. It was noted as well that the spinal stenosis observed in the postoperative patient is very similar to that seen in the nonoperated spine. Both central canal stenosis and lateral recess narrowing were found.

There were a few patients whose findings were indeterminate by CT (criteria discussed above). As noted, these were probably due to spinal stenosis accompanied by some fibrous "perithecal" scarring in the epidural space.

More importantly, a large number of levels were found by CT to be without evidence of herniated disc when the myelograms at the same levels were abnormal. The abnormal myelograms ranged from single unfilled root sleeves to multiple, bilateral areas of irregular filling of the thecal sac and root sleeves. The changes on these myelograms were nonspecific. This group was especially important because unnecessary reoperation was avoided.

In the patients demonstrating spinal stenosis, the findings were confirmed operatively. Of those that demonstrated indeterminate radiographic findings preoperatively, three demonstrated spinal stenosis at operation. The fourth patient had findings that were unclear even at operation. Obviously, in the final analysis, it must be the operating surgeon who determines the degree of spinal stenosis and other findings as well. A certain lack of clarity may be a problem at operation in general. It is often difficult for the individual performing an operation to explore the spine with the same degree of precision that CT findings indicate should be possible. It is likely that the numerous subtleties seen by CT examination cannot be readily perceived through a small and deep operative wound. In addition, a combination of bulging annulus, small spinal canal, and "tight nerve roots" may be found at operation with no single component predominating.[73] Hence, there arises some difficulty correlating diagnostic and operative findings in a few cases. It would be ideal if CT routinely demonstrated root tension or root relaxation as well as anatomical changes.

There is evidence that a good result after spinal surgery tends to decrease in frequency with an increasing number of operations. The data supporting this, however, were gathered prior to the days of CT scanning and often prior to extensive utilization of water-soluble contrast material. It would appear, therefore, that some improvement in the operative results might follow identification of more specific pathologic alterations now made possible by refined diagnostic techniques. For this reason, detailed and thorough examination of the postoperative spine is essential in bringing about better results.

In conclusion, evaluation of the postoperative lumbar spine has been made much easier by the advent of CT scanning, especially accompanied by CT scanning with metrizamide. These newer diagnostic techniques accompanied by improved surgical techniques, better patient selection, and decreasing use of oily contrast material should cause a marked decrease in the morbidity involved in the evaluation and treatment of the postoperative lumbar spine.

REFERENCES

1. Elkington J.ST.C.: Meningitis serosa circumscripta spinalis (spinal arachnoiditis). *Brain* 59:181–203, 1936.
2. Knutsson E.: The myelogram following operation for herniated disc. *Acta Radiol.* 32:60–65, 1947.
3. Smolik E.A., Nash F.P.: Lumbar spinal arachnoiditis: A complication of the intervertebral disc operation. *Ann. Surg.* 133:490–495, 1951.
4. Hurteau E.F., Baird W.C., Sinclair E.: Arachnoiditis following the use of iodized oil. *J. Bone Joint Surg.* 36:393–400, 1954.
5. Teng P., Rudner N.: Multiple arachnoid diverticula. *Arch. Neurol.* 2:348–356, 1960.
6. Cronqvist C.: The post-operative myelogram. *Acta Radiol.* 52:45–51, 1959.
7. Lombardi G., Passerini A., Migliavacca F.: Spinal arachnoiditis. *Br. J. Radiol.* 35:314–320, 1962.
8. Fisher R.L.: An experimental evaluation of Pantopaque and other recently developed myelographic contrast media. *Radiology* 85:537–545, 1965.
9. Howland W.J., Curry J.L.: Experimental studies of Pantopaque arachnoiditis. *Radiology* 87:253–261, 1966.
10. Bergeron R.T., Rumbaugh C.L., Fang H., et al.: Experimental Pantopaque arachnoiditis in the monkey. *Radiology* 99:95–101, 1971.
11. Smith R.W., Loeser J.D.: A myelographic variant in lumbar arachnoiditis. *J. Neurosurg.* 36:441–446, 1972.
12. Jakobsen J.K.: Clinical evaluations of a histologic examination of the side effects of myelographic contrast media. *Acta Radiol. Diag.* 14:638–646, 1973.
13. Moseley I.: The oil myelogram after operation for lumbar disc lesions. *Clin. Radiol.* 28:267–276, 1977.
14. Quencer R.M., Tenner M., Rothman L.: The postoperative myelogram. *Radiology* 123:667–679, 1977.
15. Picard L., Roland J., Blanchot P., et al.: Scarring of the theca and the nerve roots as seen at radiculography. *J. Neuroradiol.* 4:29–48, 1977.
16. Castan P., Bourbotte G., Herail J.P., et al.: Follow-up and post-operative radiculography. *J. Neuroradiol.* 4:49–93, 1977.
17. Auld A.W.: Chronic spinal arachnoiditis: A post-operative syndrome that may signal its onset. *Spine* 3:88–92, 1978.
18. Nainkin L.: Arachnoiditis ossificans: Report of a case. *Spine* 3:83–86, 1978.
19. Skalpe I.O.: Adhesive arachnoiditis following lumbar myelography. *Spine* 3:61–64, 1978.
20. Brodsky A.E.: Cauda equina arachnoiditis: A correlative clinical and roentgenologic study. *Spine* 3:51–60, 1978.
21. Quiles M., Marchisello P.J., Tsairis P.: Lumbar adhesive arachnoiditis: Etiologic and pathologic aspects. *Spine* 3:45–50, 1978.
22. Benner B., Ehni G.: Spinal arachnoiditis: The postoperative variety in particular. *Spine* 3:40–44, 1978.
23. Johnston J.D.H., Matheny J.B.: Microscopic lysis of lumbar adhesive arachnoiditis. *Spine* 3:36–39, 1978.
24. Burton C.V.: Lumbosacral arachnoiditis. *Spine* 3:24–30, 1978.
25. Benoist M., Ficat C., Baraf P., et al.: Post-operative lumbar epiduroarachnoiditis: Diagnostic and therapeutic aspects. *Spine* 5:432–436, 1980.
26. Barsoun A.H., Cannillo K.L.: Thoracic constrictive arachnoiditis after Pantopaque myelography: Report of two cases. *Neurosurgery* 6:314–316, 1980.
27. Mooij J.J.A.: Spinal arachnoiditis: Disease or coincidence? *Acta Neurochir.* 53:151–160, 1980.
28. Compere E.L.: Arachnoiditis confusion. *Int. Surg.* 65:305–307, 1980.
29. Epstein F., Allen J.: Segmental arachnoiditis after posterior fossa operation: Differentiation from metastatic tumor deposit. *Neurosurgery* 9:183–184, 1981.
30. Skalpe I.O., Sortland O.: Adhesive arachnoiditis in patients with spinal block. *Neuroradiology* 22:243–245, 1982.
31. Naidich T.P., King D.G., Moran C.J., et al.: Computed tomography of the lumbar thecal sac. *J. Comput. Assist. Tomogr.* 4:37–41, 1980.
32. Sheldon J.J., Leborgne J.: Computed tomography of the lumbar vertebral column, in Post M.J.D. (ed.): *Radio-*

graphic Evaluation of the Spine: Current Advances with Emphasis on Computed Tomography. New York, Masson Publishing Company, 1980, pp. 56–87.

33. Ulrich C.G., Kieffer S.A.: Computed tomographic evaluation of the lumbar spine: Quantitative aspects and sagittal-coronal reconstruction, in Post M.J.D. (ed.): Radiographic Evaluation of the Spine: Current Advances with Emphasis on Computed Tomography. New York, Masson Publishing Company, 1980, pp. 88–107.

34. Glenn W.V., Rhodes J.L., Altschuler E.M.: Multiplanar computerized tomography of lumbar disc abnormalities: The proponent's viewpoint, in Post M.J.D. (ed.): Radiographic Evaluation of the Spine: Current Advances with Emphasis on Computed Tomography. New York, Masson Publishing Company, 1980, pp. 108–138.

35. Dorwart R.H., deGroot J., Sauerland E.K.: Computed tomography of the lumbosacral spine: Normal anatomy and normal variants, in Genant H.K. (ed.): Computed Tomography of the Lumbar Spine. Berkeley, Calif., University of California Printing Company, 1982, pp. 53–66.

36. Haughton V.M., Syvertsen A., Williams A.L.: Soft-tissue anatomy within the spinal canal as seen on computed tomography. Radiology 134:649–655, 1980.

37. Livingston P.A., Grayson E.V.: Computed tomography in the diagnosis of herniated discs in the lumbar spine, in Post M.J.D. (ed.): Radiographic Evaluation of the Spine: Current Advances with Emphasis on Computed Tomography. New York, Masson Publishing Company, 1980, pp. 308–319.

38. Coin C.G., Ying-Sek C., Keranen V., et al.: Computer assisted myelography in disk disease. J. Comput. Assist. Tomogr. 1:398–404, 1977.

39. Federle M.P., Moss A.A., Margolin F.R.: Role of computed tomography in patients with "sciatica." J. Comput. Assist. Tomogr. 4:335–341, 1980.

40. Carrera G.F., Williams A.L., Haughton V.M.: Computed tomography in sciatica. Radiology 137:433–437, 1980.

41. Gulati A.N., Weinstein R., Studdard E.: CT scan of the spine for herniated discs. Neuroradiology 22:57–60, 1981.

42. Muller H.A., Sachsenheimer W., van Kaick G.: Die Wertigkeit der CT bei der praoperativen Diagnostik von Bandscheibenvorfallen. Fortschr. Rontgenstr. 135:535–540, 1981.

43. Junges R., Zwicker H.: Die Wertigkeit der CT-Untersuchung bei Bandscheibenvorfallen. Fortschr. Rontgenstr. 136:166–170, 1982.

44. Williams A.L., Haughton V.M., Daniels D.L., et al.: CT recognition of lateral lumbar disk herniation. A.J.N.R. 3:211–213, 1982.

45. Williams A.L., Haughton V.M., Meyer G.A., et al.: Computed tomographic appearance of the bulging annulus. Radiology 142:403–408, 1982.

46. Raskin S.P., Keating J.W.: Recognition of lumbar disk disease: Comparison of myelography and computed tomography. A.J.N.R. 3:215–221, 1982.

47. Williams A.L., Haughton V.M., Syvertsen A.: Computed tomography in the diagnosis of herniated nucleus pulposus. Radiology 135:95–99, 1980.

48. Haughton V.M., Eldevik O.P., Magnaes B., et al.: A prospective comparison of computed tomography and myelography in the diagnosis of herniated lumbar disks. Radiology 142:103–110, 1982.

49. Claussen V.C., Grumme T., Treisch J., et al.: Die diagnostic des lumbalen bandscheibenvorfalls—computertomographische und myelographische engebnisse. Fortsch. Rontgenstr. 136:1–8, 1982.

50. Haughton V.M., Williams A.L.: Computed Tomography of the Spine. St. Louis, C.V. Mosby Co., 1982.

51. Ciappetta P., Delfini R., Cantore G.P., et al.: CT evaluation of epidural scars following multiple operations of lumbar disc arthrosis. Eur. Neurol. 21:129–135, 1982.

52. Schubiger O., Valavanis A.: CT differentiation between recurrent disc herniation and postoperative scan formation: The value of contrast enhancement. Neuroradiology 22:251–254, 1982.

53. Mall J.C., Kaiser J.A.: Computed tomography of the post-operative spine, in Genant H.K. (ed.): Computed Tomography of the Lumbar Spine. Berkeley, Calif., University of California Printing Department, 1982, pp. 245–260.

54. Meyer J.D., Latchaw R.E., Roppolo H.M., et al.: Computed tomography and myelography of the post-operative lumbar spine. A.J.N.R. 3:223–228, 1982.

55. Meyer J.D.: CT myelography of the post-operative spine, in Post M.J.D. (ed.): Computed Tomography of the Spine. Baltimore, Williams & Wilkins Co., (to be published).

56. Kirkaldy-Willis E., McIvor G., (eds.): Symposium: Spinal stenosis. Clin. Orthop. 115:2–144, 1976.

57. Quencer R., Murtach F., Post J., et al.: Post-operative bony stenosis of the lumbar spinal canal: Evaluation of 164 symptomatic patients with axial radiography. A.J.R. 131:1059–1064, 1978.

58. Ciric I., Mikhael M., Tarkington J., et al.: The lateral recess syndrome, a variant of spinal stenosis. J. Neurosurg. 53:433–443, 1980.

59. McAfee P.C., Ullrich C.G., Yuan H.A., et al.: Computed tomography in degenerative spinal stenosis. Clin. Orthop. 161:221–234, 1981.

60. Lancourt J.E., Glenn W.V. Jr., Wiltse L.L.: Multiplanar computerized tomography in the normal spine and in the diagnosis of spinal stenosis—a gross anatomic-computerized tomographic correlation. Spine 4:379–390, 1979.

61. Burton C.V., Heithoff K.B., Kirkaldy-Willis W., et al.: Computed tomographic scanning and the lumbar spine: II. Clinical considerations. Spine 4:356–368, 1979.

62. Risius B., Modic M.T., Hardy R.W., et al.: Sector computed tomographic spine scanning in the diagnosis of lumbar nerve root entrapment. Radiology 143:109–114, 1982.

63. Brodsky A.E.: Post-laminectomy and post-fusion stenosis of the lumbar spine. Clin. Orthop. 115:130–139, 1976.

64. Levy W.J., Dohn D.F., Duchesneau P.M.: Recurrence

of lumbar canal stenosis a decade after decompressive laminectomy. *Surg. Neurol.* 17:96–98, 1982.

65. Frymoyer J.W., Hanley E.N. Jr., Howe J., et al.: A comparison of radiographic findings in fusion and non-fusion patients ten or more years following lumbar disc surgery. *Spine* 4:435–440, 1979.

66. Reynolds A.F., Weinstein P.R., Wachter R.D.: Lumbar monoradiculopathy due to unilateral facet hypertrophy. *Neurosurgery* 10:480–486, 1982.

67. Beamer Y.B., Garner J.T., Shelden C.H.: Hypertrophied ligamentum flavum—clinical and surgical significance. *Arch. Surg.* 106:289–292, 1973.

68. Pagni C.A., Cassinari V., Bernasconi V.: Meningocele spurius following hemilaminectomy in a case of lumbar discal hernia. *J. Neurosurg.* 18:709–710, 1961.

69. Miller P.R., Elder R.W.: Meningeal pseudocysts (meningocele spurius) following laminectomy—report of 10 cases. *J. Bone Joint Surg.* 50A:268–276, 1968.

70. Borgesen S.E., Vang P.S.: Extradural pseudocysts—a cause of pain after lumbar-disc operation. *Acta Orthop. Scand.* 44:12–20, 1973.

71. Cilluffo J.M., Miller R.H.: Post-traumatic arachnoidal diverticula. *Acta Neurochir.* 54:77–87, 1980.

72. Patronas N.J., Jafar J., Brown F.: Pseudomeningoceles diagnosed by metrizamide myelography and computerized tomography. *Surg. Neurol.* 16:188–191, 1981.

73. Paine K.W.E., Huang P.W.H.: Lumbar disc syndrome. *J. Neurosurg.* 37:75–82, 1972.

30

Tumors and Inflammatory Conditions of the Spine and Spinal Cord

WILLIAM E. ROTHFUS, M.D.
RICHARD E. LATCHAW, M.D.
JOSEPH A. HORTON, M.D.

COMPUTED TOMOGRAPHIC SCANNING has become a vital tool in the evaluation of infectious and neoplastic lesions of the spinal column and intraspinal contents. Scanning allows precise evaluation of bone destruction, the presence and size of a paraspinal mass, and the degree of cord and/or nerve root compression. Because the radiographic appearance may be similar, infectious and neoplastic lesions are considered together in this chapter. Bone destruction with an epidural mass may have a similar appearance whether caused by infection or neoplasm and may be distinguishable only by defining whether the lesion appears to originate in the vertebral body (neoplasm) or in the disc space (infection). Following a brief discussion of techniques of examination, this chapter will be divided into neoplasms originating in bony structures, intraspinal tumors, and infectious lesions.

TECHNIQUES OF EXAMINATION

The plain CT scan may be all that is necessary for the evaluation of a single focus of bone destruction such as a bony metastasis, a primary neoplasm of bone, or a disc space infection with contiguous destruction of vertebral bodies. High-resolution scanners afford good definition of the epidural spread of such neoplastic and infectious processes, and the paraspinal component can be well defined. Generally, all that is necessary is contiguous scans of 5-mm thickness through the area of interest. Better definition is given by contiguous thinner cuts. The latter is advocated so that good coronal and sagittal reformatted images may be obtained. Five-millimeter cuts spaced every 3 mm also give excellent reformatted images. Scanning should be performed at

0° angulation of the gantry to speed the reformatting computations.

Intravenously administered contrast media serve multiple functions, including enhancement of the dura for better definition of the margins of the thecal sac. In addition, they give added information in certain disease processes. Inflammatory tissue will enhance, providing sharper definition between the epidural mass and the thecal sac than is present on unenhanced CT. Certain primary bone tumors may enhance markedly, such as hemangioma, plasmacytoma, and aneurysmal bone cyst. The presence of marked enhancement of a bony neoplasm may shift the differential diagnosis to these lesions. Enhancement is also present with a number of the primary intraspinal tumors. Schwannoma and meningioma are characterized by well-circumscribed masses with uniform contrast enhancement. Primary intramedullary tumors such as astrocytoma may have spotty enhancement.

It is obviously impossible to scan the complete spine or even major segments of the spine when multiple lesions are suspected or when the exact level of an intraspinal lesion is unknown. In addition, tumor or infection may obscure the soft-tissue planes within the spinal canal. Myelography serves the important functions of localizing the particular levels to be evaluated with CT and defining the margins of the thecal sac. Once the appropriate levels have been determined, CT scanning with either contiguous 5-mm or 3-mm slices is generally sufficient for evaluation. The necessity for reformatted images will dictate the need for thinner or overlapping cuts.

Delayed CT scanning following the intrathecal placement of a water-soluble contrast agent may show movement of the contrast agent into the lesion within the spinal cord ("imbibition"). This has been classically described with syringomyelia/hydromyelia,[1] although movement of contrast into the cystic portion(s) of an intramedullary tumor has also been commonly visualized.[2] The difference in appearance is one of volume and sharpness of the imbibed contrast media, with that in tumors being of lesser volume and less well circumscribed than that in syringomyelia. Contrast material has also been noted to move in a diffuse fashion into an injured cord and slightly into the normal spinal cord, similar to diffusion throughout the brain following myelography. Therefore, the movement itself of contrast material into the spinal cord is a nonspecific finding. We generally obtain delayed scans at 6 and 24 hours after the myelogram. A good study of the transit times of contrast media into varying lesions has yet to be performed, and therefore the efficacy of scanning at 6, 12, or 24 hours has not been defined.

Reformatting of images is occasionally of value. If plain films and/or tomograms of the spine are not available to demonstrate the site of origin of a bony lesion, i.e., originating in a disc space (infection) or in a vertebral body (neoplasm), the reformatted image may serve this purpose. Reformatted images are also useful in the evaluation of changes within the canal, with the sagittal and coronal images representing second and third views to the axial images.

TUMORS OF BONE

Hemangioma

Hemangiomas represent the most common neoplasm of the bony spine and occur most often in the lower thoracic and upper lumbar segments.[3] Like soft-tissue hemangiomas in other portions of the body, they may be of either the capillary or cavernous type and produce thinning of vertebral trabeculae by constant pressure and slow expansion. The remaining trabeculae become thickened as a response to the decrease in overall number of trabeculae and increased stress on those remaining, producing the classic "stippled" appearance of the vertebral body on the axial image (Fig 30–1,A).

The majority of hemangiomas are confined to the vertebral body, but they may spread along the contiguous bony structures to involve the rest of the neural arch (Fig 30–1,B). They may break through the cortex to extend into the epidural and/or paraspinal regions; epidural extension may produce cord compression.

The stippled appearance on a CT scan is classic for hemangioma, although thickened trabeculae may occur with other infiltrating neoplasms such as multiple myeloma. Paget's disease likewise produces thickened trabeculae, but there is also thickening of the cortex and overall enlargement of a vertebral segment. Enhancement of a hemangioma with intravenous contrast material may be dramatic, although the degree of enhancement may be less than expected for the degree of vascularity of the lesion, secondary to dilution by the "blood pool."

Osteochondroma

Osteochondroma is an unusual tumor of the spine and most commonly involves the spinous process (Fig 30–2). The CT characteristics are similar to those of plain films and include a margin of cortical bone surrounding an inner, less dense component of chondroid tissue that may or may not be calcified.

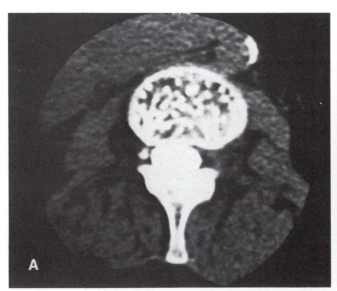
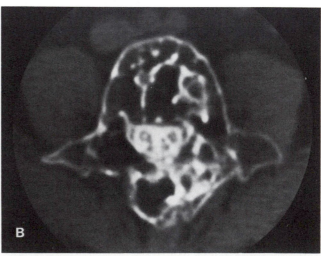

Fig 30–1.—Vertebral hemangiomas. **A,** note typical stippled appearance of the vertebral body. **B,** more extensive involvement, extending into the transverse processes and posterior arch, is a less frequent finding. Hemangioma was confirmed by biopsy.

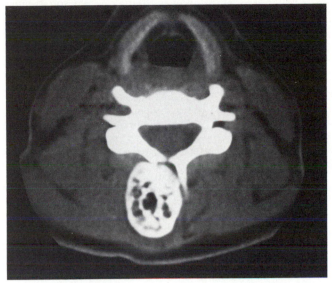

Fig 30–2.—Osteochondroma. The pedunculated mass protrudes from the spinous process. The pattern of calcification is typical of a chondroid lesion.

Osteoid Osteoma and Osteoblastoma (Giant Osteoid Osteoma)

The classic location of an osteoid osteoma is the pedicle or other portions of the neural arch in the thoracic or upper lumbar spine of a young male presenting with back pain. Typically, the pain is worse at night and is relieved with aspirin. Plain films and CT scan demonstrate a sclerotic segment of bone with slight expansion. Plain film tomography[4] or bone windows of the CT image may demonstrate the radiolucent nidus of the osteoma.

The spine is involved in close to one half of all osteoblastomas. The radiographic appearance differs from osteoid osteoma in that there is a diffuse lytic expansion of a portion of the neural arch, particularly in the cervical spine, with thinning of the cortex. There is expansion into the intraspinal and paraspinal soft tissues far more commonly than with osteoid osteoma, producing compression of the spinal cord and/or nerve roots. The radiographic appearance is similar to that of aneurysmal bone cyst, and pathologically the two entities may be found contiguously, suggesting that aneurysmal bone cyst is a "secondary" lesion.[5]

Aneurysmal Bone Cyst

Aneurysmal bone cysts are comprised of large blood-filled cavities and are not true neoplasms. They are expansile lesions, and one fifth involve the spine, particularly the posterior elements. Because of this, they closely resemble the radiographic appearance of osteoblastoma. Because aneurysmal bone cysts are found in association with a number of neoplasms, many authorities do not consider them to be primary lesions, but simply "secondary" to the presence of a neoplastic expansion.[5]

The CT scan characteristics are those of a multiloculated, expansile lesion generally involving the posterior elements of a vertebral segment, but commonly extending into the vertebral body. Contrast enhancement is a prominent feature following intravenous infusion. Cord compression may occur, requiring decompression. Angiography and embolization may be of value preoperatively.

Plasmacytoma

Neoplasia involving plasma cells results in plasmacytoma in the isolated form and multiple myeloma in the diffuse form. Many of the patients presenting with solitary plasmacytoma will be found in later years to have multiple myeloma. Solitary plasmacytoma is characterized by diffuse expansion of a vertebral body or the neural arch, and contrast enhancement may be prominent (Fig 30–3). The appearance may be indistinguishable from aneurysmal bone cyst. Angiography may likewise give a similar appearance, and preoperative embolization is extremely useful, as with aneurysmal bone cysts.

Giant Cell Tumor

The majority of giant cell tumors are histologically benign, but they may progress to malignancy. Giant cell tumors generally involve the sacrum, with a presentation in other portions of the spine distinctly uncommon.[6] While a giant cell tumor may produce expansion, bone erosion and destruction are typically present. The giant cell tumor commonly has poorly defined margins, whereas aneurysmal bone cyst and plasmacytoma tend to have a more expansile, multilocular appearance. Giant cell tumor is rare before the age of 20, whereas aneurysmal bone cyst commonly occurs

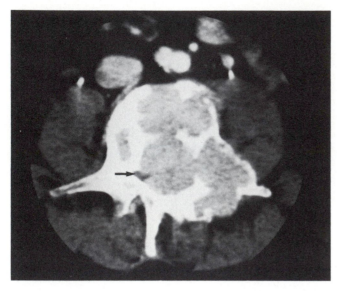

Fig 30–3.—Plasmacytoma. Following intravenous contrast administration, the interstices of this expansile lesion enhance homogeneously. The tumor fills most of the spinal canal; only a very compressed portion of the thecal sac can be identified *(arrow).*

before the age of 20 and usually involves the spine rather than the sacrum.[6]

Scanning by CT is important in the evaluation of giant cell tumor, both for evaluation of the paraspinal mass and the degree of intraspinal extension. Surgical resection may be curative, although local recurrence and/or progression to malignancy is common, as it is in other locations in the body.

Chordoma

The chordoma arises from notochordal cell rests within a disc space, thereby providing the mechanism

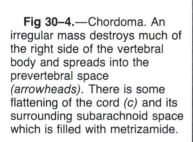

Fig 30–4.—Chordoma. An irregular mass destroys much of the right side of the vertebral body and spreads into the prevertebral space *(arrowheads).* There is some flattening of the cord *(c)* and its surrounding subarachnoid space which is filled with metrizamide.

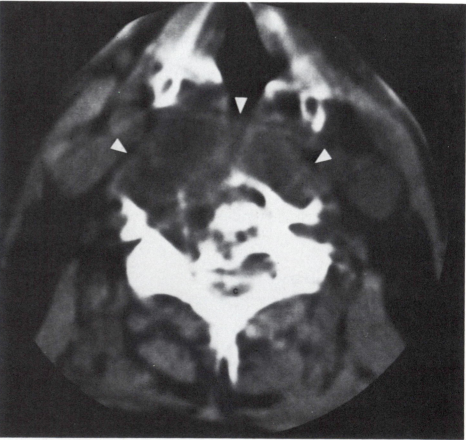

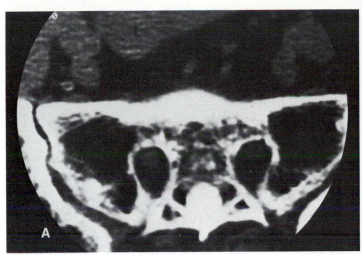

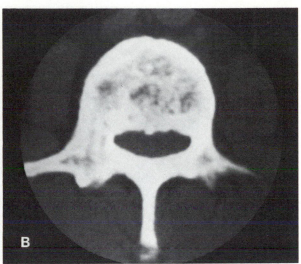

Fig 30–5.—Paget's disease. **A,** the cortex of the sacrum is thickened, and the sacral trabecular pattern is accentuated. **B,** more severe involvement causes much denser trabecular pattern and compromise of the canal because of bony expansion (diagnosis proved by biopsy).

to spread into contiguous vertebral bodies. In this sense, it mimics disc space infection. The most common locations for the chordoma are the sphenoid bone and clivus, with the sacrum the next most common. Vertebral involvement accounts for only 15% or less of cases.

Poorly marginated destruction is typically seen by CT, with large paraspinal and intraspinal components (Fig 30–4). Calcifications are common (approximately 50%[7]) and there may be contrast enhancement.

Paget's Disease

Paget's disease is not a form of neoplasia, but is considered here because of differential diagnosis. Paget's disease classically has three phases, including an initial lytic phase, a second phase characterized by mixed osteolytic and osteoblastic components, and a tertiary diffuse osteoblastic phase. When a vertebral segment is involved, there is enlargement of that segment, with thickening of the cortex and prominence of the trabecular pattern (Fig 30–5,A). There may be sufficient enlargement of both the vertebral body and neural arch to produce compression of the spinal cord and/or nerve roots, although this is uncommon (Fig 30–5,B).

Metastatic Tumor

Metastases to bone may be either osteolytic or osteoblastic. The most common osteolytic metastases are carcinoma of the breast, lung, and kidney; lymphoma/leukemia; and multiple myeloma. The most common osteoblastic metastasis is carcinoma of the prostate (Fig 30–6), with carcinoma of the breast also causing an osteoblastic response.

A single focus of disease seen on plain films may be well evaluated with CT scanning without myelography.

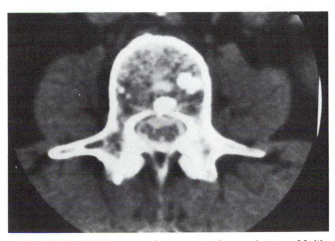

Fig 30–6.—Metastases from prostatic carcinoma. Multiple well-defind blastic metastatic deposits dot the medullary cavity of the vertebral body.

The degree of intraspinal extension and the paraspinal component may be well demonstrated (Fig 30–7). However, because of the possibility of multiple levels of involvement and the need to define the level(s) producing neurologic compression when multiple segments are involved, myelography with a water-soluble contrast agent is generally the first examination of choice. The myelogram will dictate the levels to be further evaluated with CT scanning. It is also much easier to define the thecal sac when it is filled with metrizamide than it is on the plain CT scan, particularly in the thoracic region, and especially in the presence of bony abnormalities and distorted intraspinal soft tissues (see Fig 30–6,B and C).

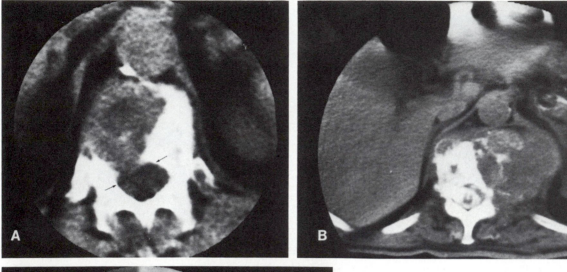

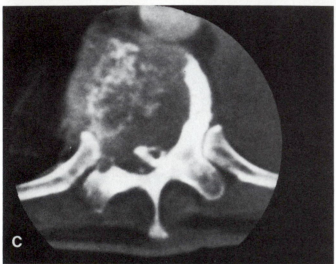

Fig 30–7.—Metastases from lung carcinoma, three different patients. **A,** a large lytic lesion destroys much of the vertebral body, but bulges only slightly into the epidural space. A thin rim of cerebrospinal fluid (*arrows*) separates the tumor from the thecal sac. **B,** this metastatic lesion is growing away from the vertebral body, causing a large, partially calcified paravertebral mass. There is only minimal impingement on the thecal sac. **C,** in contrast to **B,** this tumor has a significant extradural component with only a small paravertebral portion. The tumor has completely destroyed the right pedicle, but preserved the costal articulation.

INTRASPINAL TUMORS

Intraspinal tumors classically have been divided into the following categories depending upon their location: epidural, intradural extramedullary, and intramedullary neoplasms. This classification allows for specific differential diagnoses, because certain tumors characteristically occur in each of the three locations. There are also classic myelographic appearances for each of the categories. Epidural tumors produce displacement of the entire thecal sac and obtuse margins to the filling defect. If a complete block is present, there is a horizontal margin to the contrast column representing the compressed spinal cord. Below the cord, the block has a characteristic "feather edge," which is due to the presence of contrast material around nerve roots that are compressed in a diffuse manner through the relatively thick dura. Intradural extramedullary tumors are sharply marginated masses that displace the spinal cord in a contralateral direction, enlarging the subarachnoid space in the region of the mass. The sharp margination is due to the close contiguity between the contrast material and the mass, separated only by the thin arachnoid. The differentiation in appearance between epidural and intradural masses, therefore, is a function of the interposed dura. Intramedullary neoplasms, on the other hand, are characterized by diffuse enlargement of the spinal cord itself in all projections, producing a "cigar" shape. A single view on a myelogram may suggest cord enlargment typical of an intramedullary expansion, whereas the cord is simply being displaced in an anteroposterior fashion by an extramedullary mass; it is therefore important to obtain two views on any myelogram.

Scanning by CT is able to define the position of the mass in a more exquisite fashion than is myelography. Cord enlargement, mass density contiguous to the cord, and/or bone involvement are easily evaluated by

CT, especially following water-soluble myelography. The myelogram is important, because the exact position of a suspected intraspinal neoplasm is difficult to predict. Without a myelogram, CT scanning over many segments is time consuming and gives a high dose of radiation. More importantly, definition of the subarachnoid space, which may be distorted by neoplasm, is extremely helpful for accurate diagnosis.

This section will describe the typical CT scan appearances of the three classes of intraspinal neoplasms. Congenital tumors such as lipoma, dermoid, epidermoid, and teratoma are discussed more extensively in Chapter 33.

Epidural Neoplasms

The majority of epidural neoplasms are extensions into the epidural space of tumors affecting the bony structures, particularly the vertebral body. The most common lesions are metastatic tumors, and the CT scan appearances of these neoplasms have been presented earlier in this chapter under Tumors of Bone. Scanning by CT with or without preceding myelography is extremely important to evaluate the degree and type of bone involvement, paraspinal extension, and involvement of intraspinal structures, including compression of the thecal sac. Two categories of tumors not previously discussed are lymphoma and neoplasms involving a neural foramen.

Lymphoma

Lymphoma may be present in the epidural soft tissues without discernible bone involvement.[8] When bone is affected, marginal erosion may be secondary to the chronicity of lymphomatous masses, or there may be frank destruction from ingrowth of tumor. The characteristic myelographic appearance is that of a long segment of diffuse circumferential narrowing and irregularity of the thecal sac (Fig 30–8). Subsequent CT scanning typically shows a small, irregularly marginated collection of contrast material with surrounding soft-tissue density and ablation of the normal soft-tissue planes.

Neoplasms Involving a Neural Foramen

Neuroblastoma.—Neuroblastoma and ganglioneuroblastoma originate in the paraspinal sympathetic chain in addition to the adrenal medulla and other sites of sympathetic nervous tissue. These tumors frequently grow in "dumbbell" fashion through a neural foramen to produce an intraspinal epidural mass.[9] Not infrequently, the compression of the spinal cord is the presenting symptom in these children.[10] Bony metastases

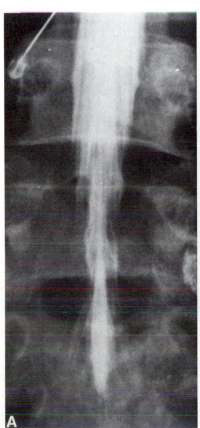

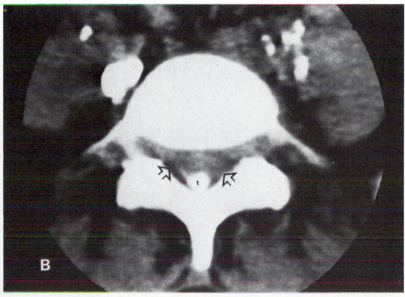

Fig 30–8.—Lymphoma. **A,** a long extradural mass concentrically constricts the thecal sac. **B,** on scan, the homogeneous extradural lymphoma *(arrows)* displaces the thecal sac *(t)* and extends along the neural foramina bilaterally.

are also common. Neuroblastoma originating within the spinal canal is rare.[10]

Scanning by CT generally shows a paraspinal mass, commonly with punctate calcification, and extension of neoplasm into the spinal epidural space. Myelography with water-soluble contrast material and postmyelographic CT scanning will adequately evaluate the extent of the paraspinal and intraspinal involvement, along with any bone destruction.

EXTRADURAL SCHWANNOMA AND NEUROFIBROMA.— Schwannomas and neurofibromas classically originate in the intradural extramedullary space along nerve roots. Extension into the extradural space and subsequent growth through a neural foramen into the paraspinal tissues is a common sequela. Occasionally, the neural tumors may be strictly extradural/extraspinal in location. Neurofibromas may be well circumscribed or plexiform in nature with poor margination and growth into surrounding tissue, simulating a malignant tumor (Fig 30–9). Multiplicity of schwannomas or neurofibromas is common.

Myelography with subsequent CT scanning defines the compressed or displaced thecal sac and/or nerve root sleeve. If the tumor is strictly extradural, the appearance may simulate a herniated disc. Enlargement of a neural foramen with extension into the paraspinal soft tissues gives evidence for its true nature, however. It is important to totally evaluate the extraspinal extension for complete removal of such a lesion. Separate intravenously enhanced CT scan is extremely helpful in the definition of the paraspinal component.

Intradural Extramedullary Lesions

The classic differential diagnosis of intradural extramedullary lesions includes the schwannoma/neurofibroma and the meningioma, with metastatic tumors being much less common in this location. Nonneoplastic cysts are rare.

Intradural Schwannoma and Neurofibroma

The intradural schwannoma or neurofibroma is generally located in the anterolateral portion of the spinal canal, and its relationship to the spinal cord is exquisitely demonstrated with CT scanning following myelography. The lesion is separated from the cord only by a thin layer of arachnoid (Fig 30–10), and the subarachnoid space in the region of the expansion is enlarged because of the contralateral displacement of the cord. Below the level of the cord, nerve roots are seen to be displaced around the mass. The margins of the tumor are sharply defined on the postmyelographic CT scan

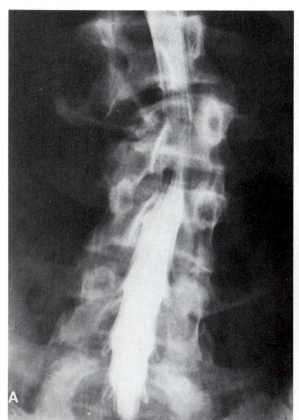

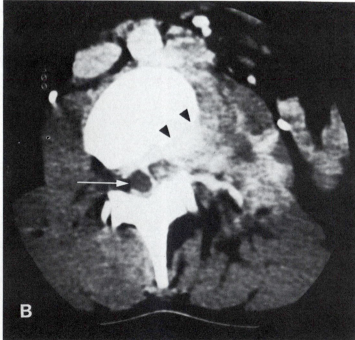

Fig 30–9.—Plexiform neurofibroma. **A,** in the region of most bony deformity and scoliosis, the thecal sac is narrowed by an extradural mass. **B,** CT with intravenous contrast shows an irregularly enhancing mass wrapping around the thecal sac (arrow), expanding the neural foramen (arrowheads), and infiltrating the psoas muscle.

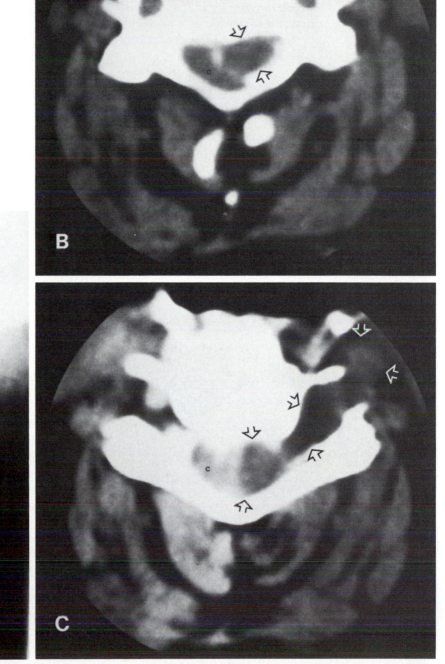

Fig 30–10.—Neurofibroma. **A,** typical myelographic appearance with a well-defined intradural extramedullary mass *(arrows)* displacing the spinal cord. **B,** with intrathecal contrast, the neurofibroma *(arrows)* is easily separated from the cord *(c)* because of a thin layer of surrounding metrizamide. **C,** contiguous section allows demonstration of the "dumbbell" shape of the tumor *(arrows),* which expands the neural foramen and extends into the paravertebral tissues. (*c* = cord)

because of the contiguity of contrast to the mass. Extension into the epidural and paraspinal soft tissues has been previously discussed. Diffuse enlargment of nerve roots, along with a nodular appearance characteristic of small neurofibromas along nerve roots, may occasionally be seen on the postmyelographic scan. These latter findings are much better appreciated on the preceding myelography, however.

Myelography preceding the CT scan is encouraged because it is impossible to accurately predict on a clinical basis the exact location of an extramedullary mass, and it is impossible to adequately "survey" the entire spinal canal or long segments of the canal by CT scanning. In addition, schwannomas and neurofibromas may be multiple, and such multiplicity is easily evaluated with complete myelography. If myelography is not possible because of contrast allergy or myelographic difficulties, CT evaluation of the intraspinal space following intravenous contrast infusion may define a solitary lesion to good advantage (Fig 30–11). In addition, an intravenous study is important to evaluate the extraspinal component of such a lesion.

Meningioma

Meningiomas account for approximately 40% of all spinal tumors. They are by far more common in women than in men and generally involve the thoracic spine. They have myelographic and CT scan characteristics

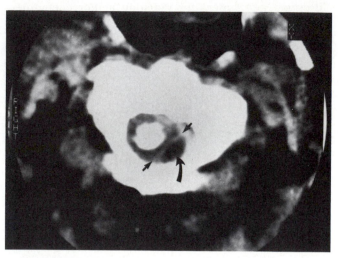

Fig 30–12.—Meningioma. The large calcified meningioma occupies most of the spinal canal. A thin rim of metrizamide (small arrows) separates the meningioma from the cord (curved arrow).

that are similar to those of the schwannoma and neurofibroma, but differ in a few important ways. First, meningiomas tend to be located in the posterior portion of the spinal canal, whereas schwannomas and neurofibromas tend to be placed anterolaterally. Second, meningiomas are commonly calcified, either with punctate psammomatous or with more globular deposits (Fig 30–12). Finally, while "dumbbell" meningiomas extending through a neural foramen do occur, this appearance is much more characteristic of schwannoma/neurofibroma.

Metastases

Most hematogenously disseminated metastases spread to a vertebral body or pedicle. Occasionally, metastases from primary neoplasms outside the nervous system may be found in an intradural location, particularly along nerve roots, such as melanoma and carcinoma of the breast or lung. "Dropped metastases" are nodular implants that are present along the outer aspect of the spinal cord, along nerve roots, or along the inner margins of the arachnoid secondary to seeding of the cerebrospinal fluid (CSF) by intracranial tumors. The most common primary tumors are medulloblastoma and glioblastoma multiforme,[11] but seeding has been reported for most classes of intracranial neoplasms.

Myelography with a water-soluble contrast agent is essential for the evaluation of the majority of these lesions, particularly the small nodular implants that could not otherwise be detected on the CT scan. Even when shown myelographically, they may be exceedingly difficult to demonstrate on a CT scan. Once demonstrated by myelography, there is little reason for persisting in extensive scanning, because the implications of

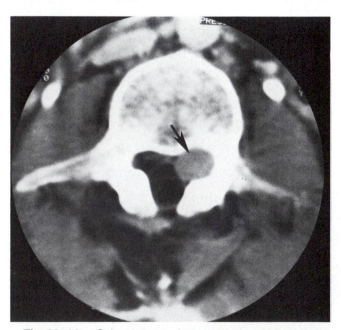

Fig 30–11.—Schwannoma. Intravenously enhanced CT scan of the L-2 segment demonstrates a well-circumscribed, homogeneously enhancing schwannoma (arrow) involving the left side of the spinal canal. The tumor produces local deformity of the lateral recess, and there is displacement of the thecal sac, the margins of which are slightly thickened by scar tissue from previous surgery.

"dropped metastases" for radiation and/or chemotherapy are apparent.

Cysts

NEURENTERIC CYST.—The neurenteric cyst is a congenital anomaly in which there is a connection between the gut or lung and the spinal column and intraspinal contents. The fistulous connection may be patent or atretic and is lined with respiratory or bowel epithelium. The abnormal connection passes through a vertebral segment, producing anomalies of bony structures and giving a clue to the congenital origin of the lesion.[12] When the fistulous connection is patent, there may be a chemical meningitis that draws attention to the need for investigation. Evaluation is best obtained by a combination of water-soluble myelography and subsequent CT scanning.

The intraspinal cyst is usually intradural and extramedullary in position, but may be firmly adherent to the pia so that it appears to be intimately related to the spinal cord (Fig 30–13). The patient presenting with symptoms of spinal cord compression may not initially have the vertebral anomaly appreciated on the plain films of the spine; the appearance of the intraspinal lobulated mass may suggest some type of congenital neoplasm. However, appreciation of the anomalous bony structures should lead to the appropriate diagnosis. The bony anomaly may be as subtle as a simple cleft in a vertebral body (see Fig 30–13).

ARACHNOID CYST.—The intraspinal arachnoid cyst most commonly involves the intradural space, although it may herniate through a dural defect into the extraspinal space or may be present in both compartments. The cyst generally communicates with the subarachnoid space through a narrow neck, although that neck may be so narrow that a ball-valve type of communication is present. While these lesions are generally congenital in nature, they, like their intracranial counterparts, may be acquired as a result of meningeal adhesions from trauma or infection. Chronic CSF pulsations and slow expansion may produce spinal cord compression and/or bony deformity and erosion.[13]

Because of the variability with which arachnoid cysts communicate with the subarachnoid space, there is a spectrum of CT appearances. At least initially, the cyst may be isolated from intrathecal contrast, presenting a

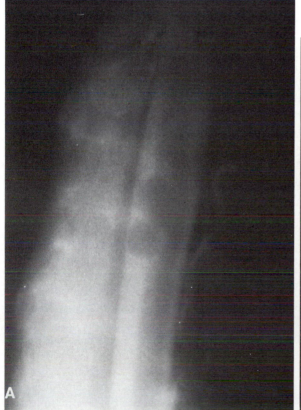
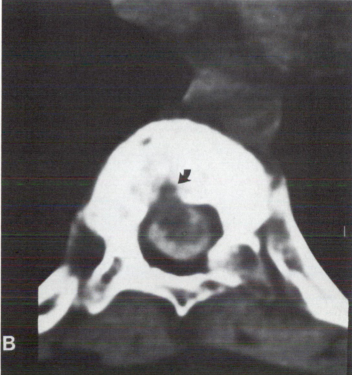

Fig 30–13.—Neurenteric cyst. **A,** a bilobed intradural extramedullary mass displaces the cord, but cannot be separated from it. **B,** CT scan following the myelogram shows the mass abutting directly on the cord *(c)*. It extends into a defect in the posterior vertebral body *(arrow)*, a finding characteristic of neurenteric cyst.

well-defined CSF-density mass. With time, the density of the cyst will usually increase as contrast percolates into it. Occasionally, the cyst may be directly punctured at the time of contrast instillation, thus giving a density collection separated from the subarachnoid space (Fig 30–14). Because an arachnoid cyst can be multicompartmental, separate punctures may be necessary to demonstrate it in its entirety.

Intramedullary Expansions

The differential diagnosis of an intramedullary expansion includes the two common gliomas, astrocytoma and ependymoma; hemangioblastoma; syringomyelia/hydromyelia; and rarely, metastatic tumor, which is usually direct extension of a neoplasm involving the cerebellum and/or brain stem. The characteristic of all of these expansions is that of an enlarged cord on myelography. Radiographic differentiation of these lesions may be difficult and is usually dependent upon CT scan density characteristics, the degree of enhancement with intravenous contrast material, and the appearance and location within the mass of "imbibed" water-soluble myelographic contrast media. The extent of the lesion is not a good differentiating characteristic, particularly when attempting to separate intramedullary glioma from syringomyelia/hydromyelia. We have seen a number of patients with long histories who have expansions involving the entire length of the cord that have been histologically proved to be neoplasms; likewise, syringomyelia has been seen in patients who have relatively short histories and involvement of a lesser length of cord than many slow-growing neoplasms.

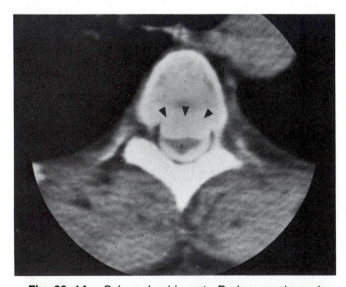

Fig 30–14.—Subarachnoid cyst. During myelography, the cyst was directly injected, causing dense accumulation within the cyst *(arrowheads)*, distinctly separate from the spinal cord *(c)* and the generalized subarachnoid space.

Intramedullary Glioma

Astrocytomas are the most common intramedullary neoplasms involving the spinal cord, while ependymomas commonly involve the lower spinal cord, conus medullaris, and filum terminale.[14] On both the myelogram and the subsequent CT scan, these expansions are characterized by diffuse symmetric enlargement of the cord. When the expansion is large enough to produce a complete myelographic block, CT scanning may well show small amounts of contrast extending diffusely around the enlarged cord, thereby more accurately defining the length of the expansion.

The scan performed close to the time of myelography shows the diffuse expansion within the opaque contrast medium (Fig 30–15,A and B). A delayed scan, however, may show "imbibition" of a water-soluble contrast agent into the spinal cord neoplasm, particularly into cystic portions of the tumor (Fig 30–15,C). Whereas imbibition of contrast media was originally thought to occur exclusively with syringomyelia/hydromyelia, this phenomenon is nonspecific. It certainly occurs with neoplasms, particularly with partially cystic tumors. Contrast material likewise moves into areas of cord damage, such as from infection, infarction, and demyelinating disease. Finally, water-soluble myelographic contrast material may permeate the normal spinal cord in an analogous fashion to penetration of the brain and may be detected on delayed scans. However, the density increase is usually subtle, requiring measurements of attenuation coefficients.

The important differentiating points in the appearances of the imbibed contrast material within an intramedullary neoplasm vs. syringomyelia/hydromyelia are the concentration of the contrast media, the single or multiple foci of the contrast, and the margination of the contrast. In syringomyelia/hydromyelia, the contrast material is usually well circumscribed and is generally of very high concentration (Fig 30–16). Syringomyelia/hydromyelia may have multiple septations and may be multicompartmental, but the contrast collections are generally quite dense and well circumscribed, with each focus well demarcated and/or confluent with contiguous compartments. On the other hand, the contrast material within a solid intraspinal neoplasm is poorly marginated and of a lesser concentration than with syringomyelia. The contrast material within a cyst(s) of a tumor varies in concentration from low to moderately dense, but the margins are usually irregular. The combination of poorly defined enhancement in a solid component and an irregularly marginated cystic collection favors tumor.

Scanning by CT following the intravenous injection of iodinated contrast material may be extremely helpful

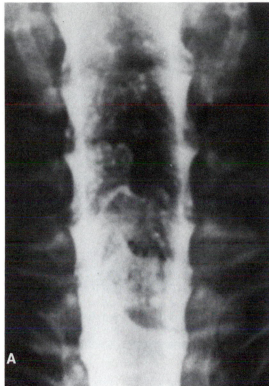

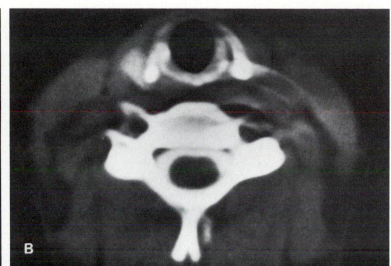

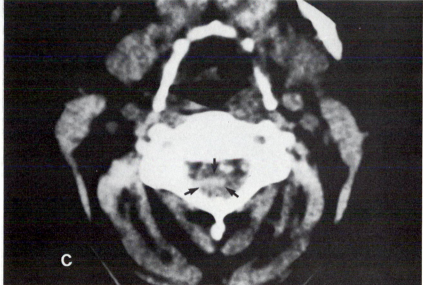

Fig 30–15.—Cervical cord astrocytoma. **A,** myelography with metrizamide shows mild cord expansion over several cervical segments. **B,** CT scan soon after myelogram confirms diffuse cord enlargement, but with relative preservation of normal topography. **C,** follow-up scan 24 hours after **B** demonstrates eccentric accumulation of metrizamide within the tumor *(arrows).* Other densities represent residual Pantopaque from a previous myelogram (see **A**).

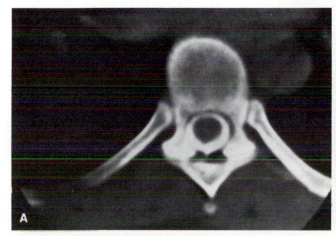

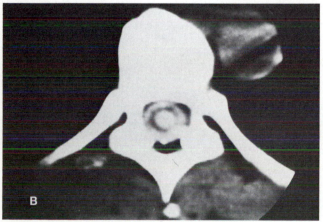

Fig 30–16.—Thoracic syringomyelia. **A,** the cord is diffusely expanded in the immediate postmyelogram study. **B,** delayed scan shows typical well-defined dense metrizamide accumulation within the cord. Compare with Figure 30–15, C.

in cases where it is difficult to differentiate between an intramedullary neoplasm and syringomyelia/hydromyelia (Fig 30–17). Neoplasms may enhance slightly, with irregularly marginated areas of enhancement, whereas syringomyelia/hydromyelia does not enhance. It may be important preoperatively to make as accurate a distinction between intramedullary glioma and syringomyelia as is possible, because the surgical therapy may be entirely different. Commonly, however, a surgeon would prefer to biopsy the wall of a cystic expansion to absolutely exclude its neoplastic origin.

Ependymomas originating from the filum terminale or conus medullaris extend into the extramedullary space, simulating an intradural extramedullary lesion. The differentiation of such a lesion from a meningioma or neurofibroma is based on the appearance of the lesion relative to the cord, nerve roots, and filum. Occasionally, short, lobulated ependymomas of the filum may have myelographic and CT scan appearances identical to other intradural tumors, requiring pathologic differentiation. Extension along the filum, however, is commonly seen on the CT scan even with well-localized lesions, thereby giving the important preoperative clue to the appropriate diagnosis.

Hemangioblastoma

Approximately one third of hemangioblastomas of the spinal cord are associated with the von Hippel-Lindau syndrome, which also consists of retinal angioma, intracranial hemangioblastomas that usually involve the posterior fossa, pancreatic and renal cysts, and hypernephroma. As with most of the intracranial tumors, the lesion is characterized by a very vascular nodule with accompanying cyst.

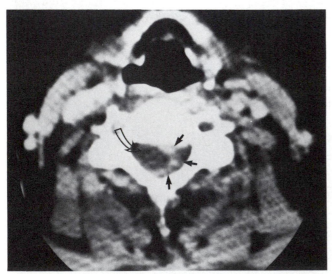

Fig 30–17.—Cervical glioma with cyst. A thin rim of enhancement *(short arrows)* surrounds a large eccentric cyst *(curved arrow)* within the enlarged cord.

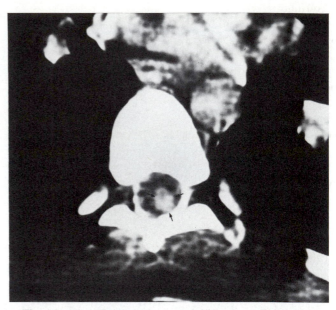

Fig 30–18.—Thoracic hemangioblastoma. Following intravenous contrast, a dense enhancing nodule *(arrows)* stands out. The remainder of the expanded cord (surrounded by intrathecal metrizamide) is lucent, representing cyst.

Myelography may demonstrate a diffuse intramedullary expansion representing the combination of solid tumor and cyst, and subsequent CT scanning may simply pass through the cystic portion of the expansion. A preoperative diagnosis of hemangioblastoma in such a case may not be possible. Enlargement of spinal cord vasculature, however, may suggest the appropriate diagnosis. In such a case, CT scanning following a bolus of intravenous contrast material may show the nodular portion of the expansion (Fig 30–18). Spinal cord angiography is definitive. All patients with spinal cord hemangioblastoma should undergo extensive intracranial evaluation, along with appropriate radiographic studies of the abdominal viscera, particularly the kidneys for the possibility of hypernephroma.

Syringomyelia/Hydromyelia

There will be no attempt in this chapter to discuss the very controversial theories regarding the origins of hydromyelia and syringomyelia. Briefly, however, hydromyelia is considered to be an expansion of the central canal and is generally associated with the Chiari malformation. Syringomyelia is thought by most to represent a cystic expansion that originates outside of the central canal and may either be congenital in origin or secondary to myelopathic processes such as trauma or infarction. There is obviously a great deal of overlap between the two entities and great controversy regarding their origin, differentiation, and therapy. The reader is referred to Chapters 32 and 33.

Syringomyelia/hydromyelia classically presents with an enlarged cord, and a low-density "cyst" may be seen on the premyelographic CT scans. However, long-standing expansion of the cyst produces atrophy of the surrounding cord. Therefore, the cord shadow may appear normal or small on a preceding myelogram or subsequent CT scan. A high level of clinical suspicion for the diagnosis must therefore be present, so that delayed CT scans may be obtained even in the face of a small or normal-sized cord. Scanning at 6 and 24 hours is generally obtained in this institution, although good studies of contrast media transport into such lesions have not been done, and the efficacy of scanning at 6, 12, 18, or 24 hours has yet to be well evaluated. The appearance of the contrast collections within the syrinx has been described previously, along with the differential diagnostic points for distinguishing between syr-

inx and neoplasm. Distinction may also be aided by appropriate scanning at the foramen magnum to detect an underlying Chiari malformation. The appearance of tonsils extending through the foramen magnum, along with the CT scan characteristics of either an enlarged or normal-sized cord with contrast media imbibition, gives evidence for a diagnosis of syringomyelia/hydromyelia (Fig 30–19).

Metastases

Hematogenous metastasis to the cord parenchyma is quite rare. Most intramedullary metastatic tumors are direct extensions of neoplasm originating within the posterior fossa, particularly medulloblastoma.[15] Such intracranial neoplasms may produce both direct extension into the cord and "dropped metastases" along the outer surface of the cord and meninges (Fig 30–20).

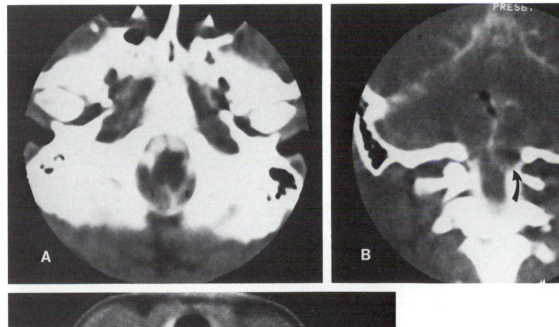

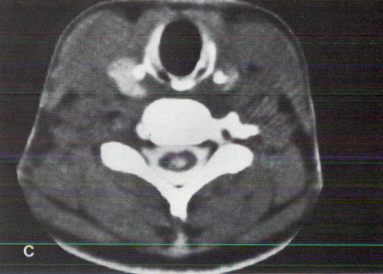

Fig 30–19.—Chiari malformation with hydromyelia. **A,** axial scan at the foramen magnum shows caudally situated tonsils *(t)* asymmetrically rotating the medulla. **B,** coronal section delineates the caudal bulge of the tonsil *(curved arrow)* below the foramen magnum. **C,** a well-defined central collection of metrizamide accumulates within the cervical cavity on delayed scan.

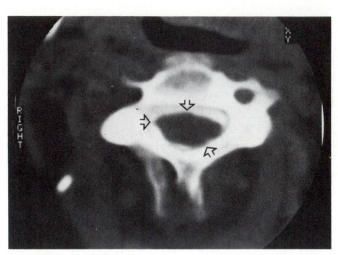

Fig 30–20.—Metastatic medulloblastoma. Not only is the cervical cord expanded by intramedullary metastasis, but nodular excrescences are seen on the cord surface from metastases coating it (arrows).

SPINAL INFECTION

Spinal infection, whether it relates to the bony vertebral column or its enclosed soft-tissue spaces, is usually diagnosed by clinical findings—backache, muscle spasm, fever, constitutional symptoms, and elevated sedimentation rate. Radiologic techniques are utilized in localizing and characterizing the infection; as such, CT is an exquisite tool for defining the site and spread of the infection. The use of CT adds important information to standard radiography, allowing direct assessment of the intervertebral discs, paravertebral tissues, and epidural space, as well as the bony structures. As emphasized previously, it is not a screening tool, but is best utilized in conjunction with conventional radiographs, nuclear medicine scans, or myelogram.

Disc-Related Infections

So-called disc space infections represent the most common type of spinal infection. There are three basic syndromes of disc space infection, only two of which actually originate from the disc. A complicating factor in considering these syndromes is the fact that infectious agents have not been isolated in all instances. Even with newer methodology for isolating anaerobic bacteria and fungi, a specific etiologic agent is not always found. Thus, it seems more appropriate to speak in terms of the exact inflammatory syndrome rather than including them in a catch-all phrase like "disc space infection," even though their radiographic manifestations are quite similar.

The first syndrome is that of vertebral osteomyelitis (also called infectious spondylitis). Primarily a disease of adults, it may be pyogenic or nonpyogenic, acute or chronic.[16–18] Osteomyelitis is believed to be a result of hematogenous seeding of infection into the subchondral region of the vertebral body. Although spread through Batson's plexus of paravertebral veins provides a means of explaining the association of infectious spondylitis with pelvic infection and instrumentation,[19] arterial seeding is more plausible as a mode of spread in the spondylitis associated with distant infections of the skin, indwelling catheters, and other sites.[20–23] Bacteria lodge and grow in the low-flow subchondral vascular arcades, causing destruction of the vertebral body. The disc is only secondarily involved, while the subjacent vertebral body is infected by contiguous infection or through small collateral channels.[16] *Staphylococcus aureus* is the most common infecting organism; however, a wide variety of anaerobic and aerobic bacteria have been isolated.

The second syndrome is postoperative disc space infection, which includes any exposure of the disc to the outside environment, including lumbar puncture, myelography, discography, chemonucleolysis, lumbar sympathectomy, epidural anesthesia, or laminectomy.[24–28] The infective agent is introduced directly into the disc and spreads through the avascular disc and subsequently into the contiguous subchondral bone. Clinically, there is usually a lag of several weeks between the time of operation and the development of symptoms or radiographic findings. Again, *Staphylococcus* species are the most common offending agents.[28]

The third syndrome is childhood discitis. This is an inflammatory, but not infectious, condition of the spine causing a wide spectrum of symptoms, including leg or back pain, tenderness, or toxemia. Although the symptoms and radiographic changes suggest a pyogenic etiology, only 30% to 40% of patients are found to have positive cultures, and antibiotics do not necessarily alter the course of disease; there is a wide spectrum of virulence.[29–33] The presumed cause is hematogenous spread of bacteria or virus to the disc (the disc is vascularized for the first three decades, after which vascularity regresses.[34] Secondary involvement of the adjacent vertebral endplates (osteomyelitis) leads to bony weakening and herniation of the disc into the vertebral body.

The conventional radiographic hallmark of these syndromes is irregularity of the subchondral vertebral body. The disc space is narrowed to a variable degree. However, there can be considerable lag between the onset of symptoms and the radiographic demonstration of disease; therefore, a normal plain film may not necessarily exclude osteomyelitis.[16, 18, 22] High-resolution CT, being more sensitive to bony destruction than conventional radiography, helps improve detection in the early stages of disease.[33, 35, 36] As disease progresses, it becomes important in defining the amount of intraspinal and extraspinal soft-tissue involvement.

Scans by CT in the early phases of osteomyelitis or discitis show rarefaction of the subchondral bone (Fig 30–21). Irregular areas of local erosion appear, which may coalesce into large areas of destruction (Fig 30–22).[33, 37] On axial scans, the destruction becomes more apparent closer to the disc, a feature that helps distinguish infection from tumor. Another characteristic that differentiates the two is the tendency for contiguous vertebral body involvement in infection, while tumor usually affects only one side of the disc space.[37] Sagittal or coronal reformatted images are particularly useful in demonstrating the location of bony destruction in relation to the disc (see Fig 30–22).

Collapse of the weakened vertebral body results in fragmentation near the disc (Fig 30–23).[37, 38] The cortical margins of the body fracture outward, giving an expanded appearance. The infected disc loses density[36] and blends into the lucency of the eroded vertebrae, especially when disc space narrowing is severe. The periphery of the disc blends with soft-tissue masses if cellulitis or abscess spreads into the pre- or paravertebral regions. Posteriorly, the disc blends with epidural mass as infection extends under or through the posterior longitudinal ligament. The resultant abscess or granulation tissue may present as a well-defined mass displacing the thecal sac or as a large mass that totally obscures the sac. Paravertebral and epidural masses are accentuated by use of intravenous contrast enhancement (see Fig 30–24).[35] Definition of a large epidural mass is usually

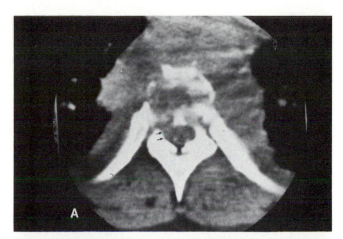

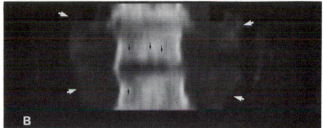

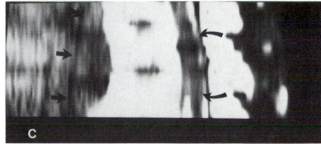

Fig 30–22.—Vertebral osteomyelitis. **A,** much of the vertebral body is destroyed on this section near the disc. The large paravertebral abscess is obvious; anterolateral epidural abscess *(arrows)* displaces the slightly opacified thecal sac and spinal cord *(c)*. **B,** coronal reconstruction at wide window setting defines areas of subchondral destruction *(black arrows)* and bilateral paravertebral abscesses *(white arrows)*. **C,** sagittal reconstruction at narrow window setting allows visualization of the compressed spinal cord *(curved arrows)* and prevertebral abscess *(arrows)*.

facilitated by scanning after the introduction of intrathecal metrizamide.

In the chronic or healing phase of infectious spondylitis, CT reflects the reparative response of the bones and soft tissues. New bone formation occurs at the vertebral body margins, causing increased bony density and peripheral bony bridges (see Fig 30–23).[39] Paravertebral abscesses organize and become better defined.

The radiographic changes of postoperative infectious discitis must be distinguished from benign changes that may occur as a normal response to disc surgery. Occa-

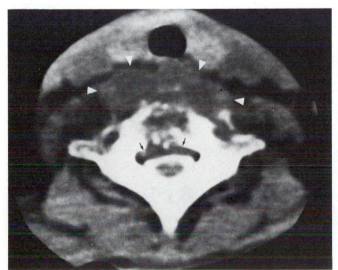

Fig 30–21.—Vertebral osteomyelitis. The subchondral portion of the vertebral body shows irregular destruction. A contiguous prevertebral abscess obscures the retropharyngeal soft-tissue planes *(arrowheads)*. There is a small epidural mass displacing the thecal sac *(arrows)*.

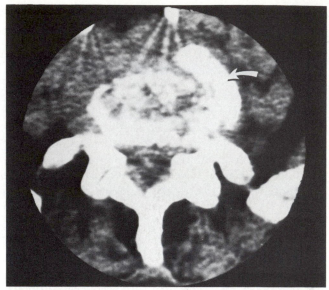

Fig 30–23.—Postoperative disc space infection. The vertebral body is severely fragmented; a large bony bridge has developed along the anterolateral aspect of the disc space *(arrow)*.

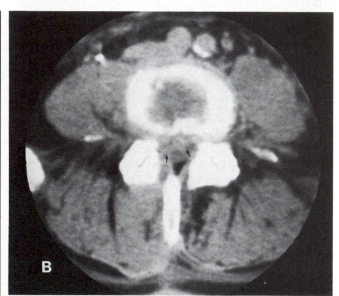

A

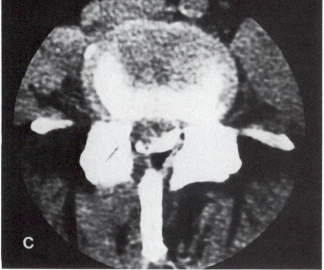

Fig 30–24.—Postoperative disc space infection. **A,** conventional tomogram shows destruction of the vertebral body cortical margin *(arrow)*. **B,** following intravenous contrast administration, an irregularly enhancing epidural abscess *(arrows)* is seen deforming the thecal sac and protruding along the right neural foramen. **C,** similar section following myelogram accentuates the deformed sac. Without intravenous contrast, the abscess is lucent.

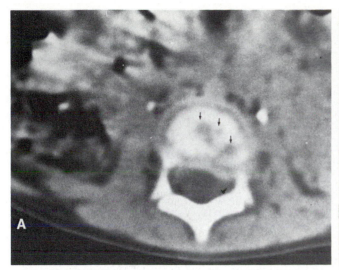
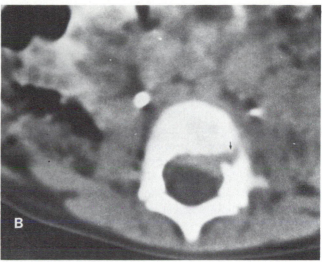

Fig 30–25.—Childhood discitis. **A,** focal areas of destruction *(arrows)* involve the subchondral bone. **B,** a contiguous section through the pedicles shows greater involvement of the left side *(arrow).* The small homogeneously enhancing epidural component asymmetrically bulges into the spinal canal. Biopsy sample was sterile.

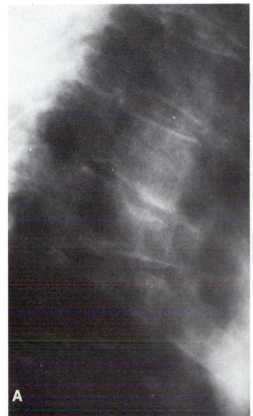
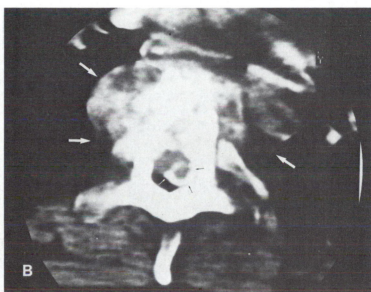

Fig 30–26.—Tuberculous spondylitis. **A,** there is destruction of the anterosuperior margin of a midthoracic vertebral body, without significant diminution of the disc space. **B,** anterolateral vertebral body destruction is accompanied by a moderate-sized paravertebral abscess *(large arrows)* and an epidural abscess displacing the opacified thecal sac *(small arrows).*

sionally, the disc space collapses, and adjacent sub-chondral margins rarefy, presumably a result of ischemic changes (analogous to osteitis pubis).[40] However, involvement is limited to those areas and does not extend significantly into the epidural or paravertebral regions as it does in infection. So, too, discitis of childhood has limited spread away from the disc and endplates. In the usual case, involvement of the epidural and paravertebral spaces is mild (Fig 30–25).[32, 33] Extensive involvement usually indicates one of the more virulent (usually pyogenic) types of discitis.

Although CT cannot reliably be used to predict the specific agent causing the spondylitis or discitis, certain characteristics help suggest nonpyogenic (tuberculosis, fungus) agents. Tuberculous spondylitis can be distinguished by its tendency to involve the anterior third of the vertebral body, its slowly progressive course, and its relative preservation of the disc space (Figs 30–26 and 30–27).[41–44] Involvement of the posterior elements is more characteristic of tuberculous than pyogenic osteomyelitis. Defects of the anterior aspects of several

vertebral bodies (subligamentous spread), especially when associated with a paravertebral abscess, is very suggestive of tuberculosis.[42] Although both pyogenic and tuberculous infections may have paraspinal abscesses, tuberculous abscesses have a greater tendency for calcification, thick enhancing rims, and extensive spread (see Fig 30–27).[41] Fungal infections can be indistinguishable from pyogenic or tuberculous infections. Occasionally, when multiple well-defined vertebral body and posterior element lytic lesions are seen without disc space involvement, a diagnosis of coccidioidal or cryptococcal spondylitis may be made.[44, 45]

Definitive diagnosis of the disc-related infections usually requires biopsy. The use of CT is not only useful in localizing the abnormalities, but may be utilized in guiding the biopsy needle to an optimum site (Fig 30–28).[35]

Other Spinal Infections

Extraosseous epidural abscesses may arise from direct hematogenous seeding or from extension of a para-

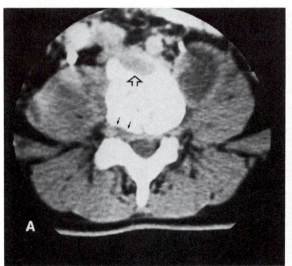
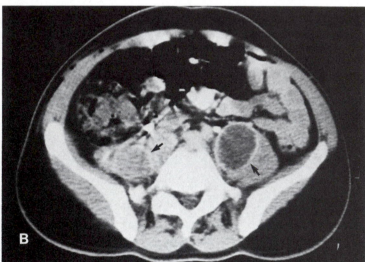
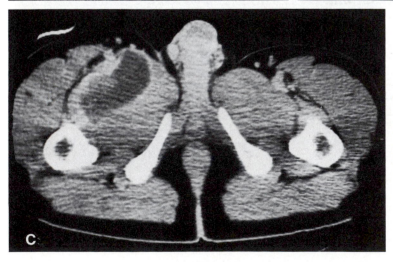

Fig 30–27.—Tuberculous spondylitis. **A,** there is focal destruction of the anterior vertebral body *(large arrow)*. An epidural abscess *(small arrows)* fills the right neural foramen. Note bilateral psoas abscesses. **B,** the thick-walled abscesses *(arrows)* can be followed to a lower level. **C,** the right abscess tracks into the leg below the femoral inlet.

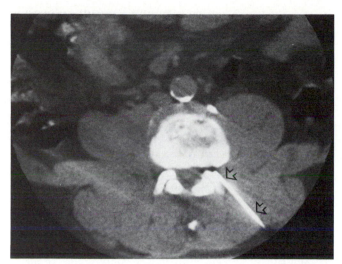

Fig 30–28.—CT-guided biopsy. The biopsy needle *(arrows)* has been directed through the paravertebral muscles to obtain a specimen near the posterior aspect of the disc.

vertebral (psoas) abscess through the neural foramen.[34] The abscess may be focal or extend over multiple segments (Fig 30–29). The CT appearance is indistinguishable from epidural abscess associated with disc-related infection. Unless there is gas within the abscess mass, it usually enhances homogeneously, surrounding or displacing the thecal sac. Lumbar abscesses are more easily distinguished than cervical or thoracic abscesses because of the larger size of the lumbar canal. By CT alone, it may be impossible to differentiate between abscess and infiltrating metastatic or lymphomatous tumor. Most extraosseous extradural abscesses are pyogenic, but a few cases of tuberculous abscesses have been reported.[46]

Empyemas of the subdural space are rarely encountered. They are not associated with osteomyelitis, but result from metastatic seeding (usually *S. aureus*) from distant infected sources.[47] Myelographically, they present as single or multiple defects simulating epidural masses or arachnoid adhesions. No CT characteristics of these empyemas have been reported. Intramedullary abscesses are similarly rare. Myelographically, they are indistinguishable from other intramedullary lesions, causing fairly focal cord widening. The thoracic cord is most commonly affected.[48] The CT features have not been delineated, but enhancement of the enlarged cord would be expected on contrast-enhanced scan.

REFERENCES

1. Aubin M.L., Vignaud J., Jardin C., et al.: Computed tomography in 75 clinical cases of syringomyelia. *A.J.N.R.* 2:199–204, 1981.
2. Pinto R.S., Kricheff I.I., Epstein F., et al.: A practical approach to the neuroradiologic investigation of spinal

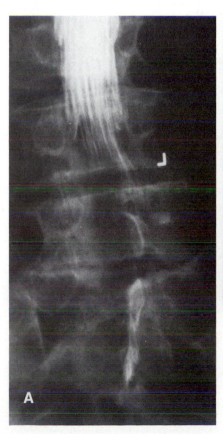

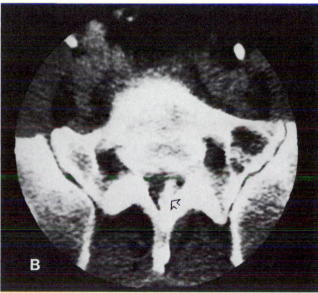

Fig 30–29.—Epidural abscess. **A,** a large epidural abscess obscures much of the thecal sac over several levels. **B,** scan at the level of the sacrum following myelogram demonstrates the thecal sac *(arrow),* pushed posterolaterally by the epidural abscess.

cord cysts. Presented at the 21st Annual Meeting of the American Society of Neuroradiology, San Francisco, June 5–9, 1983.

3. Schmorl G., Junghanns H.: *The Human Spine in Health and Disease*, ed. 2, Beseman E.F. (trans.-ed.). New York, Grune & Stratton, 1971.

4. Freiberger R.H.: Osteoid osteoma of the spine: A cause of backache and scoliosis in children and young adults. *Radiology* 75:232–235, 1960.

5. Levy W.M., Miller A.S., Bonakarpour A., et al.: Aneurysmal bone cyst secondary to other osseous lesions: A report of 57 cases. *Am. J. Clin. Pathol.* 63:1–8, 1975.

6. Dahlin D.C.: *Bone Tumors: General Aspects and Data on 6,221 Cases*, ed, 3. Springfield, Ill., Charles C Thomas, Publisher, 1978.

7. Firooznia H., Pinto R.S., Lin J.P., et al.: Chordoma: Radiologic evaluation of 20 cases. *A.J.R.* 127:979–805, 1976.

8. Epstein B.S.: *The Spine*, ed. 4. Philadelphia, Lea & Febiger, 1976.

9. Fagan C.J., Swischuk L.E.: Dumbbell neuroblastoma or ganglioneuroma of the spinal canal. *A.J.R.* 120:453–460, 1974.

10. Latchaw R.E., L'Heureux P.R., Young G., et al.: Neuroblastoma presenting as central nervous system disease. *A.J.N.R.* 3:623–630, 1982.

11. Polmeteer F.E., Kernohan J.W.: Meningeal gliomatosis: A study of forty-two cases. *Arch. Neurol. Psychiatry* 57:593–616, 1947.

12. Bentley J.F.R., Smith J.R.: Developmental posterior enteric remnants and spinal malformations: The split notochord syndrome. *Arch. Dis. Child.* 35:76–86, 1960.

13. Kendall B.E., Valentine A.R., Keis B.: Spinal arachnoid cysts: Clinical and radiological correlation with prognosis. *Neuroradiology* 22:225–234, 1982.

14. Haft H., Ransohoff J., Carter S.: Spinal cord tumors in children. *Pediatrics* 23:1152–1159, 1959.

15. Deutsch M., Reigel D.H.: The value of myelography in the management of childhood medulloblastoma. *Cancer* 45:2194–2197, 1980.

16. Stauffer R.N.: Pyogenic vertebral osteomyelitis. *Orthop. Clin. North Am.* 6:1015–1027, 1975.

17. Bonfiglio M., Lange T.A., Kim Y.M.: Pyogenic vertebral osteomyelitis: Disk space infections. *Clin. Orthop.* 96:234–247, 1973.

18. Digby J.M., Kersley J.B.: Pyogenic non-tuberculous spinal infection: An analysis of thirty cases. *J. Bone Joint Surg. [Br.]* 61:47–55, 1979.

19. Batson O.V.: The function of the vertebral veins and their role in the spread of metastases. *Ann. Surg.* 112:138–149, 1940.

20. Wiley A.M., Trueta J.: The vascular anatomy of the spine and its relationship to pyogenic vertebral osteomyelitis. *J. Bone Joint Surg. [Br.]* 41:796–809, 1959.

21. Sapico F.L., Montgomerie J.Z.: Vertebral osteomyelitis in intravenous drug abusers: Report of three cases and review of the literature. *Rev. Infect. Dis.* 2:196–206, 1980.

22. Musher D.M., Thorsteinsson S.B., Minuth J.N., et al.: Vertebral osteomyelitis: Still a diagnostic pitfall. *Arch. Intern. Med.* 136:105–110, 1976.

23. Waldvogel F.A., Vasey H.: Osteomyelitis: The past decade. *N. Engl. J. Med.* 303:360–370, 1980.

24. Baker A.S., Ojemann R.G., Morton M.D., et al.: Spinal epidural abscess. *N. Engl. J. Med.* 293:463–468, 1975.

25. Stern W.E., Crandall P.H.: Inflammatory intervertebral disc disease as a complication of the operative treatment of lumbar herniations. *J. Neurosurg.* 16:261–276, 1959.

26. Pilgaard S.: Discitis (closed space infection) following removal of lumbar intervertebral disc. *J. Bone Joint Surg. [Am.]* 51A:713–716, 1969.

27. Lindholm T.S., Pylkkanen P.: Discitis following removal of intervertebral disc. *Spine* 7:618–622, 1982.

28. Rawlings C.E., Wilkins R.H., Gallis H.A., et al.: Postoperative intervertebral disc space infection. *Neurosurgery* 13:371–375, 1983.

29. Smith R.F., Taylor T.K.: Inflammatory lesions of intervertebral discs in children. *J. Bone Joint Surg. [Am.]* 49:1508–1520, 1967.

30. Pritchard A.E., Thompson W.A.L.: Acute pyogenic infections of the spine in children. *J. Bone Joint Surg. [Br.]* 42:86–89, 1960.

31. Menelaus M.B.: Discitis: An inflammation affecting the intervertebral discs in children. *J. Bone Joint Surg. [Br.]* 46:16–23, 1964.

32. Grunebaum M., Horodniceanu C.H., Mukamel M., et al.: The imaging diagnosis of nonpyogenic discitis in children. *Pediatr. Radiol.* 12:133–137, 1982.

33. Sartoris D.J., Moskowitz P.S., Kaufman R.A., et al.: Childhood diskitis: Computed tomographic findings. *Radiology* 149:701–707, 1983.

34. Conventry M.B., Ghormley R.K., Kernohan J.W.: The intervertebral disc: Its microscopic anatomy and pathology. I. Anatomy, development, and pathology. *J. Bone Joint Surg.* 27:105–112, 1945.

35. Golumbu C., Firooznia H., Rafii M.: CT of osteomyelitis of the spine. *A.J.N.R.* 4:1207–1211, 1983.

36. Larde D., Mathiew D., Frija J., et al.: Vertebral osteomyelitis: Disc hypodensity on CT. *A.J.R.* 139:963–967, 1982.

37. Price A.C., Allen J.H., Eggers F.M., et al.: Intervertebral disk-space infection: CT changes. *Radiology* 149:725–729, 1983.

38. Hermann G., Mendelson D.S., Cohen B.A., et al.: Role of computed tomography in the diagnosis of infectious spondylitis. *J. Comput. Assist. Tomogr.* 7:961–968, 1983.

39. Kattapuran S.V., Phillips W.C., Boyd R.: CT in pyogenic osteomyelitis of the spine. *A.J.R.* 140:1199–1201, 1983.

40. Lowman R.M., Robinson F.: Progressive vertebral interspace changes following lumbar disk surgery. *A.J.R.* 97:664–671, 1966.

41. Whelan M.A., Naidich D.P., Post J.D., et al.: Computed tomography of spinal tuberculosis. *J. Comput. Assist. Tomogr.* 7:25–30, 1983.

42. Chapman M., Murray R.O., Stoker D.J.: Tuberculosis of the bones and joints. *Semin. Roentgenol.* 14:266–282, 1979.

43. Allen E.H., Cosgrove D., Millard F.J.C.: The radiologi-

cal changes in infections of the spine and their diagnostic value. *Clin. Radiol.* 29:31–40, 1978.

44. Goldman A.B., Freiberger R.H.: Localized infectious and neuropathic diseases. *Semin. Roentgenol.* 14:19–31, 1979.

45. McGahan J.P., Graves D.S., Palmer P.E.S.: Coccidioidal spondylitis: Usual and unusual radiographic manifestations. *Radiology* 136:5–9, 1980.

46. Chin D., Barrow D., Edis R., et al.: Extraosseous extra-dural tuberculous granuloma of the spine. *Surg. Neurol.* 19:428–430, 1983.

47. Fraser R.A.R., Ratzan K., Wolpert S.M., et al.: Spinal subdural empyema. *Arch. Neurol.* 28:235–238, 1973.

48. Brant-Zawadzki M.: *Infections in Computed Tomography of the Spine and Spinal Column,* Newton T.H., Potts D.G. (eds.). San Anselmo, Calif., Clavadel Press, 1983, pp. 205–221.

31

Traumatic Lesions of the Spinal Column

MICHAEL BRANT-ZAWADZKI, M.D.

THE RADIOLOGIC EVALUATION of acute trauma to the spinal column is often a trying experience. Multiple radiographic views and techniques are often necessary, the affected patient is usually suffering from severe pain and has difficulty cooperating with the technician, and the accurate diagnosis of his injuries is critical to appropriate therapeutic management. Missing a fracture or the presence of significant instability may lead to irreparable neurologic consequences for the patient. Within this context, the diagnostic radiologist must not only choose the appropriate imaging modality, but must also combine such a choice with a thorough knowledge of the varied anatomy in the different spinal regions and an understanding of the interplay between the traumatic vectors of force and their effect, which may differ among the major spinal levels.

The traditional radiographic techniques used in the evaluation of spinal trauma include plain films, multidirectional tomography, and, occasionally, myelography. Recently, CT has found a major role in the evaluation of spinal trauma.[1-5] This role is one that has been the traditional province of multidirectional tomography and myelography. Namely, in cases where the initial screening plain films fail to provide a thorough evaluation of spinal injury, a more definitive modality is necessary to elucidate equivocal injuries, to unravel complex fractures, to detect the presence of significant spinal instability from ligamentous disruption, and, finally, to depict the compromise of vital neural structures within the bony spinal canal. The usefulness of any particular imaging modality is judged in terms of its performance in these important categories. However, the ultimate value of any imaging modality rests on its ability to translate its diagnostic information toward more appropriate therapeutic management of the patient.

This last contribution of imaging is difficult to judge in the setting of spine trauma, because considerable controversy still exists regarding the appropriate treatment of such injuries as spinal instability and spinal cord and nerve root damage in the early stages of injury. Although a discussion of controversies in management of acute spinal injury is not possible in this chapter, a brief understanding of the major areas of debate will help the reader's perspective and may serve to underscore some of the advantages that CT offers in this setting.

The two major areas of therapeutic controversy in treatment of spinal injuries are the therapy of spinal instability and the treatment of the patient with acute trauma to the spinal cord or nerve roots. Spinal instability may result from purely ligamentous damage unassociated with bony disruption, or it may be the result of significant disruption of the posterior elements of the vertebral bodies, which are directly involved with intervertebral articulation. The two modes of therapy available are either a conservative immobilization or some form of surgical fusion. The choice of one therapy or the other depends on the type and degree of disruption, the potential for the body's own mechanisms to provide stability through bony fusion, the potential for nonunion and subsequent malalignment and possible neurologic compromise, the needs of the patient for early rehabilitation, and, finally, the therapeutic philosophy of the responsible physician.

The controversy regarding management of injury to the neural structures is even more difficult. Neurologic symptoms may result following injury to the cord from several mechanisms. Mild cord contusion, more severe degrees of compression and edema, frank laceration with hematoma, and even transection may be indistinguishable in the first few hours following injury. However, mild contusion and even more severe forms of edema may spontaneously resolve, given enough time. Occasionally, cord compression from bony or disc fragments may need surgical intervention, and such treatment may lead to resolution of neurologic symptoms and signs. However, all too often the initial neurologic signs are caused by an irreversible process. The managing physician is faced with the choice of deciding in the first several hours whether acute surgical decompression of the spinal cord or affected nerve roots will have any effect on the patient's outcome, especially in view of the inherent risks in such an aggressive approach.

The traditional imaging modalities have been part of this controversy, and although some improvement in their diagnostic ability has occurred, the controversies persist. By virtue of its accuracy and efficiency, CT may be more helpful than the more traditional imaging modalities in helping to resolve at least some components of the therapeutic dilemmas faced in this patient population. We will illustrate the usefulness of CT in each of the major areas that imaging is used for evaluating the spinal trauma patient, namely, the assessment of instability, the evaluation of complex fractures, and the compromise of neural structures within the spinal canal. Let us first briefly describe the general technique factors used in scanning patients with spine trauma in our institution.

TECHNIQUE

Having sufficient personnel greatly facilitates transfer of the patient onto the scanning couch. If traction has been applied, maintenance of traction during the study is critical (see following). Next, a lateral digital radiograph is obtained in the region of interest for the purpose of accurate localization of the subsequent axial sections.

Next, the slice thickness, spacing, and exposure factors are selected. Thin CT sections are critical for optimal resolution of spine injury, especially if image reformation is anticipated. We generally employ 5-mm thick sections with only 3 mm of table motion between adjacent sections, yielding 2 mm of overlap. This provides adequate detail of subtle structures both on axial and reformatted views. In the cervical region, where the architecture of the spine is both the smallest and most complex, the thinnest possible sections (we employ 1.5-mm sections) should be obtained for thorough evaluation of bony structures and their relationships.

The efficiency of CT in diagnosing spinal trauma is one of the major virtues of this modality. Such efficiency is optimized by use of rapid-sequence scanning, a capability present on several current generation scanners. This technique allows constant serial scanning of the sequential sections, with the only interruption being automatic table incrementation between each succeeding slice. Low mAs technique is necessary to

prevent buildup of excessive heat in the x-ray tube with such a rapid scan sequence. However, the exquisite sensitivity of CT to objects of high contrast allows the use of such low mAs factors (160 to 310 mAs) without the risk of significant degradation in spatial resolution. The entire (up to 45-slice) study can take less than 12 minutes of patient time and aids in preventing patient motion between slices. This, in turn, optimizes registration of contiguous sections on reformatted images. Occasionally, low mAs technique is suboptimal in the C6-7 region, where the shoulder girdle severely increases attenuation of the x-ray beam. Higher exposure factors may be necessary in this particular region of the spine. Also, it must be remembered that the appearance of soft-tissue structures such as disc material, viscera, etc., is somewhat degraded with low mAs technique; hence higher exposure factors might be opted for in selected cases. However, when searching for bony disruption, the low mAs factors suffice for all practical purposes.[6] After the administration of metrizamide, the subarachnoid space gains sufficient contrast that the low mAs factors allow definitive assessment of any cord compromise by bony fragments or epidural hematomas and also allow depiction of cord enlargement caused by edema or contusion. The contrast agent can be introduced via the C1-2 approach with the patient supine, obviating unnecessary motion. Sufficient angulation of a tiltable gurney will ensure distribution of the contrast agent down to the desired level. Approximately 5 ml of metrizamide in a concentration of 170 to 200 mg/ml will suffice for opacification of the thecal sac for CT purposes. We only use metrizamide in those cases of acute spine trauma that are associated with neurologic signs or symptoms. We also encourage liberal hydration of the patient following the procedure.

Following the CT study, image reformations of the axial sections are routinely obtained. This requires approximately 5 to 15 minutes of postprocessing time by an experienced radiologist. In general, a midsagittal reformation and parasagittal reformations through the facets are all that is needed, although occasional injuries necessitate more diverse image manipulation.

Having discussed the technical aspects of the study, we now return to the clinical role of CT in the setting of spine trauma.

Spinal Instability

The stability of the spinal column depends largely on the integrity of the strong spinal ligaments that bind the adjacent bony vertebral bodies and their elements together. The anterior and posterior longitudinal ligaments strengthen the column of vertebral bodies, whereas the capsular ligaments and ligamentum flavum bind the articular facets and laminae respectively. The interspinous ligaments connect and fix the spinous processes of adjacent vertebral levels. Disruption of the ligamentous complex in the spine cannot be visualized directly. However, severe damage to the ligamentous complex can be suspected when a paraspinal hematoma is seen. The damage is manifest by malalignment of the spine, which becomes especially evident with motion. Because either flexion and/or extension views will exaggerate any malalignment, these are key to making the radiographic diagnosis. Occasionally, cinefluorography is necessary to delineate the type of instability present. Clearly, any static imaging modality, including CT, will have difficulty detecting instability from ligamentous disruption unless some malalignment is present with the patient supine. Nevertheless, even subtle malalignment of bony structures can be detected with CT. Occasionally, axial views are insufficient for illustrating abnormal facet relationships, because the disturbance may be vertical in nature (Fig 31–1). The most common type of violence that produces ligamentous disruption is one that includes flexion and rotation vectors.[7] Sufficient ligamentous disruption may actually lead to facet "locking," which occurs when the inferior facet jumps over and finally rests anterior to the superior facet, reversing the usual orientation. Such an event can easily be recognized on axial CT sections, provided careful attention is paid to the sequence of scans. Image reformation along the facets is useful in illustrating this entity in a sagittal plane (Fig 31–2).

If insufficient malalignment is present with the patient supine, CT or other static image modalities will not detect instability. However, the presence of actual fracture of the posterior vertebral elements strongly suggests the presence of instability, and such fracture is easily detected with the high-resolution capabilities of current generation CT scanners (see following). Overall, facet or vertebral body subluxation is more common in the cervical region, where the ligamentous structures play a more significant role in providing spinal stability, because the articulating facets relate in a relatively horizontal fashion without much overlap, and the weight of

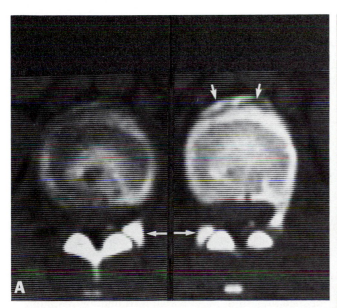

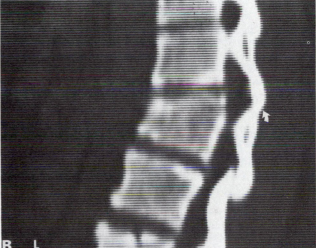

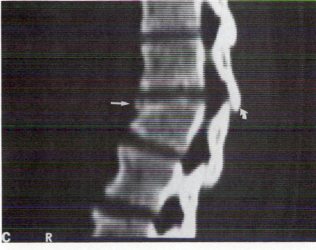

Fig 31–1.—Facet subluxation, thoracolumbar junction. **A,** contiguous axial CT sections (*left* and *right,* 3 mm apart) at the T12-L1 level of a 26-year-old woman who jumped 30 feet show evidence of L-1 vertebral compression *(upper arrows, right).* Note that the facet relationships appear undisturbed, the anterolaterally positioned superior facets of L-2 *(lower arrows)* "hugging" the inferior facets of L-1. **B, C,** image reformations in the sagittal plane of the facet joints show "perching" of the left **(B)** and right **(C)** facets *(curved arrows)* with slight gibbous deformity, and define the vertebral body compression **(C,** *arrow)* to better advantage. (*L* = left facets, *R* = right facets.)

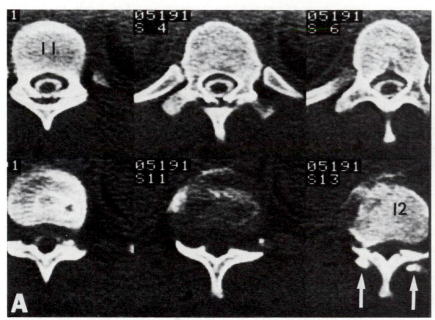

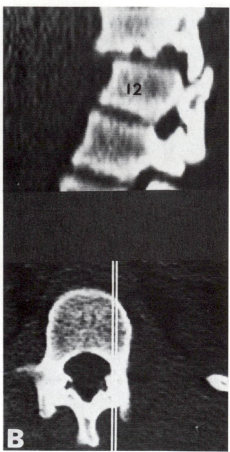

Fig 31–2.—Locked facets, lower thoracic region ("seat-belt" fracture). **A,** axial CT sections of the lower thoracic spine show the eventual appearance of superior facets of T-12 *(arrows)* behind the inferior facets of T-11 *(11)* in this young man thrown out of a jeep while wearing a lap belt. Note the normal facet relationship at the T10-T11 level (first section) and the progressive disappearance of metrizamide in the contiguous sections (indicating block). Also seen is a fractured superior end-plate of T-12 *(12)*. **B,** sagittal image reformation delineates the "locked" inferior facet of T-11, in front of the superior facet of T-12 *(12)*.

the head provides a pendulum-like action in any acceleration or deceleration force.

The sturdiness and marked overlap of the thoracic articulations and the stability provided by the bony and muscular elements of the rib cage tend to make instability in the thoracic region appear only with the gravest injuries. Instability in the lumbar spine following trauma is probably more frequent than is realized; however, its consequences are relatively less significant than those of instability in the cervical region, because the spinal cord is not at risk with injuries at this level. Nevertheless, such instability predisposes to subsequent degenerative facet disease and possibly disc herniation, and thus its recognition and proper management is of some clinical importance.

From the above discussion, the reader can infer that although spinal stability may not always be directly evaluated with CT, sufficient information may be gleaned from an appropriately performed study to make the diagnosis. Again, thin CT sections are critical for the optimal resolution of traumatic injury, especially so if image reformation is necessary. It must be remembered, however, that despite the most meticulous CT technique, proof of spinal instability can only be pro-

vided by flexion-extension views or cinefluorography in occasional instances.

Fractures

The detection of fracture following spinal trauma usually begins with the screening plain films. If the findings on plain films are equivocal or if the fracture is sufficiently complex to necessitate a more thorough evaluation, a tomographic modality is indicated. Plain films have been shown to underestimate the presence of spinal fracture; indeed, the introduction of high-quality conventional tomography changed the mode of therapy in up to 35% of spinal trauma cases.[8, 9] The mode of CT has achieved a comparable spatial resolution capability to that of conventional tomography.[10] The additional advantages it offers for improving the efficiency of the study while minimizing patient discomfort are making it the procedure of choice for the evaluation of complex spinal fracture in many institutions. Obviously, optimal resolution of certain fractures necessitates thin CT slices. Recent innovations have allowed the radiologist to "target" a certain region for high-resolution analysis. This is done by placing the entire pixel matrix within a small section of the scanning circle. The advantages of this technique for delineation of subtle bony anatomy such as exists in the middle ear cannot be denied; however, the aplication of such high-resolution bone reconstruction algorithms in the spine has limited advantages (Fig 31–3). In most instances, conventional reconstruction algorithms provide sufficient detail to define bony fractures even when minimal displacement occurs (Fig 31–4).

Image reformation is especially helpful in cases where horizontal fractures (those parallel to the original beam orientation) exist, such as fractures through the base of the odontoid process (see Fig 31–3). Image reformation also helps the radiologist to understand fracture lines in a three-dimensional sense and helps in orienting the inexperienced observer. Another advantage of image reformation is one already mentioned in the discussion of ligamentous disruption. Namely, the rearrangement of axial information into a vertical orientation is quite important when fractures distort vertical relationships; for instance, when vertebral body compression exists, its degree is difficult to appreciate on axial views (see Fig 31–1).

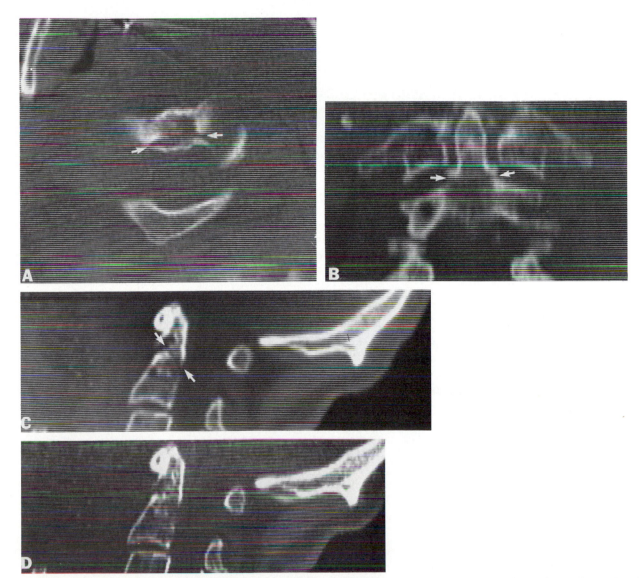

Fig 31–3.—Fracture of the odontoid process. **A,** axial CT section at the level of the C-2 vertebral body in this motor vehicle accident victim shows a linear fracture in back of the C-2 plateau *(arrows)*; however, orientation regarding the particular level and type of fracture is difficult. **B,** coronal reformation depicts a horizontal fracture *(arrows)* through the base of the dens. Note the normally aligned C-1 and C-2 lateral masses. The rest of the facet relationships are out of the plane of this reformation. **C,** sagittal reformation defines the fracture at the base of the dens to better advantage *(arrows)* and shows the integrity of the spinal canal at this level. **D,** midsagittal plane reformation of CT sections obtained following "target" reconstruction using a high-resolution bone algorithm. Note relatively little difference between the "target" reconstruction image vs. the original image **(C)**, which used conventional reconstruction algorithms.

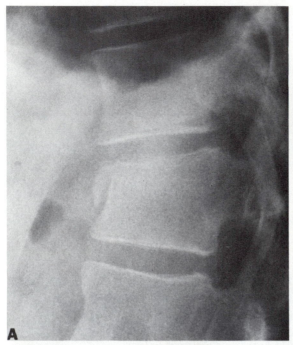

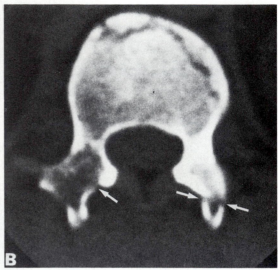

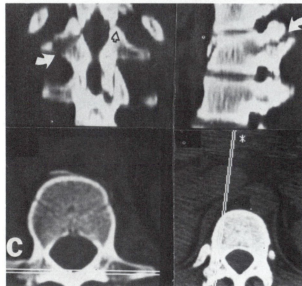

Fig 31–4.—L-1 fracture, blunt trauma. **A,** initial lateral film at the L-1 level shows compression of the vertebral body. No definite posterior element injury was noted; unfortunately, the facets were coned off the film because of technical error. **B,** axial CT section shows the irregularity of the superior part of the vertebral body, indicating compression fracture. Note the section also suggests fractures in the lateral facets *(arrows),* as evidenced by discontinuity of the cortical bone and linear lucencies on both sides. **C,** coronal *(left)* and sagittal *(right)* image reformations define a fracture through the lateral mass on the *right* and show it extending into the pedicle *(curved arrows).* The coronal view also shows blunting of the "Scotty dog ear" on the *left (open arrow),* corresponding to the fracture seen on the axial section in **B.**

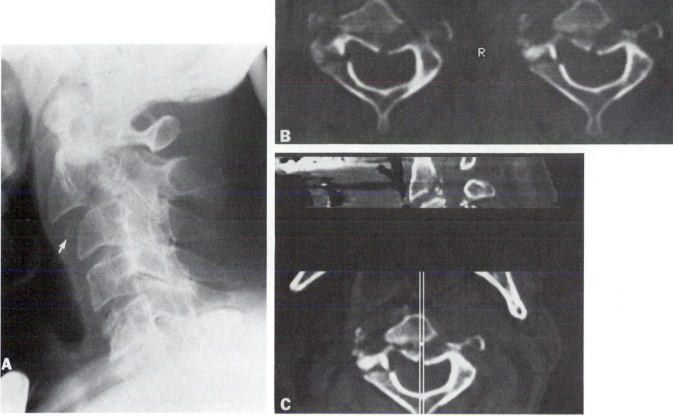

Fig 31–5.—Pseudo "hangman's" fracture. **A,** lateral cervical spine film of a middle-aged man following a car accident shows subluxation of C-2 anterior to C-3. The normal alignment of the posterior elements and evidence of bony disruption at the levels of the pedicles led to the diagnosis of a bipediculate fracture or so-called hangman's fracture. Also, note the chip fracture of the superoanterior aspect of C-3 *(arrow)* and an old compression of C-5. **B,** axial CT sections through the C-2 vertebral body show that the fracture line actually spares the left pedicle, affecting instead the vertebral body itself through its entire extent, the right *(R)* pedicle. **C,** midsagittal image reformation shows that the fracture also involves the posteroinferior aspect of the vertebral body. No significant compromise of the spinal canal is seen (patient had no neurologic symptoms). The apparent fragmentation depicted between the C-2 and C-3 spinous processes is due to misregistration artifact.

Also, axial sections may include osteophytes or even normal bony projections for only a portion of their true volume, occasionally simulating fragmentation from trauma. The availability of multiple projections from image reformation is clearly helpful in such instances.

The advantages of CT discussed above have made it exceedingly useful in studying fractures even in instances where plain films seem to have made the definitive diagnosis (Fig 31–5). Fractures of the cervical spine are especially dangerous, because damage to the cervical spinal cord may lead to a devastating neurologic deficit. Trauma to the lower cervical segments causes neurologic deficits more commonly than does trauma to the cranial cervical junction.[11–13] In addition, up to 40% of patients with fractures in the thoracolumbar junction and lumbar region may develop neurologic deficits; thus, a tomographic evaluation of fractures in

this region is often justified.[1] Fractures of the thoracic region are less common than those of the cervical or lumbar spine. The gentle kyphosis of the thoracic spine, its sturdy bony elements, and the stability afforded by the rib cage translate most vectors of force into flexion. The most common fracture seen in the thoracic spine is, therefore, an anterior compression of the vertebral body. When sufficient force occurs to produce hyperextension of the thoracic spine, a very severe injury with spinal cord damage usually results (Fig 31–6).

After the evaluation of traumatic injury to the spine, the radiologist may be asked to assess the results of therapy. Most often, the question of sufficient realignment is one that is addressed. This can be easily answered with axial sections and image reformation in the midsagittal plane, even when metallic fixation devices are in place (Fig 31–7). Although metal can give off suf-

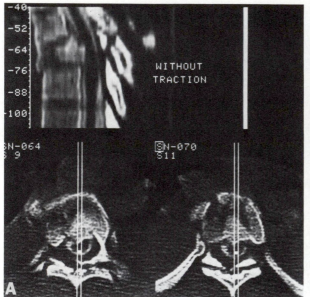

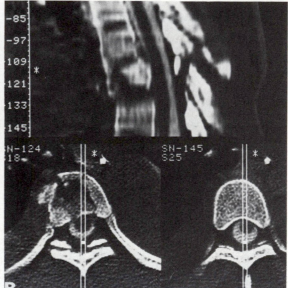

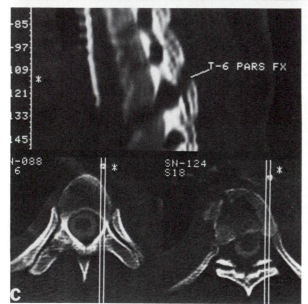

Fig 31–6.—Effects of traction on spinal cord compromise. **A,** the initial CT study of this young girl rendered paraplegic after a fall suggested compromise of the spinal cord by bony fragments at the T-6 level. Note the effacement of the metrizamide column anteriorly and posteriorly on the midsagittal reformation. Evidence of posterior element injury is likewise seen. **B,** following institution of traction, the patient was immediately rescanned. Note the increase in the width of the metrizamide column posteriorly on the subsequent study. Her continuing symptoms could not, therefore, be attributed to persistent compression of the spinal cord, and surgery was delayed. **C,** image reformations helped to define the associated fractures, including a pars interarticularis fracture at T-6 shown here.

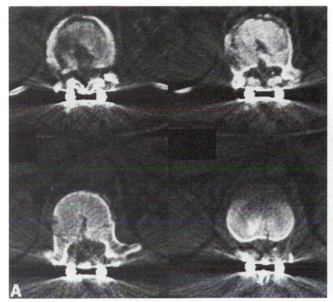

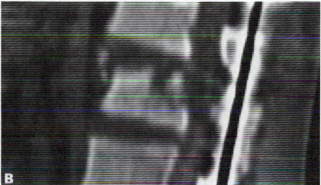

Fig 31–7.—CT scan for spinal alignment following introduction of metallic fixation devices. **A,** axial CT sections in the lumbar region show marked streak artifact from metallic structures in back of the posterior elements. Note that the vertebral bodies and the facets themselves can be distinguished despite the presence of the artifacts. **B,** midsagittal plane reformation shows relative realignment of the spinal canal following the marked compression of the L-2 vertebral body. Spinal canal integrity is depicted. The streak artifacts are summed to produce the black vertical bar seen in the region of the posterior elements.

ficient streak artifacts to grossly degrade the imaging of soft tissues, bony structures suffer less from such image degradation, and enough information is generally provided to answer the question at hand.

Neurologic Compromise

Although damage to neural structures within the spinal cord can be suggested with plain films and CT, direct visualization of the nature of the injury necessitates the presence of an intrathecal contrast agent. Those patients with a neurologic deficit of recent onset, and especially those in whom incomplete or progressive neurologic deficits occur, should be evaluated with some form of myelographic technique, because the correct diagnosis of such lesions is crucial to proper patient management. Myelography has a long tradition in the investigation of acute spinal trauma and has been used to guide specific therapy.[14–16] When there is clinical evidence of cord or cauda equina compression, the level of such compression may be demonstrated by myelography (Fig 31–8). However, conventional myelography has several disadvantages. It is difficult to perform a sterile and careful puncture in the setting of acute spinal trauma, and sufficient patient manipulation is necessary to position the dye and obtain proper views so that a significant risk of aggravating existing neurologic deficits or inducing new ones exists.

The introduction of water-soluble contrast agents has allowed CT to assume a myelographic role as well. Intrathecal introduction of metrizamide for CT scan purposes can be performed with the patient supine, using a cervical approach. The contrast agent can be positioned at the level necessary by having the patient on a gurney that can tilt. Because the agent is water-soluble, it quickly distributes itself evenly within the subarachnoid space, thus obviating the necessity for significant patient manipulation. As discussed previously, relatively low volumes and concentrations of the agent adequately opacify the subarachnoid space and still allow the use of the rapid-sequence, low mAs technique discussed above.

The controversies discussed earlier regarding management of patients with acute cord compromise make it critical that those patients evaluated for such an injury be studied with appropriate traction devices in place. What appears to be continuing compression of the spinal cord with the patient out of traction may be seen to resolve with this conservative form of therapy if the scan is performed during active traction, thus staying the hand of the surgeon who believes emergency surgical decompression may help to free the cord (see Fig 31–6). Also, vertical reformation of images is important in more accurately delineating the relationships of the neural structures to the surrounding bony canal,

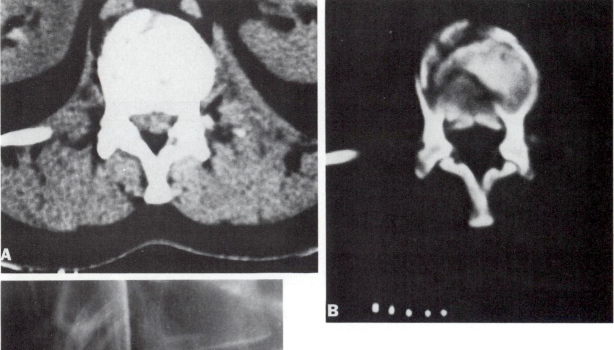

Fig 31–8.—Aggravation of neurologic deficit following conventional myelography. **A, B,** this 28-year-old woman had decreased anal sphincter tone following a fall off a roof. Plain films showed a comminuted fracture of L-1. Axial CT sections with soft-tissue **(A)** and bone **(B)** windows revealed significant comminution of the vertebral body with a retropulsed bony fragment compromising the thecal sac. **(C)** myelography was performed and verified the compromise of the thecal sac. Soon after this examination, however, she developed a left foot drop, possibly caused by movement necessary for the study.

because axial sections may not necessarily show the narrowest point in the canal, depending on the beam angulation.

Another advantage of metrizamide is that it can delineate dural tears. Such dural laceration may allow the herniation of nerve roots in the lumbar region and their subsequent entrapment within bony fragments. Such an injury is sometimes associated with vertical load fractures in the lumbar region, and because instability is often produced by these fractures, early stabilization may be attempted.[1, 17] The unwary surgeon may transect viable nerve roots if presence of herniation of the

structures beyond their dural confines is not recognized. In addition, although nerve root contusion can heal spontaneously, continued compression of nerve roots within bony fragments after they have herniated beyond the dura may prevent return of normal neurologic function. The use of CT with metrizamide can show such dural laceration and aid the surgeon both in planning his approach and in making the decision to operate in the presence of multiple radiculopathies (Figs 31–9 and 31–10).

Finally, the use of intrathecal contrast agents can detect delayed consequences of trauma. For instance, the

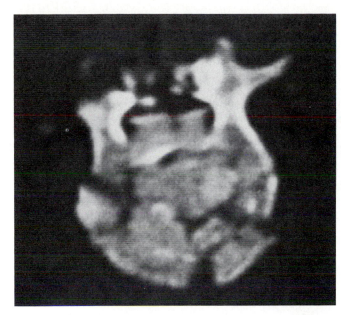

Fig 31–9.—Lumbar compression with nerve root herniation. Severe comminution of the L-2 vertebral body is seen in this young man following a jump. Symptoms referable to the cauda equina were present. Emergency surgical stabilization was elected, and nerve roots were found posterior to the bony spinal canal, having herniated through a dural laceration and the fragmented bony canal. Metrizamide might have shown the site of the dural tear (see Figure 31–10).

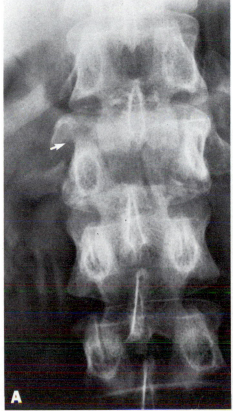

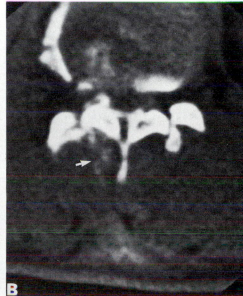

Fig 31–10.—CT demonstration of metrizamide leak. **A,** this young man suffered a compression injury of L-1 vertebral body *(arrow)* and had a lower lumbar radiculopathy. The initial plain films suggested posterior element injury. **B,** axial CT section at the T12-L1 level shows anterior subluxation of the inferior facets of T-12 in respect to the facets of L-1. Additionally, metrizamide within the spinal canal is compressed, and some is seen leaking posteriorly *(arrow)* into the paraspinal musculature. Because of this finding, the surgeon performing the stabilization was careful to avoid any herniated nerve roots. None were found, but a dural laceration was confirmed.

presence of a post-traumatic syrinx can be depicted with CT scanning obtained several hours after the introduction of intrathecal metrizamide. The development of such cysts within the spinal cord is thought to be secondary to focal myelomalacia, and subsequent extension of the cavity caused by the straining associated with coughing, sneezing, etc., may cause extension of the lesion above and below the level of injury. Because the preservation of as much neurologic function as possible is optimal in the neurologically handicapped individual, the detection and treatment of such lesions is important and is permitted with CT (Fig 31–11).

SUMMARY

The intent of this chapter is to acquaint the reader with the potential uses of CT in the evaluation of the spine injury patient. Over the past several years, our experience with CT in a major trauma center has left us feeling quite confident of the capabilities of this imaging modality. Our use of more traditional techniques such as myelography and conventional tomography has

become almost nonexistent. The capability of CT to detect even subtle fractures, to orient these fractures in a three-dimensional sense with the use of image reformation, to allow the depiction of compromise of neural structures within the spinal canal, and even to suggest the presence of spinal instability has made it the procedure of choice following plain film evaluation when a more definitive assessment of spinal injury is necessary. The fact that a simple spine fracture evaluation lasts less than 12 minutes of patient's time, and that even the more complex studies that require introduction of intrathecal metrizamide last not much longer, only enhances the utility of this technique. We believe the added risks posed by conventional tomography and myelography do not warrant their use in this setting, because they offer minimal, if any, additional information in the vast majority of cases.

REFERENCES

1. Brant-Zawadzki M., Jeffrey R.B., Minagi H., et al.: High-resolution CT of thoracolumbar fractures. *A.J.N.R.* 3:69, 1982.

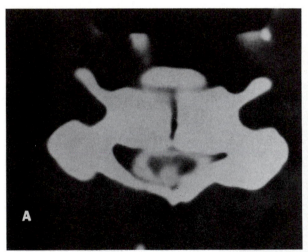

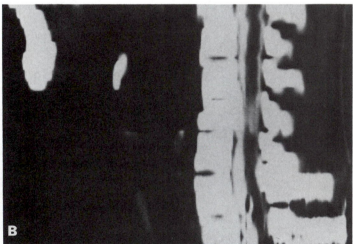

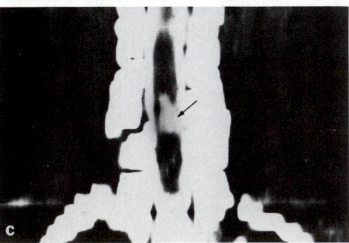

Fig 31–11.—Post-traumatic syrinx. **A,** progression of neurologic symptoms in this victim of cervical spine injury led to a metrizamide CT study. The axial section shown here demonstrates a sagittal cleavage of the vertebral body, the cervical cord outlined by metrizamide, and a focal collection of metrizamide apparently within the substance of the cord itself. **B, C,** coronal and sagittal image reformations verify the presence of the syrinx (*arrow,* **C**) and define its extent. (Courtesy of Dr. Judith Post, Miami.)

2. Brant-Zawadzki M., Miller E.M., Federle M.P.: CT in the evaluation of spine trauma. *A.J.R.* 136:369, 1981.

3. Coin C.G., Pennink M., Ahmad W.D., et al.: Diving-type injury of the cervical spine: Contribution of computed tomography to management. *J. Comput. Assist. Tomogr.* 3:362, 1979.

4. Faerber E.N., Wolpert S.M., Scott R.M., et al.: Computed tomography of spinal fractures. *J. Comput. Assist. Tomogr.* 3:657, 1979.

5. Colley D.P., Dunsker S.B.: Traumatic narrowing of the dorsolumbar spinal canal demonstrated by computed tomography. *Radiology* 129:95, 1978.

6. Brown B.M., Brant-Zawadzki M., Cann E.: Dynamic CT of spinal column trauma. *A.J.R.* 139:1177–1180, 1982.

7. Holdsworth F.W.: Fractures, dislocations, and fracture-dislocations of the spine. *J. Bone Joint Surg.* 45B:6, 1963.

8. Maravilla K.R., Cooper P.R., Sklar F.H.: The influence of thin-section tomography on the treatment of cervical spine injuries. *Radiology* 127:131, 1978.

9. Binet E.F., Moro J.J., Marangola J.P., et al.: Cervical spine tomography in trauma. *Spine* 2:162, 1977.

10. Blumenfeld S.M., Glover G.: Spatial resolution in computed tomography, in Newton T.H., Potts D.G. (eds.): *Radiology of the Skull and Brain: Technical Aspects of Computed Tomography.* St. Louis, C.V. Mosby Co., 1981, pp. 1119–1142.

11. Gehweiler J.A. Jr., Clark W.M., Schaaf R.E., et al.: Cervical spine trauma: The common combined conditions. *Radiology* 130:77, 1979.

12. Calenoff L., Chessare J.W., Rogers L.F., et al.: Multiple level spinal injuries: Importance of early recognition. *A.J.R.* 130:665, 1978.

13. Jefferson G.: Discussion of spinal injuries. *Proc. R. Soc. Med.* 8:625, 1927.

14. Carol M., Ducker T.B., Byrnes D.P.: Minimyelogram in cervical spinal cord trauma. *Neurosurgery* 7:219, 1980.

15. Leo J.S., Bergeron R.T., Kricheff I.I., et al.: Metrizamide myelography for cervical spinal cord injuries. *Radiology* 129:707, 1978.

16. Laasonen E.M.: Myelography for severe thoracolumbar injuries. *Neuroradiology* 13:165, 1977.

17. Miller C.A., Dewey R.C., Hunt W.E.: Impaction fracture of the lumbar vertebrae with dural tear. *J. Neurosurg.* 53:765, 1980.

32

The Detection and Characterization of Post-traumatic Spinal Cord Cysts

ROBERT M. QUENCER, M.D.

INTRADURAL AND EXTRADURAL adhesions, subarachnoid cysts, myelomalacia, spinal cord atrophy, and intramedullary cysts may occur as a late sequela to a spinal cord injury. In a patient who is experiencing a progressive worsening of his neurologic status, the presence of an expanding post-traumatic spinal cord cyst (PTSCC) is most likely. The early recognition of the clinical features and the proper radiologic detection and characterization of these intramedullary cysts are important, because treatment of these cysts by shunting the cyst into the subarachnoid space may reverse recent neurologic deficits and halt further neurologic deterioration. The object of this chapter is to describe the clinical presentations of PTSCC, the techniques used in its detection, the pathogenesis of its formation, its radiographic characteristics, and the results of surgical treatment. This data is based on the observation of 20 cases of proved PTSCC.

CLINICAL PRESENTATION

Although there are variable circumstances under which PTSCC presents, these patients typically have suffered a severe spinal cord injury associated with a fracture/dislocation of the cervical or thoracic spine. In the most common situation, their neurologic status remains fixed (either complete or incomplete quadriplegia or paraplegia) for months to years following the original injury. Following this, they begin to notice new symptoms, of which neck/back pain, increasing spasticity, ascending motor and/or sensory loss, and hyperhidrosis are most frequent.[1, 2] Less commonly, there is a progressive deterioration of the patient's neurologic status right from the time of the original injury. Although once believed to be an unusual sequela of spinal cord trauma,[3-6] PTSCC is, in my experience, a frequent late consequence of spinal trauma. The increased detection of PTSCC will relate to a high degree of clinical suspicion of this problem and the widespread use of metrizamide computed tomography (MCT).

DETECTION

There are two crucial points concerning the radiographic detection of PTSCC: (1) A water-soluble myelographic agent must be used, and (2) delayed CT following myelography is the only reliable method of cyst detection.

Prior to the widespread use of water-soluble myelographic contrast agents (specifically metrizamide), the diagnosis of a PTSCC was made when, under the proper clinical setting, an air or Pantopaque myelogram outlined an enlarged spinal cord.[3, 6, 7] My experience with metrizamide myelography and CT has shown that the majority of PTSCC are *not* present in enlarged cords, but rather in normal-sized (70% of cases, 14 patients) or atrophic spinal cords (20% of cases, 4 patients). This means that 90% of PTSCC will be missed if Pantopaque or air myelography is used.

The clear benefit of metrizamide over Pantopaque or air is the fact that this water-soluble agent can diffuse through the parenchyma of the damaged spinal cord via enlarged Virchow-Robin spaces and collect within the cysts. Because the amount of metrizamide within the cysts gradually increases with time, it is crucial that a delayed rather than an immediate CT scan be obtained. In *normal* patients, there is entry of metrizamide along perivascular channels into the extracellular space of the spinal cord, following which intracellular concentration may occur;[8] however, visual detection of this is difficult. Nonetheless, this phenomena can be confirmed by taking absorption coefficient measurements of the spinal cord premyelography and comparing them with values obtained a few hours postmetrizamide myelography.

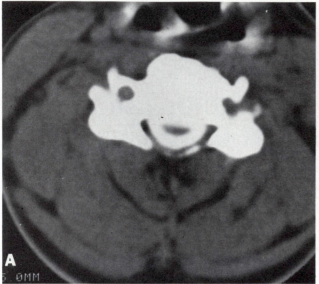

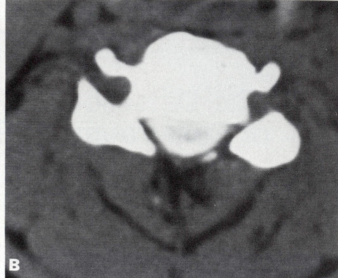

Fig 32–1.—MCT in the midcervical region. When performed 30 minutes following the introduction of metrizamide into the subarachnoid space **(A)**, MCT shows no evidence of an intramedullary cyst. However, a 4-hour delayed scan **(B)** at the same level shows a large central PTSCC. Note that the cord is not enlarged despite the presence of the cyst. Without the use of a water-soluble myelographic contrast agent and a delayed CT scan, the proper diagnosis could not have been made.

Using the data of Dubois and coworkers,[9] which showed that in *normal* dogs the time to maximum cord concentration ranges from 5 to 8 hours following myelography, and the probability that metrizamide would penetrate a severely traumatized cord more rapidly than this, a delayed CT scan 4 hours postmyelography was the time interval believed to be most efficacious in scanning PTSCC. The importance of a delayed CT scan following metrizamide myelography (MCT) is illustrated in Figure 32–1, in which an MCT performed 30 minutes following the myelogram showed no evidence of a cyst, but the 4-hour scan clearly demonstrated the cyst.

We routinely scan suspected cases of PTSCC with contiguous 5-mm thick sections both below and above the injury level. This allows us to see not only the cyst, but also the surrounding noncyst-bearing areas of the spinal cord that may show areas of significant atrophy (Fig 32–2). Sagittal and coronal reformatted images are evaluated along with the axial images in order to characterize the cysts.

There are two conditions that may mimic an intramedullary cyst on MCT: (1) a post-traumatic fissure of the cord (Fig 32–3,A–C) and (2) altered cord permeability (Figs 32–4 and 32–5). Post-traumatic cord fissures are usually found incidentally in patients in whom the surgeon is trying to rule out a bone or disc fragment within the canal. In such patients, an MCT is performed immediately following myelography and will show a dense accumulation of contrast within the cord (see Fig 32–3,C) that is greater than the density of con-

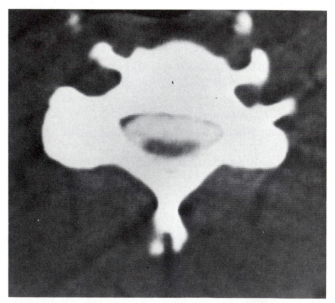

Fig 32–2.—An atrophic cervical cord with flattening of its ventral surface, present at a level above a PTSCC.

trast within the subarachnoid space. An altered permeability of the cord may be manifested by either a hazy increase in cord density (see Fig 32–4) or a diffuse, dense opacification of the cord (see Fig 32–5). In neither situation is a well-defined cyst present. This radiographic picture results from the fact that an abnormal amount of metrizamide penetrates into an injured cord that has no significant-sized cystic cavities in which the metrizamide may collect.

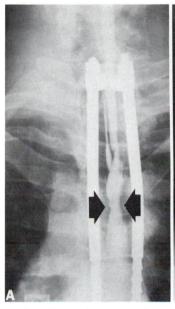
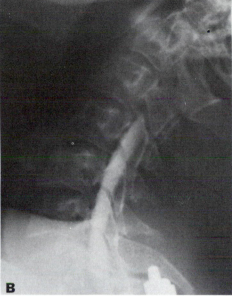
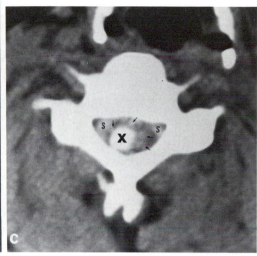

Fig 32–3.—A metrizamide myelogram showing irregularities of the contrast at T-4 (*arrows,* **A**). In the upper thoracic and cervical **(B)** regions, there is a smooth column of contrast in the center of the spinal canal. These films clearly indicate that there has been a direct entrance of contrast from the subarachnoid space into the substance of the cord, i.e., a spinal cord fissure. The MCT done immediately post-myelography **(C)** shows the extremely dense contrast *(X)* within the cervical cord, which has tracked superiorly from its entrance into the cord fissure at T-4. The immediate appearance of a dense contrast collection distinguishes this from the typical PTSCC (compare with Figures 32–1,B, 32–8 to 32–10). Notice that the contrast in the cervical subarachnoid space *(S),* which is too faint to be imaged on plain radiographs, is outlining an enlarged spinal cord. Areas of increased density within the cord *(arrows)* may result from intramedullary penetration of metrizamide from *X* because of an altered state of cord permeability (see Figures 32–4 and 32–5).

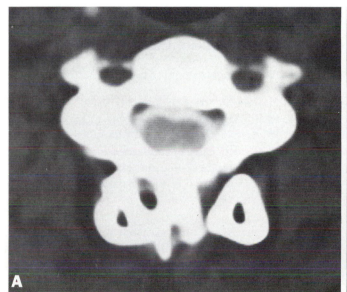
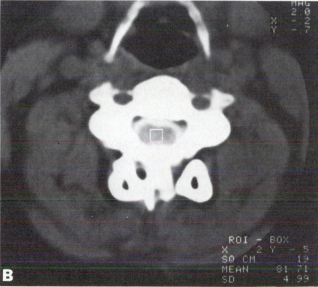

Fig 32–4.—A subtle visual increase in cord density **(A)** confirmed by absorption coefficient measurements **(B).** The value of 81.71 within the region-of-interest box **(B)** is approximately twice the value of the normal spinal cord tissue density 4 hours following metrizamide myelography. This reflects the altered permeability of an injured cord, which has allowed an excessive amount of metrizamide to penetrate the cord. There was no well-defined collection of contrast to suggest the presence of a PTSCC.

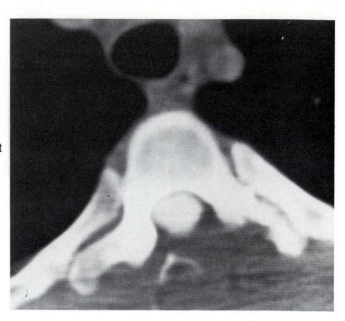

Fig 32–5.—Dense opacification of the thoracic cord reflecting an even more pronounced state of altered permeability than seen in Figure 32–4. At this and adjacent cord levels, there was no discernible cystic cavity, and it was not possible to separate contrast in the subarachnoid space from contrast within the cord. These facts help distinguish a large cyst from a state of altered cord permeability.

PATHOGENESIS

There are two basic theories used to explain the initial development of PTSCC. The first theory assumes that an area of hematomyelia breaks down and later becomes cystic.[3, 7] The second theory ascribes the development of a cystic cavity to cord ischemia[10] and the release of cellular enzymes,[11] the result of which is a myelomalacic core of tissue that undergoes necrosis and then becomes cystic.

Following the formation of this initial cavity, whether it is due to hemorrhagic or ischemic factors, the cyst will gradually enlarge because of the combined effect of increasing intracavitary fluid volume and pressure changes transmitted to the cyst from the subarachnoid space. The cerebrospinal fluid (CSF)-equivalent fluid that fills the slowly expanding cyst either is produced by the gliotic cells that surround the cyst,[3] or the fluid enters the cyst from enlarged Virchow-Robin spaces.[12, 13] The forces that cause cyst expansion relate to the fact that there is significant leptomeningeal thickening and adhesions around the cord at the level of injury. In a *normal* person, straining or Valsalva maneuvers cause an increase in pressure in the epidural veins that in turn compress the dura, and there is then, as a result, an evenly distributed increase in pressure throughout the entire subarachnoid space. However, in an *injured* patient, the adhesions effectively tether the cord at the level of original trauma, and the increased CSF pressure will then be directed to that area rather than being evenly dispersed. This abnormal pressure will be transmitted through the substance of the spinal cord to the cyst. A gradually enlarging cyst will then result.

As will be seen in the discussion that follows, the majority of cysts will be found in the dorsal portion of the spinal cord. This radiographic finding correlates well with the fact that an intramedullary hemorrhage is most likely to occur in the dorsal gray matter, because it has a rich capillary blood supply.[3] The cyst subsequently is most likely to spread dorsally along the length of the cord because of the presence in that area of a relatively poor connective tissue framework.[10, 14] In addition, the constraining effect of the more lateral rigid fibers of the posterior columns[3] means cyst expansion must occur in anterolateral directions.

RADIOGRAPHIC CHARACTERISTICS

Any radiographic description of PTSCC should include the following information: (1) the number of cysts present, (2) the position of the cyst within the cord, (3) the length of each cyst and whether it extends above and/or below the injury site, and (4) the width of each cyst relative to the width of the cord at that level. Each of these considerations has a bearing on the surgical planning.

Although the majority of patients will have a single cyst (Fig 32–6), multiple cysts (Fig 32–7) are not infrequent, and the routine axial and reformatted images should be closely evaluated for evidence of multiplicity. Of our cases, 75% (15 patients) had a single cyst, while 25% (5 patients) had multiple cysts. The existence of multiple cysts has been previously reported only on pathologic specimens;[3, 4, 15] however, increased physician awareness of this possibility means that multiplicity will be more frequently searched for and found. When more than one cyst is found, and each is of suitable

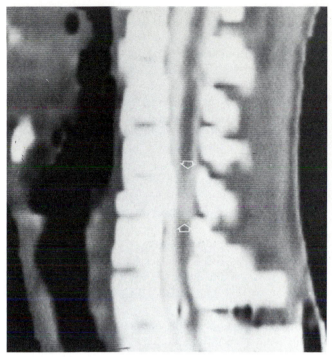

Fig 32–6.—Sagittal reformatted MCT showing a single cyst (between *open arrows*) extending superiorly from the C5-6 level (site of the original fracture/dislocation) to the C4-5 level. The cyst measured 2 cm in length and was present in a normal-sized cord.

length and width for shunting, separate shunts may be used.

The majority of cysts will be found in the dorsal portion of the cord (Fig 32–8), with central cysts (Fig 32–9) and ventral cysts (Fig 32–10) being less common. As

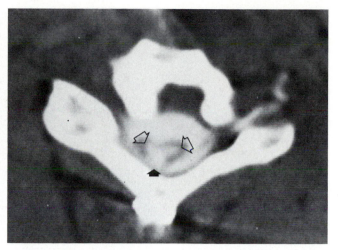

Fig 32–8.—A wide cyst present directly beneath the pial surface in the dorsal portion of the spinal cord *(arrow)*. According to the presumed pathogenesis of cyst formation and enlargement (see text), the original cavity started in the dorsal cord, and then because of the constraining effect of the posterior columns, the cyst could expand only in an anterolateral direction *(open arrows)*. This patient has had a previous anterior decompression.

discussed above, the dorsal location of PTSCC correlates well with the known microscopic anatomy of the spinal cord and the pathophysiology of cyst enlargement. Knowing the exact position of the cyst within the cord is important to the surgeon, because a dorsal cyst located directly under the pial surface will be technically easier to shunt than cysts in a ventral or central location. To reach either of these latter locations, dis-

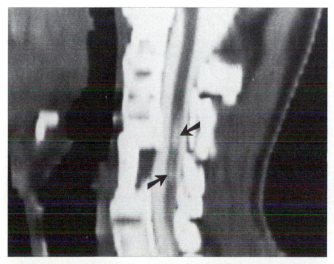

Fig 32–7.—Sagittally reformatted MCT demonstrating two separate cysts within the cord *(arrows)*. Between these two cysts is an area of spinal cord in which no cyst is present. Note that both cysts are superior to the old injury site. An anterior interbody fusion is present from C-4 to C-6.

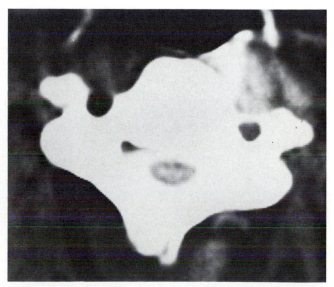

Fig 32–9.—A wide central cyst seen in the cervical spinal cord. In these central cysts and in ventral cysts (see Figure 32–10), surgical dissection through cord tissue will be required before the cyst is reached.

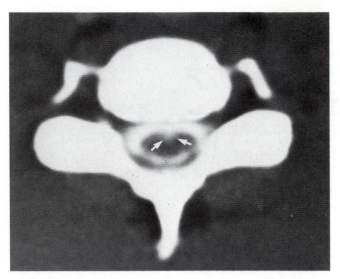

Fig 32–10.—A narrow midline ventral cyst outlined by *arrows*. Those cysts identified in the ventral cord tend to be shorter and narrower than dorsal cysts. Their small size and ventral location makes them much less accessible to surgical intervention than the more common dorsal cyst (see Figure 32–8).

section through the cord may be required, and this factor may persuade the surgeon not to perform a shunting procedure. Because the position and width of a cyst may vary along its length, these parameters should be described relative to the spinal cord segments. Note should also be made of whether the cyst is in a midline or eccentric position, because this will determine whether the cyst will be accessible at the level of the median raphe or whether a paramidline incision will be necessary.

Extension of PTSCC only above the level of the original injury site is most common (see Figs 32–6 ad 32–7). However, in one third of patients, there is inferior extension also (Fig 32–11). The superior extension of a cyst clearly can result in continuing loss of neurologic function; however, cyst extension inferior to the original injury site may rob those patients with an incomplete cord lesion of important neurologic functions or be the cause of increasing pain. This is the reason that MCT above and below the injury site is recommended. As a general rule, short cysts (2 cm or less) extend superiorly only, while longer cysts tend to have both a superior and inferior extension. Radiographically detectable cysts range in size from 0.5 cm to the entire length of the cord and even may extend into the medulla. Pathologic and surgical reports[3, 13, 15–17] have confirmed this variability in the length and potential for superoinferior cyst expansion.

Careful note should also be made of the width of the cyst relative to the width of the cord, because this may have a bearing on the operability of the cyst. If cysts are designated either narrow (less than one half the cord width) or wide (greater than one half the cord width), the majority will fall into the "wide" category (see Figs 32–1,B, 32–8, and 32–9). Narrow cysts most commonly are ventral in location (see Fig 32–10).

An example of a proper radiologic description of a typical PTSCC would be as follows: "A single 5-cm cyst extending superiorly from the level of fracture/dislocation at C5-6 is noted. From C5-6 to C-4, the cyst is dorsal and midline in position and is greater than one half the width of the cord. The upper 1.5 cm of the cyst, from C-4 level to the superior border of C-3, is central in location and narrow, measuring less than one half the cord width." This report will inform the surgeon that only a single shunt is needed, that he need operate only above the level of the original injury, and that at its maximum width the cyst will be located directly beneath the pial surface of the cord. As a general rule, patients with cysts that are less than 1.0 cm in length and patients with narrow cysts, particularly when they are located in the ventral cord, are not good candidates for shunting. These patients are followed clinically, and if there are signs of neurologic deterioration, reevaluation with MCT may show sufficient cyst enlargement to justify a shunting procedure.

SURGICAL TREATMENT AND RESULTS

In the shunting procedure, a straight Cordis ventricular catheter with multiple side holes is passed into the cyst, following which it is secured to the pial surface. The distal 1.5 cm of the tubing drains the cyst into the adjacent subarachnoid space. Recently, we have made use of intraoperative ultrasonography to determine the

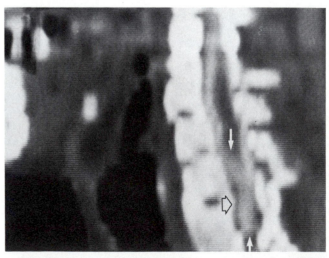

Fig 32–11.—A 3.5-cm cyst (between *arrows*) seen on this sagittally reformatted MCT, extending superiorly and inferiorly from the original injury site *(open arrow)*.

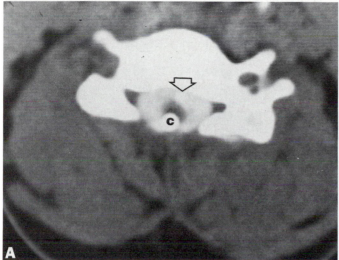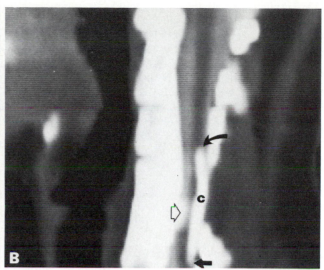

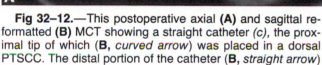

Fig 32–12.—This postoperative axial **(A)** and sagittal reformatted **(B)** MCT showing a straight catheter *(c)*, the proximal tip of which (**B,** *curved arrow*) was placed in a dorsal PTSCC. The distal portion of the catheter (**B,** *straight arrow*) is draining the cyst into the subarachnoid space. The dense collection of contrast (**A, B,** *open arrows*) anterior to the cord is in a small subarachnoid cyst.

exact size and position of the cyst during surgery. A postshunting MCT is demonstrated in Figure 32–12.

Postoperative evaluation of the patient's clinical status has allowed determination of the efficacy of the shunting procedures performed, and in every patient except one there was an improvement in at least one or more of their symptoms. All patients with neck/back pain and hyperhidrosis improved following the shunting procedure; however, spasticity was the one symptom that did not uniformly respond to this surgical treatment. At this time, a long-term clinical follow-up of greater than 1 year has been obtained in two patients, and in neither of them has there been a recurrence of the preoperative PTSCC symptoms.

SUMMARY

1. In a patient who suffered a severe spinal cord injury in the past, a progressive deterioration of his neurologic status strongly suggests the presence of a PTSCC.

2. The majority of cases of PTSCC will be detected only if a water-soluble myelographic agent in conjunction with a delayed CT is employed.

3. The proposed pathogenesis for the formation and expansion of PTSCC correlates well with the radiographically demonstrable position of the cyst.

4. Cases of PTSCC *most frequently* are single, occur in the dorsal portion of the cord, extend superiorly from the injury site, and are wider than half the width of the spinal cord. However, exceptions to these "typical"

characteristics are common and must be searched for carefully.

5. Shunting of these cysts into the subarachnoid space will result in neurologic improvement.

REFERENCES

1. Quencer R.M., Green B.A., Eismont J.: Posttraumatic spinal cord cysts: Clinical features and characterization with metrizamide computed tomography. *Radiology* 146:415–423, 1983.
2. Seibert C.E., Dreisbach J.M., Swanson W.B., et al.: Progressive posttraumatic cystic myelopathy. *A.J.N.R.* 2:115–119, 1981.
3. Barnett H.J.M., Jousse A.T., Ball M.J.: Pathology and pathogenesis of progressive cystic myelopathy as a late sequel to spinal cord injury, in *Major Problems in Neurology: Syringomyelia.* London, W.B. Saunders Co., 1973, vol. 1, pp. 179–219.
4. Watson N.: Ascending cystic degeneration of the cord after spinal cord injury. *Paraplegia* 19:89–95, 1981.
5. Griffiths E.R., McCormic C.C.: Posttraumatic syringomyelia (cystic myelopathy). *Paraplegia* 19:81–88, 1981.
6. Rossier A.B., Foo D., Shillito J., et al.: Progressive late posttraumatic syringomyelia. *Paraplegia* 19:96–97, 1981.
7. Williams B., Terry A.F., Jones F., et al.: Syringomyelia as a sequel to traumatic paraplegia. *Paraplegia* 19:67–80, 1981.
8. Isherwood I., Fawcitt R.A., Forbes W., et al.: Computer tomography of the spinal canal using metrizamide. *Acta Radiol. Suppl.* 355:299–305, 1977.
9. Dubois P.J., Drayer B.P., Sage M., et al.: Intramedullary penetrance of metrizamide in the dog spinal cord. *A.J.N.R.* 2:313–317, 1981.

10. Turnbull I.M., Breig A., Hassler O.: Blood supply of the cervical spinal cord in man: A microangiographic cadaver study. *J. Neurosurg.* 24:951–965, 1966.

11. Kao C., Chang L.W.: The mechanism of spinal cord cavitation following spinal cord transection: I. A correlated histo-chemical study. *J. Neurosurg.* 46:197–209, 1977.

12. Durward Q.J., Rice G.P., Ball M.J., et al.: Selective spinal cordectomy: Clinicopathological correlation. *J. Neurosurg.* 56:359–367, 1982.

13. Ball M.J., Dayan A.D.: Pathogenesis of syringomyelia. *Lancet* 2:794–801, 1972.

14. Gillilan L.A.: The arterial blood supply of the human spinal cord. *J. Comp. Neurol.* 110:75–103, 1958.

15. Feigen I., Ogata J., Bodzilovich G.: Syringomyelia: The role of edema in its pathogenesis. *J. Neuropathol. Exp. Neurol.* 30:216–232, 1971.

16. Jensen F., Roske-Nielsen E.: Post-traumatic syringomyelia: Review of the literature and two new autopsy cases. *Scand. J. Rehabil. Med.* 9:35–43, 1977.

17. Oakley J.C., Ojemann G.A., Alvord E.C.: Posttraumatic syringomyelia. *J. Neurosurg.* 55:276–281, 1981.

33

Congenital Anomalies of the Spine and Spinal Cord

CHARLES R. FITZ, M.D.

Use of CT

Abnormalities that run in the axis of the CT image plane, such as narrowing of the disc space, fracture, or lack of fusion of the odontoid, are difficult to see in the axial CT image. For such abnormalities, plain films or conventional sagittal or coronal tomography are usually preferable. The use of CT in such a case is not unlike trying to estimate the depth of water in the bottom of a glass by looking into it from above rather than from the side. Dynamic studies requiring bending of the spine are generally unsuitable for CT, though the relationship of cord to spine in a particular level may be best seen by CT.

When intrathecal contrast is needed, the digital radiograph of CT is not yet equivalent to plain film myelography. As the cord is a long structure, plain films have the advantage of showing a large segment of the cord in a single radiograph. Cross-sectional detail in an abnormal area is obviously the realm of CT. While one can do thin-section CT of the whole spine and reconstruct it, this would be a very time-consuming procedure for the patient and the computer with even the best of current equipment.

One must also keep in mind that in children up to age 7 or 8 years, anesthesia or sedation is likely to be used. One does not want to prolong anesthesia, and sedation wears off, so the ethical radiologist must, in the best interests of the child, sometimes try for the best reasonable study rather than the ideal study. Even the older child, with whom one is less concerned about time, may rebel when you have exceeded his or her tolerance for cooperation.

The sequence of radiographic investigations at the author's hospital is noted in Fig 33–1. Plain films still form the base level of investigation and determine the next step in diagnostic investigation. While the large

majority of cases go on to myelography followed by CT, not all cases do, and it is unwise to pour the entire diagnostic load through the CT gantry.

Technical Aspects

Very often, high-detail CT is another name for high radiation dose. In most cases, this is not needed when dealing with the high-contrast anatomy of the bony spine and metrizamide-filled subarachnoid space (Fig 33–2). While there are no proved harmful effects to doses of diagnostic radiation, it is common sense to keep the dose as low as possible in a child.

When using water-soluble contrast or examining the bone, the target reconstruction technique (such as the General Electric ReView) further enhances the sharpness of interfaces and clearly delineates small structures. Such techniques should be used routinely.

Direct coronal imaging is possible and occasionally useful. Infants and small children can sometimes undergo coronal CT by having them lie on their side. Older children are best examined in machines adapted for this technique with a bicycle seat apparatus.[1] Direct sagittal examination is currently feasible in only the largest-diameter gantrys with the smallest patients. The major problem with these techniques in children is image degradation in the thoracic and cervical spine caused by respiratory motion, which may also allow acquisition of noncontiguous slices.

NORMAL ANATOMY

Axial CT is ideally suited to reveal the size and ossification of the *child's* bony spinal canal. In the infant, the small size of the patient means less anatomical detail than in the older child in most scanners, but it is nonetheless sufficient for clearly revealing the contour

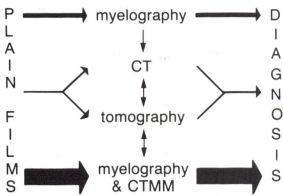

Fig 33–1.—Protocol for examination of the spine in the author's hospital.

and ossification centers of the various portions of the spine.

In spite of the lesser thickness of the bone relative to the older child and adult, visualization of the cord is quite unreliable without intrathecal contrast, with the exception of the C-1 level. In the infant, the bony canal is straighter than in the older child, making the cord more central within the canal throughout its length. The cord takes a relatively straight course within the canal, so that as the child grows the cord moves closer to the inside of each curve, leaving it posterior in the midcervical, anterior in the upper and midthoracic, and again posterior in the lumbar area.

In early infancy, the posterior elements of the bony canal are open, but curve so that if a line were drawn to continue the arc of the bone, it would complete a circle. The vertebral bodies at each level are small relative to the size of the canal and in comparison to the size in the adult. The vertebral bodies grow proportion-

ately more in childhood than does the spinal canal diameter. In infancy, the spinal canal is relatively round, though variations are visible in each area.

In the newborn, both the anterior arch of C-1 and the odontoid may have one or two ossification centers that are unfused, as are the posterior arches, which also have open neurocentral junctions (Fig 33–3). The arches are usually closed by age 2 to 3 years, but may remain open as a normal variant, especially at C-1.

The neurocentral synchondroses begin to fuse at age 2 years in the cervical region, with the line of fusion being visible into later childhood. Fusion of the odontoid to its base and the height of the process itself are difficult to ascertain in infancy on axial CT, but they are clearly visible on coronal head sections in which the upper cervical spine is also extended into the coronal plane (Fig 33–4). The spinous processes of the cervical spine are not visible until about age 2 years. Until the fusion of the posterior elements, the cervical canal is

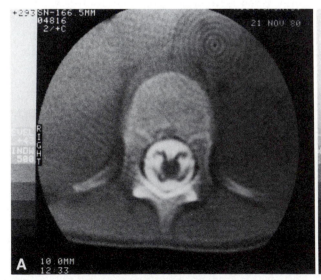

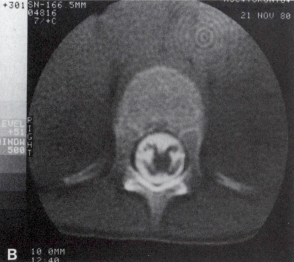

Fig 33–2.—Radiation dose. **A,** 500-mR slice through normal conus. **B,** repeat slice using 200 mR. Both images have had target reconstruction, which has caused a slight ring artifact. Though the lower radition dose image is minimally more grainy, there is no information lost in this high-contrast image.

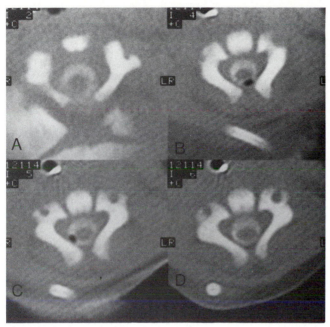

Fig 33–3.— Normal newborn cervical spine. **A,** C-1. **B–D,** C-2. The slices are 5 mm thick. Both the anterior ossification center of C-1 and the odontoid are unfused to the laminae, which are in turn open posteriorly. A small bubble of air is present in the subarachnoid space. A shunt tube courses through the posterior subcutaneous tissue.

often somewhat triangular in shape, slowly progressing to the ovoid shape of later childhood and adulthood.

The cervical cord cross section is also slightly rounder in infancy than in the older child and shows less change with growth than do the vertebral bodies and the bony canal. With intrathecal contrast, the cord is seen to be round at C-1. The remainder of the cervical cord is nearly round during the first year, but becomes more ovoid, greater in the transverse diameter, by the end of the first year (Fig 33–5). Dorsal and ventral rootlets are visible, especially with 5-mm thick slices. In the first

few months of life, the cord is less than 50% of the spine diameter. Later, it is slightly greater than 50% of the entire transverse diameter of the bony canal in the midcervical region. As the cord approaches the thoracic level, it again becomes round.

The thoracic cord is nearly uniform in size and shape throughout its length from infancy onward. In both absolute size and size relative to the surrounding subarachnoid space and bony canal, it is smaller than the cervical cord. It occupies approximately one third of the transverse diameter of the subarachnoid space

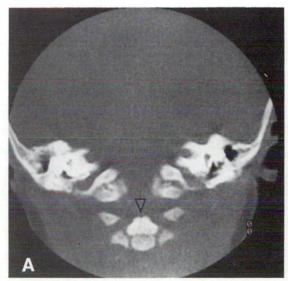

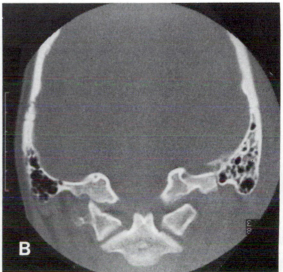

Fig 33–4.—Odontoid process, coronal view. **A,** in a 3-month-old child, the odontoid *(arrow)* is unfused to its base or the laminae. The separation of the base and odontoid was not visible in axial slices. **B,** complete fusion of the odontoid to its base in an 8-year-old child.

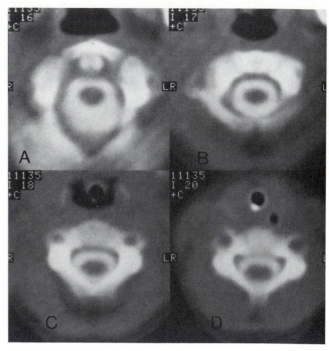

Fig 33–5.—Normal cervical cord and spine, 1½-year-old boy. **A–D,** sequential slices from C-1 through C-4. The cord shape is slightly more ovoid than in Figure 33–3, the cord and subarachnoid space take a larger volume of the canal, and the canal is less triangular in shape than in Figure 33–3.

and approximately one quarter of the transverse diameter of the canal (Fig 33–6), enlarging slightly with growth.

The thoracic bony canal is round to slightly ovoid in outline, being largest anteroposteriorly. Even in early infancy, the posterior arches approximate themselves closely at the site of the future spinous processes. With growth, both the pedicles and the laminae expand in equal proportions.

The lumbar canal is rounder in infancy than in the older child, but even in infancy becomes more trian-

gular further caudally, being wider across its base and shorter sagittally (Fig 33–7). The cord is round and widest at the T12-L1 conus expansion, tapering to the central filum, which is the size of the nerve roots that surround it in a symmetric ^V_W pattern in the upper canal (Fig 33–8).

The ring apophyses that are visible on plain film radiographs in later childhood are not easily seen on the routine 5- or 10-mm CT slices. Because the apophyses are so close to the vertebral bodies, the space between them is averaged into the image.

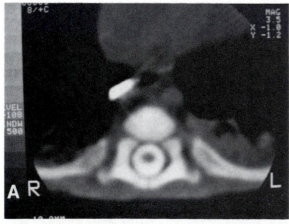

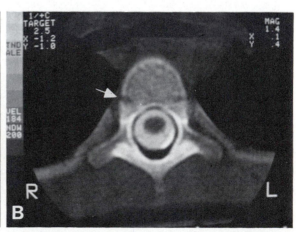

Fig 33–6.—Normal mid-thoracic spine and cord. **A,** 3-month-old child. **B,** 2½-year-old child. The cords are approximately equal in shape, with the younger patient having a slightly smaller and more centrally placed cord. In **A,** the neurocentral synchondroses are unfused. Though in close approximation, the laminae are also posteriorly unfused. In **B,** a spinous process is visible. A visible notch remains at the fusing neurocentral synchondroses *(arrow).* The bony canal is proportionately larger in the sagittal direction in **B.**

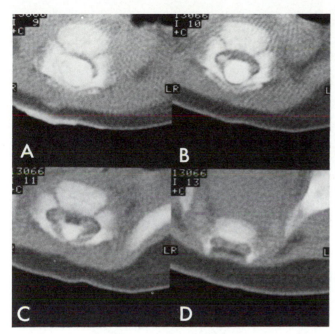

Fig 33–7.—Normal lumbosacral canal in a 1-month-old child. **A-C,** lower lumbar levels below the tip of the conus. **D,** upper sacral canal. The canal gradually becomes more triangular in cross section as it approaches the sacrum. As visible in **D,** the normal infant sacral canal is open posteriorly.

BONY ANOMALIES

The craniovertebral junction is a common site for bony anomalies. As noted, fusions of C-1 to the occiput or dens anomalies without displacement are not ideally seen by CT in the axial plane. Examination in the coronal plane or sagittal reformations may be extremely helpful in such cases (Fig 33–9).

Many isolated abnormalities such as hypoplasia of the arch or pedicle of C-1 or other cervical level are of minor consequence. They are often discovered incidentally to other symptoms,[2] though a "syndrome" of pain with weakness or numbness is described.[3] Because such absence often brings up the question of erosion

from tumor, CT is done and is definitive in its findings. The lack of pedicle or arch is well demonstrated along with hypertrophy of the adjacent or contralateral structures that bear the added stress (Fig 33–10).[4, 5]

The Klippel-Feil anomaly with multiple cervical fusions probably does not warrant investigation by CT if asymptomatic. While CT may reveal unsuspected aspects of the condition (Fig 33–11), it is often less revealing than plain film examination.

Bony anomalies without dysraphism are often discovered incidentally or may be a cause of scoliosis. While the anomalies themselves may not be significant, they should be a flag to do a complete neurologic examina-

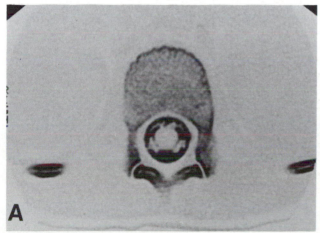

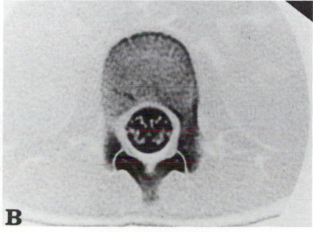

Fig 33–8.—Normal conus and cauda equina, reversed gray scale. **A,** at L-1 the conus is widest. Dorsal and ventral nerve roots are visible exiting from the conus. **B,** at the next lower vertebral body level, the small central filum is surrounded by nerve roots in a symmetric pattern.

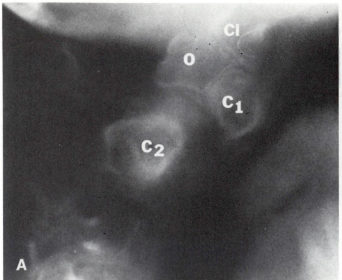

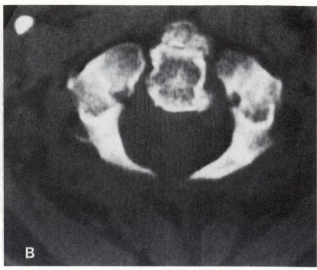

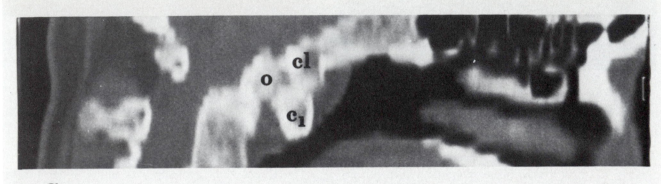

Fig 33–9.—Os odontoideum. **A,** lateral tomography demonstrates the anatomy. The os *(O)* is the odontoid ossification center that fails to fuse to the body of C-2 *(C₂)*. There is a bony mound, or "hillock deformity," along the superior margin of C-2. The os is fused to both the anterior arch of C-1. *(C₁)* and the clivus *(Cl)*. **B,** an axial CT slice through C-1 does not give a true appreciation of the degree of canal narrowing at this level. **C,** sagittal CT reformation is comparable to plain tomography **(A)** in anatomical clarity and shows the canal narrowing and soft-tissue compromise to good advantage. *(o = os, c₁ = C-1, cl = clivus.)* (Courtesy of Richard E. Latchaw, M.D., University Health Center of Pittsburgh.)

Fig 33–10.—Absent pedicle, 3-year-old boy. CTMM shows absent right pedicle, hemivertebrae, and thickening of the left pedicle in compensation. The cord is asymmetrically positioned to the right because of mild scoliosis.

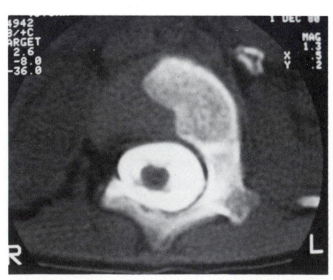

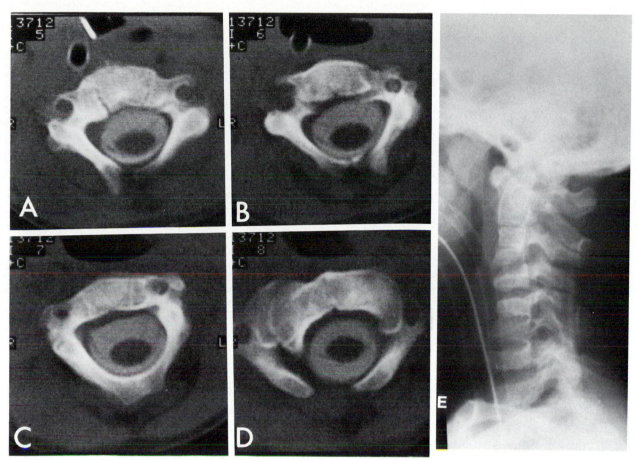

Fig 33–11.—Klippel-Feil anomaly. Axial CT slices at C-4 **(A),** C-3 **(B, C),** and C1-2 **(D)** show posterior spina bifida, irregularity of the vertebral bodies, and "rotation" of C-2 on C-1. **E,** lateral plain film shows fusion of C-2 through C-4 not visible on CT.

tion, which may discover minimal deficits that then are reasons to pursue further studies.

Basilar invagination is an uncommon anomaly of the craniocervical junction. Although multiple methods have been devised for measuring basilar invagination, McRae,[6] the originator of one of these, states they must be used with care. A measured mild invagination without clinical symptoms probably means nothing.

In childhood, the causes of basilar invagination are few. Though the entity is said to occur in 25% of patients with Chiari malformation,[7] it is not a significant cause of childhood symptoms in the author's experience. It is also said to be common among the Dutch.[8] Rare symptomatic diseases such as osteogenesis imperfecta, cleidocranial dysostosis, and acro-osteolysis may cause a significant amount of basilar impression. Such systemic diseases are accompanied by other signs. The degree of a marked basilar impression is not easily seen on plain films, being hidden by the skull base itself. Either plain film tomography or CT will demonstrate the amount of disease well, though slices no less than

3 mm apart are needed for any reconstruction of the CT image in a sagittal or coronal plane (Fig 33–12).

DYSRAPHIC STATES

Tethered Conus

According to postmortem studies of infants by Barson,[9] the conus tip is at the L1-2 space 2 months after birth. Reimann and Anson[10] in much earlier studies indicated the conus tip might normally be as low as mid-L-2, and this was more likely in females. Work by Fitz and Harwood-Nash[11] used a practical compromise of L2-3 at age 2 years and the middle of the L-2 level by age 12 years at the lower limits of normal. A conus ending below those levels is considered abnormal by the author.

The embryology of the abnormality has not been examined, but is presumed to be secondary to a halt in or slowing of the normal upward regression of the cord that progresses from sacrum to lumbar canal in utero. Because nearly all other forms of dysraphism have a

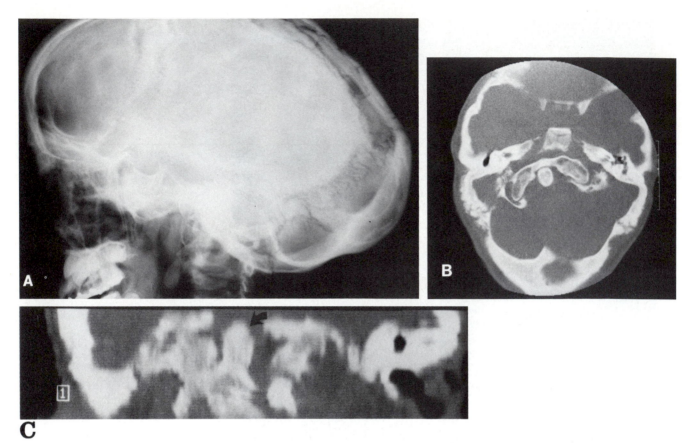

Fig 33–12.—Basilar invagination in an 11-year-old child with unclassified dysostosis and cranial nerve weakness. **A,** lateral skull x-ray shows the marked upward displacement of C-1 into the skull. **B,** axial CT shows the upward invagi-nation of C-1 into the foramen magnum. **C,** coronal reconstruction accurately reveals the amount of displacement of the cervical spine into the skull vault. Odontoid is identified by *arrow.*

tethering as part of their pathology, and even the mildest isolated tethering has at least an occult spina bifida, the interruption of the normal regression appears to be part of a process that may be very complicated.

The clinical presentation is variable and has been dealt with by several authors.[12–14] There may be leg weakness or shortening, enuresis, back pain, or sensory changes, to name a few symptoms. Skin abnormalities such as a hairy patch or hemangioma are common. In addition to the spina bifida that is always present, there may be a widened interpediculate distance and other dysraphic abnormalities on the plain films.

The need for CT varies with the complexity of the disease. In the simplest type, there is only a conus that ends a half to a whole vertebral body low and a filum that is thickened (greater than 1.5-mm diameter) as seen on a supine myelographic film. No other abnormalities are present, and the CT is usually not necessary or helpful.

In the second type, the filum is thicker through part or all of its length, and CT of the filum indicates if it contains fatty tissue (Fig 33–13). The third type is quite

dependent on CT for accurate diagnosis of the many facets of the disease. The conus may not be evident, with the cord gradually narrowing into a tube of variable diameter, but often 5 to 8 mm in size (Fig 33–14). This tube may be a true filum surrounded by fat, but most frequently is cord neural tissue, and there is no true filum. Large lipomas are common in this type of tethering. Axial slices indicate the relationship of the lipomas to the cord and the circumference of the spinal canal, and sagittal reconstruction reveals the longitudinal extent of the abnormalities for surgical repair.

The lipoma is primarily on the posterior aspect of the cord. While it may simply lie dorsal to the cord, it does occasionally invade the cord itself as seen on CT and become intramedullary in position. With this latter type of involvement, it can be quite difficult to tell a tethered cord from a lipomyelomeningocele (LMMC). Two CT findings are helpful. First is that the dysraphism of a tethered conus is less severe than that of a meningocele, and the laminae, though dysraphic, still tend to be arcuate in shape. Second, the lipoma is

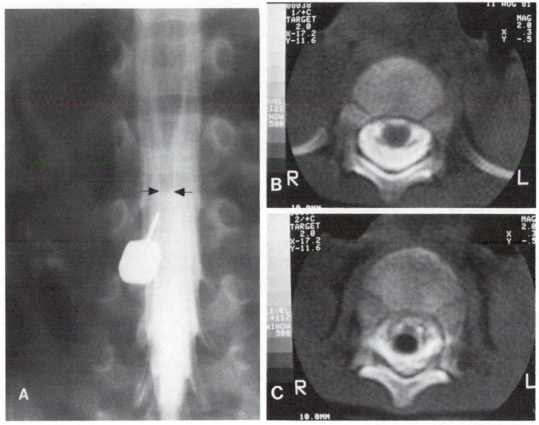

Fig 33–13.—Tethered conus, type II. **A,** plain film myelogram reveals thickening of the conus *(arrows).* **B,** CT through the conus is normal. **C,** CT at the junction of the conus and filum shows enlargement with fatty infiltration.

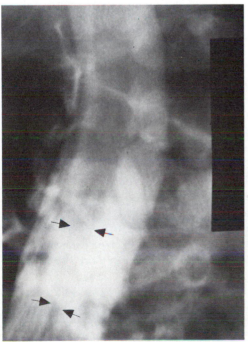

Fig 33–14.—Tethered conus, type III-A, 1-year-old girl. Plain myelogram shows a cord with no conus enlargement that gradually narrows to its tip at the end of the lumbar canal *(arrows).* Nerve roots are coming off the cord at a wider angle than is normal. CT showed no fat within the cord.

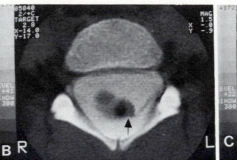

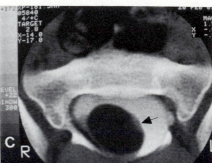

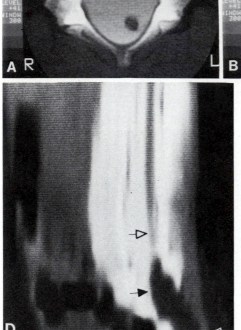

Fig 33–15.—Tethered conus, type III-B, 5-year-old girl. **A,** CTMM through lower lumbar level. The narrow cord is eccentric within the widened canal. Nerve roots are not visible because of their horizontal exiting from the cord. **B,** 10 mm lower, fat visible and infiltrating the cord *(arrow)*, from which dorsal nerve roots are seen exiting. Because of averaging with surrounding metrizamide, much of the fat appears denser than the cord. Note the mild spina bifida. **C,** sacral level. The lipoma is large and distorts the cord tip *(arrow)* that surrounds the lipoma. The lipoma clearly remains in the spinal canal. **D,** sagittal reconstruction showing cord *(open black arrow)* entering large lipoma *(solid black arrow)* and separation between the lipoma and the more posterior subcutaneous fat by muscle and connective tissue *(open white arrowheads).*

likely to remain within the bony spinal canal in the tethered conus (Fig 33–15).

Meningocele, Myelomeningocele

The spectrum of these lesions seems to be less of a continuum than does the tethered conus. This is especially so in comparing the myelomeningocele (MMC) with a simple meningocele or LMMC. The MMC is almost always associated with a Chiari II malformation of the brain and upper cervical cord and has more severe neurologic deficits. Similar-appearing abnormalities of the cord occur with LMMC, which is usually far less symptomatic. The main structural difference of the two lesions is the presence of fat in the LMMC. Plain meningocele, protrusion of the meninges without neural elements within, is about one tenth as common as the other varieties.

Causes of these dysraphic states is unknown, with the main theories for MMC formation being that of abnormal distension and rupture of the neural tube[15] and abnormal closure of the neural tube at an even earlier time.[16] Discovery of myeloschises of the unclosed tube in aborted fetuses by Osaka and colleagues[17] gives strength to a later theory, even though variations of the severity of the distended neural tube give a more uni-

fied theory to explain associated abnormalities such as diastematomyelia. Simple meningocele, with only a herniation of the dura through a dysraphic bony canal, presumably occurs later or by a somewhat different mechanism.

In all of these protrusions, CT clearly shows a marked posterior abnormality of the laminae, which tend to be nearly parallel and sagittally oriented. In MMC especially, the dysraphism usually extends over a long segment, sometimes involving the entire lumbar canal or even more. Vertebral body abnormalities may also be present.

Because MMC is routinely repaired immediately after birth, neuroradiologic studies are often not done. The main goal in these operations is to cover the neural placode with dura and skin and prevent or stop any CSF leakage. The patients may return several years later with deterioration and undergo more thorough investigation at that time.[18]

Adequate investigation includes metrizamide in the subarachnoid space with a preliminary plain film myelogram and high-quality CT. Lumbar puncture can usually be done either above or below the surgical repair. The canal may be wide and shallow, so an off-midline puncture with the needle angled at about 45° cranially is easily accomplished if the spinous processes are deficient. Because of scarring and adhesions, the subarachnoid space may be loculated and prevent successful puncture, in which case lateral C1-2 puncture should be carefully done, keeping in mind that nearly all MMC patients will have a Chiari malformation.

In an MMC, the cord structure changes gradually over two or more vertebral levels until it reaches the placode area, which can be short, very disorganized, and difficult to evaluate. Contiguous 10-mm sections through the region of gradual change and 5-mm sections through the placode are the most efficient ways to examine the patient, using preliminary plain myelographic film and the CT digital radiograph as guides. Target reconstruction or its equivalent is necessary to adequately see the structural detail. Sagittal reconstruction can be enlightening to the surgeon (Fig 33–16).

The anatomy of such cases is complicated, and it is only since CT that such investigations have been worthwhile. The patients are often symptomatic, because the placode has become retethered to the dura, but the association of congenital abnormalities should also be verified. The cord is often split, either above or uncommonly at the placode. The flattened placode, if tethered to the dura, blends with it and is barely visible (see Fig 33–16). Because the placode is a cord that has been

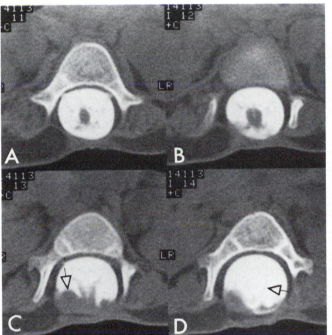

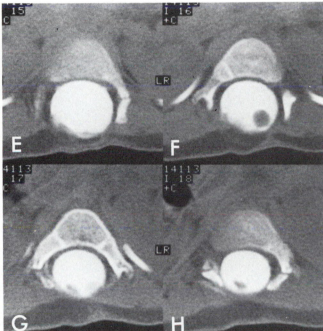

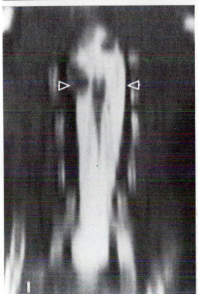

Fig 33–16.—Repaired MMC, 5-year-old girl. Serial 5-mm sections through the placode start inferiorly. **A,** midlumbar section showing thickened reconstituted cord. **B,** end of cleft of the cord. **C,** unusual diastematomyelic splitting of the cord in the placode, which extends across the posterior canal. A rare inclusion dermoid is visible *(arrow).* **D,** a ventral nerve root *(arrow)* visible arising from the center of the placode. **E,** the placode remaining adherent to the posterior aspect of the subarachnoid space. **F,** a second dermoid visible. **G, H,** the placode reforming into a dysplastic cord superiorly. **I,** coronal reconstruction revealing the two epidermoids and a portion of the splitting. As the coronal slice cannot follow the curvature of the spine, the entire lumbar cord is not visible on a single slice. The *arrows* indicate the level of axial slice **(C).**

sagittally split and opened from the back, the posterior surface of the placode is in fact the inside of the open cord plastered to the skin (or dura if already repaired). The anterior side of the placode is the entire outer surface of the cord. This means that the nerve roots visible off the ventral surface of a normal cord are now coming off the central portion of the placode (see Fig 33–16,D). The dorsal nerve roots exit at the lateral edges of the placode.

There can be distortions of the shape of the placode on axial projection. If the placode is at the upper lumbar level or above, the cord may also reconstitute inferiorly into a conus (see Fig 33–16,A).

Lipomyelomeningocele

Lipomyelomeningoceles are radiologically more complicated and surgically more of a challenge. Having less neurologic symptomatology, the abnormality is in part cosmetic, but because there is much better preservation of neurologic function even with deterioration, the patient is usually fully evaluated before any surgery. There is a need to give as radical but careful a treatment as can be done to improve both function and appearance. Diagnosis can be accomplished only with a high-quality metrizamide myelogram with CT (CTMM).

The lipoma of the lower back that is the signal lesion is not different from surrounding subcutaneous fat. In fact, if the patient lies on his back, the external mass may be flattened and unrecognizable by CT. The mass generally blends laterally with the surrounding normal fat. It enters the wide spinal canal and affixes to the neural placode in one or two general ways. The placode itself is like that in MMC. The lipoma may attach centrally to the placode within the widened dysraphic canal, usually across the full width of the placode. In such a case, there is usually not herniation of the sub-

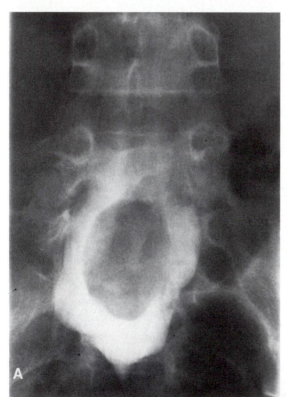

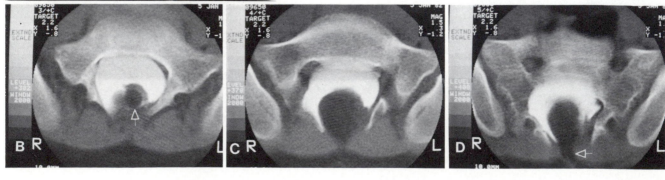

Fig 33–17.—LMMC, 11-year-old boy. **A,** plain film myelogram. There is a large lipoma in the sacral canal at the end of the spinal cord. **B,** CTMM through the upper portion of the lipoma showing its infiltration *(arrow)* into the neural tissue. **C,** slice through the middle of the lipoma showing infiltration similar to Figure 33–14, except the laminae are much more widely dysraphic. **D,** further inferiorly, the lipomatous tissue *(arrow)* exiting from the canal to enter the subcutaneous fat.

arachnoid space dorsal to the placode (Fig 33–17). If the lipoma is more laterally placed on the placode, it may rotate the placode, and there is often a subarachnoid herniation sac on the side of the canal where there is no lipoma (Fig 33–18). The lipoma is said to fix to the placode by a layer of fibrous tissue. This cannot be separated from neural tissue on CT. Although the physical distortion of the cord is precisely defined by CT, the densities of neural and fibrous tissue are alike and cannot be separated.

As in MMC, sagittal reconstruction is useful in picturing the full longitudinal extent of the lipoma and also the metrizamide-filled sac. Unless the back is unusually straight, coronal reconstruction is of limited value. Careful analysis of the axial sections is the most important factor in diagnosis. Except for the absence of the Chiari II malformation and its associated syringomyelia, the possible cord pathology of LMMC is the same as that of MMC. Tethering of the conus is present.

Meningocele

Simple meningoceles, posterior protrusions of the meninges without neural elements, are uncommon compared with MMC and LMMC and are easily recognizable on plain film myelography or CTMM. No special analysis or techniques are needed to see that the sac contains no neural elements.

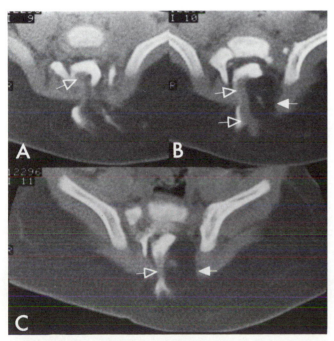

Fig 33–18.—LMMC, 2-month-old girl. **A–C,** sequential CTMM slices progressing inferiorly. The laterally placed lipoma (*solid arrows*) blends with the subcutaneous fat. The cord (*open arrows*) is lateral to the portion of the lipoma that enters the spinal canal and also herniates posteriorly to form a placode.

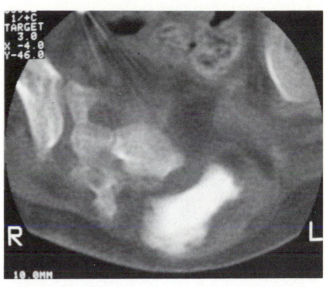

Fig 33–19.—Anterior sacral meningocele, 2-year-old girl. CTMM reveals absence of the left side of the sacrum and a small meningocele protruding through the defect into the pelvis.

Anterior sacral meningoceles, though rare, constitute a more serious problem, but one ideally suited to examination by CTMM. Patients usually have constipation from the mass itself, sphincter weakness, and mild neurologic dysfunction from sacral nerve pressure. Headaches from subarachnoid fluid shifts with positional changes may also occur.

Plain film x-rays usually show the typical dysplastic "scimitar" or hook-shaped sacrum on the AP view. Posterior spina bifida may be present.

Intrathecal metrizamide is necessary to distinguish the meningocele from other cystic pelvic masses. There may be a neck with the meningocele protruding flask-like into the pelvis, or the base may be wide (Fig 33–19). While the sac is reportedly empty of neural tissue in most cases, nerves may pass into it[19] and should be carefully looked for on CT and distinguished from septations that are often in the sac.

Diastematomyelia

Diastematomyelia is a longitudinal splitting of the cord and a relatively common anomaly that is almost always in combination with other dysraphic conditions, especially tethering of the conus, MMC, and LMMC. Two types occur, one being a split within a single dural sac, and the other associated with a double dural sac and having a spur that is usually bony.

The development of the condition has been explained by Gardner[15] as an anterior and posterior splitting of an abnormally dilated fetal cord. Another theory by Herren and Edwards[20] suggests an abnormal closure of the neural canal within the two dorsal halves of the neural plate falling ventrally without touching, thereby making two tubes. Bremer[21] suggested the possible abnormal persistence of the temporary neurenteric canal that normally exists between the yolk sac and amniotic sac through Hensen's node.

A single sac variety was ignored and probably not recognized by most authors before the availability of water-soluble contrast and CT, though Emery and Lendon[22] found a 31% incidence in a careful autopsy series on infants with MMC and probably LMMC. The fact that it occurs more commonly than the spur variety was noted by Scotti and coworkers.[23] In my experience, it is about twice as common as the other type. While often visible on plain film myelography, it may be obscured by contrast dilution or close proximity of the two cord parts. Therefore, CT is most important to secure the diagnosis. The split usually is present over several vertebral segments of the lower thoracic or lumbar cord, but may extend an even shorter distance. The majority of cases occur in association with a tethered conus, especially the milder type I or II tethers. The two cord parts are usually approximately equal in size, but vary somewhat. Likewise, the two parts tend to be round on axial section, but may be flattened medially, especially if in close approximation (Fig 33–20). There is occasionally a bridge between the two halves, presumably of neural tissue (Fig 33–21). The nerve roots are visible laterally, and sometimes more medially, most likely as a result of cord rotation. The two halves usually rejoin before forming the filum, but occasionally remain separate, and it is the presence of a second filum that may be the most important radiologic find-

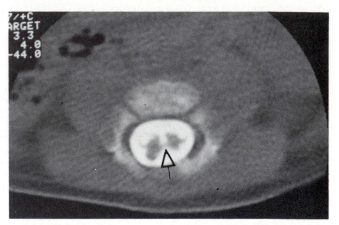

Fig 33–21.—Diastematomyelia, 1-month-old girl. A thin bar of tissue *(arrow)* joins the two unequal halves in this single sac variety.

ing, because the split itself seems to be nonsymptomatic.

If there is no associated complicated anomaly, 10-mm axial CT sections are adequate to define this type of diastematomyelia. The exact location of its beginning and end are much less important than whether or not it ends and whether or not other pathology is also present.

When in association with LMMC or MMC, it is the author's experience that the split is above the placode in most cases. Emery and Lendon[22] found 22% to be in the placode, but no other series has found this high an incidence. They also noted a 9% incidence of one half of the cord forming a placode and the other half in a normal position within the neural canal. I believe this to be a much less common finding, though it certainly does occur.

Diastematomyelia with associated dural splitting has been well described in the radiologic literature since Neuhauser and colleagues[24] first noted the plain film findings. An excellent review of these findings and the plain film myelography was also undertaken by Hilal and coworkers.[25] Most significant findings are spina bifida, a widened spinal canal, vertebral body and laminar anomalies, and a narrowing or absence of the disc space at the level of the spur, plus visualization of the spur itself. Clinical symptoms are similar to those of the tethered conus. External skin markers such as dimples or hemangiomas are very common, and Winter and associates[26] reported hairy patches to be present in 75% of patients.

The use of CTMM has been extremely helpful in dissecting the various parts of the sometimes complex disease, and sagittal or coronal reconstructions may be very helpful (Fig 33–22). When the bony spur is oblique, it is sometimes difficult or impossible to see on

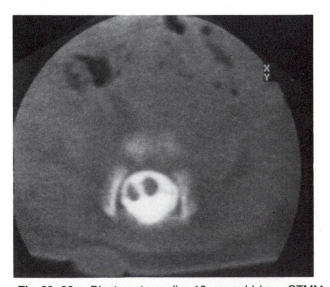

Fig 33–20.—Diastematomyelia, 10-year-old boy. CTMM in lumbar region shows two cord halves in a single dural sac with some medial flattening of each half. The halves are slightly unequal.

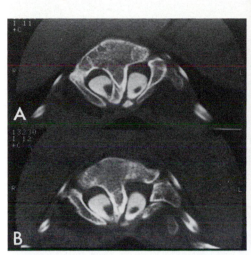

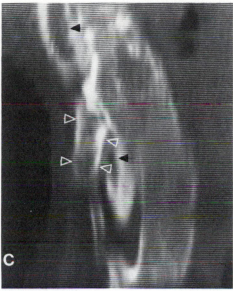

Fig 33–22.—Diastematomyelia, 10-year-old girl. **A, B,** axial CTMM showing bony spur, dysraphism, and segmentation of the vertebra. **C,** sagittal reconstruction of 5-mm slices. The spur *(white arrowheads)* attaches to the back of the vertebral body rostral to its posterior tip. The intact cord above and a portion of the split cord at the spur are visible *(black arrows).*

plain film, as is the split cord itself on myelography. The use of CTMM defines the spur, the bony anomaly, and the cord parts, which are often unequal (Fig 33–23). If scoliosis is present, as it commonly is, CT is even more valuable, because the scoliosis may be locally severe and distort the diastematomyelia. Sections of 5 mm or less may be needed to analyze such cases, and it may be necessary to do extra slices with the angle adjusted perpendicular to the curve after collecting continuous parallel slices that are needed for reconstruction. Cartilaginous spurs have not been encountered by the author, with the possible exception of one case. Partial spurs with an incomplete cleft indenting the dura are occasionally picked up by CT and are virtually impossible to find by any other method.

Diplomyelia, or true duplication of the cord with full

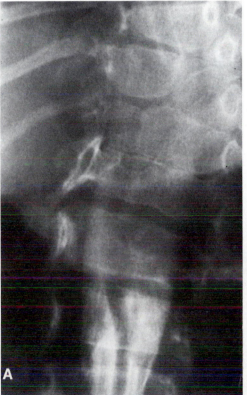

Fig 33–23.—Diastematomyelia with oblique bony spur, 5-year-old girl. **A,** plain film myelogram with marked widening of the spinal canal, dysraphism, and loss of disc spaces in the area of the bony spike, which is not seen. **B,** CTMM, reversed gray scale. Large obliquely oriented spike is easily seen running through the spinal canal and dividing the subarachnoid space into two separate compartments in a somewhat anteroposterior manner. The cord parts are of uneven size.

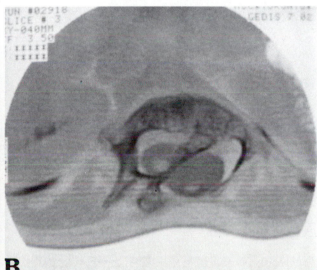

sets of nerve roots from both sides of both hemicords, is described in a report by Herren and Edwards,[20] but there is some doubt as to the authenticity of any of the cases in that report. No well-documented case has since been reported, and it seems likely that the entity only exists, if it does at all, in the rare occasion where there is a complete duplication of a portion of the bony spine.

Chiari Malformation

In children, the Chiari II malformation with MMC, hindbrain malformation, and displacement of the cervical canal is much more common than the Chiari I (tonsillar displacement only), or Chiari III (hindbrain malformation with occipital encephalocele). Postulated causes for the malformation are overgrowth of the developing brain[27] and herniation of the hindbrain from delayed opening of the fourth ventricular foramina.[5]

The anatomical changes are complex. While axial CT easily identifies the abnormality, even with multiplanar reconstructions the exact components may be unclear. The cervical cord is inferiorly displaced. This is sometimes demonstrable by visualizing the nerve roots and lower cranial nerves traversing upward in the cervical canal. There is herniation of the brain stem, usually only the medulla, downward and dorsally over the cervical cord. Though the fourth ventricle is carried down with the medulla, it more often than not does not fill with metrizamide. The kink or fold that the medulla makes atop the cord may be identifiable, especially in sagittal reconstruction (Fig 33–24). On top of the medulla is the cerebellum, pulled down to a peg-like tip. This may be tonsil or vermis. The medulla may be more inferior, or the cerebellum may be more inferior.[28] At times, all three components—cord, medulla,

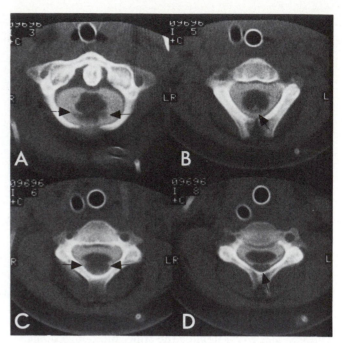

Fig 33–25.—Chiari II, same patient as in Figure 33–23. **A–D,** axial CTMM progressing inferiorly showing cerebellum in **(A)** and **(B)** *(arrows)* and, below that, herniated medulla in **(C)** and **(D)** *(arrows)* with flattened cervical cord anterior to the displaced medulla.

and cerebellum—may be identifiable (Fig 33–25). The cord and the medulla are often rectangular in cross section because of compression. The cervical level varies, but it is uncommon to visualize these defects below the midcervical region on CT.

Given the associated myelomeningocele, it is unlikely that a Chiari II malformation will be mistaken for anything else. A Chiari I with only tonsillar displacement is much more an incidental finding and not reliably different in appearance from tonsillar herniation secondary to an intracranial mass. In such a case, one should do a CT scan of the head to rule out the possibility of a secondary cause. In the author's experience, no Chiari I malformations have required decompression.

Hydrosyringomyelia

Hydromyelia, enlargement of the central canal of the cord, is commonly associated with MMC. Its exact incidence is unknown, because asymptomatic patients are usually not examined. Emery and Lendon[22] found a 20% incidence in their autopsy series, which again might be greater than the true incidence. Syringomyelia is a dissection of fluid out of the central canal or completely separate from the canal as a result of cord damage. As hydromyelia itself might promote damage, it is not possible to distinguish one from the other un-

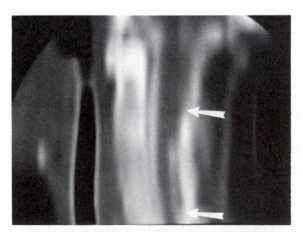

Fig 33–24.—Chiari II malformation, 12-year-old boy. Sagittal reconstruction of 5-mm slices with 2-mm overlap. The cerebellar tip extends down to the level of C-3 *(upper arrow),* and the medulla itself is herniated all the way down to C-6 *(lower arrow).*

less the dissection or separation can be seen in the axial sections. The general term syringomyelia is usually used to cover both entities. While it is inaccurate in the pediatric setting, I will use the term, even though hydromyelia is almost always the primary entity.

Although Bonafe and coworkers[29] reported the diagnosis of cervical syringomyelia without the use of contrast by using a specially modified CT scanner, I believe the most reliable method of diagnosis is with water-soluble contrast. As the search for syringomyelia in children is usually accompanied by the evaluation of MMC and Chiari II pathology, contrast is already in place.

The diagnosis is best made with axial sections, and reconstruction in other planes generally adds little to the diagnosis. The most apparent finding is the collapsed (ribbon-like) cord, seen with or without metrizamide, in the flattened canal (Fig 33–26). The cord is flattened anteroposteriorly. Immediate entry of contrast media into the central canal suggests communication with the fourth ventricle. At the author's hospital, delayed studies are not done on collapsed syrinxes, though a point could be made for such an examination if it altered the type of treatment.

The enlarged cord, which is round in cross section, may be seen with or without contrast in the central canal. Delayed examination 6 to 24 hours later may show delayed filling of the central canal with metrizamide (Fig 33–27). The canal may be relatively small, or may be large with only a thin shell of cord tissue. Aubin and coworkers[30] reported that the vast majority of syrinxes have delayed filling. In children, about half do not fill. Aubin and coworkers[30] noted that cases with active hydrocephalus did not fill, and because most patients with MMC have hydrocephalus, this is the probable ex-

planation for a much lower rate of central canal filling in children.

Whether delayed filling occurs via the fourth ventricle or through the cord is not clear. Even delayed filling is not conclusive evidence of syringomyelia, because Kan and associates[31] have shown this also occurs in tumor cysts. However, the knowledge of an existing Chiari malformation is strong supportive evidence of a syrinx, whereas its absence combined with a widened canal without dysraphism is equally strong support for the diagnosis of a tumor. Bonafe and colleagues[32] suggest that a small cord is evidence of a syrinx, but I believe this is more likely part of the MMC dysgenesis.

CONGENITAL TUMORS

Dermoid and Epidermoid

Dermoid and epidermoid cysts are considered together in this section, because there is little radiologic difference between them. Both are presumed to arise from cell rests, possibly secondary to incomplete separation of the cutaneous and neural ectoderm at the time of neural tube closure.[33] Epidermoids contain only superficial skin elements, while dermoids have glandular follicular elements. This may have some practical significance in that the dermoid may contain enough fatty material to give a low-density CT reading. Rarely, these lesions may be secondary to implantation from lumbar puncture or MMC repair. While epidermoids are evenly distributed throughout the spine, the majority of dermoids are lumbosacral.[33] The tumors may be extra- or intramedullary. Not all cysts are connected to a sinus tract, and likewise not all sinus tracts connect to a cyst. It is estimated that about 30% of the cysts are connected to sinuses,[34, 35] and about half the sinuses

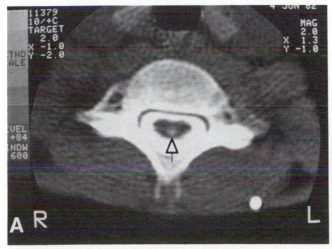

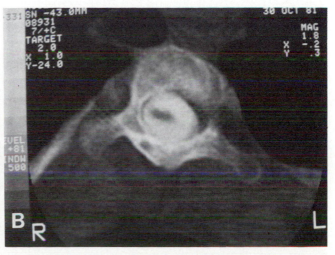

Fig 33–26.—Syringomyelia with flattened cord. **A,** 10-year-old girl. CTMM through cervical cord reveals partial flattening and metrizamide in enlarged central canal (arrow).

B, 11-year-old boy. CTMM through thoracic region shows collapsed cord without visualization of the central canal.

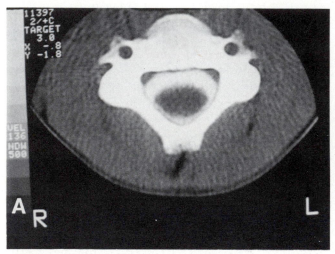 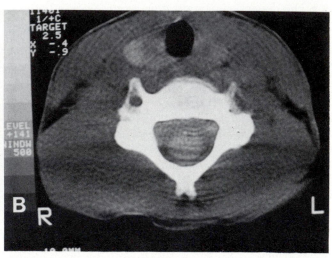

Fig 33–27.—Syringomyelia, enlarged cord, 12-year-old boy. **A,** initial CTMM showing dilated cervical cord surrounded by metrizamide. **B,** delayed study at 18 hours. Metrizamide has left the subarachnoid space, but some has entered the large central canal, which is now denser than the surrounding cord and subarachnoid space.

end in tumors.[36] The incidence is reported to vary from 7% of pediatric spinal tumors[37] to 2.2% of all spinal tumors.[34] Epidermoids and dermoids may present with symptoms because of their mass effect or meningitis. The meningitis may be chemical from release of the contents of the cyst or infectious if there is a sinus connected to the skin.

Plain films usually will show hypoplasia of the spinous process or spina bifida, especially if there is a sinus. If meningitis is present, it is safer to do the spinal puncture cervically if the infection is in the lumbar region or vice versa. Use of CTMM, especially with reconstruction in the sagittal plane, is the best method of preoperative investigation. While any sinus tract is partially visible on axial slices, sagittal reconstructions reveal the rostral course that it takes going from skin to dura and show to better advantage the cord expansion caused by the intramedullary lesions (Fig 33–28). As the tumors vary from a few millimeters to 1 to 2 vertebral body segments in size and usually have accompanying radiologic and clinical signs, they are not often confused preoperatively with other diagnoses.

In my limited experience with two infected tumors in which a total block to contrast has occurred, CTMM was much less precise. While the visible sinus tract and abnormal spine denoted the site, limits of the tumor could not be determined, and intravenous contrast did not add further information.

Teratoma

Teratomas, having tissue from all three germ layers, are less common, making up 7% or less of pediatric intraspinal masses.[37] Their origin is less clear than dermoids, possibly arising from rests of abnormal germ cells,[38] or more likely primitive somatic cells.[39] Because they are occasionally associated with diastematomyelia, the abnormal retention of the temporary neurenteric canal[21] has been proposed as a cause. More often, there are no vertebral anomalies. Enlargement of the spinal canal is common.

The mass is most often small and involves one or two vertebral segments. Rarely, they have been reported to occupy the entire cord.[40] They may be intramedullary, extramedullary, or combined.

Their character on CTMM is variable. They may be solid or cystic and may have fatty components or even calcification. If the nonsolid elements are identifiable, the diagnosis can be made with relative certainty. If the tumor is solid, it may be impossible to distinguish it from an acquired tumor such as astrocytoma, which will also expand the spinal canal. Because astrocytomas are frequently cystic, a cystic tumor containing no fat that expands the spinal canal may be either of these lesions. In general, astrocytomas are larger, both in cord expansion and length of cord involved, but as noted by Pickens and coworkers,[40] the whole cord may be involved with teratoma. The limits of the tumor are visible by CTMM if there is not a complete obstruction to the flow of the contrast.

Lipoma

The subject of intraspinal lipomas is difficult, because they occur both as isolated lesions and in conjunction with a variety of dysraphic states, especially the tethered conus and LMMC. The isolated lipoma is uncommon, occurring in less than 1% of all spinal tumors.[41]

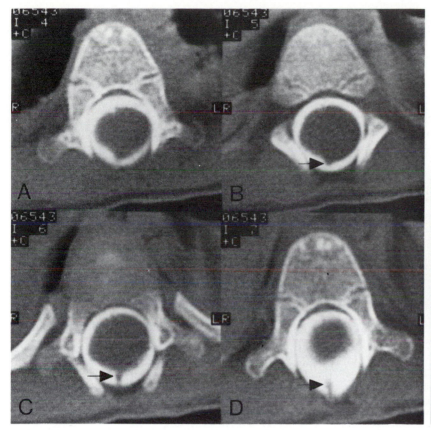

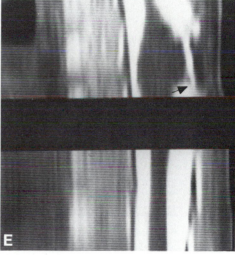

Fig 33–28.—Thoracic dermoid, 4-year-old girl. **A–D,** inferiorly progressing sequential 5-mm sections. Posterior spina bifida and cord enlargement are clearly visible. The dermoid tract *(arrows)* enters the cord from behind. **E,** sagittal reconstruction. The complete area of cord enlargement and upward passage of the tract *(arrow)* is well seen. The *black bar* in the middle of the reconstruction is due to software error that would not allow reconstruction of some of the slices.

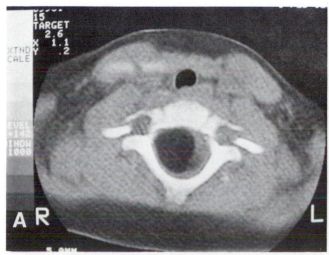

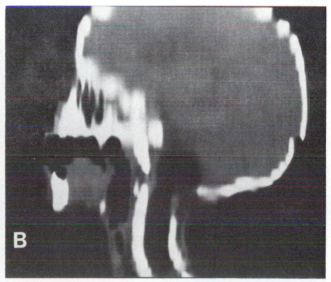

Fig 33–29.—Lipoma, 1-year-old girl. **A,** axial CT slice through cervical region. A large low-density lipoma has infiltrated the cord and enlarged the spinal canal. **B,** sagittal reconstruction. The lipoma occupies nearly the entire cervical canal and extrudes into the posterior fossa.

The mass is most often cervical or thoracic in location,[42] and there is no dysraphism. The mass is dorsally placed within the spinal canal and may invade the cord. The author has experience with only one such lesion, which extended into the posterior fossa. Scans by CT, especially the sagittal reconstruction, gave a remarkable picture that, because of the low density of the fat, was pathopneumonic (Fig 33–29). As the cord expansion or compression occurs only at the site of the lipoma itself, it is not likely to be confused with a fat-containing tumor that is of larger dimensions.

Lipomas associated with tethering and LMMC are discussed in those sections. It is worth noting that Emery and Lendon[43] found 49 intrathecal lipomas of the filum, 26 dural lipomas, and 8 leptomyelolipomas mixed with neural tissue in 100 autopsied meningomyeloceles. The leptomyelolipomas are most likely cases of LLMC, as are perhaps some of the other lesions. Scans by CT of many true cases of MMC by the author have not substantiated the numbers found by Emery and Lendon, suggesting such lipomas, if present, must be quite small.

SPLIT NOTOCHORD SYNDROME

There are several rare gastrointestinal duplications combined with vertebral and cord anomalies that fall under the general term of split notochord syndrome. The syndrome usually includes some gut duplication or cyst with an attachment to or connection through an anomalous vertebral body. It can extend through the canal to the posterior wall or rarely be entirely posterior in location.[44] The origins are obscure, but theories include adhesion between the endoderm and ectoderm

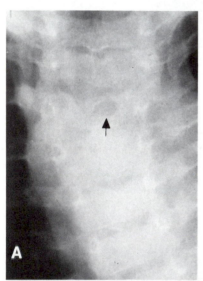

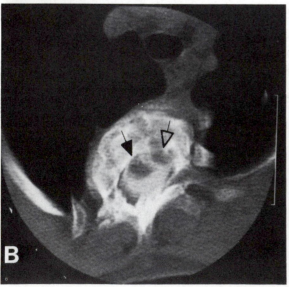

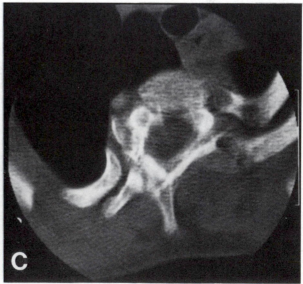

Fig 33–30.—Neurenteric cyst, 14-year-old boy. **A,** plain film of the thoracic spine at age 3 showing the typical cleft *(arrow)* through a vertebral body, which is not visible by age 14 because of progressive kyphosis. **B,** axial CTMM at age 14. The vertebrae are deformed. The cord *(solid arrow)* is deformed by the adjacent cyst *(open arrow)* that has entered the subarachnoid space. **C,** adjacent higher slice. Cord and cyst have merged into a single large mass almost completely blocking the flow of metrizamide. The cyst was thought to be intramedullary at operation.

that is normally separated by the advancing notochord tissue,[45] splitting of the notochord,[44] or persistence of the neurenteric canal.[21]

The majority of these lesions are neurenteric cysts that present as intrathoracic masses with associated vertebral anomalies, usually a canal through a vertebral body. The chest mass contains gut elements at pathology. Computed tomography has the advantage of visualizing the extraspinal mass if it has not been resected, the tract through the vertebral body, and the intraspinal component. This spinal component is variable and not easily seen even with the best CT or CTMM. After it has passed through the vertebral body, the cyst may end at the dura, pass through the dura and end in an extramedullary location, or extend into the cord itself. While the extradural type is identifiable because of the normal subarachnoid space on CTMM, the cyst that ends in an intradural extramedullary location attaches to the cord surface, making it difficult to determine intramedullary invasion. In either the intradural-extramedullary or intramedullary types, the cord and cyst make up a single "mass" that looks like an expanded and distorted cord on axial slices (Fig 33–30).

The adherence of the tissue to the cord allows no contrast material to pass between them.

SACRAL AGENESIS

Sacral agenesis is a very rare lesion. The plain film findings of partial or total sacral agenesis are obvious. Motor and sensory deficits and gait disturbances from abnormal hip anatomy are common symptoms that may be progressive. Maternal diabetes appears to be a strong factor in the occurrence of the disease, and perhaps paternal diabetes may also be causative.[46]

Two types of agenesis occur, and they can be investigated and distinguished by CTMM.[47] The stenotic type has a narrow lumbar subarachnoid space that ends above the sacrum with compression of the cauda equina (Fig 33–31). This type may benefit from a duraplasty. The second variety is identical to a tethered conus and may benefit from release of the conus. Both types can be distinguished by plain film myelography. The conditions have been reported in association with MMC and other abnormalities, so each case must be individually assessed.

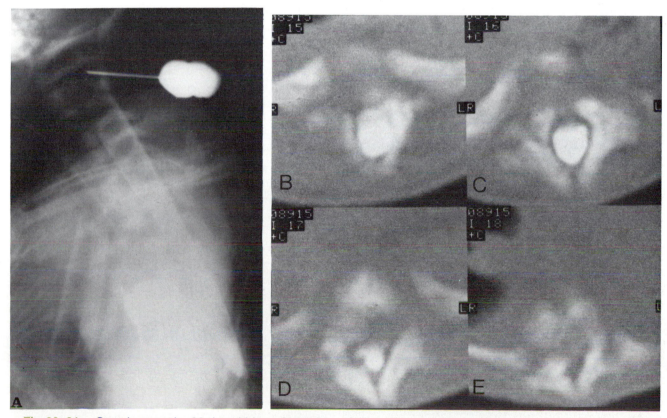

Fig 33–31.—Sacral agenesis, 20-day-old boy. **A,** lateral plain film myelogram done by cervical puncture shows the short subarachnoid space ending in the lower thoracic spine. The vertebral bodies are dysplastic. **B–E,** sequential CTMM slices through the lower thoracic spine. The inferior subarachnoid space contains no nerve roots. The spinal canal progressively narrows as the metrizamide-filled subarachnoid space ends.

NONDYSRAPHIC ABNORMALITIES

Neurofibromatosis

This is one of the most complicated and diverse diseases in its manifestations. The spine is involved in both the central and mixed forms of the disease, but, unlike the brain, has relatively few types of abnormalities, though they occur in a high frequency of patients. Scoliosis is the most common finding, occurring in about one half of the patients.[48] Scoliosis is clinically obvious and sometimes severe over a relatively short length of vertebrae. It often has a rotatory component. The challenge to the neuroradiologist is to decide if the scoliosis is from bony or intraspinal abnormalities. While the bony abnormalities can be fairly well documented by plain film tomography, the need for CTMM to examine the subarachnoid space diminishes the need and usefulness for the former study. If a curve is severe, one may obtain a sagittal projection from an axial slice through part of the curve. The seeming distortion caused by the slicing of different parts of adjacent vertebral bodies may be confusing and require reconstructions in obliquely oriented planes. The cord, if stretched tightly along the curve, will be somewhat flattened, even though normal (Fig 33–32).

Minor abnormalities such as scalloping of the posterior aspects of the vertebral bodies, dural ectasia, and bulging of the subarachnoid space through the foramina are easily recognized (Fig 33–33). Though these pa-

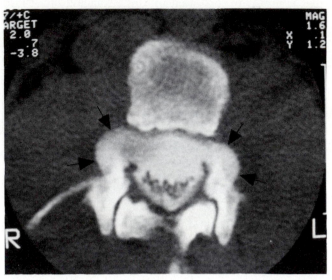

Fig 33–33.—Neurofibromatosis in a 15-year-old boy, CTMM through lumbar spine. Bulging of the subarachnoid space through the vertebral foramina *(arrows)*, presumed to be part of the "dural ectasia," is common in this disease. The vertebra is somewhat dysplastic.

tients develop schwannomas of nerve roots in about 20% of cases,[49] this is rare in childhood.

Achondroplasia

Achondroplastic dwarfs have the misfortune of a normal-sized spinal cord in a narrowed spinal canal. The cross-sectional area of the canal throughout the spine is decreased by a combination of early fusion of the neurocentral synchondroses and abnormally thick pedicles from hypertrophic periosteum.[50] These abnormalities especially narrow the lumbar canal, which does not have the usual physiologic widening (Fig 33–34). Further aggravating the compromised canal is the prominence of the intervertebral discs and a small "key-hole" foramen magnum (Fig 33–35). About 30% of these patients also have kyphosis with vertebral body wedging.[51] All of these features are easily seen on CTMM, though plain film myelography will in fact identify the spinal canal changes fairly well. Cord compression by kyphosis is best visualized by CTMM.

Mucopolysaccharidosis

The inherited group of diseases called mucopolysaccharidoses (MPS), although having similar enzymatic defects interfering with mucopolysaccharide metabolism, have marked variations in clinical severity and radiographic abnormalities. These abnormalities are primarily due to the deposition of mucopolysaccharides in bones, cartilage, ligaments, and dura. Four of the diseases have been reported to have myelographic abnormalities; these are Hurler's syndrome (MPS-I), Hurler-

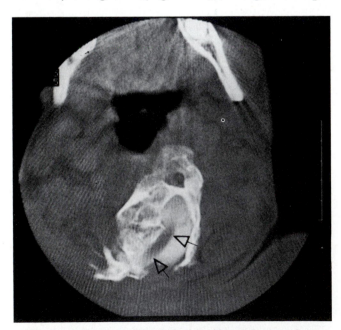

Fig 33–32.—Neurofibromatosis with scoliosis, 18-year-old male. Axial CTMM is oblique through dysplastic cervical vertebrae in a patient with a severe cervicothoracic scoliosis. The cord *(arrows)* is flattened against the vertebral body through the apex of the curve.

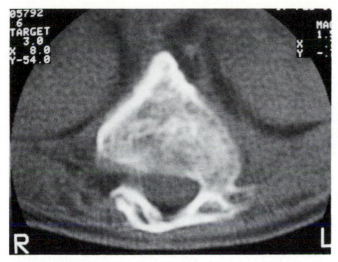

Fig 33–34.—Achondroplasia in an 11-year-old girl, CT through a lumbar vertebra. The vertebral body is anteriorly pointed. The right pedicle is thickened, and the canal is small, especially in the sagittal plane. The slice is partially through the foramen on the right.

Scheie syndrome (MPS-I H/S), Morquio's syndrome (MPS-IV), and the Maroteaux-Lamy syndrome (MPS-VI).

The best-known anomalies are the flattened thoracolumbar "bullet" vertebral bodies of MPS-I and MPS-IV. Potentially more dangerous are the abnormalities that affect the cervical spine. Kennedy and colleagues[52] described a case of MPS-I H/S with compression of the cervical canal caused by dural deposits and ligamentous thickening, and Sostrin and coworkers[53] added another case plus one with MPS-VI.

Cervical abnormalities in MPS-IV[54] are especially severe. These neurologically threatening abnormalities require CTMM for full evaluation. The full extent of the disease in MPS-IV was described by Edwards and coworkers.[55] There is a small cervical canal with thick laminae and odontoid hypoplasia. The small C-1 arch may be trapped on the posterior lip of the foramen

magnum. Hypoplasia of the odontoid combined with ligament laxity causes subluxation of C-1 on C-2, which is further complicated because of the narrow cervical canal and dural deposits of the MPS. The same findings are also seen in MPS-I (Fig 33–36).

Spondylolisthesis

Spondylolisthesis, the forward slippage of one vertebral body on another, usually L-5 on S-1 or L-4 on L-5, is a fairly common pediatric entity. Its true cause is unknown. The review of McKee and colleagues[56] of 63 pediatric cases suggested most are caused by nonunion of stress fractures, a congenital weakness of the pars, or a combination of factors. The first theory is supported by the very uncommon occurrence before children walk, and the second by a strong familial correlation.

Very few cases are truly congenital, and these are usually due to facet anomalies. The use of CT does not

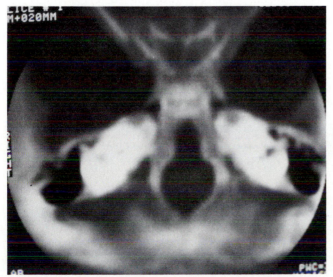

Fig 33–35.—Achondroplasia in a 9-month-old boy. CT through the skull base reveals the small key-hole shaped foramen magnum.

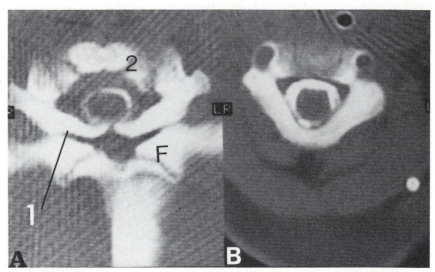

Fig 33–36.—MPS-I, 2½-year-old boy. A, CTMM at foramen magnum shows laminae of C-1 (1) caught against the foramen magnum (F). The slice also includes the base of C-2 (2). The subarachnoid space is thought to be displaced posteriorly by dural deposits. B, C-4 slice shows better the small cervical canal and markedly thick laminae.

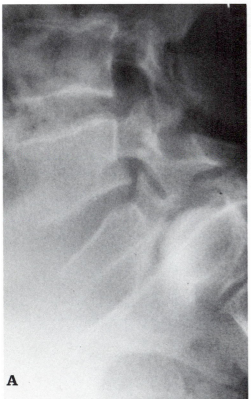

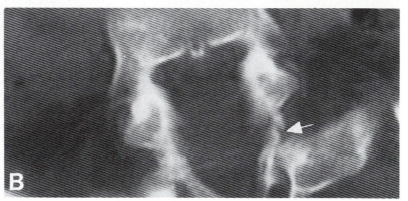

Fig 33–37.—Spondylolisthesis, 13-year-old boy. A, lateral spine film shows grade IV displacement of L-5 on S-1. B, CT through plane of laminae of L-5 shows elongated hypoplastic laminae with probable congenital fracture (arrow) on the right.

improve the understanding of the causations of spondylolisthesis, but is well suited to the differentiation of the idiopathic and congenital types when plain films do not adequately do so. This may be combined with myelography when compression of the cauda equina causes neurologic symptoms.

The common idiopathic type of spondylolisthesis has a similar appearance on both CT and plain films. The rare congenital types are extremely difficult to analyze by plain film, and axial or near axial CT is a much more informative imaging technique for such anomalies (Fig 33–37).

REFERENCES

1. Kaiser M.C., Veiga-Pires J.A.: Evaluation de nouvelles techniques en tomodensitometrie. *Ann. Radiol.* 23:559–563, 1980.
2. Brugman E., Palmers Y., Staelens B.: Congenital absence of a pedicle in the cervical spine: A new approach with CT scan. *Neuroradiology* 17:121–125, 1979.
3. Oestreich A.E., Young L.W.: The absent cervical pedicle syndrome: A case in childhood. *A.J.R.* 107:505–510, 1969.
4. Maldague B.E., Malghem J.J.: Unilateral arch hypertrophy with spinous process T1H: A sign of arch-deficiency. *Radiology* 121:567–574, 1976.
5. Lauten G.J., Wehunt W.D.: Computed tomography in absent cervical pedicle. *A.J.N.R.* 1:201–203, 1980.
6. McRae D.L.: The significance of abnormalities of the cervical spine. *Am. J. Roentgenol. Rad. Ther. Nucl. Med.* 84:3–25, 1960.
7. McRae D.L.: Roentgenologic findings in syringomyelia and hydromyelia. *A.J.R.* 89:695–703, 1966.
8. Caetano de Barros M., Farias W., Ataide L., et al.: Basilar impression and Arnold-Chiari malformation. *J. Neurol. Neurosurg. Psychiatry* 31:596–605, 1968.
9. Barson A.J.: The vertebral level of termination of the spinal cord during normal and abnormal development. *J. Anat.* 106:489–497, 1970.
10. Reimann A.F., Anson B.J.: Vertebral level of termination of the spinal cord with report of a case of sacral cord. *Anat. Rec.* 88:127–138, 1944.
11. Fitz C.R., Harwood-Nash D.C.: The tethered conus. *Am. J. Roentgenol. Rad. Ther. Nucl. Med.* 125:515–523, 1975.
12. Hendrick E.B., Hoffman H.J., Humphreys R.P.: Tethered cord syndrome, in McLaurin R. (ed.): *Myelomeningocele*. New York, Grune & Stratton, 1977.
13. Hoffman H.J., Hendrick E.B., Humphreys R.P.: The tethered spinal cord: Its protean manifestations, diagnosis and surgical correction. *Childs Brain* 2:145–155, 1976.
14. Garceau G.J.: The filum terminale syndrome. *J. Bone Joint Surg.* 35:711–716, 1953.
15. Gardner W.J.: Etiology and pathogenesis of the development of myelomeningocele, in McLaurin R. (ed.): *Myelomeningocele*. New York, Grune & Stratton, 1977.
16. Lichtenstein B.W.: Spinal dysraphism. *Arch. Neurol. Psychiatry* 44:742–810, 1940.
17. Osaka K., Matsumoto S., Tanimura T.: Myeloschisis in early human embryo. *Childs Brain* 4:347–359, 1978.
18. Heinz E.R., Rosenbaum A.E., Scarff T.B., et al.: Tethered spinal cord following meningomyelocele repair. *Radiology* 131:153–160, 1979.
19. Dyck P., Wilson C.B.: Anterior sacral meningocele. *J. Neurosurg.* 53:548–552, 1980.
20. Herren R.Y., Edwards J.E.: Diplomyelia (duplication of the spinal cord). *Arch. Pathol.* 30:1203–1214, 1940.
21. Bremer J.L.: Dorsal intestinal fistula; accessory neurenteric canal; diastematomyelia. *A.M.A. Arch. Pathol.* 54:132–138, 1952.
22. Emery J.L., Lendon R.G.: The local cord lesion in neurospinal dysraphism (meningomyelocele). *J. Pathol.* 110:83–96, 1973.
23. Scotti G., Musgrave M.A., Harwood-Nash D.C., et al.: Diastematomyelia in children: Metrizamide and CT metrizamide myelography. *A.J.N.R.* 1:403–410, 1980.
24. Neuhauser E.B.D., Wittenborg M.H., Dehlinger K.: Diastematomyelia: Transfixation of the cord or cauda equina with congenital anomalies of the spine. *Radiology* 54:659–664, 1950.
25. Hilal S.K., Marton D., Pollack E.: Diastematomyelia in children. *Neuroradiology* 112:609–621, 1974.
26. Winter R.B., Haven J.J., Moe J.H., et al.: Diastematomyelia and congenital spine deformities. *J. Bone Joint Surg.* 56A:27–39, 1974.
27. Barry A., Patten B.M., Stewart B.H.: Possible factors in the development of the Arnold-Chiari malformation. *J. Neurosurg.* 14:285–301, 1957.
28. Peach B.: The Arnold-Chiari malformation. *Arch. Neurol.* 12:527–535, 1965.
29. Bonafe A., Ethier D., Melancon D., et al.: High resolution computed tomography in cervical syringomyelia. *J. Comput. Assist. Tomogr.* 4:42–47, 1980.
30. Aubin M.L., Vignaud J., Jardin C., et al.: Computed tomography in 75 clinical cases of syringomyelia. *A.J.N.R.* 2:199–204, 1981.
31. Kan S., Fox A.J., Vinuela F., et al.: Delayed CT metrizamide enhancement of syringomyelia secondary to tumor. *A.J.N.R.* 4:73–78, 1983.
32. Bonafe A., Manelfe C., Espagno J., et al.: Evaluation of syringomyelia with metrizamide computed tomographic myelography. *J. Comput. Assist. Tomogr.* 4:797–802, 1980.
33. List C.F.: Intraspinal epidermoids, dermoids and dermal sinuses. *Surg. Gynecol. Obstet.* 73:525–538, 1941.
34. Guidetti B., Gagliardi F.M.: Epidermoid and dermoid cysts. *J. Neurosurg.* 47:12–18, 1977.
35. Bailey I.C.: Dermoid tumours of the spinal cord. *J. Neurosurg.* 33:676–681, 1970.
36. Cardell B.S., Laurence B.: Congenital dermal sinus associated with meningitis: A report of a fatal case. *Br. Med. J.* 2:1558–1561, 1951.
37. Harwood-Nash D.C., Fitz C.R.: *Neuroradiology in Infants and Children*. St. Louis, C.V. Mosby Co., 1976.

38. Newcastle N.B., Francouer J.: Teratomatous cysts in the spinal canal. *Arch. Neurol.* 11:91–99, 1964.

39. Kaplan C.G., Askin F.B., Benirschke K.: Cytogenetics of extragonadal tumours. *Teratology* 19:261–266, 1979.

40. Pickens J.M., Wilson J., Myers G.G., et al.: Teratoma of the spinal cord. *Arch. Pathol.* 99:446–448, 1975.

41. Rubinstein L.J.: *Tumours of the Central Nervous System.* Atlas of Tumour Pathology, Armed Forces Institute of Pathology, 1972, series 2, fasc. 6.

42. Giuffre R.: Intradural spinal lipomas. *Acta Neurosurg.* 14:69–95, 1966.

43. Emery J.L., Lendon R.G.: Lipomas of the cauda equina and other fatty tumours related to neurospinal dysraphism. *Dev. Med. Child Neurol.,* suppl 20, 1969, pp. 62–70.

44. Bentley J.F.R., Smith J.R.: Developmental posterior enteric remnants and spinal malformations. *Arch. Dis. Child.* 35:76–86, 1960.

45. Beardmore H.E., Wiglesworth F.W.: Vertebral anomalies and alimentary duplications. *Pediatr. Clin. North Am.* 5:457–473, 1958.

46. Pang D., Hoffman H.J.: Sacral agenesis with progressive neurological deficit. *Neurosurgery* 7:118–126, 1980.

47. Brooks B.S., El Gammal T., Hartlage P., et al.: Myelography of sacral agenesis. *A.J.N.R.* 2:319–323, 1981.

48. Casselman E.S., Mandell G.A.: Vertebral scalloping in neurofibromatosis. *Radiology* 131:89–94, 1979.

49. Casselman E.S., Miller W.T., Lin S.R., et al.: Von Recklinghausen's disease: Incidence of roentgenographic findings with a clinical review of the literature. *C.R.C. Crit. Rev. Diagn. Imaging* 9:387–419,, 1977.

50. Duvoisin R.C., Yahr M.D.: Compressive spinal cord and root syndromes in achondroplastic dwarfs. *Neurology* 12:202–207, 1962.

51. Galanski M., Herrmann R., Knoche U.: Neurological complications and myelographic features of achondroplasia. *Neuroradiology* 17:59–63, 1978.

52. Kennedy P., Swash M., Dean M.F.: Cervical cord compression in mucopolysaccharidosis. *Dev. Med. Child Neurol.* 15:194–199, 1973.

53. Sostrin R.D., Hasso A.N., Peterson D.I., et al.: Myelographic features of mucopolysaccharidosis: A new sign. *Radiology* 125:421–424, 1977.

54. Lipson S.J.: Dysplasia of the odontoid process in Morquio's syndrome causing quadriparesis. *J. Bone Joint Surg.* 59A:340–344, 2977.

55. Edwards M.K., Harwood-Nash D.C., Fitz C.R., et al.: CT metrizamide myelography of the cervical spine in Morquio syndrome. *A.J.N.R.* 3:66–69, 1982.

56. McKee B.W., Alexander W.J., Dunbar J.S.: Spondylolysis and spondylolisthesis in children: A review. *Journal de L'Association Canadienne des Radiologistes* 22:100–109, 1971.

Therapeutic Techniques

34

Stereotaxy and the Role of CT in Morphological and Functional Surgery of the Human Brain

L. Dade Lunsford, M.D.

Historical Perspective

Stereotaxy, or guided brain surgery, has been revitalized by the major radiologic imaging advances generated by CT. Guided brain surgery first was introduced into the English scientific literature in 1908 by Horsley and Clark,[1] who constructed a stereotaxic device to study the structure and function of the monkey cerebellum. Although guiding devices were employed successfully for electrode coagulation of the trigeminal ganglion by Kirschner[2] in 1933, intracranial surgery remained dormant until Spiegel and Wycis[3] developed human stereotaxy in 1947. The technique was refined and expanded by many contributors in Europe and the United States, including Leksell,[4] Riechert,[5] Talairach,[6] Cooper,[7] and Van Buren.[8] For many years, the major usage involved functional surgery of the brain, especially that of Parkinson's disease and other dyskinesias. Radiologic definition of the brain was dependent upon contrast encephalography or cerebral angiography and the usage of anatomical landmarks as reference points for the determination of intracranial targets. To many surgeons, the technique remained too abstruse, highly sophisticated, and impractical to use in routine neurosurgical practice. Nonetheless, instruction in stereotaxic technique by major teaching programs in the United States was widespread throughout the 1950s and 1960s. After the introduction of dopaminergic agents to treat Parkinson's disease, the number of cases referred for stereotaxic surgery declined rapidly, and interest in the technique as a whole waned. The development of sophisticated new imaging techniques, with the promise of early recognition of intracranial pathology and the direct visualization of intracranial targets, mandated the current resurgent interest in stereotaxy.

Seeing the promise of even early CT diagnostic units, several intrepid investigators demonstrated that CT could be used to visualize appropriate targets for neurosurgical intervention and to guide catheters or biopsy instruments to these lesions. In 1977, Maroon and coworkers[9] used the first generation scanner to provide freehand guidance in the biopsy of deep diencephalic tumors. At the Karolinska Hospital in Stockholm, Bergström and Greitz[10] constructed an interchangeable base ring adapted to the EMI scanner and a Leksell stereotaxic frame, permitting true stereotaxic procedures.

The first major problem encountered by early workers in the field of CT-guided intracranial surgery was the need to relate the target shown on a horizontal CT image to external skull landmarks or skull radiographs. Accordingly, a series of localizing grids was developed by various workers,[11–13] which could then be used to orient the target in space. Evolution of the scanners resulted in evolution of surgical technique. Enlargement of the scanner aperture, reduction in imaging and reconstruction time, improvement in resolution, and accurate electronic radiographic localization using the scanner x-ray tube have all eliminated the problems encountered by early workers.[14] With increasingly earlier recognition of lesions, as well as more detailed assessment of the relationship of that lesion to the normal brain, the need for accurate guiding devices fully compatible with CT has been demonstrated convincingly. Accumulated evidence has shown that CT stereotaxis is safer, more accurate, and more reliable than CT-guided techniques that do not rely on stereotaxic instrumentation. The mode of CT has become an important imaging device to the stereotaxic surgeon, replacing other radiographic imaging techniques in many cases.

Technical Achievements

The conceptual problem in CT stereotaxis was the need to convert two-dimensional horizontal images into three-dimensional stereotaxic targets. Coordinates identified on the CT scan required conversion to stereotaxic frame coordinates. The need to transpose stereotaxic coordinates visualized by CT into lateral skull x-rays has been eliminated by the usage and development of entirely new devices for stereotaxis or the modification of existing devices for CT. Devices that have been modified for CT stereotaxis include the Leksell (Fig 34–1),[15] Riechert-Mundinger,[16] and Todd-Wells[17] frames. Entirely new devices integrated with sophisticated computer programs for coordinate determination include those developed by Brown, Robert, and Wells,[18] Perry, Rosenbaum, and Lunsford,[19] Glenn and co-workers,[20] and Koslow and associates.[21] Each device possesses its own relative merits, but the choice of instruments ultimately depends on both the surgeon's needs and the goals of the procedures to be performed. The choice of instruments should be made after review of several pertinent questions:

1. Is it *complete* system (i.e., are the necessary instruments for imaging, biopsy, or lesioning fully integrated within the system)?

2. Is it *simple* (i.e., does the user understand the concept of coordinate determination and the manipulations that are necessary to obtain the surgical coordinates)?

3. Is it *versatile* (i.e., are multiple approach trajectories available, including temporal, posterior fossa, and transsphenoidal routes)?

4. Is it *accurate?**

5. Is it *compatible only with CT* (i.e., can the same instrument be used with other radiographic techniques, including contrast encephalography and angiography)?

6. Is it *computer dependent* (i.e., can coordinate determination be obtained only with the usage of sophisticated computer programs)?

7. Is it *adaptable for the future* (i.e., will the device be useful in the burgeoning study of human brain function determined by nuclear magnetic resonance [NMR] and positron emission tomography [PET])?

Requirements of Stereotaxic Devices

Table 34–1 demonstrates the requirements of CT stereotaxic systems. The completion of any CT stereotaxic procedure requires coordination of a sophisticated and precise stereotaxic surgical instrument and an evolving and sophisticated x-ray imaging device. Stereotaxic instruments must be constructed of rigid, low atomic number material to maintain image quality. Firm skull fixation must be provided by pins placed into the outer table of the skull, immobile and strong. The pins should be constructed of materials to reduce image degradation (e.g., carbon fiber) or be adjustable in order to place them out of the region of interest containing the intracranial target.

The instrument should provide full access to the head

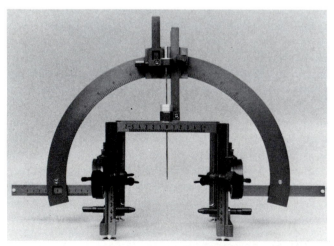

Fig 34–1.—Leksell model CT stereotaxic frame. The tip of the biopsy probe is at the X, Y, and Z = 0 point of the frame. Four pins are used to fix the coordinate frame to the skull. Plastic supports are used for the carbon fiber pins to reduce CT artifacts and are adjustable in location. The frame is centered on the head using ear bars placed in the external auditory canal.

TABLE 34–1.—CT STEREOTAXY:
SYSTEM REQUIREMENTS

STEREOTAXIC INSTRUMENT
  Rigid skull fixation
  Low atomic no. construction (image compatibility)
  Mechanical accuracy: ± 0.6 mm
  Rapid detachability
  Smooth mechanisms
  Completely sterilizable
COMPUTER HARDWARE
  High spatial resolution (0.75 mm)
  Variable collimation (slice thickness: 1.5–10 mm)
  Low image noise
  Low radiation dosage per slice (2–5 rad)
  Accurate remote controlled bed assembly (0.1 mm)
  Megabyte disc storage
  High-speed computer
  Laser localization
  Sagittal electronic radiographic localization
  High matrix display (360 × 360)
COMPUTER SOFTWARE
  Multiplanar reconstruction
  Target coordinate calculation
  Probe trajectory preview

*Voluntary guidelines for worst condition target accuracy mandated by the Standards for Testing Materials, Committee F4-5, Neurosurgical Instrumentation, Philadelphia, state that worst condition target accuracy should be less than or equal to 0.6 mm.

in order for the surgeon to manipulate the frame satisfactorily under sterile conditions and still to allow the supporting nursing and anesthesia staffs full access to the patient. The frame should be rapidly detachable. The instrument should be easily cleaned, smooth in mechanism, and readily sterilizable by conventional steam or gas autoclaving techniques.

Advanced generation CT scanners have the necessary requirements for CT stereotaxis. Increased spatial resolution brought about by increasing the quality and number of detectors has pushed spatial resolution to the virtual theoretical limit. Compatible frames do not degrade image resolution (Fig 34–2). Collimation can be reduced to 1.5 mm if necessary for accurate coordinate determination and detailed reconstructed images. Megabyte disc storage and a high-speed computer allow the necessary image manipulation to fully define the lesion or target. Laser localization and sagittal electronic radiographic techniques have fully oriented the surgeon to his standard domain, the extracranial topography and lateral skull x-rays with which he is most familiar.

Computer software techniques are of paramount importance during all of the procedures. Multiplanar reconstructions and reformatted images in the oblique planes have provided minute detail of the lesion, permitted subsequent verification of the target coordinate calculations, and allowed previews of trajectories prior to the actual passage of the instruments.

The team approach must be emphasized, with the surgeon working hand-in-hand with the radiologist to maximize image quality and clinical safety. Whether surgery is performed within the CT scanner, in the operating room, or shared between these two units becomes the personal option of the surgeon and the radiologist, the facilities available, and the time required.

Cost

The expense of commercially available CT stereotaxic devices remains high. Three competitive units available in the United States can be purchased for between $30,000 and $40,000. Most devices are freely adaptable to commercially available CT scanners. Comparable neurosurgical devices currently in widespread use, including lasers, ultrasonic aspirators, and counterbalanced operating microscopes, are all considerably more expensive than CT stereotaxic devices.

Use of the Leksell Stereotaxic System

Because of its utility and versatility in both morphological and functional neurosurgery, the usage of the Leksell model CT stereotaxic device will be described in detail. This frame is constructed of low atomic number, lightweight aluminum and can be used without modification for CT as well as standard stereotaxic procedures requiring ventriculography and angiography.[22] Additional modifications for CT usage were made:

1. Skull fixation pins (two frontal, two suboccipital) are adjustable in location to minimize the image artifacts (Fig 34–3). Four steel drills with accompanying drill sleeves are used to penetrate the scalp and anchor the frame to the external table of the skull. The steel sleeves and drills are replaced subsequently by four carbon fiber pins, which fit snugly into the small drill holes placed in the external table. Low atomic number carbon fiber is ideal for CT usage.

2. The "chucks" used to house the pins are constructed of low-artifact plastic.

3. Plastic earplugs are used for precise application of this frame, but are removed during the CT localization and surgical aspects of the procedure.

The operation of the Leksell system is simple: The

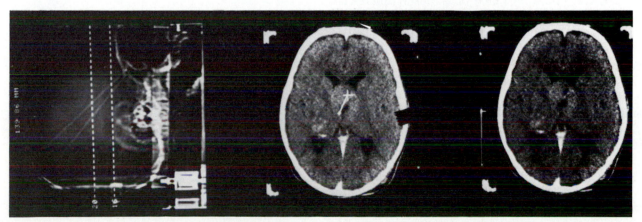

Fig 34–2.—Artifact-free CT images. These can be obtained using the electronic sagittal radiograph, and the computer software can be used to determine the coordinates of the target. The site for a biopsy of this deep midline lesion is indicated by the *large cross hair.*

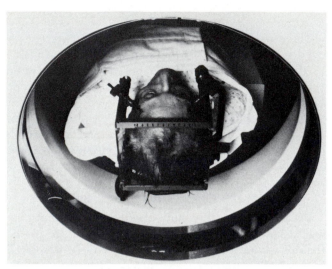

Fig 34–3.—The patient in position in the aperture of the CT scanner after placement of the stereotaxic frame.

chosen target is placed at the center of a semicircular arc, which is attached to the coordinate frame at the chosen target coordinates. The target selected is defined by three-dimensional rectilinear coordinates, where X is defined as the patient's anterior-posterior coordinate, Y as the patient's superior-inferior coordinate, and Z as the patient's left-right coordinate. This coordinate system was based on the standard stereotaxic viewing of a lateral skull x-ray where the patient's anterior-posterior coordinate was chosen as X (the abscissa) and the patient's superior-inferior coordinate was chosen as Y (the ordinate). It should be noted that CT terminology, which increasingly has been adopted for stereotaxic orientation, has chosen the coordinate system based on the axial or horizontal image, where the patient's left-right coordinate is X (the abscissa) and the patient's anterior-posterior coordinate is Y (the ordinate). This is a semantic problem, but users and readers should be aware of this difference in terminology. In the Leksell system, the target can be approached by any anatomically and functionally safe trajectory described by the semicircular arc in the probe holder.

The Leksell coordinate frame is applied under local anesthesia after prepping the entire head with antiseptic solution. It is generally easier to apply the frame with the patient sitting comfortably in a chair. Prior CT images are reviewed to assess the general region of interest. This allows the surgeon to place the skull fixation pins above or below the general region of interest to further reduce image artifacts. The frame is centered on the head using plastic ear bars, which are positioned without anesthesia in the external auditory canals. The ear bars are adjusted so that the Z = 0 coordinate of the frame roughly corresponds to the midline of the pa-

tient. The earplugs are rotated to lock them firmly in position, and the stereotaxic frame can then be angled up or down to select the needed and desired relationship to the orbitomeatal plane.

The four steel sleeves and pins are advanced under local anesthesia through the scalp until they rest against the outer table of the skull. A hand or battery-powered drill is used to insert the pins into the outer table of the skull. After all four steel pins are placed suitably, they are removed sequentially and replaced with carbon fiber pins. After proper tension has been assured and the frame has been checked for secure application to the head, the earplugs are removed. The frame is extremely lightweight and is supported easily by the patient, who is free to sit or ambulate with the frame attached. After transporting the patient to the CT table, the steel footplates of the coordinate frame are attached to the CT adaptor, which substitutes for the standard headrest available on the bed of the CT scanner (Fig 34–4). The frame remains attached to the adaptor by magnetic footplates, allowing rapid detachment if necessary.

Intravenous contrast can be administered during the application of the frame. The gantry is not tilted, because the horizontal CT images should be taken parallel to the Y = 0 plane. Collimation size is selected so that each slice thickness provides sufficient anatomical detail. The CT image reconstructed should be sufficiently large to include the patient's head and the stereotaxic frame (using the CT/T 8800 scanner, General Electric Corp., Milwaukee, infant mode should be selected).

During CT imaging, two plastic sideplates are attached to the CT coordinate frame (Fig 34–5). These

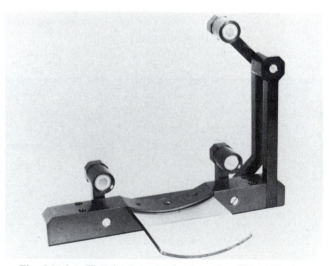

Fig 34–4.—The frame attached to the CT pallet by removing the usual headrest and replacing it with a stereotaxic frame adaptor. The stereotaxic frame fixes to the three footplates by magnetic adaptors. This allows rapid detachability, but firm fixation.

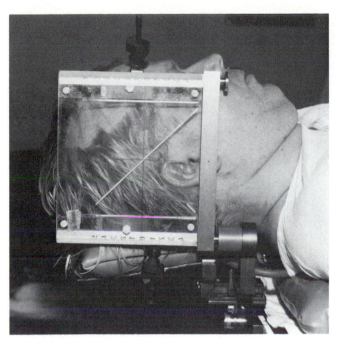

Fig 34–5.—Fixation of the frame, shown to the magnetic adaptor. A small inflatable pillow supports the occipital region during stereotaxic CT imaging. A localization plate is attached to the stereotaxic frame. The center of the diagonal aluminum 2-mm bar that runs from posterior/superior to anterior/inferior is at the Y = 0 and X = 0 (stereotaxic coordinates) point of the frame.

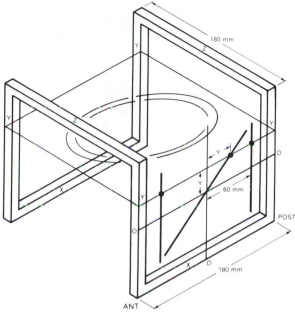

Fig 34–6.—A diagram depicting the stereotaxic coordinates. In the Leksell stereotaxic system, which was initially based on looking at a lateral skull x-ray, the abscissa represents the anterior-posterior coordinate of the patient *(X),* and ordinate represents the superior-inferior coordinate of the patient *(Y),* whereas the left-right coordinate of the patient is Z. CT scanner coordinates, based upon looking at the axial image where the abscissa is the left-right coordinate of the patient *(X)* and the ordinate is the anterior posterior coordinate *(Y),* should be noted. Axial images will show three small dots, which represent the intersection of the vertical and descending bars. The Y coordinate can be determined by measuring the distance from the most posterior dot on the scan to the middle dot and subtracting this value from 60 mm when the target is *superior* to the Y = 0 plane. This provides the Y^1 value, which is equal to the *actual* Y value. Similarly, when the target plane is inferior to the Y = 0 plane, 60 mm should be subtracted from the value to provide the actual Y coordinate millimeters *inferior* to the Y = 0 plane. The coordinate frame is a cube 180 mm in diameter. The distance between the two vertical aluminum bars on the side plates is 120 mm.

sideplates are used for coordinate determination, whether using the CT scanner computer software or a specially scaled grid for determining the coordinates of the target.[15] Each plastic coordinate indicator plate has two vertical 2-mm aluminum strips connected by a diagonal horizontal bar, which is attached to the frame so that the diagonal bar always descends from posterior frame to anterior frame (Fig 34–6). The distance between the two vertical bars is 120 mm. The middle of the diagonal bar, 60 mm from each vertical bar, represents the center of the stereotaxic frame (Y = 0, X = 0). All axial CT images will demonstrate three small radiopaque indicators on each side, which are used to determine the X, Y, and Z coordinates.

Software options on currently available CT scanners differ between manufacturers. However, simple distance measurements using a cursor are generally included. No additional computer software must be added to the system in order to determine the coordinates of the target located on the horizontal CT image. It is important to remember that CT body scanners have images reversed so that the patient's left is right on the CT image. General principles of computer coordinate determination using the Leksell CT system involve identification of the center or origin of the stereotaxic frame from the CT image. Figure 34–6 shows a

schematic representation of the coordinate determination. It should be noted that the patient's superior-inferior coordinate (Y) can be determined by simply measuring with the cursor the distance between the posterior indicator and the middle indicator. When the target lies in a plane *superior* to the Y = 0 plane, the value can be subtracted from 60 mm (Y^1), giving the *actual* Y coordinate, because $Y^1 = Y$ (Fig 34–7). Similarly, when the target is noted in a Y plane *inferior* to the Y = 0 plane, the distance between the posterior indicator and the middle indicator will be greater than 60 mm. Subtracting 60 from this value will give the actual Y coordinate inferior to the Y = 0 plane.

Because the superior-inferior coordinate values will

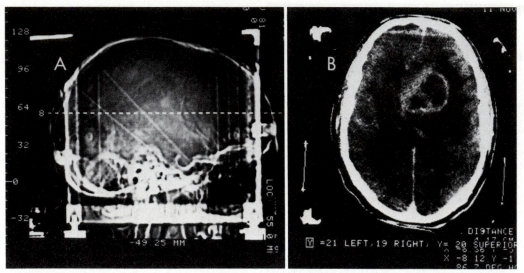

Fig 34–7.—A, sagittal computed radiograph showing the target plane and the fact that the axial images are parallel to the base. The gantry is not tilted during CT imaging. **B,** determination of the Y coordinate in a 55-year-old patient prior to a biopsy of a deep left frontal mass. Using the software installed in GE 8800 CT/T scanner (General Electric Corp., Milwaukee), a cursor measures the distance from the posterior dot to the middle dot, and the value subtracted from 60 to note that the Y coordinate on the left was 21. A similar measurement is made on the Y coordinate on the right. Often, a 2- to 3-mm difference is noted because of some angulation of the frame when it is placed on the head. For midline targets, the average of the two values may be determined. For most tumor work, this is insignificant. For tumor localizations, 5-mm slice thickness images are taken.

vary slightly between the two sides selected because of frame angulation, an average of the two values can be used for targets near the midline. Variability between the two Y coordinates is rarely of practical significance using collimation 5 mm or less.

The X coordinate (anterior-posterior) and the Z coordinate (left-right) can be determined in the following way. The center of the stereotaxic frame on the horizontal CT image containing the target is determined by defining the center of the rectangle formed by the four radiopaque indicators created by the vertical aluminum bars on the side plates (Fig 34–8). The center of the frame is identified and stored, and the cursor is then moved to the desired target seen on the image, and the coordinate of the target is defined in reference to the center of the frame. Using the General Electric 8800 scanner, two values for X (Z in the Leksell system) are given by the scanner. If the signs of these two values are the same (either both positive or negative), the values are *subtracted* from each other to give the actual *stereotaxic* Z coordinate. If the signs of these two values are different, the values are *added* numerically, disregarding the signs themselves. The *stereotaxic* X coordinate (Y in CT) is similarly defined by appropriately adding the two values when they are of different signs or subtracting the two values (regardless of their signs) when they are either both positive or both negative.

The Leksell stereotaxic frame is equipped with a target coordinate indicator grid scaled for each user's own CT scanner and resultant image size. This grid can be used to read off the coordinates directly, allowing the targets to be determined from only one CT image containing the target and without requiring any usage of the computer software. Both techniques can be used to verify the accuracy of target determination.

After CT imaging has been completed and the coordinates determined and checked, the surgical procedure can begin. The procedure can be performed in the scanner, or alternatively the patient can be transported to the operating room. The plastic sideplates are removed and kept in the CT scanner suite. The magnetic adaptor for the stereotaxic frame can be used on the operating room table itself. The stereotaxic frame and the patient's head are prepped with antiseptic solution, with care taken to prep the entire frame (including the pins). In the operating room, the surgeon sits or stands at the head of the operating room table, whereas in the scanner the surgeon sits at the back of the CT aperture.

After suitable prepping and draping, the semicircular arc is attached to the side bars, which have been set at the determined X and Y coordinates. The Z coordinate is set on the spherical arc. The site of the burr hole is selected. Because the target is the center of the spherical arc, any functionally safe trajectory can be selected. However, in the lateral approach to lesions in the temporal lobe, it is important to place the burr hole virtually in the center of the spherical rings that attach the arc to the side bars of the frame. Because of the location

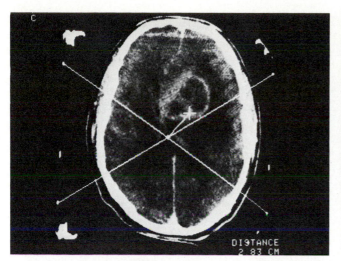

Fig 34–8.—The target point for biopsy of this enhancing lesion, shown by the *cross hairs*. The actual coordinates can be determined by first defining the center of the stereotaxic frame. This is done by drawing diagonal lines from the dots shown. The intersection of these lines represents the center of the stereotaxic frame, from which coordinates are chosen for the target. By storing the center of the stereotaxic frame and placing the cursor on the final target for the biopsy site, and measuring the distance between these two, the software of the GE 8800 scanner provides four values. When the two X values have the same sign (Z coordinate in stereotaxis), the values are *subtracted* regardless of their signs. Thus, the actual stereotactic Z coordinate represents the difference between 3.08 and 1.16, which is 1.92 cm, or 19 mm to the patient's *left*. Similarly, the X coordinate in stereotaxis (CT Y coordinate) is determined by *adding* two values when they are of different signs, regardless of their signs. In this case, the actual stereotaxic X coordinate represents 1.8 cm + 0.2 cm = 20 mm *anterior* to the center of the stereotaxic frame.

of certain targets and the relationship of the pins, the coordinate frame, and the semicircular arc, it may be necessary to reverse the semicircular arc on the side bars. The appropriate Z values must be switched accordingly so that the correct side is selected. This allows a full range of trajectories to reach targets from supraorbital and low frontal to coronal, vertex, parietal, occipital, suboccipital, temporal, and even transsphenoidal approaches. The radius of the Leksell spherical arc is 190 mm. When the probe stop is set at 0, the probe tip will be at the target. The probe stop on the spherical arc can be set between 50 mm above the target and 20 mm below the target and serial biopsies, for example, taken in the line of that trajectory (Fig 34–9).

Intraoperative Imaging

The desire to reimage the patient with CT during the stereotaxic procedure[23] stemmed from the need to (1) confirm target accuracy by visualizing the probe tip at the target site; (2) assess the results of therapeutic in-

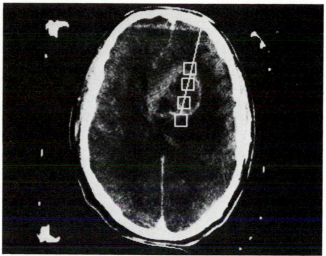

Fig 34–9.—Preplotting the path of the biopsy probe by CT software. The biopsies at each site (indicated by *squares*) can be correlated with the histologic findings.

tervention, such as biopsy or aspiration; and (3) immediately assess the possibility of operative complications, such as postoperative hemorrhage.

Because the spherical arc of the Leksell system produces intolerable image artifacts, a probe holder was constructed that allows removal of the spherical arc for intraoperative CT (Fig 34–10). This device anchors the stereotaxic probe in position, allowing the spherical arc to be totally removed as well as the side bars. Artifact-free CT images can then be taken during the procedures.

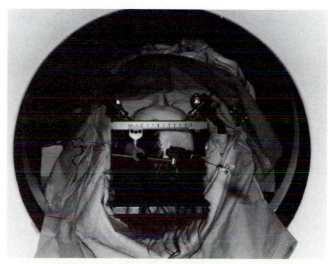

Fig 34–10.—A probe holder (AB Elekta Instruments, Stockholm), which has been designed to hold a stereotaxic probe in position at the target site, allowing the spherical arc to be removed. This permits intraoperative CT imaging to verify target accuracy and therapeutic results with minimal image artifacts (54-year-old patient with a colloid cyst of the third ventricle undergoing evacuation).

MORPHOLOGICAL SURGERY OF THE BRAIN

Both diagnostic exploration of various brain lesions and individual therapy can be provided by stereotaxic technique. Such procedures can be described as explorative (biopsy procedures), decompressive (puncture or aspiration techniques), or therapeutic (injection or implantation of specific therapeutic agents), as shown in Table 34–2.

Explorative Stereotaxic Surgery

The need to accurately biopsy brain lesions recognized by CT has stimulated renewed interest in stereotaxic surgery more than any other single feature. Tumor biopsy has been proved to be an accurate, precise, and safe method to obtain correct histologic diagnoses and to appropriately direct subsequent therapy.[24–26] Introduction of CT guidance in stereotaxic technique has increased not only the volume of cases, but also reduced patient morbidity and mortality. Centers that have long relied upon stereotaxic biopsy technique for tumor diagnosis have demonstrated that mortality should be less than 1% and significant morbidity less than 3%.[27, 28]

Biopsy Technique

Patients are referred after prior CT evaluations have disclosed the brain abnormality. The need for cerebral angiography is based on the location and the size of the tumor. At the present time, we still regard angiography as a valuable adjunct in the evaluation of deep midline, intraventricular, pineal region, or parasellar masses. We have found little correlation between the "vascular-

TABLE 34–2.—CT STEREOTAXY: MORPHOLOGICAL SURGERY OF THE BRAIN

PROCEDURE TYPE	CONDITIONS
Explorative (Biopsy)	Primary glial neoplasms
	Metastasis
	Pituitary adenoma
	Degenerative diseases
	Leukemia infiltrate
	Sarcoidosis
	Lymphoma
	Pineal region tumors
	Acoustic neurinomas
	Herpes simplex encephalitis
Decompressive (Puncture, aspiration)	Brain abscess
	Arachnoid cysts
	Colloid cysts
	Intracerebral hematoma
Therapeutic (Injection, implantation)	Intracystic irradiation
	Interstitial irradiation
	Tumor chemotherapy or immunotherapy

ity" demonstrated by either contrast-enhanced CT scans or angiography and the occurrence of a hemorrhagic complication after tumor biopsy.

The patient is brought to the CT scanner, and the Leksell frame is applied to the head after prepping the entire scalp with alcohol. Serial axial CT images are taken to determine the target slice and to obtain the necessary coordinates. Contrast enhancement is performed in all cases. Patients with iodine allergies are treated in advance with intravenous corticosteroids and antihistamines. Five-millimeter slice thickness images are taken to localize the target area and preplot the probe trajectory and biopsy sites (Fig 34–11,A). Both sagittal and coronal reconstructions are then performed to further define the lesion and preplot the pathway of a phantom probe (see Fig 34–11,B). Multiplanar reconstructions have been very helpful not only to define the lesion fully, but also to select a probe trajectory that appears the safest. Serial biopsies of various regions of the tumor can be correlated histologically with the site of the biopsy demonstrated by CT scan (Fig 34–12).[29, 30] These reconstructed CT images can then also be compared with the scout image to demonstrate the location of a preselected burr hole and probe pathway (Fig 34–13). After transporting the patient to the operating room, the scalp and frame are prepped, draped, and the side bars are attached at the chosen coordinates. Serial biopsies are taken in the trajectory of the probe shown by the CT scans. Multiple biopsy instruments have been created for stereotaxic devices and include suction or aspiration devices[31] and microforceps.[27] We prefer to use a "corkscrew" spiral instrument developed by Backlund.[32] Using this technique, a corkscrew spiral (inner cannula) is advanced 1 cm beneath the tip of the probe (outer cannula, 2.1-mm outer diameter). The outer probe is then advanced over the spiral to amputate tissue within the spiral. Both the spiral and the outer cannula are removed, and a small 10 mm × 0.2 mm core of the lesion is unscrewed between the thumb and forefinger of the surgeon. These specimens are placed immediately in formalin. Frozen sections are not performed, having proved frustrating to both the surgeon and the pathologist. Aspiration specimens also are taken, smeared directly on slides, and immersed in ethyl alcohol prior to histologic staining. On the day after surgery, the surgeon reviews the case and x-rays with the neuropathologist. This has resulted in a strong working relationship with the neuropathologic team and allowed a highly positive diagnostic biopsy rate.

Results

The spectrum of diseases treated by CT explorative techniques can be seen in Table 34–2. Primary glial

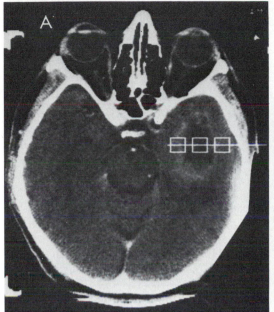

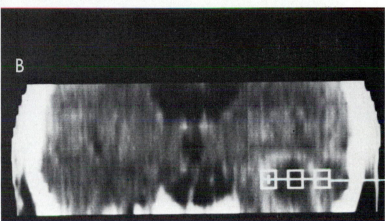

Fig 34–11.—A, stereotaxic CT of a left dominant hemisphere temporal lobe lesion, demonstrating the lateral approach using the Leksell stereotaxic instrument and the sites of the three biopsy specimens (indicated by *squares*). **B,** biopsy sites *(squares)* also can be visualized in the coronal plane following reconstruction.

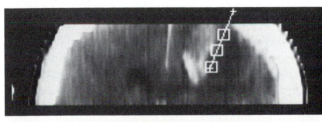

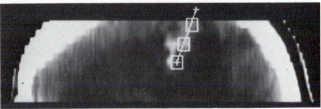

Fig 34–12.—Coronal *(top)* and sagittal *(bottom)* reconstructions, both of which are useful in preplotting the path of the biopsy probe (patient with a left parietal calcified mass, which on biopsy proved to be a mixed glioma). At the site of the second biopsy, cystic fluid was encountered, and 5 cc of tumor cyst were evacuated. CT imaging had suggested that this was edema rather than true cyst formation. (*squares* = biopsy sites.)

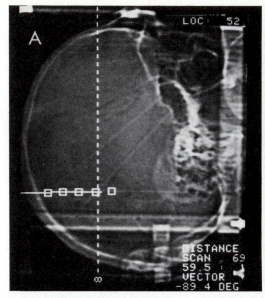 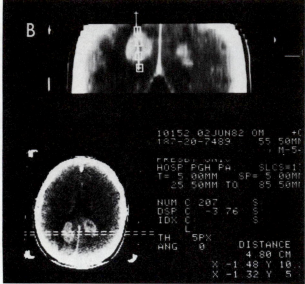

Fig 34–13.—A, the site of a biopsy *(square)*, projected on the lateral electronic radiograph prior to biopsy in a 61-year-old patient with a butterfly glioblastoma of the splenium of the corpus callosum. **B,** coronal scan displaying the sites of biopsy *(squares).*

neoplasms, including glioblastomas and astrocytomas, were the most frequently encountered tumors (19 of 50) in a series of 50 patients who underwent CT stereotaxic surgery between February 1981 and July 1982 at Presbyterian-University Hospital in Pittsburgh. Firm histologic diagnosis was made in 92% of the overall series. Two additional patients (4%) were believed to have a "probable glial neoplasm" on histologic grounds. Definite histologic diagnosis was not possible in two cases. Appropriate postoperative therapy based on biopsy results was directed in 31 of 34 positive biopsy cases. Revisions in therapy were required after biopsy in three cases (unsuspected brain abscess, cerebral infarct, and leukemic infiltrate of brain respectively). Stereotaxic intervention resulted in immediately improved neurologic condition in five cases. Preoperative diagnostic and therapeutic dilemmas were resolved by biopsy alone in 14 cases (39%).

This technique has been useful in the demonstration of typical findings in Alzheimer's disease, the recognition of intracranial lymphoma or leukemia and sarcoidosis, and especially valuable and accurate in the rapid diagnosis of herpes simplex encephalitis. As herpes encephalitis is a highly treatable and frequently fatal intracranial disease, frozen sections have been performed on these cases. Four patients with suspected herpes encephalitis underwent stereotaxic biopsy. All four patients had positive frozen sections showing typical signs of encephalitis, and all four rapidly grew out herpes simplex virus within 48 hours after the biopsy procedure.

Pineal region tumors can be diagnosed successfully by this technique, allowing postoperative irradiation to be given in cases of pineal region germinoma[33, 34] or providing further impetus for direct intracranial attack on those lesions that may be extirpated by open surgical techniques.

Complications

Intracranial hemorrhage after stereotaxic biopsy occurs with surprising rarity. The high morbidity associated with freehand biopsy techniques can be traced to several features:

1. Poor localization of the lesion prior to CT scanning.

2. Multiple attempts to reach the target, fostered by multiple probe passages using different trajectories.

3. Attempts to secure large pieces of tumor tissue in order to "increase" the positive biopsy rate, fostered by the frustrating experience of frozen sections and the mistaken belief that large specimens of tissue are required to reach a diagnosis.

These complications can be avoided by stereotaxic technique, which provides precise target identification, allows multiple biopsies in a single trajectory, and has rigid probe and skull fixation. In 50 consecutive cases undergoing stereotaxic biopsy at this institution between February 1, 1981, and July 1982, no patient suffered an operative mortality. Three patients had transient worsening of neurologic signs, including hemiparesis or aphasia. These signs resolved in all three cases over several days after temporarily increasing the dosage of corticosteroids. No patient sustained a clinically significant intracerebral hematoma. This complication has been reduced by eliminating multiple probe passages to the target. Percutaneous techniques through high-risk areas such as the lateral temporal lobe and Sylvian fissure may also increase morbidity.[35] Percutaneous techniques not requiring open burr hole and exposure of the cortex have been reserved in the present series for those patients with either frontal or occipital polar lesions, where the likelihood of encountering major arterial feeders is reduced. In all other cases, an appropriately located burr hole is placed in order to visualize the cortex and to allow coagulation of the arachnoidal vessels prior to passage of the biopsy probe. After the last biopsy specimen is obtained, the probe is left at the deepest site with the stylet removed to observe for any bleeding. The probe is left in position until all bleeding ceases, which suggests that any hemorrhage has coagulated at the tip of the probe. Applying coagulating current to the biopsy probe itself is not advocated, because uncontrolled current spread is dangerous and may provoke unwanted rupture of nearby small tumor vessels. Intraoperative CT has allowed rapid identification of postoperative hematoma formation. Postoperative CT scans often have shown small hematomas at the biopsy site. In addition, a tiny air defect introduced by the probe can be used to confirm accurate location of the biopsy target site.[23]

DECOMPRESSIVE STEREOTAXIC INTERVENTION

Puncture or aspiration of various brain cysts and abscesses has been possible using stereotaxic technique (Fig 34–14).[36–39] Aspirations of such lesions have identified the responsible organism, immediately reduced mass effect, allowed catheter drain placement, and appropriately directed antibiotic therapy. Multiple abscesses can be aspirated at the same operation. Stereotaxic aspiration for diagnosis and bacteriologic culture is preferable to empirical therapy with antibiotics alone.[36]

Benign Brain Cysts

Arachnoid cysts have been successfully aspirated, and intracystic pressure has been measured as a guide to the need for extirpation or shunting.[23] Colloid cysts of the third ventricle are especially amenable to stereotaxic intervention, because simple cyst aspiration alone may be curative.[40] Figure 34–15 demonstrates the technique for CT stereotaxic aspiration of a colloid cyst at the foramen of Monro. This cyst had produced intermittent ventricular obstruction and hydrocephalus. With the patient in the CT scanner and the probe placed at the target site, a 1.8-mm outer diameter probe is advanced in and out of the cyst (Fig 34–16). Suction is applied with a 5-cc syringe. Intraoperative imaging can be used to demonstrate the probe tip at the center of the colloid cyst. After aspiration of the colloid material, reduction in the cyst wall and replacement of the cyst contents with air can be seen (Fig 34–17). After introduction of contrast into the ventricle, ventriculography can be performed to demonstrate a now patent ventricular system and to visualize resolution of the ventricular obstruction.[23]

Intracerebral Hematoma

Rapid recognition of deep post-traumatic or hypertensive hematomas has been promoted by CT. The pos-

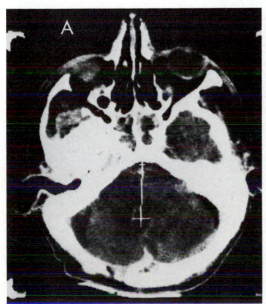
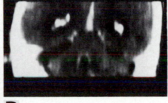
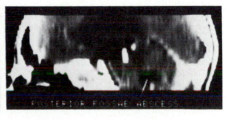

Fig 34–14.—A, target for aspiration in a 47-year-old patient with a cerebellar infarction followed by development of a postsurgical cerebellar abscess. **B,** coronal *(left)* and sagittal *(right)* reconstructions performed at the time of CT stereotaxic localization, disclosing the lesion and its proximity to the roof of the fourth ventricle.

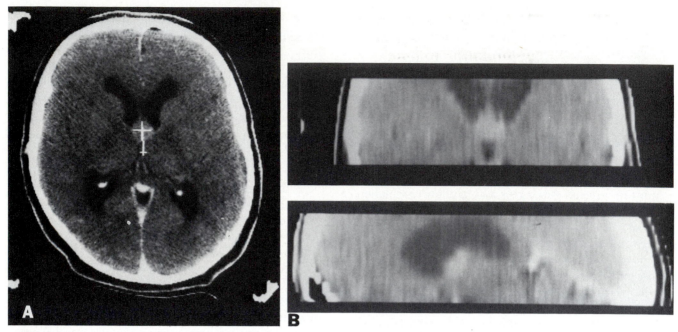

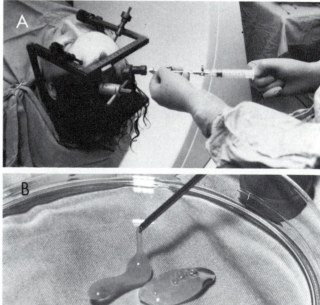

Fig 34–15.—A, stereotaxic CT localization of a midline third ventricular mass prior to stereotaxic aspiration. **B,** reconstructed coronal *(top)* and sagittal *(bottom)* views disclose the location of the radiodense lesion at the foramen of Monro associated with clinical evidence of intermittent ventricular obstruction.

Fig 34–16.—A, demonstration of intraoperative percutaneous stereotaxic aspiration of the colloid cyst of the third ventricle performed in the CT scanner. **B,** 2 cc of viscous colloid material were removed.

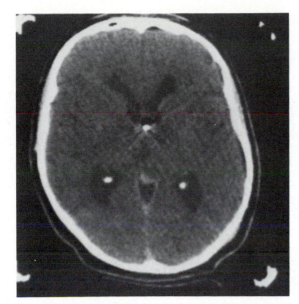 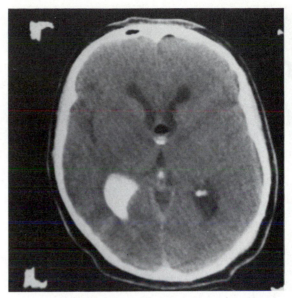

Fig 34–17.—Immediately after aspiration of the colloid cyst of the third ventricle. The patient is reimaged with the probe tip in the cyst *(left)*, demonstrating a small bubble of air in the remaining cyst. Partial withdrawal of the probe followed by instillation of metrizamide (170 mg I/ml) *(right)* demonstrates metrizamide within the right lateral ventricle and partial entry of metrizamide into the colloid cyst remnants. Subsequent images demonstrated free flow of metrizamide into the contralateral ventricle.

sibility of partial or incomplete removal of such lesions has been afforded by stereotaxic technique.[41, 42] Early stereotaxic aspiration of such hematomas may allow reduction in patient mortality and morbidity by simply reducing the volume of intracerebral blood and intracranial pressure.[43] Whether such surgery will improve the quality of survival remains unknown. The removal of putaminal, thalamic, cerebellar, and pontine hemorrhages has been contemplated by CT stereotaxic technique.

THERAPEUTIC STEREOTAXIC TECHNIQUE

In addition to biopsy diagnosis and aspiration, CT stereotaxis can be used for a variety of interventional procedures, which include implantation of radioactive agents and intratumoral chemotherapy.[44]

Intracystic Irradiation

Backlund[32, 45–47] has pioneered the use of intracystic irradiation in the treatment of craniopharyngioma. Over the last 15 years, more than 100 cases of craniopharyngioma have been treated by a program of stereotaxic irradiation. The majority of tumors were solitary cystic or occasionally multicystic lesions, which were treated by the stereotaxic implantation of a beta-emitting isotope (yttrium 90 colloid) into the cyst. The use of CT has promoted early recognition of these tumors and allowed accurate volume determinations of the cyst size to be performed prior to surgery.[48] Using stereotaxic

techniques, the craniopharyngioma cyst is punctured, after which 1 ml of fluid is removed for examination and confirmation of the nature of the cyst. One ml of technetium 99 colloid then is injected and repeatedly aspirated. A 1-ml sample of cyst-isotope fluid is aspirated and a scintillation count performed. Using a tube dilution technique, the volume of the cyst can be calculated and compared with that determined by CT technique. The isotope injected is designed to provide an optimal dose of 20,000 rads of irradiation to the cyst wall. The cyst is aspirated approximately 2 weeks later in order for decompression. Yttrium 90 has a half-life of 2.3 days, and essentially the full dose of irradiation has been delivered at 2 weeks. Yttrium 90 colloid is not available in the United States. Neither the FDA nor the manufacturer of yttrium 90 (Amersham-Searle) wish to investigate its usage in the United States because of the expense involved. Phosphorus 32 colloid has been used in the United States instead. Yttrium 90 colloid has some theoretical advantages, including a half-value tissue penetration of 1.1 mm compared with 0.6 mm for phosphorus 32 and a much shorter half-life.[48] Intracystic irradiation is designed to eliminate cyst secretion. Gradual involution of the cyst is shown by serial CT examinations (Fig 34–18). The greatly reduced mortality and morbidity of this procedure have contrasted with the results after frontal craniotomy and radical or subtotal tumor excision. Stereotaxic technique is associated with a reduced incidence of postoperative visual loss, endocrine dysfunction, or development of diabetes

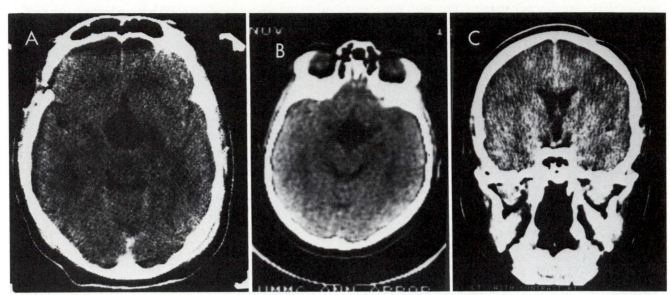

Fig 34–18.—A, stereotaxic CT in a 25-year-old patient with a craniopharyngioma prior to stereotaxic treatment by injection of yttrium 90 colloid into the cyst for cyst wall irradiation. **B,** follow-up CT image performed 3 months after delivering 20,000 rad to the cyst wall (beta irradiation, yttri- um 90). The tumor cyst is smaller. **C,** coronal CT image performed 1 year after treatment disclosing complete reso- lution of the cyst, with herniation of the cyst remnants into the region of the sella turcica.

insipidus.[49] These results warrant the more widespread usage of this technique in the treatment of craniopharyngioma and in the exploration of newer roles for intracystic stereotaxic irradiation.

Interstitial Irradiation

Stereotaxic technique has been used in multiple centers throughout the world for the biopsy of various malignant brain tumors and the subsequent implantation of radioactive isotopes for interstitial irradiation (brachytherapy).[50–52] Isotopes that have been used include gold 198, iridium 192, and iodine 125. Radium has proved difficult to work with, because it is toxic to the person performing the implantation. Iodine 125 seeds have been shown to possess attractive features that have allowed the development of both afterloading techniques using "high-dose" or "low-dose" iodine 125 seeds (less than 1 mCi).[53] The use of CT stereotaxis has been shown to be a necessary adjunct for accurate isotope implantation.[54]

Volume implantation of intracranial tumors using low-dose iodine 125 seeds is under evaluation at the University of Pittsburgh. Based upon concepts similar to that used with the treatment of prostate carcinoma, patients with malignant glial or metastatic neoplasms have been selected for therapy after being declared a failure of conventional treatment techniques that include surgery, external beam radiation therapy, and/or chemotherapy provided under protocol by the brain tumor study group program. Such patients undergo ste-reotaxic CT scanning with the Leksell frame attached, after which the center of the tumor is determined. Multiplanar reconstruction has permitted a volume determination of the lesion. The sites of implantation of the iodine 125 seeds are selected to provide a volume coverage of the entire tumor, and isodose curves are constructed. After transporting the patient to the operating room, a craniotomy is performed. The stereotaxic probe is placed into the lowest and deepest part of the center of the tumor, and a template constructed for the estimated volume of the tumor is placed in a geometric configuration around the central probe. Iodine 125 seeds are extruded to provide a volume irradiation of the tumor.

The results demonstrated by Mundinger and colleagues,[50] Ostertag and coworkers,[27] and Hosobuchi and associates[52] have been promising enough to warrant continued development of interstitial irradiation as a treatment for malignant brain tumors. Volume implantation techniques using low-dose irradiation seeds, thereby reducing hazards to the patient, operating surgeon, and radiation therapist, remain unproved at present, but are an exciting frontier in the field of tumor therapy as well as CT stereotaxic technique.

FUNCTIONAL SURGERY OF THE BRAIN

Surgical treatment of symptoms caused by neurologic disease and treated at a site remote from the origin or source of the disease constitutes the field of functional neurosurgery. Marino has stated, "The aim and objective of functional neurosurgery are to treat, correct, or balance the functions of the brain that are altered toward either hyperfunctional or hypofunctional states."[55] Intracranial functional neurosurgery has long relied upon presumed stable anatomical landmarks such as the posterior-anterior commissural (intercommissural) line to define the sites or targets for surgical intervention. These targets have been carefully defined in various neurosurgical atlases of the brain and were derived from the study of pooled anatomical specimens.[56] The target sites themselves, not visualizable by conventional radiographic techniques, have been defined in relationship to the intercommissural line. At the time of actual surgery, the target area has been precisely defined by electrophysiologic recording or stimulating to confirm or adjust the target site. Radiographic anatomical detail has been insufficient to successfully delineate the target. The integration of CT and functional neurosurgery has become one of the remaining frontiers for radiographic-neurosurgical interaction.[57] High-resolution images on advanced generation scanners have provided graphic anatomical detail of the brain, enabling the recognition of normal ventricular landmarks as well as depiction of the important white matter tracks (e.g., the internal capsule). At last, CT has provided sufficient radiographic detail to recognize the target, although physiologic monitoring has remained necessary to understand and treat the disordered physiology studied by functional neurosurgery.

The ability to obtain artifact-free CT scans with a stereotaxic frame attached, coupled with advanced CT software programming, has improved resolution sufficiently to define the known anatomical landmarks of the brain. Serial 1.5-mm high-resolution scans (600 mAs) can be used for sagittal reconstruction of the midline third ventricle. Oblique reformatted images (Arrange,® General Electric Corp., Milwaukee) have permitted definition of the intercommissural plane from midline sagittal reconstructions of the third ventricle and identification of the anterior and posterior commissures. From this reconstructed image, the target coordinates of, for example, a ventral lateral nucleus thalamotomy for dyskinesia can be derived (Fig 34–19). Alternatively, the actual axial images containing the posterior commissure and the anterior commissure can be used to reconstruct the oblique plane containing, for example, both anterior and posterior commissures (Fig 34–20). The reconstructed image can be performed at different angles to define a target plane containing the pineal and anterior commissure (Fig 34–21). When stereotaxis is performed within the CT scanner itself, the probe may initially be placed into the third ventricle and metrizamide injected (1 ml, 170 mg I/ml). A sagittal computed radiograph (Scoutview,® General Electric Corp., Milwaukee) can be used to define the anterior and posterior commissures, after which the appropriate axial CT images can be performed superior or inferior to the intercommissural plane.[22]

One major advantage of intracranial stereotaxis based on CT lies in the identification of the internal capsule. Stereotaxic targets can be selected to avoid this critical pathway, which represents the lateral border of the thalamus. Ventriculography techniques used conventionally have relied upon the width of the third ventricle as a guide to the lateral location of the target site within the brain. The use of CT has demonstrated no clear relationship between the width of the third ventricle and the thalamic width. Kelly and coworkers[17] at the State University of New York at Buffalo have pioneered the software digitization of the Schaltenbrand and Bailey stereotaxic atlas within the CT scanner. The

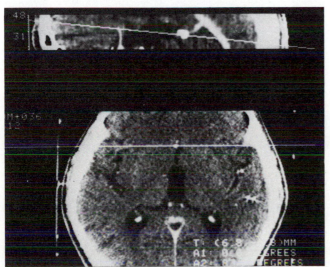

Fig 34–19.—During CT imaging of a patient with Parkinson's disease. The 1.5-mm axial CT images are "stacked" on top of one another, after which a midline sagittal reconstruction is performed to identify the anterior and posterior commissures. An oblique reformatted image can be generated by the CT scanner (Arrange® software program, General Electric Corp., Milwaukee). Excellent detail of the brain anatomy can be obtained.

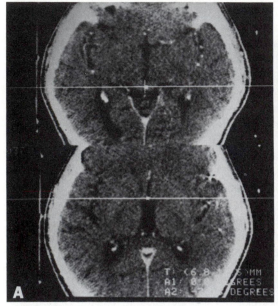
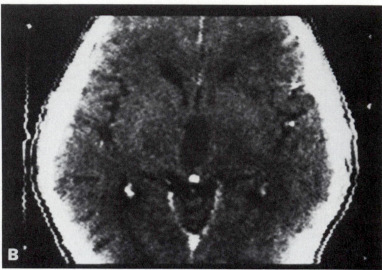

Fig 34–20.—A, both the posterior commissure *(upper)* and the anterior commissure *(lower)* can be identified in axial CT images in a patient undergoing CT stereotaxic thalamotomy. **B,** the oblique reformatted image reconstructed between these two points to define the intercommissural plane, from which all necessary coordinates can be chosen to determine the target point for stereotaxic thalamotomy (ventrolateral thalamic nucleus). The third ventricle is wide and has been found to have little clear relationship to the thalamic width distance from the wall of the third ventricle to the internal capsule.

Fig 34–21.—Reformatted image of a plane drawn from the anterior commissure to the pineal region.

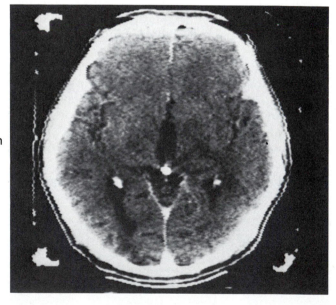

TABLE 34–3.—CT STEREOTAXY: FUNCTIONAL SURGERY OF THE BRAIN

PROCEDURE TYPE	CORRELATION	TARGET SITE
Neuroablative (Lesion)	Dyskinesias Parkinson's tremor, rigidity Cerebellar outflow, tremor Dystonia	Ventrolateral thalamus
	Psychiatric Anxiety, obsessive-compulsive or depressive neuroses	Anterior internal capsule Cingulum
Neurostimulative (Electrode implantation)	Pain	Periaqueductal gray Medial thalamus Thalamic sensory nuclei Postlimb internal capsule
	Dyskinesias	Dentate nuclei, pulvinar
Neurorecording (Depth electrodes)	Epilepsy	Temporal, frontal, occipital, parietal lobes

digitized atlas can be scaled for each patient's CT images, allowing a specific labeling of the various brain nuclei and tracts.

The usage of CT stereotaxic and functional surgery of the brain can be subdivided into neuroablative, neurostimulative, and neurorecording techniques (Table 34–3).

Neuroablative Techniques

The introduction of dopaminergic agents in the treatment of Parkinson's disease resulted in an immediate and profound reduction in the number of patients referred for stereotaxic surgery. Recent evidence has rekindled interest in stereotaxic treatment for dyskinesias, based on the recognition that dopaminergic precursors often fail to significantly improve tremor or rigidity, and long-term dopa treatment may result in excessive dyskinesias.[58] Stereotaxic thalamotomy again may become a first-line treatment for unilateral Parkinson tremor and rigidity, cerebellar outflow tremor related to benign essential tremor or multiple sclerosis, and dystonia.[59, 60] The common target site for these disparate diseases is the ventrolateral nucleus of the thalamus.[61] This target site, as well as its relationship to the internal capsule, is demonstrated in Figure 34–22. Multiplanar reconstruction allows identification of the intercommissural line and depiction of the target in the sagittal and coronal plane (Fig 34–23). The effects of a right ventrolateral nucleus thalamotomy are demonstrated in Figure 34–24 (bipolar lesion, 6-mm exposed tips, interelectrode distance of 6 mm, 65° lesion for 30 seconds). The use of CT has shown that these lesions are not just simple pale areas of a coagulation, but instead hemorrhagic.

The use of CT has afforded the recognition of precise areas for intervention in patients with profound psychi-

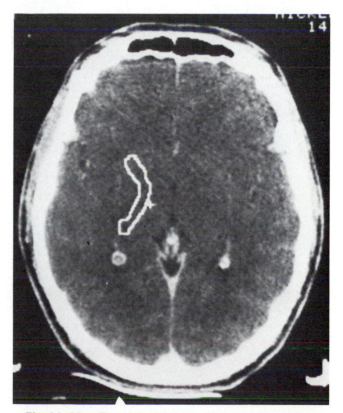

Fig 34–22.—Target localization of the ventrolateral nucleus of the thalamus and its relationship to the internal capsule, which has been highlighted for pictorial purposes using the software.

atric neurosis unresponsive to conventional psychiatric or medical intervention. Both the anterior limb of the internal capsule and the cingulum have been ablated in the treatment of severe depression and obsessive compulsive and anxiety neurosis.[62] Psychotic behavior is not treated at the present time by behavioral surgery.

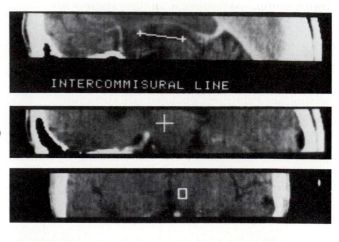

Fig 34–23.—Multiplanar reconstruction of the third ventricle, which provides good definition of the intercommissural line *(top)* and allows display of the thalamic target in sagittal *(middle)* and coronal *(bottom)* planes.

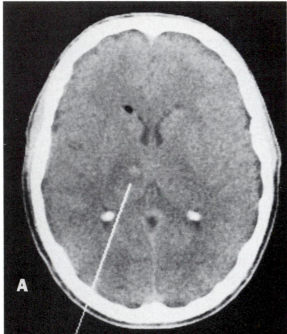
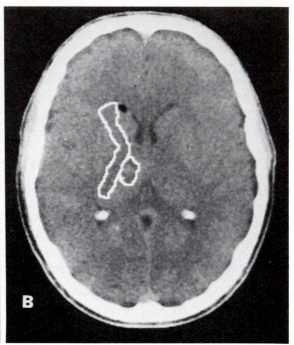

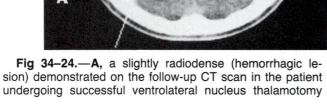

Fig 34–24.—A, a slightly radiodense (hemorrhagic lesion) demonstrated on the follow-up CT scan in the patient undergoing successful ventrolateral nucleus thalamotomy for parkinsonian tremor and rigidity. B, the size of the lesion and its relationship to the internal capsule have been highlighted.

Neurostimulative Procedures

Electrode implantation for the purpose of chronic deep brain stimulation has been used primarily in the treatment of both nociceptive (somatic) and deafferentation pain syndromes. Implantation of bipolar platinum electrodes into the medial thalamus and periaqueductal gray has been used in the treatment of patients with somatic pain, especially those having cancer involving upper extremity, head and neck, or midline structures.[63, 64] The target site is visualized well by CT alone, because the periventricular target area has been identified as 2 mm anterior to the posterior commissure and 2 mm lateral to the wall of the third ventricle.[65] The ability to define this target using CT alone has demonstrated that functional neurosurgery can be performed without the need for ventriculography. Follow-up CT scans have shown that the electrode has been placed successfully at the target site.

The thalamic sensory nuclei and posterior limb of the internal capsule have been used for electrode implantation in patients suffering such deafferentation pain syndromes as thalamic pain and anesthesia dolorosa.[66, 67] Although the site of implantation can be recognized by CT alone (e.g., the posterior limb of the internal capsule target is 15 mm lateral to the posterior commissure), confirmation of the appropriate target area still depends upon appropriate intraoperative stimulation findings as well as subsequent poststimulation pain relief. Surgery has been more successful in the treatment of somatic pain than deafferentation pain, which is notoriously difficult to treat by neurosurgical technique. Pain relief obtained with deep brain stimulation has been related to enhanced production of endogenous morphine-like substances (endorphins) as well as augmentation of descending serotonergic inhibitory pathways.[68, 69]

Implantation of electrodes for the treatment of dyskinesia has been reported.[59] Target sites for implantation have been identified in the dentate nuclei and the pulvinar nucleus of the thalamus. Thus far, the long-term results of deep brain stimulation for movement disorders have not proved so gratifying as to warrant widespread adoption of this technique in the treatment of dyskinesias.

Neurorecording

Long-term depth recording has been shown to be a valuable modality in the treatment and identification of epileptogenic foci within the brain. Using stereotaxic technique coupled with angiography, multiple electrodes have been inserted into various cortical and subcortical areas of the brain.[70] We have placed bilateral temporal lobe electrodes to study patients with temporal lobe epilepsy, prior to consideration of surgical resection, temporal lobectomy, or stereotaxic intervention for intractable seizure disorders (Fig 34–25). The target sites for electrode implantation can be identified by CT and the pathway of a phantom probe plotted on the CT images prior to actual stereotaxic implantation in the brain. Such depth recordings have allowed differentiation between primary and "mirror" epileptogenic foci.

CT STEREOTAXIS: THE FUTURE

Radiologic vs. Surgical Sites?

The mode of CT-guided stereotaxis has been performed entirely in the scanner or begun in the scanner prior to performing the actual surgery in the operating room. The time constraints imposed by busy radiologic imaging sites often have made it impractical to reserve large blocks of time for stereotaxic surgery. If surgery is performed in the CT scanning suite, the unit must be fully equipped with all necessary anesthesia and life support facilities. The traditional aseptic environment of the operating room must be maintained in the scanner suite. The additional time required for intermittent electrophysiologic monitoring and testing has reduced further the likelihood that extensive time can be devoted to CT stereotaxis in the diagnostic scanner. To circumvent these problems, a surgical CT unit dedicated to CT stereotaxis has been developed at the University of Pittsburgh.[22] In this new operating room concept, the CT scanner has been reversed in location so that the rear of the scanner opens onto the larger part of the room. The patient is placed supine on the scanner bed and advanced through the scanner aperture after attachment of the stereotaxic frame. In this way, the surgeon has free access to the head of the patient. At

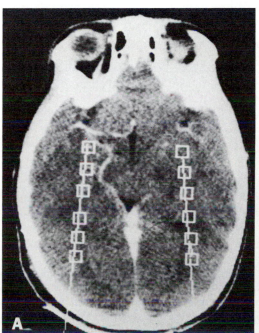

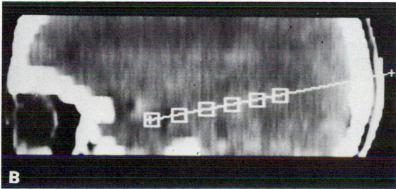

Fig 34–25.—A, stereotactic CT scan demonstrating the preplotted pathway of bilateral 6-pole deep brain recording electrodes and the position of each electrode pole *(squares)*. An 11-year-old child with intractable epilepsy of the Lennox-Gasteau variety was implanted with depth electrodes for recording purposes prior to consideration of temporal lobectomy. **B,** the pathway of the probe and the position of each electrode pole, which can be demonstrated on the sagittal reconstructed image.

any time during the procedure, CT images can be taken by retracting the patient into the scanner aperture. The potential development of other surgical procedures guided by images performed in body scanners is intriguing. Percutaneous cervical cordotomy represents one spinal procedure during which CT guidance may provide superior definition of the spinal cord. Xenon-enhanced CT for determining cerebral blood flow can be performed during surgical revascularization of the brain or during particulate embolization of arteriovenous malformations. Surgical treatment of extracranial carotid vascular disease (endarterectomy) and even the results of intracranial aneurysm surgery can be assessed by CT scanners dedicated solely to surgical procedures. It has become incumbent upon neurosurgeons to fully grasp and use the advanced radiologic imaging techniques currently available to diagnostic radiologists, lest neurosurgeons remain dependent upon outmoded, inadequate radiographic imaging techniques.

Certainly not all centers reasonably can be expected to finance the cost of surgical CT units. A diagnostic unit, with allowances for specific times for surgical study and intervention, will remain an option in many centers. Alternatively, Glenn[71] has proposed that mobile CT units housed in motorized vans might be sufficiently equipped to perform neurosurgical procedures. The violation of the brain for the purpose of a "simple" tumor biopsy must be respected always as a precise and potentially risky surgical procedure, which warrants all facilities of the standard neurosurgical operating rooms currently available.

New Applications?

The role of stereotaxic technique in brain surgery has been enhanced by the increasing acceptance of the technique, the elimination of "mysterious" methods for coordinate determination, and by the simplicity of systems readily understandable to both surgeons and radiologists. Development of new applications for guided brain surgery has forecast a bright future for CT stereotaxis.

Newer roles for stereotaxic technique include its use in reconstructive surgical techniques. Backlund and colleagues[72] have demonstrated the safety and feasibility of opening an occlusion of the aqueduct of Sylvius by stereotaxic implantation of a small shunt prosthesis from the caudal third ventricle to the rostral fourth ventricle. While CT identification of the target area seems to offer little advantage over contrast ventriculography performed in the standard fashion in such cases, both the resultant reduction in ventricular size and the position of the aqueductal prosthesis can be confirmed best by CT scanning.

Stereotaxis promises to be one of the necessary tools to study further the biochemistry of the brain and perhaps to allow new treatments in the field of neurochemical disorders. Animal experimentation has demonstrated the successful transplantation of neurosecretory cells from the adrenal gland to the brain.[73] At the Karolinska Institute, an experimental protocol has been approved for the transplantation of an adrenal tissue into the head of the caudate nucleus in an attempt to restore dopamine production in parkinsonian patients (Dr. E. O. Backlund, personal communication). While the results of such intervention are not predictable in advance, it is clear that stereotaxic surgery will be one of those tools that will permit new understanding of the biochemistry and physiology of the brain.

The use of CT stereotaxis has spawned the development of a variety of new instruments for tumor resection, biopsy, and treatment. Microdissection probes and hyper- or hypothermia induction devices have been combined with CT stereotaxic intervention.[74] The method of CT-guided stereotaxic tumor vaporization using the carbon dioxide laser has been performed by Kelly and Alker.[75] Stereotaxic tumor "resectoscopes" using laser technology have been developed by Shelden and coworkers[76] in Long Beach, Calif. Future stereotaxis will be enhanced by the exciting combination of advanced CT imaging and precise neurosurgical instrumentation. Radiologists and surgeons together must strive to develop new usages that will sustain the value of CT stereotaxic technique well into the future.

Acknowledgment

This work was supported in part by American Cancer Society Grant no. IN-58T. The author thanks Phyllis Shoemaker for preparation of this manuscript.

REFERENCES

1. Horsley V., Clark R.H.: The structure and functions of the cerebellum examined by a new method. *Brain* 31:45–124, 1908.
2. Kirschner M: Die Punktionstechnik und elektrokoagulation des ganglion gasseri: Uber "gezielte" operationionen. *Arch. Klin. Chir.* 176:581–620, 1933.
3. Spiegel E.A., Wycis H.J., Marks M., et al.: Stereotaxic apparatus for operations on the human brain. *Science* 106:346–350, 1947.
4. Leksell L.: *Stereotaxis and Radiosurgery: An Operative System.* Springfield, Ill., Charles C Thomas, Publisher, 1971, p. 69.
5. Riechert T.: *Stereotactic Brain Operations, Methods, Clinical Aspects, Indications.* Bern, Switzerland, Stuttgart, Germany, Vienna, Hans Huber, 1980, p. 387.
6. Talairach J., David M., Tournoux P.: *L'exploration Chirurgicale Stereotaxique du Lobe Temporal dans L'epilepsie Temporale.* Paris, Masson, 1958, p. 136.
7. Cooper I.S.: *Parkinsonism: Its Medical and Surgical*

Therapy. Springfield, Ill., Charles C Thomas, Publisher, 1961, p. 239.

8. Van Buren J.M., MacCubbin D.A.: An outline atlas of the human basal ganglia with estimation of anatomical variants. *J. Neurosurg.* 19:811–839, 1962.

9. Maroon J.C., Bank B.O., Drayer B.P., et al.: Intracranial biopsy assisted by computerized tomography. *J. Neurosurg.* 46:740–744, 1977.

10. Bergström M., Greitz T.: Stereotaxic computed tomography. *A.J.R.* 127:167–170, 1976.

11. Levinthal R., Winter J., Bentson J.R.: Technique for accurate localization with the CT scanner. *Bull. Los Angeles Neurol. Soc.* 41:6–8, 1976.

12. Piskun W.S., Stevens C.A., LaMorgese J.R., et al.: A simplified method of CT assisted localization and biopsy of intracranial lesions. *Surg. Neurol.* 11:413–417, 1979.

13. Hahn J.F., Levy W.J., Weinstein M.J.: Needle biopsy of intracranial lesions guided by computerized tomography. *Neurosurgery* 5:11–15, 1979.

14. Lunsford L.D., Maroon J.C.: CT localization and biopsy of intracranial lesions, in Schmidek H.H., Sweet W.H. (eds.): *Operative Neurosurgery.* New York, Grune & Stratton, 1982, pp. 403–418.

15. Leksell L., Jernberg B.: Stereotaxis and tomography: A technical note. *Acta Neurochir.* 52:1–7, 1980.

16. Birg W., Mundinger F.: Direct target point determination for stereotactic brain operations from CT data and evaluation of setting parameters for polar-coordinate stereotactic devices. *Appl. Neurophysiol.* 45:387–395, 1982.

17. Goerss S., Kelly P.J., Kall B., et al.: A computed tomographic stereotactic adaptation system. *Neurosurgery* 10:375–379, 1982.

18. Brown R.A.: A computerized tomography-computer graphics approach to stereotactic localization. *J. Neurosurg.* 50:715–720, 1979.

19. Perry J.E., Rosenbaum A.E., Lunsford L.D., et al.: CT guided stereotactic surgery: Conception and development of a new methodology. *Neurosurgery* 7:376–383, 1980.

20. Rhodes M.L., Wong S.H., Glenn W.V., et al.: Stereotactic neurosurgery using 3-D image data from computer tomography. *Proceedings of the 14th Hawaii International Conference on System Sciences,* 16:399–408, 1981.

21. Koslow M., Abele M.G., Griffith R.C., et al.: Stereotactic surgical system controlled by computerized tomography. *Neurosurgery* 8:72–82, 1981.

22. Lunsford L.D.: A dedicated CT system for the stereotactic operating room. *Appl. Neurophysiol.* 45:374–378, 1982.

23. Lunsford L.D., Rosenbaum A.E., Perry J.: Stereotactic surgery using the "therapeutic" CT scanner. *Surg. Neurol.* 18:116–122, 1982.

24. Boëthius J., Bergström M., Greitz J.: Stereotactic computerized tomography with a GE 8800 scanner. *J. Neurosurg.* 52:794–800, 1980.

25. Bosch D.A.: Indications for stereotactic biopsy in brain tumors. *Acta Neurochir.* 54:167–179, 1980.

26. Lobato R.D., Rivas J.J., Cabello A., et al.: Stereotactic biopsy of brain lesions visualized with computed tomography. *Appl. Neurophysiol.* 45:426–430, 1982.

27. Ostertag C.B., Mennel H.D., Kiessling M.: Stereotactic biopsy of brain tumors. *Surg. Neurol.* 14:275–283, 1980.

28. Edner G.: Stereotactic biopsy of intracranial space occupying lesions. *Acta Neurochir.* 57:213–234, 1981.

29. Boëthius J., Collins V.P., Edner G., et al.: Stereotactic biopsies and computerized tomography in gliomas. *Acta Neurochir.* 40:223–232, 1978.

30. Levander R., Bergström M., Boëthius J., et al.: Stereotactic computer tomography for biopsy of gliomas. *Acta Radiol. Diagn.* 19:867–888, 1978.

31. Shelden C.H., McCann G., Jacques S., et al.: Development of a computerized microstereotaxic method for localization and removal of minute CNS lesions under 3-D vision. *J. Neurosurg.* 52:21–27, 1980.

32. Backlund E.O., Johansson L., Sarby B.: Studies on craniopharyngiomas: II. Treatment by stereotaxis and radiosurgery. *Acta Chir. Scand.* 138:749–759, 1972.

33. Backlund E.O.: Stereotactic radiosurgery in intracranial tumors and vascular malformations, in Krayenbuhl H. (ed.): *Advances and Technical Standards in Neurosurgery.* Wien, New York, Springer-Verlag, 1979, vol. 6, pp. 1–37.

34. Backlund E.O., Rähn J., Sarby B.: Treatment of pinealomas by stereotaxic radiation surgery. *Acta Radiol. Diagn.* 13:368–376, 1974.

35. Patil A.A.: Computed tomography-oriented stereotactic system. *Neurosurgery* 10:370–374, 1982.

36. Lunsford L.D., Nelson P.B.: Stereotactic aspiration of a brain abscess using the "therapeutic" CT scanner. *Acta Neurochir.* 62:25–29, 1982.

37. Gildenberg P.L., Kaufman H.H., Murthy K.S.K.: Calculation of stereotactic coordinates from the computed tomographic scan. *Neurosurgery* 10:580–586, 1982.

38. Moran C.J., Naidich T.P., Gado M.H., et al.: Central nervous system lesions biopsied or treated by CT-guided needle placement. *Radiology* 131:681–686, 1979.

39. Wise B.L., Gleason C.A.: CT-directed stereotactic surgery in the management of brain abscess. *Ann. Neurol.* 6:467, 1979.

40. Bosch D.A., Rähn T., Backlund E.O.: Treatment of colloid cysts of the third ventricle by stereotactic aspiration. *Surg. Neurol.* 9:15–18, 1978.

41. Backlund E.O., Von Holst H.: Controlled subtotal evacuation of intracerebral hematomas by stereotactic technique. *Surg. Neurol.* 9:99–101, 1978.

42. Higgins A.C., Nashold B.S., Cosman E.: Stereotaxic evacuation of primary intracerebral hematomas: New instrumentation. *Appl. Neurophysiol.* 45:438–442, 1982.

43. Broseta M., Gonzalez-Dareler J., Barcia-Salorio J.L.: Stereotactic evacuation of intracerebral hematomas, *Appl. Neurophysiol.* 45:443–448, 1982.

44. Bosch D.A., Hindmarsh T., Larsson S., et al.: Intraneoplastic administration of bleomycin in intracerebral gliomas: A pilot study. *Acta Neurochir.,* suppl. 30, 1980, pp. 441–444.

45. Backlund E.O.: Stereotaxic treatment of craniopharyngiomas. *Acta Neurochir.,* suppl. 21, 1974, pp. 177–183.

46. Backlund E.O.: Studies on craniopharyngiomas: III. Ste-

reotaxic treatment with intracystic yttrium[90]. *Acta Chir. Scand.* 139:237–247, 1972.

47. Backlund E.O.: Studies on craniopharyngiomas: IV. Stereotactic treatment with radiosurgery. *Acta Chir. Scand.* 139:344–351, 1972.

48. Kobayashi T., Kageyama N., Ohara K.: Internal irradiation for cystic craniopharyngioma. *J. Neurosurg.* 55:896–903, 1981.

49. Backlund E.O.: Stereotactic treatment of craniopharyngiomas—15 years' experience (abstracted). Presented at the 32nd Annual Meeting of the Scandinavian Neurosurgical Society, Linköping, Sweden, September 5, 1980.

50. Mundinger F., Birg W., Ostertag C.B.: Treatment of small cerebral gliomas with CT aided stereotaxic curie therapy. *Neuroradiology* 16:564–567, 1978.

51. Kelly P.J., Olson M.H., Wright E.A., et al.: CT localization and stereotactic implantation of iridium 192 into CNS neoplasms, in G. Szikla (ed.): *Stereotactic Cerebral Irradiation.* INSERM symposium no. 12. New York, Elsevier North-Holland Pub. Co., 1979, pp. 123–128.

52. Hosobuchi Y., Phillips T.L., Stupar T.A., et al.: Interstitial brachytherapy of primary brain tumors: Preliminary report. *J. Neurosurg.* 53:613–617, 1980.

53. Gutin P.H., Dormandy R.: A coaxial catheter system for afterloading radioactive sources for interstitial irradiation of brain tumors. *J. Neurosurg.* 56:734–735, 1982.

54. Mackay A.R., Gutin P.H., Hosobuchi Y., et al.: Computed tomography-directed stereotaxy for biopsy and interstitial irradiation of brain tumors: Technical note. *Neurosurgery* 11:38–42, 1982.

55. Marino R.: Introduction: Functional neurosurgery as a speciality, in Rasmussen T., Marino R. (eds.): *Functional Neurosurgery.* New York, Raven Press, 1979, pp. 1–5.

56. Schaltenbrand G., Wahren W.: *Atlas for Stereotaxy of the Human Brain.* Chicago, Year Book Medical Publishers, 1977.

57. Rosenbaum A.E., Lunsford L.D., Perry J.H.: Computerized tomography guided stereotaxis: A new approach. *Appl. Neurophysiol.* 43:172–173, 1980.

58. Kelly P.J., Gillingham F.J.: The long-term results of stereotaxic surgery and L-dopa therapy in patients with Parkinson's disease. A 10-year follow-up study. *J. Neurosurg.* 53:332–337, 1980.

59. Cooper I.S.: Twenty-five years of experience with physiological neurosurgery. *Neurosurgery* 9:190–200, 1981.

60. Matsumoto K., Asano J., Baba J., et al.: Long-term follow-up results of bilateral thalamotomy for Parkinsonism. *Appl. Neurophysiol.* 39:257–260, 1977.

61. Passerini A., Broggi G., Giorgi G.: CT studies in patients operated with stereotaxic thalamotomies. *Neuroradiology* 16:561–563, 1978.

62. Meyerson B.A., Bergstrom M., Greitz T.: Target localization in stereotactic capsulotomy with the aid of computed tomography, in Hitchcock E.R., Ballantine H.J. Jr., Meyerson B.A. (eds.): *Modern Concepts in Psychiatry Surgery.* Amsterdam, Elsevier, 1979, pp. 217–224.

63. Richardson D.E., Akil H.: Pain reduction by electrical brain stimulation in man: I. *J. Neurosurg.* 47:128–183, 1977.

64. Richardson D.E., Akil H.: Pain reduction by electrical stimulation in man: II. *J. Neurosurg.* 47:184–194, 1977.

65. Boive J., Meyerson B.A.: A correlative anatomical and clinical study of pain suppression by deep brain stimulation. *Pain* 13:113–126, 1982.

66. Hosobuchi Y., Adams J.E., Rutkin B.: Chronic thalamic stimulation for the control of facial anesthesia dolorosa. *Arch. Neurol.* 29:158–161, 1973.

67. Hosobuchi Y., Adams J.E., Fields H.L.: Chronic thalamic and internal capsular stimulation for the control of facial anesthesia dolorosa and dysesthesia of thalamic syndrome. *Adv. Neurol.* 4:783–787, 1974.

68. Meyerson B.A.: Biochemistry of pain relief with intracerebral stimulation: Few facts and many hypotheses. *Acta Neurochir. Suppl.* 30:229–237, 1980.

69. Hosobuchi Y.: The current status of analgesic brain stimulation. *Acta Neurochir. Suppl.* 30:219–227, 1980.

70. Talairach J., Szikla G.: Stereotactic neuroradiological concepts applied to surgical removal of cortical epileptogenic areas, in Rasmussen T., Marino R. (eds.): *Functional Neurosurgery.* New York, Raven Press, 1979, pp. 219–242.

71. Glenn W.H.: Stereotaxis and CT (abstracted). Presented at the seminar of Contemporary Stereotactic Techniques. Buffalo, N.Y., June 4, 1982.

72. Backlund E.O., Grepe A., Lunsford L.D.: Stereotaxic reconstruction of the aqueduct of Sylvius. *J. Neurosurg.* 55:800–810, 1981.

73. Perlow M.J., Freed W.J., Hoffer B.J., et al.: Brain grafts reduce motor abnormalities produced by destruction of nigrostriatal dopamine system: Behavioral and histochemical evidence. *Science* 204:643–647, 1979.

74. Jacques S., Shelden C.H., McCann G.D.: Computerized three-dimensional stereotaxic removal of small central nervous system lesions in patients. *J. Neurosurg.* 53:816–820, 1980.

75. Kelly P.K., Alker G.J.: A stereotactic approach to deep-seated central nervous system neoplasms using the carbon dioxide laser. *Surg. Neurol.* 15:331–334, 1981.

76. Shelden C.H., Jacques S., McCann G.D.: The Shelden CT-based microneurosurgical stereotactic system: Its application to CNS pathology. *Appl. Neurophysiol.* 45:341–346, 1982.

Index